Nephrology Worldwide

José A. Moura-Neto
José Carolino Divino-Filho • Claudio Ronco
Editors

# Nephrology Worldwide

Springer

*Editors*
José A. Moura-Neto
Brazilian Society of Nephrology
Salvador
Bahia
Brazil

José Carolino Divino-Filho
Division of Renal Medicine, CLINTEC
Karolinska Institutet
Stockholm
Sweden

Claudio Ronco
DIMED - University of Padova
Department Nephrology Dialysis &
Transplantation
International Renal Research Institute (IRRIV)
San Bortolo Hospital
Vicenza
Italy

More information on the Nephrology Worldwide initiative can be found at http://www.nephrologyworldwide.com.

ISBN 978-3-030-56889-4     ISBN 978-3-030-56890-0 (eBook)
https://doi.org/10.1007/978-3-030-56890-0



This Springer imprint is published by the registered company Springer Nature Switzerland AG
The registered company address is: Gewerbestrasse 11, 6330 Cham, Switzerland

*To my beloved wife, Ana Flavia, and my parents, Moura and Socorro, for their support.*
*To my children, Thor and Maya – my reason for everything. May the Nephrology Worldwide mission inspire you to aim for a world 'without borders', more integrated and with equitable healthcare access*

*José A. Moura-Neto*

*To my family, Sandra, José, Felipe and Pedro, my beloved parents, José and Rita, and mentors, Ricardo Germano, Tore Lindholm, Ulla Bengtsson and Jonas Bergström*

*José Carolino Divino-Filho*

*To all my IRRIV fellows who came to Vicenza in the last 20 years with enthusiasm and strong interest in research. May this book represent an inspiration for personal engagement in the fight against kidney diseases*

*Claudio Ronco*

# Foreword

In combining the challenges of long-term pastoral care and the highly technical, often costly, medicine that is implicit in maintenance treatment of chronic kidney disease, Nephrology is one of the most demanding, if not the most demanding medical specialty. *Nephrology Worldwide* provides fascinating insights into how these challenges have, so far, been met in different parts of the world.

With chapters written by authorities from every corner of the globe, the reader is given a perspective on both the widely differing epidemiology and aetiology of renal disease in different countries and the strategies for renal health-care provision.

Most accounts detail the history how the challenge of providing renal replacement therapy for those patients reaching end-stage renal failure has to date been met and how the profession has organized itself.

Both the failings and the successes are outlined in a way that should make this book a compelling read, not just for the well-informed renal physician, but also for planners and policy makers whose thinking and actions are integral to the way we practice medicine.

I commend it to all.

United Kingdom
February 2020

Peter J. Ratcliffe

# Preface

The original idea for this book first emerged at some point between 2013 and 2015 during my nephrology fellowship in Rio de Janeiro. The idea came and went from my mind constantly in the following years – a sign to invest time and effort to make it happen. During the embryonic stage of this project, every time I shared the idea with friends and colleagues at conferences, their excitement and genuine demonstration of interest encouraged me.

A few years after finishing the fellowship in nephrology and kidney transplantation, I ended up editing a book on renal replacement therapy, which was finally published in 2018. During this extraordinary and unexpected experience, I had the opportunity to connect and collaborate with competent nephrologists around the world. Many of them became good friends and naturally were invited to join this endeavor. Two of them coedited this book: José Carolino Divino-Filho and Claudio Ronco.

José Divino was more than a partner of this project. Despite our age difference, we have developed a close friendship. As a young medical student, he lived in my hometown, Salvador, and coincidentally was a friend of my father, who is now a retired nephrologist. Right after completing his medical degree, José Divino started a unique international journey, living in many different countries: Sweden, Belgium, Mexico, Switzerland, and Germany. His successful (and somewhat nomadic) career has made him a complete nephrologist – a mix of an academic and a practitioner – and one of the most international professionals in the field: the "right guy" for the *Nephrology Worldwide* project.

Claudio Ronco needs no introduction. In the past years, he has established himself as one of the most iconic scientists in the field, known for addressing controversial and important topics of nephrology. It was an honor when he accepted the invitation to join this project – his "*joie de vivre*," kindness, and humble brilliance were a constant education during this process.

By putting together "the guy who knows the world" and "the guy who the world knows," we were prepared to face the challenge of making the *Nephrology Worldwide* project happen. Over the course of several months, we carefully curated a selection of nephrologists around the world to take on the daunting task of providing a comprehensive description of the nephrology field in their respective countries.

The selected corresponding authors were asked to join a diverse team of coauthors, with different backgrounds, able to fully describe the field in their country, such as kidney transplantation, maintenance hemodialysis, peritoneal dialysis, pediatric nephrology, acute kidney injury and critical care nephrology, nephrology practice, and job market. We meticulously elaborated an editor's guideline and a chapter template in order to avoid the missing of key information and to create a didactic pattern throughout the book, which would make the life of the readers easier since they could become familiar with the book once they read one of its chapters. In the first chapter, we detail the project in all its stages, as well as the Editors' vision of *Nephrology Worldwide*, its mission, and a selection of some highlights from the book.

One central premise of this project was the representation of all regions and continents, so that the book would be legitimately international. Sixty-two countries had initially agreed to participate, but some authors were not able to deliver their chapters by the final deadline and therefore could not be included in this first edition. In the end, 53 chapters and more than 300 authors, from 51 different nationalities, contributed to this book. This makes *Nephrology Worldwide* one of the most international books in nephrology. The great diversity of nationalities made this book unique and occasionally posed additional challenges, such as political instability, cultural barriers, and linguistic difficulties.

The countries represented in the book embrace a population of about 5.7 billion people, representing around three-quarters of the world population. Another point that stands out in the project is the involvement of the nephrology societies around the world; many corresponding authors hold leadership positions in their societies, although most of them were not contacted through their organizations. The International Society of Nephrology (ISN) was also invited to contribute; they wrote Chap. 2.

We believe this project has fulfilled its goals. It is international, representative, and unique. The reader will be able to travel through *Nephrology Worldwide*, a pleasant reading experience with not only relevant information and updated data, but also a comprehensive look at the history, countries' peculiarities, and a critical analysis of the scenario of nephrology and renal replacement therapy.

Finally, we felt we opened a box of new opportunities. More than a book, *Nephrology Worldwide* will become a living document – to be updated periodically. We believe this project will survive through its multiple missions and ultimate goal: "to connect nephrology around the world."

Salvador, Bahia, Brazil José A. Moura-Neto
May 2020

# Acknowledgment

We sincerely thank Springer Nature for believing in this project, especially the Editorial Director Richard Lansing and the Associate Editor Vanessa Shimabukuro. We also greatly appreciate Anila Vijayan and Arul Viveaun for their support during this process. A special recognition to our personal editorial assistants, Lara Schmertmann and Anya Carrasco.

Finally, we acknowledge Jorge Filipe Santana Santos and Vinícius Silva Carvalho for their amazing work in developing the Nephrology Worldwide website – http://www.nephrology-worldwide.com. It has been designed as a user-friendly platform connecting editors and readers, allowing them to get additional information about the project, share their feedback and 'apply' to contribute as reviewer or author in future editions of *Nephrology Worldwide*.

# Contents

## Part V Oceania

# Editors and Contributors

## Editors

**José Carolino Divino-Filho, MD, PhD** Division of Renal Medicine, CLINTEC, Karolinska Institutet, Stockholm, Sweden

**José A. Moura-Neto, MD, MBA, MS, FASN** Brazilian Society of Nephrology (SBN), Salvador, Bahia, Brazil

**Claudio Ronco, MD** DIMED - University of Padova, Department Nephrology Dialysis & Transplantation, International Renal Research Institute (IRRIV), San Bortolo Hospital, Vicenza, Italy

## Contributors

**Aliyu Abdu, MBBS, MSc, FMCP** Department of Medicine, Aminu Kano Teaching Hospital/ Bayero University, Kano, Nigeria

**Adrian Liew, MBBS, MRCP, FAMS, FRCPE, FASN** The Kidney & Transplant Practice, Mount Elizabeth Novena Hospital, Singapore, Singapore

**Afiatin, MD, FINASIM** Division of Nephrology and Hypertension, Department of Internal Medicine, Faculty of Medicine Universitas Padjadjaran – Dr. Hasan Sadikin General Hospital, Bandung, West Java, Indonesia

**Maria Alejandra Aguilar-Kitsu, MD** Department of Nephrology, Hospital de Pediatría, Centro Medico Nacional Siglo XXI, Instituto Mexicano del Seguro Social, Mexico City, Mexico

**G. Ahmad, MBBCh Hons (National University of Ireland), MMed (UKM), FRCP (Ireland)** Department of Cardiology, National Heart Institute, Kuala Lumpur, Malaysia

**Momina M. Ahmed** Renal Unit, Saint Paul Millenium Medical College (SPMMC), Addis Abeba, Ethiopia

**Shamim Ahmed, FCPS, FRCP (E), FRCP (G)** Department of Nephrology, Kidney Foundation Hospital and Research Institute, Dhaka, Bangladesh

**Intisar Al-Alawi, PhD** The National Genetic Centre, The Royal Hospital, Muscat, Oman

**Kazi Shahnoor Alam, MBBS, FCPS (Medicine), MD (Nephrology)** Department of Nephrology, National Institute of Kidney Diseases & Urology, Dhaka, Bangladesh

**Mohammad Rafiqul Alam, MBBS, MD (Nephro), FCPS (Med)** Department of Nephrology, BSMMU-Bangabandhu Sheikh Mujib Medical University, Dhaka, Bangladesh

**Carlo Alfieri** Nephrology, Dialysis and Renal Transplantation, Fondazione IRCCS Ca Granda Ospedale Maggiore Policlinico, Milan, Italy

Department of Clinical Sciences and Community Health, University of Milan, Milan, Italy

**Jorge Alfonzo, PhD** Instituto de Nefrología, La Habana, Cuba

**Medhat Ali, MD** The Renal Medicine Department, Nizwa Hospital, Nizwa, Oman

**Zubaida Al Ismaili** Pediatric Institute, Sheikh Khalifa Medical City, Abu Dhabi, United Arab Emirates

**Zulkhair Ali, MD, PhD, FINASIM** Division of Nephrology and Hypertension, Department of Internal Medicine, Faculty of Medicine Universitas Sriwijaya – Dr. Mohammad Husein General Hospital, Palembang, Indonesia

**Miguel Almaguer, MD** Instituto de Nefrología, La Habana, Cuba

**Yaqoub Al-Maymmani** The Renal Medicine Department, The Royal Hospital, Muscat, Oman

**Manuela Almeida** Nephrology Department, Centro Hospitalar e Universitário do Porto, Porto, Portugal

**Ali Alobaidli, MB, BCh, BAO, MPH** Department of Medicine, Nephrology, Sheikh Khalifa Medical City, Abu Dhabi, United Arab Emirates

**Evelyn Alonzo, MSc** Hospital Universitario de Caracas, Caracas, Venezuela

National Organization of Transplant of Venezuela, Valencia, Venezuela

**Fatma Al-Rahbi, RN** The Renal Medicine Department, The Royal Hospital, Muscat, Oman

**Waleed Al-Rajhi, PhD** College of Pharmacy and Nursing, Nizwa, Oman

**Soud Al Rasheed, MD, FRCP** King Saud Bin Abdulaziz University for Health Sciences, Riyadh, Saudi Arabia

**Mohammed Al-Riyami, MD** The Renal Medicine Department, The Royal Hospital, Muscat, Oman

**Mona Al-Rukhaimi, BSc,MBBCh, MRCP(UK), FRCP, FRCPE** Department of Medicine, Dubai Medical College, Dubai, United Arab Emirates

**Issa Al-Salmi, MD, BA, MB, Bch, BAO (Trinity College), FRCPI, MRCP (UK), FRCP, MIPH (AUS), PhD (AUS), FASN (USA)** The Renal Medicine Department, The Royal Hospital, Muscat, Oman

**Abdullah Al Sayyari, MBA, MD, FRCP** King Saud Bin Abdulaziz University for Health Sciences, Riyadh, Saudi Arabia

**J. Emilio Sánchez Alvárez** Department of Nephrology, University Hospital of Cabueñes, Gijón, Asturias, Spain

**Yanet Alvarez, PhD** Instituto de Nefrología, La Habana, Cuba

**Ruqiya Al-Za'abi, PHD, BSN (VU, USA), Msc (Uclan, England), PhD (UOG, Scotland), RN, BSN, MSsc, PhD (MoH, Oman)** Nurse Tutor, Muscat, Oman

**Pablo Amair, MD** Venezuelan Society of Nephrology, Caracas, Venezuela

**Patrice Ambühl, MD** Service of Nephrology, Stadspital Waid, Zürich, Switzerland

**Samaya J. Anumudu, MD, FASN** Baylor College of Medicine, Houston, TX, USA

**Yu An** National Clinical Research Center of Kidney Diseases, Jinling Hospital, Nanjing University School of Medicine, Nanjing, China

**Leopoldo Ardiles, MD, FACP** Hospital Regional, Facultad de Medicina, Universidad Austral de Chile, Valdivia, Chile

**Shakib Uz Zaman Arefin, MBBS, MCPS, FCPS (NEPHRO)** Department of Nephrology, Kidney Foundation Hospital and Research Institute, Dhaka, Bangladesh

**Mustafa Arıcı** Hacettepe University Faculty of Medicine, Department of Nephrology, Ankara, Turkey

**Marcos Ariza, MD** Hospital de Niños, Caracas, Venezuela

**Fatiu Abiola Arogundade, MBBS, FMCP, FWACP, FRCP (Edin), FRCP (London)** Department of Medicine, Obafemi Awolowo University/Teaching Hospitals Complex, Ile-Ife, Osun State, Nigeria

**Ricardo Silvestre Arze Arze, MD** NEFRODIAL (CENTRO DEL RIÑON), Cochabamba, Bolivia

**Suheir Assady, MD, PhD** Rambam Health Care Campus, Haifa, Israel

Technion – Israel Institute of Technology, Haifa, Israel

The Israeli Society of Nephrology and Hypertension, Ramat Gan, Israel

**Kenan Ateş** Ankara University Faculty of Medicine, Department of Nephrology, Ankara, Turkey

**David Atuhe** St Francis Hospital Nsambya, Kampala, Uganda

**Ana Azevedo** Nephrology Department, Hospital Vila Franca de Xira, Vila Franca de Xira, Portugal

**Peace Bagasha** Makerere University College of Health Sciences, Kampala, Uganda

Mulago National Referral Hospital, Kampala, Uganda

**Ingretta Bagdasarova, MD, Prof. of Medicine** Ukrainian Association of Nephrologists & Kidney Transplant Specialists, Kyiv, Ukraine

State Institution «Institute of Nephrology of the National Academy of Medical Sciences», Department of Pediatric Nephrology, Kyiv, Ukraine

**Rasheed Abiodun Balogun, MBBS, FACP, FMCP, HP(ASCP)** Division of Nephrology, Department of Medicine, University of Virginia, Charlottesville, VA, USA

**Ebun Ladipo Bamgboye, MBBS, FWACP, FRCP (London), FNAN** St. Nicholas Hospital, Lagos Island, Lagos State, Nigeria

**Ria Bandiara, MD, PhD, FINASIM** Division of Nephrology and Hypertension, Department of Internal Medicine, Faculty of Medicine Universitas Padjadjaran – Dr. Hasan Sadikin General Hospital, Bandung, West Java, Indonesia

**José Diogo Barata** Nephrology Department, Hospital da Luz, Lisbon, Portugal

**Myftar Barbullushi, MD, PhD, FERA** Service of Nephrology, University Hospital Center "Mother Teresa", Tirana, Albania

**Katherine Barraclough, MBBS(Hons), FRACP, PhD** Nephrology, Royal Melbourne Hospital, Parkville, VIC, Australia

**Anthony Batte** Makerere University College of Health Sciences, Kampala, Uganda

**S. Bavanandan, MBBS, FRCPE** Department of Nephrology, Kuala Lumpur Hospital, Kuala Lumpur, Malaysia

**B. C. Bee, MD (UKM), FRCP (Edin)** Department of Nephrology, Selayang Hospital, Kepong, Selangor, Malaysia

**Nura Afza Salma Begum, MBBS, MSc, MRCP (UK), Specialty Certified in Nephrology (UK)** Department of Nephrology, Kidney Foundation Hospital and Research Institute, Dhaka, Bangladesh

**Antonio Bellasi, MD, PhD** Department of Research, Innovation, Brand Reputation, Ospedale di Bergamo, ASST Papa Giovanni XXIII, Bergamo (BG), Italy

**Max Bell, MD, PhD** Perioperative Medicine and Intensive Care Medicine, Karolinska University Hospital, Stockholm, Sweden

**Ezequiel Bellorin-Font, MD** Saint Louis University, St. Louis, MO, USA

**Milka Bengochea, MD** Instituto Nacional de Donación y Trasplantes. Hospital de Clínicas, Facultad de Medicina, Universidad de la República, Montevideo, Uruguay

**Joyita Bharati** Postgraduate Institute of Medical Education and Research, Chandigarh, India

**Boris T. Bikbov, MD, PhD** Academician V.I.Shumakov Federal Research Center of Transplantology and Artificial Organs, Moscow, Russian Federation

**Peter G. Blake, MB, MSc, FRCPC** Western University, London, Ontario, Canada

London Health Sciences Centre, London, Ontario, Canada

Ontario Renal Network, Toronto, Ontario, Canada

**Boris Iliev Bogov, MD, PhD** University Hospital "Alexandrovska" Sofia, Sofia Medical University, Sofia, Bulgaria

**Raúl Bohorques, MD** Instituto de Nefrología, La Habana, Cuba

**Ioannis Boletis** Department of Nephrology & Renal Transplant Unit, Laiko General Hospital, University of Athens Medical School, Athens, Greece

**Geoffrey Boner, MBBCh** Rabin Medical Center, Petah Tikva, Israel

Tel Aviv University, Tel Aviv, Israel

**Olivier Bonny, MD, PhD** Department of Pharmacology and Toxicology, University of Lausanne, Lausanne, Switzerland

**Behrooz Broumand, MD, FACP** Pars Hospital, Tehran, Iran

Iranian Society of Nephrology (IrSN), Tehran, Iran

Iran University of Medical Sciences, Tehran, Iran

**Michel Burnier, MD** Service of Nephrology and Hypertension, Departments of Medicine, University Hospital, Lausanne, Switzerland

**Vilma Cadri** Service of Nephrology, University Hospital Center "Mother Teresa", Tirana, Albania

**Guang-Yan Cai, MD, PhD** Department of Nephrology, Chinese PLA General Hospital, State Key Laboratory of Kidney Diseases, National Clinical Research Center for Kidney Diseases, Beijing, China

**Bernard Canaud, MD, PhD** Montpellier University, School of Medicine, Montpellier, France

Global Medical Office, Fresenius Medical Care, Bad Homburg, Germany

**Raul G. Carlini, MD** Venezuelan Society of Nephrology, Caracas, Venezuela

**Nicolas Carlson, BA, MD, PhD** Department of Nehrology, Righshospitalet, Copenhagen, Denmark

**Fernanda Carvalho** Nephropathology Department, Nefrolab-Clara Saúde, Paço de Arcos, Portugal

**Eduardo Celia** Argentine Society of Nephrology, Buenos Aires, Argentina

**Cynthia Gabriela Cervantes-Sanchez, MD** Nephrology Service, Hospital Civil de Guadalajara Fray Antonio Alcalde, University of Guadalajara Health Sciences Center, Guadalajara, Mexico

**Jonathan Samuel Chavez-Iñiguez, MD, MSc** Nephrology Service, Hospital Civil de Guadalajara Fray Antonio Alcalde, University of Guadalajara Health Sciences Center, Guadalajara, Mexico

**Jiang-Hua Chen** Kidney Disease Center, The First Affiliated Hospital, College of Medicine, Zhejiang University, Hangzhou, China

National Key Clinical Department of Kidney Diseases, Institute of Nephrology, Zhejiang University, Hangzhou, China

**Titi Chen, MBBS, FRACP** The University of Sydney, The Westmead Institute for Medical Research, Department of Renal Medicine, Westmead Hospital, Westmead, NSW, Australia

**Wei Chen** Department of Nephrology, The First Affiliated Hospital, Sun Yat-sen University, Guangzhou, Guangdong, China

Key Laboratory of Nephrology, National Health Commission and Guangdong Province, Guangzhou, Guangdong, China

**Xiang-Mei Chen, MD, PhD, CAE academician** Department of Nephrology, Chinese PLA General Hospital, State Key Laboratory of Kidney Diseases, National Clinical Research Center for Kidney Diseases, Beijing, China

**Liliana Chifflet, MD** Fondo Nacional de Recursos, Montevideo, Uruguay

**Mogamat-Yazied Chothia, FCP(SA), MMed, Cert Nephrol(SA)** Division of Nephrology, Stellenbosch University and Tygerberg Hospital, Cape Town, South Africa

**Gabriel Choukroun, MD, PhD** Internal Medicine, Dialysis and Transplantation Department, CHU Amiens-Picardie, Amiens, France

Society Francophone of Nephrology, Dialysis and Transplantation (SFNDT), CHABANIERE, France

**Rolando Claure-Vallejo, MD** Unidad de Atención al Enfermo Renal (UNAER S.R.L.), Cochabamba, Bolivia

**Arturo Cornejo-Cordero, MD** Instituto de Nefrología, La Paz, Bolivia

**Zhao Cui, MD** Renal Division, Peking University First Hospital, Beijing, China

**Jarosław Czerwiński, MD, PhD** Department of Emergency Medicine, Medical University of Warsaw and Polish Transplant Coordinating Center Poltransplant, Warsaw, Poland

**Damon Tan, MBBS** Lee Kong Chian School of Medicine, Nanyang Technological University, Singapore, Singapore

**Miriam Davidovits, MD** Tel Aviv University, Tel Aviv, Israel

Schneider Children's Medical Center, Petah Tikva, Israel

**Mogamat Razeen Davids, FCP(SA), MMed, PhD** Division of Nephrology, Stellenbosch University and Tygerberg Hospital, Cape Town, South Africa

**Bianca Davidson, FCP(SA), MMed, Cert Nephrol(SA)** Division of Nephrology and Hypertension, University of Cape Town and Groote Schuur Hospital, Cape Town, South Africa

**Pablo Dávila-Erquicia, MD** Hospital Infantil "Manuel Ascencio Villarroel", Cochabamba, Bolivia

**Alicja Dębska-Ślizień, MD, PhD** Department of Nephrology Transplantology and Internal Medicine, Medical University of Gdańsk, Gdańsk, Poland

**Biagio Di Iorio** Department of Nephrology and Dialysis AORN San Giuseppe Moscati, Avellino (AV), Italy

**Luca Di Lullo** Department of Nephrology and Dialysis, "L. Parodi – Delfino" Hospital, Colleferro (RM), Italy

**Ian Dittmer, MB.ChB, FRACP** Department of Nephrology, Auckland City Hospital, Auckland, New Zealand

**José Carolino Divino-Filho** Division of Renal Medicine, CLINTEC, Karolinska Institutet, Stockholm, Sweden

**Marcelo Mazza do Nascimento, MD, PhD** Brazilian Society of Nephrology (SBN), São Paulo, Brazil

Federal University of Paraná (UFPR), Curitiba, PR, Brazil

**Iryna Dudar, MD, Prof. of Medicine** Ukrainian Association of Nephrologists & Kidney Transplant Specialists, Kyiv, Ukraine

State Institution «Institute of Nephrology of the National Academy of Medical Sciences», Department of Efferent Technology, Kyiv, Ukraine

**Ahmet Duraku** Service of Nephrology, University Hospital Center "Mother Teresa", Tirana, Albania

**Tevfik Ecder** Demiroglu Bilim University Faculty of Medicine, Department of Internal Medicine, Division of Nephrology, Istanbul, Turkey

**Emmanuel Edet Effa, MBBCh, MSc, FMCP** Department of Internal Medicine, University of Calabar, Calabar, Cross River state, Nigeria

**Somchai Eiam-Ong, MD** Department of Medicine, Chulalongkorn University, Bangkok, Thailand

**Addisu M. Ejigu** Renal Unit School of Medicine, College of Health Sciences, Addis Ababa University, Addis Ababa, Ethiopia

**Pépé Mfutu Ekulu, MD, PhD** Department of Pediatrics, Kinshasa University Hospital, University of Kinshasa, Kinshasa, Democratic Republic of the Congo

**Susana Elgueta, MD** Histocompatibility Laboratory, Instituto de Salud Publica, Santiago, Chile

**Christopher I. Esezobor, MBBS, FMCPaed, FWACP (Paed)** Department of Paediatrics, College of Medicine University of Lagos, Lagos, Lagos, Nigeria

**Simon Peter Eyoku** Mulago National Referral Hospital, Kampala, Uganda

**Stephen Z. Fadem, MD, FASN** Baylor College of Medicine, Houston, TX, USA

**Aníbal Ferreira** Nephrology Department, Centro Hospitalar e Universitário de Lisboa Central, Lisbon, Portugal

Nova Medical School, Universidade Nova de Lisboa, Lisbon, Portugal

**Alejandro Ferreiro, MD** Centro de Nefrología, Hospital de Clínicas, Facultad de Medicina, Universidad de la República, Montevideo, Uruguay

**José Florín, MD** Hospital Pediátrico de Centro Habana, La Habana, Cuba

**Svitlana Fomina, MD, PhD** Ukrainian Association of Nephrologists & Kidney Transplant Specialists, Kyiv, Ukraine

State Institution «Institute of Nephrology of the National Academy of Medical Sciences», Department of Pediatric Nephrology, Kyiv, Ukraine

**Renato Demarchi Foresto, MD** Hospital do Rim, Oswaldo Ramos Foundation, Federal University of São Paulo (UNIFESP), São Paulo, SP, Brazil

**Victor Frajewicki, MD** Carmel Medical Center, Haifa, Israel

The Israeli Society of Nephrology and Hypertension, Ramat Gan, Israel

**Marco Franchin** Vascular Surgery Unit, Department of Medicine and Surgery, University of Insubria School of Medicine, ASST Settelaghi University Teaching Hospital, Varese (VA), Italy

**Liliana Gadola, MD** Centro de Nefrología, Hospital de Clínicas, Facultad de Medicina, Universidad de la República, Montevideo, Uruguay

**Guillermo Garcia-Garcia, MD, FACP, FASN, FNKF** Nephrology Service, Hospital Civil de Guadalajara Fray Antonio Alcalde, University of Guadalajara Health Sciences Center, Guadalajara, Mexico

**Maria Simeonova Gaydarova, MD, PhD** University Pediatric Hospital Sofia, Sofia Medical University, Sofia, Bulgaria

**Ryszard Gellert, MD, PhD** Department of Nephrology and Internal Medicine, Center of Postgraduate Education, Warsaw, Poland

**Marin Ivanov Georgiev, MD, PhD** University Hospital "Alexandrovska" Sofia, Sofia Medical University, Sofia, Bulgaria

**José Manuel Gil-Cunquero** Department of Nephrology, University Hospital of Jaén, Jaén, Spain

**Albana Gjyzari, MD, PhD** Service of Nephrology, University Hospital Center "Mother Teresa", Tirana, Albania

**Helmuth Goecke, MD** Hospital Naval Almirante Nef – Universidad de Valparaíso, Viña del Mar, Chile

**Pedro Henrique Franca Gois, MD, PhD, FRACP, FASN** Nephrology Department, Royal Brisbane & Women's Hospital, Brisbane, QLD, Australia

University of Queensland School of Clinical Medicine - Royal Brisbane Clinical Unit, Brisbane, QLD, Australia

**Eliezer Golan, MD** The Israeli Society of Nephrology and Hypertension, Haifa, Israel

Tel Aviv University, Tel Aviv, Israel

**María Carlota Gonzalez-Bedat, MD** Registro Uruguayo de Diálisis. Sociedad Uruguaya de Nefrología, Montevideo, Uruguay

**Francisco Gonzalez-Martinez, MD** Facultad de Medicina, Universidad de la República, Montevideo, Uruguay

**Miguel González-Molina Alcaide** Department of Nephrology, Carlos Haya Regional University Hospital, Málaga, Spain

**Rolando Claure-Del Granado, MD, FASN** Servicio de Nefrología, Hospital Obrero No 2 - C.N.S., Universidad Mayor de San Simón, School of Medicine, Cochabamba, Bolivia

**Ryszard Grenda, MD, PhD** Department of Nephrology, Kidney Transplantation & Hypertension, The Children's Memorial Health Institute, Warsaw, Poland

**Guillermo Guerra, MD** Instituto de Nefrología, La Habana, Cuba

**Joseph Ogavu Gyagenda** St Francis Hospital Nsambya, Kampala, Uganda

**Margarita Halty, MD** Clínica Pediátrica, Centro Hospitalario Pereira Rossell, Facultad de Medicina, Universidad de la República, Montevideo, Uruguay

**Norio Hanafusa, MD, PhD** Department of Blood Purification, Tokyo Women's Medical University, Tokyo, Japan

**Chuan-Ming Hao, MD, PhD** Huashan Hospital Fudan University, Shanghai, China

**David Harris, AM, MD, MBBS, FRACP** International Society of Nephrology, The University of Sydney, The Westmead Institute for Medical Research, Department of Renal Medicine, Westmead Hospital, Westmead, NSW, Australia

**Seema Hashmi, MBBS, FCPS (Pediatrics), Fellow ISN (Pediatric Nephrology)** Department of Pediatric Nephrology, Sindh Institute of Urology and Transplantation (SIUT), Karachi, Pakistan

**James Heaf, MD, DMSc** Department of Medicine, Zealand University Hospital, Roskilde, Denmark

**Helen G. Healy, MBBS, PhD, FRACP** Nephrology Department, Royal Brisbane & Women's Hospital, Brisbane, QLD, Australia

**Olof Heimbürger, MD, PhD** Division of Renal Medicine, CLINTEC, Karolinska Institutet, Stockholm, Sweden

Department of Nephrology, Karolinska University Hospital, Stockholm, Sweden

**Fayez Hejaili, MD, FRCP** King Saud Bin Abdulaziz University for Health Sciences, Riyadh, Saudi Arabia

**Kelly Hendricks** International Society of Nephrology, Global Operations Center, Brussels, Belgium

**Domingo Hernández Marrero** Department of Nephrology, Carlos Haya Regional University Hospital, Málaga, Spain

**Eka Laksmi Hidayati, MD** Division of Nephrology and Hypertension – Department of Child Health, Faculty of Medicine Universitas Indonesia – Dr. Cipto Mangunkusumo General Hospital, Jakarta, Indonesia

**L. S. Hooi, MA, MBBChir, FRCPE, FAMM, FASN** Johor Bahru, Malaysia

**Junichi Hoshino, MD, MPH, PhD** Nephrology Center, Toranomon Hospital, Tokyo, Japan

**Fan-Fan Hou** Division of Nephrology, Nanfang Hospital, Southern Medical University, State Key Laboratory of Organ Failure Research, National Clinical Research Center for Kidney Disease, Guangzhou, China

**Chanseila Hy** Cambodian Association of Nephrology, Phnom Penh, Cambodia

**Toru Hyodo** Cambodian Association of Nephrology, Phnom Penh, Cambodia

NGO Ubiquitous Blood Purification International, Yokohama, Japan

**Christos Iatrou** Center for Diagnosis, Treatment and Research on Kidney Diseases, Hygeia Hospital, Athens, Greece

**Alma Idrizi, MD, PhD** Service of Nephrology, University Hospital Center "Mother Teresa", Tirana, Albania

**Matilda Imeraj, MD** Service of Nephrology, University Hospital Center "Mother Teresa", Tirana, Albania

**Nazrul Islam, MBBS, MRCP (UK), FRCP (Edin)** Department of Nephrology, Dhaka Medical College and Hospital, Dhaka, Bangladesh

**Helena Jardim** Pediatric Nephrology Department, Hospital CUF Porto, Porto, Portugal

**Vivekanand Jha, MD, DM, FRCP, FAMS** International Society of Nephrology, Brussels, Belgium

George Institute for Global Health, UNSW, New Delhi, India

Faculty of Medicine, Imperial College, London, UK

Manipal Academy of Higher Education, Manipal, India

**David W. Johnson, MBBS, FRACP, DMed, FASN, PhD** Department of Nephrology, University of Queensland at Princess Alexandra Hospital, Brisbane, QLD, Australia

**Robert Kalyesubula** Makerere University College of Health Sciences, Kampala, Uganda

MRC/UVRI & London School of Hygiene and Tropical Medicine Research Unit, Entebbe, Uganda

Departments of Physiology and Medicine, Makerere University College of Health Sciences, Kampala, Uganda

**John Kanellis, MBBS, PhD, FRACP** Department of Nephrology, Monash Health and Centre for Inflammatory Diseases, Department of Medicine, Monash University, Monash Medical Centre, Clayton, VIC, Australia

**Grace Kansiime** Mulago National Referral Hospital, Kampala, Uganda

**Tasnuva Sarah Kashem, MBBS(UK), BSc Physiology (UK), MRCP (UK)** Department of Nephrology, Kidney Foundation Hospital and Research Institute, Dhaka, Bangladesh

**Kea Keng** Cambodian Association of Nephrology, Phnom Penh, Cambodia

**Peter G. Kerr, MB, BS, PhD, FRACP** Nephrology, Monash Health and Monash University, Clayton, VIC, Australia

**Petar Kes, MD, PhD, FERA** School of Medicine, University of Zagreb, and Academy of Medical Sciences of Croatia, Zagreb, Croatia

**Asia Khanam, MBBS, MD (Nephrology)** Department of Nephrology, BSMMU-Bangabandhu Sheikh Mujib Medical University, Dhaka, Bangladesh

**Daniel Kiggundu** Mulago National Referral Hospital, Kampala, Uganda

**Gianna Mastroianni Kirsztajn, MD, PhD** Brazilian Society of Nephrology (SBN), São Paulo, Brazil

Federal University of São Paulo (UNIFESP), São Paulo, SP, Brazil

**Mykola Kolesnyk, MD, Prof. of Medicine** State Institution «Institute of Nephrology of the National Academy of Medical Sciences», Department of Nephrology and Dialysis, Kyiv, Ukraine

Ukrainian Association of Nephrologists & Kidney Transplant Specialists, Kyiv, Ukraine

**Daniel Landau, MD** Tel Aviv University, Tel Aviv, Israel

Schneider Children's Medical Center, Petah Tikva, Israel

**Andrew J. P. Lewington, BSc (Hons), MBBS, MEd, MD, FRCP** Renal Department, St. James's University Hospital, Leeds Teaching Hospitals Trust, Leeds, UK

**Christian Leyva, MD** Instituto de Nefrología, La Habana, Cuba

**Monika Lichodziejewska-Niemierko, MD, PhD** Department of Nephrology Transplantology and Internal Medicine, Medical University of Gdańsk, Gdańsk, Poland

**Erjola Likaj, MD, PhD** Service of Nephrology, University Hospital Center "Mother Teresa", Tirana, Albania

**Vadhana Lim** Cambodian Association of Nephrology, Phnom Penh, Cambodia

**Y. N. Lim, MBBS (Malaya), FRCPCH (UK)** Prince Court Medical Centre, Kuala Lumpur, Malaysia

**Bi-Cheng Liu, MD** Institute of Nephrology, Zhong Da Hospital, Southeast University School of Medicine, Nanjing, China

**Zhi-Hong Liu** National Clinical Research Center of Kidney Diseases, Jinling Hospital, Nanjing University School of Medicine, Nanjing, China

**Raúl Lombardi, MD** Centro de Nefrología, Hospital de Clínicas, Facultad de Medicina, Universidad de la República, Montevideo, Uruguay

**José António Lopes** Nephrology and Renal Transplantation Department, Centro Hospitalar e Universitário de Lisboa Norte, Lisbon, Portugal

**Abel Lucero Ruiz, MD** Hospital Obrero N° 1 – C.N.S., La Paz, Bolivia

**Torbjörn Lundgren, MD, PhD** Swedish Renal Registry, Jönköping County Hospital, Jönköping, Sweden

Department of Transplantation Surgery, Karolinska University Hospital, Stockholm, Sweden

Department of Clinical Science, Intervention and Technology, Karolinska Institute, Stockholm, Sweden

**Aida Lydia, MD, PhD, FINASIM** Division of Nephrology and Hypertension, Department of Internal Medicine, Faculty of Medicine Universitas Indonesia – Dr. Cipto Mangunkusumo General Hospital, Jakarta, Indonesia

**Kelvin Lewis Lynn, MB.ChB, FRACP** Department of Nephrology, Christchurch Hospital, Christchurch, New Zealand

**Fernando Macário** Chief Medical Officer, Diaverum, Portugal

**Charles Magrans, PhD** Instituto de Nefrología, La Habana, Cuba

**Gyaviira Makanga** Bank of Uganda, Kampala, Uganda

**Andrew John Mallett, MBBS, MMed, PhD, CF, AFRACMA, FASN, FRACP** Department of Renal Medicine, Townsville University Hospital, Douglas, QLD, Australia

**Jolanta Małyszko, MD, PhD, FERA, FASN** Department of Nephrology, Dialysis and Internal Medicine, Warsaw Medical University, Warsaw, Poland

**Smaragdi Marinaki** Department of Nephrology & Renal Transplant Unit, Laiko General Hospital, University of Athens Medical School, Athens, Greece

**Belén Marrón, MD, PhD** Corporate Diaverum Home Therapies, Diaverum Madrid Clinic, Madrid, Spain

**Juan Carlos Martínez-Ocaña** Department of Nephrology, Parc Tauli University Hospital, Sabadell, Barcelona, Spain

**Carmen Tzanno Branco Martins, MD, PhD** Brazilian Society of Nephrology (SBN), São Paulo, Brazil

**La Salete Martins** Nephrology Department, Centro Hospitalar e Universitário do Porto, Porto, Portugal

**Ikuto Masakane, MD, PhD** Department of Nephrology, Yabuki Hospital, Yamagata, Japan

**Mignon McCulloch, DCH(SA), FRCPCH(UK), FCPaed(SA)** Division of Paediatric Nephrology, University of Cape Town and Red Cross War Memorial Children's Hospital, Cape Town, South Africa

**Mara Medeiros, MD, PhD** Unidad de Investigación y Diagnóstico en Nefrologia y Metabolismo Mineral Óseo, Hospital Infantil de México Federico Gómez, Mexico City, Mexico

**Yewondwossen T. Mengistu** Renal Unit School of Medicine, College of Health Sciences, Addis Ababa University, Addis Ababa, Ethiopia

**Piergiorgio Messa** Nephrology, Dialysis and Renal Transplantation, Fondazione IRCCS Ca Granda Ospedale Maggiore Policlinico, Milan, Italy

Department of Clinical Sciences and Community Health, University of Milan, Milan, Italy

Incoming president of the Italian Society of Nephrology (SIN), Rome (RM), Italy

**Carmen Luisa Milanés, MD** National Organization of Transplant of Venezuela, Valencia, Venezuela

**Andromachi Mitsioni** Department of Nephrology, Children's Hospital "P. & A. Kyriakou", Athens, Greece

**Mariko Miyazaki, MD, PhD** Department of Nephrology, Endocrinology, and Vascular Medicine, Tohoku University Graduate School of Medicine, Sendai, Japan

**Raúl Mizraji, MD** Instituto Nacional de Donación y Trasplantes. Hospital de Clínicas, Facultad de Medicina, Universidad de la República, Montevideo, Uruguay

**Ehab Abul Raziq Mohammed, MD** The Renal Medicine Department, The Royal Hospital, Muscat, Oman

**Z. Morad, MBBS (Malaya), FAMM, FRCP (Edin)** Ampang Puteri Hospital, Kuala Lumpur, Malaysia

**Gustavo Lorenzo Moretta** Northwest Nephrological Center, National University Northwest Buenos Aires, Buenos Aires, Argentina

**Mamun Mostafi, MBBS, MACP (USA), MRACP (Australia), FCPS (Med), FRCP (I)** Department of Nephrology, Gonoshathaya Nagar Hospital Dhanmondi, Dhaka, Bangladesh

**Conceição Mota** Pediatric Nephrology Department, Centro Hospitalar e Universitário do Porto, Porto, Portugal

**Ana Flavia Moura, MD, PhD** Department of Internal Medicine, Bahiana School of Medicine and Public Health, Salvador, Bahia, Brazil

**José A. Moura-Neto, MD, MBA, MS, FASN** Brazilian Society of Nephrology (SBN), Salvador, Bahia, Brazil

**Suela Mumajesi** Service of Nephrology, University Hospital Center "Mother Teresa", Tirana, Albania

**Ricardo Muñoz-Arizpe, MD** Unidad de Investigación y Diagnóstico en Nefrologia y Metabolismo Mineral Óseo, Hospital Infantil de México Federico Gómez, Mexico City, Mexico

**Rubina Naqvi, MBBS, MD (Nephrology), Fellow ISN (Research), PGD Bioethics** Department of Nephrology, Sindh Institute of Urology and Transplantation (SIUT), Karachi, Pakistan

**Beata Naumnik, MD, PhD** 1st Department of Nephrology and Transplantation with Dialysis Unit, Medical University of Białystok, Białystok, Poland

**Hayato Nishida, MD, PhD** Department of Urology, Yamagata University Faculty of Medicine, Yamagata, Japan

**Qing-Yu Niu, MD, PhD** Department of Nephrology, Peking University People's Hospital, Beijing, China

**Oscar Noboa, MD** Centro de Nefrología, Hospital de Clínicas, Facultad de Medicina, Universidad de la República, Montevideo, Uruguay

**Michał Nowicki, MD, PhD** Department of Nephrology, Hypertension and Kidney Transplantation, Medical University of Łódź, Central University Hospital, Łódź, Poland

**Nazaire Mangani Nseka, MD, PhD** Renal Unit, Kinshasa University Hospital, University of Kinshasa, Kinshasa, Democratic Republic of the Congo

**Pringgodigdo Nugroho, MD, FINASIM** Division of Nephrology and Hypertension, Department of Internal Medicine, Faculty of Medicine Universitas Indonesia – Dr. Cipto Mangunkusumo General Hospital, Jakarta, Indonesia

**Shaikh A. Nurmohamed** Department of Nephrology, Amsterdam University Medical Center, Amsterdam, The Netherlands

**Gregorio T. Obrador, MD, MPH** Universidad Panamericana School of Medicine, Mexico City, Mexico

**Henrietta Uchenna Okafor, MBBS, FMCPaed** Department of Paediatrics, University of Nigeria Teaching Hospital, Enugu, Enugu, Nigeria

**Sergio Orihuela, MD** Instituto de Nefrología y Urología - Trasplante Renal, Hospital Italiano, Montevideo, Uruguay

**Alberto Ortíz** Department of Nephrology and Hypertension, Fundación Jiménez Díaz University Hospital, Madrid, Spain

**Ana Ortiz, MD** Facultad de Medicina, Pontificia Universidad Católica de Chile, Santiago, Chile

**Janusz Ostrowski, MD, PhD** Department of the History of Medicine, Centre of Postgraduate Medical Education, Warsaw, Poland

**Nestor Muyulu Pakasa, MD, PhD** Department of Pathology, Kinshasa University Hospital, University of Kinshasa, Kinshasa, Democratic Republic of the Congo

**Ramón Paniagua, MD, PhD** Unidad de Investigación Médica en Enfermedades Nefrológicas, UMAE Hospital de Especialidades, Centro Médico Nacional Siglo XXI, Instituto Mexicano del, Seguro Social, Mexico City, Mexico

**Mauricio Paredes-Fernández, MD** Seguro Social Universitario, Cochabamba, Bolivia

**Nevi Pasko, MD, PhD** Service of Nephrology, University Hospital Center "Mother Teresa", Tirana, Albania

**Ploumis Passadakis** Department of Nephrology, University Hospital of Alexandroupolis, Democritus University of Thrace Medical School, Alexandroupolis, Greece

**Jacqueline Pefaur, MD** Facultad de Medicina, Universidad de Chile Hospital Barros Luco Trudeau, Santiago, Chile

**Jorge Perez-Oliva, PhD** Instituto de Nefrología, La Habana, Cuba

**José Osmar Medina Pestana, MD, PhD, FRCS** Hospital do Rim, Oswaldo Ramos Foundation, Federal University of São Paulo (UNIFESP), São Paulo, SP, Brazil

**Elin Phon** Cambodian Association of Nephrology, Phnom Penh, Cambodia

**Liam Plant, BSc, MB, FRCPI, FRCPE** Department of Renal Medicine, Cork University Hospital and University College Cork, Cork, Ireland

Irish Nephrology Society (INS), Cork, Ireland

**Raul Plata-Cornejo, MD** Instituto de Nefrología, La Paz, Bolivia

**Daniela Ponce, MD, PhD** Botucatu School of Medicine, University of São Paulo (UNESP), Botucatu, SP, Brazil

**Pedro Ponce** Renal Unit and Intensive Care Unit, Hospital Cuf Infante Santo, Lisbon, Portugal

Fresenius Medical Care, Lisbon, Portugal

**Joyce Popoola, MBChB, PhD, FRCP, FEBTM** Department of Renal Medicine and Transplantation, St George's University Hospitals NHS Foundation Trust, London, UK

**Johan V. Povlsen, MD** Department of Nephrology, Aarhus University Hospital, Aarhus, Denmark

**Kearkiat Praditpornsilpa, MD** Department of Medicine, Chulalongkorn University, Bangkok, Thailand

**Ruth Rachamimov, MD** The Israeli Society of Nephrology and Hypertension, Ramat Gan, Israel

Tel Aviv University, Tel Aviv, Israel

The Israeli Transplantation Society, Ramat Gan, Israel

Rabin Medical Center, Petah Tikva, Israel

**Sanjin Rački, MD, PhD** Department of Nephrology, Dialysis and Transplantation, Rijeka University Hospital Centre, and School of Medicine, University of Rijeka, Rijeka, Croatia

**M. Muhibur Rahman, MBBS(DMC), FCPS(Medicine), MRCP(UK), PhD Nephrology (London)** Department of Nephrology, Popular Medical College Hospital, Dhaka, Bangladesh

**Dwarakanathan Ranganathan, MD, DM, FRCP, FRACP, FASN** Nephrology Department, Royal Brisbane & Women's Hospital, Brisbane, QLD, Australia

School of Medicine, Griffith University, Brisbane, QLD, Australia

**Harun Ur Rashid, PhD, FCPS, FRCP** Department of Nephrology, Kidney Foundation Hospital and Research Institute, Dhaka, Bangladesh

**Anabella Rebori, MD** Unidad de Nefrología pediátrica de ASSE, Hospital Pereira Rossell, Montevideo, Uruguay

**Rafael Reyes-Acevedo, MD** Department of Surgery, Centenario Hospital Miguel Hidalgo de Aguascalientes, Aguascalientes, Mexico

**Pablo Rios, MD** Programa de Salud Renal. Fondo Nacional de Recursos, Montevideo, Uruguay

**Roberto Rivas, MD** Instituto de Nefrología, La Habana, Cuba

**Israel D. Rivas-Salazar, MD** Hospital Obrero No 2 - C.N.S., Cochabamba, Bolivia

**Anabela Rodrigues** Nephrology Department, Centro Hospitalar e Universitário do Porto, Porto, Portugal

**Eric Roessler, MD** Hospital Clínico Pontificia Universidad Católica de Chile, Santiago, Chile

**Claudio Ronco** DIMED - University of Padova, Department Nephrology Dialysis & Transplantation, International Renal Research Institute (IRRIV), San Bortolo Hospital, Vicenza, Italy

**Pía Rosati, MD** San Juan de Dios, Santiago, Chile

**Dimitar Lubomirov Roussinov, MD, PhD** University Pediatric Hospital Sofia, Sofia Medical University, Sofia, Bulgaria

**Merita Rroji, MD, PhD** Service of Nephrology, University Hospital Center "Mother Teresa", Tirana, Albania

**Ximena Rubilar-Araya, RN, MSc** Universidad Panamericana School of Nursing, Mexico City, Mexico

**Ivan Rychlík** Czech Society of Nephrology (CSN), Prague, Czech Republic

Department of Medicine, Third Faculty of Medicine, Charles University and Faculty Hospital Kralovské Vinohrady, Prague, Czech Republic

**Helena Rydell, MD, PhD** Swedish Renal Registry, Jönköping County Hospital, Jönköping, Sweden

Division of Renal Medicine, CLINTEC, Karolinska Institutet, Stockholm, Sweden

Department of Nephrology, Karolinska University Hospital, Stockholm, Sweden

**Jose Scapuzzi** Internal Medicine Academic Unit, Ezeiza Hospital Buenos Aires University, Buenos Aires, Argentina

**Staffan Schön, MD** Swedish Renal Registry, Jönköping County Hospital, Jönköping, Sweden

**Saimir Seferi, MD, PhD** Service of Nephrology, University Hospital Center "Mother Teresa", Tirana, Albania

**Mårten Segelmark, MD, PhD** Swedish Renal Registry, Jönköping County Hospital, Jönköping, Sweden

Department of Clinical Sciences, Division of Nephrology, Skane University Hospital and Lund University, Lund, Sweden

**Ana Maria Sesin** National Hospital of Clinics, National University of Córdoba, Córdoba, Argentina

**Faissal A. M. Shaheen, MD, FSM (Neph), FRCP(UK), FACP** Suleiman Fakeeh Hospital, Jeddah, Saudi Arabia

**Nelson Orta Sibu, MD** Universidad de Carabobo, Valencia, Venezuela

**Cassiano Augusto Braga Silva** Grupo CSB, Salvador, BA, Brazil

**Laura Sola, MD** Comisión Asesora del Programa de Salud Renal, Montevideo, Uruguay

**Søren Schwartz Sørensen, MD, DMSc** H.C. Andersen's Children's Hospital, Odense University Hospital, Odense, Denmark

**Edison Souza, MD, PhD** Clinical and Academic Unit of Nephrology, Hospital Universitário Pedro Ernesto, Faculty of Medical Sciences, Universidade do Estado do Rio de Janeiro (UERJ), Rio de Janeiro, RJ, Brazil

**Oğuz Söylemezoğlu** Gazi University Faculty of Medicine, Department of Pediatric Nephrology, Ankara, Turkey

**Nereida Spahia, MD, PhD** Service of Nephrology, University Hospital Center "Mother Teresa", Tirana, Albania

**Nattachai Srisawat, MD** Department of Medicine, Chulalongkorn University, Bangkok, Thailand

**Emmanuel Ssekasanvu** Panorama Medical Center, Kampala, Uganda

**Maria Stendahl, MD, PhD** Swedish Renal Registry, Jönköping County Hospital, Jönköping, Sweden

**Natalia Stepanova, MD, Prof. of Medicine** State Institution «Institute of Nephrology of the National Academy of Medical Sciences», Department of Nephrology and Dialysis, Kyiv, Ukraine

Ukrainian Association of Nephrologists & Kidney Transplant Specialists, Kyiv, Ukraine

**Ariana Strakosha, MD, PhD** Service of Nephrology, University Hospital Center "Mother Teresa", Tirana, Albania

**José Hermógenes Rocco Suassuna, MD, PhD** Brazilian Society of Nephrology (SBN), São Paulo, Brazil

Clinical and Academic Unit of Nephrology, Hospital Universitário Pedro Ernesto, Faculty of Medical Sciences, Universidade do Estado do Rio de Janeiro (UERJ), Rio de Janeiro, RJ, Brazil

**Gültekin Süleymanlar** Akdeniz University Faculty of Medicine, Department of Nephrology, Antalya, Turkey

**Sylvie Dusilová Sulková** Czech Society of Nephrology (CSN), Prague, Czech Republic

Hemodialysis Center, University Hospital, Hradec Králové, Czech Republic

**Ernest Kiswaya Sumaili, MD, PhD** Renal Unit, Kinshasa University Hospital, University of Kinshasa, Kinshasa, Democratic Republic of the Congo

**Qi-Quan Sun** Third Affiliated Hospital of Sun Yat-sen University, Guangzhou, China

**Kamonwan Tangvoraphonkchai, MD** Mahasarakham University, Maha Sarakham, Thailand

**Maiko A. Tavera-Díaz, MD** Hospital Elizabeth Seton, Cochabamba, Bolivia

**Pieter M. Ter Wee** Department of Nephrology, Amsterdam University Medical Center, Amsterdam, The Netherlands

**Vladimír Tesař** Czech Society of Nephrology (CSN), Prague, Czech Republic

Department of Nephrology, First Faculty of Medicine, Charles University and General Faculty Hospital, Prague, Czech Republic

**Pichthida Thim** Cambodian Association of Nephrology, Phnom Penh, Cambodia

**Khajohn Tiranathanagul, MD** Department of Medicine, Chulalongkorn University, Bangkok, Thailand

**Natavudh Townamchai, MD** Department of Medicine, Chulalongkorn University, Bangkok, Thailand

**Matteo Tozzi** Vascular Surgery Unit, Department of Medicine and Surgery, University of Insubria School of Medicine, ASST Settelaghi University Teaching Hospital, Varese (VA), Italy

**Desiré Tshala-Katumbay, MD, PhD** Department of Neurology, University of Kinshasa, Democratic Republic of the Congo and Oregon Health & Science University, Portland, OR, USA

**Kriang Tungsanga, MD** Department of Medicine, Chulalongkorn University, Bangkok, Thailand

**Aydın Türkmen** Istanbul University Faculty of Medicine, Department of Internal Medicine, Division of Nephrology, Istanbul, Turkey

**Douglas Urbina, MD** Venezuelan Society of Nephrology, Caracas, Venezuela

**Rafael Valdez-Ortiz, MD, PhD** Nephrology Service, Hospital General de Mexico Dr. Eduardo Liceaga, Mexico City, Mexico

**Johanna A. E. Van Wijk** Department of Paediatrics, Section of Paediatric Nephrology, Amsterdam University Medical Center, Amsterdam, The Netherlands

**Evgueniy Stefanov Vazelov, MD, PhD** University Hospital "Alexandrovska" Sofia, Sofia Medical University, Sofia, Bulgaria

**Armando Vazquez-Rangel, MD, MSc** Department of Nephrology, Instituto Nacional de Cardiología Ignacio Chavez, Mexico City, Mexico

**Ondřej Viklický** Czech Society of Nephrology (CSN), Prague, Czech Republic

Nephrology Department, Institute for Clinical and Experimental Medicine, Prague, Czech Republic

**José Vinhas** Nephrology Department, Centro Hospitalar de Setúbal, Setúbal, Portugal

**Marina Wainstein, MBBS, FRACP, MA (bioethics)** Nephrology Department, Royal Brisbane & Women's Hospital, Brisbane, QLD, Australia

**Robert James Walker, MB.ChB, MD, FRACP, FASN, FAHA** Department of Medicine, University of Otago, Dunedin, New Zealand

**Angela Yee-Moon Wang, MD, PhD, FRCP** Department of Medicine, Queen Mary Hospital, The University of Hong Kong, Hong Kong Special Administrative Region, China

**Ren-Ding Wang** Kidney Disease Center, The First Affiliated Hospital, College of Medicine, Zhejiang University, Hangzhou, China

National Key Clinical Department of Kidney Diseases, Institute of Nephrology, Zhejiang University, Hangzhou, China

**Nicola Wearne, FCP(SA), Cert Nephrol(SA)** Division of Nephrology and Hypertension, University of Cape Town and Groote Schuur Hospital, Cape Town, South Africa

**Angela C. Webster, MBBS, MM(Clin Epi), PhD, FRCAP, FRCP** Centre for Transplant and Renal Research, Westmead Hospital, Westmead, NSW, Australia

**Talia Weinstein, MD, PhD** The Israeli Society of Nephrology and Hypertension, Haifa, Israel

Tel Aviv University, Tel Aviv, Israel

Sourasky Medical Center, Tel Aviv, Israel

**Jose R. Weisinger, MD** International University of Florida, Gainesville, FL, USA

**Gunilla Welander, MD** Swedish Renal Registry, Jönköping County Hospital, Jönköping, Sweden

Nephrology Unit, Central Hospital Karlstad, Karlstad, Sweden

**I Gde Raka Widiana, MD, PhD, FINASIM** Division of Nephrology and Hypertension, Department of Internal Medicine, Faculty of Medicine Universitas Udayana – Sanglah General Hospital, Bali, Indonesia

**Andrzej Więcek, MD, PhD, FRCP(Edin), FERA, FASN** Department of Nephrology, Transplantation and Internal Diseases, Medical University of Silesia, Katowice, Poland

**Rebecca Winzeler, MSc** Service of Nephrology and Hypertension, Departments of Medicine, University Hospital, Lausanne, Switzerland

Service of Nephrology, Stadspital Waid, Zürich, Switzerland

**Per Wittenhagen, MD, DMSc** H.C. Andersen's Children's Hospital, Odense University Hospital, Odense, Denmark

**Damin Xu** Renal Division, Peking University First Hospital, Beijing, China

**Chao Yang** Renal Division, Peking University First Hospital, Beijing, China

**Li Yang** Renal Division, Peking University First Hospital, Beijing, China

**Xue-Qing Yu** Department of Nephrology, The First Affiliated Hospital, Sun Yat-sen University, Guangzhou, Guangdong, China

Key Laboratory of Nephrology, National Health Commission and Guangdong Province, Guangzhou, Guangdong, China

**Vasileios Zavvos** Center for Diagnosis, Treatment and Research on Kidney Diseases, Hygeia Hospital, Athens, Greece

**Luxia Zhang, MD, MPH** Renal Division, Peking University First Hospital, Beijing, China

National Institute of Health Data Science at Peking University, Beijing, China

**Ming-Hui Zhao, MD, PhD** Renal Division, Peking University First Hospital, Beijing, China

Peking Tsinghua Center for Life Sciences, Beijing, China

**Li Zuo, MD, PhD** Department of Nephrology, Peking University People's Hospital, Beijing, China

# Nephrology Worldwide: the Vision, the Project, and the Mission

1

José A. Moura-Neto, José Carolino Divino-Filho, and Claudio Ronco

## Introduction

Nephrology as a specialty was established in the early decades of the twentieth century, after centuries of scattered scientific and clinical observations. Its true expansion, however, only occurred in the years following the Second World War due to the application of hemodialysis, peritoneal dialysis, and kidney transplantation, as well as the utilization of renal biopsy to identify different forms of nephropathies. The important contributions from the pharmaceutical and dialysis industries spurred new interest in innovative technology and novel therapies, allowing dissemination of information through international conferences and publications in scientific journals.

Nephrology was then recognized as an independent specialty by various universities and medical schools, with the creation of a specific core curriculum for physicians who wanted to focus their careers on the area of kidney disease. In the final decades of the last century, nephrologists concentrated their attention on the technological advances in dialysis and the new approach to diagnosis of clinical syndromes through histopathological techniques of electron microscopy and immunofluorescence. In the meantime, new drugs and protocols were developed for the treatment of specific kidney diseases, both primitive and secondary to systemic disease. Further developments have occurred in the area of kidney transplant, where studies on genetics together with clinical trials on new immunosuppressive drugs have allowed for the expansion of transplant programs while concurrently reducing the rate of organ rejection.

J. A. Moura-Neto (✉)
Brazilian Society of Nephrology (SBN), Salvador, Bahia, Brazil
e-mail: moura@nephrologyworldwide.com

J. C. Divino-Filho
Division of Renal Medicine, CLINTEC, Karolinska Institutet, Stockholm, Sweden

C. Ronco
DIMED - University of Padova, Department Nephrology Dialysis & Transplantation, International Renal Research Institute (IRRIV), San Bortolo Hospital, Vicenza, Italy

When compared to the establishment of Nephrology as an organized specialty, kidney diseases have had a longer history, transcending the medical discipline. Furthermore, it also poses a global public health concern, affecting more than 750 million people in the world [1–3]. Currently, more than three million patients are estimated to be on renal replacement therapy worldwide.

The burden of kidney diseases varies significantly among countries. Socioeconomic, cultural, and political factors influence both the prevalence of kidney diseases and the provision of health care, leading to significant inequality in the disease burden, even in developed countries [4–6]. These disparities exist across the spectrum of kidney disease – ranging from preventive efforts to access to subspecialty health care and treatment of kidney failure with renal replacement therapy [1].

More than a medical discipline, field of study, and public health problem, nephrology (especially renal replacement therapy) is also an organized sector, or industry, directly and indirectly responsible for creating jobs for millions of people worldwide, often called stakeholders. With all this in mind, we designed the book "Nephrology Worldwide". This introductory chapter goes beyond concepts and data and addresses the initiative behind the book, in all its spheres: the vision, the project, and the mission. In addition, we also curated a selection of nephrology highlights in the countries from local nephrologists' view. Finally, we summarize our vision on education and future perspectives for nephrology.

## Nephrology Worldwide

### The Vision

The central idea that guided our vision for this book is quite simple: to answer the first question colleagues usually ask us when we meet at international conferences – "What is Nephrology like in your country?". Prior to this project, we were already aware of the vast differences in



J. A. Moura-Neto et al. (eds.), *Nephrology Worldwide*, https://doi.org/10.1007/978-3-030-56890-0_1

Nephrology among regions and countries in many aspects, such as the prevalence and incidence of kidney diseases, access to renal care, local guidelines, clinical management of kidney patients, nephrology practice, reimbursement, patients' and professionals' preferences, availability of renal replacement therapy, workforce in the nephrology setting, etc.

The response to this book's central question requires not only objective numbers and cold data, but also a critical analysis of the scenario and future perspectives for nephrology in the country. By the end of each chapter, readers should have a clear and general idea of the field in the country. We expect this book will help integrate nephrologists and stakeholders around the world and eliminate the still-standing frontiers of nephrology; this is our vision.

## The Project

To fulfill our ultimate goal for "Nephrology Worldwide", we had to design a project, in all its stages, capable of providing the answers and information we were seeking. We also had to conceive this book in such a way that it would have credibility among our peers and stakeholders. Therefore, our first challenge was selecting the leading authors, also called corresponding authors, and the countries to be included in this first edition.

One of the premises of the "Nephrology Worldwide" project was to include countries from all regions and continents, so the book would be legitimately international. Although 62 countries had initially agreed to participate, some authors were not able to deliver their chapters by the final deadline and thus were not included in the first edition. Ultimately, 51 countries are represented in this book, encompassing around 5.7 billion people (Fig. 1.1). In addition to our concern with geographic representation, the final selection included, among others, the most populated countries, as well as countries with the highest Growth Domestic Products (GDP) and Human Development Index (HDI).

| |
|---|
| The 10 most populated countries |
| 22 of the 25 highest GDP |
| 8 of the 10 highest HDI |

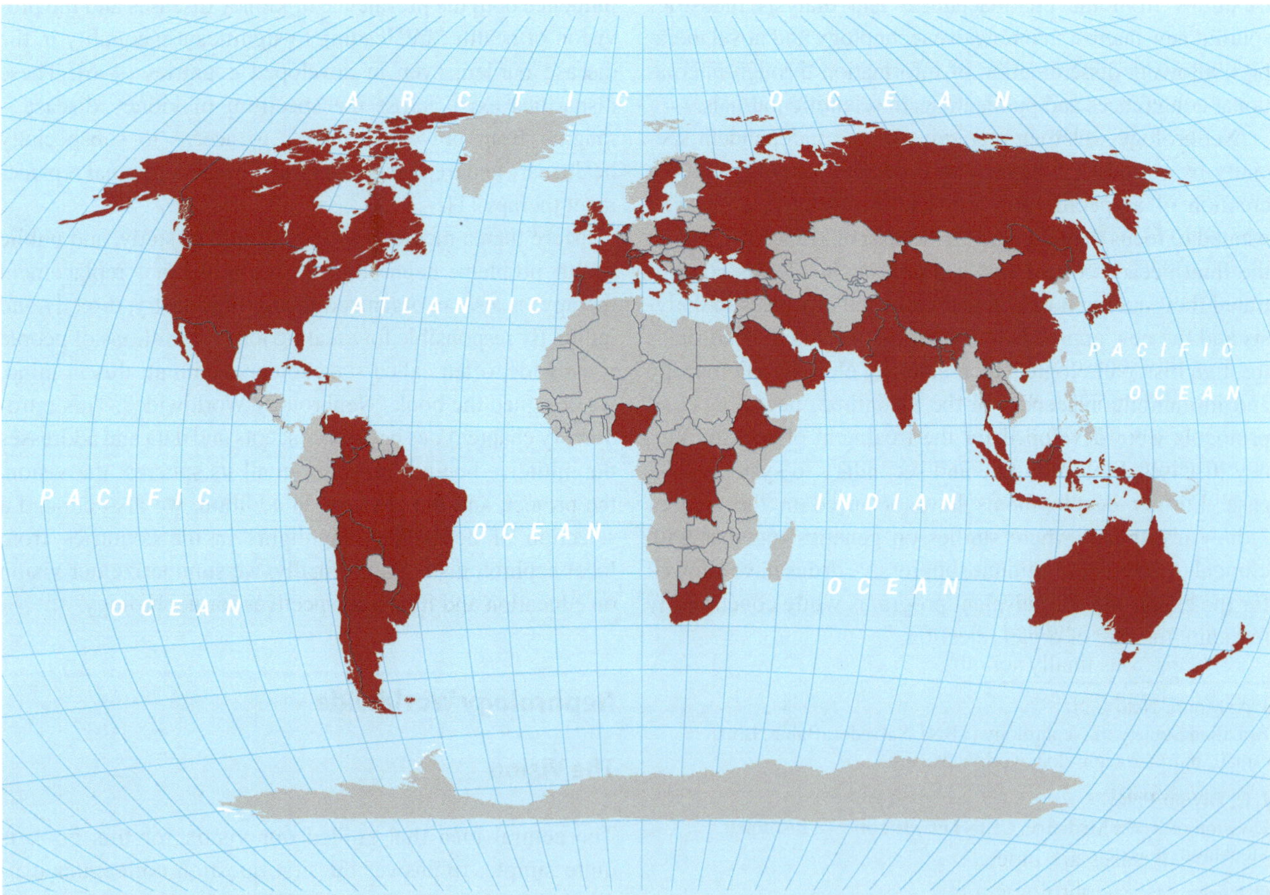


**Fig. 1.1** Map highlighting the 51 countries included in "Nephrology Worldwide". About 5.7 billion people are represented, covering all continents and regions of the world

We carefully chose each leading author based on their background, nephrology practice, and leadership in the national nephrology society. To do so, we searched on the Internet and contacted colleagues around the world in order to hear their opinions. The leading authors were responsible for putting together a diverse team of co-authors, with different professional experiences, able to fully describe the field in their country. More than 300 authors, from 51 different nationalities, contributed to this book, which makes "Nephrology Worldwide" probably the most international book in nephrology.

Our second challenge in this project was to provide a chapter template and adequate guidelines to the selected authors. We did so in order to avoid missing key information and to create a didactic pattern throughout the book, with the goal of making the life of readers easier, since they would become familiar with the layout of chapters after reading just one. In these guidelines and template, we requested authors to provide a full overview of nephrology in the country, in their diverse fields and areas, such as kidney transplantation, maintenance hemodialysis, peritoneal dialysis, pediatric nephrology, acute kidney injury, and critical care nephrology. We stressed the importance of using the most up-to-date information and to consider including unpublished data, if relevant. We also asked the authors to address the history of nephrology in the country, reimbursement, nephrology practice, and job market, not only for physicians but also for nurses and the multidisciplinary team, when applicable. To make the book friendly and easier for readers, we deliver a kind reminder to the authors at the end of the guidelines: "be aware you will be presenting your country to a foreign audience, unfamiliar with the specificities of nephrology practices and healthcare in your country".

The third phase of the project was the review of the manuscripts. In this stage, we meticulously reviewed the chapters and sent the authors a checklist asking to provide missing information and also anticipating questions that readers might have. Each chapter was first reviewed by two editors and the revised version was carefully looked over once more by one of the three editors. Our goal was to complete the revision in a timely fashion in order to avoid information and data becoming outdated. After concluding this stage, the manuscript was finally submitted to Springer Nature to finalize the editing process.

## The Mission

Kidney diseases are indeed a global public health problem that we, as a nephrology community, must prioritize in the coming decades. Its prevalence will probably steadily rise in the next years due to the population aging and an increasing prevalence of diseases such as hypertension and diabetes [7, 8]. To make an already concerning scenario worse, estimates have suggested that 2.3–7.1 million patients die per year due to an inability to access dialysis or sustain the treatment, which is called "the renal replacement therapy gap" [9–11]. We are now, more than ever, convinced that this a major issue, and the global nephrology community should shift its focus to this gap and the inequalities that contributed to it.

Editing this book was a transformative process for the editors in many ways, we hope readers will have a similar experience. It changed our view and perspective on the (Nephrology) World and it raised several important questions, not only medical, but also socioeconomic and political, that surround the field. Questions of a nature quite different than the one the book initially posed, now asking "Why?" in the place of "What?". While we feel our original query has been responded, we finished this first edition with more questions than answers. More than that: although we feel we have finished the project, a book, we have only just started the "Nephrology Worldwide" mission.

## Nephrology Worldwide Highlights

When this book was planned, it was agreed that each chapter would have a section entitled Highlights, in which authors could write about any special feature, story, history, project, or program specific to their country and considered worthy of sharing with the Nephrology community worldwide. Here, we address some of these highlights, most of them excerpts taken directly from the chapters. Please be aware you will find spoilers from the book in the following paragraphs.

### History

The history of the local nephrology societies gives us a true perspective of how nephrology has developed around the world. It is not uncommon for local doctors to be sent abroad for nephrology training, often to faraway places for long periods of time, in order to come back home and propagate what was learned abroad. Each history includes many stories of real colleagues and events that contributed to the development of Nephrology in each one of the 51 countries represented in this first edition of this book. Schumlansky, Yu Voronoy, Richard Bright, Nils Alwall, Peter Kolff, Murray, Van Rood, Fred Boen, Belding Scribner, John Merril, Jean Hamburger, Cimino-Brescia, Iversen & Claus Brunn, Giordano & Giovannetti, Moncrief & Popovich, Dimitris Oreoupolous, Priscila Kincaid-

Smith, Gianantonio, and many others – names that have contributed to the position where Nephrology stands today.

## Diseases and the Kidney

This book will also provide an insight on different diseases and conditions, unknown to many, that pose a potential burden to acute kidney injury (AKI) and/or chronic kidney disease (CKD) and nephrologists around the world may face: Plasmodium malaria, dengue, HIV, traditional medicines – for example, Callilepis laureola (locally referred to as "impila"), potassium dichromate, Cape Aloe, high altitude-polycythemia, star fruit, snake bites, scorpion stings, fish gallbladder toxicity, cutaneous leishmaniasis, Nipah virus, leptospirosis, scrub typhus, melioidosis, use of poisonous substances (PPD, methanol, organo phosphorous compounds, paraquat, copper sulfate, rat killer), nephrotoxic drug exposure, etc.

In Bolivia, for example, more than four million people (38% of total population) currently live at high altitude (2500 meters above sea level); 8–10% of this population develops high altitude polycythemia. In a study, 40% of total screening polycythemia healthy subjects had some degree of proteinuria, so we estimate that roughly more than three hundred thousand peoples are at risk for kidney disease.

Another interesting story worth reading relates to Balkan endemic nephropathy, originally described in 1956. This is a unique familial form of interstitial nephritis, encountered with a high prevalence rate in Bulgaria, Serbia, Romania, Croatia, and Bosnia-Herzegovina, that leads to kidney failure.

## Chronic Kidney Disease

CKD is a significant cause of morbidity and mortality globally, but in certain regions and countries communicable diseases impose an extra burden in the prevalence of CKD. Unfortunately, the reasons for this increased burden are most likely due to factors such as poverty, health care relegated as non-priority, and poor governance. For many of us, it may be a surprise to learn that serum creatinine test is not provided for hospitalized patients in many corners of the world. This book cites several concrete examples of the effect of socioeconomic disparities on the epidemiology of kidney diseases. CKD is mainly a disease of the young population in many developing countries, especially on the African continent; however, this is in sharp contrast with the older age groups seen in the developed world. Moreover, in most countries there are a great number of CKD patients diagnosed in later stages; over half of patients with CKD in India seek medical attention only after they have developed advanced kidney failure, often requiring dialysis.

Also of note, the Chronic REnal Disease In Turkey – CREDIT Study – described a higher CKD prevalence than found in many industrialized western countries. Associations between CKD and several cardiovascular risk factors emphasize that CKD is a major public health problem and a major predictor of overall morbidity and mortality.

## Nephrologists Worldwide

Shortages of nephrologists and renal nurses are not uncommon in several countries. Uganda, for example, has only ten nephrologists for a population of 45 million people, resulting in a ratio of one nephrologist per approximately 4.5 million people. Since the needs of these professionals are not met, emigration of nephrologists and nurses to other countries where they are better paid and which fully provide the working resources required is a common occurrence. This phenomenon is called "brain drain" and there may be countries where the number of emigrated nephrologists is higher than the number practicing in the country. Additionally, there is low availability or lack of local training in several African countries for aspiring professionals in the field. On the other hand, there are countries, like South Africa, contributing to the training of nephrologists from other countries on the continent through different Fellowship programs. This phenomenon is also observed on other continents, for example, some Cambodian nephrologists have been trained in France, Australia, Japan, and Thailand.

In Oman, most nephrologists are non-Omani and mostly from Egypt and Indian Subcontinent countries. Nephrology training for Omani clinicians was done entirely abroad in North America, Europe, and Australia. However, recently the Oman Medical Specialty Board approved the Nephrology fellowship program of at least 2 years following 4 years of Internal Medicine training. The Renal Dialysis Nurse Specialty program, launched in 1997, is one of the major accomplished nursing education programs in Oman with 344 nephrology nurses graduating from this program.

The vast majority of the 50 Irish Consultants accredited in Nephrology will have had some of their Nephrology Training outside of Ireland; some will have held Consultant, Attending, or other Faculty positions in other countries. These countries are typically, but not exclusively, English-speaking, such as England & Wales, Scotland, Canada, Australia, New Zealand, or the USA.

An important issue faced by many countries is the lack of appeal of the nephrology discipline, which ultimately may result in a shortage of nephrologists. A positive and different example from the global trend that needs to be highlighted comes from France, where Nephrology has become quite an attractive discipline for trainees and interns. It has been ranked among the first medical specialties selected from interns over the last few years for its attractiveness. Diversity of activities (clinical nephrology, dialysis, transplantation, laboratory) is one of its positive aspects. The image of the discipline has been changed due to the University College of Nephrology Teachers (CUEN), dynamism of university nephrology departments and scientific societies and development, and creation of various clubs and platforms where trainees and young nephrologists can meet and exchange ideas. In addition to its attractiveness, recent changes in intern fellowship program rules also permitted a significant increase in the number of nephrology fellows in France. The outcomes from all of this are becoming clear and, due to the potential of this new, younger working force, it appears that nephrology needs will be covered adequately in the foreseeable future in France.

## Dialysis

There are important gaps in CKD policies and renal replacement therapy availability among countries and regions. Renal replacement therapy is available to a very small number of end-stage renal disease (ESRD) patients in only a few urban centers in several countries, with rates inferior to 10 dialysis patients per million population (pmp) whereas countries like the USA and Japan have an overall prevalence of renal replacement therapy over 2000 pmp. Many other contrasts are expressed in the chapters, such as the fact that in Uganda there are only 52 HD machines in the entire country, 21 of which belong to the public sector, providing both acute and chronic HD.

In countries in development, such as the Democratic Republic of the Congo, the lack of financial resources forces patients either to reduce dialysis frequency, withdraw from dialysis, or use alternative treatment which results in higher mortality with a median survival of 17 months or 78 per 1000 patient-years. In contrast, the survival rate of dialysis patients in Japan has been excellent; the annual crude death rate was 10% in 2018, and it has hovered between 9% and 10% since 1983. Although the reasons for this have not been fully clarified, it is believed that could be related to the unique dialysis system and to the concept of chronic dialysis in Japan. Another curious fact regarding Japanese dialysis, which is also seen in other Asian countries, is the low dialysis blood flow rate (200–220 ml/min) – very different than that observed in many western countries (300–450 ml/min).

Besides blood flow rate, other dialysis practices such as dialysis frequency and average time per session are also addressed. In addition, regulatory issues are also discussed in "Nephrology Worldwide"; we would like to highlight dialyzer reuse, which may still be a matter of debate in some countries. While reuse is forbidden by law in several countries, it is widely used in others. There is yet another group of countries where reuse is permitted, but is rarely used, such as Canada, Switzerland, Russia, China, South Africa, and USA. In the latter, for example, reuse of dialyzers was once popular – in 1997, 82% of dialysis facilities participated in a reuse program – but currently it is rarely, if ever, used. Table 1.1 shows examples found in this book of countries where reuse is performed and countries where it is not performed as of 2019.

**Table 1.1** Countries where dialyzer reuse is performed and not performed (2019)

| Reuse allowed | No reuse |
|---|---|
| Argentina | Albania |
| Bangladesh | Australia |
| Bolivia | Czech Republic |
| Brazil | Denmark |
| Cambodia | France |
| Canada (rare) | Greece |
| Chile | Iran |
| China (rare) | Israel |
| Cuba | Italy |
| India | Japan |
| Malaysia | Netherlands |
| Mexico | New Zealand |
| Nigeria | Poland |
| Oman | Portugal |
| Pakistan | Saudi Arabia |
| Russia (rare) | Singapore |
| South Africa (rare) | Spain |
| Switzerland (rare) | Sweden |
| Thailand | Turkey |
| USA (rare) | Ukraine |
| Uruguay | United Arab Emirates |
| | Venezuela |

As a global trend, the number of patients on dialysis is steadily rising. In keeping with the increase in the incidence and prevalence of ESRD around the world, the burden of ESRD is on the rise in the Chinese Mainland. The number of ESRD patients receiving dialysis treatment has drastically increased from 261,877 in 2011 to 610,811 by the end of 2017.

This book also explores the differences between private and public healthcare for nephrology patients. In Portugal, considering the 2018 prevalent HD population, 91% were being treated in an outpatient dialysis unit run by the private sector, while 9% were dialyzed in public hospitals. In stark contrast to this scenario, in Cuba all of the HD centers are state-owned and operated.

Several different models of dialysis reimbursement exist globally and were discussed in the chapters. While in Brazil there is a huge difference in reimbursement for one HD session depending on the source of payment (the government or private health insurance), in Greece the reimbursement price per HD session is almost equivalent for the public and the private sector, and the increasing number of private HD units does not increase the state expenses and health budget.

The medical workforce present in HD centers is also very different among countries. In Turkey, for example, most HD centers have general practitioners or internists who are continuously taking care of patients. These HD practitioners receive a special certificate following 3–6 months of education for HD practice. HD certificate education is given by the nephrology training centers in Turkey.

While peritoneal dialysis (PD) is not practiced in some countries due to the lack of financial resources, other countries have a PD-first program policy. For countries with an underrepresentation of PD in chronic renal replacement therapy provision, new models of renal services are being implemented. In some countries, PD patients are only followed in PD units integrated into nephrology departments in public hospitals.

When mentioning successful PD-first programs, Mexico is the first country that comes to mind. A contributing and decisive factor for its success was the 1985 earthquake in Mexico City, during which a large number of public HD facilities were damaged, thus requiring the use of PD on a larger scale. Following in Mexico's steps, other countries successfully applied the PD-first program. In 1985, PD-first policy was adopted by the Hospital Authority of Hong Kong, in which PD was reimbursed by the government as a first-line dialysis modality for patients with ESRD; Thailand and Indonesia were the latest to adopt it.

Finally, the last dialysis highlight comes from the Japanese PD program: the combination therapy, or hybrid therapy, with in-center HD. Out of 9445 PD patients in Japan, 1863 (19.7%) patients were under the combination therapy in 2018, with 1505 (16.6%) being treated with at least one HD session per week.

## Renal Transplantation

The transplant project in many countries is faced with several challenges, the most important of which are very limited resources on budgeting and provision of health care facilities, the precarious continuity of supplies, and the underdeveloped infrastructure. The successful transplant project in Ethiopia, which was a result of a collaborative effort between a local Medical College and an American university, is an exemplary model that can be replicated in other developing countries.

Two well-established transplantation programs also deserve mention. Brazil has the largest publicly funded transplantation program in the world, with a fair organ allocation system and no social or cultural privileges. The numbers are expressive, but still far below the growing demands of the country. Spain is the country that should perhaps be looked to as the role model for renal transplantation. It is considered the renal replacement therapy of choice in Spain since it generally provides better quality of life and survival at a lower cost. Therefore, a large public policy effort is aimed at increasing renal transplantation rates and acceptance of donation by the population.

Nephrology Worldwide will also offer readers the possibility to understand the obstacles and opportunities faced when creating and/or improving the necessary legislation for development or enhancement of organ transplantation. The example of Croatia shows that development of surgical transplant techniques, long-term transplant tradition, and the existence of a national transplant organization are not, neither together nor individually, a guarantee for a successful transplant system if they are not accompanied by a set of appropriate legal, financial, and primarily organizational measures. It is interesting to note that kidney health and nephrology are of particular interest to the governments of some countries, such as in the United Arab Emirates, since the founder and first president of the country, Sheikh Zayed Al Nahyan, received a kidney transplant in 2000.

## Home Dialysis

Regarding home dialysis, we would like to highlight three examples: New Zealand, Denmark, and Canada. New Zealand has one of the highest rates worldwide of home dialysis, with 1291 (47%) of the 2768 individuals on dialysis therapy. Of the patients on home dialysis, 34% are on home HD and the rest of them are on PD. In Denmark, there is also a high prevalence of home dialysis therapies (28% of dialysis patients), with 21% on PD and 7% on HD.

The proportion of Canadian patients treated with home dialysis modalities remains relatively high by international standards. However, it is much lower than it was in the 1980s and early 1990s when CAPD was being used in over 35% of prevalent patients. There has recently been an increase in home dialysis prevalence back up toward 25%, in part related to efforts by provincial renal agencies. This places Canada in the top 12 countries in the world for home dialysis use. About 20% of home dialysis in Canada is accounted for by home HD, less than is the case for Australia, New Zealand, and Denmark, but much more than in the USA and most of Europe.

Of note, the chapter on Australia, a country in which about 10% of the HD patients are under HD at home, provides a brief yet comprehensive description of their home HD program, addressing the history, epidemiology, selection of patients and training, equipment, barriers, and outcomes of home HD.

## Health Care Services, Registries, and Programs

Examples of health care services and nephrology care are also reported in each chapter. For instance, Cuba has a unique health system that ensures universal and free coverage, with 56 nephrology centers distributed throughout the country offering specialized nephrology care and renal replacement therapy coverage. Similarly, in Uruguay, Nephrology has gradually developed, and yet has allowed for providing full, universal nephrology care to all inhabitants, both children and adults, across the nation.

National Registries are of utmost importance when targeting improvement in the different areas of activities and assuring a continuous quality control of the nephrology care in each country. Renal biopsy, glomerular diseases, CKD, renal transplantation, and dialysis registries (pediatric and adult), both national and regional, are also part of Nephrology Worldwide. Malaysia is one of many excellent examples. The Dialysis and Transplant Register was started in 1992, the first report of the Malaysian Dialysis and Transplant Registry was published in 1993, and it is still reporting today. The Malaysian Registry of Renal Biopsy started reporting in 2005 and the deceased donor kidney transplant waiting list linked to the Malaysian Organ Sharing System started in 1999. Data on renal replacement therapy are shared with the USRDS, and with the Global Observatory on Donation and Transplantation.

Exciting programs are being launched in several developing countries. Thailand, an endemic area of several tropical illnesses, has been gradually overshadowed by non-communicable diseases. The prevalence of pre-dialysis CKD in Thailand was greater than the global prevalence and this became a concerning issue. This could be linked to the upward trend of dialysis patients and centers, which resulted in catastrophic national health expenditure. In an attempt to overcome this burden, the Thai government released several campaigns and issued policies to slow down CKD progression. The model in CKD clinics is a multidisciplinary approach, implemented in all levels of public hospitals in order to improve health promotion and increase access of health care even in remote areas. The introduction of the Universal Health Coverage Scheme and the PD-First policy are laudable initiatives to narrow the gap between the wealthy and the poor in relation to access to health services. In order to avoid financial burden, any project aiming to decelerate CKD progression or providing economical renal replacement therapy with comparable outcomes to international standards is deemed a priority.

The Indonesian Society of Nephrology has developed short- and long-term programs in conjunction with the Ministry of Health including: unleashing the PD preferred program for the endorsement of CAPD; early detection and preventive program for CKD in the community and primary health care; and development of kidney transplantation in some tertiary hospitals.

Some of the success stories described in the book are summarized here. Nephrology in Albania has achieved great improvement in the twenty-first century. The possibility of treating every ESRD patient with renal replacement therapy became a reality in the last decade, and this is considered their greatest success. Academic nephrologists on the Chinese Mainland also play an increasingly important role in conducting global clinical trials that impact the development of global clinical practice guidelines.

In the 1980s, Poland had limited access to the modern methods of treatment of AKI and CKD, and only a limited number of patients with ESRD had access to renal replacement therapy. For many of our Polish colleagues, a trip to the western countries at that time was, in their own words, "like a journey to a different planet". Thirty years later, however, the situation in Poland has changed dramatically and, nowadays, nephrology in Poland has developed almost to the level of many western European countries and the access to all types of renal replacement therapy is unlimited for those who need them.

On the concerning side, we must pay special attention to the Venezuelan chapter and the current sociopolitical landscape, which contrasts with its beautiful history and role in Latin American Nephrology. They finalize their chapter: *"Actions to retake a path towards stabilization or growth of the attention to kidney disease in all expressions have to be rethought within policies to rebuild the national health system; no simple or individual remedies seem possible at this time. But we are also certain that the country will at some point start retaking the route towards political stability, economic growth, and social development."* The Nephrology Worldwide community should be ready to assist them however possible when this becomes a reality.

## Acute Kidney Injury

There has been a reborn interest in acute renal failure, recently renamed acute kidney injury (AKI). The UK has a long history of recognizing and furthering the clinical management of AKI, dating back to the first descriptions of crush injury during the bombing of London in the Second World War. It was during the bombing of London in World War II that Eric Bywaters at the Hammersmith Hospital became interested in the histopathology of the AKI caused by crush injury. Due to military conflicts, nephrologists in Israel have also gained expertise in management of casualties with crush injuries and subsequent devastating AKI, hemodynamic, and electrolyte disturbances.

Since the Second World War and the first description of acute renal failure and Hemolytic Uremic Syndrome in 1962, extensive developments in renal replacement therapy as a means of treating AKI have occurred. However, the disparity in the access to basic prevention measures and these technical developments, when comparing developed and underdeveloped countries, is an important warning sign and rescue alert to the nephrology community worldwide. The predominant causes of AKI in many countries are still acute gastroenteritis (related to sub-optimal sanitation and water quality), inadvertent use of drugs, tropical infections, sepsis, poor obstetric care, and insufficient monitoring after major surgeries. In Bangladesh, for example, the incidence of AKI increases by 18–24% during monsoon season, secondary to an increase in new cases of acute gastroenteritis, dengue, leptospirosis, and bacillary dysentery.

## Final Remarks on Nephrology Worldwide Highlights

Nephrology Worldwide will provide unique information on topics from kidney disease/renal replacement therapy and natural disasters – such as earthquakes (Chile, Iran, Turkey, Italy), monsoons – to the dialyzer crisis in Croatia. It will also discuss exciting projects like "Kidney in Health and Disease", Green Nephrology, the Swiss Transplantation Cohort, the Swiss Kidney Stone Cohort, as well as interesting themes like "Fasting during the month of Ramadan and kidney disease". Furthermore, the reader will learn about the Chernobyl tragedy and its impact on children born in the compromised zone after 1995, consanguinity rates in different countries, and genetic kidney diseases and congenital anomalies of the kidney and urinary tract.

It is our humble belief and firm objective that Nephrology Worldwide will fill a void within the nephrology community by allowing each and every country represented in this book to tell their history, stories, actions, and accomplishments, both past and present, hopefully reserving the future for new editions of this project with even more countries represented. Here all countries are equal and have the opportunity to tell everyone involved in Nephrology their realities, strengths, weaknesses, priorities, goals, and dreams.

## Nephrology Education and the "Open Nephrology" Culture

Nephrology, like other disciplines, has been mostly separated from other specialties and disciplines for several reasons. The focus of postgraduate medical training has not typically been multidisciplinary or problem-oriented, but rather specialty-oriented, often leading to the development of an adversarial "them and us" mentality. Thus, specialists were consulted for specialty-related problems or for the performance of procedures and tests with which they were familiar with and had the particular required skills. Such an approach was often deleterious to patient care because it led to fragmentation and conflicts. In addition, while some nephrologists endeavored to take a global view of the patient's condition, their familiarity with intensive care technology, current management, and pathophysiology was often limited. As a consequence, the global perception of the patient was often out of touch with reality. This limited understanding of critical care medicine or, in several cases, the limited interest in considering the critically ill patient a target for innovation and special interest in nephrology then resulted in inadequate training and capacity to share decision-making and therapeutic strategies with the critical care colleagues. Such action, in turn, fueled the fire of antagonism rather than cooperation. The same process has occurred with cardiology in the area of hypertension and heart failure, urology in the area of kidney stones, rheumatology in the area of systemic diseases affecting the kidney and finally diabetology and science of nutrition. The clash of these "cultures" significantly impeded the development of a combined strategy in the management of patients with specific kidney problems, but at the same time combined syndromes where other organs and functions were involved. Other obstacles, such as financial incentives, competition in research, political strategies, and control of patient care, have further impeded the development of an "open nephrology" culture.

The vision of illuminated scientists and physicians belonging to the new generation allowed for the opening of nephrology as a specialty to other disciplines, favoring the development of a multidisciplinary culture. In this direction, scientific societies have tried to merge knowledge and information and, at the same time, scientific journals have started new policies to accept interdisciplinary papers. With this new wave, the era of cardionephrology began with a shared definition and classification of the cardiorenal syndromes. Critical care nephrology has become a new subspecialty with an enormous amount of publications. Currently, acute kidney injury represents one of the most interesting areas of common research from the pathophysiological mechanisms to the extracorporeal organ therapies and the world of regenerative medicine. Immunology and genetics are involved in the advanced research for immunetolerance to permit safe and effective kidney transplantation. New drugs have been utilized or are under evaluation for onconephrology, hemolytic uremic syndromes, and glomerulonephritis.

## Future Perspectives for Nephrology Worldwide

Overall, we can say that the future of nephrology will impact the future of the whole medical discipline. We think the future is *GREEN*. This is an acronym that describes the initials of the sciences that are likely to characterize the future of nephrology. *G for genetics*: patient genotyping will allow for the expansion of the application of precision medicine solutions in different kidney disorders in the future. *R for robotics*: the mechanical actuation of operations normally carried out by a caregiver will permit taking maximum advantage of bidirectional interactions between the patient and the dialysis equipment. *E for E-health and information communication technology*: remote monitoring as well as enhanced human intelligence by computers will provide the basis for specific diagnostic algorithms or research programs on big data that can be further improved by artificial intelligence networks. This will provide support in the decision-making process and will even provide the basis for automated feedback operations. *E for eco-compatibility*: water sparing technologies and home therapies with remote monitoring will contribute to save natural resources and will provide environment-friendly solutions. *N for nanosciences*: this interesting area of research will offer a new spectrum of biomaterials and will enable possible uses of nanofluids and therapeutic nanoparticles, drugs, and vaccines.

The GREEN approach to nephrology will provide new directions for investigators and physicians to achieve an equal distribution of care among individuals of various areas of the planet, cost reduction with possibility to expand the interventions to vast populations that today may be undertreated or segregated, early detection and resolution of problems, as in the case of virus dissemination and pandemics, improved treatment compliance and automatic feedback on results, reduction of patient's access to hospital center for technical and clinical complications, increased confidence of patients treated at home, with higher incidence and prevalence of home therapies, and consequent improvement in patient's quality of life.

We must work together to achieve a common pace of progress and advancement of science in different areas of the planet, concomitantly dealing with the global inequalities and disparities in access to kidney health care worldwide. We are all part of a big family in this small world that must collectively strive to fulfill the "Nephrology Worldwide" mission.

**Note:** More information on the Nephrology Worldwide initiative can be found at http://www.nephrologyworldwide.com. Readers will find a friendly platform where they can send feedback, suggestions and also 'apply' to contribute as author or reviewer in future *Nephrology Worldwide* editions.

## References


1. Crews DC, Bello AK, Saadi G. 2019 World Kidney Day Editorial – burden, access, and disparities in kidney disease. Kidney Int. 2019;95:242–8.
2. GBD 2015 DALYs and HALE Collaborators. Global, regional, and national disability-adjusted life-years (DALYs) for 315 diseases and injuries and healthy life expectancy (HALE), 1990–2015: a systematic analysis for the Global Burden of Disease Study 2015. Lancet. 2016;388:1603–58.
3. Bikbov B, Perico N, Remuzzi G, On Behalf of the GBD Genitourinary Diseases Expert Group. Disparities in chronic kidney disease prevalence among males and females in 195 countries: analysis of the global burden of disease 2016 study. Nephron. 2018;139:313–8.
4. Crews DC, Liu Y, Boulware LE. Disparities in the burden, outcomes, and care of chronic kidney disease. Curr Opin Nephrol Hypertens. 2014;23:298–305.
5. Nicholas SB, Kalantar-Zadeh K, Norris KC. Socioeconomic disparities in chronic kidney disease. Adv Chronic Kidney Dis. 2015;22:6–15.
6. Crews DC, Pfaff T, Powe NR. Socioeconomic factors and racial disparities in kidney disease outcomes. Semin Nephrol. 2013;33:468–75.
7. Lozano R, Naghavi M, Foreman K, et al. Global and regional mortality from 235 causes of death for 20 age groups in 1990 and 2010: a systematic analysis for the Global Burden of Disease Study 2010. Lancet. 2012;380:2095–128.
8. White SL, Chadban SJ, Jan S, Chapman JR, Cass A. How can we achieve global equity in provision of renal replacement therapy? Bull World Health Organ. 2008;86:229–37.
9. Liyanage T, Ninomiya T, Jha V, et al. Worldwide access to treatment for end-stage kidney disease: a systematic review. Lancet. 2015;385:1975–82.
10. Anand S, Bitton A, Gaziano T. The gap between estimated incidence of end-stage renal disease and use of therapy. PLoS One. 2013;8:e72860.
11. Luyckx VA, Miljeteig I, Ejigu AM, Moosa MR. Ethical challenges in the provision of dialysis in resource-constrained environments. Semin Nephrol. 2017;37(3):273–86.

# Nephrology Worldwide: A Perspective from the International Society of Nephrology

2

Titi Chen, Rolando Claure-Del Granado, Kelly Hendricks, Vivekanand Jha, and David Harris

## Overview of Global Nephrology

### Epidemiology and Burden of Kidney Disease Worldwide

Over the last few decades, there has been a dramatic shift in the spectrum of disease worldwide, with a reduction in the burden of communicable disease and an increase in that of non-communicable disease [1]. Rising life-expectancy and ever-increasing global epidemic of diabetes and hypertension, the major causes of chronic kidney disease (CKD), have led to a marked rise in the burden of CKD [2]. Since the standardization of the definition of stages of CKD in 2002, overwhelming evidence from epidemiological studies has reinforced that CKD is now an enormous public health problem. According to the Global Burden of Disease Study 2017, the global incidence, prevalence, death, and disability-adjusted life years (DALYs) due to CKD increased dramatically from 1990 to 2016. In 2016, the global incidence of CKD was 21 million per year (increased by 89%), prevalence was 276 million (increased by 87%), 1.2 million deaths were attributable to CKD (increased by 98%), and attributable DALYs were 35 million years (increased by 62%) [2]. From 18th position in the list of leading causes of death in 1990, CKD rose to 11th place in 2016 [1], and is predicted to become the 5th leading cause of years of life lost in 2040 [3]. The economic burden of CKD is also enormous and disproportional to the size of population with the condition. High-resource nations are estimated to spend more than 3% of their healthcare budget on treating end-stage renal disease (ESRD) patients who represent under 0.03% of the total population [4]. The total cost of treating other CKD patients is estimated to be even greater than that of treating ESRD patients [5].

There is substantial variation in the epidemiology and burden of CKD across the globe. For example, aging is found to be the main driver of increasing DALYs in high-resource nations, while population growth is the main driver in low-resource nations [2]. The contribution of diabetes and hypertension to increased CKD DALYs is more marked in high-resource nations than low-resource nations [6]. The age-adjusted burden of CKD is more pronounced in low–resource nations where CKD develops and causes death at a younger age compared with high-resource nations [4]. Low-resource nations are less equipped to provide life-saving treatment such as dialysis and transplant to patients who progress to ESRD. The morbidity and mortality due to CKD is increasing in most world regions, with the most concerning trend in Central America where CKD has the highest death rate in the world, and has tripled over the past 20 years [1, 6].

Acute kidney injury (AKI) is associated with high morbidity and mortality, and has been increasingly recognized as a global concern, especially in developing countries. AKI affects 13.3 million people and causes 1.7 million deaths per year worldwide [7]. As with CKD, there is large geographical variation in the epidemiology of AKI and its outcome. The

T. Chen (✉)
The University of Sydney, The Westmead Institute for Medical Research, Department of Renal Medicine, Westmead Hospital, Westmead, NSW, Australia
e-mail: titi.chen@sydney.edu.au

R. Claure-Del Granado
Servicio de Nefrología, Hospital Obrero No 2 - C.N.S., Universidad Mayor de San Simón, School of Medicine, Cochabamba, Bolivia

K. Hendricks
International Society of Nephrology, Global Operations Center, Brussels, Belgium
e-mail: khendricks@theisn.org

V. Jha
International Society of Nephrology, Brussels, Belgium

George Institute for Global Health, UNSW, New Delhi, India

Faculty of Medicine, Imperial College, London, UK

Manipal Academy of Higher Education, Manipal, India
e-mail: vjha@georgeinstitute.org.in

D. Harris
International Society of Nephrology, The University of Sydney, The Westmead Institute for Medical Research, Department of Renal Medicine, Westmead Hospital, Westmead, NSW, Australia
e-mail: david.harris@sydney.edu.au



J. A. Moura-Neto et al. (eds.), *Nephrology Worldwide*, https://doi.org/10.1007/978-3-030-56890-0_2

burden of AKI is particularly high in low-income countries (LIC) where the annual incidence is as high as 11.3 million and the death rate is estimated to be 1.4 million per year [8]. This contrasts with high-income countries (HIC) where AKI mainly occurs in hospital and patients are usually older with multiple co-morbidities, whereas in LIC, AKI mainly occurs in the community as a result of dehydration, infection, pregnancy-related events, and poor access to care [9]. Children and women in these countries are particularly susceptible to AKI [10]. The overall cost of AKI care has not been well quantified. In one English study, inpatient AKI care was estimated to cost 1.72 billion USD (1% of the National Health Service budget) per year [11]. In addition to the costs of AKI itself, AKI is a well-known risk factor for the development of CKD. Compared with matched patients without AKI, the risk of developing CKD is nine times higher and the risk of premature death is two times higher in patients with AKI [12]. In the USA, CKD as a result of AKI accounts for 3% of all ESRD [13]. The societal burden associated with providing care for these long-term effects of AKI is enormous.

## Current State of Kidney Care and Challenges

To assess the status and capacity for kidney care across the globe, the International Society of Nephrology (ISN) launched the Global Kidney Health Atlas (GKHA) in 2017. As one of the largest health-related country-level capacity reviews, GKHA describes the capacity for kidney care according to the World Health Organization (WHO) Universal Health Coverage domains [14]. It captured data from 160 countries, comprising >98% of global population. The following sections will discuss the current state of care as well as the challenges according to the key building blocks of healthcare system as described by the WHO.

### Health Finance and Service Delivery

GKHA identified lack of funding as a major barrier for detection and early management of CKD in large parts of the world. Less than half (48%) of the countries responding to the GKHA survey provide public funding for non-dialysis CKD care, lower in LIC (22%) than HIC (68%) [15]. Detection and early management of CKD is the most common element excluded from public funding coverage (52% of countries), followed by early management to reduce progression of CKD (43%) (Table 2.1) [16]. Early detection and management is essential to prevent progression of CKD, and appropriate management of non-dialysis CKD is crucial to prevent progression to ESRD. One of the important aspects of early detection and management is the reduction of risk factors, which includes both traditional risk factors such as diabetes, hypertension, and obesity as well as nontraditional risk factors such as nephrotoxin exposure, kidney stones, fetal and maternal factors, infections, environmental factors, and AKI. These nontraditional risk factors have been increasingly recognized as major threats to global kidney health especially in LIC [17]. Lack of funding in these areas may lead to higher CKD and ESRD burden due to the progression of kidney disease and the cost associated with treating more severe kidney disease is likely to be much higher.

More countries (64%) provide public funding for renal replacement therapy (RRT) than non-dialysis CKD care [18]. Public funding for RRT is less prevalent in LIC (48%) than HIC (78%) [19]. RRT is unaffordable for many people, especially in LIC where public funding is limited. Annually, approximately 188 million people experience catastrophic health expenditure in LIC and low- and middle-income countries (LMIC) due to this condition, more than that for any other health condition [20]. In middle and eastern Africa, only 1–3% of those in need of RRT receive it [21]. Therefore, in these countries, effective population-based early detection and management programs as well as low-cost RRT techniques are needed.

In terms of service delivery, there is significant regional variation in ESRD care delivery and management. Forty percent of countries report within-country variation in ESRD care delivery, with the variation being greater in LIC (65%) [18]. In addition, 13% of LIC do not have structured ESRD management systems [18]. All of these factors contribute to inequitable and suboptimal CKD care.

### Health Workforce

GKHA documented a global shortage of nephrology workforce, particularly in LIC (Fig. 2.1). The median number of nephrologists is 9.95 per million population (pmp) worldwide, while in LIC, this number is only 0.2 pmp [16]. South Asia, which accounts for a quarter of the world population, has only 1.17 nephrologists pmp [16]. A similar trend was observed for nephrology trainees. The trainee density in LIC is 30 times lower than that of HIC, with all countries in Southeast Asia having trainee density below the global average [22]. Paradoxically, nephrologists trained in LIC or LMIC often cover the manpower shortage in many HICs [22]. One of the limiting factors for training adequate numbers of nephrologists is the lack of nephrology training programs. More than half of LIC do not have a nephrology training program [16]. In addition, declining interest in nephrology among trainees, lack of exposure to nephrology among medical students, erosion of the scope of nephrology practice by other specialists, and inflexible work schedules have been mentioned to play a role in the shortage of nephrologists [23].

There is also a shortage of all other nephrology care providers worldwide regardless of income group. The most commonly reported shortage is of renal pathologists (86%) followed by vascular access coordinators (81%) [16]. This

**Table 2.1** Aspects of kidney care excluded from public funding in different regions

| | Dialysis N (%) | Transplantation N (%) | Management of CKD complications[a] N (%) | Management to reduce risk of CKD progression[b] N (%) | Early management to reduce risk of CKD progression[b] N (%) | Early detection in individuals at risk N (%) | Management of AKIN (%) | None – all aspects funded N (%) |
|---|---|---|---|---|---|---|---|---|
| Overall | 33 (29) | 42 (37) | 46 (40) | 48 (42) | 49 (43) | 60 (52) | 29 (25) | 40 (35) |
| *ISN regions* | | | | | | | | |
| Africa | 12 (38) | 19 (59) | 19 (59) | 14 (44) | 12 (38) | 18 (56) | 9 (28) | 6 (19) |
| Eastern & Central Europe | 1 (6) | 1 (6) | 1 (6) | 3 (19) | 4 (25) | 3 (19) | 1 (6) | 12 (75) |
| Latin America | 5 (31) | 8 (50) | 6 (38) | 8 (50) | 9 (56) | 9 (56) | 5 (31) | 5 (31) |
| Middle East | 2 (17) | 1 (8) | 2 (17) | 3 (25) | 4 (33) | 6 (50) | 1 (8) | 5 (42) |
| NIS & Russia | 0 (0) | 0 (0) | 2 (40) | 3 (60) | 3 (60) | 4 (80) | 2 (40) | 1 (20) |
| North America | 1 (50) | 1 (50) | 2 (100) | 2 (100) | 2 (100) | 2 (100) | 1 (50) | 0 (0) |
| North & East Asia | 2 (33) | 2 (33) | 3 (50) | 1 (17) | 2 (33) | 3 (50) | 2 (33) | 2 (33) |
| Oceania & Southeast Asia | 7 (54) | 7 (54) | 7 (54) | 7 (54) | 7 (54) | 8 (62) | 5 (38) | 4 (31) |
| South Asia | 2 (40) | 2 (40) | 3 (60) | 4 (80) | 3 (60) | 3 (60) | 2 (40) | 1 (20) |
| Western Europe | 1 (13) | 1 (13) | 1 (13) | 3 (38) | 3 (38) | 4 (50) | 1 (13) | 4 (50) |
| *World Bank income groups* | | | | | | | | |
| Low-income | 9 (56) | 12 (75) | 11 (69) | 10 (63) | 8 (50) | 11 (69) | 8 (50) | 2 (13) |
| Lower-middle-income | 9 (27) | 16 (48) | 18 (55) | 19 (58) | 20 (61) | 20 (61) | 8 (24) | 7 (21) |
| Upper-middle-income | 8 (27) | 8 (27) | 11 (37) | 10 (33) | 11 (37) | 14 (47) | 7 (23) | 12 (40) |
| High-income | 7 (19) | 6 (17) | 6 (17) | 9 (25) | 10 (28) | 15 (42) | 6 (17) | 19 (53) |

Reproduced from GKHA 2017 with permission
[a]Anemia, bone disease, malnutrition
[b]Risk factor control

shortage of other nephrology care providers further compounds the huge adverse impact of workforce shortage on public health.

## Essential Medicine and Technology

Besides high morbidity and mortality, kidney disease is associated with enormous healthcare costs for both the individual and society. Providing equitable access to affordable and safe essential medicines and technologies is crucial in addressing the healthcare needs of these patients [24]. Early detection, management, and monitoring of AKI and CKD are vital to slow down their progression and can yield significant clinical and economic benefit [25]. Essential laboratory tests, including serum creatinine and proteinuria testing, are not available in many countries, especially LIC (Fig. 2.2) [24]. None of the LIC has the ability in primary care settings to do these simple and low-cost tests, that have been shown to improve the detection and management of CKD [16].

Patients with ESRD usually require phosphate binders, vitamin D supplements, calcimimetics, antihypertensives, erythropoiesis-stimulating agents, and iron supplements [26]. The high cost of these medications is frequently a major barrier for patients and most of these medications are not covered by public funding.

Timely access to RRT is essential to reduce the morbidity and mortality associated with ESRD. However, access to dialysis services can be as low as 5% in LIC [18] and patients often die from life-threatening complications such as hyperkalemia and metabolic acidosis because dialysis is not accessible. Providing hemodialysis (HD) is usually not realistic in low-resource settings due to lack of electricity and water supply, high cost of HD machines and consumables as well

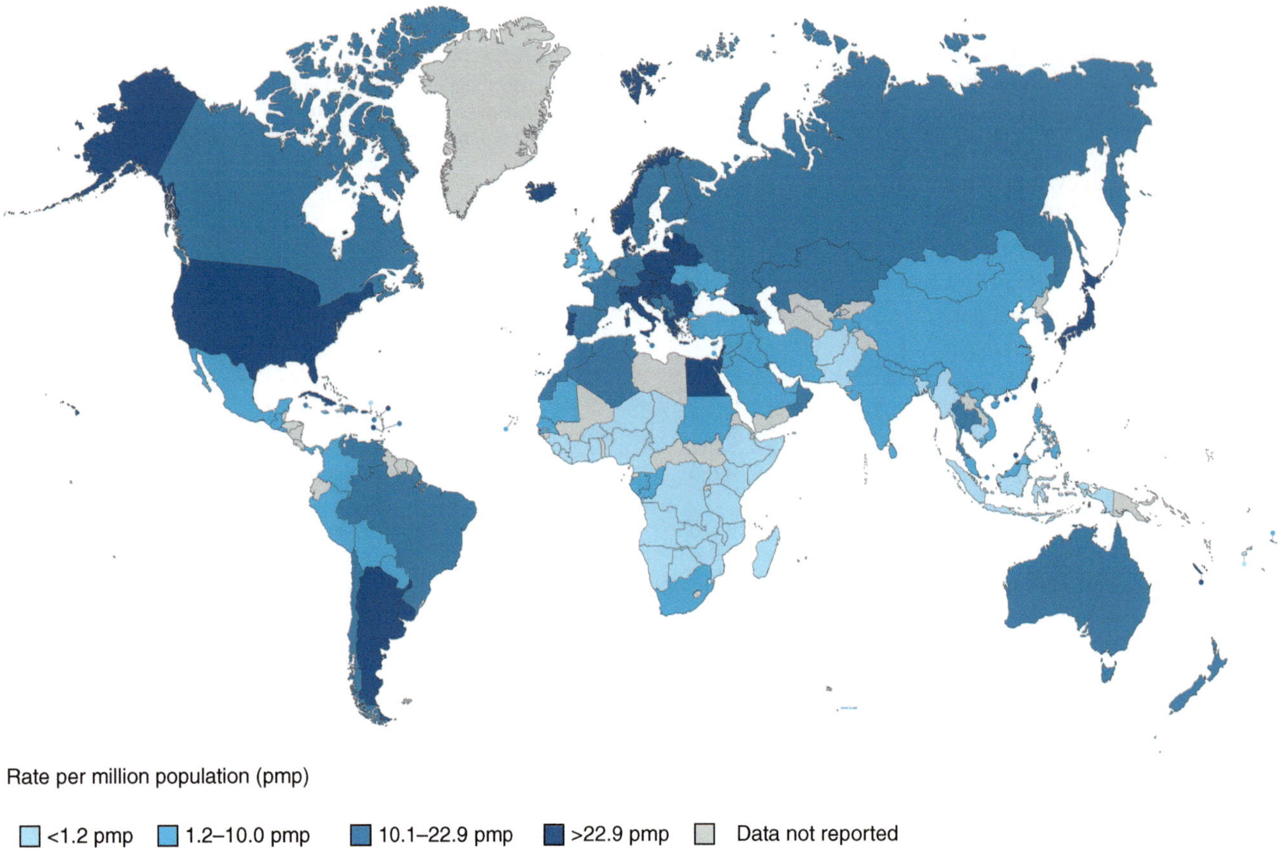


**Fig. 2.1** Prevalence of nephrologists worldwide. (Reproduced from GKHA 2019 with permission)

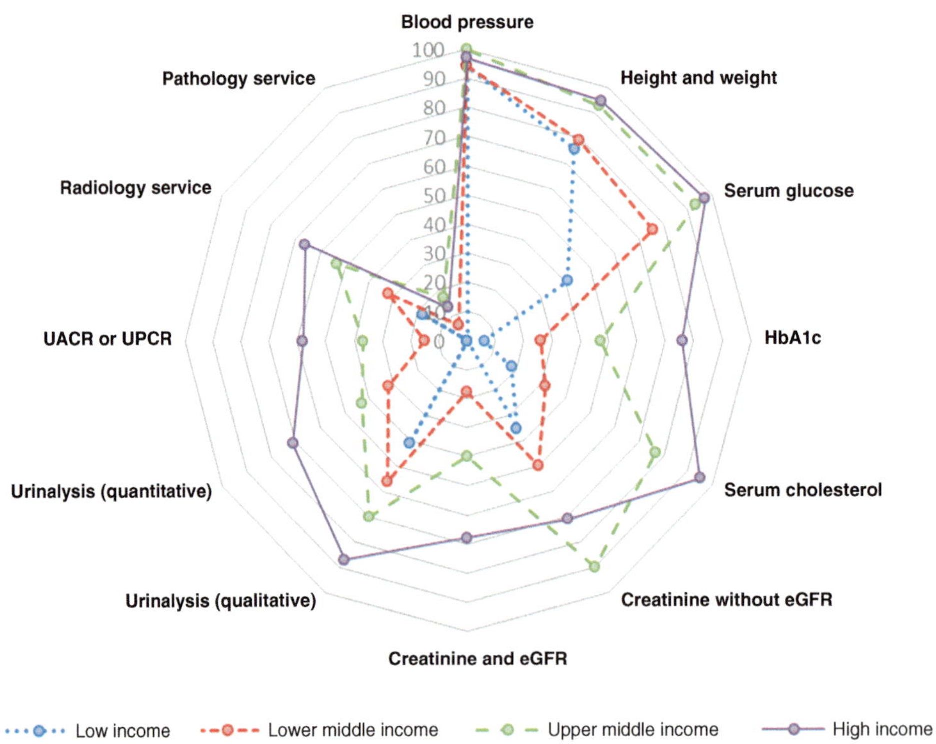


**Fig. 2.2** Healthcare services for the identification and management of CKD at primary care level by World Bank income group. Capacities of primary healthcare services for CKD care are reported as percentages of countries with particular services in each income group. eGFR, estimated glomerular filtration rate; HbA1c, glycated hemoglobin; UACR, urine albumin to creatinine ratio; UPCR, urine protein to creatinine ratio. (Reproduced with permission from Htay et al. [24])

as lack of expertise in managing this type of RRT. In this setting, peritoneal dialysis (PD), which is generally less expensive to run, may be preferable in LIC. Paradoxically, acute and chronic PD are less available in these countries (18% and 23% respectively) than HD [18].

Access to kidney transplantation is also very low, being available in only 23% of LIC [18]. Even in countries with transplantation services, accessibility to this service may be low, particularly in LIC [18]. Low access to transplantation in these regions is due to a number of factors that are related to an individual country's health system characteristics such as shortage of personnel, lack of infrastructure, absence of system coordination, limited financing, and lack of expertise to perform the surgery. In addition, other factors such as cultural reasons, pubic and professional attitudes to transplantation, legislations, and political barriers may obstruct organ donation [27]. Low rates of deceased donation and utilization of organs are also very common due to ineffective organ procurement networks, lack of facilities for taking care of potential donors, religion, and poor public education [28, 29].

Given that dialysis or transplantation is not feasible for all patients with ESRD, conservative care is an important alternative. It refers to the management of health conditions using noninvasive practices, with the goal to maintain health as much as possible and lessen adverse events [30]. Conservative care should be considered as a valid option for ESRD care in some settings due to its lower costs, the benefits on quality of life, and the lack of evidence that dialysis leads to better outcomes [31]. However, access to medically advised conservative care is low (33%) in LIC, with none of the LIC providing training in conservative care for nephrology healthcare providers [18]. In order to optimize the care and quality of life of patients with ESRD, efforts need to be made to increase awareness and standardization of conservative care particularly in LIC and LMIC.

## Health Information Systems

Information systems are critical for healthcare service planning and development. Registries are a fundamental tool in supporting the planning and regulation of public health systems as well as for research purposes [32]. Globally, there is a lack of registries for AKI and non-dialysis CKD, with only 13 AKI registries and 19 non-dialysis CKD registries worldwide [16]. Transplantation and dialysis registries are more common with 66% of countries having dialysis registries and 57% having transplantation registries [16]. This is unsurprising as dialysis and transplantation patients are usually registered into the system for resource allocation purposes. However, there are significant disparities in the availability of registries among income groups. Most HIC have dialysis and transplantation registries while only 18% of LIC have dialysis registries and none have transplantation registries [18]. As a result of deficiency in registry data, most countries were unable to estimate the prevalence of AKI and one-third of countries were unable to estimate the prevalence of CKD [33]. Challenges in developing registries include limited financial and material resources, lack of trained personnel and support, insufficient understanding from government and policy makers, as well as cultural and religious constraints [34]. Given the importance of registries for resource allocation and predicting future resource requirements, effort needs to be made in developing and implementing these registries since any investment will lead to long term returns that will more than offset the initial costs (Table 2.2).

**Table 2.2** Prevalence of renal registries

| | AKI N (%) | Non-dialysis CKD N (%) | Dialysis N (%) | Transplantation N (%) |
|---|---|---|---|---|
| Overall | 13 (8) | 19 (12) | 101 (66) | 88 (57) |
| *ISN regions* | | | | |
| Africa | 4 (10) | 3 (7) | 18 (44) | 6 (15) |
| Eastern & Central Europe | 2 (11) | 1 (5) | 17 (89) | 17 (89) |
| Latin America | 1 (6) | 5 (28) | 14 (78) | 13 (72) |
| Middle East | 1 (9) | 1 (9) | 6 (55) | 8 (73) |
| NIS & Russia | 1 (14) | 2 (29) | 5 (71) | 6 (86) |
| North America | 0 (0) | 0 (0) | 4 (44) | 3 (33) |
| North & East Asia | 1 (14) | 2 (29) | 7 (100) | 7 (100) |
| Oceania & Southeast Asia | 1 (7) | 2 (13) | 10 (67) | 8 (53) |
| South Asia | 0 (0) | 0 (0) | 2 (29) | 1 (14) |
| Western Europe | 2 (10) | 3 (15) | 18 (90) | 19 (95) |
| *World Bank income groups* | | | | |
| Low-income | 2 (9) | 2 (9) | 4 (18) | 0 (0) |
| Lower-middle-income | 4 (11) | 4 (11) | 18 (51) | 10 (29) |
| Upper-middle-income | 2 (5) | 2 (5) | 31 (76) | 27 (66) |
| High-income | 5 (9) | 11 (20) | 48 (86) | 51 (91) |

Reproduced from GKHA 2019 with permission
*AKI* acute kidney injury, *CKD* chronic kidney disease

## Leadership and Governance

Leadership and governance are crucial for developing, overseeing, and regulating healthcare systems [14]. Effective leadership and governance ensure these conditions receive priority through properly framed policies and effective implementation framework. Globally, there is a lack of advocacy and priority for kidney diseases. The percentage of countries recognizing AKI, CKD, and ESRD as health priorities are only 13%, 51%, and 58% respectively [35]. Similarly, the percentage of countries with advocacy groups for AKI, CKD, and ESRD are 14%, 63%, and 39% [35]. The prevalence of advocacy groups for CKD and ESRD is lower in LIC, with resulting failure to recognize these conditions as health priorities [18]. Less than half (44%) of countries have national strategies for CKD care and only 34% have CKD-specific policies [18]. Notably, none of the LIC has CKD-specific policies [18].

Due to the global shortage of nephrologists, primary care physicians play an important role in the management of CKD. However, the awareness of AKI and CKD was rated as low or extremely low among primary care physicians (by 57% and 64% of countries respectively) [35]. This figure is even higher in LIC. This low awareness leads to poor adoption of guidelines among non-nephrologists. Only 7% of countries have national AKI guidelines and 27% have CKD guidelines [16]. Despite the freely available evidence-based international guidelines developed by KDIGO which are translated into many languages, access is limited – only 45% for AKI and 52% for CKD [35]. In countries that have their own guidelines, the rate of adoption of AKI and CKD guidelines is only 65% and 66% respectively [35]. Other barriers to adoption of guidelines include workforce or resource shortage, lack of support from policy makers, and physician factors such as lack of accountability related to specific outcomes [36].

## ISN's Response to Major Problems Facing Global Nephrology

The ISN is dedicated to advancing kidney health worldwide. The organisation's activities focus on bridging gaps in care, building capacity, and connecting communities, and aim to address the burden of AKI, CKD, and ESRD, in addition to the many other facets of kidney disease (Fig. 2.3). The following section provides a brief outline of the ISN's broader actions to improve the state of kidney health worldwide, focusing especially on the ISN's response to tackle major challenges in AKI, CKD, and ESRD.

## Bridging the Gaps, Building Capacity, and Connecting Communities

The ISN bridges the gaps of available care through advocacy and collaborations with global partners. It builds capacity with healthcare professionals via granting programs, and supporting education and research relevant to global nephrology. The ISN works with other stakeholder communities to develop a stronger understanding of how to manage kidney diseases and engage in a collaborative effort to improve prevention, diagnosis, and treatment [37].

To effectively work toward bridging the gaps, the ISN entered into official relations as a non-state actor with the WHO in 2012. Relations are governed by a joint action plan, and the ISN is invited to participate and provide input into official WHO meetings such as the WHO General Assembly, the WHO Executive Board, and relevant civil society meetings organized by the United Nations [38]. The ISN is the only kidney organization currently in official relations with the WHO.

Global awareness building also has an important role to play in both bridging gaps and connecting communities. In addition to its annual World Kidney Day campaign which creates global awareness about the importance of kidney health, the ISN and The Lancet launched The Lancet Kidney Campaign (http://www.thelancet.com/campaigns/kidney) on World Kidney Day 2016. This initiative aims to raise awareness about acute and chronic kidney diseases, bring together the best available evidence to inform strategy making, and set the stage for future advocacy. The campaign published

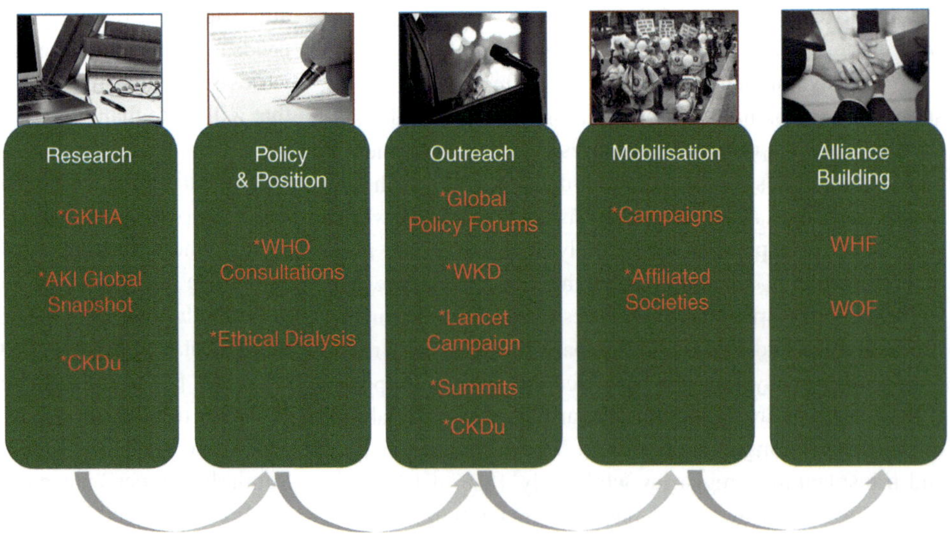


**Fig. 2.3** ISN's advocacy activities in addressing the burden of kidney disease. GKHA, Global Kidney Health Atlas; AKI, acute kidney injury; CKDu, chronic kidney disease of unknown etiology; WHO, World Health Organization; WKD, World Kidney Day; WHF, World Heart Federation; WOF, World Obesity Federation

many updates on recent advances in nephrology and expert commentaries on relevant issues in kidney health and policies. Eight international nephrology society partners joined the campaign in 2016. The campaign was a great success and received broad public exposure [39].

The ISN regularly brings together high-level decision-makers and stakeholders to connect communities and address the burden of kidney disease. The first ISN Global Kidney Policy Forum was held in Mexico at the World Congress of Nephrology 2017 [40]. The second meeting took place at the World Congress of Nephrology 2019 in Melbourne (Australia). Participants included representatives from national health ministries, international and regional health organizations, key opinion leaders, and representatives of the wider health community [40]. These meetings aim to improve understanding of regional issues related to delivering kidney care and its funding, highlight and address the gaps identified in the ISN GKHA, and share information and best practices at a regional and global level [40]. The meetings culminate in clear calls to develop policy proposals which support the improvement of kidney health management [40].

Building evidence is important in all of the ISN's advocacy efforts to improve awareness of the burden of AKI, CKD, and ESRD among health policy makers and funders. For this, products such as the Global Kidney Health Atlas are crucial, as well as supporting renal registries worldwide. Renal registry data can provide critical information to support the planning, delivery, and evaluation of renal services, as well as highlight discrepancies in service provision within and between countries. Unfortunately, many low-resource countries (and some HIC) do not have renal registries. Therefore, to support the establishment of renal registries in these countries, the ISN partnered with a group of international organizations to create the team "SHARing Expertise to support the set-up of Renal Registries (SharE-RR)" to help develop resources that kidney health advocates can use to assist the development of a renal registry in their countries [41].

Bringing together the expertise of its members, the ISN builds capacity for better prevention and effective treatments to reduce the impact of kidney and associated diseases in the world, through a wide range of educational programs. The Sister Centers Program aids in building the capacity of renal centers in developing countries with educational support and guidance from other more advanced centers, with the goal of the emerging centers ultimately becoming self-sufficient and improving the services available for their patients. The Fellowship Program supports nephrologists from disadvantaged parts of the world to receive training abroad in an advanced host institute of their choice. The fellows are then required to return to their home country after the fellowship and use the knowledge and skills they acquired to improve the education and kidney care provision in their home countries upon their return. According to a recent survey, most of the fellows who completed the program are now working in local academic centers, directly contributing to the provision of care and teaching [42]. The Educational Ambassador Program supports visits of experts to emerging centers to deliver high quality and relevant hands-on training, and the Continuing Medical Education (CME) Program supports expert speakers to provide teaching at regional conferences in emerging countries. The Clinical Research Program, Mentorship Program, and Scientific Writing course provide financial support as well as mentorship from highly experienced nephrologists on clinical research projects and manuscripts in the developing world. To ensure access to education regardless of location, the ISN offers an eLearning portal, the ISN Academy, with a plethora (8000+) of training resources which allow nephrologists worldwide to have one-click access to knowledge on the prevention, diagnosis, and management of kidney diseases.

These various training and education activities position the ISN to be more impactful in its projects tackling the specific burdens of AKI, CKD, and ESRD.

## Tackling AKI

### 0by25 Initiative

Recognizing AKI as a growing global problem, the ISN in 2013 launched the ISN AKI 0by25 human rights initiative with the ambitious goal of *eliminating preventable deaths* from AKI worldwide by 2025 [9]. The aim of this initiative is to call for globally applicable strategies that permit timely diagnosis and treatment of AKI for patients with potentially reversible diseases. Its emphasis is on developing countries in Africa, Asia, and Latin America with disadvantaged populations and poor access to care.

The first project of this initiative was the AKI Global Survey, which aimed to gain a better understanding of the way AKI is managed globally. Launched in 2014, the AKI Global Survey sent out surveys in eight different languages, asking more than 10,000 nephrologists around the world to report how AKI is diagnosed and treated in their respective countries [43].

The Survey laid the groundwork for future 0by25 research projects, specifically the AKI Global Snapshot. The Global Snapshot recorded information on over 4000 pediatric and adult patients with AKI encountered in their regular practice by 372 physicians from 72 countries over a 10-week period in the last quarter of 2014 [10, 44]. It provided a prospective, cross-sectional understanding of the growing burden of AKI, including how it is identified, managed, and treated in different settings around the world [10]. In 2015, it culminated in The Lancet AKI Commission Report [10].

The important work from these first two research projects paved the road for the 0by25 Pilot Feasibility Study in 2016–2017. This study was the first to evaluate the feasibility and impact of a comprehensive education and training program for management of community-based AKI in low-resource settings [45]. Working in three selected clusters located in Africa, Asia, and Latin America, it identified the barriers for the recognition and management of AKI in different settings and compared outcomes from AKI before and after interventions. In parallel, it enabled the establishment of a network of stakeholders across the world to raise public awareness of AKI [45].

The ISN 0by25 AKI human rights initiative matured into its action phase with the Kidney Care Network (KCN), a project which focuses on locally led education and training in LMIC sites (initially in Bolivia, Brazil, Nepal, and South Africa) to achieve sustainable, affordable improvement in routine AKI detection and management. It was launched in July 2017 and tested whether the successful intervention from the 0by25 Pilot Feasibility Study could be incorporated into routine care in LMIC [46]. These project sites provide education and training in AKI care given by local experts using materials evaluated as successful during the Pilot Feasibility Study [46]. Working in full collaboration with local institutions, the project aims to improve the standard of care in AKI detection and management in a way that is appropriate and sustainable in the local setting [46].

### Saving Young Lives Project

Together with International Pediatric Nephrology Association, International Society for Peritoneal Dialysis, the European Society for Peritoneal Dialysis, and the Sustainable Kidney Care Foundation, ISN started the Saving Young Lives (SYL) project in 2012 with the aim of developing sustainable programs for treating AKI in low-resource health settings. The project focuses on hospital development, provides hands-on training and education in order to establish a proof-of-principle sustainable acute PD program in very low-resource settings in sub-Saharan Africa and Southeast Asia. It also provides a template for the extension of such a model across the world with the ultimate goal to save lives of people with severe AKI [47, 48]. The program has supported the development of acute PD in ten centers where dialysis was in the past unavailable. Between January 2013 and September 2015, 175 children and adults received acute PD; complete renal recovery was achieved in 33% of patients reflecting that 58 "young lives" (mean age 12 ± 13 years) were saved. With these encouraging results demonstrating sustainability and reproducibility, the SYL program is being expanded to other ISN regions. However, real sustainability of the SYL program can only be achieved with local government support. For this reason SYL has also begun collecting data in its centers to demonstrate to local authorities that providing acute PD for patients with severe AKI is possible, affordable, and deliverable and will save lives in low-resource settings.

## Tackling CKD

### ISN Global Kidney Health Summit 2016

The 2016 ISN Global Kidney Health Summit brought together 85 individuals with diverse expertise and professional backgrounds from around the globe to identify and prioritize key activities for the next 5–10 years in the domains of clinical care, research, and advocacy and to create an action plan and performance framework to improve CKD care worldwide. The summit discussions were divided into ten themes: (1) strengthen CKD surveillance; (2) tackle major risk factors for CKD; (3) reduce AKI – a special risk factor for CKD; (4) enhance understanding of the genetic causes of CKD; (5) establish better diagnostic methods in CKD; (6) improve understanding of the natural course of CKD; (7) evaluate and implement established treatment options in patients with CKD; (8) improve management of symptoms and complications of CKD; (9) develop novel therapeutic interventions to slow CKD progression and reduce CKD complications; and (10) increase the quantity and quality of clinical trials in CKD. Each group produced a prioritized list of goals, activities, and a set of key deliverables for each of the themes [49]. Gaps in research, care, and policy relevant to CKD were identified during this Summit and a comprehensive plan was developed to address them [49]. The plan covered activities in education, research, policy creation, and involved collaboration across academic and healthcare institutions, government agencies, industry partners, research funding agencies, clinicians, researchers, policy makers, and patients [49]. An initial high-level performance measurement framework was proposed by which activities would be documented, timelines and responsible parties identified, and the impact on specific metrics anticipated [49]. All of these were published in a post-summit declaration in The Lancet in 2017.

In addition to The Lancet publication, additional manuscripts elaborating on the individual themes described above were published in October 2017 in Kidney International Supplements [16, 17, 50–55].

### GKHA 2016

In response to the identified gaps in knowledge about the prevalence and incidence of CKD, the ISN initiated the GKHA in 2016. The first edition was published in April 2017 [16, 56], and gave a high-level overview of the current state of CKD care, and how it was organized and structured worldwide. It showed trends in the burden of CKD and its consequences across the world [16]. It made key recommendations, which included the need to: extend healthcare financing and access to treatment; increase capacity by addressing workforce shortages; enhance consistency of care through national strategies and guidelines; and increase support for prevention [16]. The GKHA acted as a platform for championing the cause using the identified gaps modeled on Universal Health Coverage domains and built the foundation for a global CKD care surveillance network [40]. The findings for each domain were published in February 2018, which included guidelines, policies, and barriers to kidney care [35]; health systems oversight and financing for kidney care [15]; the nephrology workforce [22]; access to health technologies and medications [24]; health information systems [33]; and capacity for clinical research in nephrology [15].

Complementing the GKHA, the ISN formalized a relationship with the Global Network of CKD Cohort Studies in 2015, thereafter called the International Network of Chronic Kidney Disease Cohort Studies (iNET-CKD), with the aim of enhancing the understanding of CKD progression and its consequences through collaboration among study investigators and implementing observational research studies.

### CKDu

CKD of unknown etiology (CKDu) is a new form of CKD which emerged over the last two decades and which is attributable to nontraditional CKD risk factors including extreme physical exertion, heat stress, water quality, and exposure to agrochemicals. There are currently significant challenges in the identification and management of CKDu due to factors such as lack of concordant approaches in individual-level diagnosis and detection at the population level, and lack of treatment or preventative strategies. Therefore, it is of critical importance to have a broad collaboration and multidisciplinary approach with the ultimate goal of strengthening health services, workforce training, access to health technology, medications, and medical surveillance through international cooperation. ISN will play key in the whole process. For example, in parallel with its broader work on CKD, the ISN has become increasingly involved in efforts related to the issues surrounding CKDu as part of its collaboration plan with the WHO. ISN started facilitating this issue by supporting collaboration and information sharing of an International Consortium of Collaborators on CKDu (i3C) to encourage information exchange. ISN is also coordinating the development of a CKDu Observatory documenting ongoing local research projects to foster collaboration and exchange of information.

## Tackling ESRD

### Affordable Dialysis Machine

Providing dialysis is expensive, and every year millions of people die because they cannot afford or do not have access to this life saving treatment. In order to inspire innovation in designing an affordable dialysis machine which can be used in resource-poor regions, the Affordable Dialysis Prize was set up in 2015 by The George Institute for Global Health with the support of the ISN, the Asian Pacific Society of Nephrology, and the Farrell Family Foundation [57]. Irish engineer Vincent Garvey won the prize to design an innovative system, which is reliable, safe, cheap (cost less than 1000 USD and provide treatment for less than 5 USD a day), and able to run on solar power using any water source. This invention has now taken out global patent protection and Ellen Medical Devices was set up to commercialize the system. It is anticipated that clinical trials using this system will start enrolling volunteer patients in 2020 [57].

### Global Kidney Health Summit 2018

To commence tackling the growing problem of ESRD especially in emerging economies, the ISN focused its 2018 Global Kidney Health Summit on integrated ESRD care. The meeting provided opportunities to define gaps in knowledge and clinical practice, to design concrete strategies to fill those gaps, and to create a performance framework to demonstrate progress over time. Summit participants developed a plan to address four important aspects of ESRD care: advocacy, sustainability, equity, and integration. Participants emphasized the need to individualize and tailor the implementation of proposed action steps in each of these four domains according to local needs, culture, and available resources [58].

The Global Kidney Health Summit on ESRD was the first step in the process of developing an overall strategic plan for integrated ESRD care (Fig. 2.4) [58]. To continue development of the plan, the ISN held a workshop during the World Congress of Nephrology in Melbourne, April 2019. Identified activities from the Summit's eight working group themes were reorganized into the following four domains: resources (training, workforce, financing); dialysis (service, standards, organization, delivery); support (pre-ESRD care, supportive care, and transplantation); and monitoring (data, monitoring, audit and quality assurance). An overall approach to develop the strategic plan was defined. Completion of the plan will include representatives of all relevant stakeholder groups who will be involved in implementing the strategy over the next 5–10 years.

### Collaboration with WHO

As part of its official relations with the WHO and a joint collaboration plan, the ISN is currently working on developing a Guidance Package on How to Set Up Dialysis in low-resource settings, to be made available to local healthcare managers [38]. The Package is expected to be published as an official ISN-WHO publication in 2020. As a first intelligence gathering step, ISN developed the ISN Kidney Collection Survey, which collected and collated many original documents and guidelines from a number of countries in

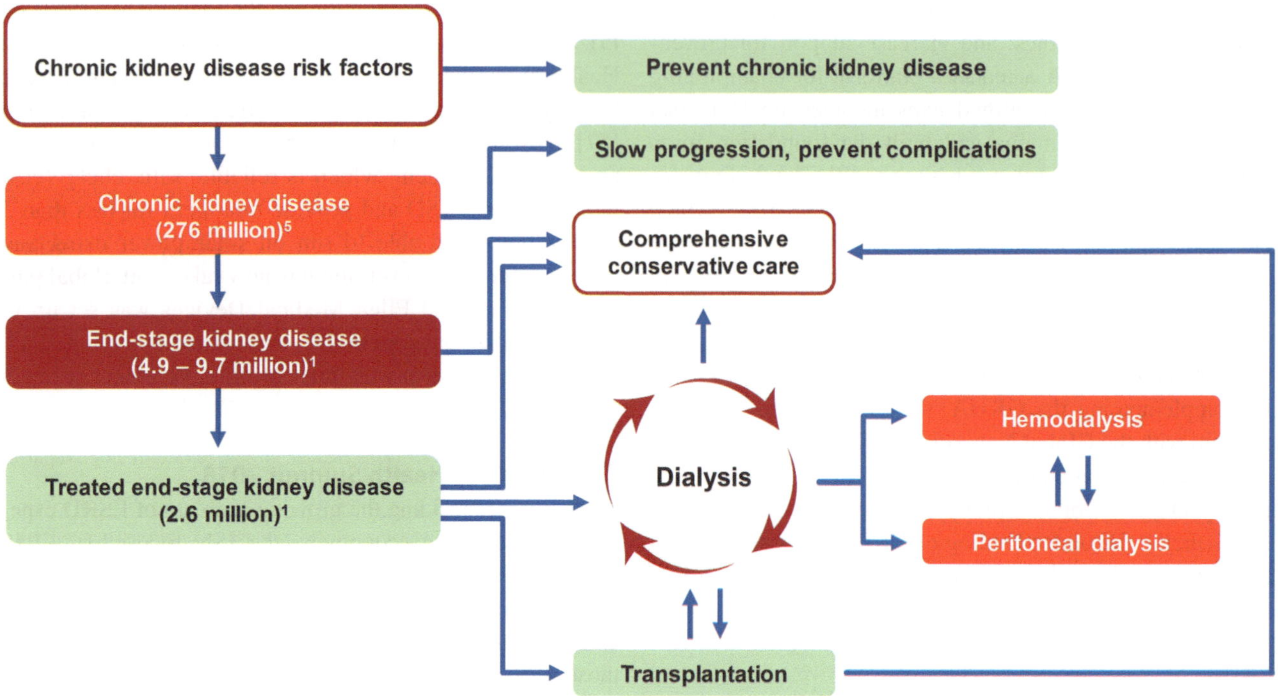


**Fig. 2.4** End-stage renal disease pathway. (Reproduced with permission from Harris et al. [58])

the areas of dialysis eligibility, procurement, care, and outcomes monitoring [38].

### Ethical Issues in Nephrology

Another parallel project is a series of papers on major ethical issues in provision of nephrology care worldwide, the first of which in The Lancet focused on dialysis, identifying priorities for further investigation and management, and presenting preliminary recommendations to guide practice and policy [59]. The ISN aims to publish reviews and position statements on ethical nephrology care relevant to emerging and developed countries. This project aims to bring awareness and advocacy for the removal of perverse financial incentives, developing minimum global quality standards and defining principles for equitable access where resources are scarce.

### GKHA 2019

A second edition of the GKHA was released in April 2019 in conjunction with the ISN's World Congress of Nephrology in Melbourne. Based on survey results of 160 nations comprising over 98.6% of the world population, this version included questions targeted at ESRD care worldwide, thus helping the ISN to determine the capacity and readiness of nations to provide ESRD patients with universal access to equitable integrated care, including dialysis, transplantation, and conservative care [18]. It will inform local and international bodies about key activities to improve healthcare policy within the global health agenda. Future work of the GKHA will include developing tools and implementing regional and national strategies, and continuing to track progress in each region and country.

## Concluding Remarks

There are many challenges faced by the current healthcare system worldwide in meeting the rising burden of AKI, CKD, and ESRD. Through its work, the ISN has identified many gaps in the current state of kidney care globally in the areas of finance and service delivery, nephrology workforce, essential medicines and technology, information systems, leadership, and governance. There are significant healthcare inequalities and inter- and intra-regional variability in the capacity for kidney care provision. In collaboration with its partners, the ISN aims to meet the global challenges in care of patients with AKI, CKD, and ESRD, through a wide range of activities involving advocacy, education, and research.

**Acknowledgment** The authors wish to thank Charu Malik (ISN Executive Director), Sophie Dupuis (ISN Capacity Building Director), Jo-Ann Donner (ISN Project Manager), Luisa Strani (ISN Advocacy Director), and Sandrine Damster (ISN Research Programs Manager) who provided details of the ISN's activities.

## References


1. GBD 2016 Disease and Injury Incidence and Prevalence Collaborators. Global, regional, and national incidence, prevalence, and years lived with disability for 328 diseases and injuries for 195 countries, 1990–2016: a systematic analysis for the Global Burden of Disease Study 2016. Lancet. 2017;390(10100):1211–59.
2. Xie Y, Bowe B, Mokdad AH, et al. Analysis of the Global Burden of Disease study highlights the global, regional, and national trends of chronic kidney disease epidemiology from 1990 to 2016. Kidney Int. 2018;94(3):567–81.
3. Foreman KJ, Marquez N, Dolgert A, et al. Forecasting life expectancy, years of life lost, and all-cause and cause-specific mortality for 250 causes of death: reference and alternative scenarios for 2016–40 for 195 countries and territories. Lancet. 2018;392(10159):2052–90.
4. Couser WG, Remuzzi G, Mendis S, et al. The contribution of chronic kidney disease to the global burden of major noncommunicable diseases. Kidney Int. 2011;80(12):1258–70.
5. Luyckx VA, Tonelli M, Stanifer JW. The global burden of kidney disease and the sustainable development goals. Bull World Health Organ. 2018;96(6):414–22D.
6. Jager KJ, Fraser SDS. The ascending rank of chronic kidney disease in the global burden of disease study. Nephrol Dial Transplant. 2017;32(Suppl_2):ii121–8.
7. Lewington AJ, Cerda J, Mehta RL. Raising awareness of acute kidney injury: a global perspective of a silent killer. Kidney Int. 2013;84(3):457–67.
8. Lameire NH, Bagga A, Cruz D, et al. Acute kidney injury: an increasing global concern. Lancet. 2013;382(9887):170–9.
9. Mehta RL, Cerda J, Burdmann EA, et al. International Society of Nephrology's 0by25 initiative for acute kidney injury (zero preventable deaths by 2025): a human rights case for nephrology. Lancet. 2015;385(9987):2616–43.
10. Mehta RL, Burdmann EA, Cerda J, et al. Recognition and management of acute kidney injury in the International Society of Nephrology 0by25 Global Snapshot: a multinational cross-sectional study. Lancet. 2016;387(10032):2017–25.
11. Kerr M, Bedford M, Matthews B, et al. The economic impact of acute kidney injury in England. Nephrol Dial Transplant. 2014;29(7):1362–8.
12. Coca SG, Singanamala S, Parikh CR. Chronic kidney disease after acute kidney injury: a systematic review and meta-analysis. Kidney Int. 2012;81(5):442–8.
13. Waikar SS, Winkelmayer WC. Chronic on acute renal failure: long-term implications of severe acute kidney injury. JAMA. 2009;302(11):1227–9.
14. World Health Organization. Monitoring the building blocks of health systems: a handbook of indicators and their measurement strategies. Geneva: World Health Organization; 2010. xii, 92 p.
15. Okpechi IG, Alrukhaimi M, Ashuntantang GE, et al. Global capacity for clinical research in nephrology: a survey by the International Society of Nephrology. Kidney Int Suppl (2011). 2018;8(2):82–9.
16. Bello AK, Levin A, Tonelli M, et al. Global kidney health atlas: a report by the International Society of Nephrology on the current state of organization and structures for kidney care across the globe. Brussels: International Society of Nephrology; 2017.
17. Luyckx VA, Tuttle KR, Garcia-Garcia G, et al. Reducing major risk factors for chronic kidney disease. Kidney Int Suppl (2011). 2017;7(2):71–87.
18. Bello AK, Levin A, Lunney M, et al. Global kidney health atlas: a report by the International Society of Nephrology on the global burden of end-stage kidney disease and capacity for kidney replacement therapy and conservative care across world countries and regions. Brussels: International Society of Nephrology; 2019.
19. Bello AK, Alrukhaimi M, Ashuntantang GE, et al. Global overview of health systems oversight and financing for kidney care. Kidney Int Suppl (2011). 2018;8(2):41–51.
20. Essue BM, Laba M, Knaul F, et al. Economic burden of chronic ill health and injuries for households in low- and middle-income countries. In: rd, Jamison DT, Gelband H, Horton S, Jha P, Laxminarayan R, et al., editors. Disease control priorities: improving health and reducing poverty. Washington, DC; The International Bank for Reconstruction and Development / The World Bank, 2017.
21. Liyanage T, Ninomiya T, Jha V, et al. Worldwide access to treatment for end-stage kidney disease: a systematic review. Lancet. 2015;385(9981):1975–82.
22. Osman MA, Alrukhaimi M, Ashuntantang GE, et al. Global nephrology workforce: gaps and opportunities toward a sustainable kidney care system. Kidney Int Suppl (2011). 2018;8(2):52–63.
23. Sharif MU, Elsayed ME, Stack AG. The global nephrology workforce: emerging threats and potential solutions! Clin Kidney J. 2016;9(1):11–22.
24. Htay H, Alrukhaimi M, Ashuntantang GE, et al. Global access of patients with kidney disease to health technologies and medications: findings from the Global Kidney Health Atlas project. Kidney Int Suppl (2011). 2018;8(2):64–73.
25. Wouters OJ, O'Donoghue DJ, Ritchie J, et al. Early chronic kidney disease: diagnosis, management and models of care. Nat Rev Nephrol. 2015;11(8):491–502.
26. Ghimire S, Castelino RL, Lioufas NM, et al. Nonadherence to medication therapy in haemodialysis patients: a systematic review. PLoS One. 2015;10(12):e0144119.
27. Muralidharan A, White S. The need for kidney transplantation in low- and middle-income countries in 2012: an epidemiological perspective. Transplantation. 2015;99(3):476–81.
28. Muller E. Transplantation in Africa – an overview. Clin Nephrol. 2016;86(2016)(13):90–5.
29. Jha V. Current status of end-stage renal disease care in South Asia. Ethn Dis. 2009;19(1 Suppl 1):S1-27–32.
30. Davison SN, Levin A, Moss AH, et al. Executive summary of the KDIGO Controversies Conference on Supportive Care in Chronic Kidney Disease: developing a roadmap to improving quality care. Kidney Int. 2015;88(3):447–59.
31. Morton RL, Kurella Tamura M, Coast J, et al. Supportive care: economic considerations in advanced kidney disease. Clin J Am Soc Nephrol. 2016;11(10):1915–20.
32. Morsy A, Lim T, Varatharajan S, et al. National registries in developing countries: understanding construction challenges and implementation steps. 5th Cairo International Biomedical Engineering Conference; December 16–18, 2010; Cairo, Egypt; 2010.
33. See EJ, Alrukhaimi M, Ashuntantang GE, et al. Global coverage of health information systems for kidney disease: availability, challenges, and opportunities for development. Kidney Int Suppl (2011). 2018;8(2):74–81.
34. Valsecchi MG, Steliarova-Foucher E. Cancer registration in developing countries: luxury or necessity? Lancet Oncol. 2008;9(2):159–67.
35. Lunney M, Alrukhaimi M, Ashuntantang GE, et al. Guidelines, policies, and barriers to kidney care: findings from a global survey. Kidney Int Suppl (2011). 2018;8(2):30–40.
36. van der Veer SN, Tomson CR, Jager KJ, et al. Bridging the gap between what is known and what we do in renal medicine: improving implementability of the European Renal Best Practice guidelines. Nephrol Dial Transplant. 2014;29(5):951–7.
37. International Society of Nephrology. ISN Position Paper on Universal Health Care. Brussels, Belgium; 2019.
38. International Society of Nephrology. ISN Biennial Report 2017–2018. Brussels, Belgium; 2019.

39. International Society of Nephrology. The Lancet Kidney Campaign 2017. Available from: https://www.theisn.org/focus/ckd – publications.
40. International Society of Nephrology. ISN Biennial Report 2015–2017. Brussels, Belgium; 2017.
41. International Society of Nephrology. Sharing expertise to support the set-up of renal registries 2019. Available from: https://www.theisn.org/advocacy/share-rr – resources.
42. International Society of Nephrology. ISN fellowship program 2019. Available from: https://www.theisn.org/all-articles/546-fellowship-program-committee.
43. International Society of Nephrology. AKI global snapshot 2019. Available from: https://www.theisn.org/0by25 – aki-global-snapshot.
44. Macedo E, Cerda J, Hingorani S, et al. Recognition and management of acute kidney injury in children: the ISN 0by25 Global Snapshot study. PLoS One. 2018;13(5):e0196586.
45. International Society of Nephrology. 0by25 pilot feasibility study 2019. Available from: https://www.theisn.org/0by25 – 0by25-pilot-feasibility-study.
46. International Society of Nephrology. ISN kidney care network 2019. Available from: https://www.theisn.org/programs/isn-kidney-care-network.
47. Kilonzo KG, Ghosh S, Temu SA, et al. Outcome of acute peritoneal dialysis in Northern Tanzania. Perit Dial Int. 2012;32(3):261–6.
48. Carter M, Kilonzo K, Odiit A, et al. Acute peritoneal dialysis treatment programs for countries of the East African community. Blood Purif. 2012;33(1–3):149–52.
49. Levin A, Tonelli M, Bonventre J, et al. Global kidney health 2017 and beyond: a roadmap for closing gaps in care, research, and policy. Lancet. 2017;390(10105):1888–917.
50. Coresh J, Hu JR, Bello AK, et al. Action plan for determining and monitoring the prevalence of chronic kidney disease. Kidney Int Suppl (2011). 2017;7(2):63–70.
51. Obrador GT, Schultheiss UT, Kretzler M, et al. Genetic and environmental risk factors for chronic kidney disease. Kidney Int Suppl (2011). 2017;7(2):88–106.
52. Pena MJ, Stenvinkel P, Kretzler M, et al. Strategies to improve monitoring disease progression, assessing cardiovascular risk, and defining prognostic biomarkers in chronic kidney disease. Kidney Int Suppl (2011). 2017;7(2):107–13.
53. Bello AK, Alrukhaimi M, Ashuntantang GE, et al. Complications of chronic kidney disease: current state, knowledge gaps, and strategy for action. Kidney Int Suppl (2011). 2017;7(2):122–9.
54. Perkovic V, Craig JC, Chailimpamontree W, et al. Action plan for optimizing the design of clinical trials in chronic kidney disease. Kidney Int Suppl (2011). 2017;7(2):138–44.
55. Jardine MJ, Kasiske B, Adu D, et al. Closing the gap between evidence and practice in chronic kidney disease. Kidney Int Suppl (2011). 2017;7(2):114–21.
56. Bello AK, Levin A, Tonelli M, et al. Assessment of global kidney health care status. JAMA. 2017;317(18):1864–81.
57. International Society of Nephrology. Affordable dialysis machine. 2019. Available from: https://www.theisn.org/news/item/3331-affordable-dialysis-project-gains-funding-to-move-forward.
58. Harris DCH, Davies SJ, Finkelstein FO, et al. Increasing access to integrated ESKD care as part of universal health coverage. Kidney Int. 2019;95(4S):S1–S33.
59. Jha V, Martin DE, Bargman JM, et al. Ethical issues in dialysis therapy. Lancet. 2017;389(10081):1851–6.

# Part I

# Africa

# Nephrology in the Democratic Republic of the Congo

3

Ernest Kiswaya Sumaili, Pépé Mfutu Ekulu, Nestor Muyulu Pakasa, Desiré Tshala-Katumbay, and Nazaire Mangani Nseka

## Abbreviations

| | |
|---|---|
| AA | African American |
| ACPMAR | Congolese renal failure patient association |
| AKI | Acute kidney injury |
| CAPD | Continuous ambulatory peritoneal dialysis |
| CKD | Chronic kidney disease |
| CKD-EPI | Chronic kidney disease epidemiology |
| DFMSA | Diplômes de Formation Médicale Spécialisée Approfondie |
| DRC | Democratic Republic of the Congo |
| ESRD | End-stage renal disease |
| FAS | Full age spectrum |
| FSGS | Focal segmental glomerulosclerosis |
| GFR | Glomerular filtration rate |
| HBV | Hepatitis B virus infection |
| HCV | Hepatitis C virus infection |
| HD | Hemodialysis |
| ISN | International Society of Nephrology |
| KUL | Katholieke Universiteit Leuven (Catholic University of Leuven) |
| KT | Kidney transplantation |
| mGFR | Measured GFR (mGFR) |
| MPGN | Membranoproliferative glomerulonephritis |
| PD | Peritoneal dialysis |
| RRT | Renal replacement therapy |
| SOCONEPH | Congolese Society of Nephrology |
| SSA | Sub-Saharan Africa |
| USA | United State of America |
| USD | United State dollars |
| VLIR | Vlaamse (Flemish) Interuniversitaire Raad |

E. K. Sumaili (✉) · N. M. Nseka
Renal Unit, Kinshasa University Hospital, University of Kinshasa, Kinshasa, Democratic Republic of the Congo
e-mail: ernest.sumaili@unikin.ac.cd

P. M. Ekulu
Department of Pediatrics, Kinshasa University Hospital, University of Kinshasa, Kinshasa, Democratic Republic of the Congo

N. M. Pakasa
Department of Pathology, Kinshasa University Hospital, University of Kinshasa, Kinshasa, Democratic Republic of the Congo

D. Tshala-Katumbay
Department of Neurology, University of Kinshasa, Democratic Republic of the Congo and Oregon Health & Science University, Portland, OR, USA
e-mail: tshalad@ohsu.edu

| | |
|---|---|
| Area[1] | 2,345,410 km$^2$ |
| Population[2] | 82,366,228 (2018) |
| Capital | Kinshasa |
| Three most populated cities (2018) | Kinshasa (12,071,463)<br>Mbuji-Mayi (3,367,582)<br>Lubumbashi (2,096,961) |
| Official language | French |
| Gross Domestic Product (GDP)[3] | 47.23 billion USD (2018) |
| GDP per capita[3] | 561.8 USD (2018) |
| Human Development Index (HDI)[4] | 0.459 (179th position, 2018) |
| Official currency | Congolese Franc (CDF) |
| Total number of nephrologists | 23 |
| National society of nephrology | Congolese Society of Nephrology (Societé Congolese de Néphrologie-SOCONEPH)<br>www.soconeph.org |
| Incidence of end-stage renal disease | 2018 – Unknown |
| Prevalence of end-stage renal disease (on dialysis) | 2018 – 3 pmp |
| Total number of patients on dialysis (all modalities) | 2017 – 200<br>2018 – 242<br>2019 – 235 |
| Number of patients on hemodialysis | 2017 – 190<br>2018 – 240<br>2019 – 230 |


J. A. Moura-Neto et al. (eds.), *Nephrology Worldwide*, https://doi.org/10.1007/978-3-030-56890-0_3

| | |
|---|---|
| Number of patients on peritoneal dialysis | 2017 – 10<br>2018 – 12<br>2019 – 5 |
| Number of renal transplantations per year | 2017 – 0<br>2018 – 0<br>2019 – 0 |

1. Institut National de la Statistique (INS) en République Démocratique du Congo. Accessed in February 2019. Available on https://undp.org/content/dam/dem-rep-congo/docs/MDG/anuaire
2. Current World Population-Worldometers. Accessed in March 2018. Available on https://www.worldometers.info/world-population/
3. Data World Bank. https://data.worldbank.org/country/congo-dem-rep
4. Human development index (HDI). Accessed in December 2019. Available on http://hdi.undp.org/in/countries/profiles (COD)

## Introduction

Kidney diseases are a major health concern worldwide but mostly in low- and middle-income countries where access to health care is limited. Black Africans, including those in the Democratic Republic of the Congo (DRC), are disproportionally affected.

The DRC is a vast mineral-rich central Africa country with 2,345,410 km$^2$ [1], including a total of 26 provinces. Despite its wealth of natural resources, DRC remains one of the poorest countries on Earth. The most vital natural resources encompass the country's arable land, minerals, forests, and wildlife.

Health infrastructures are minimally developed and most people lack basic services, including but not limited to, diagnosis and treatment of kidney diseases. Shortage in healthcare resources forces those who can afford to seek medical attention overseas. There is no coverage for health benefits whether private or public and the trained nephrology workforce is still in its infancy stage of development, with only 26 certified nephrologists for a population of ~82 million [2, 3].

Until now, chronic kidney disease (CKD) has not received the needed government attention. The lack of detection programs and data on CKD including dialysis are sparse. Prevention remains the only recourse to save lives.

## History of Nephrology in the Democratic Republic of the Congo

Although DRC is a vast country, there is only one Renal Unit (RU) that has been operating at the Kinshasa University Hospital. Nephrology education and training was first under the supervision of internists until 1974 when André Kalatanda Tshiani (MD, PhD) who trained as nephrologist in Scotland returned home. In this regard, Professor André Kalatanda Tshiani was considered the father of the Congolese Nephrology (the beginning of a formal nephrology training program). He worked together with Professor Corneille Ntumba Tshipeta (Urologist) who introduced in 1972 the first artificial kidney treatment for acute kidney injury (AKI). Unfortunately, due to financial constraints, this renal replacement therapy (RRT) was discontinued in its infancy stage. However, peritoneal dialysis (PD) was still performed since the beginning of the 1960s and renal biopsy was occasionally practiced by internists. Renal biopsy practice has become an exclusive task to be carried out by nephrologists starting 1974 and papers by Tshiani et al. on CKD and hypertension in Blacks have regularly been published in peer-reviewed journals [4–8].

In 1986, the RU experienced a kind of revival thanks to the return of Professor Nazaire Mangani Nseka (graduated from the Catholic University of Leuven, KUL Belgium) and close collaboration with Professor François Bompeka Lepira in diagnostic and therapeutic management of kidney diseases.

With the expertise of Professor Nestor Muyulu Pakasa (renal pathologist graduated from KUL), the interpretation of renal biopsies has significantly improved. The treatment protocols of different glomerular lesions were established and an outpatient follow-up clinic was organized for patients with KD.

For the first time, a continuous ambulatory peritoneal dialysis (CAPD) program was initiated using locally produced consumables before resorting to commercially available products. This has allowed dialysis in end-stage renal disease (ESRD) to be performed even for patients from remote provinces. In 1985, Professor Prosper Binda Ki Muaka (graduated from KUL) started pediatric nephrology but died few years later. Then, pediatric patients were taken care of by two pediatric nephrologists (Michel Ketani Aloni and Pépé Mfutu Ekulu) in collaboration with adult nephrologists. Since then, the pediatric renal unit has been growing up.

At the end of 1980s, a new hemodialysis (HD) center (with only two HD machines) was set up at the private "Presidential Clinic" in Kinshasa. The facility was, unfortunately, ransacked during a widespread looting that took place in 1991 in the midst of a political turmoil, leaving CAPD as the only form of RRT (both for AKI and ESRD) for nearly 16 years. HD has resumed only in private clinics; currently, there are 15 functional HD centers for the whole country, of which eight are located in Kinshasa, the capital city.

Acting within the framework of the World Kidney Day developed by the International Society of Nephrology (ISN), mass campaigns for raising awareness about early detection and prevention of kidney diseases and their main risk factors (hypertension, diabetes, and obesity) are yearly conducted since 2006 [9, 10].

By the end of 2019, a total of in-country certified 26 nephrologists, for either adult (23) or pediatric care (3), have been trained locally. In addition, fellowships from Belgian technical cooperation, Catholic University of Louvain, Diplômes de Formation Médicale Spécialisée Approfondie (DFMSA), Vlaamse (Flemish) Interuniversitaire Raad (VLIR), and ISN were awarded to six nephrologists (including two pediatricians) for hands-on training in renal centers in Belgium and/or France. Upon their return home, the care of kidney diseases has significantly improved. Their input has contributed substantially to a better knowledge of histologically proven kidney diseases [11, 12] as evidenced in several high-quality publications [10, 13–16].

## Epidemiology of Chronic Kidney Disease and Other Important Renal Diseases

The full magnitude of kidney diseases (e.g., AKI, CKD as well ESRD) in the Democratic Republic of the Congo is presumably high, but remains unknown due to the lack of reliable census and national registries. Most studies have focused on selected cities, including Kinshasa [10, 17], Kisantu [18], Lubumbashi [19], and Bukavu [14, 20]. It is estimated that 2–3% of hospital admissions in tropical countries, including the Democratic Republic of the Congo, are due to kidney diseases [21]. In the general population, the prevalence of CKD varies from 12.4% in the Kinshasa [10] to 7.3% in Bukavu [20]. It appears significantly much higher in urban Bukavu residents (15.3%, $p = 0.01$) relative to rural settings (10%). Moreover, CKD affects mainly young adults in their productive years. In contrast to the USA where CKD appears to predominate in older, rather than younger subjects, there is a distinct overrepresentation of CKD in younger people in our Country (Fig. 3.1) [10].

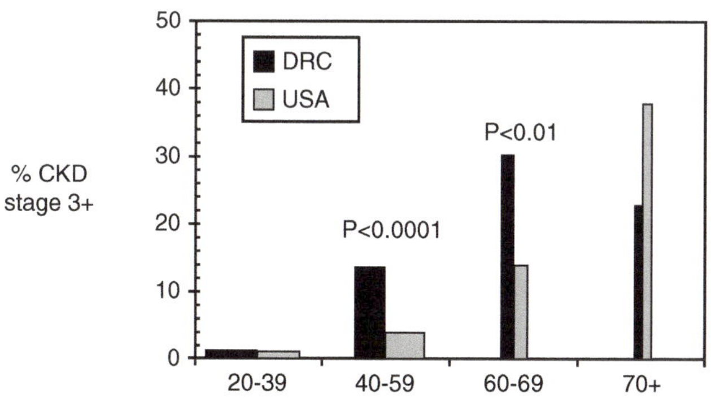


**Fig. 3.1** Prevalence of CKD stage 3 or higher, according to age range and country. The width of the columns is proportional to the percentage of subjects in that age bracket, by cohort. There is a distinct overrepresentation of CKD in younger people in the Democratic Republic of the Congo cohort, in contrast to the US cohort. This difference in distribution is highly significant for the two middle age ranges ($P < 0.01$, chi-square test). (The data for the USA were taken from Coresh et al. [43])

Furthermore, unlike in developed countries where, more than 50% of ESRD patients are over 60 years old, data in Congolese series indicate that only 9% of ESRD patients are above 60 years of age. According to the latest WHO data published in 2018 [3], life expectancy in the DRC (58.9 years for men, 62 for women, and 60.5 overall) remains significantly low compared to that of the USA (76 years for men, 81 for women, and 78.7 overall). Reasons for this discrepancy have yet to be determined. A recent genetic study found a prevalence of 12.7% for two *APOL 1* risk alleles in the CKD population of Kinshasa [22], explaining partially the younger age of the Congolese individual with CKD. This observation is consistent with the findings of Kanji [23] and Tzur [24] from the USA showing that African Americans (AA) with non-diabetic ESRD carrying two *APOL 1* risk alleles initiated dialysis at a mean age that was 9 years younger that of those without *APOL 1* risk alleles. CKD affects also Congolese people at school age. Indeed, the prevalence of CKD among adolescents and young adults (16–24 years old) of Kinshasa is 1.5% [25]. In this school environment, the prevalence of qualitative and quantitative proteinuria was 7.4% versus 1%, respectively.

In the voluntary mass screening of the 2007 World Kidney Day for proteinuria and risk factors associated with CKD, we found the prevalence of proteinuria to be 17%. To identify one case of proteinuria, it would need to screen four persons with diabetes, four subjects having metabolic syndrome, five persons with hypertension, five persons aged more than 72 years old, and nine persons without any of the conditions mentioned above [26].

CKD is also a significant cause of death in our Country [17], resulting from kidney and/or cardiovascular disease. Adverse outcomes of CKD such as ESRD, cardiovascular disease, and premature death can be prevented or delayed when treatment is initiated in the early stages. Hence, prevention is of paramount importance in our Country with no or limited access to RRT. In this context, glomerular filtration rate (GFR) is the best quantitative renal function marker, as it may be measured or estimated. Measurement of GFR by using reference methods is not easily feasible, especially in developing countries. In clinical practices, GFR is estimated from endogenous biomarkers such as creatinine. In this regard, Bukabau et al. [27] reported that serum creatinine in Black Africans is closer to Caucasian subjects than AA. Therefore, the AA race-ethnicity factor is not appropriate in Black Africans and the performance of the CKD epidemiology (CKD-EPI) and full age spectrum (FAS) equations is satisfactory and equivalent for measured GFR (mGFR) ≥60 ml/min/1.73 m$^2$, when ethnic factor is omitted. The inadequacy of the AA race-ethnicity factor for the equations is probably because they have been developed in populations with different anthropometrical characteristics. Indeed, by contrast to Fernandes et al. [28] who showed a significantly higher creatinine levels in Brazilian Black patients relative to Caucasians, Black Africans have low muscle mass compared to AA, probably due to poor diet and/or overall health, otherwise partially explained by the preponderance of HIV infection or other chronic diseases [27]. Nevertheless, the difference between creatinine levels in Black subjects from different continents may also have specific causes that require closer genomic ancestry scrutiny. For example, studies from Brazil [29, 30] have suggested that each Brazilian has singular proportions of American, European, and African ancestries in their mosaic genome.

In the Democratic Republic of the Congo, the burden of CKD reflects typically the interaction of genetic, socioeconomic, cultural and environmental factors, as well as the multiple deficiencies of the healthcare system (Fig. 3.2). CKD is likely due to the double burden of communicable diseases (e.g., malaria, filariasis, onchocerciasis, schistosomiasis, tuberculosis, HIV, HCV, and HBV) as well non-communicable diseases such as hypertension, diabetes, sickle cell disease, obesity, heart disease, collagen vascular disease, and APOL 1 nephropathy.

While glomerular disease (35%) remains the primary cause of ESRD, hypertensive kidney disease (30%) and diabetic nephropathy (25%) are currently important additional causes of CKD [31]. Other CKD that are important causes of ESRD include obstructive uropathy (e.g., renal calculi, benign prostatic hyperplasia, prostate disease), autosomal dominant polycystic disease, lupus nephritis, chronic interstitial nephritis, amyloidosis secondary to chronic infection (e.g., tuberculosis, HIV, HCV), herbs nephropathy, HIV nephropathy, and sickle cell nephropathy. During the 1970s, the country experienced the decline of parasitic causes of the nephrotic syndrome with colonial and post-colonial eradication campaigns. Unfortunately, this effort has been lost overtime due to poor governance, lack of political will, civil war, and poverty in the country, resulting in persistence and re-emergence of tropical diseases (e.g., chronic parasitic, bacterial, fungal, and viral infections) [32], explaining the preponderance of glomerular diseases. Other plausible explanations include those related to the genetic adaptation of microbial agents, occupational exposures, inappropriate use of antibiotic, and environmental factors (climate and weather variations, economic development, and changes in land use). Currently, focal segmental glomerulosclerosis (FSGS) remains the leading cause of nephrotic syndrome; with virus human infection accounting for 30% of the cases, the remainder was idiopathic. Pakasa et al. [32] showed that CKD secondary to tropical parasites are heterogenous. Indeed, FSGS occur during various filariasis infections, *Schistosoma mansoni* is responsible for membranoproliferative glomerulonephritis (MPGN) and amyloidosis whereas human African trypanosomiasis is associated with cryoglobulinemic MPGN.

While *Plasmodium falciparum* infection may lead to acute pattern of AKI (acute tubular necrosis or acute post-infectious glomerulonephritis), *Plasmodium malariae* is mainly responsible for CKD due to membranous glomerulopathy. Several other viral (i.e., HCV, HBV), parasitic (onchocerciasis), bacterial (leprosy and tuberculosis) infections, which are still highly prevalent in DRC may affect also the kidney. A variety of renal injuries associated with sickle cell disease is also encountered [32, 33].

The second cause of CKD in our Country is hypertension-attributed nephropathy, which accounts for 25% of the subjects in the dialysis facilities of Kinshasa [16]. It is unclear whether the high frequency of hypertensive kidney disease is a result of damage from severe essential hypertension, potentiated by environmental nephrotoxins such as the use of herbal remedies, illicit or prescribed drugs or other factors. Our recent study [22] identified a significantly elevated odds ratio (OR) for hypertension-attributed CKD among carriers of two risk alleles, which could partly explain the heavy burden of CKD and hypertension in Kinshasa [22]. Hypertension, in general, occurs earlier and is more severe in Black Africans than it is in AA [34].

Although diabetic kidney disease is still the third cause of ESRD, its incidence is increasing mainly among those in RRT. The continuing rise in the incidence of diabetic ESRD may be due to a combination of increasing incidence rate of diabetes and ineffective therapy to retard progression of diabetic renal disease in the early stages. For example, a screening for diabetes in the general population of semi-rural area of Kisantu (at 120 km from Kinshasa) yielded the prevalence of microalbuminuria and macroalbuminuria in 45.2% and 12%, respectively [18]; intervening early in the course of the disease would be more effective than after the disease has been established.

Persisting public health issues such as inadequate sanitation, lack of safe drinking water, suboptimal infection control and reproductive health, and environmental hazards continue to generate a large and preventable burden of CKD and AKI [35]. There is also a striking difference between the etiologies of AKI in the developed world compared to that of developing countries.

AKI in Western societies is now largely the consequence of cardiovascular surgery, drugs, multi-organ failure, consequences of traffic and industrial accidences. In the developing world including the DRC, medical causes remain the dominant subgroup of AKI [36]. In this context, most cases are probably community-acquired AKI in which infections, hypovolemia, and herbal medicines remain the most common etiological factors.

AKI is also common in hospitalized patients, particularly in critically ill patients. In this regard, a more recent survey [13] indicated that more than half of critically ill Congolese patients developed AKI, which substantially

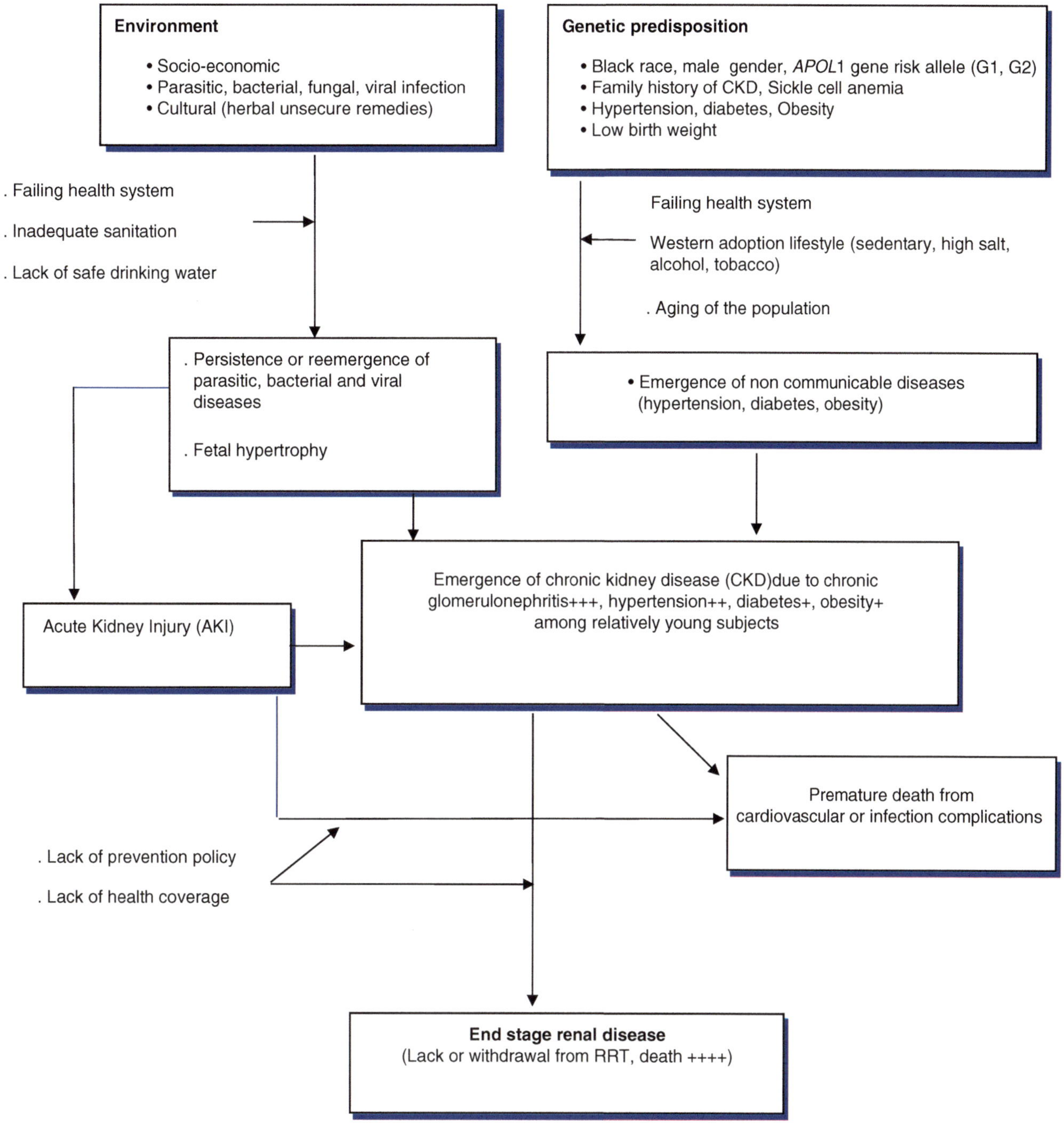


**Fig. 3.2** Epidemiological peculiarities of kidney diseases (AKI, CKD) in DRC

contribute to short-term mortality. According to Oluwo et al. [36], most patients in sub-Saharan Africa (SSA) presented with severe AKI, with 70% of adults and 66% of children needing dialysis (stage 3 AKI), suggesting that it is a more aggressive disorder in SSA than elsewhere, due probably to late admission and inability to pay for dialysis. AKI is an important independent risk factor for CKD and ESRD, death, and other non-renal outcomes. This situation prompted the ISN through the 0by25 initiative to make the fight against one of its priorities, by recognizing a reduction in preventable death due to AKI a "human right" issue and called for stakeholder engagement, public awareness, and education of general practitioners and non-physician healthcare workers on causes of AKI (e.g., infections, herbs, contamination waters, over-the-counter medicines, and obstetric care) and the importance of its prevention [35]. Through the ISN program for developing countries, some Congolese physicians have received nephrology training which has impacted our country improving the standards of care and the developing acute PD for AKI.

## Renal Replacement Therapy

RRT for ESRD in DRC encompasses HD and PD modalities as well as kidney transplantation (both living and deceased are not available). The majority of the 230 prevalent patients are undergoing HD. Of note, the majority of HD centers offer both diffusive (HD) as well as convective therapy (hemodiafiltration, hemofiltration). Since patients are sometimes treated by one or the other method, depending on the patient's condition as well as the availability of equipment, it seems difficult to determine the exact number of patients undergoing only convective therapy.

With regards to vascular access, only 9.3% of patients use arteriovenous fistulas for HD. 60.5% of patients have tunneled catheters and 30.2% temporary vascular access. Our standard HD prescription has a dialysate flow of 500 ml/min and a blood flow rate that varies from 250 to 400 ml/min, depending on the patient's condition and vascular access. The conventional in-center HD is done for 4 hours, three-weekly sessions for patients who can afford the cost of long-term HD treatment. We do not reuse the same dialyzer in DRC.

A recent survey [37] showed that the overall prevalence of hepatitis C virus infection (HCV) in six HD centers of Kinshasa was 17.3% (only two centers had a low prevalence). Determinants of HCV infection were as follows: multiple blood transfusions (>4), lack of erythropoietin (EPO) therapy, HD duration >14 months, temporary catheter, and/or treatment in charitable HD centers. Currently, there are no patients with hepatitis B virus or HIV in HD.

Although the total number of subjects with ESRD and requiring RRT remains unknown, Sumaili et al. [10] reported a prevalence of stage 5 CKD of 0.2% in Kinshasa. This suggests that 164,000 Congolese people should present ESRD requiring RRT. Our data [38] indicate also that more than three-quarters of patients admitted in the renal unit at the University of Kinshasa were already at stage 5 CKD, and only 11% of them could afford RRT. For example, currently, only 230 patients are on HD in the country. Indeed, access to dialysis in the Democratic Republic of the Congo is limited by insufficient infrastructure and catastrophic out-of-pocket expenses [39].

Limitations to regular maintenance dialysis include paucity of dialysis units (currently there are only 15 HD centers and 3 other PD centers (with currently five patients on CAPD, automated DP is not available)), restriction of these units to urban centers, and absence of government funding or health insurance to cover the high costs. Lack of financial resources forces patients either to reduce dialysis frequency, withdraw from dialysis, or use alternative treatment responsible for the higher mortality with a median survival of 17 months or 78 per 1000 patient-years (17 per 1000 in preserved versus 61 per 1000 in reduced residual urine volume (<500 ml/day) [40]. Mokoli et al. [40] found also that in Kinshasa, 18.4% died from withdrawal of HD due to financial constraints. In two HD centers funded by the provincial government of Kinshasa "called charitable HD center" at 75% (direct cost of HD per session is about 60 USD compared to more than 200 USD in the other Congolese HD centers [41]). Withdraw from dialysis supplies is more frequent, contributing to poor quality of life and all-cause mortality in ESRD patients.

We also observed that about 80% of all patients with AKI, despite indications, did not receive dialysis, due to lack of resources and inability to afford the prohibitive cost of the therapy. Considering that a single HD session costs at least 200 USD (2500–3000 USD per month) versus 100 USD for PD (3000 USD per month, hence the monthly cost of CAPD is nearly similar to HD), it becomes clear that long-term dialysis will not be an option for most Central Africans with renal failure except in some countries such as Angola, Chad, Cameroon, and Gabon where governmental RRT expenditure coverage exceeds 95% (Table 3.1). Medications are funded solely by private and out-of-pocket money.

In all central African countries including ours, there are no kidney transplantation (KT) as well renal registries which may provide a standardized method to collect data on disease burden, treatment, and outcomes, and monitor disease progression over time.

Finally, there are specific barriers to optimal kidney diseases care such as geographic locations (distance from care or prolonged travel time), physician-related limits (availability, access, knowledge, and attitude), patient knowledge and attitude, limited availability of nephrologists, and poor healthcare system (poor availability, access, capability).

## Kidney Transplantation

Despite the fact that KT would be the only viable alternative for long-term survival of Congolese ESRD patients, KT is not performed in DRC. Until now, legislations for regulation of organ transplantation do not exist. A regulatory KT law has already been drafted and is awaiting acceptance by the parliament and promulgation by the President of the DRC.

More recent unpublished data show that few privileged ESRD patients are transplanted from living-related donors elsewhere, especially in India (86%) where the cost of KT operation is relatively cheaper ~28,000 USD than ~50,000 USD in South Africa (6.8%) and 54,000 USD in Belgium (6.8%). A third of them had never been followed by

**Table 3.1** Country-wise distribution of population, resource, CKD prevalence, type of RRT, dialysis centers, and dialysis patients in Central Africa

| Country | Population in millions 2017 [3] | GDP USD | Total health expenditure as % GDP | CKD prevalence in general population in % | Type of RRT available | Number of nephrologists | Number of renal pathologists | Number of dialysis centers | Number of dialysis patients | Average cost of hemodialysis session USD | Governmental RRT expenditure coverage in % |
|---|---|---|---|---|---|---|---|---|---|---|---|
| Angola | 26,655 | 102,627 | 3.8 | Unknown | HD | 4 | Unknown | 4 | Unknown | Unknown | 100 |
| Cameroon | 24,513 | 28,416 | 5.1 | 10–13 | HD | 21 | 0 | 9 | 961 | 185 | 95.6 |
| Central African Rep. | 5,098 | 1,584 | 3.9 | Unknown | HD | Unknown | Unknown | Unknown | Unknown | Unknown | Unknown |
| Chad | 14,965 | 10,889 | 3.5 | Unknown | HD | 3 | 0 | 2 | Unknown | 322 | 98 |
| Congo, Rep | 4,866 | 8,853 | 4.1 | Unknown | HD | 7 | 0 | 3 | Unknown | 270 | 0 |
| Congo, Dem Rep | 82,242 | 35,238 | 3.5 | 9–12 | HD,DP | 26 | 2 | 15 | 350 | 184 (50–250) | 0% in the majority of centers/75% in two centers |
| Gabon | 1,919 | 14,262 | 8.9 | Unknown | HD | 8 | 0 | 6 | 306 | 225 | 100[a] |
| Equatorial guinea | 0,894 | 12,202 | 3.4 | Unknown | – | Unknown | Unknown | Unknown | Unknown | Unknown | Unknown |
| Sao Tome and Principe | 0,198 | 318 | 6.9 | Unknown | – | Unknown | Unknown | Unknown | Unknown | Unknown | Unknown |

www.worldometers.info/world-population/population-by-country/accessed on March 27th, 2018

[a]Health insurance providers

Congolese nephrologists before the KT. Among those who have returned home, the follow-up is irregular. As a result, almost half of them resumed dialysis (after chronic rejection) and 24% died. The median survival of all the KT patients is low (but, little better for those who came from Belgium), estimated to be as low as 4 years. Patients have no access to immunosuppressive therapy or any kind of government support once they return home.

## Pediatric Nephrology

Pediatric nephrology is also an emerging discipline even though it is not yet quite developed in the different provinces of the country. In a country of approximately 82 million inhabitants, half of which are children, there is only one well-organized pediatric nephrology ward, located in the University Hospital of Kinshasa. As mentioned above, this pediatric nephrology ward was implemented around the 1980s by one of the first pioneers of pediatric nephrology in SSA, Professor Prosper Binda Ki Muaka. From 1999 to 2001, the unit experienced a significant decrease in its activities following the death of its founder. In 2001, the pediatric nephrology activities resumed thanks to a renewed staff which remained since then extremely devoted to the development of this discipline throughout the country.

Being established in a teaching and referral hospital, the activities of pediatric nephrology ward are focused on a triple mission namely: care, teaching, and research. Treated patients come from peripheral hospitals and all other provinces of the country. Led by two qualified physicians in pediatric nephrology with the collaboration of six nurses, this unit has eight hospital beds with an average monthly occupation of 85% and approximately 80 outpatient consultations per month.

Before 2018, most children with AKI who required RRT were treated with the collaboration of adult nephrologists. Since December 2017, a pediatric acute PD program, using home-made fluids and bedside catheter insertion technique, has been established in the Department of Pediatric. The main areas of research in this pediatric nephrology unit are kidney and sickle cell disease, kidney and HIV infection, kidney and heart diseases, kidney and malaria, kidney and malignant diseases, urinary tract infections, AKI and CKD including nephrotic syndrome. With regard to education, undergraduate and postgraduate courses are offered across the country. Furthermore, kidney health promotion activities in the community are frequently held.

The major challenge in running pediatric nephrology activities is the lack of financial commitment from the government. Parents, most of them of very low income, are responsible for all costs related to the care of their children including all laboratory tests and dialysis. Ignorance and cultural beliefs are also among the many challenges to face. Indeed, many parents in our society as in neighboring countries believe that kidney diseases cannot affect children since the kidney is a genital organ of the adult male. This justifies the community awareness strategies implemented by the pediatric nephrology team.

## Reimbursement and Health Policies

In this country, there is a lack of government or employer reimbursement or health insurance. In only two HD centers, the direct cost of HD (not PD) is supported by the provincial government of Kinshasa at 75%. Currently, one of these two charitable HD centers has been closed for 6 months due to financial constraints. This situation forces patients to attend other more expensive HD centers. Maintenance of immunosuppression cost is not supported by state or insurance in the majority of patients, and self-financed patients are forced to decrease or discontinue costly immunosuppressants. However, the government is responsible for salaries of health professionals working in public hospitals.

## Brief Overview of the Job Market for Professionals in the Sector, Member of Nephrology, and Their Roles in Health Care

Current estimates indicate that there are more than 10,000 physicians in the country, for a population of 82 million, i.e., a ratio of 1 physician per 8200 [3]. This number is low compared to many high-income countries including the USA which has more than a million physicians in a country of 325 million people [42].

The overall workforce needed to address CKD is similarly very limited (Table 3.1). In general, Central African countries have less than 40 nephrologists (~0.22/million inhabitants). That number is much less than the ratio of nephrologists to population in most other countries, which is 17/million in Belgium, 20/million in the USA, and 10/million in Egypt [31]. There is also a shortage of renal pathologists, vascular access coordinators, dialysis nurses, dialysis technicians, dietitians, social workers, etc.

Only two countries in central Africa, i.e., Cameroon and the Democratic Republic of the Congo have a Nephrology training program. In these contexts, general practitioners and non-physician healthcare workers will still need to be involved in CKD prevention and care. As mentioned above, challenges in care are compounded not only by shortage of workforce but also poor infrastructure and lack of medical coverage.

In most developing countries and in the Democratic Republic of the Congo in particular, the few trained nephrologists are involved with CKD care in both public and private clinics working low-pay strenuous hours in public sectors, compensating for lost income via what is commonly known as "extramural" attendance in numerous private clinics, several times a week. With such limited and overextended workforce, it will be difficult to implement programs to detect, prevent, or treat CKD.

## National Nephrology Society

The Congolese Society of Nephrology (SOCONEPH) was founded in 2016 at Kinshasa. SOCONEPH comprises nephrologists, other physicians, nurses, dietitians, clinical psychologists, social workers, dialysis maintenance technicians, and other employees interested in kidney diseases.

This national society collaborates closely with the Congolese renal failure patient association (ACPMAR). The vision is the following: "A future where all Congolese people, at risk or having acute or chronic kidney disease, benefit an equitable access to realistic and achievable prevention, sustainable care and support interventions focused on the individual.

The mission statement reads that by acting in collaboration and in synergy with all partners involved in the promotion of kidney health, the SOCONEPH will support kidney research through all aspects of basic research, clinical, healthcare services, and the health of population; promote and organize high-quality continuing medical education for physicians, nurses, biomedical engineers, researchers, and all partners involved in the health kidney promotion and in the fight against kidney disease.

Finally, SOCONEPH hopes to promote high quality of health care offered to people at risk or already kidney disease carriers and their families. Our values include permanent research for excellence, collaboration (partnership) and inclusiveness, transparency and integrity; medical practice based on evidence or facts, and advocacy for equity and diversity.

## Future Perspectives of Nephrology in the Democratic Republic of the Congo

Pediatric as well as adult nephrology seek an expansion of the PD program throughout the country and promote CKD early detection and prevention programs in the country. A large national network for CKD management in children as well as in adults is essential. In addition, as part of the ongoing training projects in Pediatric Department, the Pediatric Nephrology Service has committed to train, at least, three experts in each of the above-mentioned research areas for the full development of this discipline in the country. Further studies regarding the epidemiology of KD (AKI, CKD), and outcomes, are urgently required.

Sustained efforts from governmental agencies, international societies, the pharmaceutical industry, and philanthropic bodies remain of paramount importance.

**Acknowledgments** The authors thank François Kaze (Cameroon), Ibrahim Hamat (Chad), Théophane Nzame Ze (Gabon), and Pamela Armella Ondele (Congo) for their contribution to collect data from their own country. They also thank François Lepira Bompeka for his contribution.

**Conflict of Interest Statement** None declared

## References

1. Institut National de la Statistique (INS) en République Démocratique du Congo. Accessed in February 2019. Available in https://undp.org/content/dam/dem-rep-congo/docs/MDG/anuaire.
2. Human development index (HDI). Accessed in December 2019. Available in http://hdi.undp.org/in/countries/profiles (COD).
3. Current World Population-Worldometers. Accessed in March 2018. Available in https://www.worldometers.info/world-population/.
4. Tshiani AK, Nseka NM, Musuamba M, Lutete K. Epidémiologie de l'hypertension artérielle au Zaire: résultat d'une enquête préliminaire chez 4988 sujets. Med Afr Noire. 1979;26(1):67–75.
5. M'Buyamba-Kabangu JR, Fagard R, Lijnen P, Staessen J, Ditu MS, Tshiani KA, Amery A. Epidemiological study of blood pressure and hypertension in a sample of urban Bantu of Zaire. J Hypertens. 1986;4(4):485–91.
6. M'Buyamba-Kabangu JR, Fagard R, Lijnen P, Staessen J, Lissens W, Ditu M, Lepira B, Tshiani KA, Amery A. Calcium entry blockade or beta-blockade in long-term management of hypertension in blacks. Clin Pharmacol Ther. 1987;41(1):45–54.
7. M'Buyamba-Kabangu JR, Lepira B, Lijnen P, Tshiani K, Fagard R, Amery A. Intracellular sodium and the response to nitrendipine or atenolol in African blacks. Hypertension. 1988;11(1):100–5.
8. Nseka M, Tshiani KA. Chronic renal failure in tropical Africa. East Afr Med J. 1989;66(2):109–14.
9. Sumaili EK, Cohen EP. Screening for chronic kidney disease in Sub-Saharan Africa. Lancet. 2010;376(9739):418.
10. Sumaili EK, Krzesinski JM, Zinga CV, Cohen EP, Delanaye P, Munyanga SM, Nseka NM. Prevalence of chronic kidney disease in Kinshasa: results of a pilot study from the Democratic Republic of Congo. Nephrol Dial Transplant. 2009;24(1):117–22.
11. Pakasa M, Mangani N, Dikassa L. Focal and segmental glomerulosclerosis in nephrotic syndrome: a new profile of adult nephrotic syndrome in Zaire. Mod Pathol. 1993;6(2):125–8.
12. Pakasa NM, Nseka NM, Nyimi LM. Secondary collapsing glomerulopathy associated with Loa loa filariasis. Am J Kidney Dis. 1997;30(6):836–9.
13. Masewu A, Makulo JR, Lepira F, Amisi EB, Sumaili EK, Bukabau J, Mokoli V, Longo A, Nlandu Y, Engole Y, et al. Acute kidney injury is a powerful independent predictor of mortality in critically ill patients: a multicenter prospective cohort study from Kinshasa, the Democratic Republic of Congo. BMC Nephrol. 2016;17(1):118.
14. Masimango MI, Sumaili EK, Jadoul M, Wallemacq P, Mubagwa DK, Makulo RJ, Lepira FB, Nseka NM. Prevalence of microalbuminuria and diagnostic value of dipstick proteinuria in outpatients

from HIV clinics in Bukavu, the Democratic Republic of Congo. BMC Nephrol. 2014;15:146.

15. Bukabau JB, Sumaili EK, Cavalier E, Pottel H, Kifakiou B, Nkodila A, Makulo JRR, Mokoli VM, Zinga CV, Longo AL, et al. Performance of glomerular filtration rate estimation equations in Congolese healthy adults: the inopportunity of the ethnic correction. PLoS One. 2018;13(3):e0193384.
16. Nlandu Y, Lepira F, Makulo JR, Engole Y, Sumaili E, Wameso MN, Mokoli V, Luse J, Longo A, Zinga C, et al. Reverse epidemiology of elevated blood pressure among chronic hemodialysis black patients with stroke: a historical cohort study. BMC Nephrol. 2017;18(1):277.
17. Sumaili EK, Cohen EP, Zinga CV, Krzesinski JM, Pakasa NM, Nseka NM. High prevalence of undiagnosed chronic kidney disease among at-risk population in Kinshasa, the Democratic Republic of Congo. BMC Nephrol. 2009;10:18.
18. Makulo R Jr, Nseka MN, Jadoul M, Mvitu M, Muyer MT, Kimenyembo W, Mandja M, Bieleli E, Mapatano MA, Lepira FB, et al. Albuminuria during the screening for diabetes in a semi-rural area (Kisantu City, DR Congo). Nephrol Ther. 2010;6(6):513–9.
19. Tshamba HM, Van Caillie D, Nawej FN, Kapend FM, Kaj FM, Yav GD, Nawej PT. Risk of death and the economic accessibility at the dialysis therapy for the renal insufficient patients in Lubumbashi city, Democratic Republic of Congo. Pan Afr Med J. 2015;19:61.
20. Masimango MI, Sumaili EK, Wallemacq P, Jadoul M. Prevalence and risk factors of chronic kidney disease in South-Kivu, Democratic Republic of Congo: a population-based study. Nephrol Dial Transplant. 2018;33(Suppl 1):i325.
21. Naicker S. End-stage renal disease in Sub-Saharan and South Africa. Kidney Int Suppl. 2003;83:S119–22.
22. Sumaili EK, Shemer R, Kruzel-Davila E, Cohen EP, Mutantu PN, Bukabau JB, Makulo JRR, Mokoli VM, Luse JL, Pakasa NM, et al. G1 is the major APOL1 risk allele for hypertension-attributed nephropathy in Central Africa. Clin Kidney J. 2019;12(2):188–95.
23. Kanji Z, Powe CE, Wenger JB, Huang C, Ankers E, Sullivan DA, Collerone G, Powe NR, Tonelli M, Bhan I, et al. Genetic variation in APOL1 associates with younger age at hemodialysis initiation. J Am Soc Nephrol. 2011;22(11):2091–7.
24. Tzur S, Rosset S, Skorecki K, Wasser WG. APOL1 allelic variants are associated with lower age of dialysis initiation and thereby increased dialysis vintage in African and Hispanic Americans with non-diabetic end-stage kidney disease. Nephrol Dial Transplant. 2012;27(4):1498–505.
25. Bukabau JB, Makulo JR, Pakasa NM, Cohen EP, Lepira FB, Kayembe PK, Nseka NM, Sumaili EK. Chronic kidney disease among high school students of Kinshasa. BMC Nephrol. 2012;13:24.
26. Sumaili EK, Nseka NM, Lepira FB, Krzesinski JM, Makulo JR, Bukabau JB, Nkoy JB, Mokoli VM, Longokolo MM, Owandjalola JA, et al. Screening for proteinuria and chronic kidney disease risk factors in Kinshasa: a World Kidney Day 2007 study. Nephron Clin Pract. 2008;110(4):c220–8.
27. Bukabau JB, Yayo E, Gnionsahe A, Monnet D, Pottel H, Cavalier E, Nkodila A, Makulo JRR, Mokoli VM, Lepira FB, et al. Performance of creatinine- or cystatin C-based equations to estimate glomerular filtration rate in sub-Saharan African populations. Kidney Int. 2019;95(5):1181–9.
28. Fernandes NM, Hoekstra T, van den Beukel TO, Tirapani L, Bastos K, Pecoits-Filho R, Qureshi AR, Dekker FW, Bastos MG, Divino-Filho JC. Association of ethnicity and survival in peritoneal dialysis: a cohort study of incident patients in Brazil. Am J Kidney Dis. 2013;62(1):89–96.
29. Pena SD, Bastos-Rodrigues L, Pimenta JR, Bydlowski SP. DNA tests probe the genomic ancestry of Brazilians. Braz J Med Biol Res. 2009;42(10):870–6.
30. Pena SD, Di Pietro G, Fuchshuber-Moraes M, Genro JP, Hutz MH, Kehdy Fde S, Kohlrausch F, Magno LA, Montenegro RC, Moraes MO, et al. The genomic ancestry of individuals from different geographical regions of Brazil is more uniform than expected. PLoS One. 2011;6(2):e17063.
31. Krzesinski JM, Sumaili KE, Cohen E. How to tackle the avalanche of chronic kidney disease in Sub-Saharan Africa: the situation in the Democratic Republic of Congo as an example. Nephrol Dial Transplant. 2007;22(2):332–5.
32. Pakasa NM, Sumaili EK. Pathological peculiarities of chronic kidney disease in patient from Sub-Saharan Africa. Review of data from the Democratic Republic of the Congo. Ann Pathol. 2012;32(1):40–52.
33. Aloni MN, Mabidi JL, Ngiyulu RM, Ekulu PM, Mbutiwi FI, Makulo JR, Sumaili EK, Gini-Ehungu JL, Nsibu CN, Nseka NM, et al. Prevalence and determinants of microalbuminuria in children suffering from sickle cell anemia in steady state. Clin Kidney J. 2017;10(4):479–86.
34. Agodoa L. End-stage renal failure in African Americans. In: Nahas ME, editor. Kidney diseases in the developing world and ethnic minorities. New York: Taylor and Francis Group, LLC; 2005. p. 563.
35. Mehta RL, Burdmann EA, Cerda J, Feehally J, Finkelstein F, Garcia-Garcia G, Godin M, Jha V, Lameire NH, Levin NW, et al. Recognition and management of acute kidney injury in the International Society of Nephrology 0by25 Global Snapshot: a multinational cross-sectional study. Lancet. 2017;387(10032):2017–25.
36. Olowu WA, Niang A, Osafo C, Ashuntantang G, Arogundade FA, Porter J, Naicker S, Luyckx VA. Outcomes of acute kidney injury in children and adults in Sub-Saharan Africa: a systematic review. Lancet Glob Health. 2016;4(4):e242–50.
37. Kadima E, Makulo JR, Ngilibuma M, Mokoli V, Ilunga C, Engole Y, Lepira F, Nseka MN, Sumaili EK. Déterminants de l'infection par le virus de l'hépatite C dans les centres d'hémodialyse. Néphrol Ther. 2019;15(5):308.
38. Pakasa NM, Sumaili EK. The nephrotic syndrome in the Democratic Republic of Congo. N Engl J Med. 2006;354(10):1085–6.
39. Ashuntantang G, Osafo C, Olowu WA, Arogundade F, Niang A, Porter J, Naicker S, Luyckx VA. Outcomes in adults and children with end-stage kidney disease requiring dialysis in Sub-Saharan Africa: a systematic review. Lancet Glob Health. 2017;5(4):e408–17.
40. Mokoli VM, Sumaili EK, Lepira FB, Makulo JR, Bukabau JB, Osa Izeidi PP, Luse JL, Mukendi SK, Mashinda DK, Nseka NM. Impact of residual urine volume decline on the survival of chronic hemodialysis patients in Kinshasa. BMC Nephrol. 2016;17(1):182.
41. Izeidi PPM, Nlandu YM, Lepira FB, Makulo JR, Engole YM, Mokoli VM, Bukabau JB, Kwilu FN, Nseka NM, Sumaili EK. Cost estimate of chronic hemodialysis in Kinshasa, the Democratic Republic of the Congo: a prospective study in two centers. Hemodial Int. 2020;24:121–28.
42. Young A, Chaudhry H, Pei X, Arnhart K, Dugan M, Snyder G. A census of actively licensed physicians in the United States, 2016. J Med Regul. 2017;103(2):7–21.
43. Coresh J, Selvin E, Stevens LA, Manzi J, Kusek JW, Eggers P, et al. Prevalence of chronic kidney disease in the United States. JAMA. 2007;298(17):2038–47.

# Nephrology in Ethiopia

4

Addisu M. Ejigu, Momina M. Ahmed,
and Yewondwossen T. Mengistu

| | |
|---|---|
| Area | 1,104,300 km$^2$ |
| Population | 112 million (2019) |
| Capital | Addis Ababa |
| Three most populated cities: | 1. Addis Ababa<br>2. Dire Dawa<br>3. Makalle |
| Official language | Amharic |
| Gross Domestic Product (GDP)[1] | 80 billion USD (2016/17) |
| GDP per capita[1] | 863 USD (2016/17) |
| Human Development Index (HDI)[2] | 0.463 (2017) |
| Official currency | Birr |
| Total number of nephrologists | 26 |
| National society of nephrology | Not formed |
| Incidence of end-stage renal disease | 2018 – Unknown |
| Prevalence of end-stage renal disease | 2018 – ~7 pmp |
| Total number of patients on dialysis (all modalities) | 2017 – Unknown<br>2018 – ~800 |
| Number of patients on hemodialysis | 2017 – Unknown<br>2018 – ~800 |
| Number of patients on peritoneal dialysis | 2017 – 0<br>2018 – 0 |
| Number of renal transplantations per year | 2017 – 32<br>2018 – 38 |

Table references:

1. Ethiopia key economic and social indicators, UNDP- https://www.et.undp.org/content/ethiopia/en/home/library/UNDPEthiopia/Ethiopia_Key_Economic_Indicators_May20181.html, Accessed on 23 July 2019
2. UNDP Human development indices & indicators: 2018 statistical update, Ethiopia http://hdr.undp.org/sites/all/themes/hdr_theme/country-notes/ETH.pdf, Accessed on 23 July 2019

A. M. Ejigu · Y. T. Mengistu (✉)
Renal Unit School of Medicine, College of Health Sciences, Addis Ababa University, Addis Ababa, Ethiopia

M. M. Ahmed
Renal Unit, Saint Paul Millenium Medical College (SPMMC), Addis Abeba, Ethiopia

## Introduction

Ethiopia is a country located in the horn of Africa, which occupies part of the North-Eastern part of the continent. It borders with six countries: Eritrea, Djibouti, Somalia, Kenya, South Sudan, and Sudan. It occupies an area of 1.1 million km$^2$ with geographical diversity ranging from 4620 meters above sea level down to 148 meters below sea level. More than half of the country lies above 1500 m. The predominant climate type is tropical monsoon, with temperate climate on the plateau and hot in the lowlands.

It is the second-most populous country in Africa with a projected population of 112 million in the year 2019. The population is predominately young; with 40.3% under the age of 15 years and 56.1% in the age group between 15 and 64 years. The population in the age group 65 and above accounts for only 3.5% of the population [1].

Ethiopia is one of the least urbanized countries in the world; only 16% of the population lives in urban areas. The majority of the population lives in the highland areas. The main occupation of the settled rural population is farming, while the lowland areas are mostly inhabited by pastoral or partially pastoral people, who move from place to place in search of grazing grounds and water.

Ethiopia is a federal parliamentary republic. It is home to a variety of nations, nationalities, and peoples with more than 80 different languages spoken. The working language of the federal government is Amharic. The country has a rich history, unique cultural heritage with a diverse population mix of ethnicity and religion. It is the oldest independent state and served as a symbol of African independence throughout the colonial period. It is a founding member of the United Nations (UN), the African Union (AU), and hosts several international organizations, including the headquarters of the AU and the UN Economic Commission for Africa.

Although Ethiopia is one of the poorest countries in the region, with a per capita income of $790, the country's economy has been growing very fast in the last decade with an annual average of 9.9% (2007/08 to 2017/18), compared to a


J. A. Moura-Neto et al. (eds.), *Nephrology Worldwide*, https://doi.org/10.1007/978-3-030-56890-0_4

regional average of 5.4% [2]. Ethiopia has implemented successive Health Sector Development Plans (HSDPs) in four phases since 1997. During this period, huge advances have been made in improving access to primary health care services and health outcomes. Ethiopia's health indicators have remarkably improved from one of the worst in Sub-Saharan Africa to among the outstanding performers.

## Brief History of Nephrology in Ethiopia

The first organized renal care facility in Ethiopia was established in 1980 at the Tikur Anbessa Hospital, which is the main teaching hospital of the Addis Ababa University School of Medicine. The service was started with the assistance of a Nephrology team from the Institute of Nephrology, Havana, Cuba. The first hemodialysis (HD) was performed in 1980 and the first peritoneal dialysis (PD) in 1981 in the same unit. The unit provided dialysis for patients with presumed acute kidney injury (AKI) on an on-and-off basis depending on the availability of supplies. It remained the only dialysis providing unit in the country until maintenance HD was started in 2001 in a private hospital in Addis Ababa. Since then, a growing number of dialysis units have cropped up in Addis Ababa and other major cities in the country with all providing only HD. There is as yet no PD service in the country. The first kidney transplant (KT) was done in Ethiopia in September 2015 at the Saint Paul Millenium Medical College (SPMMC), the National Kidney Transplant Center designated by the Federal Ministry of Health [3]. Just over 100 KT, all living-related donor transplants have been done until July 2019.

The first Ethiopian nephrologist returned from training in the United Kingdom in 1982 and took over the Renal Unit at the Tikur Anbessa Hospital, from the Cuban team that started the first dialysis service in the country. The number of nephrologists in Ethiopia remained low until the 2000s when a number of physicians were able to get scholarships from the International Society of Nephrology (ISN). A total of six physicians received training through the ISN. These nephrologists were subsequently instrumental in the expansion of renal services and the launching of two local nephrology fellowship programs. There is not yet a National Society of Nephrology in Ethiopia.

## Renal Diseases in Ethiopia

There are no national data on kidney diseases in Ethiopia based on epidemiological studies or registry data. Hence, the information available is from hospital-based studies from a few urban centers and estimates from international sources. It is generally assumed that kidney diseases, both acute and chronic, are common in Ethiopia given the double burden of diseases of poverty that continue to plague the population and the rising tide of non-communicable diseases (NCD).

## Acute Kidney Injury and Critical Care Nephrology

Hospital-based studies in the 1990s indicated that the main causes of AKI among patients referred to tertiary care were septic abortion, severe malaria, and nephrotoxic medications [4, 5]. In a 4-year-long prospective observational study done between 1989 and 1992 among hospitalized patients in a teaching hospital in the capital Addis Ababa, septic abortion was the leading cause of AKI (52%). Falciparum malaria (21%) and nephrotoxic agents (9%) were the second and third most common causes. In this study, 86% of the patients required dialysis [4]. Another study done in 1990 in the same hospital showed that one-third of the patients with severe *P. falciparum* malaria developed AKI and 38% of them required dialysis [5].

In contrast to the reports from the 1990s, we have observed a significant change in the causes of AKI in the last two decades. A retrospective observational study of 151 patients, who were dialyzed in a teaching hospital in Addis Ababa between 2013 and 2015, demonstrated these changes. In this study, the vast majority of patients with AKI were young, less than 40 years of age, in contrast to the older population with AKI in Western country studies. Hypovolemia, acute glomerulonephritis (GN), and obstetric causes (mainly driven by preeclampsia and puerperal sepsis) were the three major causes of AKI. Malaria contributed to a much lower proportion of causes (7.3%) compared to the observations in the 1990s and septic abortion was a very rare cause of AKI (0.7%). The in-hospital mortality was 29%. This shift in epidemiology is likely to be due to the marked reduction in the incidence of malaria in Ethiopia and changes in the abortion law and practice [6].

Serum creatinine is not universally done among all hospitalized patients in the country, with the exception of a few teaching referral hospitals. This practice might be a result of lack of awareness, clinical inertia, cost, and limited access to the test. Two cross-sectional studies done a few years ago have confirmed this practice [7, 8]. The first study, done in three hospitals in different parts of the country, showed that patients admitted to medical wards are more likely to have their renal function tests checked when compared to those admitted to surgical or obstetrics-gynecology wards. Urine output monitoring was also not routinely done in most medical and surgical wards [7]. The second study, which was done in a single hospital in northwest Ethiopia, indicated that 32% of the patients admitted had no record of renal function measurement during their hospitalization. These data indicate that there are lots of missed opportunities in detecting AKI among hospitalized patients in Ethiopia [8].

Intensive care units (ICU) are being established in most regions of the country but the majority of the hospitals where these units are located do not have any dialysis service. At best, patients in these ICUs may have a very limited access to a dialysis unit in a hospital in a nearby town. Continuous renal replacement therapy (CRRT) is not available in the entire country. For critically ill patients with AKI, intermittent HD with prolonged duration is occasionally used by some practitioners.

## Chronic Kidney Disease

There is a huge information gap regarding chronic kidney disease (CKD) in Ethiopia. There are no population-based studies done on the prevalence, causes, and outcomes of CKD. Nonetheless, population-based surveys on non-communicable diseases and their risk factors indicate that the prevalence of the major risk factors of CKD, i.e., diabetes and hypertension is growing [9].

Using the WHO's STEPwise approach to Surveillance (STEPs), a nationwide, community-based survey was conducted in 2015 among 10,000 respondents aged 15–69 years. In this survey, the prevalence of raised blood pressure as defined by SBP >140 and/or DBP >90 mmHg was 15.6%. Additionally, 6% of the study population had increased blood glucose, as defined by a fasting capillary whole blood glucose level of ≥110 mg/dl or being on treatment for diabetes. The prevalence of diabetes mellitus (FBS >126 mg/dl), including those on medication, was 3.2% (3.5% males and 3.0% females) [9].

An old hospital-based observational study done in 1980 in a referral hospital in Addis Ababa reported the commonest cause of CKD to be chronic glomerulonephritis [10]. A recent cross-sectional study done in the same hospital with 247 CKD patients, in order to assess the management practice of CKD showed that hypertension, diabetes, and ischemic heart disease were present in 91%, 41.6%, and 13.4% respectively. Although this study was not specifically designed to investigate the causes of CKD, the findings indicate that diabetes and hypertension are very common comorbidities, and likely etiologies, among Ethiopian CKD patients [11]. The authors' observations in their regular clinical practice concur with the findings in the above-cited study. Diabetes and hypertension are presumed to be the leading causes of CKD in older adults while CKD of unknown etiology is common in younger adults.

The pre-dialysis care of patients with CKD in Ethiopia mainly constitutes management of proteinuria, high blood pressure, fluid overload, and cardiovascular risk reduction [11]. Treatment of anemia is generally inadequate due to inconsistency in the availability and the high cost of erythropoiesis-stimulating agents and intravenous iron. Oral iron is the most commonly used pharmacologic intervention for anemia. Management of CKD-MBD is also suboptimal due to limited availability of laboratories, which determine serum calcium, phosphorus, and PTH, besides the lack of access to calcium-based phosphate binders outside Addis Ababa. The only non-calcium-based phosphate binder, sevelamer chloride, has been made available in the Ethiopian market only in 2019 and yet its prohibitive costs prevent most patients from using it.

It has been observed that CKD awareness among patients at risk of kidney disease is quite low [12]. However, the authors believe that there is excessive fear among the public regarding kidney diseases. This is believed to be due to the influence of the media. Movies have been made based on stories of poor patients with end-stage renal disease (ESRD). Several calls for contributing money for individuals with ESRD, particularly for famous individuals, have been advertised by the media. As this is the commonest type of message passed through the media and as the diagnosis of ESRD is associated with catastrophic out-of-pocket health care expenditure, it has resulted in excessive fear of kidney disease among the general public. Counseling patients and family members about any kidney disease is, hence, a difficult exercise as it causes a lot of anxiety.

## Other Kidney Diseases

Although glomerular diseases have not been very well characterized by systematically performed studies, they are common in the nephrology practice in the country. Referrals of patients to nephrologists by general practitioners or internists carrying a diagnosis of "clinical rapidly progressive GN", "acute GN", or "GN" are common. Unfortunately, we have not done studies to examine the causes of these glomerular diseases. In the few kidney biopsies we manage to do from time to time, we have seen all kinds of primary glomerular diseases including minimal change disease, focal & segmental glomerulosclerosis, IgA nephropathy, membranous nephropathy, and membranoproliferative GN. Lupus nephritis is a very common secondary glomerular disease that we see in our practice. Although HIV infection is quite common, we do not see the classic HIV-associated nephropathy clinical presentation in our population, i.e., massive proteinuria with big kidneys and normal blood pressure. This might be due to genetic reasons; a study among Ethiopian Jews in Israel has demonstrated the lack of the high-risk APOL1 variants [13].

An old light microcopy series of adult patients with the nephrotic syndrome treated in one hospital in Addis Ababa reported membranoproliferative pathology to be the most common histopathology pattern. Amyloidosis was also reported in a substantial proportion of patients. Nonetheless, this report should be interpreted cautiously as no immunofluorescence or immunohistochemistry studies were done [14].

Urolithiasis is a common problem in Ethiopia. Stone kidney disease requiring urologic intervention accounts for 13.6–22% of the urologic admissions. Many of these patients have established CKD and stone kidney disease appears to contribute substantially to the CKD burden in Ethiopia [15, 16].

### Pediatric Nephrology

Pediatric nephrology services are available in three hospitals in Ethiopia and there are five pediatric nephrologists certified.

### AKI in Pediatrics

In a study in the early 2000s with 30 pediatric patients, post-diarrheal hemolytic uremic syndrome (HUS) diagnosed in 23 children was the leading cause of AKI. The mortality was very high at 46.7% [17].

A prospective, hospital-based study showed an AKI incidence of 12.7/1000. The presence of sepsis, heart failure, and cancer were the major risk factors identified [18].

In a recent retrospective review of the pattern of renal diseases in pediatric patients in Addis Ababa, kidney disease accounted for 3.3% of the 14,521 admissions. The three most common renal diseases observed were congenital anomalies of the kidney and urinary tract (CAKUT) seen in 127 children (26.8%), followed by nephrotic syndrome in 80 children (16.9%) and acute GN in 58 children (12.2%). Other renal diseases observed were urinary tract infection 8.0%, urolithiasis 6.7%, Wilms' tumor 6.3%, AKI 4.2%, and CKD 4.0%. Other less frequently detected diseases were bladder exstrophy, lupus nephritis, Henoch Schönlein purpura nephritis, and prune belly syndrome [19].

## Renal Replacement Therapy in Ethiopia

### Hemodialysis

HD has been available to a very small number of patients with ESRD in a few urban centers in the country for the last 20 years or so. There are about 800 patients on maintenance HD, spread across 25 small centers in the country. This makes the rate of HD at 7 per million population (pmp). Most of the centers are private facilities with a few government facilities providing the services. Patients pay out of pocket for the services as there are no insurance schemes or government funding that cover the costs of dialysis. The average cost of HD per session is 65 USD and that does not include the cost of medications.

The majority of the centers cater for patients with ESRD, with only a few providing dialysis for patients with AKI. The dialysis centers, in the few public hospitals where dialysis is available, provide dialysis for patients with presumed AKI at a very subsidized rate or free of charge depending on the patient's income. There are no use of convective therapies in Ethiopia.

### Peritoneal Dialysis

There are no patients with ESRD on PD in Ethiopia. PD has been used for the management of patients with AKI, particularly children in the distant past and also recently at the Tikur Anbessa Hospital. The Saving Young Lives (SYL) initiative of the International Society of Nephrology (ISN) provided supplies and PD training during a few years. Services could not be maintained as there is no consistent supply of consumables.

### Renal Transplantation

With the increasing burden of ESRD and public pressure, the government of Ethiopia decided to pilot a living donor kidney transplantation (KT) program in 2013 and selected Saint Paul's Hospital Millennium Medical College (SPMMC) in Addis Ababa for the implementation of the project. The University of Michigan from the United States of America became the external partner for the project. The project was started with the understanding that transplantation is a better and cheaper option for the management of ESRD. The project aimed to provide KT as a first option for the management of patients age 14 and above with ESRD, having hemodialysis as a bridge for transplantation. The collaboration with the University of Michigan was designed to build local competence in performing KT. After painstaking planning and preparation, the first-ever KT in Ethiopia was performed in September 2015. From September 2015 until July 2019, a total of 118 living-related KT have been performed. The 1-year graft and patient survival are 96% and 98%, respectively, while overall outcome to date is 92% graft and 95% patient survival. The standard immunosuppressive protocol used is a combination of tacrolimus, mycophenolate mofetil, and steroids after induction with basiliximab or antithymocyte globulin depending on the immunologic risk assessment [3].

The center is able to do basic laboratory tests, drug levels, and has a renal pathology service that can process and interpret transplant biopsies. However, neither the center itself nor other labs in the country have the capacity to do HLA typing and crossmatch. Samples are, therefore, sent abroad for these tests. The center has succeeded in training transplant surgeons and supports the training of nephrologists, and has therefore reached self-sufficiency in terms of manpower.

The legal framework governing organ transplantation was established in January 2014 with the Federal Ministry of Health as the authority to prepare directives for organ transplantation. The current directive restricts donations among individuals related by blood or marriage and an independent national organ transplant committee approves each recipient–donor pair before surgery. To date, the government covers all the cost of pre-transplant evaluation, transplant surgery, and perioperative care while transplant patients must be able to pay for immunosuppressive medications that are provided to them at subsidized cost. All the immunosuppressive drugs available are generic medications. The social workers of the hospital provide help to needy patients by finding sponsors to assist the patients meet the cost of medications.

The transplant project is faced with several challenges, the most important of which are the precarious continuity of supplies and the underdeveloped infrastructure. Shortage of kidney donors is another major challenge as the regulations restrict donors to members of the family. The program is unable to offer transplant to sensitized patients and blood group incompatible pairs because of limited facilities and experience. To alleviate the shortage of donors, the option of paired kidney donations is being considered and the possibility of developing a deceased donor program is being explored.

Because the national transplant center cannot care for all patients who need KT, many patients still travel abroad with their donors for KT. There are currently an estimated 350 KT recipients nationwide.

## Nephrology Practice in Ethiopia

Although big strides have been made in the provision of renal care in Ethiopia in the last few decades, there is no comprehensive national renal care program in Ethiopia and the service is provided in a policy vacuum and with no national financing plan in place.

There are 26 nephrologists in Ethiopia, including five pediatric nephrologists; and only five nephrologists work outside Addis Ababa, the capital city. There are two nephrology fellowship programs and one KT fellowship program in place. Most nurses in the dialysis units are not certified dialysis nurses, as there are no formal training programs in the country. Most of them get a few weeks of hands-on training during employment by those who have had some experience. Diagnostic services are quite limited including renal pathology, but recently a renal pathology service has been established at the SPMMC.

The few private hospitals and clinics with dialysis units as well as the stand-alone dialysis centers employ nephrologists on a part-time basis. Some dialysis units have no nephrologist to supervise and direct patient care. In those centers where there are no nephrologists, internists or general medical practitioners supervise. Full-time employment for nephrologists is available in public and, particularly, in teaching hospitals but not in the private sector. The average salary, in the public hospitals, for a nephrologist is 5500 USD per year. Due to the high living expenses almost all nephrologists work part-time in the private sector. The average salary for a dialysis nurse is 3100 USD per year. There are no dialysis provider companies operating dialysis units or group practices by nephrologists in Ethiopia, as is common in the developed countries. There is a market for experienced/trained dialysis nurses and technicians as such professionals are generally difficult to find.

## Highlight of Nephrology in Ethiopia

The successful transplant project in Ethiopia that was a result of a collaborative effort between the SPMMC and the University of Michigan is an exemplary collaborative model that can be replicated in other developing countries. In a time span of just about 6 years, the collaboration made it possible to transplant over a hundred patients, to develop local workforce to do transplants, and to provide general nephrology service.

## Future Perspectives of Nephrology in Ethiopia

Renal care is very likely to grow rapidly in Ethiopia given the increasing burden of kidney disease, the public demand for services, and the government's increasing attention to NCD. There is already an NCD policy expected to be implemented through programs that address NCDs in general as well as programs specific to each NCD. The Ministry of Health's determination to start a KT center and maintain it as well as its efforts to expand dialysis services is a testimony to the government's commitment. This, of course, should be directed by a well thought out comprehensive renal care policy and program as well as a financing strategy. The private (for-profit sector) has been in the lead in the provision of dialysis services and in the years and decades to come, it is likely to continue as a major provider in the big urban areas.

Regarding the development of human resources for health care, there are already two nephrology fellowship training programs and the number of nephrologists is going to increase. There are also efforts underway to form the Ethiopian Society of Nephrology and this may become a reality very soon.

## Conclusion

Although information on kidney disease which is based on well-designed studies or registry data is lacking in Ethiopia, kidney diseases of all types are common. There is a growing prevalence of NCD that are risk factors for CKD and so the incidence of CKD is expected to rise. The services available for patients with kidney disease are far from optimal but there is a significant improvement in the provision of services in the last two decades. This includes the establishment of a national KT program.

## References

1. United Nations, Department of Economic and Social Affairs, Population Division. World Population Prospects 2019, Volume II: demographic profiles (ST/ESA/SER.A/427). https://population.un.org/wpp/. Accessed 19 Jan 2020.
2. The World Bank in Ethiopia. https://www.worldbank.org/en/country/ethiopia. Accessed 18 Jan 2020.
3. Ahmed MM, Tedla FM, Leichtman AB, Punch JD. Organ transplantation in Ethiopia. Transplantation. 2019;103(3):449–51.
4. Zewdu W. Acute renal failure in Addis Ababa, Ethiopia: a prospective study of 136 patients. Ethiop Med J. 1994;32(2):79–87.
5. Habte B. Acute renal failure due to falciparum malaria. Ren Fail. 1990;12(1):15–9.
6. Ibrahim A, Ahmed MM, Kedir S, et al. Clinical profile and outcome of patients with acute kidney injury requiring dialysis—an experience from a haemodialysis unit in a developing country. BMC Nephrol. 2016;17:91. https://doi.org/10.1186/s12882-016-0313-8.
7. Phillips L, Allen N, Phillips B, Abera A, Diro E, Riley S, Tadesse Y, Williams J, Phillips A. Acute kidney injury risk factor recognition in three teaching hospitals in Ethiopia. S Afr Med J. 2013;103(6):413–7.
8. Riley S, Diro E, Batchelor P, Abebe A, Amsalu A, Tadesse Y, Williams J, Phillips AO. Renal impairment among acute hospital admissions in a rural Ethiopian hospital. Nephrology. 2013;18:92–6.
9. Gebreyes YF, Goshu DY, Geletew TK, Argefa TG, Zemedu TG, Lemu KA, et al. Prevalence of high blood pressure, hyperglycemia, dyslipidemia, metabolic syndrome and their determinants in Ethiopia: evidences from the National NCDs STEPS Survey. PLoS One. 2018; https://doi.org/10.1371/journal.pone.0194819.
10. Habte B, Teklu B. Chronic renal failure in Ethiopians. Ethiop Med J. 1980;18(2):37–44.
11. Kefale B, Tadesse Y, Alebachew M, Engidawork E. Management practice, and adherence and its contributing factors among patients with chronic kidney disease at Tikur Anbessa Specialized Hospital: a hospital-based cross-sectional study. PLoS One. 2018; https://doi.org/10.1371/journal.pone.0200415.
12. Goro KK, Wolide AD, Dibaba FK, Fufa FG, Garedow AW, Tufa BE, Bobasa EM. Patient awareness, prevalence, and risk factors of chronic kidney disease among diabetes mellitus and hypertensive patients at Jimma University Medical Center, Ethiopia. BioMed Research International. 2019. https://doi.org/10.1155/2019/2383508.
13. Behar DM, Kedem E, Rosset S, Haileselassie Y, Tzur S, Kra-Oz Z, Wasser W, Shenhar Y, Shahar E, Hassoun G, Maor C, Wolday D, Pollack S, Skorecki K. Absence of APOL1 risk variants protects against HIV-associated nephropathy in the Ethiopian population. Am J Nephrol. 2011;34:452–9.
14. Guerra JP, Landells JW, Mengistu M. Nephrotic syndrome in adult Ethiopians. Ethiop Med J. 1982;20(3):125–30.
15. Andualem D, Gidena G. Admission patterns and management of urolithiasis: a hospital based study in Tikur Anbessa Specialized Hospital (TASH), Addis Ababa, Ethiopia. East Cent Afr J Surg. 2014;19(3):29–34.
16. Alemu MH. Pattern of urinary tract stone diseases in Mekelle, Ethiopia. Ethiop Med J. 2008;46(3):237–41.
17. Shimelis D, Tadesse Y. Clinical profile of acute renal failure in the Department of Pediatrics, Tikur Anbessa Hospital. Ethiop Med J. 2004;42:17–22.
18. Shimelis D, Abebe B, Deyessa N. Incidence of acute kidney injury and determinant factors in children admitted to a tertiary hospital. IOSR J Dent Med Sci (IOSR-JDMS). 2018;17(3):48–53.
19. Mola K, Shimelis D. Pattern and outcome of renal diseases in hospitalized children in Tikur Anbessa Specialized Teaching Hospital, Addis Ababa, Ethiopia. Ethiop Med J. 2016;54(3):117–23.

# Nephrology in Nigeria

**5**

Fatiu Abiola Arogundade, Christopher I. Esezobor, Henrietta Uchenna Okafor, Aliyu Abdu, Rasheed Abiodun Balogun, Emmanuel Edet Effa, Joyce Popoola, and Ebun Ladipo Bamgboye

| | |
|---|---|
| Area[1] | 923,768 $Km^2$ |
| Population[1] | 203.5 million (2018) |
| Capital | Abuja |
| Three most populated cities[1] | 1. Lagos (13.5 million)<br>2.Kano (3.8 million)<br>3.Ibadan (3.4 million) |
| Official language[1] | English |
| Gross Domestic Product (GDP)[2] | 375.8 billion USD (2017) |
| GDP per capita[2] | 1968.6 USD (2017) |
| Human Development Index (HDI)[3] | 0.532 (2017) |
| Official currency | Naira |
| Total number of nephrologists | 188 |
| National society of nephrology | Nephrology Association of Nigeria (NAN) |
| Incidence of end-stage renal disease | 2018 – not available |
| Prevalence of end-stage renal disease | 2018 – ~15 pmp |
| Total number of patients on dialysis (all modalities) | 2017 – ~2000<br>2018 – ~3000 |
| Number of patients on haemodialysis | 2017 – ~2000<br>2018 – ~3000 |
| Number of patients on peritoneal dialysis | 2017 – <10<br>2018 – <10 |
| Number of renal transplantations per year | 2017 – 117<br>2018 – 142 |

General information on Nigeria

1. CIA. The World Factbook: Nigeria2019 June 2019. Available from: https://www.cia.gov/library/publications/the-world-factbook/attachments/summaries/NI-summary.pdf
2. WorldBank. Country Profile: Nigeria2018 June 2019. Available from: https://data.worldbank.org/country/nigeria
3. UNDP. Human Development Indices and Indicators: 2018 Statistical Update7th May 2019. Available from: http://hdr.undp.org/en/data#

## Introduction

Nigeria is situated in the West African sub-region with a total area of 923,768 $Km^2$ and a current population of 203.5 million, making it the 32nd largest but the 7th most populous country in the world [1]. It is believed that one out of every five Black people in the world is a Nigerian. Nigeria is the most populous country in Africa and has the largest economy in the continent [2]. The economy is diverse but the largest revenue earner for the country is crude oil with the 10th largest reserves of crude oil in the world. The federal capital was moved to Abuja in 1984 from the coastal city of Lagos; however, Lagos remains the financial capital and the most populous city in the country.

Even though a democracy since its independence from Britain 59 years ago, Nigeria was bedevilled with a civil war and multiple military insurgences and regional conflicts for the first 39 years after its independence from the UK. This is partly responsible for the emigration of many of its professionals to many parts of the western world and the Middle East, such that there are possibly more nephrologists practicing outside the country than there are currently practicing in the country. Fortunately, however, it has had more than 20 consistent years of democracy to date and it is hoped that this will lead to sustained economic growth and development.

F. A. Arogundade
Department of Medicine, Obafemi Awolowo University/Teaching Hospitals Complex, Ile-Ife, Osun State, Nigeria

C. I. Esezobor
Department of Paediatrics, College of Medicine University of Lagos, Lagos, Lagos, Nigeria

H. U. Okafor
Department of Paediatrics, University of Nigeria Teaching Hospital, Enugu, Enugu, Nigeria

A. Abdu
Department of Medicine, Aminu Kano Teaching Hospital/Bayero University, Kano, Nigeria

R. A. Balogun
Division of Nephrology, Department of Medicine, University of Virginia, Charlottesville, VA, USA

E. E. Effa
Department of Internal Medicine, University of Calabar, Calabar, Cross River state, Nigeria

J. Popoola
Department of Renal Medicine and Transplantation, St George's University Hospitals NHS Foundation Trust, London, UK

E. L. Bamgboye (✉)
St. Nicholas Hospital, Lagos Island, Lagos State, Nigeria
e-mail: ebamgboye@saintnicholashospital.com


J. A. Moura-Neto et al. (eds.), *Nephrology Worldwide*, https://doi.org/10.1007/978-3-030-56890-0_5

The population growth rate is 2.6%. The population is young with 42.5% and 3.3% of the country younger than 15 years and >65 years, respectively [1]. About 60.9% of this population are adjudged as being below the poverty line, although there is a marked disparity with its distribution around the country. While in the southwestern part of the country only 20% of the populations live below this poverty line, in some states in the northern part of the country, over 80% of the citizens live below the poverty line [3]. This skewed wealth distribution is also reflected in the distribution of Nephrology capacity around the country. While the southwest part of the country has as many as 62 dialysis units, the Northeast consisting of 6 states and a population of 19 million (by 2006 census) has only 10 dialysis units (Figs. 5.1 and 5.2). Regardless of the geopolitical zone, none of these units are located in the rural areas where 49.7% of the population resides.

The disease pattern is reflective of a developing economy and features a double burden of both communicable and non-communicable diseases. While still battling with the scourge of malaria, tuberculosis and HIV, there is a rising prevalence of hypertension (now 28.9% of the adult population) and type 2 diabetes mellitus [4, 5]. These reflect strongly on the prevalence and aetiology of kidney diseases in the country. In addition, 20–30% of the population carry the sickle cell gene and 23–28% have the high-risk APOL1 genotype – two recognised genetic markers of non-diabetic chronic kidney disease [6–8].

Despite this double burden of disease, the allocation to health in the national budget is just 3.7% of the GDP. In addition, less than 5% of the population is covered by the National Health Insurance Scheme [9]. Consequently, most of the spending on health by individuals is out of pocket and, with the prevailing poverty index in the country, many resort to alternative health practitioners, faith healers, herbalists and complementary medicines in the pursuit of cures for their various ailments [10]. This partly explains why the number of patients with CKD receiving standard care is low and very few patients initiating dialysis are able to sustain long-term care (Table 5.1).

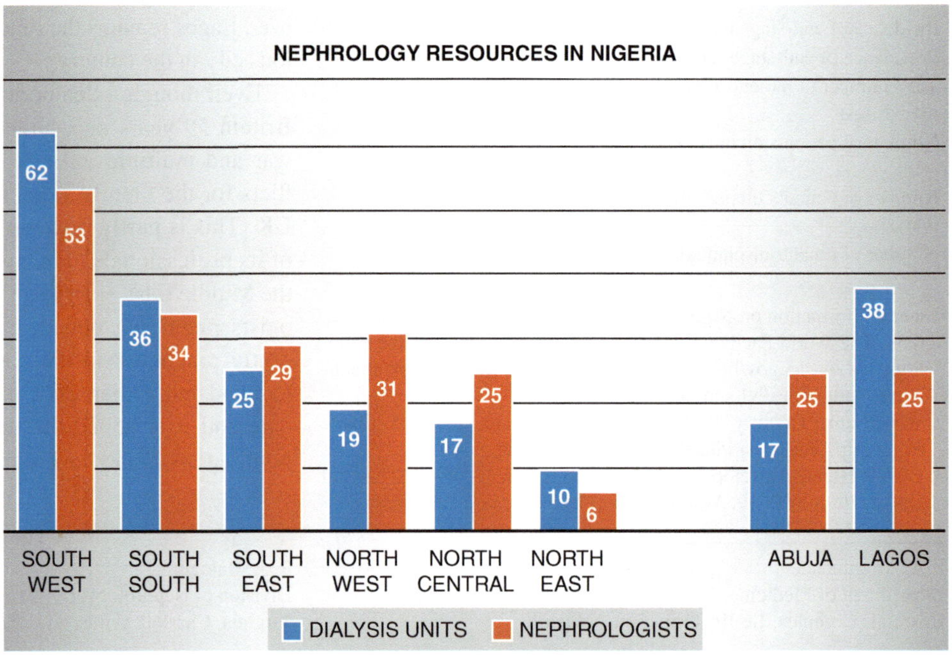


**Fig. 5.1** Distribution of haemodialysis units and nephrologists in Nigeria

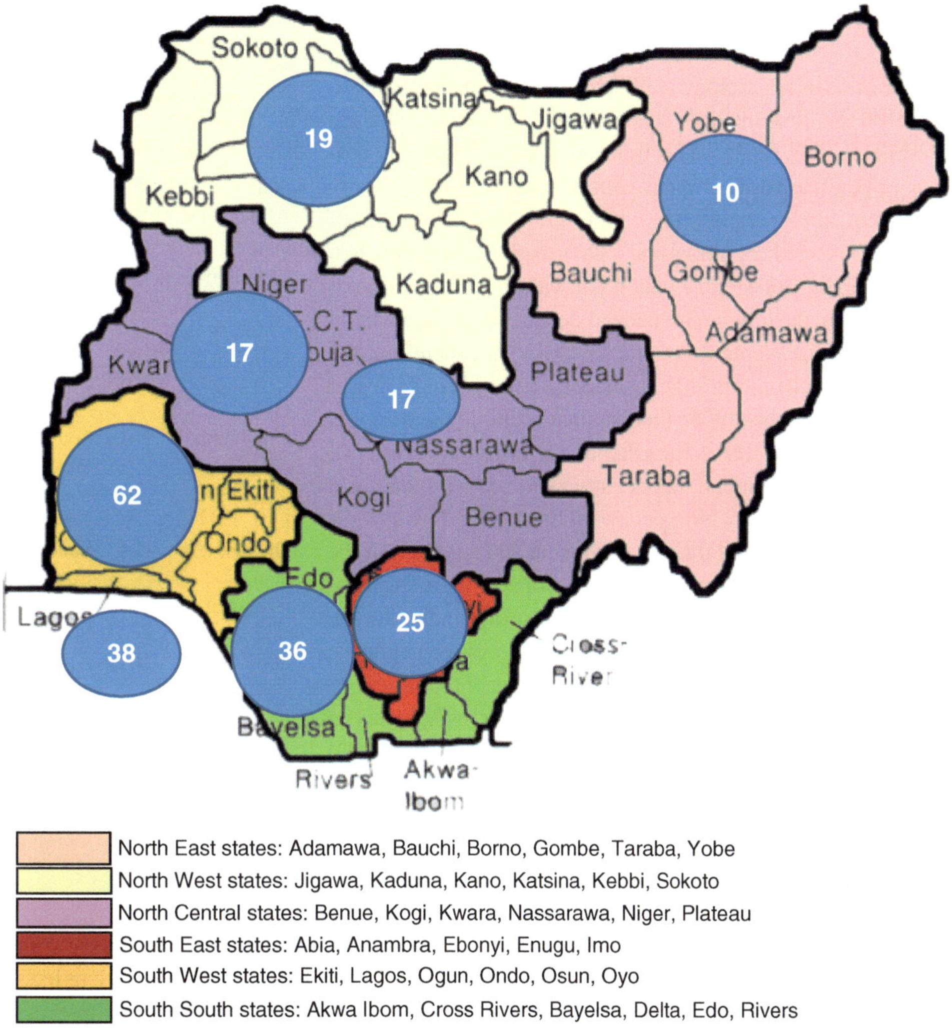


**Fig. 5.2** Map of Nigeria with the numbers of dialysis centres in each of the six geopolitical zones, Lagos and Abuja

North East states: Adamawa, Bauchi, Borno, Gombe, Taraba, Yobe

North West states: Jigawa, Kaduna, Kano, Katsina, Kebbi, Sokoto

North Central states: Benue, Kogi, Kwara, Nassarawa, Niger, Plateau

South East states: Abia, Anambra, Ebonyi, Enugu, Imo

South West states: Ekiti, Lagos, Ogun, Ondo, Osun, Oyo

South South states: Akwa Ibom, Cross Rivers, Bayelsa, Delta, Edo, Rivers

**Table 5.1** Analysis of publications on haemodialysis treatments for ESRD in Nigeria

| Author | Year | Region | Number studied | Number that could not afford HD | Duration of haemodialysis | | | |
|---|---|---|---|---|---|---|---|---|
| | | | | | <1 Month | 1–<3 Months | 3–12 Months | >12 Months |
| Arije et al. [28] | 2008 | South West | 158 | 14 (8.9%) | 112 (70.8%) | 0 | 29 (18.4%) | 3 (1.9%) |
| Ulasi et al. [27] | 2010 | South East | 1538 | 624 (40.6%) | 715 (46.5%) | 116 (7.5%) | 63 (4.1%) | 15 (1.0%) |
| Arogundade et al. [26] | 2011 | South West | 760 | 188 (24.7%) | 503 (66.2%) | 40 (5.3%) | 28 (3.7%) | 0 (0.0%) |
| Alebiosu et al. [31] | 2006 | South West | 180 | 146 (81.1%) | 34 (18.8%) | 0 | 0 | 0 |
| Oluyombo et al. [44] | 2014 | South West | 150 | NA | 111 (73.8%) | 29 (19.4%) | 10 (6.8%) | 0 |
| Total prevalence | | All region | 2786 | 972 (34.9%) | 1475 (52.9%) | 205 (7.4%) | 110 (3.9%) | 18 (0.6%) |

*NA* not available. This study focused on only those who received a session of haemodialysis

## History of Nephrology in Nigeria

The practice of nephrology in Nigeria began with the establishment of the first medical school in the University College Hospital (UCH), Ibadan. This was one of the first teaching hospitals in the British Commonwealth and was at a time designated the 4th best hospital within the Commonwealth of Nations. The medical school was established first as a branch of the University College of London but with the inauguration of UCH Ibadan, the training of medical doctors took place wholly in Nigeria. The Nephrology unit in UCH was, therefore, the first-ever of such units in Nigeria under the headship of Professor Oladipo Akinkugbe, the first indigenous nephrologist who was trained in the UK. He is regarded as the doyen and father of nephrology in Nigeria and was recently awarded the International Society of Nephrology pioneers award for Africa.

The unit carried out the first peritoneal dialysis (PD) in the country in 1965 and along with other pioneers in the hospital published seminal works on tropical nephrology including the role of *Plasmodium malariae* in the aetiology of the nephrotic syndrome – the so-called quartan malaria nephropathy [11–13]. Ever since, several other units have been established in different parts of the country. The first haemodialysis (HD) unit in the country was established at the Lagos University Teaching Hospital in Lagos, under Professors Mabadeje and Odutola. This unit spurred on and helped with training staff for the over 180 other different dialysis units now in existent in different parts of the country. The first private dialysis unit was established in 1987 by Dr Okey Onuzo in Lagos. Renal transplantation was first carried out successfully at St Nicholas hospital in Lagos in March 2000. This unit remains the most active renal transplantation centre, but has been joined by 14 other centres in different parts of the country.

The distribution of the dialysis and transplant units based on the six geopolitical zones in the country is outlined in Fig. 5.1. Although most of the units are in public hospitals, the most active ones are in private hospitals. Unfortunately, however, these units are restricted to the urban parts of the country where there is a concentration of personnel to run these units.

There has been a rapid increase in the numbers of nephrologists, dialysis nurses and technologists trained to run these units since the commencement of postgraduate training in Nigeria by the National Postgraduate Medical College of Nigeria in 1969 and the West African Postgraduate Medical College in 1976.

## Renal Diseases in Nigeria

Kidney diseases are now very common and their prevalence has now assumed epidemic proportions globally. Though the true prevalence figure of end-stage renal disease (ESRD) in Nigeria is unknown, it is assumed to be high. However, several community and hospital studies have reported rates from 7.8% to 23.5% and an increase of 300% in the prevalence of CKD in the last three decades [14–26]. Awobusuyi et al. [23], in the largest community study involving ten urban communities in ten state capitals distributed among all the six geopolitical zones of the country, found a CKD crude prevalence of 23.47% (1896 out of 8077 participants). An analysis of all the available publications on prevalence of CKD from all geopolitical zones of Nigeria revealed that 20.4% of 14,253 screened participants had overt or covert CKD (Table 5.2). Advanced CKD and ESRD are also recognised to be quite common constituting about 8–23% of medical admissions in different tertiary hospitals [26, 27].

**Table 5.2** An analysis of population studies on prevalence chronic kidney disease (CKD) in Nigeria

| Author | Year | Region of Nigeria | Number studied | Number with kidney damage or CKD (*n*) | Prevalence of kidney damage or CKD (%) |
|---|---|---|---|---|---|
| Afolabi et al. [15] | 2009 | South West | 250 | 26 | 10.4 |
| Oluyombo et al. [3] | 2009 | South West | 454 | 56 | 12.3 |
| Okoye et al. [17] | 2009 | South South | 520 | 126 | 24.3 |
| Ulasi et al. [18] | 2013 | South East | 1941 | 221 | 11.4 |
| Oluyombo et al. [16] | 2013 | South West | 1084 | 154 | 14.2 |
| Abene et al. [20] | 2017 | North Central | 510 | 128 | 25 |
| Okwuonu et al. [21] | 2017 | South East | 328 | 44 | 13.4 |
| Egbi et al. [22] | 2014 | South South | 179 | 14 | 7.8 |
| Awobusuyi et al. [23] | 2015 | All six regions | 8077 | 1896 | 23.47 |
| Nalado et al. [24] | 2016 | North West | 454 | 117 | 26 |
| Oyebisi et al. [25] | 2018 | South West | 456 | 126 | 27.6 |
| Total prevalence | | All six regions | 14,253 | 2916 | 20.4 |

CKD is mainly a disease of the young and middle-aged (20–50 years) in Nigeria and this compares favourably with what is reported in other developing countries in Africa; however, it is in sharp contrast with the older age groups seen in the developed world [14, 26, 27]. A large proportion of CKD patients are males who are in the most economically productive age group [14, 26, 27]. The causes of CKD in Nigeria, though similar to what have been reported from different countries in sub-Saharan Africa, differ remarkably from that in the developed world [14, 26–28]. Hypertension and glomerulonephritis remain the most common causes of CKD with diabetic nephropathy being a distant third, though with the rising prevalence of diabetes mellitus, this is expected to increase [5, 26, 27, 29]. The traditional infectious causes of CKD still abound and HIV-associated nephropathy (HIVAN) remains a major contributor to the CKD burden [14, 26, 30]. Other important causes include obstructive uropathy, sickle cell nephropathy and chronic tubulointerstitial nephritis [27, 31].

The outcome of ESRD in Nigeria remains gloomy as majority of our patients cannot afford renal replacement therapy (RRT) and are thus placed on conservative management. Even those that are able to start RRT are unable to sustain RRT beyond a few sessions. Mortality is thus very high among patients presenting with ESRD with majority dying within the first year of presentation. This poor outlook has been attributed to a number of additional reasons including late presentation to healthcare facilities, associated co-morbidities, limited capacity for RRT, the exorbitant cost of managing patients, limited capacity of health workers particularly non-nephrologists in kidney disease prevention, and poor awareness of kidney disease as well as poor health-seeking attitude in the community [14, 26–28].

Acute kidney injury (AKI) in adults occurs mainly from prerenal and intrinsic renal causes and is principally community-acquired. The incidence established as a percentage of medical admissions is 3–5%, though figures as high as 19–24% of AKI have been reported following intensive care and surgical admissions (Table 5.3) [32–42]. The principal causes are gastroenteritis whether cholera related or not, nephrotoxins, sepsis from various infections, glomerulonephritis, malaria especially in non-immune visitors, obstructive uropathy in the elderly and drugs including radiocontrast agents. Pregnancy-related causes also abound and these include septic abortion, ante or postpartum haemorrhage and eclampsia among others [32–36, 38–41]. RRT modalities used in the management of AKI in Nigeria include acute or intermittent PD and acute HD. Continuous therapies are generally unavailable but are gradually being introduced in the last 5–10 years. Overall mortality varies remarkably between centres (18–45%) with differing patient populations but on the average hovers around 36% [32–36, 38–41].

**Table 5.3** Studies on acute kidney injury (AKI) in adult patients in Nigeria

| Author | Year | Region of the country | Number studied | Mortality (%) |
|---|---|---|---|---|
| Kadiri et al. [32] | 1992 | South West | 40 | 25 |
| Bamgboye et al. [33] | 1993 | South West | 175 | 39.4 |
| Arogundade et al. [34] | 2007 | South West | 58 | 43.5 |
| Emem Chioma et al. [35] | 2012 | South South | 62 | 43.5 |
| Okunola et al. [36] | 2012 | South West | 80 | 28.8 |
| Oluseyi et al. [37] | 2016 | South West | 91 | 38.5 |
| Makusidi et al. [38] | 2016 | North West | 38 | 45 |
| Bello et al. [39] | 2017 | South West | 54 | 29.8 |
| Awowole et al. [40] | 2018 | South West | 43 | 18 |
| Total | | | 641 | 35.9% |

## Haemodialysis in Nigeria

HD was first used in the management of ESRD at the Lagos University Teaching Hospital in 1981. Subsequently, the number of HD centres has grown remarkably and now stands at about 186 in the entire country (Figs. 5.1 and 5.2). It is the most commonly prescribed modality of RRT. Most of the patients (60–90%) are commenced on HD with very few patients (<1%) being initiated on PD and only about 1–2% being offered kidney transplantation [26, 27, 43]. The majority of ESRD patients are first offered HD, usually as an emergency lifesaving procedure, because many of them present with severe complications even at first visit. It is estimated that there are currently about 3000 patients accessing HD services yearly across the 186 units spanning the country. Many of these are, however, unable to sustain HD beyond a few sessions particularly in most of the public hospital run centres.

A review of HD publications use in the management of ESRD revealed that about 38.6% of the patients were unable to pay for any session of dialysis while 53.2% could only support it for less than 1 month. Only 0.6% of our ESRD patients are able to support the treatment for longer than 1 year (Table 5.3) [26–28, 31, 44, 45]. National Health Insurance Scheme (NHIS) now covers dialysis care for AKI, offering six sessions to enrollees with no support for chronic dialysis or transplantation. In addition, the relatively exorbitant cost of HD (about 100–200 US dollars per session) leads to withdrawal from dialysis care and eventual uremia and death. Even for those patients who are able to commence dialysis, adequacy is another major challenge as some may opt for once- or twice-weekly session on account of financial constraints. An audit of RRT in five public dialysis units in Lagos metropolis revealed financial constraints, 30.9% dialyse twice weekly, 43.6% once weekly even though the standard prescription is 4-hour sessions thrice weekly. This is at variance with the experience at St Nicholas hospital, a privately run unit, where 87% of the patients adhered to a twice-weekly scheduling, 10% to a thrice-weekly scheduling and just 3% to a once-weekly scheduling, a reflection of the different mix of patients seen in the unit differs from those in the publicly run units. This differential is also reflected in the various access routes employed by patients in these public units where 10% had AV fistulae as access, 81.8% temporary femoral catheters and just 7.3% long-term internal jugular catheters, as opposed to the SNH private unit where 10% had AV fistulae, 2% temporary catheters and 88% long-term internal jugular catheters in place. These statistics also consequently reflect on the outcomes of the patients managed in the public and private settings. While mortality is high in many of the public dialysis units with mortality at 1 year characteristically being in excess of 70% in contra-distinction to the mortality at the SNH unit which is just 5.3% in 1 year. This unit has a patient who has been on dialysis for over 20 years (as he has declined a kidney transplant being a Jehovah's witness) along with 5.3% others on maintenance HD for more than 5 years. This is likely replicated in many of the units all around the country, but more likely in the privately run units that are more likely to manage patients with the capacity to sustain the costs involved.

Reuse of dialysers is not common but a few of the public units recycle patient-specific dialysers for up to five times in an attempt to limit costs. There is no applied ratio of nurses to HD patients but units generally have one nurse to 2–4 patients. Haemodiafiltration/haemofiltration are available in a few units particularly the privately run units but costs of running these limit their usage.

Incidence of the various viral infections, routinely screened for, varies but at the SNH unit in the year 2018 this was: HIV 4%, HCV 2.6% and HBsAg 2.6%. All units screen patients at presentation and most would repeat the screens after every 6 months if the patient remains on HD. Most units isolate viral positive patients when they are accepted for HD.

Erythropoietin-stimulating agents are generally available as are all other drugs used routinely in the care of patients with ESRD on dialysis. These are however often beyond the capacity of the patients to access them routinely as they often have to pay for these out-of-pocket. Consequently, uncontrolled hypertension, anaemia and poor control of mineral and bone disorder are not infrequent among these patients, contributing to the poor outcomes often encountered in these patients.

There are currently no Government regulations for the sector but the Nephrology Association of Nigeria (NAN) has developed guidelines, which are followed by its members staffing the various dialysis units.

## Peritoneal Dialysis in Adult Nigerians

PD has been employed in the management of renal failure in Nigeria since 1967, when it was first used in patients with AKI secondary to post-abort sepsis [11]. Since then, several reports on the use of acute and intermittent PD in the country have been published [46, 47]. However, continuous ambulatory peritoneal dialysis (CAPD) is used infrequently [48].

Fewer than ten renal centres offer PD mainly in the form of acute or intermittent PD; none of them perform automated PD (APD). Only one centre performed CAPD but stopped because of daunting challenges, which included irregular supply of PD fluids and catheters and the exorbitant cost of these consumables; these consumables are not manufactured locally. In one earlier publication, PD consumables were a major challenge and frequently improvised [48]. Expectedly, peritonitis was a major setback and complicated 60–65% of acute PD [48, 49]. Several centres still practice acute PD, particularly in the management of AKI in adults and children, though it is more commonly used in the paediatric population [46, 47, 49]. In summary, PD practice is still largely suboptimal in Nigeria with CAPD being very irregular and APD virtually unavailable; there are thus less than ten patients on CAPD or APD in the whole country. If, however, the forementioned challenges are surmounted, CAPD would contribute to the capacity to manage ESRD patients in the country.

## Kidney Transplantation in Nigeria

Kidney transplantation became available in the country since 2000, first at St. Nicholas Hospital, a private facility in Lagos, and subsequently in two public facilities in 2002 [50]. Thereafter, 11 more facilities have been established (Table 5.4). By December 2018, about 550 patients have been transplanted within Nigeria with over 80% performed

**Table 5.4** List of kdney transplant centres and dates of commencement of transplant activity in Nigeria

| S/No | Name of hospital | Region | Commencement date (year) |
|---|---|---|---|
| 1 | St Nicholas Hospital, Lagos | South West | 2000 |
| 2 | Aminu Kano Teaching hospital, Kano | North West | 2002 |
| 3 | Obafemi Awolowo University Teaching hospital, Ile Ife | South West | 2002 |
| 4 | Garki Hospital, Abuja | North Central | 2010 |
| 5 | Lagos University Teaching Hospital, Lagos | South West | 2010 |
| 6 | University of Maiduguri Teaching Hospital, Maiduguri | North East | 2010 |
| 7 | University College Hospital, Ibadan | South West | 2011 |
| 8 | University of Ilorin Teaching Hospital, Ilorin | North Central | 2011 |
| 9 | View Point Hospital, Abuja | North Central | 2012 |
| 10 | Delta State University Teaching Hospital, Oghara | South South | 2012 |
| 11 | Lagos State University Teaching Hospital | South West | 2015 |
| 12 | Zenith Medical and Kidney Centre Abuja | North Central | 2015 |
| 13 | Babcock University, Ilishan Ogun State | South West | 2017 |
| 14 | Federal Medical Centre Umuahia, Abia State | South East | 2017 |

in two private-funded centres. Logistics, bureaucratic and funding challenges have impeded the development of the services in public-funded health institutions. Despite the availability of this service in Nigeria, quite a number of patients still travel abroad for transplantation [50, 51]. The total number of kidney transplants performed in Nigeria in all the units in 2017 was 117 and in 2018 142. All of these were living-related transplants and almost all were carried out by the two private units located in Lagos and Abuja.

Kidney transplantation in Nigeria received legal backing in 2014 by an act of the National Assembly [50]. This provided a legal framework for transplantation activities in Nigeria, although its implementation has been rather sporadic and inadequate. For example, only living donor kidney transplantation is available in the country, at the moment [50]. The majority of the organs are donated by genetically related individuals with a few from emotionally related persons. Kidney donation is usually reviewed by an independent committee, which provides ethical guidance. Pre-transplant investigations are mainly done within the centres, but there is limited availability of HLA typing and crossmatch services with only one centre, the Obafemi Awolowo University Teaching Hospital Complex, currently providing this service [52]. None provides flow cytometry crossmatch and testing for donor-specific antibodies. As a result, most centres still send their samples abroad with its attendant delays and increased cost of service.

Maintenance immunosuppressants are available and the majority of patients are on calcineurin inhibitor-based triple therapies. However, cost considerations limit the options available to patients with several patients opting for azathioprine rather than mycophenolate mofetil, for instance. Also, induction regimen is guided by HLA match and affordability. Measurement of drug levels for the calcineurin inhibitors is only available in a few centres. However, post-transplantation follow-up is available in many centres in Nigeria as there are nephrologists with locally and internationally acquired experience caring for kidney transplant patients. Although there is no countrywide transplant registry available, one publication that reviewed data from the various centres reported a 1-year graft and patient survival of 83.2% and 90.2%, respectively [53]. The 5-year graft and patient survival were 58.7% and 73.4% respectively. Post-transplant complications reported include acute rejection episodes, chronic allograft nephropathy, CMV infection, and malignancies especially Kaposi's sarcoma.

## Challenges of Renal Replacement Therapy

The challenges of RRT are mainly those of availability, affordability and accessibility, which are closely linked with the myriads of problems prevalent in a region bedevilled by widespread poverty, ineffective public policies, high unemployment, poor planning and mismanagement of available resources [54].

Funding remains a major challenge as most patients have to provide the cost of RRT from out of pocket in a country where the cost of a session of HD (which is 100–200 USD) is higher than the minimum wage of even the gainfully employed individuals. The implication of this is that the cost of an HD session is out of the reach for most of the population needing RRT [30]. Most patients are unable to afford more than a week of dialysis in government-owned facilities. Only a few private dialysis centres have affluent patients that are able to sustain for longer periods [26–28, 30]. Also, a few corporate patients have employers that provide healthcare support including dialysis.

The phenomenon termed "brain drain" has contributed to the dearth of nephrology personnel in Nigeria. The quest for economic greener pastures has favoured an emigration to developed countries much to the detriment of the developing countries such as Nigeria where there is dire need for their skills and expertise. There are several Nigerian trained medical personnel practicing as Nephrologists round the globe and their numbers may actually be more than the numbers practicing in Nigeria.

Challenges to the applicability and usefulness of CAPD in the sub-region include non- availability of PD cyclers, PD fluids and catheters, which have to be imported. Others include high peritonitis rates, and more recently, dearth of skilled manpower in peritoneal dialysis [14, 26, 27, 43]. The challenges of kidney transplant in Nigeria include funding concerns, and paucity of laboratories able to perform tissue typing, drug levels and transplant kidney histology.

## Paediatric Renal Diseases in Nigeria

Renal diseases in children are frequent and common reasons for hospitalisation (Table 5.5). From a prevalence of 1.1% of all paediatric admissions in the 1980–90s, kidney diseases now account for 3.8–8.9% of all paediatric admissions into public-funded tertiary hospitals [55–58]. The increase in the frequency of kidney diseases in hospitalised children may reflect a true increase, better recognition and/or as a result of refinement in the definitions of some these diseases to include milder forms. The changes in the definition of AKI and CKD to more sensitive ones are notable examples [59–61].

Nephrotic syndrome (NS) is the most commonly reported kidney disease in children. In most series, it accounted for 20–30% of all kidney diseases in children outside the neonatal period [57, 58, 62]. Its dramatic presentation with generalised oedema makes it easier to be recognised. Unlike in the period between 1970 and 2000 which was characterised by

**Table 5.5** Pattern of paediatric kidney diseases in Nigeria

| Study | Eke 1994 [55] | Etuk 2006 [56] | Ibasdin 2003 [57] | Adedoyin 2012 [67] | Ugwu 2014 [62] | Ladapo 2014 [58] | Anigilaje 2019 [68] |
|---|---|---|---|---|---|---|---|
| Region of Nigeria | South South | South South | South South | North Central | South South | South West | North Central |
| Year of study | 1986–1991 | 1991–2000 | 1997–2002 | 1995–2008 | 2010–2012 | 2008–2011 | 2013–2016 |
| No of children with kidney disease | 699 | 182 | 250 | 164 | 110 | 320 | 163 |
| No of children with kidney disease/year | 46.6 | 18.2 | 50 | 12.6 | 55 | 80 | 54.3 |
| Kidney disease as % of admissions | 1.1 | 3.2 | 4.5 | | 1.6 | 8.9 | 3.8 |
| Common kidney disease, % | | | | | | | |
| Nephrotic syndrome | 14.6 | 30.7 | 24.4 | 42.1 | 30 | 22.8 | 11.7 |
| Acute glomerulonephritis | 11.4 | 36.9 | 20 | 28.7 | 18.2 | 10 | 7.9 |
| Acute kidney injury | 4.7 | 6.7 | 4.1 | 11.6 | 10.9 | 20 | 30.7 |
| Chronic kidney disease | 2.1 | 3.9 | 24 | 0.6 | 7.3 | 4.2 | 6.7 |
| Obstructive uropathy & other CAKUT | 2.7 | 6.7 | 5.8 | 11.6 | 7.3 | 17.5 | 9.7 |
| Urinary tract infection | 68.9 | 8.9 | 32.8 | – | 16.3 | 3.1 | 30.7 |
| Wilms tumour | 1.6 | 6.2 | 6.8 | – | | 22.2 | 3.7 |

the predominance of steroid-resistant nephrotic syndrome, most recent reports of childhood nephrotic syndrome in Nigeria indicate that about 60–80% of children with idiopathic nephrotic syndrome have steroid-sensitive NS [13, 55, 63, 64]. The reason for the increased steroid responsiveness is not known, however, children are now developing nephrotic syndrome at a much younger age than in the past decades [63, 65, 66]. On the other hand, the frequency of acute glomerulonephritis is on the decline as would be expected with increase in the standard of living, access to antibiotics and health care [67, 68].

Following the adoption of AKI consensus definitions, which recognise milder forms, AKI is now reported among the top most common kidney diseases in children in Nigeria. Since 2012, AKI accounts for 20–30% of cases of kidney diseases among hospitalised children outside the neonatal period [58, 68]. In addition, congenital anomalies of the kidneys and urinary tract (CAKUT), with or without urinary tract infection, are also commonly reported in hospitalised children in Nigeria [58, 68]. Because most of the published studies focused on hospitalised children, it is likely that the frequency of CAKUT would be higher than currently reported as most cases of CAKUT seen only in outpatient settings are not included in these studies. Consistently, CKD accounts for less than 10% of kidney diseases [58, 68]. The near absence of symptoms until marked reduction in glomerular filtration rate (GFR) means that milder forms of CKD would be missed. Wilms tumour is the most common kidney tumour reported, accounting for 1.6–6.8% of cases of kidney disease [57, 68]. In one large tertiary hospital, Wilms tumour accounted for one-fifth of kidney diseases reported in hospitalised children [58].

## Paediatric Chronic Kidney Disease Epidemiology

The true burden of CKD in children in Nigeria is largely unknown. The absence of a national registry means reliance on reports from single centres to estimate the prevalence of CKD. Yearly incidence and prevalence of CKD in children in Nigeria is put between 3.0 to 11 and 12.5 to 48 cases per million children per year, respectively [69–72]. Although it does appear that CKD is less prevalent in children in Nigeria compared with children in the developed world, reliance on data from large urban hospitals means that the true burden of CKD in Nigeria is largely unknown, and most likely underreported [73, 74].

Chronic glomerulonephritis, either primary or secondary, is the leading cause of CKD in children. In a recent study of children in a southwest city, about 77% of the 53 children with ESRD had chronic glomerulonephritis; a third of which initially presented as nephrotic syndrome [71]. In another study involving 45 children with CKD defined as GFR <30 ml/min/1.73 m$^2$, chronic glomerulonephritis was the cause of the CKD in 56% of the children [69]. The secondary causes of chronic glomerulonephritis include HIV, hepatitis B infection, and systemic lupus erythematosus [69, 70]. In one study, these secondary causes made up about a quarter of causes of CKD [70]. With a prevalence of sickle cell disease (SCD) of 1.5–3%, and an estimated 100,000 children born each year with sickle cell anaemia [75, 76], its contribution to CKD is expected to be higher than currently reported. In addition, as more children with SCD survive into adolescence, the prevalence of SCD-related chronic kidney disease is expected to increase.

CAKUT is the second most common causes of CKD in children. They accounted for 20–30% in most series [69, 71]. Posterior urethral valves (PUV) were the most common CAKUT reported, which partly explained the over-representation of males in most published studies [71, 72]. The predominance of chronic glomerulonephritis as the leading cause of CKD in children in Nigeria contrasts with the picture in most developed countries, where CAKUT, including aplasia, hypoplasia and dysplasia, are the leading causes [77, 78]. It is possible that with the high neonatal and under-5 mortality rates in Nigeria, mostly from prematurity, neonatal sepsis, pneumonia and malaria, younger children with undiagnosed CAKUT die before detection and are underrepresented in series of children with CKD, which feature mostly adolescents. It is not unusual in Nigeria for cases of PUV to be diagnosed in children older than 5 years [79, 80].

Management of children with CKD in Nigeria is largely suboptimal and frustrating to health workers and the affected families. The majority of children with ESRD in Nigeria do not get dialysis due to the family's inability to pay for the care and the near-absence of any form of health insurance that provides coverage for dialysis [71, 72]. As with reimbursement for dialysis in adults, payment for RRT is out of pocket. Those that get dialysis do so infrequently and for only a few weeks or months at most, again, largely as a result of its costs [72, 81]. Chronic PD is not an established modality for ESRD both in children as well as in adults in Nigeria. Vascular access is mostly via acute femoral catheters; occasionally some children get tunnelled lines [82]. Not unexpected, management of anaemia, hypertension, fluid overload, metabolic acidosis, hyperkalemia, bone and mineral disease, and growth impairment is suboptimal.

As a result of suboptimal care, mortality from CKD is disproportionately high. Not uncommonly, mortality at 1 year after diagnosis of ESRD is in excess of 50% [71, 83].

## Paediatric Haemodialysis in Nigeria

HD is generally not accessible to most African children [84]. This is largely due to the lack of facilities, lack of trained workforce and cost implications to the patient. In the few children who received HD with good outcome, the most common indication for HD was AKI [82]. Most children needing chronic HD receive it for only a short period because of the inability to pay for it [45]. Unavailability of size-appropriate dialysis consumables such as bloodlines and dialysers means that only bigger children get access to HD; for smaller children priming of the bloodlines is an option commonly used [82].

## Peritoneal Dialysis in Children in Nigeria

PD, as a form of RRT, is a distant second option to HD for most persons needing dialysis in Nigeria. It is only available in large tertiary hospitals in urban centres of the country [85, 86]. When used, PD is administered manually rather than with automated cyclers in Nigeria [85, 86]. In some cases, nasogastric tubes and intercostal drains are used as improvised PD catheters [86]. In addition, it is not unusual for non-commercial PD fluids to be used because the cost of PD fluids is exorbitant [86]. These improvisations are needed because of the non-availability or exorbitant cost of the consumables and consequently PD in Nigeria is currently limited to children with AKI.

## Paediatric Acute Kidney Injury and Critical Care Nephrology

AKI is a common kidney disease among children presenting to emergency hospital services in the country. In most recent studies, AKI ranks as high as nephrotic syndrome in terms of prevalence [58, 68]. Unlike in developed countries, most cases of AKI in children in Nigeria are community-acquired rather than hospital-acquired [87]. Sepsis is now commonly reported as the leading cause of AKI in the post-neonatal age group [88, 89]. Other common causes of AKI include primary kidney diseases and malaria [88, 90, 91]. The primary kidney diseases reported include nephrotic syndrome, posterior urethral valves and acute nephritic syndrome from post-streptococcal glomerulonephritis. Gastroenteritis as sole cause of AKI is less commonly encountered [88, 90]. Among the neonates, perinatal asphyxia and neonatal sepsis are the leading causes of AKI [91, 92].

AKI in children in Nigeria is characterised by the predominance of severe forms and high attendant mortality. In most series, children with stage 3 or RIFLE-F AKI made up more than 50% of the children with AKI [88, 90], and in-hospital mortality rate reached up to 30% [87, 89, 91]. The high mortality rate often stems from late presentation, predominance of more severe forms of AKI and poor availability of paediatric ICU services and dialysis [87, 93].

## Approaches to Prevention of Kidney Diseases in Nigeria

With health insurance coverage clearly excluding chronic kidney care, most patients in Nigeria are unable to bear the cost of care. This makes prevention of CKD an imperative strategy. More so, awareness of kidney diseases in the general population is low [94]. There are no established prevention programs for CKD in Nigeria. However, many nephrologists have leveraged the opportunity presented by the annual World Kidney Day to raise awareness, educate and screen the population for kidney diseases. This has led to many prevention-related activities across the country [20, 21]. Kidney disease prevention activities in Nigeria can be categorised into programs aimed at:

- Increasing awareness among the general population
- Early detection and management of at-risk individuals
- Timely referral for specialist care

Kidney disease awareness-raising activities have largely involved the use of mass media such as radio, television, online and print media. Face-to-face campaigns target places with large numbers of people such as markets, worship centres such as churches and mosques as well as schools, and densely populated work environments. Lately, social media platforms such as *WhatsApp* and *Facebook* are being used by kidney disease practitioners to raise awareness of kidney diseases. Given that CKD may be asymptomatic in the early phases, screening activities need to be sustained. However, large population screenings are not logistically possible in Nigeria as it involves enormous costs. It would be more appropriate to make the activities more efficient and cost-effective by embedding in the process a prescreening phase. This would involve an initial clinical history, blood pressure and anthropometric checks in which at-risk persons are identified for further screening with blood and urine testing [95]. It seems reasonable to offer this service as part of an integrated screening for prevention of both communicable and non-communicable diseases packages at primary and secondary care level. Nigeria's three-tier health system has been designed to facilitate referrals from the primary to secondary to tertiary level of care and vice versa. However, due to a dearth of human resources for health and inadequate healthcare financing, this referral system has been suboptimal. In practice, primary care physicians refer patients with suspected or definite kidney diseases to specialists mostly practicing at tertiary centres.

## Nephrology Practice in Nigeria

As stated earlier, renal care units were first established in the early 1960s and situated in the teaching hospitals in Ibadan (UCH), Lagos, Zaria, Ile-Ife and Enugu as part of internal medicine and paediatric services offered by these hospitals. The early specialists in these units, most of whom were trained abroad, were responsible for care of patients with renal diseases in addition to their responsibilities of care for patients with other non-communicable and communicable illnesses. At that time, PD and an attempt at HD using a coil dialysis machine were made at the University College Hospital, Ibadan. There was also a lot of research into the aetiology of nephrotic syndrome done at these early teaching hospitals including the association of steroid-resistant form of childhood nephrotic syndrome and *Plasmodium malariae* [12, 13].

The first dedicated HD unit was established at the Lagos University Teaching Hospital in 1981 and following this other units have been opened in almost every teaching hospital and federal tertiary hospital all over the country. Several state government hospitals also have established units.

Many of these units are bedevilled with various challenges faced by the public-funded institutions in Nigeria today, consequent on poor funding, poor administration of these units, inter-professional rivalry and rather frequent industrial disputes within these establishments. As a result of this, there are now many private renal care units that currently outnumber the public institutions in numbers and capacity. Generally, private units tend to be larger in capacity and attend to much larger numbers of patients than most public-funded units. Almost invariably, however, these renal units are situated in the urban centres and almost none in any of the rural areas where almost 50% of the population live. In addition, these private units are less likely to be involved in strikes and generally have better outcomes as they are more likely to see privately funded patients who have the capacity to sustain the costs associated with renal care by any of the various modalities. This would explain why the most active kidney transplant units in the country are in the private-funded hospitals and just two of these are responsible for over 80% of more than the 500 kidney transplants that have been carried out in the country till date. The costs involved in renal care in Nigeria are not covered by the National Health Insurance Scheme (NHIS) although advocacy by the NAN has led to a policy by government for the NHIS to cover the costs of the first six sessions of dialysis. With less than 5% of the population covered by the NHIS, most patients have to pay the costs for their care, out of pocket.

Majority of the nephrology specialists are engaged by the public institutions but many in their spare time also make their services available in many of the private institutions. Altogether there are over 180 nephrologists (over 150 adults and about 30 paediatric nephrologists) practicing in the country.

Currently, between 10 and 15 adult and paediatric nephrologists are certified each year by two postgraduate medical colleges through over a 6-year period. Each trainee passes through a similar three-stage examination process (Primary, Part 1 and Part 2 examinations) before certification as a nephrologist. Graduates of these training programs are appointable as consultant nephrologists. There are currently

188 consultant adult and paediatric nephrologists practicing in Nigeria, with the majority working in public hospitals where most of the nephrology and dialysis centres are located. There are estimated to be about 788 nurses and 295 renal technicians practicing in these units. The training for these nurses and technicians, after the initial training the pioneers of these professions received abroad, has also been done locally in the various units.

The NAN is the official professional body of nephrologists, renal nurses, renal technicians and other professionals involved in the care of the renal patient. It was established in 1987 in Ibadan, Oyo State, and currently boasts over 500 members. Yearly, it holds its scientific and general meeting with the venue rotated to different parts of the country with active nephrology practice. The themes and sub-themes of these meetings focus on relevant aspects of renal care in Nigeria. The Association accepts all physicians involved in the care of renal patients as ordinary members while nurse practitioners, nephrology nurses, dialysis technicians and dietitians are accepted as associate members. Through its members, the NAN is active in research and advocacy, and is in the process of setting up a national renal registry.

The Association is affiliated to both ISN and AFRAN. NAN has enjoyed an excellent collaboration with ISN that has led to significant development of capacities in most renal units across the country. Several nephrologists have benefitted from the Fellowship program of ISN and many centres have graduated from the Sister Renal Centre (SRC) relationship with several others still benefitting at different stages. NAN continues to benefit from the ISN Continuous Medical Education Committee with sponsorship of 3–4 resource persons to our annual scientific conference held in the second week of February every year. Many of our centres are also involved in the Educational Ambassador Program (EAP) and Library Enhancement Program (LEP). The attendance at the World Congress of Nephrology (WCNs) from Nigeria has improved remarkably in the last three decades. NAN now undertakes advocacy with the government and their agencies with a view to improving nephrology practice in the country, thereby engendering excellent outcomes to our patients as well as influencing policy decisions of the government.

There are job opportunities available around the country for all cadre of professionals engaged in the care of renal patients, more so in the northern parts of the country where the number of these specialists remains inadequate. The average starting salary for a young nephrologist would be in the region of $2000 per month. This relatively low pay when compared with similarly skilled professionals in the developed world is a major driver of the exodus of the Nigerian renal care professionals to various countries in the western world. An additional reason for the exodus is the suboptimal outcome of renal patients in the country, which is tied closely to poor funding.

## Nephrology Practice by Nigerians in the Diaspora

Emigration, for a variety of reasons, has been an increasingly common practice among medical professionals from Nigeria [96]. The trend, part of a larger process colloquially known as the "Brain Drain" is largely believed to have started in the late 1980s and is considered to have reached levels where, by some accounts, majority of licensed physicians are either themselves considering emigration or know several colleagues who are [97].

The reasons for emigration vary according to the time of graduation. There are three common time frames for emigration: immediately following completion of pre-registration year and national youth service, during or when seeking middle-grade training or once established as a consultant. For earlier time points, movement seems to be a combination of training opportunities, family ties and socioeconomic opportunities. Movement of the established consultant seems more geared to socioeconomic opportunities. This may be reflected in the tendency of more mature practitioners to choose the Middle East as an emigration destination and the younger to seemingly favour the UK and the USA. The UK and USA are unarguably the two most desired countries for emigrant Nigerian physicians [97]. This is partly as a result of the convenience of the language and culture. English is the lingua franca (official language) in Nigeria. The UK is often the first relocation point for younger trainees even if they plan the USA to be their final destination. This may be due to historical ties to the UK existing since the colonial times (1914–1960). Another likely reason for the predilection to the UK is pre-existing family and social ties of would-be emigrants, easing the stress of the move and settling into a foreign and potentially hostile environment. Opportunities for progression in the UK in selected medical specialities such as Nephrology for the International Medical Graduate (IMGs) appear limited compared to those available in the USA potentially due to the relative size of the USA and varied perception of IMGs in the UK and the USA. This may explain the disproportionately high number of Nigerian IMGs registered with the General Medical Council versus only seven attaining certification in Nephrology in the UK. This is in contrast to the USA where there are 124 board-certified Nephrologists who received their initial medical degree from a Nigerian medical school. Other countries where Nigerian trained professionals are known to practice include the various countries in the Middle East, Australia,

South Africa and Canada. Altogether, there are possibly more Nigerian nephrologists practicing outside the country than there are within.

## Conclusion

In Nigeria, kidney diseases are very common in adults and children and the outcome of patients with ESRD is dismal because of suboptimal care. The suboptimal care is mainly driven by the inability of most families to meet the financial cost of care. Illiteracy, underdevelopment, dearth of personnel and infrastructure are additional major barriers mitigating against access to healthcare and RRT by the vast majority of the population domiciled largely in the rural areas. The true prevalence of CKD, though still largely speculative, is expected to rise markedly with the predicted increase in the prevalence of non-communicable diseases such as diabetes mellitus, and the continued scourge of infectious diseases. There is an ongoing concerted effort to develop a Nigerian renal registry and this is expected to assist in determining the true prevalence of ESRD and provide a firm basis for policies aimed at preventing and treating affected patients. Targeted screening of at-risk populations should be developed and aggressively implemented as well as measures to ensure sustainable financing of RRT. There is the need to develop effective monitoring systems that would ensure judicious utilisation of available resources while the health personnel need to be sufficiently motivated to mitigate the effects of brain drain.

## References

1. CIA. The World Factbook. Nigeria; 2019.
2. World Bank. Country Profile. Nigeria; 2018.
3. OPHI. Nigeria Country Briefing, Multidimensional Poverty Index Data Bank; 2017.
4. Adeloye D, Basquill C, Aderemi AV, Thompson JY, Obi FA. An estimate of the prevalence of hypertension in Nigeria: a systematic review and meta-analysis. J Hypertens. 2015;33(2):230–42. https://doi.org/10.1097/HJH.0000000000000413.
5. Adeloye D, Ige JO, Aderemi AV, Adeleye N, Amoo EO, Auta A, et al. Estimating the prevalence, hospitalisation and mortality from type 2 diabetes mellitus in Nigeria: a systematic review and meta-analysis. BMJ Open. 2017;7(5):e015424. https://doi.org/10.1136/bmjopen-2016-015424.
6. Tayo BO, Kramer H, Salako BL, Gottesman O, McKenzie CA, Ogunniyi A, et al. Genetic variation in APOL1 and MYH9 genes is associated with chronic kidney disease among Nigerians. Int Urol Nephrol. 2013;45(2):485–94. https://doi.org/10.1007/s11255-012-0263-4.
7. Ulasi II, Tzur S, Wasser WG, Shemer R, Kruzel E, Feigin E, et al. High population frequencies of APOL1 risk variants are associated with increased prevalence of non-diabetic chronic kidney disease in the Igbo people from South-Eastern Nigeria. Nephron Clin Pract. 2013;123(1–2):123–8. https://doi.org/10.1159/000353223.
8. Fleming AF, Storey J, Molineaux L, Iroko EA, Attai ED. Abnormal haemoglobins in the Sudan savanna of Nigeria. I. Prevalence of haemoglobins and relationships between sickle cell trait, malaria and survival. Ann Trop Med Parasitol. 1979;73(2):161–72. https://doi.org/10.1080/00034983.1979.11687243.
9. Hafez R. Nigeria health financing system assessment. 2018.
10. Chukwuneke FN, Ezeonu CT, Onyire BN, Ezeonu PO. Culture and biomedical care in Africa: the influence of culture on biomedical care in a traditional African society, Nigeria, West Africa. Niger J Med. 2012;21(3):331–3.
11. Akinkugbe OO, Abiose P. Peritoneal dialysis in acute renal failure, West Afr Med J 1967;16:165–168.
12. Hendrickse RG, Gilles HM. The nephrotic syndrome and other renal diseases in children in Western Nigeria. East Afr Med J. 1963;40:186–201.
13. Hendrickse RG, Adeniyi A, Edington GM, Glasgow EF, White RH, Houba V. Quartan malarial nephrotic syndrome. Collaborative clinicopathological study in Nigerian children. Lancet. 1972;1(7761):1143–9.
14. Arogundade FA, Barsoum RS. CKD prevention in Sub-Saharan Africa: a call for governmental, nongovernmental, and community support. Am J Kidney Dis. 2008;51(3):515–23. https://doi.org/10.1053/j.ajkd.2007.12.006.
15. Afolabi MO, Abioye-Kuteyi EA, Arogundade FA, Bello IS. Prevalence of chronic kidney disease in a Nigerian family practice population. S Afr Fam Pract. 2009;51(2):132–7.
16. Oluyombo R, Ayodele OE, Akinwusi PO, Okunola OO, Akinsola A, Arogundade FA, et al. A community study of the prevalence, risk factors and pattern of chronic kidney disease in Osun State, South West Nigeria. West Afr J Med. 2013;32(2):85–92.
17. Okoye OCA, Oviasu E, Ojogwu L. Prevalence of chronic kidney disease and its risk factors amongst adults in a rural population in Edo State, Nigeria. J US China Med Sci. 2011;8(8):471–81.
18. Ulasi II, Ijoma CK, Onodugo OD, Arodiwe EB, Ifebunandu NA, Okoye JU. Towards prevention of chronic kidney disease in Nigeria: a community-based study in Southeast Nigeria. Kidney Int Suppl. 2013;3:195–201.
19. Oluyombo R, Olamoyegun MA, Ayodele OE, Akinwusi PO, Akinsola A. Clustering of chronic kidney disease and cardiovascular risk factors in South-West Nigeria. J Nephropathol. 2017;6(3):196–203. https://doi.org/10.15171/jnp.2017.33.
20. Abene EE, Gimba ZM, Agaba PA, Uchendu DG, Olaniru OB, Ocheke IE, et al. Chronic kidney disease screening: results of the 2013 World Kidney Day activities conducted at the Jos University Teaching Hospital. Highl Med Res J. 2017;17(1):1–5.
21. Okwuonu CG, Chukwuonye II, Adejumo OA, Agaba EI, Ojogwu LI. Prevalence of chronic kidney disease and its risk factors among adults in a semi-urban community of South-East Nigeria. Niger Postgrad Med J. 2017;24(2):81–7. https://doi.org/10.4103/npmj.npmj_34_17.
22. Egbi OG, Okafor UH, Miebodei KE, Kasia BE, Kunle-Olowu OE, Unuigbe EI. Prevalence and correlates of chronic kidney disease among civil servants in Bayelsa state, Nigeria. Niger J Clin Pract. 2014;17(5):602–7. https://doi.org/10.4103/1119-3077.141426.
23. Awobusuyi JO, Bakare O, Dada A, Adamu U, Abasi-Ekong U, Effa E, et al. Indices of kidney damage in Nigeria: a survey of 8077 subjects in the six geopolitical zones of the country. Trop J Nephrol. 2015;10(2):95–105.
24. Nalado A, Abdu A, Adamu B, Aliyu MH, Arogundade FA, Sanusi AA, et al. Prevalence of chronic kidney disease markers in Kumbotso rural Northern Nigeria. Afr J Med Med Sci. 2016;45(1):61–5.
25. Oyebisi OO, Okunola OO, Jaiyesimi AE, Arogundade FA, Adelaja MA, Erohibe CE, et al. Prevalence and pattern of chronic kidney disease and its associated risk factors in a rural community in South Western Nigeria. West Afr J Med. 2018;35(2):109–16.

26. Arogundade FA, Sanusi AA, Hassan MO, Akinsola A. The pattern, clinical characteristics and outcome of ESRD in Ile-Ife, Nigeria: is there a change in trend? Afr Health Sci. 2011;11(4):594–601.
27. Ulasi II, Ijoma CK. The enormity of chronic kidney disease in Nigeria: the situation in a teaching hospital in South-East Nigeria. J Trop Med. 2010;2010:501957. https://doi.org/10.1155/2010/501957.
28. Arije A, Kadiri S, Akinkugbe OO. The viability of hemodialysis as a treatment option for renal failure in a developing economy. Afr J Med Med Sci. 2000;29(3–4):311–4.
29. King H, Aubert RE, Herman WH. Global burden of diabetes, 1995–2025: prevalence, numerical estimates, and projections. Diabetes Care. 1998;21(9):1414–31. https://doi.org/10.2337/diacare.21.9.1414.
30. Naicker S. Burden of end-stage renal disease in Sub-Saharan Africa. Clin Nephrol. 2010;74 Suppl 1:S13–6. https://doi.org/10.5414/cnp74s013.
31. Alebiosu CO, Ayodele OO, Abbas A, Olutoyin AI. Chronic renal failure at the Olabisi Onabanjo University Teaching Hospital, Sagamu, Nigeria. Afr Health Sci. 2006;6(3):132–8. https://doi.org/10.5555/afhs.2006.6.3.132.
32. Kadiri S, Ogunlesi A, Osinfade K, Akinkugbe OO. The causes and course of acute tubular necrosis in Nigerians. Afr J Med Med Sci. 1992;21(1):91–6.
33. Bamgboye EL, Mabayoje MO, Odutola TA, Mabadeje AF. Acute renal failure at the Lagos University Teaching Hospital: a 10-year review. Ren Fail. 1993;15(1):77–80.
34. Arogundade FA, Sanusi AA, Okunola OO, Soyinka FO, Ojo OE, Akinsola A. Acute renal failure (ARF) in developing countries: which factors actually influence survival. Cent Afr J Med. 2007;53(5–8):34–9.
35. Emem-Chioma PC, Alasia DD, Wokoma FS. Clinical outcomes of dialysis-treated acute kidney injury patients at the University of Port Harcourt teaching hospital, Nigeria. ISRN Nephrol. 2013;2013:540526. https://doi.org/10.5402/2013/540526.
36. Okunola OO, Ayodele OE, Adekanle AD. Acute kidney injury requiring hemodialysis in the tropics. Saudi J Kidney Dis Transpl. 2012;23(6):1315–9. https://doi.org/10.4103/1319-2442.103587.
37. Oluseyi A, Ayodeji A, Ayodeji F. Aetiologies and short-term outcomes of acute kidney injury in a tertiary centre in Southwest Nigeria. Ethiop J Health Sci. 2016;26(1):37–44. https://doi.org/10.4314/ejhs.v26i1.8.
38. Makusidi AM, Liman HM, Yakubu A, Hassan M, Isah MD, Chijioke A. Hemodialysis among pregnancy related acute kidney injury patients: a single center experience in North-Western Nigeria. Indian J Nephrol. 2016;26(5):340–2. https://doi.org/10.4103/0971-4065.171224.
39. Bello BT, Busari AA, Amira CO, Raji YR, Braimoh RW. Acute kidney injury in Lagos: pattern, outcomes, and predictors of in-hospital mortality. Niger J Clin Pract. 2017;20(2):194–9. https://doi.org/10.4103/1119-3077.183258.
40. Awowole IO, Omitinde OS, Arogundade FA, Bola-Oyebamiji SB, Adeniyi OA. Pregnancy-related acute kidney injury requiring dialysis as an indicator of severe adverse maternal morbidity at a tertiary center in Southwest Nigeria. Eur J Obstet Gynecol Reprod Biol. 2018;225:205–9. https://doi.org/10.1016/j.ejogrb.2018.04.041.
41. Okunola OO, Arogundade FA, Sanusi AA, Akinsola A. Acute renal failure in the intensive care unit: aetiological and predisposing factors and outcome. West Afr J Med. 2009;28(4):240–4.
42. Raji YR, Ajayi SO, Ademola AF, Lawal TA, Ayandipo OO, Adigun T, et al. Acute kidney injury among adult patients undergoing major surgery in a tertiary hospital in Nigeria. Clin Kidney J. 2018;11(4):443–9. https://doi.org/10.1093/ckj/sfx144.
43. Arogundade FA, Ishola DA Jr, Sanusi AA, Akinsola A. An analysis of the effectiveness and benefits of peritoneal dialysis and haemodialysis using Nigerian made PD fluids. Afr J Med Med Sci. 2005;34(3):227–33.
44. Oluyombo R, Okunola OO, Olanrewaju TO, Soje MO, Obajolowo OO, Ayorinde MA. Challenges of hemodialysis in a new renal care center: call for sustainability and improved outcome. Int J Nephrol Renovasc Dis. 2014;7:347–52. https://doi.org/10.2147/IJNRD.S65835.
45. Bello BT, Raji YR, Sanusi I, Braimoh RW, Amira OC, Mabayoje OM. Challenges of providing maintenance hemodialysis in a resource poor country: experience from a single teaching hospital in Lagos, Southwest Nigeria. Hemodial Int. 2013;17(3):427–33. https://doi.org/10.1111/hdi.12024.
46. Akinsola A, Arije A. Peritoneal dialysis in Nigerian patients with a short history of advanced renal failure. West Afr J Med. 1987;6:205–9.
47. Ojogwu LI. Peritoneal dialysis in the management of hypertensive acute oliguric renal failure. Trop Geogr Med. 1983;35(4):385–8.
48. Akinsola A, Adelekun A, Arogundade FA. Continuous ambulatory peritoneal dialysis (CAPD) practice in OAUTHC Ile-Ife., Nigeria, a preliminary experience. Dial Transplant. 2000;29(12):774–82.
49. Arogundade FA, Olatunde LO, Ishola DA Jr, Bappa A, Sanusi AA, Akinsola A. PD (peritoneal dialysis) peritonitis: still a major limiting factor in peritoneal dialysis management today. Afr J Nephrol. 2004;8:52–6.
50. Ulasi II, Ijoma CK. Organ transplantation in Nigeria. Transplantation. 2016;100(4):695–7. https://doi.org/10.1097/TP.0000000000001149.
51. Okafor UH. Kidney transplant in Nigeria: a single centre experience. Pan Afr Med J. 2016;25:112. https://doi.org/10.11604/pamj.2016.25.112.7930.
52. Bolarinwa RA, Oyekunle AA, Arogundade FA, Sanusi AA, Salawu L, Togun RA, et al. Preliminary report of HLA (DNA) typing of Nigerians using sequence-specific primer technique. Niger Postgrad Med J. 2014;21(4):285–9.
53. Arogundade FA. Kidney transplantation in a low-resource setting: Nigeria experience. Kidney Int Suppl (2011). 2013;3(2):241–5. https://doi.org/10.1038/kisup.2013.23.
54. Bamgboye EL. Barriers to a functional renal transplant program in developing countries. Ethn Dis. 2009;19(1 Suppl 1):S1-56–59.
55. Eke FU, Eke NN. Renal disorders in children: a Nigerian study. Pediatr Nephrol. 1994;8(3):383–6.
56. Etuk IS, Anah MU, Ochighs SO, Eyong M. Pattern of paediatric renal disease in inpatients in Calabar, Nigeria. Trop Dr. 2006;36(4):256. https://doi.org/10.1258/004947506778604968.
57. Michael IO, Gabriel OE. Pattern of renal diseases in children in Midwestern Zone of Nigeria. Saudi J Kidney Dis Transpl. 2003;14(4):539–44.
58. Ladapo TA, Esezobor CI, Lesi FE. Pediatric kidney diseases in an African country: prevalence, spectrum and outcome. Saudi J Kidney Dis Transpl. 2014;25(5):1110–6.
59. Kidney Disease: Improving Global Outcomes (KDIGO) Acute Kidney Injury Work Group. KDIGO clinical practice guideline for acute kidney injury. Kidney Int Suppl. 2012;(2):1–138.
60. Kidney Disease: Improving Global Outcomes (KDIGO) Glomerulonephritis Work Group. KDIGO clinical practice guideline for glomerulonephritis. Kidney Int Suppl. 2012;2:139–274.
61. Bellomo R, Ronco C, Kellum JA, Mehta RL, Palevsky P, Acute Dialysis Quality Initiative w. Acute renal failure – definition, outcome measures, animal models, fluid therapy and information technology needs: the Second International Consensus Conference of the Acute Dialysis Quality Initiative (ADQI) Group. Crit Care. 2004;8(4):R204–12. https://doi.org/10.1186/cc2872.
62. Ugwu GI, Nwajei G, Chinemelu U. Pattern of renal diseases among children in the Niger Delta Region, Nigeria. Arab J Nephrol Transplant. 2014;7(1):49–50.

63. Ladapo TA, Esezobor CI, Lesi FE. High steroid sensitivity among children with nephrotic syndrome in Southwestern Nigeria. Int J Nephrol. 2014;2014:350640. https://doi.org/10.1155/2014/350640.
64. Anochie I, Eke F, Okpere A. Childhood nephrotic syndrome: change in pattern and response to steroids. J Natl Med Assoc. 2006;98(12):1977–81.
65. Ibadin MO, Abiodun PO. Epidemiology and clinicopathologic characteristics of childhood nephrotic syndrome in Benin-City, Nigeria. J Pak Med Assoc. 1998;48(8):235–8.
66. Okoro BA, Okafor HU, Nnoli LU. Childhood nephrotic syndrome in Enugu, Nigeria. West Afr J Med. 2000;19(2):137–41.
67. Adedoyin OT, Adesiyun OA, Mark F, Adeniyi A. Childhood renal disorders in Ilorin, North Central Nigeria. Niger Postgrad Med J. 2012;19(2):88–91.
68. Anigilaje EA, Adesina TC. The pattern and outcomes of childhood renal diseases at University of Abuja Teaching Hospital, Abuja, Nigeria: a 4 year retrospective review. Niger Postgrad Med J. 2019;26(1):53–60. https://doi.org/10.4103/npmj.npmj_174_18.
69. Anochie I, Eke F. Chronic renal failure in children: a report from Port Harcourt, Nigeria (1985–2000). Pediatr Nephrol. 2003;18(7):692–5. https://doi.org/10.1007/s00467-003-1150-0.
70. Olowu WA, Adefehinti O, Aladekomo TA. Epidemiology and clinicopathologic outcome of pediatric chronic kidney disease in Nigeria, a single center study. Arab J Nephrol Transplant. 2013;6(2):105–13.
71. Asinobi AO, Ademola AD, Ogunkunle OO, Mott SA. Paediatric end-stage renal disease in a tertiary hospital in South West Nigeria. BMC Nephrol. 2014;15:25. https://doi.org/10.1186/1471-2369-15-25.
72. Odetunde OI, Okafor HU, Uwaezuoke SN, Ezeonwu BU, Adiele KD, Ukoha OM. Chronic kidney disease in children as seen in a tertiary hospital in Enugu, South-East, Nigeria. Niger J Clin Pract. 2014;17(2):196–200. https://doi.org/10.4103/1119-3077.127553.
73. Ardissino G, Dacco V, Testa S, Bonaudo R, Claris-Appiani A, Taioli E, et al. Epidemiology of chronic renal failure in children: data from the ItalKid project. Pediatrics. 2003;111(4 Pt 1):e382–7.
74. Harambat J, van Stralen KJ, Kim JJ, Tizard EJ. Epidemiology of chronic kidney disease in children. Pediatr Nephrol. 2012;27(3):363–73. https://doi.org/10.1007/s00467-011-1939-1.
75. Piel FB, Hay SI, Gupta S, Weatherall DJ, Williams TN. Global burden of sickle cell anaemia in children under five, 2010–2050: modelling based on demographics, excess mortality, and interventions. PLoS Med. 2013;10(7):e1001484. https://doi.org/10.1371/journal.pmed.1001484.
76. Adedoyin OT, Adesiyun OO, Adegboye OA, Bello OA, Fatoye OP. Sickle cell nephropathy in children seen in an African Hospital – case report. Niger Postgrad Med J. 2012;19(2):119–22.
77. Wong CJ, Moxey-Mims M, Jerry-Fluker J, Warady BA, Furth SL. CKiD (CKD in children) prospective cohort study: a review of current findings. Am J Kidney Dis. 2012;60(6):1002–11. https://doi.org/10.1053/j.ajkd.2012.07.018.
78. Lewis MA, Shaw J, Sinha MD, Adalat S, Hussain F, Castledine C, et al. UK Renal Registry 12th Annual Report (December 2009): chapter 14: demography of the UK paediatric renal replacement therapy population in 2008. Nephron Clin Pract. 2010;115(Suppl 1):c279–88. https://doi.org/10.1159/000301237.
79. Orumuah AJ, Oduagbon OE. Presentation, management, and outcome of posterior urethral valves in a Nigerian tertiary hospital. Afr J Paediatr Surg. 2015;12(1):18–22. https://doi.org/10.4103/0189-6725.150937.
80. Ikuerowo SO, Balogun BO, Akintomide TE, Ikuerowo AO, Akinola RA, Gbelee HO, et al. Clinical and radiological characteristics of Nigerian boys with posterior urethral valves. Pediatr Surg Int. 2008;24(7):825–9. https://doi.org/10.1007/s00383-008-2163-3.
81. Olowu WA. Renal failure in Nigerian children: factors limiting access to dialysis. Pediatr Nephrol. 2003;18(12):1249–54. https://doi.org/10.1007/s00467-003-1255-5.
82. Asinobi AO, Ademola AD, Alao MA. Haemodialysis for paediatric acute kidney injury in a low resource setting: experience from a tertiary hospital in South West Nigeria. Clin Kidney J. 2016;9(1):63–8. https://doi.org/10.1093/ckj/sfv112.
83. Odetunde OI, Okafor HU, Uwaezuoke SN, Ezeonwu BU, Ukoha OM. Renal replacement therapy in children in the developing world: challenges and outcome in a tertiary hospital in Southeast Nigeria. ScientificWorldJournal. 2014;2014:903151. https://doi.org/10.1155/2014/903151.
84. Ashuntantang G, Osafo C, Olowu WA, Arogundade F, Niang A, Porter J, et al. Outcomes in adults and children with end-stage kidney disease requiring dialysis in Sub-Saharan Africa: a systematic review. Lancet Glob Health. 2017;5(4):e408–17. https://doi.org/10.1016/S2214-109X(17)30057-8.
85. Ademola AD, Asinobi AO, Ogunkunle OO, Yusuf BN, Ojo OE. Peritoneal dialysis in childhood acute kidney injury: experience in Southwest Nigeria. Perit Dial Int. 2012;32(3):267–72. https://doi.org/10.3747/pdi.2011.00275.
86. Esezobor CI, Ladapo TA, Lesi FE. Peritoneal dialysis for children with acute kidney injury in Lagos, Nigeria: experience with adaptations. Perit Dial Int. 2014;34(5):534–8. https://doi.org/10.3747/pdi.2013.00097.
87. Olowu WA. Acute kidney injury in children in Nigeria. Clin Nephrol. 2015;83(7 Suppl 1):70–4.
88. Ademola AD, Asinobi AO, Ekpe-Adewuyi E, Ayede AI, Ajayi SO, Raji YR, et al. Acute kidney injury among paediatric emergency room admissions in a tertiary hospital in South West Nigeria: a cohort study. Clin Kidney J. 2018:1–6. https://doi.org/10.1093/ckj/sfy120.
89. Esezobor CI, Ladapo TA, Lesi FE. Clinical profile and hospital outcome of children with severe acute kidney injury in a developing country. J Trop Pediatr. 2015;61(1):54–60. https://doi.org/10.1093/tropej/fmu066.
90. Esezobor CI, Ladapo TA, Osinaike B, Lesi FE. Paediatric acute kidney injury in a tertiary hospital in Nigeria: prevalence, causes and mortality rate. PLoS One. 2012;7(12):e51229. https://doi.org/10.1371/journal.pone.0051229.
91. Anochie IC, Eke FU. Acute renal failure in Nigerian children: Port Harcourt experience. Pediatr Nephrol. 2005;20(11):1610–4. https://doi.org/10.1007/s00467-005-1984-8.
92. Airede A, Bello M, Weerasinghe HD. Acute renal failure in the newborn: incidence and outcome. J Paediatr Child Health. 1997;33(3):246–9.
93. Olowu WA, Adelusola KA. Pediatric acute renal failure in Southwestern Nigeria. Kidney Int. 2004;66(4):1541–8. https://doi.org/10.1111/j.1523-1755.2004.00918.x.
94. Oluyombo R, Ayodele OE, Akinwusi PO, Okunola OO, Gbadegesin BA, Soje MO, et al. Awareness, knowledge and perception of chronic kidney disease in a rural community of South-West Nigeria. Niger J Clin Pract. 2016;19(2):161–9. https://doi.org/10.4103/1119-3077.175960.
95. Perico N, Remuzzi G. Prevention programs for chronic kidney disease in low-income countries. Intern Emerg Med. 2016;11(3):385–9. https://doi.org/10.1007/s11739-016-1425-7.
96. Burch VC, McKinley D, van Wyk J, Kiguli-Walube S, Cameron D, Cilliers FJ, et al. Career intentions of medical students trained in six Sub-Saharan African countries. Educ Health (Abingdon). 2011;24(3):614.
97. NOIPolls. 2018. https://www.noi-polls.com/documents/Emigration_of_Medical_Doctors_Survey_Report.pdf. Accessed 28 May 2019.

# Nephrology in South Africa

6

Mogamat Razeen Davids, Mogamat-Yazied Chothia, Nicola Wearne, Bianca Davidson, and Mignon McCulloch

*General Table*. A profile of South Africa.

| | |
|---|---|
| Area[1] | 1.22 million km$^2$ |
| Population | 57,725,600 (2018) |
| Capital | Pretoria |
| Three most populated cities | 1. Johannesburg (9.17 million)<br>2. Cape Town (4.00 million)<br>3. Durban (3.66 million) |
| Official languages | English, Afrikaans, Sepedi, Sesotho, Setswana, siSwati, Tshivenda, Xitsonga, isiNdebele, isiXhosa and isiZulu |
| Gross Domestic Product (GDP)[2] | 368.3 billion USD (2018) |
| GDP per capita[2] | 6374 USD (2018)<br>13,730 USD (2018, PPP method) |
| Human Development Index (HDI)[3] | 0.699 (2017) |
| Official currency | South African Rand (ZAR) |
| Total number of nephrologists | 142 |
| National society of nephrology | South African Renal Society www.sa-renalsociety.org |
| Incidence of treated end-stage kidney disease | 2017 – 25 pmp |
| Prevalence of treated end-stage kidney disease | 2016 – 183 pmp<br>2017 – 190 pmp |
| Total number of patients on dialysis (all modalities)[4,5] | 2016 – 8832<br>2017 – 8881 |
| Number of patients on haemodialysis[4,5] | 2016 – 7525<br>2017 – 7682 |
| Number of patients on peritoneal dialysis[4,5] | 2016 – 1307<br>2017 – 1199 |
| Number of new kidney transplants per year[6] | 2016 – 254<br>2017 – 260 |

Table References:

1. Statistics South Africa. Mid-year population estimates for 2017 and 2018. http://www.statssa.gov.za/
2. The World Bank, https://data.worldbank.org/country/south-africa
3. United Nations Development Programme. Human development indicators for South Africa. http://hdr.undp.org/sites/all/themes/hdr_theme/country-notes/ZAF.pdf
4. Davids MR, Jardine T, Marais N, Jacobs JC. South African Renal Registry Annual Report 2016. Afr J Nephrol. 2018;21:61–72
5. Davids MR, Jardine T, Marais N, Jacobs JC. South African Renal Registry Annual Report 2017. Afr J Nephrol. 2019;22:60–71
6. South African Organ Donor Foundation, www.odf.org.za

M. R. Davids (✉) · M.-Y. Chothia
Division of Nephrology, Stellenbosch University and Tygerberg Hospital, Cape Town, South Africa
e-mail: mrd@sun.ac.za; yaziedc@sun.ac.za

N. Wearne · B. Davidson
Division of Nephrology and Hypertension, University of Cape Town and Groote Schuur Hospital, Cape Town, South Africa
e-mail: nicola.wearne@uct.ac.za

M. McCulloch
Division of Paediatric Nephrology, University of Cape Town and Red Cross War Memorial Children's Hospital,
Cape Town, South Africa
e-mail: mignon.mcculloch@uct.ac.za

## Introduction

The Republic of South Africa is the southernmost country in Africa, with 2,798 kilometres of coastline stretching along the South Atlantic and Indian oceans. It has nine provinces and, according to mid-year estimates for 2018, is home to nearly 58 million people [1]. Approximately 25% of the population lives in the province of Gauteng, with the next most populous provinces being KwaZulu-Natal (20%), the Eastern Cape and the Western Cape (11% each). Figure 6.1 illustrates the provinces and major cities of South Africa.

South Africa is a multi-ethnic and multilingual country, with 80.9% of citizens being Black African, 8.8% of mixed ancestry, 7.8% White and 2.5% Indian/Asian. We have 11 official languages, with the most spoken language inside the home being isiZulu (25%), followed by isiXhosa (15%) and Afrikaans (12%) [2]. English is spoken at home by 8% of South Africans. It is the second most commonly spoken language outside the home (17%) and is the dominant language used in government and the media.


J. A. Moura-Neto et al. (eds.), *Nephrology Worldwide*, https://doi.org/10.1007/978-3-030-56890-0_6

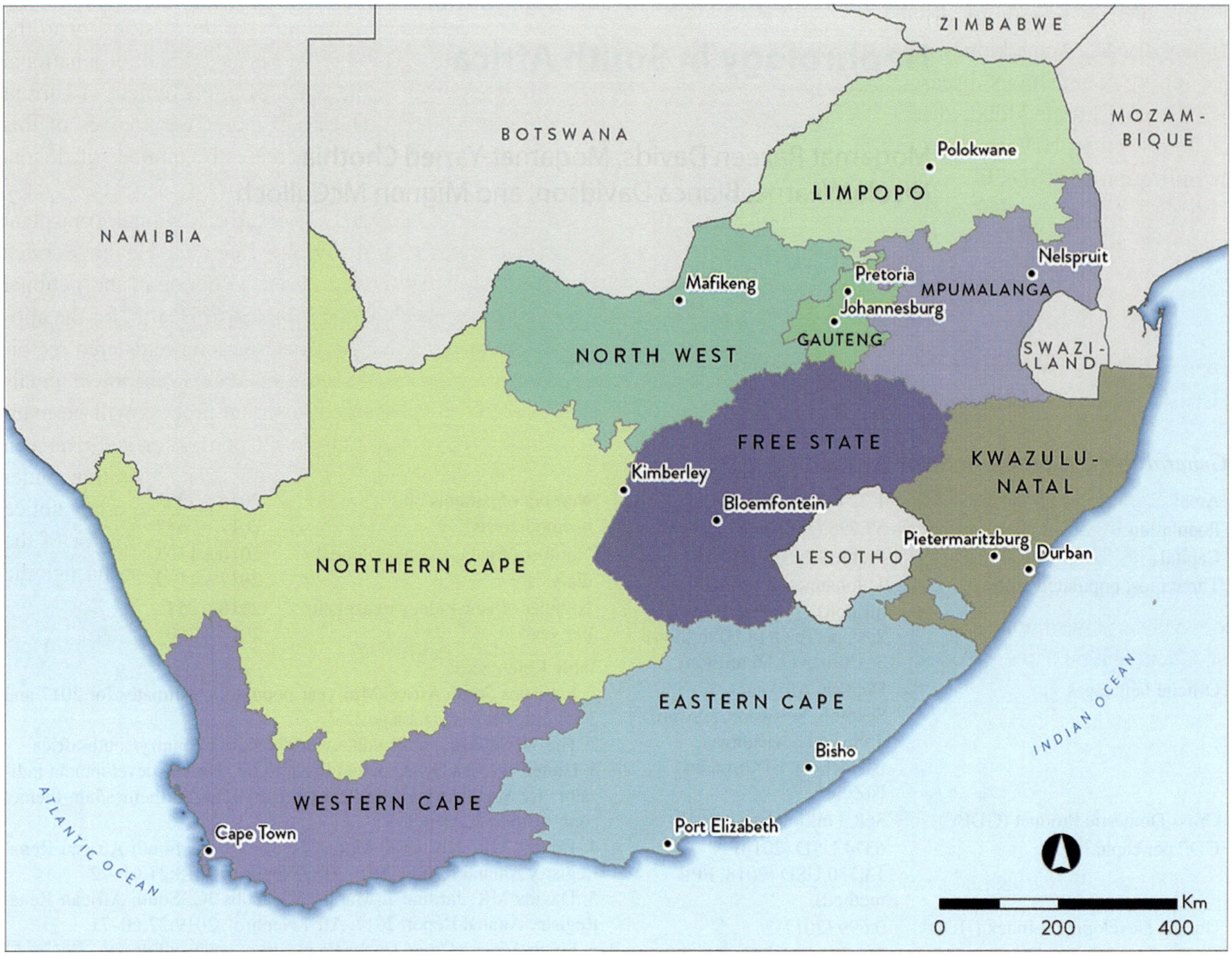


**Fig. 6.1** Provinces and major cities of South Africa

South Africa has been a democracy since 1994, but still struggles with the legacy of apartheid, which entrenched inequality on the basis of ethnicity. South Africa has one of the highest inequality rates in the world, with a Gini coefficient of 0.63 in 2015. It is classified as an upper-middle-income country by the World Bank [3] but high levels of unemployment and poverty exist among previously disadvantaged communities.

The expenditure on health as percentage of GDP was 8.1% in 2016. There is a two-tier model of healthcare: a well-resourced private healthcare sector that mainly serves the 16% of the population who are able to afford medical insurance, and a poorly resourced public sector serving mainly the 84% of the population who are uninsured [4].

Like many other African countries, South Africa labours under the quadruple burdens of infections, non-communicable diseases, pregnancy-related and injury-related disorders. While communicable diseases have long been the leading causes of death and disease burden in sub-Saharan Africa, it is estimated that non-communicable diseases (NCDs) will be the leading cause of death by 2030 [5]. Risk behaviours for NCDs such as smoking, alcohol use, physical inactivity and unhealthy diet are on the rise [6]. In young South Africans, cardiometabolic risk factors are increased, with 40.2% being overweight or obese, and the metabolic syndrome is present in 3.1% of females and 6.0% of males [7]. Injuries related to violence or road traffic accidents also contribute a substantial disease burden.

South Africa carries a heavy burden of HIV infection, with approximately 13.1% of the population (approximately 7.5 million people) living with HIV [1]. Significant improvements in mortality rates and life expectancy have been recorded following the increased availability of antiretroviral treatment (ART) but the numbers of new infections remain high, especially among young women.

All of these factors are driving the current epidemic of kidney disease. Acute kidney injury (AKI) often develops in the setting of infectious diseases, complicated pregnancies, or injuries. Chronic kidney disease (CKD) may follow AKI or be related to HIV or other infections and is a frequent complication of NCDs like diabetes mellitus and hypertension. In a review on the burden of NCDs in South Africa, Mayosi et al. [8] reported a 67% increase in deaths from kidney disease from 1999 to 2006.

## Brief History of Nephrology and Nephrology Highlights in South Africa

Despite many challenges, nephrology in South Africa has been fortunate to develop in a similar way as higher-income countries, albeit on a much smaller scale. The first haemodialysis (HD) treatment was performed in 1957 by a general practitioner in Krugersdorp, close to Johannesburg. The doctor, whose name remains unknown, had observed dialysis treatment abroad and developed his own version of the Kolff rotating drum machine. AJ (Tony) Leonsins established an acute dialysis programme at the Johannesburg General Hospital in 1958 [9] and Groote Schuur Hospital in Cape Town followed in 1959 [10]. Chronic HD clinics were established in the 1960s in Johannesburg and Cape Town, before developing in the rest of the country.

The first kidney transplant in South Africa was performed in Johannesburg, in August 1966, by Thomas Starzl and Bert Myburgh [11]. Christiaan Barnard performed the first kidney transplant in Cape Town in October 1967 and performed the world's first human heart transplant soon thereafter. His kidney transplant patient lived for more than 20 years and died with a functioning graft.

Other important milestones for South African nephrology were the establishment of national organizations for the promotion of nephrology. The South African Renal Society and the National Kidney Foundation of South Africa were established in 1967. South Africa was the second country in the world (after the USA) to form both a national kidney foundation and a national renal society. These bodies were able to lobby the authorities for recognition and the provision of facilities to treat patients with end-stage kidney disease (ESKD) [10].

The South African Transplant Society was established in 1970 and the South African Dialysis and Transplantation Registry in 1977. The registry failed due to resource constraints after it published its 1994 data. It was resurrected almost two decades later as the South Africa Renal Registry, publishing 2012 data in its first annual report. It has published reports regularly since then and provides country-wide data on all patients being treated with kidney replacement therapy (KRT) [10].

South Africans have been involved with the African Association of Nephrology (AFRAN) since its earliest days. Yackoob Seedat was the first to join, as an individual member, in 1987 and full membership of the South African Renal Society followed in 1995 when sanctions were lifted. Anthony Meyers, Sarala Naicker and Charles Swanepoel have served either as president of AFRAN or as president of the AFRAN Congress.

The African Journal of Nephrology (AJN) is the official AFRAN journal and was established in 1997, with Maher Fouad Ramzy of Egypt as the founding editor. The Journal has been run from South Africa since 2012, with Alain Assounga as editor-in-chief. Razeen Davids, Fergus Caskey and Faiçal Jarraya are the current associate editors. In 2016, Razeen Davids supervised the migration of AJN to an online, open-access publication which uses the Open Journal Systems platform and is hosted by Stellenbosch University. Papers are published as they are accepted (in a single, continuous issue annually) and articles written in English or French are considered.

The African Paediatric Nephrology Association (AFPNA) was founded in 2000 and South African paediatric nephrologists have played an active role. Mignon McCulloch is the current AFPNA president. In the last 10 years, combined AFRAN/AFPNA congresses have been very successful in reaching both the adult and paediatric nephrology communities.

South Africans have made positive contributions to global nephrology through their involvement with various organizations. Leadership roles have been played by Sarala Naicker, Anthony Meyers and Charles Swanepoel on the International Society of Nephrology (ISN) Council, and by Sarala Naicker on the ISN Executive Committee. Sarala Naicker also served as chair of the ISN Education Committee and Nominating Committee and was awarded the International Distinguished Medal of the National Kidney Foundation (USA) in 2005. In 2013, Yackoob Seedat received an ISN Pioneer Award for extraordinary contributions to nephrology in the African region. Mignon McCulloch has served on the Executive Committee of the International Paediatric Nephrology Association (IPNA), and Sarala Naicker and Brett Cullis on the International Society for Peritoneal Dialysis (ISPD) Council. Sarala Naicker also chaired the ISPD Fellowships and Awards Committee. Brett Cullis was appointed chairperson of the 'Saving Young Lives' Steering Committee in 2019. Elmi Muller is the current vice-president of The Transplantation Society (TTS) and Mignon McCulloch the president of the International Paediatric Transplantation Society (IPTA).

South Africa has also contributed to the training of nephrologists from many African countries through the ISN, IPNA and ISPD Fellowship programmes. Many of these trainees are now making major contributions to nephrology and kidney care in their home regions.

The World Congress of Nephrology was successfully hosted in Cape Town, in 2015, with Charles Swanepoel the chairperson of the local organizing committee and Mignon McCulloch co-chair of the paediatrics scientific committee. This was a huge highlight for South African and African nephrology as it was the first time that the meeting was held on the African continent.

## Kidney Diseases in South Africa

### Acute Kidney Injury and Critical Care Nephrology

In South Africa, many patients develop community-acquired AKI and present late to healthcare facilities, leading to an increased need for acute dialysis support and high mortality rates. Difficulties with transport are common, especially for patients from rural areas. With acute dialysis mostly available at tertiary centres, most patients with AKI are only referred once the healthcare practitioner at the primary or secondary level facility anticipates that dialysis may be needed.

A 2009 study from Cape Town reviewed the outcomes of 198 patients admitted to the medical intensive care unit (ICU) and reported that 23.2% of patients either had established AKI at ICU admission or developed it during their ICU stay [12]. The patients with AKI had an average age of 44 years, most were male, and more than half had comorbid conditions that included diabetes, hypertension and congestive heart failure. Acute tubular necrosis due to sepsis was the most common cause of AKI. The ICU patients with AKI had a much higher mortality compared to patients without AKI (47.8% vs. 17.5%). Predictors of mortality included high APACHE II scores, the need for dialysis, multiple organ failure and oliguria.

More recently, a few larger studies have been published. A prospective study in Cape Town included 366 patients with AKI and reported a 30-day mortality rate of 38.6% for patients admitted to the ICU [13]. The mortality rate was 40.7% in the ICU patients who required dialysis support. The patient profile was similar to the earlier study [12] but additional comorbidities included HIV infection and CKD. Mechanical ventilation was the only predictor of 90-day mortality.

A 4-year retrospective cohort study from the Free State province focused on continuous renal replacement therapy (CRRT)-requiring AKI, and reported that patients were older, predominantly male and had underlying diabetes, hypertension, heart disease and HIV [14]. The overall mortality rate was 31%. HIV infection and female sex were strong predictors of death at 90 days.

Most recently, a study from Johannesburg on 324 patients with dialysis-requiring AKI reported an overall mortality rate of 23% and a renal recovery rate of 31% [15]. Approximately 45% had long-term sequelae, including 23% with dialysis dependence, while 22% were transferred to an outpatient facility with eventual dialysis cessation.

### AKI in Human Immunodeficiency Virus Infection

With 70% of the world's HIV population living in sub-Saharan Africa, HIV-related kidney diseases have become a major burden in South Africa. Despite having the largest ART programme in the world, the first diagnosis of HIV is often made during hospitalization for complications of HIV infection [16]. AKI is common [16] and may develop due to hypovolaemia, sepsis and the use of nephrotoxic drugs. Glomerular disease can also manifest as AKI and may be the underlying condition upon which an additional insult has precipitated AKI [17–19]. AKI in hospitalized HIV-infected patients has a high risk of mortality, even after the initiation of ART [20].

Tenofovir disoproxil fumarate (TDF) may cause AKI, CKD or Fanconi syndrome, especially in patients with pre-existing renal impairment, low body weight, older age, advanced HIV disease, diabetes, hypertension, and concomitant use of other nephrotoxic drugs [20]. A prospective cohort study from the North West province found that TDF-exposed patients were more likely to have severe AKI, had higher serum creatinine concentrations at hospital discharge, and a lower rate of recovery of renal function at 3 months [21]. There were no differences regarding in-hospital or 3-month mortality. Vomiting and diarrhoea at presentation were predictors of severe AKI.

In a study from Johannesburg, 15% of patients with kidney failure were HIV-positive, with sepsis the cause of AKI in 60%. The mortality rate was 44%, as compared to 47% in the HIV-negative patients [22]. In Cape Town, sepsis and acute tubular necrosis were the most common causes of AKI in a series of 117 HIV-positive patients who received acute dialysis. The mortality rate was 41% [23]. A recent study from Bloemfontein reported a mortality rate of 60% (and 10% in HIV-uninfected patients) among HIV-infected ICU patients needing CRRT [14].

A retrospective study from Cape Town reported no difference in in-hospital mortality of AKI in HIV-infected patients as compared to those who were HIV seronegative (34.5% vs. 29.1%, respectively, $p = 0.34$) [24]. More recently, a study from Johannesburg reported higher mortality in HIV-infected patients with dialysis-requiring AKI; however, better renal recovery rates were seen in the HIV-infected patients who survived [15]. In both studies, septic acute tubular necrosis was the most common cause of AKI.

### AKI and Toxins

In sub-Saharan Africa, more than 80% of people use traditional medicines as their principle form of healthcare. Many of these medicines have been associated with kidney injury, and delayed presentation to medical care [25]. It has been estimated that one-third of AKI may be related to the use of traditional medicines [26]. However, this may be an underestimate due to the difficulty in confirming their use. In most cases, the mechanism of nephrotoxicity is unknown; however, hypovolaemia due to the vomiting and diarrhoea which may follow the use of traditional medicines is a major risk factor.

Culprit compounds that have been identified in locally used remedies include *Callilepis laureola* (locally referred to as 'impila') [27], potassium dichromate [28] and Cape aloe [29]. Table 6.1 provides examples of traditional medicines used in Southern Africa that have known nephrotoxic effects.

Animal toxins are also a major cause of AKI in Africa, which may follow snake and spider bites, and scorpion stings. South Africa has 38 venomous snake species and the most common species responsible for life-threatening envenomation is *Bitis arietans* (commonly referred to as the puff adder) [30]. The highest incidence of snake bites occurs along the north-eastern coastal belt of the KwaZulu-Natal province and is reported to be 28–96.5 per 100,000 per year [31, 32]. The rates of AKI and death due to snake bites in South Africa are very low, with the latter reported to be 0.08–2.67 per 100,000 [33]. Mechanisms for AKI may be related to intravascular haemolysis, hypotension, hyperviscosity, myoglobinuria and haemorrhage [34]. The renal pathology includes acute tubular necrosis, acute interstitial nephritis and proliferative glomerulonephritis. A recent study from KwaZulu-Natal that included 879 patients reported that cytotoxic snake bites were the most common (98%) [35]. AKI was an uncommon complication, with only 3.4% of patients having a serum creatinine concentration exceeding 115 μmol/L. None of the patients required dialysis.

Medically important spider bites in South Africa include neurotoxin- and cytotoxin-producing spiders [36]. The most common species responsible is the button or widow spider, from the genus *Lactrodectus*. These spiders produce a neurotoxin which causes an enormous release of neurotransmitters, stimulating somatic and autonomic nerves. Clinical features include profuse sweating, abdominal rigidity, hypertension, tachycardia, restlessness and agitation. This toxidrome is referred to as lactrodectism. In a South African study of 45 patients with lactrodectism, there were no reported cases of AKI [37].

**Table 6.1** Nephrotoxic effects of some traditional medicines used in Southern Africa

| Nomenclature | | | |
|---|---|---|---|
| Scientific name | Colloquial name | Common uses | Nephrotoxic effects |
| *Aloe vera species* | Cape aloe | Arthritis, burns/skin conditions, hypertension, purging/laxative, dyspepsia, anti-inflammatory, cosmetics, eye ailments, venereal diseases, infertility and impotence | Volume depletion and electrolyte imbalance<br>Acute tubular necrosis<br>Acute interstitial nephritis |
| *Cymbopogon citrullus* | Lemongrass | Diabetes, oral thrush | Volume depletion/diarrhoea<br>Chronic kidney disease secondary to chronic interstitial nephritis |
| *Crotalaria laburnifolia* | Wild sun hemp<br>Rattlepod<br>Birdflower | Enema, purging, dysmenorrhoea, dyspepsia, abortifacient, antispasmodic | Acute tubular necrosis (nephrotoxic alkaloids)<br>Hepatorenal failure |
| *Callilepsis laureola* | Ox-eye daisy<br>Impila | Dyspepsia, anti-parasitic, impotence, infertility, purging, evil spirits | Acute tubular necrosis<br>Acute interstitial nephritis<br>Hepatorenal failure<br>Chronic kidney disease<br>Hyperkalaemia |

Adapted from Stanifer et al. [25]

Scorpion stings are a significant problem in South Africa [38]. Most scorpion stings are harmless, with only *Parabuthus granulatus* causing life-threatening stings in South Africa. Children are particularly vulnerable and have a reported mortality of 20% [39]. *P. granulatus* venom contains a neurotoxin that acts on the sodium channels of excitable cells, stimulating the autonomic nervous system and causing neurological hyperexcitability. Respiratory failure, the primary cause of death, may develop within 1–2 hours following envenomation [39]. A study of 42 patients with scorpionism conducted in the Western Cape province reported no renal complications [40].

#### Pregnancy-Related AKI

Obstetric AKI remains an important cause of AKI in African countries, mainly secondary to preeclampsia/eclampsia, sepsis and haemorrhage. A study published in 1978 from the province of KwaZulu-Natal reported that the most common cause of AKI during pregnancy was septic abortion [41]; however, a decade later a report from the same centre found that this was overtaken by preeclampsia/eclampsia as the leading cause [42]. Septic abortion is now an uncommon cause of AKI, most likely due to the introduction of the Choice on Termination of Pregnancy Act (Act 92 of 1996).

A large study that included 1547 women from three South African tertiary hospitals recently described the outcomes of women with pre-eclampsia [43]. They reported that 17.6% of the pregnancies were complicated by AKI and 3% of the women with AKI died. In women with the highest blood pressure (systolic BP >200 mmHg), AKI developed in 40%. A prediction model for AKI that included admission gestational age, blood pressure and protein on urine dipsticks gave an area under the receiver operating curve value of 0.68.

A study of 58 women with eclampsia in rural KwaZulu-Natal reported that, of the 49 'booked' patients, 11 (22.4%) had risk factors which had been identified during antenatal care. Persistent proteinuria and haematuria had been identified in four patients, gestational hypertension in two patients, mild to moderate pre-eclampsia in two patients, and three patients had uncontrolled blood pressure on all antenatal visits [44].

Renal sequelae occurred in one-third (32.7%) of patients and a single death was recorded in an unbooked patient who had a cerebrovascular accident and multi-organ failure.

A study from Cape Town [45] that included 61 pregnant patients with AKI and HELLP syndrome (Haemolysis, Elevated Liver enzymes and Low Platelets) reported no difference in outcomes between patients that were at greater or less than 36 weeks gestation. Seven (11.5%) patients required dialysis support; 6 of the 7 were at <36 weeks gestation. The mortality rate was 3.3%. More stillborn foetuses occurred in woman at <36 weeks gestation.

#### 'Saving Young Lives'

'Saving Young Lives' (SYL) is a partnership between several international nephrology organizations: ISN, IPNA, ISPD and Euro PD. This initiative was launched in 2012 and aims to develop acute peritoneal dialysis (PD) programmes in low-resource settings [46, 47]. The programme focuses on developing hospital capacity and the training of staff, as well as educating people within communities about AKI so that it can be prevented and also allow earlier recognition of patients that will require hospitalization.

South Africa has played a major supporting role in the SYL programme, with hands-on training on acute PD provided at Red Cross War Memorial Children's Hospital in Cape Town to more than 75 teams of nurses and doctors. This is currently one of only two such courses offered in sub-Saharan Africa (delivered in English in Cape Town and in French in Dakar, Senegal). Physician–nurse pairs have been trained and their hospitals have pledged their support. Attendees have been taught how to use creative alternatives to commercially available cuffed catheters and PD fluids. Between January 2013 and September 2018, the SYL initiative assisted more than 300 children and adults with AKI (average age 11.6 years) [48]. Acute PD was performed for an average of 11.6 days and 64% of those treated completely recovered their kidney function (personal communication, Brett Cullis and Mignon McCulloch). Although a relatively small number of patients have benefited directly from the SYL initiatives, it is evident that the programme can work in low-resource settings by increasing awareness of the prevention and treatment of AKI within communities. For the programme to have a wider reach, it will require buy-in from governments and therefore advocacy is an important component of this initiative.

## Chronic Kidney Disease

Increases in NCDs, pregnancy-related disorders, injuries and the high burden of infectious diseases all contribute to the epidemic of CKD being experienced in South Africa.

#### Issues in the Diagnosis and Staging of CKD

The accurate estimation of glomerular filtration rate (GFR) is critically important in the diagnosis and staging of CKD. The Modification of Diet in Renal Disease (MDRD) and Chronic Kidney Disease Epidemiology Collaboration (CKD-EPI) equations are two commonly used formulae to estimate GFR in adults. The CKD-EPI equation is recommended in current guidelines unless another equation has superior accuracy in a specific population.

Four South African studies have validated GFR prediction equations against measured GFR using nuclear medicine methods. Van Deventer et al. [49] studied 100 Black South Africans, Madala et al. [50] studied 91 Black South Africans and 57 of Indian origin, Moodley et al. [51] studied 287 Black and Indian patients and Holness et al. [52] studied 80 South Africans of mixed ancestry. The van Deventer and Madala studies reported good performance of the MDRD equation in Black South Africans and concluded that the correction factor for ethnicity should not be used. Madala et al. suggested that a new correction factor, or a new equation, is needed for South Africans of Indian ancestry. Moodley et al. found better performance of the CKD-EPI equation (without the correction factor) than the MDRD equation in Black patients, and similar performance in patients of Indian ancestry. Holness et al. found that both equations, without the ethnicity factor, had good agreement with measured GFR. The MDRD equation performed marginally better than the CKD-EPI equation. Both equations tended to overestimate GFR, with bias of 1.6 and 7.9 ml/min/1.73 $m^2$ for the MDRD and CKD-EPI equations, respectively.

## CKD Prevalence

In two studies from Cape Town, Matsha et al. [53] reported a crude prevalence of 17.3% in a geographical cohort, while Adeniyi et al. [54] reported an age-adjusted prevalence of 6.4% in a cohort of teachers. The higher estimates by Matsha et al. may at least partly be explained by the very high burden of hypertension, diabetes, obesity and smoking in their study population.

## Common Causes of CKD and ESKD

In many cases of CKD or ESKD a specific diagnosis is never established because patients present late, with poor renal function, hypertension and shrunken kidneys. Data on the aetiology of CKD are available from renal registries for some African countries. The 'CKD/ESKD unknown' category was indicated as the most common renal diagnosis in reports from Sudan [55], Tunisia [56] and Morocco [57].

### Diabetic Nephropathy

Regarding South African data on renal outcomes in patients with diabetes, two prospective cohort studies with long-term follow-up have been published. In 59 patients with type 2 diabetes, Keeton et al. [58] found that kidney failure was a major cause of death. By the end of the 12-year study, 47 patients (79.7%) had died and of these deaths, 17 (28.8%) were due to kidney failure. In another study, Gill et al. [59] followed up 88 type 1 diabetic patients for 20 years and reported a crude mortality rate of 43%, with 43% of these deaths due to kidney failure. The South African Renal Registry has reported that nearly 40% of patients receiving KRT are diabetic, while diabetic nephropathy is the primary renal diagnosis in 15.3% [60].

### Glomerulonephritis

According to South African registry data, glomerular disease was the primary renal diagnosis in 10.3% of patients on KRT in 2017 [60]. South African studies on the spectrum of biopsy-proven renal disease (Table 6.2) indicate that mesangiocapillary glomerulonephritis (GN) is the most common primary glomerular disease in the Cape Town area (Western Cape province), while focal segmental glomerulosclerosis is the most common in the north of the country. The reasons for

**Table 6.2** The spectrum of biopsy-proven glomerular disease in South Africa

| Study | Region | Period | Total biopsies | PGN | SGN |
|---|---|---|---|---|---|
| [a]Patchapen (2017) [61] | Johannesburg | 2001–2010 | 1495 | FSGS 29.8%<br>MGN 19.5%<br>MCGN 18% | LN 55.8%<br>Diabetic nephropathy 9.6%<br>Post-infectious GN 6.8% |
| Vermeulen (2019) [19] | Johannesburg | 1982–2011 | 1848 | FSGS 29.6%<br>MGN 25.7%<br>MCGN 18.1% | LN 31.0%<br>HIVAN 13.3%<br>Post-infectious GN 9.1%<br>Diabetic nephropathy 6.6% |
| Okpechi (2011) [62] | Cape Town | 2000–2009 | 1753 | MCGN 20.4%<br>Mesangioproliferative GN 19.2%<br>MGN 18.5% | LN 39.0%<br>Post-infectious GN 30.1% |
| Esmail (2019) [63] | Cape Town | 1995–2017 | 2564 | MCGN 32.2%<br>FSGS 21.2%<br>MGN 15.5%<br>Mesangioproliferative GN 14.4% | LN 42.5%<br>HIVAN 20.2%<br>Diabetic nephropathy 13.7%<br>Post-infectious GN 13.3% |

*PGN* primary glomerulonephritis, *SGN* secondary glomerulonephritis, *FSGS* focal segmental glomerulosclerosis, *MGN* membranous nephropathy, *MCGN* mesangiocapillary GN, *LN* lupus nephritis, *HIVAN* HIV-associated nephropathy
[a]This series excludes HIV-positive patients

this are unclear but may include differences in the populations in terms of ethnicity or exposure to environmental triggers. IgA nephropathy is an uncommon diagnosis.

Lupus nephritis is the most common secondary glomerular disease throughout the country. HIV-associated nephropathy (HIVAN), the most commonly identified renal pathology in HIV-positive patients, and diabetic nephropathy are the other common secondary forms of glomerular disease. Post-infectious GN, which is now rare in high-income countries, remains a significant problem in South Africa.

Tannor et al. [64] examined the utility of repeat renal biopsies in South African patients with lupus nephritis. In patients with disease flares, repeat biopsies infrequently revealed changes in histological class and seldom led to changes in treatment. Outcomes in patients needing repeat biopsies were poor, with failure to respond to induction therapy in 62.2%, ESKD within 1 year in 36.3% and a mortality rate after 1 year of 23.0%. The authors suggested that repeat biopsies be considered when the initial biopsy is non-proliferative or in the case of an inadequate response to treatment changes.

#### Kidney Disease Associated with HIV Infection

HIVAN was first reported in 1984 [65–67], with the first report from South Africa published by Bates et al. in 1994 [68]. The condition occurs especially in the absence of antiretroviral therapy and in patients with markedly reduced CD4 counts and elevated viral loads [69]. Individuals of African descent have a genetic susceptibility to the development of HIVAN and certain other renal diseases that is related to polymorphisms in the apolipoprotein L1 (APOL1) gene [70]. Kasembeli et al. [71] demonstrated that HIV-positive, ART-naïve Black South Africans with two APOL1 risk alleles are at very high risk for developing HIV-associated nephropathy. Their odds of developing HIV-associated nephropathy were 89-fold higher than HIV-positive controls without the risk alleles.

In Durban, Han et al. [72] biopsied HIV-positive patients with proteinuria who were not on ART and found that 83% had HIVAN. Gerntholtz et al. [17] described their biopsy findings in the Johannesburg area: 27% showed HIVAN, 21% had HIV-related immune complex disease (HIV-ICD), and more than half had diagnoses not directly related to the HIV infection. In another biopsy series from Johannesburg, Vermeulen et al. [19] found HIVAN in 32.7% and HIV-ICD in 11.8% of cases. In Cape Town, Wearne et al. [18] reported that HIVAN was present in 57%, immune complex disease in 8.3% and a combination of HIVAN and HIV-ICD in 21.9%.

There have been conflicting reports on the benefit of ART in patients with HIV-ICD, with Szczech et al. [73] finding that renal lesions other than HIVAN did not benefit from treatment. In contrast, two South African studies [18, 74] have demonstrated benefit in both HIVAN and HIV-ICD. Against the background of earlier studies suggesting a benefit of corticosteroids for the treatment of HIVAN [75], Wearne et al. [76] conducted a clinical trial to assess the effect of corticosteroids in ART-naïve patients with HIVAN. They demonstrated an improvement in median eGFR in the corticosteroid arm (25 vs. 9 ml/min/1.73 $m^2$) but also a higher mortality rate. The routine use of corticosteroids could therefore not be recommended.

#### Glomerular Disease Associated with Hepatitis B Virus Infection

Hepatitis B virus (HBV) infection is highly endemic in Africa. Bates et al. [77] studied South African and Namibian children with HBV-associated membranous GN and found that they frequently had prominent haematuria, raised serum transaminases or low serum complement levels. Features of mesangiocapillary GN, virus-like bodies and tubuloreticular inclusion bodies were often seen on renal biopsy in addition to the typical sub-epithelial deposits. The remission rate was 57% at 4 years. Older children and those with prominent mesangial deposits on biopsy had worse renal outcomes.

Bhimma et al. [78] have documented a significant decline in the numbers of new cases of HBV-associated MGN following the introduction of routine HBV immunization in 1995. By 2000–2001, the incidence of HBV-associated MGN had declined to 12% of the pre-immunization rate. The latest data from the South African Renal Registry indicate that 2.2% of all patients on KRT are hepatitis B positive [60].

#### Hypertensive Renal Disease

In our registry data, hypertension has been reported as the aetiology of ESKD in 35.1% of patients [60]. Gold et al. [79] reviewed the renal histology in 65 Black patients on chronic HD and reported that primary malignant hypertension was the most common cause, occurring in 49%. In the largest South African renal biopsy series [63], hypertensive renal disease was diagnosed in only 2.7% of the cases despite approximately half of the patients being hypertensive.

It appears that many patients labelled as having 'hypertensive renal disease' probably have primary glomerular disease which may be related to renal-risk variants of the APOL1 gene and have secondarily elevated blood pressure [80]. The South African Renal Registry has recommended that hypertension be recorded as the primary renal diagnosis only when the following criteria are met: hypertension known to precede renal dysfunction, left ventricular hypertrophy, proteinuria <2 g/day, and no evidence of other renal diseases [81, 82].

### Genetic Disorders

The data from South African populations on genetic renal diseases are sparse. A study of autosomal recessive polycystic kidney disease (ARPKD) in the Afrikaner population estimated the live-birth rate and the carrier rate of mutations in the PKHD1 gene at 1:11,000 and 1:53, respectively [83]. Lambie et al. [84] studied a cohort of patients from 36 Afrikaner families, finding that 27 patients, from 24 families, were homozygous for the p.M627K substitution, providing strong evidence of a founder mutation.

Regarding genetic tubular disorders, new mutations of the SLC12A3 gene, which encodes the sodium-chloride cotransporter in the distal convoluted tubule, have been reported in a South African family with Gitelman syndrome who presented with hypokalaemia and unusual food cravings [85]. Mutations of the epithelial sodium channel (ENaC) have also been identified in South African patients in association with hypertension [86, 87] and pre-eclampsia [88].

## Kidney Replacement Therapy in South Africa

South Africa is the only country on the continent that has regularly reported country-wide data on KRT in recent years. In December 2017, the number of patients who were treated with chronic dialysis or kidney transplantation stood at 10,744, a prevalence of 190 pmp [60]. The treatment modality was HD in 71.5%, PD in 11.2% and transplantation in 17.3%. This is very different from the situation two decades ago when KRT was mainly delivered by government-funded public sector facilities and more than half of all patients had functioning kidney transplants [89].

The overall KRT prevalence has been increasing due to increasing numbers of patients accessing HD in the private healthcare sector, where the treatment of ESKD is a 'prescribed minimum benefit' for patients who have private medical insurance. The prevalence of treated ESKD in the private sector (855 pmp) is on par with that of many high-income countries.

In the public sector, which serves 84% of the South African population, the prevalence of KRT (66 pmp) has fallen below the level reported for 1994, so that the disparity in access continues to increase. This rate of treatment is well below that of countries with similar or lesser gross national incomes per capita. There are also large disparities in access to KRT between ethnic groups and between different provinces, with Blacks being the most underserved group and with two provinces (Limpopo and Mpumalanga) having no public sector dialysis centres at all [60]. Section 27 of the Constitution of South Africa promises the progressiverealisation of access to healthcare; however, this is not happening in the area of KRT and is a cause of great concern.

New regulations that will govern the licensing and operation of dialysis units are currently being developed by the National Department of Health. Because of the severe resource constraints, only patients who are considered transplantable, and are willing to undergo transplantation, are accepted onto public sector dialysis programmes. In many government facilities, dialysis slots are full, and a new patient can only be accommodated when an existing patient is transplanted. The South African Constitutional Court has ruled that the rationing of dialysis is appropriate, given the resource scarcity [90].

The Western Cape is the only province that has an official policy which guides the selection of patients for KRT in the public sector. These guidelines were developed through extensive consultation with stakeholders, including patient representatives and ethics experts. The 'Accountability for Reasonableness' approach and the overarching ethical principle of utilitarianism was used in this process [91]. The guidelines categorize patients into three groups. Category 1 patients are those who are excellent candidates for transplantation (e.g., younger patients, no other comorbidities) and these patients will all be accommodated on the KRT programme. Category 2 patients are those not considered as ideal candidates but who are nevertheless still transplantable. They include patients who are older than 50 years, smokers, obese patients, those with diabetes or HIV infection, etc. This category also includes patients with social circumstances that will adversely impact KRT outcomes. Patients in this category may be offered access to KRT depending on the existing capacity. Category 3 includes patients with medical or social factors making them poor transplant candidates and these patients are not offered KRT. These factors include serious major organ or mental health disease, uncontrolled HIV infection, substance abuse and non-adherence to treatment.

Kilonzo et al. reviewed the use of these selection criteria over a 4-year period, reporting that more than half (53.9%) of patients who were referred for KRT were not accepted [92]. Another centre in the same province reported that 75% of all patients considered were declined [93].

The survival of South African patients on KRT has recently been evaluated by Jardine et al. [94]. Using data from the South African Renal Registry, they found 1-year survival in incident patients ($n$ = 6,187) to be 90.4%. Higher mortality was associated with older age, province of residence and primary renal diagnosis, specifically ESKD of unknown aetiology. Overall one-year survival in prevalent patients ($n$ = 10,155) was 90.1%. There were no differences in survival rates between public and private healthcare sectors, even after adjusting for case mix, and no difference related to first treatment modality. These favourable outcomes compare well with survival rates reported from better-resourced countries [95, 96].

Recent papers on the costs of dialysis at public hospitals in the provinces of Gauteng [97] and Limpopo [98] indicate that the overall annual cost per patient (including laboratory tests and medications) is approximately USD 31,000 for HD and USD 25,000 for PD. Costs in the private sector are generally higher, with a single session of chronic HD costing around USD 150 and the monthly cost of CAPD around USD 1,600. Regarding reimbursement, in the private sector the costs of dialysis and transplantation, most medications and routine blood tests are usually fully covered by medical insurance since the treatment of ESKD is a 'prescribed minimum benefit'. In the public healthcare sector, a sliding scale (based on income) is applied and indigent patients are treated at minimal or no cost.

## Haemodialysis

In 1994, HD was the treatment modality for 29.8% of all patients on KRT (66.9% of dialysis patients) [89]. By 2017, this had changed dramatically, with 71.5% of patients on KRT being treated with HD (86.5% of dialysis patients) [60]. The median KRT vintage of the patients was 3.8 years (interquartile range (IQR) 1.8–6.5 years). The growth in the numbers of patients on HD has mainly occurred in private sector facilities. There has been a dramatic increase in the number of privately owned treatment centres over the years. In 1994, there were 31 centres contributing data to the national renal registry. Of these, 26 were public and 5 were private. By 2017, there were a total of 278 centres, with 29 of these being public and 249 being private facilities. Figure 6.2 illustrates the distribution of patients on KRT by modality in the public and private healthcare sectors in 2017.

Several public–private initiatives have been established to improve the access to KRT in the public sector and to allow patients to have their dialysis closer to home. These arrangements involve the use of spare capacity in private dialysis units for treating public sector patients at a negotiated fee per treatment.

The South African Renal Society has published guidelines for chronic dialysis (www.sa-renalsociety.org) which are widely accepted by the local nephrology community. These include guidance on the supervision and staffing of dialysis units, dialysis dose and prescription, water quality standards, infection control, and routine laboratory testing. The recommended staff (nurses and/or clinical technologists) to patient ratio is 1:4; no recommendations exist for nephrologists/physicians.

Thrice-weekly dialysis sessions for 4 hours is the usual treatment regimen. Convective therapies are not yet widely used, but this option is available at certain private sector treatment centres. High-flux membranes are routinely used, and bicarbonate is the usual buffer. While dialyzer re-use is allowed and has been practiced in the past, it is no longer done in view of the human resource requirements, the increasing costs of the reuse procedures and the decreasing costs of new dialyzers.

Patients generally have good access to erythropoiesis-stimulating agents and intravenous iron. Access to non-calcium-containing phosphate binders and cinacalcet is very limited in the public sector and in the private sector may be covered by insurance only after special motivation or may need to be paid for by the patient.

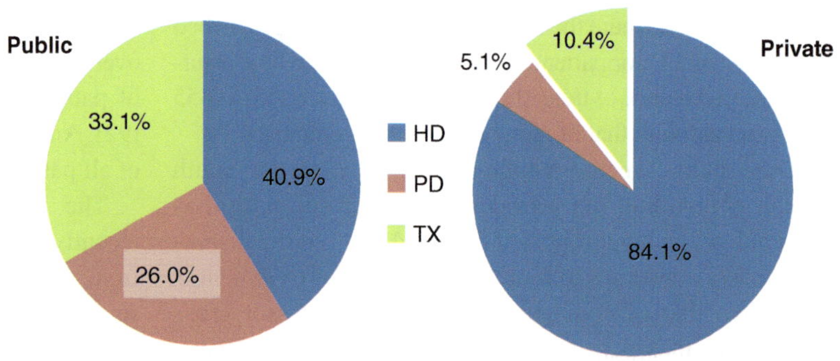


| Treatment modality | Public sector | | Private sector | |
|---|---|---|---|---|
| | Patients | % | Patients | % |
| Haemodialysis | 1,282 | 40.9 | 6,400 | 84.1 |
| Peritoneal dialysis | 814 | 26.0 | 385 | 5.1 |
| Transplant | 1,038 | 33.1 | 825 | 10.4 |

Fig. 6.2 Kidney replacement modalities in South Africa, by healthcare sector [60]

Regarding vascular access, data for 2014 from the national renal registry revealed that 54.1% of HD patients were dialyzed via an arteriovenous fistula, 32.8% via a tunnelled catheter, 7.2% via an arteriovenous graft and 5.9% via a temporary HD catheter [99].

South Africa is fortunate in having a low population prevalence of hepatitis C infection, and the hepatitis B virus carrier rate has fallen since the introduction of routine HBV vaccination. In the KRT population, the prevalence for hepatitis C seropositivity is 0.8%, for hepatitis B 2.2% and for HIV 10.8% [60]. Patients who are hepatitis B virus carriers are dialyzed in isolation.

## Peritoneal Dialysis

South Africa performs 85% of the PD in Africa [100]. Informal estimates obtained from provider companies suggest that automated PD (APD) is used by 35–50% of patients in the private sector and by around 10% of patients in the public sector. According to registry data, PD is the treatment modality for 13.5% of all dialysis patients in South Africa, and for 38.8% of dialysis patients in the public sector, where a 'PD-first' policy is often applied (Fig. 6.2) [60]. The median KRT vintage of the patients on PD was 3.5 years (IQR 1.6–6.3 years). The South African setting presents a unique set of challenges, including high rates of poverty, unemployment, lack of formal housing, running water and sanitation, as well as high crime rates which limit the ability to do home visits [101]. A recent economic analysis reported that PD costs less than HD in South Africa [97].

A number of centres have reported on their PD programmes (Table 6.3). Patient survival at 1 year is 86.7–91.3%, and at 5 years is 50.2–65.3% [101–103]. These results are comparable to those reported in other middle-income countries and in high-income countries but need to be viewed in the context of a younger cohort and the stringent selection criteria for access to KRT. Factors associated with increased mortality included diabetes [101], low BMI, low serum albumin, low haemoglobin and more than one episode of peritonitis [103].

The most common cause of technique failure was peritonitis. Black African ethnicity and increased age were strong predictors of technique failure in both cohorts from Cape Town [101, 102]. In the Groote Schuur study, 45.3% of Black patients experienced technique failure. The reasons remain unclear but may include the impact of socioeconomic status (SES). In 1994, Zent et al. [104] found that poorer SES was associated with peritonitis. Since this study, however, newer techniques (flush-before-fill) have decreased peritonitis rates. The more recent study from Limpopo echoed findings from the BRAZPD cohort and did not demonstrate an association between family income or SES and technique failure [103, 105].

The peritonitis rates reported from South African centres are generally higher than the ISPD standard of 0.67 events per patient-year [106]. It was 0.82 events per patient-year in the Limpopo study. In Cape Town, the rate was 0.87 [101] but has been steadily declining over the last 15 years [104, 107]. Ndlovu et al. [108] studied a PD cohort in the province of KwaZulu-Natal and found that HIV infection with a CD4 count <200 cells/mm$^3$ was associated with increased peritonitis risk and that HIV infection was associated with relapsing peritonitis. There was no increase in technique failure rates.

The Cape Town study by Davidson et al. [101] provides important insights into the survival of PD patients in our setting. A substantial proportion (31%) of the patients who died had technique failure but could not be offered a modality switch to HD. When a timely switch was indeed possible, survival was excellent, with no deaths recorded at 5 years.

Two studies have examined the quality of life (QOL) of patients on PD. Okaka et al. [109, 110] found that patients in Johannesburg had lower QOL scores than healthy controls, with better scores in patients under 30 years of age, those with a duration on PD of less than 4 years and those with higher incomes. In Cape Town, Tannor et al. [111] found that PD patients (as compared to patients on HD) experienced a heavier symptom burden and greater limitations related to their dialysis modality. The fear of developing peritonitis caused many patients to sacrifice social interactions to be able to do their PD exchanges at home and at the specified times.

South Africa has demonstrated that a PD-first approach can be successful in a resource-limited setting, with limited access to automated PD and icodextrin, and without home visits. This is due, at least in part, to the criteria used in rationing dialysis in the public sector, resulting in the selection of younger and healthier patients who are suitable for transplantation. Concerted efforts are required to reduce peritonitis rates as this is the leading cause of technique failure.

**Table 6.3** Patient and technique survival in PD programmes in South Africa

| | Period | *n* | Age years (mean) | DM (%) | Technique survival (%) | | | | Patient survival (%) | | | | Peritonitis rate |
|---|---|---|---|---|---|---|---|---|---|---|---|---|---|
| | | | | | 1 year | 2 year | 3 year | 5 year | 1 year | 2 year | 3 year | 5 year | |
| W Cape GSH [101] | 2008–2015 | 199 | 39 | 9.8 | 85.0 | 75.2 | – | 45.0 | 91.3 | 79.6 | – | 50.2 | 0.87 |
| W Cape TBH [102] | 2008–2014 | 170 | 36 | 1.7 | 80.0 | – | 54.0 | 39.0 | 90.0 | – | 82.0 | 63.0 | – |
| Limpopo [103] | 2007–2012 | 152 | 37 | 9.9 | 83.3 | 71.7 | – | 62.1 | 86.7 | 78.7 | – | 65.3 | 0.82 |

A notable success story is the nurse-led PD programme which was developed in the province of KwaZulu-Natal by Brett Cullis. It involved the training of local clinicians to insert PD catheters at the bedside and training a nurse to perform the dialysis procedure and assess aspects such as fluid balance, anaemia and metabolic control. After an apprenticeship of 6 months, the PD nurse took over the programme. An evaluation confirmed that all the significant medical issues were correctly identified by the nurse and that there was no difference between the management plans made by the nurse and that of the nephrologist. Ten years after its initiation, this programme continues to function, proving its sustainability. It has grown to 95 patients and has recorded peritonitis rates of approximately 1 episode in 22 patient-months.

## Kidney Transplantation

South Africa is one of only 12 countries within Africa that performs kidney transplantation, and the only African country that relies on deceased donation for the majority of its transplants [112]. Kidney transplants are performed in six public sector and nine private sector centres, located in four of the nine provinces [60]. Most public sector transplant programmes utilize immunological risk stratification protocols to reduce costs and a regimen based on cyclosporine, azathioprine and prednisone is still frequently used for low-risk patients. Transplantation in the public sector is particularly important to ensure access to new patients requiring KRT. There are currently 22 transplant coordinators in the country and these colleagues are vital to the success of our kidney transplant programmes. In areas without coordinators, local doctors or nurses assume their responsibilities [113].

The latest published renal registry data [60] (combining information from the public and private sectors) report an annual total of 260 adult and paediatric transplants, of which 50% were from deceased donation. In the private sector, most of the transplants are from living donors (62%). In comparison, the majority of public sector transplants are from deceased donation (69%). Each province has their own set of rules governing organ allocation and has their own waiting list. In provinces where transplantation is not offered, patients are added onto the list of larger provinces (e.g., patients from the Limpopo province are on the Johannesburg waiting list of Gauteng province). The waiting lists use scoring systems based on factors such as age, time on the waiting list, urgent medical indications and percentage panel-reactive antibodies. In the Western Cape, one kidney is allocated to the procuring institution and other to the first suitable patient on the common (public and private) waiting list.

Moosa [114] recently reviewed 25 years of transplantation in South Africa. During the period 1991–2015, 7191 kidney transplants were performed, the majority (58.3%) derived from deceased donors. Hospitals in Cape Town and Johannesburg performed over 75% of these transplants. The overall transplant rate was 6.4 pmp (4.8 pmp in the public sector and 15.2 pmp in the private sector) but the trend has been towards a decline in the annual number of kidney transplants performed (Fig. 6.3).

The number of deceased donor transplants has declined over the last two decades, necessitating a more flexible approach to deceased donor selection. This includes using extended criteria donors, donation after circulatory death and HIV positive-to-positive transplantation. The trend of decreasing deceased donation is not explained by the level of public awareness [115]. Poor consent rates for donation (around 33%) have been linked to education, religious beliefs, cultural traditions and a lack of transplant coordinators speaking the different local languages [114].

Muller et al. pioneered HIV-positive-to-positive transplantation in 2008, when HIV infection was still considered a contraindication to KRT. Outcomes were comparable to those of HIV-negative recipients, with a 1-year patient survival rate of 84% and 5-year survival rate of 74%. The rates of graft survival (censored for death with a functioning graft) were 93% and 84%, respectively. Rejection rates were 8% at 1 year and 22% at 3 years. The HIV infection remained well controlled, with undetectable virus in blood after transplantation [116].

A 5-year review of transplantation at Groote Schuur Hospital in Cape Town revealed that two-thirds of patients received kidneys from deceased donors and one-third from living donors. There were 7 donations after circulatory death and 11 patients were enrolled in the HIV-positive donor to HIV-positive recipient trial. Trauma accounted for 54% of deceased donations, with the vast majority of the donors being male (84%). Females accounted for 59% of the living donors [117]. Patient survival for this cohort at 1, 2 and 5 years was 90.4%, 87.9% and 83.1%, respectively. Graft survival was 89.4%, 85.8% and 80.0%, respectively.

Longer-term outcomes have been reported in a study of 100 kidney transplants from Johannesburg. The 10-year patient and graft survival rates were 80.4% and 66.8%, respectively [118]. Despite many constraints, the outcomes were comparable with international registry data.

South Africa's proud history in organ transplantation was blemished by organ trafficking involving living, non-related renal transplantation during the period 2001–2003. This practice was halted by new guidelines and safeguards. Written informed consent is obtained by dedicated transplantation coordinators from all next of kin prior to transplantation from deceased donors. All centres have signed the Declaration of Istanbul and all non-related living donor transplants require prior approval by a national Ministerial Advisory Committee.

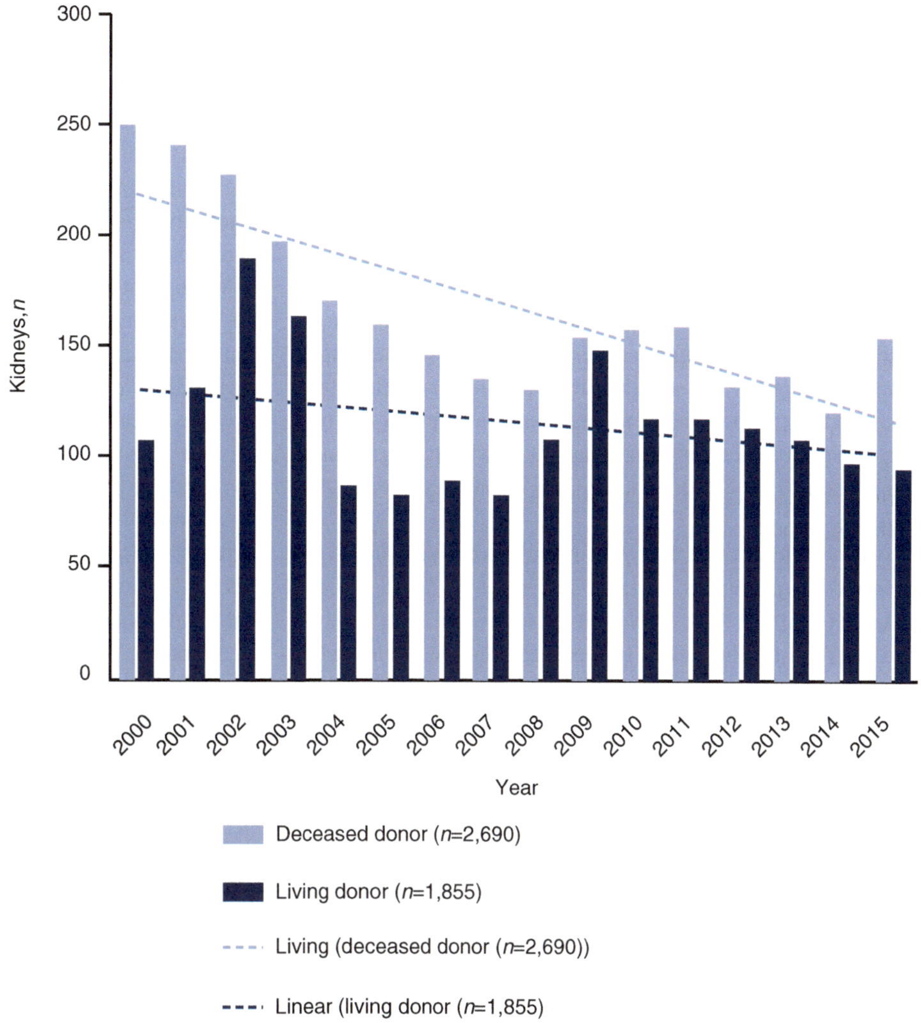


**Fig. 6.3** Numbers of deceased and living donor kidney transplants in South Africa, 2000–2015 [114]

## Paediatric Nephrology

The epidemiology of paediatric kidney disease in Africa has been largely unknown but, in South Africa, this should now improve as paediatric data is now being collected as part of the South African Renal Registry [119]. Infants commonly suffer from congenital abnormalities of the kidney and urinary tract (CAKUT) but little is described in Africa. Antenatal scans are not routinely available for all pregnant mothers thus there is often late presentation and delayed diagnosis of disorders needing urological intervention. Kidney biopsies in paediatric patients are mainly performed in larger centres where there is good radiology and anaesthesiology support, and many cases from secondary level centres therefore have to be transferred to these tertiary centres.

A recent study from Red Cross Children's Hospital in Cape Town described pelvi-ureteric junction obstruction in 100 infants and reported that the obstruction resolved spontaneously in 70% of cases, mainly in mild to moderate cases [120]. Diseases such as cystinosis, atypical haemolytic-uraemic syndrome (aHUS) and primary hyperoxaluria are being recognized in South Africa with increasing frequency and there is now a Rare Diseases Group advocating for these children (https://www.rarediseases.co.za/) as many of these conditions require expensive genetic tests and the use of expensive drugs. Genetic testing is having a major impact on paediatric nephrology and the development of inexpensive testing is likely to expand this area considerably.

HIV-associated kidney disease in children is rarely seen since the implementation of the Maternal-to-Child-Transmission Prevention programmes and the availability of ART. A study of 620 young people (9–14 years) in Cape Town who had been on ART >6 months reported that proteinuria was uncommon [121].

Post-infectious GN is a common cause of glomerular disease in South African children, with the incidence decreasing in recent years in the Johannesburg area (personal communication, Udai Kala) but remaining a problem in other parts of South Africa.

Childhood nephrotic syndrome still has minimal change disease as the predominant cause. This mostly responds to steroids during early childhood and goes into remission after adolescence. Immunosuppressive agents, including calcineurin inhibitors, are used routinely as steroid-sparing agents. Rituximab is being used more often for frequently relapsing cases. Steroid side-effects are important in growing children and have special relevance in South Africa where there are also other causes of poor growth including poor food security and a high burden of infections. Hepatitis B-related nephrotic syndrome, previously a significant problem in South African children, has all but disappeared since the introduction of routine hepatitis B immunization in 1995 [77, 78].

Vasculitides, especially Takayasu's arteritis, are well described in paediatric nephrology centres in South Africa. Takayasu's arteritis presents with hypertension, seizures and cardiac failure. The use of immunosuppressive agents (steroids, cyclophosphamide and methotrexate) and revascularization by interventional radiology or surgery has produced good outcomes [122].

AKI is often related to poverty-related diseases such as gastroenteritis and other infections. Short-term dialysis for children with AKI is available, either as acute PD or acute HD (often in adult units). The 'Saving Young Lives' initiative has contributed to the increased use of acute PD for children with AKI [46]. CRRT treatments in children and infants with AKI are becoming more accessible with the development of 'child-friendly' machines and equipment [123].

CKD is a silent killer as children may present late with fatigue, pallor and stunted growth. Chronic dialysis is mostly available in tertiary centres where paediatric surgeons are available for the insertion of dialysis catheters. PD with home-based machines is the dialysis modality of choice so that children can receive dialysis overnight and attend school during the day. HD requires the availability of a dialysis slot and also the presence of a parent to accompany the child for thrice-weekly treatment sessions. The impact of the disease on the whole family must therefore be taken into consideration [124]. Kidney transplantation in children is very successful and by far the preferred KRT modality, with pre-emptive living-related transplantation being the optimal management [125]. Children are prioritized on transplant waiting lists in view of their poor growth and loss of schooling if they remain on dialysis. Post-transplantation infections are a challenge but international guidelines have local relevance to South Africa too [126]. Paediatric palliative care is an area that has been developing recently to cater for children with ESKD who are not treated with dialysis or transplantation.

## Adolescent Nephrology

There are no published data on the prevalence or aetiologies of ESKD in adolescents in Africa. Extrapolating paediatric and adult data from South Africa, and adolescent data from the United States, Australia and New Zealand, it is likely that glomerular disease is the leading cause of ESKD in South African adolescents [127–130].

Adolescent nephrology is a growing area in South Africa and there are efforts by paediatric and adult doctors to improve the transition of patients from paediatric to adult services. However, difficulties do arise for children who may have developmental delays and fail to meet the criteria required for entry into the resource-limited adult KRT programmes.

Adolescents are a vulnerable group, due to their neurocognitive development, engagement in high-risk social activities and prevalence of mental illness [131]. Numerous challenges exist in treating adolescents with kidney disease and these challenges are amplified in settings with limited access to healthcare and KRT [132]. Paediatric units tend to have more generous staff-to-patient ratios than adult units and adult nephrologists are less familiar with the diseases of children such as CAKUT and metabolic diseases. In South African hospitals, transfer to the adult services usually occurs in the early teens but many nephrology centres are now changing their policies so that the transfers occur at older ages.

An adolescent nephrology service in Cape Town [133] reported that adolescents with CKD experience feelings of loneliness and isolation, anxiety over their illness, dissatisfaction with their physical appearance, difficulties communicating with staff (who appear not to appreciate the difficulty of the lifestyle changes required) and difficulties with remembering to take all their medication.

## Nephrology Practice in South Africa

The provision of optimal care for adults and children with renal disease requires multi-disciplinary teams of professionals which include nephrologists, nurses, renal technologists, surgeons, dieticians, psychologists and social workers. This is usually the case for KRT programmes in South Africa. In addition, some paediatric programmes involve educators and play therapists. Access to high care and intensive care facilities are important for both adult and paediatric programmes.

Practicing as a nephrologist in South Africa requires obtaining a 4-year specialist qualification in internal medicine or paediatrics, followed by 2 years of sub-speciality training in nephrology or paediatric nephrology. In the public sector, the gross annual salary for a nephrologist is approximately USD 90,000. Income is generally higher in the private sector but no published data are available on this.

Currently, there are insufficient numbers of nephrologists in South Africa, and a markedly uneven distribution among the different provinces and healthcare sectors. A recent study by Hassen et al. [134] characterized the South African nephrologist workforce and reported that there were a total of 120 adult and 22 paediatric nephrologists in 2018, an overall density of 2.5 nephrologists pmp. This is well below the median for middle-income countries of 10.8 pmp [135].

The median age was 45 years and there was a male predominance (66%). Most of the adult nephrologists (60%) are working in the private sector, while most of the paediatric nephrologists (68%) are based in the public sector. There is also a striking geographic maldistribution, with 92% of the nephrologists working in three of the nine South African provinces (Gauteng, Western Cape and KwaZulu-Natal), only one each in Limpopo and the Northern Cape, and none in the North West and Mpumalanga.

Regarding their skills, most South African nephrologists are competent at placing temporary HD catheters and performing native and allograft kidney biopsies. Approximately half report competence with respect to performing renal ultrasound and bedside PD catheter insertion, and one-quarter feel competent at placing tunnelled HD catheters [134].

Qualitative data from Hassen et al. [134] indicate that South African nephrologists generally have positive attitudes towards their chosen profession and would recommend nephrology as a career to junior doctors or students. While most are happy with their remuneration, workload and working environment, there are significant numbers who are not. In the public sector, nephrologists face considerable resource limitations, a high workload, challenging policies and unsatisfactory remuneration. In the private sector, they face a high workload, large administrative burdens and uncertainty about the potential impact of the proposed National Health Insurance. A substantial number are contemplating emigration or early retirement.

Published data on the other professionals in the nephrology team are sparse. There were 205 renal clinical technologists registered with the Health Professions Council of South Africa in March 2019.

## Nephrology Education

ISN's Commission for the Global Advancement of Nephrology (COMGAN), the forerunner of ISN's global outreach programs, was crucial in promoting nephrology education and care in many regions of the world and in Africa, in particular [136]. Sarala Naicker was invited to join COMGAN by its inaugural chairs, Barry Brenner and John Dirks, and served as chair of the Africa region, visiting many African countries, arranging and participating in educational activities, and meeting the authorities in these countries.

The ISN Fellowship Program is a noteworthy initiative which sponsors nephrology training for physicians from developing countries. To date, 214 ISN Fellowships have been awarded to Africans, including 6 to South African doctors who trained at centres in the USA, Canada, Australia and the UK. In recent years, South Africa has become an important nephrology training ground for the African continent, with 73 physicians from other African countries, and 2 from Nepal, being awarded ISN Fellowships for nephrology training at South African institutions. Yewondwossen Tadesse, from Ethiopia, was the first ISN Fellow to train in South Africa, with Sarala Naicker at the University of Natal in Durban, in 1999. Most of the fellows have been hosted at the academic hospitals linked to Stellenbosch University, the University of Cape Town and the University of the Witwatersrand and many have obtained Masters or PhD degrees during their training in South Africa.

A 25-year review of the ISN Fellowship Program reported that many ISN Fellows have gone on to assume leadership positions in their home institutions, countries and regions. Fellows who had trained at centres within their region reported fewer difficulties with obtaining visas, more hands-on clinical training, greater relevance and impact on their home units, and less 'brain drain' [137].

Fellowships from IPNA and ISPD have also allowed many health professionals from African countries to come to South Africa for training in paediatric nephrology and PD, respectively. There have been 33 trainees from African countries who have been trained as paediatric nephrologists at South African hospitals linked to the University of Cape Town (Red Cross War Memorial Children's Hospital), the University of the Witwatersrand (Charlotte Maxeke Johannesburg Academic Hospital and Chris Hani Baragwanath Hospital) and the University of Pretoria (Steve Biko Academic Hospital).

The ISN Educational Ambassadors Program, initiated by its first chairperson, Sarala Naicker, is another important educational initiative of ISN. The programme supports nephrology in the developing world through the delivery of focused, high-quality, hands-on training by experts over a period of 1–4 weeks. Razeen Davids, Mignon McCulloch, Elmi Muller and Ikechi Okpechi are South Africans who have delivered training in Kenya, Ghana, Nigeria, Zambia, Zimbabwe and Nepal as ISN Educational Ambassadors.

Apart from contributions to the training of nephrology fellows from other countries, South Africans have been involved in other important educational initiatives. Brett Cullis, Mignon McCulloch, Peter Nourse and Nicola Wearne have trained many African doctors and nurses in delivering acute PD in the 'Saving Young Lives' programme [46], while

Sarala Naicker [138–140], Brett Cullis [141] and Charles Swanepoel [139] have had leading roles in developing international nephrology guidelines and chairing workgroups and consensus conferences. Razeen Davids has contributed to a series of teaching articles [142–144] and developed an interactive e-learning resource on the topic of electrolyte and acid-base disorders [145, 146], and Mignon McCulloch has co-edited a new handbook on paediatric critical care nephrology [147].

Two South Africans have been honoured for their outstanding achievements in the field of education in nephrology via the ISN's Roscoe R Robinson Award. Sarala Naicker and Mignon McCulloch were recipients of this prestigious award in 2009 and 2017, respectively.

## Conclusions

Like many African countries, South Africa faces an epidemic of acute and chronic kidney disease. There are many competing priorities, resulting in serious resource constraints to providing comprehensive kidney care, especially in the public healthcare sector which serves most of the population. Nephrology is a well-developed speciality in the country, with active training programmes and good national organizations to carry the discipline forward. South African contributions to African and global nephrology have been substantial and should continue to grow in the future.

## References


1. Mid-year population estimates, 2018. Pretoria: Statistics South Africa; 2018.
2. General household survey, 2018. Pretoria: Statistics South Africa; 2019.
3. South Africa overview. Washington, DC: The World Bank; 2019.
4. Council for Medical Schemes Annual Report 2017/18. Pretoria: Council for Medical Schemes; 2018.
5. Marquez PV, Farrington JL. The challenge of non-communicable diseases and road traffic injuries in Sub-Saharan Africa: an overview. Washington, DC: The World Bank; 2013.
6. Noncommunicable diseases among young people in Africa. Washington, DC: Population Reference Bureau; 2015.
7. Sekokotla MA, Goswami N, Sewani-Rusike CR, Iputo JE, Nkeh-Chungag BN. Prevalence of metabolic syndrome in adolescents living in Mthatha, South Africa. Ther Clin Risk Manag. 2017;13:131–7.
8. Mayosi BM, Flisher AJ, Lalloo UG, Sitas F, Tollman SM, Bradshaw D. The burden of non-communicable diseases in South Africa. Lancet. 2009;374:934–47.
9. Keene R. Our graduates 1924–2012. Johannesburg: Adler Museum of Medicine, Faculty of Health Sciences, University of the Witwatersrand; 2013.
10. Wearne N, Okpechi IG, Swanepoel CR. Nephrology in South Africa: not yet Ubuntu. Kidney Dis. 2019;5:189–96.
11. Fabian J, Maher H, Bentley A, Gaylard P, Crymble K, Rossi B, et al. Favourable outcomes for the first 10 years of kidney and pancreas transplantation at Wits Donald Gordon Medical Centre, Johannesburg, South Africa. S Afr Med J. 2016;106:172–6.
12. Friedericksen DV, Van der Merwe L, Hattingh TL, Nel DG, Moosa MR. Acute renal failure in the medical ICU still predictive of high mortality. S Afr Med J. 2009;99:873–5.
13. Dlamini TAL, Heering PJ, Chivese T, Rayner B. A prospective study of the demographics, management and outcome of patients with acute kidney injury in Cape Town, South Africa. PLoS One. 2017;12:e0177460.
14. Camara SN, Chothia M-Y. Outcomes of critically ill adult patients with continuous renal replacement therapy-requiring acute kidney injury in the Free State province of South Africa: the impact of HIV. Afr J Nephrol. 2017;20:39–44.
15. Variava M, Mashabane M, Bentley A, Naicker S. Epidemiology and outcomes of dialysis-requiring acute kidney injury at Chris Hani Baragwanath Hospital. Wits J Clin Med. 2019;1:31–6.
16. Wyatt CM, Arons RR, Klotman PE, Klotman ME. Acute renal failure in hospitalized patients with HIV: risk factors and impact on in-hospital mortality. AIDS. 2006;20:561–5.
17. Gerntholtz TE, Goetsch SJ, Katz I. HIV-related nephropathy: a South African perspective. Kidney Int. 2006;69:1885–91.
18. Wearne N, Swanepoel CR, Boulle A, Duffield MS, Rayner BL. The spectrum of renal histologies seen in HIV with outcomes, prognostic indicators and clinical correlations. Nephrol Dial Transplant. 2012;27:4109–18.
19. Vermeulen A, Menezes C, Mashabane M, Butler O, Mosiane P, Goetsch S, et al. Patterns of renal disease: a 30-year renal biopsy study at Chris Hani Baragwanath Academic Hospital, Soweto, Johannesburg, South Africa. S Afr Med J. 2019;109:486–92.
20. Boswell MT, Rossouw TM. Approach to acute kidney injury in HIV-infected patients in South Africa. S Afr J HIV Med. 2017;18:a714.
21. Seedat F, Martinson N, Motlhaoleng K, Abraham P, Mancama D, Naicker S, et al. Acute kidney injury, risk factors, and prognosis in hospitalized HIV-infected adults in South Africa, compared by tenofovir exposure. AIDS Res Hum Retrovir. 2017;33:33–40.
22. Vachiat AI, Musenge E, Wadee S, Naicker S. Renal failure in HIV-positive patients-a South African experience. Clin Kidney J. 2013;6:584–9.
23. Arendse C, Okpechi I, Swanepoel C. Acute dialysis in HIV-positive patients in Cape Town, South Africa. Nephrology. 2011;16:39–44.
24. Chothia M-Y, Ramsunder N. In-hospital mortality of HIV-positive patients with acute kidney injury a decade after the roll-out of anti-retroviral therapy in Cape Town, South Africa. Afr J Nephrol. 2019;22:46–53.
25. Stanifer JW, Kilonzo K, Wang D, Su G, Mao W, Zhang L, et al. Traditional medicines and kidney disease in low-and middle-income countries: opportunities and challenges. Semin Nephrol. 2017;37:245–59.
26. Luyckx VA. Nephrotoxicity of alternative medicine practice. Adv Chronic Kidney Dis. 2012;19:129–41.
27. Ashuntantang G, Osafo C, Olowu WA, Arogundade F, Niang A, Porter J, et al. Outcomes in adults and children with end-stage kidney disease requiring dialysis in Sub-Saharan Africa: a systematic review. Lancet Glob Health. 2017;5:e408–17.
28. Dunn J, Krige J, Wood R, Bornman P, Terblanche J. Colonic complications after toxic tribal enemas. Br J Surg. 1991;78:545–8.
29. Luyckx VA, Ballantine R, Claeys M, Cuyckens F, Van den Heuvel H, Cimanga RK, et al. Herbal remedy-associated acute renal failure secondary to Cape aloes. Am J Kidney Dis. 2002;39:E13.11–5.
30. Müller G, Modler H, Wium C, Veale D, Marks C. Snake bite in southern Africa: diagnosis and management. Contin Med Educ. 2012;30:362–82.
31. Coetzer P, Tilbury C. The epidemiology of snakebite in Northern Natal. S Afr Med J. 1982;62:206–12.

32. Blaylock R. Epidemiology of snakebite in Eshowe, KwaZulu-Natal, South Africa. Toxicon. 2004;43:159–66.
33. Chippaux J-P. Estimate of the burden of snakebites in Sub-Saharan Africa: a meta-analytic approach. Toxicon. 2011;57:586–99.
34. Chippaux JP. Snake-bites: appraisal of the global situation. Bull World Health Organ. 1998;76:515–24.
35. Wood D, Sartorius B, Hift R. Snakebite in North-Eastern South Africa: clinical characteristics and risks for severity. S Afr Fam Prac. 2016;58:62–7.
36. Müller G, Wium C, Marks C, Du Plessis C, Veale D. Spider bite in southern Africa: diagnosis and management. Contin Med Educ. 2012;30:382–92.
37. Muller GJ. Black and brown widow spider bites in South Africa. A series of 45 cases. S Afr Med J. 1993;83:399–405.
38. Chippaux J-P, Goyffon M. Epidemiology of scorpionism: a global appraisal. Acta Trop. 2008;107:71–9.
39. Müller G, Modler H, Wium C, Veale D. Scorpion sting in Southern Africa: diagnosis and management. Contin Med Educ. 2012;30:356–61.
40. Muller GJ. Scorpionism in South Africa. A report of 42 serious scorpion envenomations. S Afr Med J. 1993;83:405–11.
41. Seedat YK. Acute renal failure among Blacks and Indians in South Africa. S Afr Med J. 1978;54:427–31.
42. Randeree IG, Czarnocki A, Moodley J, Seedat YK, Naiker IP. Acute renal failure in pregnancy in South Africa. Ren Fail. 1995;17:147–53.
43. Nathan HL, Seed PT, Hezelgrave NL, De Greeff A, Lawley E, Conti-Ramsden F, et al. Maternal and perinatal adverse outcomes in women with pre-eclampsia cared for at facility-level in South Africa: a prospective cohort study. J Glob Health. 2018;8:020401.
44. Makhanya V, Moodley J, Govender L. Eclampsia: still a major problem in rural KwaZulu-Natal Province, South Africa. S Afr J Obstet Gynaecol. 2016;22:13–7.
45. Bouwer F, Langenegger E, Moosa MR. Comparison of the outcome of patients with acute renal failure as a complication of HELLP syndrome before and after 36 weeks gestation. MMed thesis. Cape Town: Stellenbosch University; 2013.
46. Smoyer WE, Finkelstein FO, McCulloch MI, Carter M, Brusselmans A, Feehally J. "Saving Young Lives" with acute kidney injury: the challenge of acute dialysis in low-resource settings. Kidney Int. 2016;89:254–6.
47. Abdou N, Antwi S, Koffi LA, Lalya F, Adabayeri VM, Nyah N, et al. Peritoneal dialysis to treat patients with acute kidney injury-the Saving Young Lives experience in West Africa: proceedings of the Saving Young Lives session at the First International Conference of Dialysis in West Africa, Dakar, Senegal, December 2015. Perit Dial Int. 2017;37:155–8.
48. Smoyer WE, Finkelstein FO, McCulloch M, Carter M, Brusselmans A, Feehally J. Saving Young Lives: provision of acute dialysis in low-resource settings. Lancet. 2015;386:2056.
49. van Deventer HE, George JA, Paiker JE, Becker PJ, Katz IJ. Estimating glomerular filtration rate in black South Africans by use of the Modification of Diet in Renal Disease and Cockcroft-Gault equations. Clin Chem. 2008;54:1197–202.
50. Madala ND, Nkwanyana N, Dubula T, Naiker IP. Predictive performance of eGFR equations in South Africans of African and Indian ancestry compared with $^{99m}$Tc-DTPA imaging. Int Urol Nephrol. 2012;44:847–55.
51. Moodley N, Hariparshad S, Peer F, Gounden V. Evaluation of the CKD-EPI creatinine based glomerular filtration rate estimating equation in Black African and Indian adults in KwaZulu-Natal, South Africa. Clin Biochem. 2018;59:43–9.
52. Holness JL, Bezuidenhout K, Davids MR, Warwick JM. Validation of equations to estimate glomerular filtration rate in South Africans of mixed ancestry. S Afr Med J. 2020;110(3):229–34.
53. Matsha TE, Yako YY, Rensburg MA, Hassan MS, Kengne AP, Erasmus RT. Chronic kidney diseases in mixed ancestry South African populations: prevalence, determinants and concordance between kidney function estimators. BMC Nephrol. 2013;14:75.
54. Adeniyi AB, Laurence CE, Volmink JA, Davids MR. Prevalence of chronic kidney disease and association with cardiovascular risk factors among teachers in Cape Town, South Africa. Clin Kidney J. 2017;10:363–9.
55. Elamin S, Obeid W, Abu-Aisha H. Renal replacement therapy in Sudan, 2009. Arab J Nephrol Transplant. 2010;3:31–6.
56. Rapport D'Activite Des Centres et Unites D'Hemodialyse, Annee 2010. Ministere de la Sante Publique, Tunisia, 2011.
57. Insuffisance rénale chronique terminale. Moroccan Society of Nephrology and Moroccan Ministry of Health, 2013.
58. Keeton G, van Zyl SR, Bryer A. Renal outcome of type 2 diabetes in South Africa—a 12-year follow-up study. J Endocrinol Metab Diabetes S Afr. 2004;9:84–8.
59. Gill GV, Huddle KR, Monkoe G. Long-term (20 years) outcome and mortality of Type 1 diabetic patients in Soweto, South Africa. Diabet Med. 2005;22:1642–6.
60. Davids MR, Jardine T, Marais N, Zunza M, Jacobs JC, Sebastian S. South African Renal Registry Annual Report 2017. Afr J Nephrol. 2019;22:60–71.
61. Patchapen Y. A retrospective study evaluating the patterns of primary glomerular disease at Charlotte Maxeke Johannesburg Academic Hospital. MMed thesis. Johannesburg: University of the Witwatersrand; 2017.
62. Okpechi I, Swanepoel C, Duffield M, Mahala B, Wearne N, Alagbe S, et al. Patterns of renal disease in Cape Town South Africa: a 10-year review of a single-centre renal biopsy database. Nephrol Dial Transplant. 2011;26:1853–61.
63. Esmail A, Amirali MH, Jardine T, Bates WD, Davids MR. Patterns of biopsy-proven renal disease in Cape Town, South Africa, from 1995 to 2017. MMed thesis. Cape Town: Stellenbosch University; 2019.
64. Tannor E, Bates W, Moosa M. The clinical relevance of repeat renal biopsies in the management of lupus nephritis: a South African experience. Lupus. 2018;27(4):525–35.
65. Rao TK, Filippone EJ, Nicastri AD, Landesman SH, Frank E, Chen CK, et al. Associated focal and segmental glomerulosclerosis in the acquired immunodeficiency syndrome. N Engl J Med. 1984;310:669–73.
66. Pardo V, Aldana M, Colton RM, Fischl MA, Jaffe D, Moskowitz L, et al. Glomerular lesions in the acquired immunodeficiency syndrome. Ann Intern Med. 1984;101:429–34.
67. Gardenswartz MH, Lerner CW, Seligson GR, Zabetakis PM, Rotterdam H, Tapper ML, et al. Renal disease in patients with AIDS: a clinicopathologic study. Clin Nephrol. 1984;21:197–204.
68. Bates WD, Muller N, van de Wal BW, Jacobs JC. HIV-associated nephropathy-an initial presentation in an HIV-positive patient. S Afr Med J. 1994;84:223–4.
69. Rosenberg AZ, Naicker S, Winkler CA, Kopp JB. HIV-associated nephropathies: epidemiology, pathology, mechanisms and treatment. Nat Rev Nephrol. 2015;11:150–60.
70. Kopp JB, Nelson GW, Sampath K, Johnson RC, Genovese G, An P, et al. APOL1 genetic variants in focal segmental glomerulosclerosis and HIV-associated nephropathy. J Am Soc Nephrol. 2011;22:2129–37.
71. Kasembeli AN, Duarte R, Ramsay M, Mosiane P, Dickens C, Dix-Peek T, et al. APOL1 risk variants are strongly associated with HIV-associated nephropathy in black South Africans. J Am Soc Nephrol. 2015;26(11):2882–90.
72. Han TM, Naicker S, Ramdial PK, Assounga AG. A cross-sectional study of HIV-seropositive patients with varying degrees of proteinuria in South Africa. Kidney Int. 2006;69:2243–50.

73. Szczech LA, Gupta SK, Habash R, Guasch A, Kalayjian R, Appel R, et al. The clinical epidemiology and course of the spectrum of renal diseases associated with HIV infection. Kidney Int. 2004;66:1145–52.
74. Fabian J, Naicker S, Goetsch S, Venter WD. The clinical and histological response of HIV-associated kidney disease to antiretroviral therapy in South Africans. Nephrol Dial Transplant. 2013;28:1543–54.
75. Yahaya I, Uthman OA, Uthman MMB. Interventions for HIV-associated nephropathy. Cochrane Database Syst Rev. 2009;4:CD007183.
76. Wearne N, Swanepoel CR, Duffield MS, Davidson BJ, Manning K, Tiffin N, et al. The effects of add-on corticosteroids on renal outcomes in patients with biopsy proven HIV associated nephropathy: a single centre study from South Africa. BMC Nephrol. 2019;20:44.
77. Bates WD. Hepatitis-B-associated glomerular disease: a clinicopathological study of hepatitis B virus associated membranous glomerulonephritis in Namibian and South African children 1974–2005 and a comparison with hepatitis B associated membranous glomerulonephritis as well as idiopathic membranous glomerulonephritis in adults. PhD thesis, Cape Town: Stellenbosch University; 2011.
78. Bhimma R, Coovadia HM, Adhikari M, Connolly CA. The impact of the hepatitis B virus vaccine on the incidence of hepatitis B virus-associated membranous nephropathy. Arch Pediatr Adolesc Med. 2003;157:1025–30.
79. Gold CH, Isaacson C, Levin J. The pathological basis of end-stage renal disease in blacks. S Afr Med J. 1982;61:263–5.
80. Freedman BI, Murea M. Target organ damage in African American hypertension: role of APOL1. Curr Hypertens Rep. 2012;14:21–8.
81. Perneger TV, Whelton PK, Klag MJ, Rossiter KA. Diagnosis of hypertensive end-stage renal disease: effect of patient's race. Am J Epidemiol. 1995;141:10–5.
82. Schlessinger SD, Tankersley MR, Curtis JJ. Clinical documentation of end-stage renal disease due to hypertension. Am J Kidney Dis. 1994;23:655–60.
83. Lombard EH, Kromberg JG, Thomson PD, Milner LS, van Biljon I, Jenkins T. Autosomal recessive polycystic kidney disease. Evidence for high frequency of the gene in the Afrikaans-speaking population. S Afr Med J. 1989;76:321–3.
84. Lambie L, Amin R, Essop F, Cnaan A, Krause A, Guay-Woodford LM. Clinical and genetic characterization of a founder PKHD1 mutation in Afrikaners with ARPKD. Pediatr Nephrol. 2015;30:273–9.
85. van der Merwe PD, Rensburg MA, Haylett WL, Bardien S, Davids MR. Gitelman syndrome in a South African family presenting with hypokalaemia and unusual food cravings. BMC Nephrol. 2017;18:38.
86. Nkeh B, Samani NJ, Badenhorst D, Libhaber E, Sareli P, Norton GR, et al. T594M variant of the epithelial sodium channel β-subunit gene and hypertension in individuals of African ancestry in South Africa. Am J Hypertens. 2003;16:847–52.
87. Jones ES, Owen EP, Rayner BL. The association of the R563Q genotype of the ENaC with phenotypic variation in Southern Africa. Am J Hypertens. 2012;25:1286–91.
88. Dhanjal M, Owen E, Anthony J, Davidson J, Rayner B. Association of pre-eclampsia with the R563Q mutation of the β-subunit of the epithelial sodium channel. BJOG. 2006;113:595–8.
89. du Toit ED, Pascoe M, MacGregor K, Thomson PD. SADTR Report 1994. Combined report on maintenance dialysis and transplantation in the Republic of South Africa. Cape Town, South Africa: South African Dialysis and Transplantation Registry; 1994.
90. Moosa MR, Wearne N. Invited commentary: should we be rationing dialysis in South Africa in the 21st century? Perit Dial Int. 2018;38:84–8.
91. Moosa MR, Maree JD, Chirehwa MT, Benatar SR. Use of the 'Accountability for Reasonableness' approach to improve fairness in accessing dialysis in a middle-income country. PLoS One. 2016;11:e0164201.
92. Kilonzo KG, Jones ES, Okpechi IG, Wearne N, Barday Z, Swanepoel CR, et al. Disparities in dialysis allocation: an audit from the new South Africa. PLoS One. 2017;12:e0176041.
93. Moosa MR, Meyers AM, Gottlich E, Naicker S. An effective approach to chronic kidney disease in South Africa. S Afr Med J. 2016;106:156–9.
94. Jardine T, Wong E, Steenkamp R, Caskey FJ, Davids MR. Survival of South African patients on renal replacement therapy. Clin Kidney J. 2020:1–9. https://doi.org/10.1093/ckj/sfaa012.
95. Kramer A, Pippias M, Noordzij M, Stel VS, Andrusev AM, Aparicio-Madre MI, et al. The European Renal Association–European Dialysis and Transplant Association (ERA-EDTA) Registry annual report 2016: a summary. Clin Kidney J. 2019;12:702–20.
96. UK Renal registry 21st annual report – data to 31/12/2017. Bristol: UK Renal Registry; 2019.
97. Makhele L, Matlala M, Sibanda M, Martin AP, Godman B. A cost analysis of haemodialysis and peritoneal dialysis for the management of end-stage renal failure at an Academic Hospital in Pretoria, South Africa. Pharmacoecon Open. 2019;3:631–41.
98. Malatji TA, Wamukuo JT, Hyera F. An analysis of the direct cost of renal dialysis provided through a public-private partnership at a tertiary hospital in Limpopo Province, South Africa. S Afr Med J. 2019;109:577–81.
99. Davids MR, Balbir Singh GK, Marais N, Jacobs JC. South African Renal Registry Annual Report 2014. Cape Town: South African Renal Society; 2016.
100. Abu-Aisha H, Elamin S. Peritoneal dialysis in Africa. Perit Dial Int. 2010;30:23–8.
101. Davidson B, Crombie K, Manning K, Rayner B, Wearne N. Outcomes and challenges of a PD-First program, a South African perspective. Perit Dial Int. 2018;38:179–86.
102. Kapembwa KC, Bapoo NA, Tannor EK, Davids MR. Peritoneal dialysis technique survival at Tygerberg Hospital in Cape Town, South Africa. Afr J Nephrol. 2017;20:25–33.
103. Isla RAT, Mapiye D, Swanepoel CR, Rozumyk N, Hubahib JE, Okpechi IG. Continuous ambulatory peritoneal dialysis in Limpopo province, South Africa: predictors of patient and technique survival. Perit Dial Int. 2014;34:518–25.
104. Zent R, Myers JE, Donald D, Rayner BL. Continuous ambulatory peritoneal dialysis: an option in the developing world? Perit Dial Int. 1994;14:48–51.
105. de Andrade BK, Qureshi AR, Lopes AA, Fernandes N, Barbosa LM, Pecoits-Filho R, et al. Family income and survival in Brazilian Peritoneal Dialysis Multicenter Study patients (BRAZPD): time to revisit a myth? Clin J Am Soc Nephrol. 2011;6:1676–83.
106. Li PK, Szeto CC, Piraino B, Bernardini J, Figueiredo AE, Gupta A, et al. Peritoneal dialysis-related infections recommendations: 2010 update. Perit Dial Int. 2010;30:393–423.
107. Okpechi IG, Rayner BL, Swanepoel CR. Peritoneal dialysis in Cape Town, South Africa. Perit Dial Int. 2012;32:254–60.
108. Ndlovu KC, Assounga A. Continuous ambulatory peritoneal dialysis in patients with HIV and end-stage renal failure. Perit Dial Int. 2017;37:321–30.
109. Okaka EI, Naidoo S, Ahmed MM, Davies M, Naicker S. Quality of life in patients on continuous ambulatory peritoneal dialysis in an African setting. Saudi J Kidney Dis Transpl. 2015;26:631–7.

110. Okaka EI, Davies M, Ahmed M, Naidoo S, Naicker S. Impact of socio-economic factors on quality of life in patients on continuous ambulatory peritoneal dialysis in an African setting. West Afr J Med. 2014;33:125–9.
111. Tannor EK, Archer E, Kapembwa K, Van Schalkwyk SC, Davids MR. Quality of life in patients on chronic dialysis in South Africa: a comparative mixed methods study. BMC Nephrol. 2017;18:4.
112. Bello AK, Levin A, Tonelli M, Okpechi IG, Feehally J, Harris D, et al. Assessment of global kidney health care status. JAMA. 2017;317:1864–81.
113. Muller E, Thomson D, McCurdie F. Transplantation in South Africa. Transplantation. 2015;99:643–5.
114. Moosa M. The state of kidney transplantation in South Africa. S Afr Med J. 2019;109:235–40.
115. Etheredge H, Turner R, Kahn D. Public attitudes to organ donation among a sample of urban-dwelling South African adults: a 2012 study. Clin Transpl. 2013;27:684–92.
116. Muller E, Barday Z, Mendelson M, Kahn D. HIV-positive–to–HIV-positive kidney transplantation—results at 3 to 5 years. N Engl J Med. 2015;372:613–20.
117. Davidson B, Du Toit T, Jones ES, Barday Z, Manning K, Mc Curdie F, et al. Outcomes and challenges of a kidney transplant programme at Groote Schuur Hospital, Cape Town: a South African perspective. PLoS One. 2019;14:e0211189.
118. Sakajiki AM, Naidoo S, Manga P, Nazir M, Naicker S. Proteinuria, graft outcomes, and cardiovascular risk among kidney transplant recipients in a South African Public Hospital. Saudi J Kidney Dis Transpl. 2016;27:1217–23.
119. Davids MR, Eastwood JB, Selwood NH, Arogundade FA, Ashuntantang G, Benghanem Gharbi M, et al. A renal registry for Africa: first steps. Clin Kidney J. 2016;9:162–7.
120. Ocheke IE, Antwi S, Gajjar P, McCulloch MI, Nourse P. Pelvi-ureteric junction obstruction at Red Cross Children's Hospital, Cape Town: a six year review. Arab J Nephrol Transplant. 2014;7:33–6.
121. Frigati L, Mahtab S, Nourse P, Ray P, Perrazzo S, Machemedze T, et al. Prevalence of risk factors for chronic kidney disease in South African youth with perinatally acquired HIV. Pediatr Nephrol. 2019;34:313–8.
122. Ladapo TA, Gajjar P, McCulloch M, Scott C, Numanoglu A, Nourse P. Impact of revascularization on hypertension in children with Takayasu's arteritis-induced renal artery stenosis: a 21-year review. Pediatr Nephrol. 2015;30:1289–95.
123. Keenswijk W, Sinclair G, Benetton M, du Plessis M, Nourse P, Reddy D, et al. Audit of hemodialysis in children weighing less than 20 kg in an African pediatric nephrology unit. Ther Apher Dial. 2018;22:617–23.
124. Levy CS, Mudi A, Venter B, Geel J. Challenges facing children on chronic peritoneal dialysis in South Africa. Perit Dial Int. 2018;38:402–4.
125. Spearman C, McCulloch M. Challenges for paediatric transplantation in Africa. Pediatr Transplant. 2014;18:668–74.
126. L'Huillier AG, Green M, Danziger-Isakov L, Chaudhuri A, Höcker B, Van der Linden D, et al. Infections among pediatric transplant candidates: an approach to decision-making. Pediatr Transplant. 2019;23:e13375.
127. Bhimma R, Adhikari M, Asharam K, Connolly C. The spectrum of chronic kidney disease (stages 2–5) in KwaZulu-Natal, South Africa. Pediatr Nephrol. 2008;23:1841–6.
128. Anochie I, Eke F. Chronic renal failure in children: a report from Port Harcourt, Nigeria (1985–2000). Pediatr Nephrol. 2003;18:692–5.
129. ANZDATA. Paediatrics. 37th Report, Australia and New Zealand Dialysis and Transplant Registry, 2015.
130. Ferris ME, Gipson DS, Kimmel PL, Eggers PW. Trends in treatment and outcomes of survival of adolescents initiating end-stage renal disease care in the United States of America. Pediatr Nephrol. 2006;21:1020–6.
131. UNAIDS. Fact sheet. Global statistics. http://www.unaidsorg/en/resources/campaigns/2014/2014gapreport/factsheet. Retrieved 5 June 2016.
132. Liyanage T, Ninomiya T, Jha V, Neal B, Patrice HM, Okpechi I, et al. Worldwide access to treatment for end-stage kidney disease: a systematic review. Lancet. 2015;385:1975–82.
133. Davidson B, Okpechi I, McCulloch M, Wearne N. Adolescent nephrology: an emerging frontier for kidney care in sub-Saharan Africa. Nephrology. 2017;22:933–9.
134. Hassen M, Archer E, Pellizzon A, Chikte UME, Davids MR. Human resources for nephrology in South Africa: a mixed-methods study. PLoS One. 2020;15(2):e0228890.
135. Bello A, Levin A, Lunney M, Osman M, Ye F, Ashuntantang G, et al. ISN Global Kidney Health Atlas 2019. Brussels: International Society of Nephrology; 2019.
136. Dirks JH, Robinson SW. The global perspective of the International Society of Nephrology: a decade of experience with COMGAN. Kidney Int. 2005;68:1395–410.
137. Harris DC, Dupuis S, Couser WG, Feehally J. Training nephrologists from developing countries: does it have a positive impact? Kidney Int Suppl (2011). 2012;2:275–8.
138. Davison SN, Levin A, Moss AH, Jha V, Brown EA, Brennan F, et al. Executive summary of the KDIGO Controversies Conference on Supportive Care in Chronic Kidney Disease: developing a roadmap to improving quality care. Kidney Int. 2015;88:447–59.
139. Swanepoel CR, Atta MG, D'Agati VD, Estrella MM, Fogo AB, Naicker S, et al. Kidney disease in the setting of HIV infection: conclusions from a Kidney Disease: Improving Global Outcomes (KDIGO) Controversies Conference. Kidney Int. 2018;93:545–59.
140. Murtagh FE, Burns A, Moranne O, Morton RL, Naicker S. Supportive care: comprehensive conservative care in end-stage kidney disease. Clin J Am Soc Nephrol. 2016;11:1909–14.
141. Cullis B, Abdelraheem M, Abrahams G, Balbi A, Cruz DN, Frishberg Y, et al. Peritoneal dialysis for acute kidney injury. Perit Dial Int. 2014;34:494–517.
142. Davids MR, Edoute Y, Jungas RL, Cheema-Dhadli S, Halperin ML. Facilitating an understanding of integrative physiology: emphasis on the composition of body fluid compartments. Can J Physiol Pharmacol. 2002;80:835–50.
143. Davids MR, Lin SH, Edoute Y, Cheema-Dhadli S, Halperin ML. Hyponatraemia and hyperglycaemia during laproscopic surgery. QJM. 2002;95:321–30.
144. Davids MR, Edoute Y, Mallie JP, Bichet DG, Halperin ML. Body compartment volumes and composition after giving a vasopressin antagonist: changes are revealed by a tonicity balance. Nephrol Dial Transplant. 2002;17:300–3.
145. Davids MR, Chikte UME, Halperin ML. Development and evaluation of a multimedia e-learning resource for electrolyte and acid-base disorders. Adv Physiol Educ. 2011;35:295–306.
146. Davids MR, Chikte U, Halperin M. The electrolyte workshop: a multimedia case-based resource for learning about hyponatraemia. Washington, DC: MedEdPORTAL Publications; 2015.
147. Sethi SK, Raina R, McCulloch M, Bunchman TE. Critical care pediatric nephrology and dialysis: a practical handbook. Singapore: Springer; 2019.

# Nephrology in Uganda

# 7

Robert Kalyesubula, Gyaviira Makanga, Joseph Ogavu Gyagenda, David Atuhe, Grace Kansiime, Daniel Kiggundu, Simon Peter Eyoku, Anthony Batte, Peace Bagasha, and Emmanuel Ssekasanvu

| | |
|---|---|
| Area[1] | 241,550 km$^2$ |
| Population[2] | 44.7 million (2019) |
| Capital | Kampala |
| Three most populated cities | 1. Wakiso<br>2. Kampala<br>3. Kibaale |
| Official languages | English, Kiswahili, Luganda, Lunyakitala, and many others |
| Gross domestic product (GDP)[3] | 27.48 billion USD (2018) |
| GDP per capita[3] | 710 USD (2018) |
| Human Development Index (HDI) | 0.516 (2017) |
| Official currency | Ugandan shillings |
| Total number of nephrologists | 10 |
| National society of nephrology | Uganda Kidney Foundation |
| Incidence of end-stage renal disease | Not available |
| Prevalence of end-stage renal disease[4](on dialysis) | 2018 – 51.8 pmp |
| Total number of patients on dialysis[5] (all modalities) | 2017 – 176<br>2018 – 186 |
| Number of patients on hemodialysis[5] | 2017 – 173<br>2018 – 184 |
| Number of patients on peritoneal dialysis[5] | 2017 – 3<br>2018 – 2 |
| Number of renal transplantations per year | 2017 – 0<br>2018 – 0 |

Table references:

1. Uganda surface available https://www.indexmundi.com/facts/uganda/surface-area
2. WHO, 2017
3. Uganda GDP per capita, available https://tradingeconomics.com
4. Kalyesubula R, Nankabirwa et al, BMC Nephrology, 2017
5. Uganda Kidney Foundation, unpublished data

## Introduction

Uganda is one of the countries found in East Africa. It is bordered by the Democratic Republic of Congo, Kenya, Rwanda, South Sudan, and Tanzania. Uganda achieved independence from the United Kingdom in 1962. The country is located on the East African Plateau, lying mostly between latitudes 4°N and 2°S (a small area is north of 4°) and longitudes 29° and 35°E. It averages about 1100 meters (3609 ft) above sea level, sloping very steadily downward to the Sudanese plain to the north. It has 134 districts and Kampala, its capital city, sits close to Lake Victoria. The population of Uganda is currently estimated at 44,700,000 people. Uganda is called the pearl of Africa due to its evergreen nature and the lively nature of the people who live in it [1, 2].

R. Kalyesubula (✉)
Makerere University College of Health Sciences, Kampala, Uganda

MRC/UVRI & London School of Hygiene and Tropical Medicine Research Unit, Entebbe, Uganda

Departments of Physiology and Medicine, Makerere University College of Health Sciences, Kampala, Uganda

G. Makanga
Bank of Uganda, Kampala, Uganda

J. O. Gyagenda · D. Atuhe
St Francis Hospital Nsambya, Kampala, Uganda

G. Kansiime · D. Kiggundu · S. P. Eyoku
Mulago National Referral Hospital, Kampala, Uganda

A. Batte
Makerere University College of Health Sciences, Kampala, Uganda

P. Bagasha
Makerere University College of Health Sciences, Kampala, Uganda

Mulago National Referral Hospital, Kampala, Uganda

E. Ssekasanvu
Panorama Medical Center, Kampala, Uganda


J. A. Moura-Neto et al. (eds.), *Nephrology Worldwide*, https://doi.org/10.1007/978-3-030-56890-0_7

Uganda has allegiance along ethnic, religious, and political lines. With more than 56 tribes, diversity is at the heart of Uganda. However, it is easy to navigate through the country if you speak either English, Swahili, or Luganda. The official currency of Uganda is Ugandan shillings (UGSH) with a symbol of /=. One US dollar is equivalent to 3700 Ugandan shillings. One of the most attractive sites includes the Bwindi forest which is home to the world's most beautiful gorillas. We have several game parks where wild animals can be found in their natural homes. Uganda is at the equator and therefore receives sunshine throughout the year.

Uganda has had several presidents and a turbulent past. However, in 1986, President Yoweri Museveni came into power and his presidency has remained until present day (2019). The Ugandan parliament is one of the largest in the world with 426 members in the 10th parliament. It is currently headed by Hon Rebecca Kadaga.

Healthcare in Uganda is generally free across the country organized into different levels of care. We do not have health insurance in the country, and the health facilities are often ill equipped to provide adequate resources to care for the growing population. This is more pronounced when it comes to chronic diseases [3].

## Brief History of Nephrology in Uganda

Uganda has a great heritage and history in the field of nephrology with key research performed in malaria-associated nephropathy and glomerulonephritis by Kibukamusoke in the late 1960s and early 1970s [4]. Acute peritoneal dialysis (PD) using normal saline fortified with dextrose 50% was introduced by Dr Edward Kigonya in the 1970s who also introduced the concept of enteric dialysis using sorbitol in 2000 (unpublished data). Dr Amos Odiit started pediatric nephrology care services in Mulago Hospital in 2000. Since then, we have had slow progress in both research and clinical nephrology until recent years. Renal replacement therapy (RRT) in the form of hemodialysis (HD) is still new in Uganda, having been introduced to the capital, Kampala, in 2001. Dr Emmanuel Ssekasanvu working alongside Mr Moses Odongo started HD at a private center and 2 years later, in 2003, at the intensive care unit of Mulago National Referral and Teaching Hospital. Since then, dialysis has improved as explained in the different sections. As of 2019, Uganda has unfortunately not yet started kidney transplant program, and most Ugandan patients are referred to outside countries for this service.

There is a lot of enthusiasm for the field of nephrology since 2012 when the Uganda Kidney Foundation (UKF) was established by Dr Emmanuel Ssekasanvu, Dr Simon Peter Eyoku, Dr Rose Muhindo, Dr Peace Bagasha, Dr Prossy Ingabire, Dr Joseph Lunyera, and Mr Tomson Masereka under the leadership of Dr Robert Kalyesubula. In 2013, the UKF team organized the first international kidney conference in Uganda. Since then the UKF holds regular scientific meetings and celebrates the World Kidney Day together with other team players like the Uganda Kidney Psychosocial Support Organization (UKPSSO) and the Uganda Ministry of Health. Since its foundation, the UKF has screened 2160 community members for hypertension, diabetes, obesity, and kidney disease and referred them for further care [5, 6].

## Renal Diseases in Uganda

Kidney disease is a common problem worldwide with one in ten people estimated to have kidney disease. Developing countries like Uganda have the largest burden of disease due to lack of well-established infrastructure for prevention, diagnosis, and care for patients with kidney disease. The current prevalence of chronic kidney disease (CKD) in Uganda ranges from 2.5% in the general population to 14.4% among high-risk groups [7, 8]. The major risk factors driving kidney disease in adults include hypertension, diabetes mellitus, and infections, particularly HIV-AIDS. In children, the major contributors to renal disease are sickle cell disease, malaria, and other infections [9–11]. However, a large proportion of the general population with CKD (49%) is not explained by the known risk factors [12]. We do not know the prevalence of acute kidney injury (AKI) in the general population. However, one study done in a hospital care setting in Mulago National Referral Hospital, the largest hospital in Uganda, provides some information. Among the 387 patients attending an emergency unit with sepsis, 16.3% had AKI and had an inhospital mortality of 21% largely due to lack of access to dialysis and intensive care services [13].

Uganda has a large population with 55% of the people below 18 years of age and only 4% of the people above 60 years [1]. We have no national health insurance policy, and there is limited health insurance for a few employed individuals. Most of these policies exclude renal care beyond renal function tests, urinalysis, antihypertensive therapy, and diabetes treatment. Individuals pay out of pocket for renal care (biopsy, dialysis, transplant, and posttransplant care). We do not have a renal registry, and most of the data is from individual community or hospital-based studies. About 1000 patients are diagnosed with renal disease every year in Mulago National Referral Hospital. Up to 56.2% of patients who attended for the first time at the renal clinic present with CKD stage 5, and most of these are under 38 years of age [14, 15]. The leading associations with CKD are hypertension, diabetes mellitus, infections (HIV in particular), and tuberculosis [15, 16]. Diseases such as malaria and schistosomiasis are some of the endemic diseases associated with kidney disease [4, 7]. Hemorrhagic fevers like Marburg and Ebola viral infections have been associated with kidney diseases. Other causes include locally available herbal remedies often used for treatment of various ailments and among pregnant women [17].

AKI accounts for 4% of hospital admissions and is a major cause of mortality among adults, and most of the cases arise from infections and trauma [13]. Pregnancy and its related complications are a major cause of AKI among women of childbearing age. Uganda has a young population and a high fertility rate with poor health systems [3, 18].

### Renal Diseases in Pediatric Population

Glomerulopathies are among the leading causes of CKD among children. Unfortunately the lack of immunofluorescence limits our ability to confirm the exact causes of the glomerulopathies. Past studies among children attributed these glomerulopathies particularly nephrotic range proteinuria to quartan malaria [4]. Recent studies describe sickle cell disease as a cause of proteinuria among children in Uganda. About 15,000 babies are born with sickle cell disease in the country annually [19]. A cross-sectional study, among children with sickle cell anemia in a steady state attending Mulago National Referral Hospital in the years 2007 and 2008, reported the prevalence of microalbuminuria to be 28% [9]. This highlights the importance of sickle cell disease as a cause of glomerulopathies in children in Uganda. The role of *Plasmodium falciparum* malaria in causing CKD has not been well documented; however, in the past 2 years, two children have received renal transplant following *P. falciparum* infection, and a study published in 2019 has indicated an increased risk of CKD in children with severe *P. falciparum* [10].

Concerning AKI among children in Uganda, *P. falciparum* is a leading cause of AKI in these children. A recent study at the Mulago National Referral Hospital showed an AKI prevalence of 35.1% among children admitted with severe malaria [10]. The study further indicated that the risk of these children progressing to CKD is three times more than those without AKI [10]. Unfortunately, AKI is associated with an increased risk of mortality in these children with malaria [10]. Other causes of AKI in children in Uganda include gastroenteritis, malnutrition, pneumonia, and HIV [11]. Even though we have limited literature in the country concerning the epidemiology of other causes of renal diseases in children, based on observations during clinical care, idiopathic nephrotic syndrome contributes to almost 50% of our outpatient reviews. In addition, post-streptococcal glomerulonephritis, urinary tract infections, and obstructive uropathies are also prevalent causes of pediatric renal diseases in Uganda [20].

## Renal Replacement Therapy in Uganda

Renal replacement therapy (RRT) in Uganda is largely restricted to HD as initial results for PD were not optimal. We are in the early stages of setting up a national kidney transplant program. Only about 9% of the people who need RRT have access to it in Uganda, and their options are currently limited to hemodialysis [5].

### Hemodialysis

RRT in the form of HD is still new in Uganda and was initiated in early 2001 at the Mulago National Referral and Teaching Hospital located in the capital, Kampala. This is a 1500-bed teaching hospital serving a population of about 30 million Ugandans. Patients therefore had to travel several kilometers from out of Kampala city to access the service at a costly fee. With a fast-growing population, at close to 45 million currently and an increased prevalence of CKD, the number of patients needing RRT has markedly increased. In response, the number of dialysis centers has also increased from one dialysis center in early 2001 to 11 centers by 2019. Regrettably, the majority of these dialysis centers are all concentrated in the central region, the capital city, Kampala. Two dialysis centers are government owned, while the remaining nine are privately run. Only two centers are located out of the capital city (Table 7.1).

**Table 7.1** Dialysis centers in Uganda (2019)

| | Dialysis unit | Ownership | No. of HD machines | No. of pts | Male | Female | Head of the unit |
|---|---|---|---|---|---|---|---|
| 1. | Kiruddu Teaching Hospital | Government | 19 | 110 | 74 | 36 | 2 nephrologists<br>1 specialist physician |
| 2. | Nakasero Hospital | Private | 5 | 7 | 6 | 1 | 1 nephrologist |
| 3. | Norvik Hospital | Private | 6 | 22 | 13 | 9 | 1 nephrologist |
| 4. | Panorama Medical Center | Private | 4 | 8 | 4 | 4 | 1 nephrologist |
| 5. | UMC Victoria Hospital | Private | 6 | 11 | 8 | 3 | 1 nephrologist |
| 6. | Case Hospital | Private | 3 | 5 | 4 | 1 | 1 nephrologist |
| 7. | Nsambya Hospital | Private | 4 | 12 | 8 | 4 | 1 nephrologist |
| 8. | Mbarara University Teaching Hospital | Government | 2 | 2 | 2 | 0 | 1 nephrologist<br>1 specialist physician |
| 9. | DMA diagnostics and laboratory | Private | 2 | 1 | 1 | 0 | 1 nephrologist<br>1 specialist physician |
| 10. | Home dialysis | Private | 1 | 1 | 1 | 0 | 1 nephrologist |

*HD* hemodialysis, *Pts* patients

There are 52 hemodialysis machines in the country, 21 of which belong to the public sector, providing both acute and chronic HD. A total of 179 patients are undergoing chronic HD, with the largest in-center number dialyzing in a government hospital due to a government subsidized cost of about 20 US dollars. The private centers and the other government center currently provide HD at an average cost of 80 US dollars per dialysis session. Other drugs used alongside dialysis like erythropoietin, iron, calcium, vitamin D, phosphate binders, and drugs for treating comorbidity disorders are paid for by the patients in both private and government dialysis centers. There is a general male predominance in dialysis accessibility in most centers; women and children are underrepresented like in many other low-income countries [21, 22].

We neither have a national health insurance scheme nor do we have a national dialysis policy for dialysis allocation in Uganda. This means that all patients access dialysis through out-of-pocket costs. The private health insurance schemes for nongovernmental organizations (NGOs) do not cover dialysis. In comparison, neighboring countries, like Kenya, Tanzania, and Rwanda, offer short-term dialysis for AKI under their existent national health insurance schemes [21, 23]. In Uganda, dialysis is only subsidized at the main national and referral hospital (Mulago); however, the majority of the patients are dialyzed once or twice weekly due to the prohibitive long-term unsustainable costs for dialysis, medications, tests, and transport to the dialysis center. The minimal internationally recommended hemodialysis dose is 4 hours, thrice weekly. Clinicians are always faced with the dilemma of dialysis adequacy. At the government center, patients are entitled to a maximum of two sessions per week. This is because the numbers are quite overwhelming. Dialysis teams often begin work at 1:00 am in the morning, and the shifts go up to 10:00 pm in the night. Patients who can afford often get a third dialysis session from private units, while the majority (about 90%) of them gets less than two sessions a week. It is therefore a challenging situation, and some patients end up using drugs, herbal remedies, and other conservative methods of treatment, like probiotics and strict diet, in between the dialysis session. It is not uncommon for patients to present with creatinine of over 2000 umol/l (22.6 mg/dl) and hemoglobin levels of less than 5 g/dl to dialysis units. Only 9 out of 184 patients (5%) have been on dialysis for more than 5 years in the country. We also do not have any national guidelines for dialysis, and this sector is not yet regulated. As a result of this, practices vary widely across centers. For example, dialyzer reuse is only done inconsistently by one private center. Even then less than six patients overall are using this method. The dialyzer is used for a maximum of eight sessions.

With a population of 44.7 million, Uganda has only 10 nephrologists, 2 pediatric, and 8 adult nephrologists, providing a nephrologist to population ratio of 0.15 per million population (pmp). The average ratio in Europe, for example, is approximately 20 pmp [24]. This very low number of nephrologists in Uganda directly affects patient access to quality care and hence dialysis access. Additionally, dialysis access is provided only in the two major cities, Kampala and Mbarara, leaving the rest of the country out of reach for dialysis services. Some patients travel more than 300 kilometers to access dialysis, while others have had to migrate to the big cities in order to access these services.

The lack of a transplant program in the country leaves some potential transplant candidates on chronic HD. This imposes an excessive financial burden on the families of the affected patients. In many instances, it has resulted in catastrophic health expenditures, leading to the sale of family property and depletion of life savings, leaving the entire family impoverished. At the government center where costs are subsidized, a number of other major challenges include overwhelming patient numbers, inadequate dialysis, and very low fistula rates. The majority of patients use temporary catheters for long periods of time, hence presenting patients with recurrent catheter-associated infections and sepsis leading to poor dialysis outcomes. Patients suffer with high rates of anemia, while staff get fatigue and burnouts. There are occasional consumable stockouts, absence of timely machine maintenance, hence frequent machine breakdowns with limited technological support, and irregular water analysis. Similar challenges have also been observed in other low- and middle-income countries [25].

## Peritoneal Dialysis

We currently have no active PD services in Uganda. Efforts to set up PD through the Sustainable Kidney Care Foundation were hampered by lack of commitment from stakeholders and the fact that peritoneal fluid for dialysis was hard to transport across the borders. There is no champion to lead this effort of dialysis development in the country. Occasionally, some children are able to get PD through insertion of temporary catheters. The dialysis equipment and fluids have to be procured from nearby Kenya by the relatives of the children. In 2018, three adult patients were on continuous ambulatory peritoneal dialysis (CAPD); two of them passed away due to peritonitis in 2019.

We are currently looking for ways to revise this program particularly for children. The international community is welcome to support us in this effort because many children are dying from AKI, a condition which also increases their risk of developing CKD [9–11].

## Renal Transplantation

As the burden of CKD increases in sub-Saharan Africa, so does the need for renal transplantation. As of 2019, we have no transplant program in Uganda, and all our patients have undergone renal transplant outside Uganda, mostly from hospitals in India. Renal transplant in conjunction with Indian Hospitals began in 2004, and over 100 recipients from Uganda have been transplanted and are monitored in continuing consultation with the mother transplant hospitals that include Trivedi in Mumbai, Apollo Hospital in New Delhi, Yashoda in Hyderabad, and Fortis in Bangalore. A few more patients have had their transplant done in South Africa (Groote Schuur), Kenya (Nairobi), and other countries.

There is an undocumented, but worrying, rise in the number of chronic allograft loss among Ugandan renal transplant recipients noted over the past decade, but the factors associated with chronic allograft injury have not been conclusively identified. Several studies have shown different factors (both donor and recipient) to be associated with poor allograft outcome/survival rate, including underlying cause of CKD stage 5, longer time on dialysis prior to renal transplantation, creatinine level at the time of discharge, and donor age, among others [26, 27].

Though there is an increasing number of patients diagnosed with CKD stage 5 and in need of kidney transplant in Uganda, very few patients (less than 1%) can get a transplant because of the prohibitive cost. In addition, because we only rely on living-related donors, there is a problem of finding suitable donors, and this is further complicated by lack of capacity among medical institutions and lack of policies to regulate the transplantation process. These factors are not different from those encountered in most African countries [26]. However, compared to the developed world, where the biggest challenge is shortage of donated kidneys, the biggest challenge in Uganda is the cost since the patients and relatives have to pay for medical care, in addition to travel and living expenses for the donor and caretaker. Thus many patients never consider transplant an option for care once diagnosed with CKD stage 5.

All our patients who have undergone kidney transplantation have had living-related donors. The nephrologists in Uganda often collaborate with the centers abroad where the patients are transplanted and only take over care once the patients return to their home country.

Uganda is currently discussing an organ transplant bill that is under review by the parliament. We are hopeful that this will be passed and transplant resources availed to patients at a local level. This may reduce the cost of medical care and set up a system for nonliving organ donation and improve local human resources and institutions' capacity building, among others.

As we await the organ transplant bill to be passed, Mulago National Referral Hospital is currently under renovation and getting ready to start kidney transplantation. This transplant program has been spearheaded by the executive director, Dr Byarugaba Baterana, and a transplant team comprising surgeons, nephrologists, pathologists, and intensivist nurses who have been trained in anticipation of the same.

We believe when the program starts more patients will be able to undergo kidney transplant.

## Nephrology Practice in Uganda

Amid the rising tide of CKD, the global nephrology workforce has shrunk and is failing to meet the growing healthcare needs of this vulnerable patient population. Africa has the lowest number of nephrologists per million population (pmp) in the world, with no nephrologists in many parts of the continent [28]. Uganda is estimated correctly to have less than 0.15 nephrologist pmp [28] (Fig. 7.1). As a matter of fact, this global shortage of nephrologists is seen in many parts of the world [29, 30].

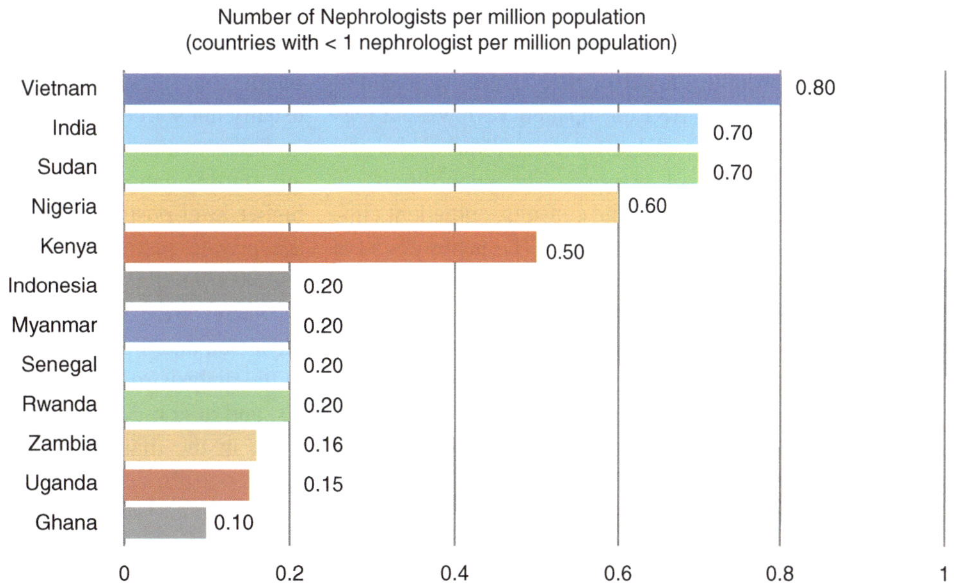


**Fig. 7.1** Number of nephrologists per million population by countries with <1 nephrologist per million population [28]

As of April 2019, Uganda had only ten nephrologists for a population of 44.71 million [1] leaving each nephrologist to take care of over four million people. The nursing arm of nephrology follows a similar trend marred by low numbers and lack of training within the nursing schools about kidney disease and its management [31]. This is mainly contributed to by the absence of in-country training opportunities for specialist nephrology practice. All specialist nephrology providers trained abroad in South Africa, the United States of America (USA), Canada, Tanzania, and India for the doctors and mostly India for the nurses. Training abroad has cost implications which must be incurred by the individual either through personal funds or through looking out for scholarship opportunities mainly offered by the International Society of Nephrology (ISN) and the host universities-hospitals.

Advanced nephrology services are distributed between two major cities; Mbarara and Kampala. Mbarara, the smaller of the two, with a projected population of 216,800 [2], only has one nephrologist who covers all the private facilities and the one public government-owned hospital. This hospital is a regional referral hospital attending most of the western region of the country and also serves as the teaching hospital for Mbarara University of Science and Technology (MUST).

Kampala, the capital city of Uganda, with a projected population of over 1.65 million people [2] hosts the 9 other nephrologists. These are also distributed between one public hospital, two private not for profit hospitals, and six private for profit hospitals. Only three of these nephrologists cover the public hospital (Mulago National Referral Hospital) which doubles as a national referral hospital and a teaching hospital for Makerere University College of Health Sciences (MakCHS). This hospital receives medical referrals from all over the country and neighboring countries like the Democratic Republic of Congo and South Sudan.

Opportunities in the private hospitals include either full coverage, as a resident nephrologist, or partial coverage, i.e., as a part-time consulting nephrologist. The most common reason for consultation is AKI for inpatient reviews, but regular outpatient clinics are also often carried out at the primary medical facilities of practice. The nephrologist is expected to be involved in inpatient consults, outpatient clinics, HD unit rounds, and ICU coverage. The nephrologist is expected to be conversant with the management of a wide range of systemic disorders, which may be responsible for malfunctioning of the kidneys, which include high blood pressure, cancers, or diabetes.

Most frequent procedures include HD catheter insertion and performing kidney biopsies, but occasionally other procedures like paracentesis for massive ascites or pleurocentesis for pleural effusions may be required. There may be an interventional radiologist to do some of these procedures, especially in the private facilities. It is most common for the nephrologist to report to the medical director or chief of specialists, depending on the institution.

Patient load has seasonal variations with each of the private facilities admitting regularly five to ten patients per week, with five to ten patients on chronic HD. Private not for profit facilities may have fewer patients due to the elevated financial costs for a population that is seen to be less economically advantaged. The public government facility has 20–30 patients in the inpatient wards, with 10–15 new patients in the inpatient clinic weekly and 100–120 HD patients on chronic hemodialysis.

Nephrologists tend to cover each other in case one is away on leave or travelling and do frequently discuss complicated cases, with the older more experienced group members giving advice and mentorship to younger members. The annual World Kidney Day celebrations mark a time for the meeting of nephrologists; the group works together to organize national celebrations often involving a community screening activity and a scientific conference. In 2019, community screening activities were organized at the parliamentary grounds, and a motion to increase funding for sustainable kidney disease care was debated by members of parliament and passed. This momentous event is aimed to be the launch pad for a proposal by the nephrology community in Uganda to increase dialysis units in the country. This proposal seeks to include hemodialysis services at all 13 regional referral hospitals in the country. There are few trained pathologists in Uganda, so most of the biopsies done are processed abroad by partnering laboratories with turnaround time of about 1–2 weeks.

Currently, there are only five intensive care units (ICUs) that offer hemodialysis, with only one offering both hemodialysis and continuous renal replacement therapy (CRRT). In places without CRRT, hemodynamically unstable patients are offered sustained low-efficiency dialysis (SLED). Intensivists often work closely with nephrologists and will usually not start dialysis without nephrology review.

Salary scales in the government/public facilities are fixed at a starting annual scale of 7500 US dollars and increase as higher-level posting is announced by the public service. In the private sector, this could range between 19,000 and 65,000 US dollars per annum.

Nurses are expected to be the coordinators between the physician and the patient. A nephrology nurse has key tasks in the dialysis room, during ward rounds, in outpatient clinics, and in non-doctor-related reviews. A dialysis nurse may work in the dialysis department of a hospital, a dialysis clinic, or a physician's office. The nurse typically operates an

HD machine, monitors patient vital signs, communicates procedure details with patients, and assesses the effectiveness of procedures, as well as being responsible for cleaning the work area. It is also the responsibility of the dialysis nurse to be sympathetic, caring, patient, positive, and responsible when caring for patients. The terms dialysis nurse and nephrology nurse are often interchangeable; however, a nephrology nurse is involved in all aspects of treatment of patients with kidney problems, including dialysis. The nursing numbers are low for the patients, ranging from three in private hospitals to 18 in the public hospitals. Nurses often work 12-hour shifts, one shift per day and up to five shifts per week with Sunday being an off day for most dialysis units. Only emergency sessions are usually scheduled on Sundays. Most chronic dialysis sessions on average last 4 hours. Exceptions lie within initiation sessions both for chronic and acute HD undertaking 2 hour sessions and very few, especially the hemodynamically unstable, lasting beyond 5 hours. The earliest nonemergency dialysis starts at 1:00 am in the public hospital. The nurse would earn between 3500 and 7000 US dollars per year. Due to a nonexistent transplant program in the country, positions such as transplant coordinator have not been started, but this would be a nephrology nurse with a transplant qualification.

The nephrology social work is usually done by the nephrologist and nurse, but we appreciate that such a position would help in activities such as evaluating for vocational rehabilitation services. This often includes employment, going to school, volunteering within the community, or returning to previously enjoyed activities, providing education and referrals to appropriate resources. Other activities include assisting with keeping or obtaining insurance coverage, assisting patients with understanding their rights and responsibilities, providing supportive counseling, and assisting in informing patients of the importance of treatment participation and advanced directive education, among others. All in all, the workforce is limited in numbers, and this creates a huge case for training, deploying, and capacity building in other areas. Collaborations with partners would go a long way in making this happen.

The Uganda Kidney Foundation – a team of doctors, health scientists, social scientists, and public health experts serving in both public and private facilities – is spearheading the advocacy arm of nephrology services in the country. We have a work plan to ensure at least one nephrologist and one nurse are trained each year to achieve numbers and continue battling the scourge of kidney disease in the country. It is also bringing multidisciplinary professionals, such as social workers, psychologists, dietitians, and physiotherapists, together with NGOs, offering psychosocial support to increase access to holistic care for kidney disease patients.

## Highlights of Nephrology in Uganda

Uganda was the first country to demonstrate that quartan malaria causes nephrotic syndrome in a landmark study by Kibukamusoke in 1967 [4]. Since 1996, in our medical school, Dr Edward Kigonya has been promoting the concept of intestinal dialysis. He believed that using laxatives and antibiotics would help in ensuring that the body got rid of some of the uremic toxins when patients could not afford dialysis (unpublished data). Probiotics have now become of great interest in delaying progression of CKD [32].

In March 2019, under the leadership of Dr Joseph Ogavu Gyagenda, the Uganda Kidney Foundation conducted screening for kidney disease at the Uganda parliament, and the healthcare bill for kidney disease was discussed by the parliamentary health committee.

## Future Perspectives of Nephrology in Uganda

The future of nephrology in Uganda very much lies in going back to the basics of prevention; screening; training; health financing; improved diagnostics; safe, affordable, and accessible dialysis; an active transplant program; and solid research.

The current annual cost of renal replacement services in Uganda ranges from 3125 to 18,720 US dollars against the average annual salary income range of 1380 to 2400 US dollars rendering renal care inaccessible for the vast majority of the Ugandan population. Worldwide, the establishment of health insurance schemes has translated into better healthcare and growth of healthcare systems. Because health financing is such a bottleneck in healthcare in Uganda, there is a more than urgent need for expedition of all measures to ensure that the country gets a health insurance scheme running in the shortest time possible. Other countries in the region are running national health insurance schemes with big benefits to tertiary care and hence kidney care. This scheme, while being applied to the entire healthcare system, would mobilize enough financial resources to fund preventive, investigative, curative, as well as rehabilitative services related to kidney health. Currently, all the nephrologists and dialysis nurses have had to pursue their specialized training outside the country. This directly translates into higher costs of training, while limiting the number of nephrology caregivers that can be trained at any one time. With the country presently only having a total of ten nephrologists, there is clearly a big need for more training among all care providers in nephrology to address the globally increasing number of patients with CKD stage 5 and those needing dialysis. This training also needs to address the big need for transplant which the country is beginning to prepare itself for.

As a country, Uganda needs to resurrect its PD services to address care for the pediatric patients as well as those that are unable to afford or take on HD as their preferred mode of RRT [33]. Whereas some locations, such as Hong Kong, have a high prevalence of PD (up to 70%) as a modality of RRT [33], Uganda presently runs absolutely no PD service due to many factors, especially unavailability of supplies and lack of training.

Summarily, the country needs to train nephrologists, transplant surgeons, transplant medical officers and nurses, dialysis nurses and technicians, renal dietitians, social workers, dialysis technical staff, transplant coordinators, clinical research leaders, as well as kidney health advocates. Developing local capacity to train these care providers is certainly the most cost-effective approach, and setting up a kidney institute is perhaps the single way of meeting all these training needs.

Globally, the established risk factors for kidney disease include diarrheal diseases, HIV infection, low birth weight, malaria, and preterm birth and also encompass life course and environmental-, infection-, and lifestyle-related risks [34]. It is also common knowledge that if these risk factors are identified early, AKI and CKD can be prevented. In addition, if CKD is diagnosed early, worsening of kidney function can be slowed or averted by inexpensive interventions, many of which are in the reach of low- and middle-income countries like Uganda. Such interventions include counseling for cardiovascular disease, diabetes, and hypertension, drug therapy, tobacco control, promotion of physical activity, and the reduction of salt intake through legislation and food labeling. The timely identification and management of AKI and CKD represent the most effective strategy to address the growing global burden sustainably [35].

The nephrology fraternity therefore needs to offer guidance to the policy-makers, Ministry of Health, medical education system, and health workers on how to effectively prevent, screen for, and manage kidney disease. We must ensure that adequate resources are allocated to the public health aspect of kidney care so as to reduce the progression to end-stage disease. The Uganda Kidney Foundation has already engaged the Parliament of Uganda in considering improved budgetary support specifically earmarked for renal care, screening being one of the primary objectives.

Our health system needs to deliver quality, safe, accessible, affordable, and sustainable dialysis as a means of managing AKI and CKD and offering an effective dialysis bridge to those being prepared to transplant. Government-led efforts should foster the establishment of more dialysis centers around the country, at least at all regional referral hospitals. This very proposal has been adapted by the Parliament of Uganda starting with the financial year 2019/2020. More dialysis centers will translate into more affordable dialysis as favored by the economies of scale. With the country only meeting a mere 0.04% of its dialysis need, it is very crucial that dialysis becomes more available in the country. An effective dialysis service will feed well-rehabilitated candidates into the transplant program and eventually cut down the cost of long-term renal care.

Despite the absence of a running PD program in the country, the barriers to policy implementation are broadly associated with government policy, economics, provider or healthcare professional education, modality-related factors, and patient-related factors; similar factors are responsible for the low HD prevalence in the country [36]. The country therefore needs to equally invest in a PD program given its comparable health outcomes and relatively cheaper cost.

Presently, the bigger part of the population is unable to access screening and diagnostic services as part of the routine healthcare checkup due to the government stratification of healthcare that puts serum creatinine and urine dipstick at health center IV level, which is at county or municipal level. At the higher level, laboratory and imaging services are sparse only best found at the tertiary facilities within the capital, Kampala. And with only two pathologists with specialized training in nephropathology, whose service provision is moreover presently only limited to light microscopy as immunofluorescence and electron microscopy are unavailable and samples cannot be shipped out due to transportation challenges, our diagnostic capability for glomerular disease is at best limited. Increasing availability and knowledge about screening at the lower-level centers while strengthening the capacity of higher-level centers will boost diagnostics related to kidney disease. The kidney institute would then serve as a one-stop superspecialized center for provision of diagnostic services receiving samples and patients referred from lower units.

With the advance of technology, the future provides more options where the advanced services of a nephrologist, nephropathologist, or other care provider, physically remote from a certain site, may provide the same service by live or recorded means in what has come to be termed telenephrology [37]. Such an approach is not new to medicine, already being employed in several disciplines like radiology, and many nephrologists worldwide are pursuing their ISN Certificate in Nephropathology via live and recorded webinars as well as shared sources.

## Conclusion

Uganda is a beautiful country with a growing burden of CKD. The lack of availability of both PD and kidney transplantation is an injustice that needs to be urgently addressed. Emphasis should be placed on disease prevention, and efforts to determine the major risk factors for CKD in this country should be prioritized.

## References


1. Uganda Population. http://worldpopulationreview.com/countries/Uganda-population/2019 [Updated 5/4/2019; cited 2019 5th April 2019]. Available from: http://worldpopulationreview.com/countries/uganda-population/.
2. Uganda Bureau of Statistics. Population of cities, Uganda. 2019 [Cited 2019 5/4/2019]. Available from: http://citypopulation.de/Uganda-Cities.html.
3. Katende D, Mutungi G, Baisley K, Biraro S, Ikoona E, Peck R, Smeeth L, Hayes R, Munderi P, Grosskurth H. Readiness of Ugandan health services for the management of outpatients with chronic diseases. Tropical Med Int Health. 2015;20(10):1385–95.
4. Kibukamusoke JW, Hutt MS. Histological features of the nephrotic syndrome associated with quartan malaria. J Clin Pathol. 1967;20(2):117–23.
5. Kalyesubula R, Odiit A, Wekesa C, Katali E, Sekasanvu E, Kotanko P, Carter M. A time to improve kidney disease care and awareness in Uganda. Dialysis Times. 2012;19(2):1–4.
6. Lunyera J, Stanifer JW, Ingabire P, Etolu W, Bagasha P, Egger JR, Patel UD, Mutungi G, Kalyesubula R. Prevalence and correlates of proteinuria in Kampala, Uganda: a cross-sectional pilot study. BMC Res Notes. 2016;9:97.
7. Kalyesubula R, Nankabirwa JI, Ssinabulya I, Siddharthan T, Kayima J, Nakibuuka J, Salata RA, Mondo C, Kamya MR, Hricik D. Kidney disease in Uganda: a community based study. BMC Nephrol. 2017;18(1):116.
8. Odongo P, Wanyama R, Obol JH, Apiyo P, Byakika-Kibwika P. Impaired renal function and associated risk factors in newly diagnosed HIV-infected adults in Gulu Hospital, Northern Uganda. BMC Nephrol. 2015;16:43.
9. Mawanda M, Ssenkusu J, Odiit A, Kiguli S, Muyingo A, Ndugwa C. Micro-albuminuria in Ugandan children with sickle cell anaemia: a cross-sectional study. Ann Trop Paediatr. 2011;31(2):115–21.
10. Conroy AL, Opoka RO, Bangirana P, Idro R, Ssenkusu JM, Datta D, Hodges JS, Morgan C, John CC. Acute kidney injury is associated with impaired cognition and chronic kidney disease in a prospective cohort of children with severe malaria. BMC Med. 2019;17(1):98.
11. Imani PD, Odiit A, Hingorani SR, Weiss NS, Eddy AA. Acute kidney injury and its association with in-hospital mortality among children with acute infections. Pediatr Nephrol. 2013;28(11):2199–206.
12. Stanifer JW, Jing B, Tolan S, Helmke N, Mukerjee R, Naicker S, Patel U. The epidemiology of chronic kidney disease in Sub-Saharan Africa: a systematic review and meta-analysis. Lancet Glob Health. 2014;2(3):e174–81.
13. Bagasha P, Nakwagala F, Kwizera A, Ssekasanvu E, Kalyesubula R. Acute kidney injury among adult patients with sepsis in a low-income country: clinical patterns and short-term outcomes. BMC Nephrol. 2015;16:4.
14. Kalyesubula R, Lunyera J, Makanga G, Kirenga B, Amukele TK. A 4-year survey of the spectrum of renal disease at a National Referral Hospital Outpatient Clinic in Uganda. Kidney Int. 2015;87(3):663.
15. Babua C, Kalyesubula R, Okello E, Kakande B, Sebatta E, Mungoma M, Mondo CK. Cardiovascular risk factors among patients with chronic kidney disease attending a tertiary hospital in Uganda. Cardiovasc J Afr. 2015;26(4):177–80.
16. Cox JA, Lukande RL, Kalungi S, Van Marck E, Van de Vijver K, Kambugu A, Nelson AM, Colebunders R, Manabe YC. Is urinary lipoarabinomannan the result of renal tuberculosis? Assessment of the renal histology in an autopsy cohort of Ugandan HIV-infected adults. PLoS One. 2015;10(4):e0123323.
17. Kiguba R, Ononge S, Karamagi C, Bird SM. Herbal medicine use and linked suspected adverse drug reactions in a prospective cohort of Ugandan inpatients. BMC Complement Altern Med. 2016;16:145.
18. Kabagenyi A, Reid A, Rutaremwa G, Atuyambe LM, Ntozi JP. Has Uganda experienced any stalled fertility transitions? Reflecting on the last four decades (1973–2011). Fertil Res Pract. 2015;1(14):1–10.
19. Ndeezi G, Kiyaga C, Hernandez AG, Munube D, Howard TA, Ssewanyana I, et al. Burden of sickle cell trait and disease in the Uganda Sickle Surveillance Study (US3): a cross-sectional study. Lancet Glob Health. 2016;4(3):e195–200.
20. Odiit A. Common childhood kidney diseases in Uganda and their prevention. Afr Health Sci. 2017;17(4):1126–9.
21. Antwi S. State of renal replacement therapy services in Ghana. Blood Purif. 2015;39(1–3):137–40.
22. Ulasi I. Gender bias in access to healthcare in Nigeria: a study of end-stage renal disease. Trop Dr. 2008;38:50–2.
23. Callegari J, Antwi S, Wystrychowski G, Zukowska-Szczechowska E, Levin NW, Carter M. Peritoneal dialysis as a mode of treatment for acute kidney injury in Sub-Saharan Africa. Blood Purif. 2013;36:226–30.
24. Sharif MU, Elsayed ME, Stack AG. The global nephrology workforce: emerging threats and potential solutions. Clin Kidney J. 2016;9:11–22.
25. Odubanjo MO, Oluwasola AO, Kadiri S. The epidemiology of end-stage renal disease in Nigeria: the way forward. Int Urol Nephrol. 2011;43:785–92.
26. Muller E. Transplantation in Africa – an overview. Clin Nephrol. 2016;1(13):90–5.
27. Courtney A, McNamee P, Maxwell A. The evolution of renal transplantation in clinical practice: for better, for worse? QJM. 2008;101(12):967–78. https://doi.org/10.1093/qjmed/hcn136.
28. Field M. Addressing the global shortage of nephrologists. Nat Clin Pract Nephrol. 2008;4(11):583.
29. Jha V. Current status of end-stage renal disease care in India and Pakistan. Kidney Int Suppl. 2013;3(2):157–60.
30. Katz IJ, Gerntholtz T, Naicker S. Africa and nephrology: the forgotten continent. Nephron Clin Pract. 2011;117(4):c320–7.
31. Naicker S. Nephrology in Africa – challenges of practice in resource-limited environment. Clin Nephrol. 2016 Supplement 1;86(2016)(13):84–9.
32. Koppe L, Mafra D, Fouque D. Probiotics and chronic kidney disease. Kidney Int. 2015;88(5):958–66.
33. United States Renal Data System. 2016 USRDS annual data report: epidemiology of kidney disease in the United States. Bethesda: National Institutes of Health, National Institute of Diabetes and Digestive and Kidney Diseases; 2016.
34. Luyckx VA, Tonelli M, Stanifer JW. The global burden of kidney disease and the sustainable development goals. Bull World Health Organ. 2018;96(6):414–422D. https://doi.org/10.2471/BLT.17.206441.
35. Levin A, Tonelli M, Bonventre J, Coresh J, Donner JA, Fogo AB, ISN Global Kidney Health Summit Participants, et al. Global kidney health 2017 and beyond: a roadmap for closing gaps in care, research, and policy. Lancet. 2017;390(10105):1888–917.
36. Liu FX, Gao X, Inglese G, Chuengsaman P, Pecoits-Filho R, Yu A. A global overview of the impact of peritoneal dialysis first or favored policies: an opinion. Perit Dial Int. 2015;35(4):406–20. https://doi.org/10.3747/pdi.2013.00204.
37. Osman MA, Alrukhaimi M, Ashuntantang GE, et al. Global nephrology workforce: gaps and opportunities toward a sustainable kidney care system. Kidney Int Suppl (2011). 2018;8(2):52–63. https://doi.org/10.1016/j.kisu.2017.10.009.

# Part II

# Americas

# Nephrology in Argentina

# 8

Gustavo Lorenzo Moretta, Ana Maria Sesin, Eduardo Celia, and Jose Scapuzzi

| | |
|---|---|
| Area[1] | 3,761,274 km$^2$ |
| Population[2] | 44,361,150 (2018) |
| Capital | Buenos Aires |
| Three most populated cities[1] | 1. Buenos Aires<br>2. Córdoba<br>3. Rosario |
| Official language[1] | Spanish |
| Gross domestic product (GDP)[3] | 912.09 billion USD (2018) |
| GDP per capita[1] | 11,653 USD (2018) |
| Human development index (HDI)[3] | 0.825 (48° position) |
| Official currency | Argentinian peso |
| Total number of nephrologists | 1200 |
| National society of nephrology | Argentinian Society of Nephrology (SAN) www.san.org.ar |
| Incidence of end-stage renal disease[4,5] | 2018 – 162 pmp<br>2019 – 160 pmp |
| Prevalence of end-stage renal disease[4,5] (on dialysis) | 2018 – 676 pmp<br>2019 – 681 pmp |
| Total number of patients on dialysis (all modalities)[4,5] | 2018 – 30,080<br>2019 – 30,610 |
| Number of patients on hemodialysis[4,6] | 2018 – 27,973<br>2019 – 28,608 |
| Number of patients on peritoneal dialysis[4,6] | 2018 – 1996<br>2019 – 2081 |
| Number of renal transplantations per year[4,7] | 2018 – 1329<br>2019 – 1576 |

1. Available from: https://www.ign.gob.ar/NuestrasActividades/Geografia/DatosArgentina
2. OPS, Argentina M de S y D de la Nación. Indicadores Básicos 2018 [Internet]. Buenos Aires; 2019. Available from: http://iris.paho.org/xmlui/handle/123456789/50802
3. Available from: https://datos.bancomundial.org/indicador/NY.GDP.PCAP.CD?locations=AR
4. Marinovich S, Lavorato C, Bisigniano L, Hansen Krogh D, Celia E, Tagliafichi V, Rosa Diez G, Fayad A, Haber V: Registro Argentino de Diálisis Crónica SAN-INCUCAI 2016. Sociedad Argentina de Nefrología e INCUCAI. Buenos Aires, Argentina. 2017
5. Available from: https://irct.incucai.gov.ar/public/centro/Show.do;jsessionid=BHLBFEGGCHIC?accion=/bridgeFromCresiToResumenEstadisticoCentroDialisis.do?click_and_list_habilitado=false&modulo=1&login=no&click_and_list_habilitado=false&
6. Available from https://cresi.incucai.gov.ar/reporte/resumenestadistico/EjecutarConsultaPre.do
7. https://cresi.incucai.gov.ar/cresi/OpenDocument.do?accion=/cresi_tx.do?CLICK_AND_LIST_HABILITADO=trueAccording

G. L. Moretta (✉)
Northwest Nephrological Center, National University Northwest Buenos Aires, Buenos Aires, Argentina

A. M. Sesin
National Hospital of Clinics, National University of Córdoba, Córdoba, Argentina

E. Celia
Argentine Society of Nephrology, Buenos Aires, Argentina

J. Scapuzzi
Internal Medicine Academic Unit, Ezeiza Hospital Buenos Aires University, Buenos Aires, Argentina

## Introduction

Argentina, officially the Argentine Republic, is a sovereign country located in the southern and southeastern corner of the Americas. It adopts the form of a republican, democratic, representative, and federal government. Argentina is organized as a decentralized federal state, composed since 1994 by 24 self-governed states, being 23 provinces and the Autonomous City of Buenos Aires (CABA), the latter designated as the federal capital of the country. Each state has its own political autonomy, constitution, flag, and security forces. The 23 provinces maintain all power not delegated to the national state and guarantee the autonomy of their municipalities. It integrates the Mercosur – a commercial block of the southern South America countries, being one of the founders in 1991 – the Union of South American Nations (Unasur), the Community of Latin American and Caribbean States (CELAC), and the Organization of American States (OAS). In 2018, its Human Development Index was 0.830 and is ranked 48th worldwide, adjusted for the inequality that is 0.714 with a Gini coefficient of 42.7. In education, it has an investment budget of 5.1% of the GDP, with a population almost fully literate [1].The Argentine economy is one of the most developed and important in South America. According to the World Bank, its nominal GDP is placed as



J. A. Moura-Neto et al. (eds.), *Nephrology Worldwide*, https://doi.org/10.1007/978-3-030-56890-0_8

21st in the world [2]. Due to its geopolitical and economic importance, it is one of the three Latin American sovereign countries that is part of the so-called Group of the Twenty and also integrates the group of the new industrialized countries (NIC). It has reached optimal levels of research and development in sciences, with five Nobel Prize winners, three of them associated to sciences. Its technological and scientific capacity has allowed to design, produce, and export satellites and build nuclear reactors. It is one of the 20 countries that have a permanent presence in Antarctica, being the one with the most permanent bases, 6 in total.

In relation to the health system, the first step was taken toward the recognition of public health as a problem of specific interest in 1943, with the creation of the National Directorate of Public Health and Social Assistance, which in 1949 became the Ministry of Health (MoH). Currently, the Argentine health system has 17,485 healthcare establishments including those managed by the public, social security, and private sectors. In Argentina there are 4.5 hospital beds per 1000 inhabitants, 3.94 doctors per 1000 inhabitants, and a total of 166,187 doctors [3].

## Brief History of Argentine Nephrology

The history of Argentine nephrology has experienced several important moments, from the study of renin-angiotensin to the first renal transplant in Latin America.

In the 1930s, in the physiology laboratory at the Medical School of the University of Buenos Aires, Nobel laureates Bernardo Houssay and Juan Carlos Fasciolo began research applying the Goldblatt kidney model. They implanted an ischemic kidney from hypertensive dogs to nephrectomized normotensive dogs, which caused an increase in blood pressure, leading them to the assumption that a hypertensive substance was being continuously produced. This was the first experience that confirmed the presence of a humoral mechanism responsible for nephrogenic arterial hypertension [4]. Subsequently, Alberto Carlos Taquini confirmed the possibility that the substance released by the kidney acted directly on the blood vessels as well as that the increase in blood pressure that was observed after restoring the blood flow in ischemic kidneys was caused by the same vasopressor substance. Fasciolo, along with Eduardo Braun Menéndez in 1939, identified the hypertensive substance from venous blood from kidneys subjected to periods of ischemia. Extracted by acetone, it was thermostable and dialyzable and had a brief hypertensive effect, characteristics that differentiated it from renin. The Argentine team named this substance hypertensin. An enzyme-substrate reaction was postulated for the formation of hypertensin, which was denominated hypertensinogen (the substrate), renin (the enzyme), and hypertensinases (the enzymes responsible for degrading hypertensin). The discovery of the Argentine team was limited to angiotensin, whereas Page and collaborators in the United States observed that a substrate was necessary for the pressor substance to be generated, the substrate being a globulin called hypertensinogen in Buenos Aires and renin activator in Indianapolis. Thus, a peptide substance was generated and named hypertensin in Argentina and in the United States angiotonin. Hypertensin and angiotonin turned out to be the same substance. In 1958, Braun Menéndez and Page agreed on a new nomenclature in Ann Arbor, so that the words angiotensin and angiotensinogen emerged [5].

In 1955, Dr. Ruiz Guiñazú performed the first hemodialysis (HD) with a machine made entirely in the country, based on the Kolff-Brigham kidney model; in 1957 Professor Alfredo Lanari performed the first renal transplant in Latin America at the Institute of Medical Research associated to the University of Buenos Aires and the First Tissue Bank created through Law 17041 [6].

Inspired by the scientific activities of this institute, so-called the kidney club, the Argentine Society of Nephrology was founded on September 15, 1960 [7].

In 1965, Ondetti and Cushman began studying ACE inhibitors, based on the research by Sergio H. Ferreira of the Ribeirão Preto School of Medicine of the University of São Paulo, Brazil. Dr. Miguel Ondetti did his PhD thesis at the University of Buenos Aires and subsequently continued his research work in the Squibb Research and Development Laboratories in Argentina in the area of natural products, isolating and characterizing alkaloids of pharmacological importance. He succeeded to characterize the most relevant peptide of these compounds studied by Ferreira that received the generic name of teprotide and that was a competitive inhibitor of the enzymatic activity of ACE. In this way, Ondetti achieved the synthesis of polypeptides and related compounds finally characterizing the structure of captopril from the structure of the teprotide molecule. The identification of this compound in the 1970s had a profound social impact, as a new and effective method of hypertension control was achieved [8].

Simultaneously in 1962, Gianantonio published in *The Journal of Pediatrics*, under the title "Acute renal failure in infancy and childhood," detailing the experience in the diagnosis, treatment, and monitoring of 41 children with acute renal failure due to a disease named hemolytic uremic syndrome (HUS), previously described by Gasser in 1955. This was also the beginning of pediatric nephrology in Argentina, by Prof. Gianantonio who contributed significantly worldwide to the study of this pathology. The following year he performed peritoneal dialysis (PD) procedures for the first time in Argentina, saving many lives of children affected by HUS [9].

César Milstein also graduated from the University of Buenos Aires, making his doctoral thesis at that university, but he had to leave the country in 1962 due to the beginning of a military dictatorship and continued his studies in

Cambrigde, where he published, in 1975 in the journal *Nature*, the article " Continuous Cultures of Fused Cells Secreting Antibody of Redefined Specificity," together with G. Köhler, which would lead to the Nobel Prize in Medicine and Physiology in 1984. Monoclonal antibodies did not exist even in the imagination of the most expert immunologists, but their work allowed the development of new techniques and equipment and the advancement in the knowledge of infectious agents, in the diagnosis of diseases, and, more recently, in their application as a therapeutic agent and their impact on the results of transplants [10].

An increase in transplants in Argentina occurred toward the end of the 1970s, due to the discovery of new immunosuppressive drugs. In 1977, Law 21.541 was passed giving birth to the Single Coordinating Center for Ablation and Implant (CUCAI) as the national procurement agency in charge of the regulation of the activity. Between 1985 and 1996, the registration of CKD patients began with voluntary information, and the provided data represented 20–30% of the prevalent patients. Between 1990 and 1996, there was a significant increase in information, through the valuable contribution of the regional registries. In 1990, with the enactment of Law 23,885, CUCAI became the National Single Central Coordination Institute for Organ Removal and Implantantion (INCUCAI), becoming a decentralized body as an autarchy and retaining its dependence on the MoH. In 1997, an agreement was established between INCUCAI and SAN that allowed the development of a patient registry with greater rigor and validity. The National Procurement and Transplant Information System of the Argentine Republic (SINTRA) is implemented in 2004, and a new stage begins in the registry era. Its implementation allowed to gather RRT information from the patients and centers (95%) and to register into a digital system [11].

In 2005, after an extensive parliamentary debate, Law 26.066 was approved incorporating the figure of the alleged donor for organ donations. The regulation, which established that every person over 18 years of age is considered a donor with the exception of those who have expressed their will not to be a donor, entered into force in 2006 and allowed the procurement activity to continue to rise. In 2010, the MoH, through INCUCAI and its procurement system, implemented the Renal Transplant Development Plan, which articulates actions at different levels to prevent, diagnose, treat, and follow-up CKD. Within this framework, the Hospital Donor Strategy was implemented, aiming to incorporate procurement as an activity of the hospitals themselves in order to increase the availability of organs and tissues for transplantation [12]. The year 2018 closed with an annual growth of 18% in terms of organ donation procedures, and this figure allowed Argentina to reach a rate of 15.75 donors per million inhabitants. Seventy-four percent of the organ donation procedures took place in public healthcare facilities. Of the 1681 organ transplants performed, 986 were renal transplants [13].

## Kidney Disease in Argentina

Few studies have published the CKD prevalence in the general population of Argentina. These epidemiological analyses establish a prevalence of CKD between 10% and 12% of the general adult population [14].

Recently, prevalence studies have been published in special groups and in certain regions, such as the Santa Fe study whose CKD prevalence rate is 11.71% and 13.1% if considering pathological proteinuria. Another recent, multicenter study has reported a slightly lower rate close to 8.10% [15].

The government in consensus with the scientific societies has been continuously developing programs that promote healthcare strategies aimed at preventing and addressing CKD in its primary stages through the PAIER (Program for the Comprehensive Approach to Renal Diseases), mentioning a special approach to the attention of the CKD stage, in order to promote registration policies on the waiting list prior to dialysis and a management model for people with advanced CKD [16]. This program has probably collaborated with the development of preemptive renal transplants, so called because these patients have never received chronic dialysis as RRT, increasing from 51 transplants in 2008 to 116 in 2017.

The number of people who submitted to RRT reached 40,899 patients, 69.8% with dialysis and 30.2% transplanted. Twenty-one percent of the patients are on renal transplant waiting list, and less than 20% of them were transplanted within 1 year of evaluation [12].

## Acute Renal Injury and Critical Care Nephrology

Acute kidney injury (AKI) data are based on epidemiological studies from developed countries, where the incidence is assessed in eminently urban environments [17]. This situation is completely different from that of developing countries in which AKI develops in eminently suburban and rural settings, where the incidence is significantly higher. The population distribution in our country according to the last census of 2010 is represented by a very marked phenomenon, where the Autonomous City of Buenos Aires is the most densely populated region with 14,185 inhabitants/Km$^2$, while the province of Santa Cruz is represented by 1.1 inhabitants/km$^2$. Given the absence of specific epidemiological data, if we projected the epidemiological figures reported in the literature, we would estimate the AKI incidence from 84,000 to 630,000 patients per year, of which approximately 22,386 to 163,800 will acutely require some type of RRT [18].

Based on the RIFLE and AKIN criteria, a multicenter study of 627 patients from 9 ICUs conducted in Argentina found that, respectively, 69.4% and 51.8% presented some degree of AKI. The overall 90-day mortality was 40.9%

(RIFLE) and a markedly increased number of patients with severe degree of renal failure (71.1%) [19].

As a relevant fact of endemic diseases causing AKI, we find *Hantavirus* infection and HUS syndrome as the most common causes in the pediatric age. In 1995, a family outbreak of pulmonary syndrome caused by *Hantavirus* in southern Argentina led to the discovery of the Andes virus. In 1998, in the city of El Bolsón and in Bariloche, interhuman transmission was documented for the first time [20]. This zoonosis is presented as (1) epidemic nephritis, (2) hemorrhagic fever with renal syndrome in Europe and Asia, whose mortality reaches 10%, and (3) cardiopulmonary syndrome caused by *Hantavirus*, the most serious of all with an average mortality of 30%, in the Americas. This last form is frequent in Argentina, and besides the severity of the cardiopulmonary component, AKI due to multi-organ failure may occur. Lethality presents a trend of decline from 60% in 1988 to 33% in 2018. More than 70% of people with *Hantavirus* infection live in rural sectors, and also approximately 70% of them carry out activities in the agricultural-forestry sector.

The latest hantavirus outbreak began on November 14, 2018, with one case with an epidemiological nexus of previous environmental exposure; this patient attended a social event, with five attendees of the same event presenting hantavirus with the onset of symptoms at week 47 and 48 epidemiological (18/11–01/12). Twenty-five total cases (23 confirmed, 2 suspects) were reported by January 10, 2019, and 9 persons died confirming interhuman contagion [21].

In relation to HUS, Argentina has the highest incidence in the world. This disease is endemic with an annual incidence of 10 cases/100,000 children under 5 years old. As a consequence, HUS is the main pediatric cause of AKI and the second of CKD in our country, in addition to being responsible for 9% of kidney transplants in children and adolescents. The toxin has been isolated from beef and its derivatives. Argentina has very high levels of meat consumption per capita, and children begin to eat meat at an early age. There is suspicion of an association between the consumption of undercooked meat and infection by the *Escherichia coli* bacteria producing Shiga toxins [22].

Treatment with a product consisting of fraction F (ab) 2 of equine immunoglobulin obtained from hyperimmune sera is currently under development in the country, generating the product INM-004 lot 3945. Preclinical studies have been conducted in vivo where no clinical alterations or side effects associated with treatment were evidenced. In the murine model, the product managed to rescue the animals from the toxic effect even when administered 48 h after administration of the toxin. Currently, the first use in human, prospective, randomized, and placebo-controlled two-stage trial is under development to assess the safety, tolerability, and pharmacokinetics. The trial is authorized to be submitted to the regulatory entity (ANMAT) awaiting its results by 2020 [23].

In the context of critical care nephrology, the RRT modality options available include conventional HD, intermittent online hemodiafiltration (HDF), veno-venous hemofiltration, and PD performed in ICUs.

## Renal Disease in Pediatric Population

There are 12,333,747 children under 18 years of age (30, 74%) in Argentina. According to the national dialysis registry, there are 559 patients under the age of 19 on chronic dialysis, 166 in PD, 185 in HD, and 13 in HDF [24].

Eighty-nine (25%) of these children are on the waiting list for kidney transplantation, and another 19 patients are on the waiting list for preemptive kidney transplantation [24].

In reference to the frequency of comorbidities in maintenance HD, 17.9% have arterial hypertension, the mean PTHi is 606 pg/ml, 20% present with normal bone remodeling (>155 < 300 pg / ml PTHi), the average albuminemia is 3.82 gr/dl with 19.1% of patients with albumin <3.50 gr/dl, and the average hemoglobin is 10.49 gr/dl [24].

It is interesting to observe that the most commonly used dialysis modality by age groups, between 0 and 4 years, is PD in 86.7%; between 5 and 9 years PD in 77.6%; between 10 and 14 years HD in 59.4%; and finally between 15 and 18 years HD in 81%.

The HD mortality when adjusted by gender and presence of diabetes was 6.47% in PD vs. 3.28% in HD between 0 and 9 years and 2.39% in PD vs. 3.20% in HD between 10 and 19 years, in 2017 [24].

The first pediatric renal transplant in Argentina was performed in 1961; since then the programs have been growing. There are 11 pediatric units that perform kidney transplants primarily in Buenos Aires. In 2017, 148 pediatric patients under 18 years of age were transplanted (105 living donors).

There are 120 pediatric nephrologists (78% women), 58% living in and around Buenos Aires. In 4 of the 23 provinces, there is no permanent pediatric nephrologist. To become a pediatric nephrologist requires complete training in clinical pediatrics, followed by a pediatric nephrology scholarship. The University of Buenos Aires also offers a scholarship program. The title of specialist is granted by the local association of doctors in each district, the Argentine Society of Pediatrics, or the University of Buenos Aires. Within the public system, the pediatric fellow receives a monthly remuneration during the full scholarship [25].

## Glomerulopathies

The SAN has developed a national registry of glomerulopathies, being the largest provider in the country the one in the areas of Buenos Aires and the Province of Buenos Aires, having together collected a total of 1714 biopsies. The clinical presentation syndromes are nephrotic syndrome (36.2%), asymptomatic urinary abnormalities (25%), rapidly evolving renal failure (9.3%), nephrotic range proteinuria (6.3%), CKD (6.7%), AKI (6.2%), nonrecurrent macroscopic hematuria (2.2%), HUS (0.3%), and unreported ones (4.7%). In relation to the distribution of the pathologies, 52.6% are primary, 37.9% secondary, 4% undetermined, 2.7% vascular, 2.6% tubular, and 0.2% miscellaneous [26].

The six most frequent primary glomerulopathies correspond to focal and segmental glomerular sclerosis (22.4%), mesangial (17.4%), membranous (13.8%), minimal change disease (8.3%), mesangial non-IgA (6.2%), and mesangiocapillary glomerulonephritis type I (6.0%), whereas within secondary glomerulopathies, most of them were grouped in the category secondary to autoimmune disease (85%) (SLE, 85%; extra GN capillary, 6%; necrotizing, 1%), secondary to gammopathy (6%), secondary to metabolic/hereditary disease (5%), secondary to non-streptococcal infection (2%), secondary to neoplastic disease (1%), and hepatopathy (1%) [26]. Currently, the practice of renal biopsies is not done routinely due to operational, economic, and/or bureaucratic difficulties.

## Renal Replacement Therapy (RRT) in Argentina

Argentina has developed a national information system (SINTRA) to collect, filter, process, create, and distribute data on donation and transplantation activities. This tool allows the whole management of the donation and transplantation procedures. Standards related to donor detection, donor maintenance with life support, procurement, selection of recipients, compatibility testing, storage and transportation of organ, tissues, and cells, as well as allocation and screening for transmissible diseases of the deceased donor have been established by national consensus.

During 2017, 7236 new patients entered maintenance dialysis corresponding to a crude rate of 164 pmp and an adjusted rate of 154.8 pmp [24]. The number of patients and the crude rate increased in relation to the values of the previous years. Almost 400 (394) patients are foreigners and their countries of origin being Paraguay, Bolivia, Chile, Italy, Uruguay, and Peru. In the last 10 years, more than 5000 patients with other nationalities have been treated with RRT in Argentina [24].

As of December 31, 2017, almost 30,000 (29,700) patients were treated with maintenance dialysis, corresponding to a crude rate of 674 pmp and an adjusted rate of 637 pmp. The number of patients has had a constant growth since 2004, but not the gross rate that stagnated between 2013 and 2016, rising again in 2017. The adjusted rate decreased from 2013 to 2017 [24].

In relation to the incident patients, fewer patients were admitted in the last 4 years, and they were in worse clinical conditions when admitted. The ESRD patients entering RRT for the first time is younger every year, more anemic, in worse nutritional conditions, has greater use of transient catheters as first access for HD (72.3% of catheter admissions in 2017, the highest percentage since 2004), and has increasing percentage of unvaccinated anti-hepatitis B.

In relation to diabetes as a cause of CKD, there is a sustained increase in incident patients reaching the maximum rate ever (four out of ten new incident patients), being the first cause of admission and with the highest growth since 2004 according to the latest published data, reaching 59 pmp with certain regional differences [24].

The percentage of insulin-dependent diabetics prior to the onset of maintenance dialysis reaches 76% of the diabetic incidents with a progressive increase in insulin prescription in recent years; only 55% received insulin at the time of admission to maintenance dialysis in 2004.

HD is the most frequent RRT modality in incident patients (94%), but PD has shown a significant growth in the last 11 years, from 3.9% to 6.5% of the total admissions. Capital Federal, Neuquén, and Chaco are the districts with the highest percentage of patients starting in PD: 15%, 12%, and 12%, respectively [24].

The average estimated initial glomerular filtration rate (GFR) was 8.7 ml/min/1.73 $m^2$, and 7.7% presented a GFR $\geq$ 15 ml/ min/1.73$m^2$ according to the 2017 data.

In relation to comorbidities, 70% present with some degree of anemia, with average hematocrit values of 27.6–27.7%. Only 35% of patients start with hematocrit ≥30%. Half of the new patients have protein malnutrition with hypoalbuminemia (<3.5 g/dL) which is a predictor of greater immediate mortality. The overweight-obesity population comprises 57% of the incident patients, and 84% of the patients present with arterial hypertension on admission [24]. Almost 40% (39%) of the incident patients are vaccinated for hepatitis B, 0.3% have positive HBsAg, 1.2% anti-HVC positive, and 0.8% anti-HIV positive. There has been a significant increase in the number of anti-HIV incident patients admitted to dialysis in the last 2 years (8 positive patients per 1000 incident patients) when compared to previous years [24].

A very significant increase in the use of the non-tunneled transient catheter, as first access to HD, has been observed, from 59% in 2004 to 72% in 2017. In contrast, the use of native fistula as first access fell very significantly in the same period (from 35% to 22%). Patients with asthma or chronic obstructive pulmonary disease accounted for 7.6% of new patients in maintenance dialysis in 2017, no difference with the previous years. Tobacco was consumed by 18% of the population admitted to maintenance dialysis in 2017, a tendency toward greater smoking, contrary to the expectations based on the implementation of active measures against smoking in Argentina. Active tuberculosis or a history of tuberculosis had a significant decrease, representing 1.1 of every 100 patients admitted to maintenance dialysis in 2017 [24].

In relation to the prevalence, diabetic nephropathy is the most frequent etiology with the highest growth since 2004, reaching 187 pmp in 2017, whereas unknown etiology is the second with 127 pmp in 2017 [24].

In relation to the dialysis modality, HD is the most frequent modality in 94% of the patients, while PD showed significant growth in the last 11 years, going from 3.9% to 6.5% of the total reflecting the data of the incident patients' data [24].

Online HDF has been performed in Argentina since 2014. The growth of this technique has been significant in the short period, from 184 patients in 2014 to 1688 patients in 2017, representing 5.7% of the prevalent population in maintenance dialysis.

In relation to comorbidities in prevalent patients, anemia is present in 61.9% of the patients, hemoglobin ≥11, and <13 g/dL in 38.1% of the patients with EPO doses up to 105 IU/Kg/week [24]. The percentage of prevalent patients with arterial hypertension increased significantly in 2016–2017, without distinction of gender, age, etiology, body mass, or dialysis modality, except for the youngest group in maintenance dialysis (0–19 years), in which it decreased. Forty percent presented values of systolic BP > 140 and diastolic BP > 90 mmHg. The percentage of patients treated with hypotensive medication increased in the last 2 years, although the percentage of hypertensive patients who do not receive antihypertensives (29%) remains high. The prevalence of positive HBsAg is 1.0%, anti-HCV 2.4%, and anti-HIV 0.9%. More than half of the population (58%) in chronic dialysis have anti-HBs values at protective levels. Cardiovascular disease presented the following frequency: coronary heart disease 8.0%, heart failure 16.0%, cerebrovascular disease 7.0%, and finally peripheral vascular disease 30.8% of the prevalent population in maintenance dialysis.

## Peritoneal Dialysis

About 2000 (1936) patients were treated with PD in 2017, achieving a growth of more than 100% in 10 years (952 patients in 2007); 471 patients out of those 1926 started PD in 2017. The annual growth was 10% for the biennium 2016–2017.

There are certain differential characteristics between patients on PD compared to HD, according to data published by the Argentine Registry. PD patients are younger (32% are 60 years or older vs. 51% in HD), consist of more female (54% s vs. 42% in HD), and have less diabetics (16% vs. 28% in HD). In relation to comorbidities, the average hemoglobin value was 10.94 g/l, albumin 3.62 g/l, and i-PTH 463, and 31.3% were hypertensive, 6.6% presented with coronary insufficiency, 10.5% have heart failure, and 18% have peripheral vascular disease. The percentage of PD patients positive for HBsAg was 1.18%, anti-HVC 2.24%, and 1.41% anti-HIV [24].

The crude mortality rate in 2017 was 10.2% (202 deaths, with 1883.6 patients' years of risk exposure) and adjusted mortality (by age and etiology by indirect standardization) of 15.16%. The crude mortality rate in diabetic patients was 16.3% in females vs. 26.6% in males.

An interesting fact to point out was the improvement of the adjusted mortality results in PD in recent years, going down from 20% in 2007 to 15.16% in 2017 [24].

The PD costs are pending, being affected by the economic crisis of the country and the devaluation of its currency, since the inputs (disposable material) reflect 60% of the cost and are imported.

## Hemodialysis

In 2017, 27,764 patients were treated with HD, achieving a growth close to 20% in 10 years (23,266 patients in 2007); almost 7000 (6765) patients entered HD (93.49% of total 2017 incident patients in dialysis). The HD growth was 3% in the biennium 2016–2017. In relation to comorbidities, the average hemoglobin value was 10.59 g/l, albumin 3.76 g/l, i-PTH 517, and 40.5% were hypertensive, 8.2% presented with coronary insufficiency, 16.5% have heart failure, and 29.4% have peripheral vascular disease. In reference to prevalence of viral infections, 0.88% were positive for HBsAg, 2.62% anti-HVC, and 0.83% anti-HIV [24].

In relation to HD adequacy, average KT/V was 1.56, whereas 76.4% presented K/TV greater than 1.3. Patients with permanent vascular access managed to reach higher average K/TV. In relation to vascular accesses distribution, 68.8% have native arteriovenous fistula, 13% grafts, 7.7% permanent tunneled catheters, and 10.4% non-tunneled transient catheters. In regard to the use of tunneled and transient catheters in different populations, there is a greater frequency of use at the extremes of life: 35.4% between 0 and 19 years and 43.7% between 65 and over 75 years [24].

The crude mortality rate was 18.16% (5038 deaths, with 27,736 patients' year of exposure to risk) in 2017. The gross mortality rate for diabetic patients was 26.6% in females vs. 26.14% in males [24].

Considering the HD population registered from January 2005 to December 2015, the probability of survival under dialysis treatment in the short (1 year), medium (5 years) and long term (10 years) is 80%, 40%, and 18%, respectively. When we select the subgroup of HD patients in the transplant waiting list, the results are 92%, 70%, and 44%, respectively [24].

The gross mortality rate of both techniques (HD and PD) decreased between 2016 and 2017, resulting in 17.7 deaths per hundred patients at risk per year. The adjusted global mortality rate also decreased last year, being 16.26 deaths per hundred patients at risk year. Adjusting for age, gender, and diabetic nephropathy, PD patients from 2011 onwards have presented significantly lower mortality than HD patients in Argentina.

In Argentina, 100% RRT coverage is guaranteed, with financing originating from the public subsector (82%) and private (18%) [24].

The financing of the admission to maintenance dialysis relies fundamentally on eight payers representing 99.4% of the total in 2017, with very similar percentages from 2004 to 2016 (always greater than 99.2%). PAMI is the largest payer in the number of incident dialysis patients per year, followed by all other institutions like Provincial Social Works, Trade Union Social Works (ex SSSAPE), provincial subsidies, Incluir Salud (ex PROFE), prepaid, other social works, and finally the public health system [24].

A recent cost study shows that the main categories and their impact on the costs of the chronic HD session are human resources (44%), disposable material (11%), real estate (8%), and transportation (8%).The cost of one chronic HD session was estimated at 2693 Argentinian pesos (170.12 USD). In the case of one HDF session, the same main cost categories were observed, although their relative magnitude changes: human resources (35%), disposable material (25%), real estate (7%), and transportation (6%). The estimated cost of the HDF session was 3372 Argentinian pesos (213.01 USD) [27].

## Kidney Transplant

In Argentina, a total of 13,185 renal transplants, performed between 1998 and December 31, 2016, have been registered. The great majority (89%) corresponds to adult donors and 11% to pediatric donors [12]. Argentina offers national and international training programs to harmonize the practices of professional staff working with organ donation and procurement activities. Several technical cooperation agreements have been signed with many countries, mainly in Latin American, and joined international forums in the field of transplantation. Public or private health institutions must be accredited for procurement and transplantation, and health professionals must be certified (Law 24,193). There are 59 centers authorized for renal transplantation distributed throughout the country but in greater number in the federal capital (17), Buenos Aires, (10) and Córdoba (6) [28].

Brain death must be certified by the criteria of complete brain death in accordance with the law. The law only allows the donation of organs from related living donors, with no additional incentives for donors. Organ trafficking is prohibited and punishable by law. The Argentine system guarantees transparency, traceability, and the quality of the procedure.

The percentage of cadaveric kidney transplant or related living donor has increased 74% in the last 14 years, from 765 in 2004 to 1329 in 2017. Considering all types of kidney transplants, the rate per million inhabitants rose from 20.0 up to 30.2 from 2004 to 2017, resulting in a 51% growth, having its maximum value (30.5) in 2013. The gross renal transplant rate in the maintenance dialysis population increased from 3.4 to 3.8 transplants per 100 patients at risk year, between 2005 and 2017. There are currently geographical differences, being Buenos Aires the city with the highest gross rate, 7/100 patients at risk year. Drawing a comparison of unadjusted rates with international data reported from the rest of the world, it will be observed that Argentina, with 28 pmp in 2016 (last year published), is placed at 34th position out of 64 countries that publish data in the USRDS Registry [29].

In the Newsletter Transplant, Argentina reported 29.8 pmp for 2017, when in reality the figure is 30.2 pmp. Argentina ranks fourth in the American continent, behind the United States, Canada, and Uruguay [30].

In relation to kidney transplants during 2019, 1576 were paid by the most important social security funders: *National Institute of Social Services for Retired and Pensioned* (PAMI) with 357 and *Incluir Salud (a federal program, public payer),* with 266 transplants [28].

## Nephrology Practice in Argentina

Annually, approximately 4000 young doctors apply for medical training positions in the different jurisdictions of the country [31].

The most frequent pathways to train as a medical specialist are the medical residence/fellowship or the university postgraduate degree. Of the 2440 professionals who have certified their specialty in the Ministry of Health of Argentina between 2008 and 2013, 57% did so at the end of an accredited medical residence/fellowship and 25% at the end of the university postgraduate degree.

In order for the degrees to have national validity, the universities which grant them must necessarily be accredited by the National Commission for University Evaluation and Accreditation (CONEAU), within the jurisdiction of the Ministry of Education and the Residency Accreditation System (SNARES) of the Ministry of Health. Both agencies are in charge of the of health specialists training programs.

The nephrologist training in Argentina requires a year of internal medicine, 3 years of nephrology, and one year of professional practice, which are articulated with different time loads in each year of the program. The internal medicine module can be incorporated into residence or certified independently. The specialty of nephrology is recognized in the 24 jurisdictions.

In order to enter medical residence in the public sector, a single medical exam is carried out concentrating the applicants of 21 states institutions dependent on the MoH. In 2018, 48 medical residence positions were offered to training in different specialties. Nephrology training is only available in 12 of the 24 states.

Among the physicians who apply for training positions by specialty, only 0.13% choose nephrology, with pediatrics (32%), general medicine (18%), and anesthesia (12%) being the most applied to [27].

The nephrologist working in a private dialysis unit earns approximately 6 USD per hour and a maximum of 1152 USD per month. In the public sector, the salary is approximately 1200 USD per month plus social benefits (paid holidays, retirement, etc.). New nephrologists entering the labor market have few opportunities in established kidney transplant programs and public nephrology services, facing great vulnerability when dealing with multinational dialysis providers or national networks. Moreover, many nephrologists own their own dialysis centers. National dialysis entrepreneurs are grouped together in the Confederation of Dialysis Associations of the Argentine Republic, which is a non-profit civil association, founded on May 8, 1997, by the Provincial Dialysis Associations of the Argentine Republic with the purpose of addressing, collectively, scientific and educational actions in nephrology and dialysis and in defense of the rights of the centers and establishments that make up the associations.

Multinational networks (Fresenius, Diaverum, and Baxter) treat the majority of patients on maintenance dialysis and are also grouped in an association called the Argentine Chamber of Renal Therapy.

According to the national dialysis center registry in 2020, there are 596 dialysis centers. There are 503 privately owned dialysis centers: 112 are owned by FMC (10,498 patients), 40 are owned by Diaverum (3515 patients), 194 are associated with the confederation of dialysis centers in Argentina (7989 patients), and 182 are independent (7006). In the public sector, there are 68 dialysis centers (1617 patients) [28].

The value of the monthly payment for the entire benefit of HD, including EPO, vascular access, and the patient transport, is 1102 USD (66,169.28 Argentinian pesos in exchange for 60 pesos for 1 USD, January 2020), and in PD, including EPO, peritoneal access, and antibiotics, it is 1186 USD (71,179.95 Argentinian pesos in exchange for 60 pesos for 1 USD, January 2020). There is a delay in reimbursement, which leads to serious difficulties in the operation of the dialysis centers (PAMI and IOMA 60 days of delay, *Incluir Salud* and MoH of the province of Buenos Aires 240 days), which results in economic difficulties for private dialysis units and the nephrologists working in these clinics.

In an HD center, the responsible medical director must be a specialist in nephrology with no less than 2 years of dialysis experience, after having obtained the title of specialist. Nephrologists must ensure that the correct dialysis prescription as well as the clinical follow-up of the patient undergoing dialysis are executed daily, at a rate of 1 every 40 patients. In case of nonavailability of a nephrologist, the acting physician must have demonstrated dialysis treatment experience for a period of at least 6 months. In relation to nursing staff, their training and education must be certified by the medical director. The ratio of staff present during each dialysis shift must not be less than one to five patients [32].

In PD, the physician responsible for the unit must have a nephrology specialist title granted by the competent authority as well as dialysis therapy experience of 2 years and not less than 3 months of experience in chronic PD in a PD service recognized by the SAN. In the case of pediatric chronic PD, the physician responsible should be a pediatric nephrologist or have a backup pediatric nephrologist for consultation, whenever needed. Nursing staff must be registered in the MoH with certified dialysis training. The nursing staff ratio should not be less than 1 nurse per 20 adult patients, whereas in pediatrics the ratio should not be less than 1 nurse per 15 patients [32]. The dialysis units must also have a psychologist, dietitian, and social worker in relation to the number of patients and at the discretion of the medical management. Each dialysis center has a continuous improvement program supported by the medical directorate and implemented by a quality committee constituted by the medical director, nursing officer, nephrologist, social worker, dietitian, psychologist, and representatives of the administrative and maintenance areas.

This quality committee evaluates, on an annual basis, the implementation of the different programs to improve vascular or peritoneal access, among others. The committee for its evaluations will take as a reference the average national results published by the Argentine Registry of Dialysis and by those suggested by the SAN [32].

The annual results obtained will be communicated to the members of the renal team in each center as well as the objectives proposed for the following period. The reports will remain available for internal and external audits.

Hemodialyzers may be reused; however, the dialyzer efficiency must be controlled by measuring the residual fiber bundle volume, which must be maintained above 80% of the initial reference value. The reference values must be included in a folded book of nonremovable sheets, although it can be kept in a computerized record, as long as it is encrypted.

In the case that it is decided to reuse the dialyzer, reprocessing must be done in a physical environment used exclusively for that purpose; anti-HCV-positive patients' dialyzers must be reprocessed in a separate, properly identified sector.

Disposal of hemodialyzers used in positive B patients is recommended, whereas in the case of patients with HIV-positive serology, discard is mandatory in each session [32].

Although the government's dialysis guidelines do not mention the number of reuses allowed for one dialyzer, it is usually discarded after 20 times of use.

## Highlights of Nephrology in Argentina

On March 28, 2015, the Favaloro Institute performed the first cross renal donation kidney transplant in Latin America. On October 12, 2017, through a resolution published in the *Official Gazette*, INCUCAI was authorized to incorporate this type of operations. The new transplant law (No. 27447, 2018) among other points incorporates the cross renal donation procedure. Before the law was enacted, there were two transplant options in Argentina: a cadaveric kidney donor or a living one. If the kidney was donated by a living donor, it should be related to the patient via a family bond, and if that link did not exist, a judicial process had to be claimed in order to authorize the transplant.

Among the different compatibilities that must exist between the patient and the donor, the most important ones are blood and tissue compatibility. Cross transplantation is a modality that allows a patient who has a potential noncompatible living donor to still receive a living donor transplant. It was reported in a paper by Rapaport in 1986 and first implemented in South Korea in 1990. The new legal framework creates a system where patients with their noncompatible living donors can be registered, and the INCUCAI is responsible for finding compatible pairs [33].

Another point to note is related to the HUS, a serious disease of great importance for our country public health and for which there is no approved medication in the world. It is the local development of an innovative biological medicine with the potential to become the first treatment to block Shiga toxin (Stx) and prevent progression to HUS.

The National Administration of Drug, Foods and Medical Devices (ANMAT) has incorporated this new drug into its "Program for Support to Innovation in Medicines and Health Products" and has also been presented to the European regulatory authorities (EMA) and United States (Food and Drug Administration, FDA) in the form of "scientific advice" and "pre-IND meeting" respectively, incorporating the suggestions of the three entities into the final design. In addition, the drug has been designated as an orphan drug in Europe and the United States. The Phase II/III clinical study is currently in progress evaluating the efficacy and safety of this drug to block Shiga toxin serum in pediatric patients at risk of developing HUS. The study is being carried out in public and private centers in different parts of the country, hoping that the results will allow to prevent HUS progress in a few years.

## Future Perspectives of Nephrology in Argentina

The main current challenge for nephrology in Argentina, as in the rest of the world, is to increase the interest among medical graduates in choosing the specialty.

Furthermore, the need to increase the reimbursement of therapies related to nephrology and repeated economic crisis conspire to the stability and development of nephrology in Argentina. The fact that a large part of the available jobs is in dialysis units facing financial problems makes it difficult for new doctors to choose this complex specialty, requiring many years of study and an inadequate salary. Access to new technologies also faces economic difficulties for everyone, including the population in need of access to them. Argentina has had several possibilities for the development of its economy and science in its past history as a country. We now hope that a new era of enlightenment may come forth and allow the development of our specialty.

## Conclusion

Nephrology in Argentina has a good organization through the various associations that regulate the nephrologist formation (CONEAU and SNARES). The SAN does an excellent job fully involved in the training of nephrologists through prestigious continuing education programs (PRONEFRO) and fundamentally being a professional pillar of the Chronic Dialysis Registry in SINTRA with INCUCAI.

Basic sciences in Argentina have demonstrated the impact of their discoveries on the renin-angiotensin system and the subsequent development of captopril and monoclonal antibodies. Today, the National Commission of Research Science and Technology (Conicet) together with a private national laboratory (Inmunova) is on its way to establish the first treatment for HUS.

The national system of organ and tissue procurement has achieved a sustained impact over time and on the perception of citizen security. Laws have accompanied this development. Quality programs have accompanied the development of dialysis units, and an improvement in the mortality of diabetic patients on chronic dialysis has been achieved.

The path of nephrology in Argentina has been paved over the past years. However, much still remains to be done, and as the tango song of Enrique Santos Discépolo [34] says, *"lleno de esperanzas el camino que los sueños prometieron a sus ansias."*

## References


1. OPS, Argentina M de S y D de la Nación. Indicadores Básicos 2018 [Internet]. Buenos Aires; 2019. Available from: http://iris.paho.org/xmlui/handle/123456789/50802.
2. OCDE et al. Perspectivas económicas de América Latina 2019: desarrollo en transición. Resumen. Paris; 2019.
3. Galli A, Pagés M, Swieszkowski S. El Sistema de Salud Argentino [Internet]. Contenidos Transversales. Buenos Aires; 2017. Available from: http://www.scielo.org.mx/pdf/spm/v53s2/06.pdf.
4. Cherne P, Young P. Historia del sistema renina angiotensina: grandes hombres, un gran descubrimiento. Revista Medica de Chile [Internet]. 2014;142:1210–6. Available from: www.scielo.org.ar/scielo.php?script=sci_ar.
5. Agrest A. La Saga de la Renina. Medicina (B Aires). 2000;60:37–45.
6. Romero L. La investigación clinica en Argentina- La tradición Lanari. Redes. 2011;17(33):63–93.
7. Gotlieb D. Síntesis histórica de los acontecimientos y circunstancias que dieron origen a la Sociedad Argentina de Nefrología. Buenos Aires; 2010.
8. Bautista RJ. Captopril, el potente agente antihipertensivo concebido y desarrollado por un investigador argentino: Miguel Ángel Ondetti. Cienc Investig Reseñas. 2016;1(66):29–33.
9. Fronteras En Medicina I, Año I. Historia de la Medicina Maestro de la Pediatría Argentina. 2017.
10. González-Fernández Á, de Espada FD. César Milstein: 35 Años de anticuerpos monoclonales. Inmunologia. Elsevier Doyma. 2011;30:30–3.
11. el Instituto Nacional Central Único Coordinador de Ablación e Implante. Incucai-Registro Nacional de Insuficiencia Renal Crónica Terminal [Internet]. 2020 [cited 2019 Dec 9]. Available from: http://sintra.incucai.gov.ar/intro/.
12. del Carmen Bacqué M, Vallejos A, Bisigniano L. Editorial. Situación del Transplante Renal y la donación de órganos en Argentina. Rev Nefrol Dial Traspl [Internet]. 2018;38(1):1–14. Available from: www.renal.org.ar.
13. Argentina. Ministerio de Salud. Noticias de Argentina, Transplantes [Internet]. Noticias. Ministerio de Salud y Desarrollo. 2019 [cited 2019 Feb 1]. Available from: Disponible en https://www.argentina.gob.ar/noticias/argentina-registro-mas-de-700-donantes-de-organos-en-2018.
14. Marinovich S, Marinovich J, Benítez ML, Baldomá S, Dohle E, del Basso L, et al. Enfermedad Renal Crónica en la Población General. Importancia de la Tasa de Filtrado Glomerular estimada absoluta Chronic Renal Disease in the General Population Importance of the Absolute Estimated Glomerular Filtration Rate [Internet]. Available from: www.renal.org.ar.
15. Suarez R, Piggiano N, Simesen G, Beatriz L, Letjam N, Pinheiro M. Estudio multicéntrico de prevalencia de Enfermedad renal crónica. Nefrología Argentina. 2019;17(1).
16. Vallejos A. Editorial: Primer Foro Global de Politicas sobre el Riñón. Nefrol Dialisis y Transpl. 2017;37:79–80.
17. Lombi F, Varela CF, Martinez R, Greloni G, Campolo Girard V, Rosa Diez G. Lesión renal aguda en Latinoamérica en la era del big data. Nefrología [Internet]. 2017 [cited 2020 Feb 13];37(5):461–4. Available from: https://linkinghub.elsevier.com/retrieve/pii/S0211699517300681.
18. Lombi F, Campolo V, Girard C, Varela F, Martinez R, Greloni G, Rosa Diez G. Epidemiología de la Injuria Renal Aguda en Argentina. Nefrología Argentina [Internet]. 2016;14. Available from: http://www.nefrologiaargentina.org.ar/numeros/2016/volumen14_3/Articulo_1.pdf.
19. Salgado G, Landa M, Masevicius D, Gianassi S, San-Román JE, Silva L, et al. Acute renal failure according to the RIFLE and AKIN criteria: a multicenter study. Med Intensiva. 2014;38(5):271–7.
20. Sosa Estani S, Salomón O, Gomez A, Esquivel M, Segura E. Diferencias regionales y Síndrome Pulmonar por Hantavirus (enfermedad emergente y tropical en Argentina). Cad Saúde Públic. 2001;17:45–57.
21. Ministerio de Salud. Hantavirosis en Epuyen, Chubut. Reporte Epidemiológico. Buenos Aires; 2019.
22. Antman J, Geffner L, Pianciola L, Rivas M. Síndrome Urémico Hemolítico en Argentina. Reporte Epidemiológico. Buenos Aires; 2014.
23. Hiriart Y, Pardo R, Bukata L, Lauché C, Muñoz L, Colonna M, Goldbaum F, Sanguineti S, Zylberman V. Desarrollo de un producto anti-toxina Shiga para la prevención del Síndrome Urémico Hemolítico. Medicina (B Aires). 2018;78:107–12.
24. Marinovich S, Lavorato C, Bisigniano L, Hansen Krogh D, Celia E, Tagliafichi V, Rosa Diez G, Fayad A, Verónica Haber V, Krogh HD, Diez RG. Registro Argentino de Diálisis Crónica- Informe 2018. Buenos Aires; 2018.
25. Exeni A. Pediatric nephrology in Argentina. 2019.
26. Liderman S. Registro Argentino de Biopsias Renales. Reporte de situación. Nefrol Dialisis y Transpl. 2008;28(2):55–60.
27. Garay OU, Palacios A, Pichon-Riviere A, Augustovski F, Martí SG, Hernández-Vásquez A, et al. The Cost-effectiveness of continuous versus intermittent renal replacement therapies in acute kidney injury: perspective of the social services for the elderly in Argentina. Value in health regional issues [Internet]. 2019 Dec 1 [cited 2020 Feb 12];20:142–8. Available from: https://www.sciencedirect.com/science/article/abs/pii/S2212109919300822?via%3Dihub.
28. INCUCAI Argentina Gobierno. Sistema Nacional de Información de Procuración y Transplante de la República Argentina [Internet]. Buenos Aires; 2020. Available from: https://irct.incucai.gov.ar/public/centro/Show.do;jsessionid=BHLBFEGGCHIC?accion=/bridgeFromCresiToResumenEstadisticoCentroDialisis.do?click_and_list_habilitado=false&modulo=1&login=no&click_and_list_habilitado=false&.
29. Saran R, Robinson B, Abbott KC, Agodoa LYC, Bragg-Gresham J, Balkrishnan R, et al. US renal data system 2018 annual data report: epidemiology of kidney disease in the United States. Am J Kidney Dis. W.B. Saunders. 2019;73:A7–8.
30. International figures on donation and transplantation 2017. Newsletter Transplant. 2018;23:3–79.
31. Duré M, Fernández Lerena M, Gilligan C. Especialidades médicas en Argentina. Reporte. Buenos Aires; 2018.
32. Santa Maria C. Directrices de organizacion y funcionamiento para los centros, servicios o unidades de dialisis [Internet]. Buenos Aires; 2019. Available from: https://www.argentina.gob.ar/sites/default/files/directrices-dialisis.pdf.
33. Rapaport F. The case for a living emotionally related international kidney donor exchange registry. Transplant Proc. 1986;18(3):5–9.
34. Enrique Santos Discépolo. Uno (Tango Song). https://youtu.be/C4fj7PKEJoY.

# Nephrology in Bolivia

9

Rolando Claure-Del Granado, Ricardo Silvestre Arze Arze, Raul Plata-Cornejo, Abel Lucero Ruiz, Arturo Cornejo-Cordero, Rolando Claure-Vallejo, Mauricio Paredes-Fernández, Pablo Dávila-Erquicia, Israel D. Rivas-Salazar, and Maiko A. Tavera-Díaz

*General Table*

| | |
|---|---|
| Area[1] | 1,098,581 km$^2$ |
| Population[1] | 11,428,245 (2019) |
| Capital | Sucre (constitutional and judicial)<br>La Paz (executive and legislative) |
| Three most populated cities[1] | 1. Santa Cruz de la Sierra<br>2. La Paz<br>3. Cochabamba |
| Official languages | Spanish and 36 indigenous languages |
| Gross domestic product (GDP)[2] | 40.288 billion USD (2018) |
| GDP per capita[2] | 2559.51 USD (2018) |
| Human Development Index (HDI)[3] | 0.703 (114th) |
| Official currency | Boliviano (BOB) |
| Total number of nephrologists[4] | 110 |
| National society of nephrology[4] | Bolivian Society of Nephrology and Hypertension<br>www.sobonefro.com |
| Incidence of end-stage renal disease[5] | 2018 – 143 pmp |
| Prevalence of end-stage renal disease[5] (on dialysis) | 2018 – 403 pmp |
| Total number of patients on dialysis[5] | 2018 – 4400; there is no data available for PD |
| Number of patients on hemodialysis[5] | 2018 – 4400 |
| Number of patients on peritoneal dialysis | No data available |
| Number of renal transplantations per year[5] | 2017 – 81<br>2018 – 76 |

1. Instituto Nacional de Estadística (INE). Accessed in January 2020. Available in: https://www.ine.gob.bo/
2. The World Bank. Accessed in January 2020. Available in: https://data.worldbank.org/country/bolivia?view=chart
3. United Nations Development Program. Human Development Reports. Accessed in January 2020. Available in: http://hdr.undp.org/sites/default/files/2018_human_development_statistical_update.pdf
4. Bolivian Society of Nephrology and Hypertension (SBNeH). Accessed in January 2020. Available in: https://sobonefro.com/
5. National Renal Health Program, Plurinational State of Bolivia Minister of Health. Available in: http://www.saludrenal.minsalud.gob.bo

## Introduction

Nephrology is closely linked to other sciences, and it involves major social, ethical, and economic implications that will be set out in this presentation, recalling some of our geography, history, and economic sociology.

R. Claure-Del Granado (✉)
Hospital Obrero No 2 - C.N.S., Universidad Mayor de San Simón, School of Medicine, Cochabamba, Bolivia

R. S. Arze Arze
NEFRODIAL (CENTRO DEL RIÑON), Cochabamba, Bolivia
e-mail: info@nefrodial.com

R. Plata-Cornejo · A. Cornejo-Cordero
Instituto de Nefrología, La Paz, Bolivia

A. Lucero Ruiz
Hospital Obrero N° 1 – C.N.S., La Paz, Bolivia

R. Claure-Vallejo
Unidad de Atención al Enfermo Renal (UNAER S.R.L.), Cochabamba, Bolivia

M. Paredes-Fernández
Seguro Social Universitario, Cochabamba, Bolivia

P. Dávila-Erquicia
Hospital Infantil "Manuel Ascencio Villarroel", Cochabamba, Bolivia

I. D. Rivas-Salazar
Hospital Obrero No 2 - C.N.S., Cochabamba, Bolivia

M. A. Tavera-Díaz
Hospital Elizabeth Seton, Cochabamba, Bolivia


J. A. Moura-Neto et al. (eds.), *Nephrology Worldwide*, https://doi.org/10.1007/978-3-030-56890-0_9

Bolivia, separated from the Pacific Ocean by the Andean Mountain Chain and from the Atlantic Ocean by the Amazon region, has an extension of 1,098,000 km$^2$ and 11 million inhabitants spread over three well-differentiated geographic areas from the climate, racial, social, and economic viewpoints – the highlands, the valleys, and the tropics (Fig. 9.1). In the past, such a layout prevented the country's integration and the implementation of national health programs.

Historically, Bolivia has stood out because of its convoluted political life. The government of the National Revolution, between 1952 and 1964, created several health insurance institutions to address the needs of salaried workers in urban areas, mineworkers, oil workers, and railroad workers. Unfortunately, the lack of coordination among such institutions was detrimental to the people, who required a more coherent and uniform healthcare, and it prevented a harmonious development of the medical specialties, including nephrology. Since 1964, the political changes prevented the creation of legal instruments to allow a regulated practice of medicine. As a result, there was no transplant law until 1996, and regulation for the provision of dialysis for patients with end-stage renal disease (ESRD) was just approved in 2014. For the same reason, not even moderately serious epidemiological studies concerning arterial hypertension, glomerular diseases, renal stones, acute kidney injury (AKI), or chronic kidney disease (CKD) among our population were carried out until the 1980s.

The drop of international mineral and oil prices in the 1980s jeopardized Bolivia's economy. However, we survived thanks to the growth of the informal economy, which encompassed an increasingly larger mass of individuals, lacking health insurance coverage. On the other hand, the increase in state bureaucracy has prevented the development of hospital laboratories and imaging technologies. In spite of such shortcomings, health insurance institutions were until 3 years ago and are still today the only possible alternative for those patients requiring sophisticated life-sustaining technology.

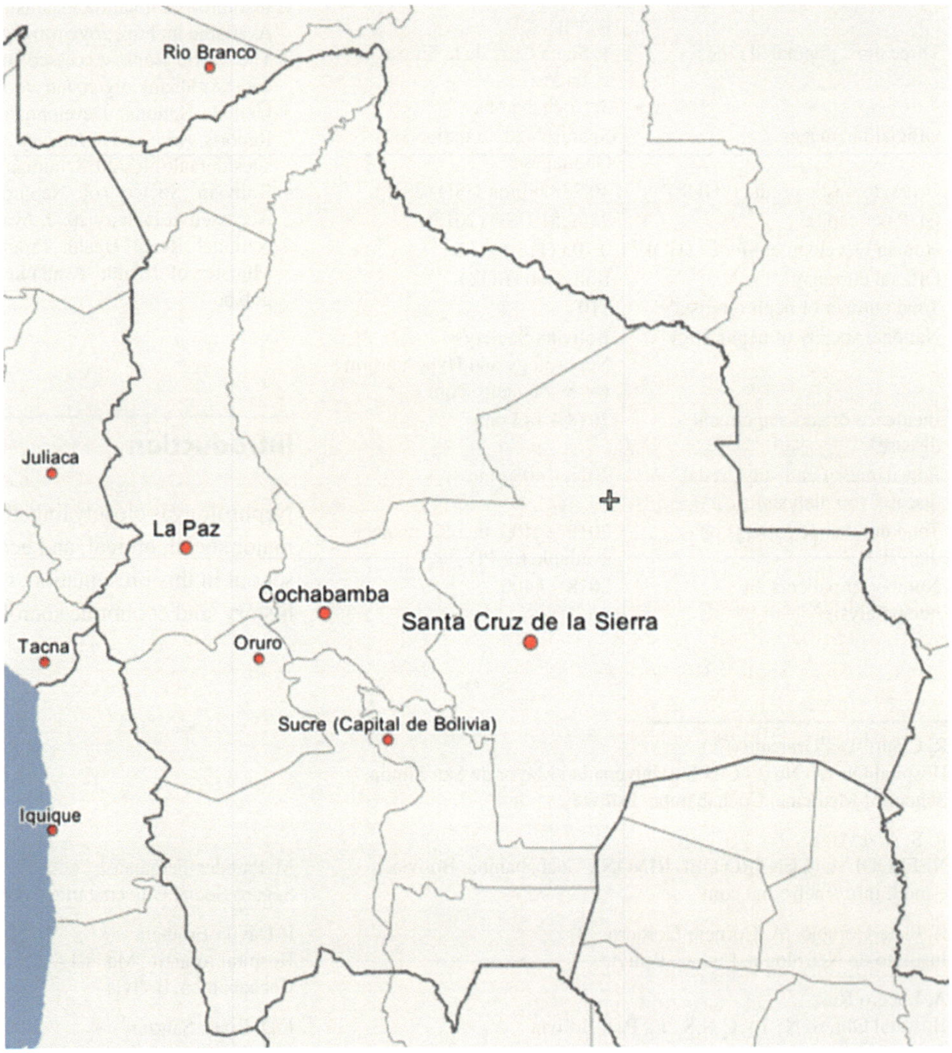


Fig. 9.1 Different regions in Bolivia; the three main cities are La Paz, Santa Cruz de la Sierra, and Cochabamba

That was the case of ESRD patients who required renal replacement therapies (RRT) until December 2014, when legislation was passed allowing patients without health insurance to receive dialysis.

We can now realize the situation being faced by nephrologists and CKD patients in Bolivia so far.

## Brief History of Nephrology in Bolivia

The history of nephrology in Bolivia started with internal medicine doctors and urologists who decided to focus on the study and treatment of kidney diseases as a joint effort. In La Paz, Dr. Guillermo Jáuregui Guachalla, professor of internal medicine, published his *Notes on Nephrology* before passing away around 1970. In the 1940s in Cochabamba, Dr. Ricardo Arze Loureiro, professor of urology, performed kidney decapsulation to restore diuresis in cases of oliguric AKI long before diuretics or dialysis was available. In the 1960s, he ventured into experimental surgery in dogs, as he was convinced of the benefits of renal transplantation as a therapy to replace the chronic loss of kidney function. In Sucre, Dr. Luis Sauma, urologist and devoted to teaching, lighted the way of his son, Alejandro, a great supporter of renal transplantation in Cochabamba (personnel communication).

In 1968, the first Bolivian nephrologist, Dr. Juan Villalba, who was trained in Mexico as a pediatric nephrologist, arrived to Bolivia. At Hospital Obrero #1 in La Paz, he exercised nephrology for the first time. Doctor Villalba is among the founders of the Latin American Society of Nephrology and Hypertension (SLANH), with an outstanding participation in international scientific events. Unfortunately, he met an early death, passing away in 1975. In the late 1970s, the first group of nephrologists arrived from Mexico, and they started the practice of nephrology in La Paz, whereas a second group arrived from Brazil and settled in Santa Cruz de la Sierra. At that time, Dr. Jorge Chávez Chajtur provided prolonged dialysis treatment with a parallel plate dialyzer to a family member affected by a familial renal disease in a small town close to Santa Cruz de la Sierra. For over 5 years, the nurse Martha Chacón offered her uremic husband home hemodialysis (HD) in Cochabamba, at a time in which there were no available nephrologists in that city (personnel communication).

In 1968, the urologist Dr. Néstor Orihuela Montero founded at "Hospital de Clinicas" in La Paz the Institute of Nephrology. He donated the first parallel plate artificial kidney, started experimental surgery in dogs, and organized the first human renal transplantation team at Hospital Obrero #1 together with Dr. Gonzalo Quiroga (nephrologist), Dr. Enrique Zubieta (vascular surgeon), and Dr. Edgar Revollo (immunologist), all of whom performed the first kidney transplant on November 2, 1979. This was the first and only deceased donor renal transplant performed in Bolivia until 1993 and took place as a consequence of a gunshot wound in the head of a curious medical student who was walking around the vicinity of Hospital Obrero #1 in La Paz during one of the many and bloody military coups d'état in such period of our history. A few days later, Dr. Orlando Canedo, also urologist, performed the first living donor kidney transplant in Cochabamba. In the next 7 years, the transplant team of Hospital Obrero #1 in La Paz performed other 24 kidney transplants; it was the most experienced team in the field of transplantation in Bolivia until 1986. One year later the transplant team of Centro Médico Quirúrgico Boliviano Belga and Caja Petrolera de Salud in Cochabamba started their transplant program performing 15 successful transplants over the next 5 years (personnel communication).

In 1982, three renal physicians from the United Kingdom and Mexico arrived in Cochabamba, and they carried out a collective work of spreading knowledge and integration with other medical specialties and with colleagues of other regions of Bolivia. They promoted a comprehensive renal care program for uremic patients in Centro Medico Quirúrgico Boliviano Belga, the Military Hospital, the Oil Workers' Health Insurance, and Hospital Obrero #2. They prospectively studied the epidemiology of AKI, glomerular diseases, lupus nephritis, arterial hypertension, kidney stones, diabetic nephropathy, hyponatremia, and the ethical, social, and economic aspects of CKD and presented the results of such observations in numerous national and international meetings (personnel communication).

The Bolivian Society of Nephrology was established in La Paz in 1978 but remained inactive for several years. The First Bolivian Congress of Nephrology was organized by the nephrologists of Cochabamba in 1984, bringing also together nephrologists from La Paz and Sucre. The society was reorganized in 1987, and Dr. Jorge Nuñez from La Paz was appointed as acting president. The Second Bolivian Congress of Nephrology organized in Cochabamba had numerous participants, with a large number of high-quality presentations from the country's three geographical regions (personnel communication).

Progress has been constant through the organization and promotion of numerous scientific events, education and clinical research has been encouraged, and the level of nephrology practice in Bolivia has increased since 1984. A greater integration occurred, not only among Bolivian colleagues but also with those from Latin American countries, who have shared experiences and similar difficulties to ours. Moreover, active work has been done with national health authorities to show them the importance of CKD as a major public health problem and to draw up guidelines for peritoneal dialysis (PD) and HD [1] and renal transplantation, as well as the renal transplant guideline and accreditation manuals [1–3].

## High-Altitude Polycythemia and Chronic Kidney Disease in Bolivia

More than 140 million people in the world currently live at high altitude, representing 2% of the world's population [4]. The Andean region of South America constitutes a third major high-altitude region, primarily inhabited by two different ethnic groups: Quechua and Aymara. Among the Andean population, the hypoxia-related increase in hemoglobin is observed starting at an altitude of 1600 me above sea level.

An increased prevalence of albuminuria and proteinuria has been reported in subjects living at high altitude [5–7]. The pathogenesis of proteinuria may relate to a variety of factors, including the effects of tissue hypoxia within kidney parenchyma, glomerular capillary hypertension, hyperviscosity, and elevated right heart pressures. Polycythemia might be an independent risk factor for renal and cardiovascular disease in people living at high altitude, which is consistent with our findings that baseline packed cell volume and hemoglobin concentration were positively correlated with arterial blood pressure, serum creatinine, blood urea nitrogen, and proteinuria [8].

In a cross-sectional study of healthy, ethnically similar participants from two regions of different altitude in South America (Bolivia, Peru), we found that individuals living at high altitude had significantly worse renal function than those living near sea level, amounting to a mean difference of estimated glomerular filtration rate (eGFR) of 30%. The worse kidney function and greater proteinuria observed at higher altitude occurred despite similar age and a lower prevalence of metabolic syndrome with respect to sea level dwellers [9].

Apparently healthy subjects living at high altitude have a remarkably higher frequency of kidney disease and proteinuria, independent of a history of hypertension or diabetes. This provides some of the strongest evidence to date that long-term living at high altitude carries an increased risk for kidney disease. The characteristics of kidney disease observed at high altitude may be a new form of CKD that might be mediated by chronic hypoxia and its effects.

More than four million Bolivians (38% of total population) currently live at high altitude (2500 m above sea level), and 8–10% of this population develops high-altitude polycythemia [10]. In our study, 40% of total screening polycythemia healthy subjects had some degree of proteinuria [5], so we estimate that roughly more than 300,000 people are at risk for kidney disease.

It is evident that diabetes, hypertension, and glomerular diseases are the leading ESRD causes in the world. However, there are specific regional conditions (e.g., high altitude-polycythemia CKD) that deserve to be studied with the main objective to reduce the exponential increase of patients requiring RRT, inaccessible to large percentage of the population in developing countries. Some of these patients are the dwellers living at high altitude in countries such as Ecuador, Peru, and Bolivia.

## Chronic Kidney Disease Epidemiology

The prevalence and incidence of renal diseases in Bolivia are not well known. This lack of knowledge is an obstacle to the adoption of preventive measures, which may be of great value in a social and economic environment where treatment options for ESRD are simply not available. A study coupled with an educational campaign on renal diseases was conducted in 21 centers from three selected areas of Bolivia (plains, tropical, and valleys regions) in 1998 [11]. In this study, urine samples were collected and screened using a dipstick for chemical analysis and microscopic urinalysis. From 14,082 subjects screened, urinary abnormalities were detected in 4261 subjects at first screening. The most common form of urinary abnormality was hematuria, which was found in 2010 (47%). Other renal abnormalities were leukocyturia (41%) and proteinuria (11%). Confirmatory tests and further clinical studies were then carried out in 1019 subjects, and the study found that 35% had no urinary abnormalities. In the remaining subjects, the following diagnoses were made: asymptomatic urinary tract infection (48.4%), isolated benign hematuria (43.9%), chronic kidney disease (1.6%), renal tuberculosis (1.6%), kidney stones (1.3%), diabetic nephropathy (1%), and polycystic kidney diseases (1.9%) [11].

According to the global burden of disease project, CKD stage 3 prevalence in the country was 40%, by 2017, and CKD was the fourth most common cause of death in Bolivia with an increase as a cause of death of 36% from 2007 to 2017 [12]. The main causes of CKD in Bolivia according to the information that the Ministry of Health has through its National Renal Health Program (NRHP) are diabetic nephropathy (47.4%) and unknown causes (13.7%). About 10% had some form of glomerulopathy. Interestingly, chronic rejection or "loss of the graft" was identified in 4% of the patients.

By March 2015 there were 2231 ESRD patients who were receiving HD, 70% (1562) of them were over 60 years old, 3% were children and adolescents, and 27% between 18 and 50 years of age. It is estimated that an increase of 68% will be observed in ESRD patients in the next 5 years [8]. Of the 2231 patients with chronic HD treatment, 44.8% have short-term health insurance that cover their treatments, 31.3% are covered by the NRHP, and 23.9% of patients pay their sessions from their own pocket [9].

Unfortunately, current policies aimed for the prevention of CKD do not have sufficient support, given that the efforts are regional and supported by local scientific societies without the involvement of the Ministry of Health through its NRHP. Most of the NRHP resources are allocated for providing HD and kidney transplant to patients with ESRD (36 million dollars), and according to the NRHP website, an investment of US$ 34,632 is made every year for providing support to the identification of CKD (creatinine blood samples and urine strips) and for training healthcare workers in the correct identification, diagnosis, treatment, and referral of CKD patients to healthcare centers [10]. Regrettably, there are no official, or up to date, data on the accurate number of CKD patients in Bolivia, and data on mortality is also not available [9].

## Renal Replacement Therapy Scenario

Free provision of HD and PD was only contemplated in the National Health Insurance system (the main state-run health insurance provider in the country) and with coverage extensible to intermittent peritoneal dialysis (IPD) until 2014 when the National Renal Health Program (NRHP) was established. After the enactment of Law no. 475 of "Integral Health Services Provision Act of the Plurinational State of Bolivia" (Ley de Prestaciones de Servicios de Salud Integral del Estado Plurinacional de Bolivia) on December 30, 2013, free treatment for patients with ESRD without health insurance started [13]. Upon review of the Ministry of Health's official page and specifically the section pertaining to the National Renal Health Program, it can be seen that all the information is limited to CKD prevention initiatives, HD, and renal transplantation. Currently there are 4400 adult patients and 31 children in Bolivia who are receiving HD treatment. Unfortunately, the NRHP could not provide us information about the number of patients who are currently receiving intermittent peritoneal dialysis (IPD). Until recently, there were no supplies to perform chronic ambulatory peritoneal dialysis (CAPD) or appropriate cyclers to perform APD. To date, the only public institution officially performing CAPD or APD with the twin-bag system, "Y" connector, and flexible 2000–6000 ml PD bags and/or a cycler is the regional National Health Insurance (Caja Nacional de Salud – CNS)'s maternal and child care unit in Santa Cruz (one patient on APD and another two on CAPD). Other patients are also treated with these modalities in private institutions in the city of Santa Cruz (three on APD and three on CAPD). IPD is the prevailing modality in the rest of the country. La Paz and Tarija still have active IPD programs in the National Health Insurance regional units. Cochabamba cancelled a similar program in mid-2018.

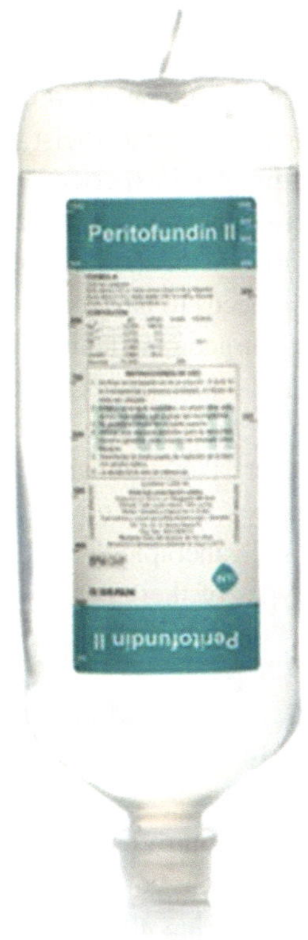


Fig. 9.2 Local production peritoneal dialysis solution (rigid bottle with 1 L volume and spike connector)

The emphasis in performing IPD is stated textually in the regulations, noting, "PD must be performed in second and third level hospitals." The regulations recommend a ratio of 1 nephrologist and 1 nurse for every 40 patients. Other guidelines provided for in such a document include a solutions' instillation time of 10–15 min, using dwell time of 30–40 min, 20 exchanges per session, 2 weekly sessions, and an exchange volume of 1000–1200 ml/m$^2$ of body surface area.

The hospitals performing IPD use locally produced solutions, sold in rigid plastic containers of 1000 ml, in 1.5%, 2.5%, and 4.25% glucose concentrations and with spike-type connectors (Fig. 9.2).

As for regulations of RRT for ESRD patients in Bolivia, there is a document entitled "Hemodialysis and Peritoneal Dialysis Regulations," which can be accessed on the Web [1]. Such regulations describe briefly HD and PD techniques, their different modalities, prescriptions, and technical aspects of each technique, like the reuse of filters which is allowed to be done up to 15 times. Most of the document is focused on administrative and technical requirements of implementing an HD unit; for example, in the case of a PD unit, the document states that for every 40 patients, the PD unit needs 1 nephrologist, 1 nurse with training and experience in PD, and 2 PD technicians for every 15 patients. The PD unit also needs to have one social worker, dietitian, psychologist, surgeon, and administrative personnel. In the case of an HD unit, it is required to have 1 nephrologist for each 40 patients and 1 nurse with training and experience in HD for no more than 4 patients, whereas the number of HD technicians is not well defined on the document, and it will depend on each HD unit workload; it also needs to have one social worker, nutritionist, psychologist, surgeon, and administrative personnel.

Convective therapies like hemodiafiltration (HDF) and hemofiltration (HF) are available in Bolivia, usually in private centers. However, the number of patients who are receiving such therapies is not known, and the number of patients placed on such therapies could be low due to the high cost of these types of therapies not reimbursed by the government.

## Peritoneal Dialysis

According to Arze's data, introduction of chronic peritoneal dialysis (PD) catheters in our country took place in the early 1980s [14]. In Bolivia, PD has always played a marginal role in relation to HD. As described by Pecoits-Filho [15], there is great variability across Latin America in the proportion of patients who receive RRT with this technique. Only Mexico provides care to a larger percentage of its ESRD population using PD (86%). Brazil has a total number of patients higher than Colombia, but proportionally Colombia ranks second in the region (46%). As mentioned by D'Achiardi [16], insufficient training in PD could be one of the causes for which such a technique is used with less frequency. An additional factor for PD not to be more widely used is the delay in the implementation of technologies that represent milestones in the provision of this type of RRT (such as the double or twin-bag system and "Y" set or the cycler machines for automated peritoneal dialysis (APD)).

An important source of information about some characteristics, particularly epidemiologic and clinical, is available through the "National Peritoneal Dialysis, Hemodialysis, and Renal Transplantation Registry," which provides information from 18 hospitals and data of 334 patients monitored until June 2007 (30.92% of all patients with RRT surveyed) [17].

Information related to PD was collected in a "National Peritoneal Dialysis Registration Form." Most of the patients on PD were elderly over 60 years old (27.4% between 61 and 70 years old and 22.3% ≥71 years old). Moreover, 49.7% were women. By ethnicity, 70.9% were mestizos, 28% white, and 1.1% Afro-Bolivian.

Almost half of the patients had completed high school (49.7%) and 32% elementary school. Only 3.4% were illiterate, and 14.3% had some university degree.

The registry also mentions some employment aspects: 44% of the patients were unemployed, 36.6% were retired, and only 14.9% were actively employed.

The eastern region of Santa Cruz had most of the patients on PD (61.1%), and when compared with the rest of the regions in the country, it had at that time one of the lowest HD percentages (17.7%).

In terms of other conditions and care received by such patients, the majority (81.7%) had high blood pressure or was on antihypertensive medication; 55.9% received erythropoietin, and 14.3% received intravenous iron. Because of the voluntary nature of the registry, it is worth mentioning that in most cases there were no data related to such prescriptions.

The adoption of this renal replacement modality was slow in the decade of the 2000s. By 2001–2002, there were records of three active patients only; by 2005, other two patients had been treated with PD. It was only in 2006 and 2007 that a significant increase in the number of patients treated with this dialysis modality was noticed (60 and 104, respectively). Most of them had short-term health insurance (59.5%) in public institutions. The main institutions that provide PD were the National Health Insurance (Caja Nacional de Salud – CNS) with 34.9% of the patients and the Oil Workers' Health Insurance (Caja Petrolera de Salud – CPS) with 18.9% of the patients. It is also noteworthy that 34.5% were private patients. Until June 2007, the two regions in the country with the most reported new cases were Santa Cruz (75 cases, 58.1%) and Oruro (30 cases, 23.5%). It is important to mention that the latter region ranks seventh in the country's GDP and that its PD patients were treated in a public institution. The latter region also contrasts with Santa Cruz, which has the most thriving economy in Bolivia. This means that the election of PD over HD was related to aspects other than economic ones, such as probably the healthcare provision (physicians and nurses), knowledge of the technique, and logistical aspects (availability or not of technology for HD, the overcrowding of HD units, etc.). Also, 77% of the patients did not exceed a year with PD. Only 61.7% had a period of less than 5 days between the IPD sessions, 22.3% had a period of 6–10 days between sessions, and 16% were treated with a latency period greater than 10 days between each session.

Physical capacity was very limited in 34.9% of the cases, 46.9% had normal activity with some limitations, only 9.1% had unrestricted normal activity, and 9.1% were unable to take care of themselves. At that time, three patients with hepatitis B (1.7% of those surveyed) and one with hepatitis C (0.57% of those surveyed) were treated in the country. No patient with HIV was treated with PD during this period. The main causes for ceasing treatment were death (31.4%) and dropping out of the technique; 6.3% were transplanted and 4% switched to HD. Here we must also take into account the considerable underreporting of mortality, which led the authors to speculate that the actual mortality figure was around 45.7%. The main causes of mortality were cardiovascular (30.9%) and multi-organ failure (29.1%). The direct percentage of mortality attributable to infectious complications related to the technique is not specified.

Colleagues from La Paz and Cochabamba (who work for the Caja Nacional de Salud – CNS) contributed data on their respective IPD programs. In La Paz, Dr. Abel Lucero is responsible for a cohort of patients receiving PD due to a formal contraindication to perform HD or the loss of vascular access. They have occasionally treated patients positive for hepatitis B. In Cochabamba, an analysis with data kindly provided by Dr. Rolando Claure-Del Granado was performed and found a total of 33 patients treated between 2014 and 2018; 48.5% were women, with a median follow-up of 21.9 months (over a period of 0.4–67.6 months). The patients received an average of 8.2 ± 1.46 sessions (or IPD days) per month and were treated for a median of 66 sessions (range, 2–145). Mortality during the follow-up was 27.3%, and the average survival with the technique was 50.1 months (CI 95% 39.9–60.3, median of 67.6 months). Survival at 12 and 48 months was 93.6% and 64.8%, respectively (Fig. 9.3); 54.5% of the patients required a switch to HD with a median follow-up of 35.6 months (CI 95% 20.6–60) until the switch (Fig. 9.4).

## Dialysis Reimbursement Policies

Until 2005, short-term health insurance companies like Caja Nacional de Salud (CNS) provided healthcare benefits to patients receiving HD up to 52 weeks; thereafter, the patient was transferred to public HD units of the Ministry of Health. In that year, the NRHP was established, and after the enactment of Law no. 475 of "Integral Health Services Provision Act of the Plurinational State of Bolivia" (Ley de Prestaciones de Servicios de Salud Integral del Estado Plurinacional de Bolivia) on December 30, 2013, free treatment for ESRD patients without health insurance started [18].

In 2008, it was estimated that 800 new cases of ESRD patients were being identified each year. The cost per HD session was estimated to be US$ 70, making a total of US$ 10,920 the cost of HD for one patient per year. Patients who did not have any type of short-term insurance like the Caja Nacional de Salud (CNS) needed to pay for their sessions. As of September 2008, 1080 HD patients were registered nationally; 40.7% corresponded to the CNS, 21.8% to private centers, and 18.6% to public hospitals. The cost per HD session at public institutions for patients who did not had any type of health insurance was approximately US$ 34.6 per session (US$ 5402 per patient per year) and was subsidized in part (around 80%) by the Minister of Health NRHP that provided some supplies for each HD treatment (i.e., filters and lines),

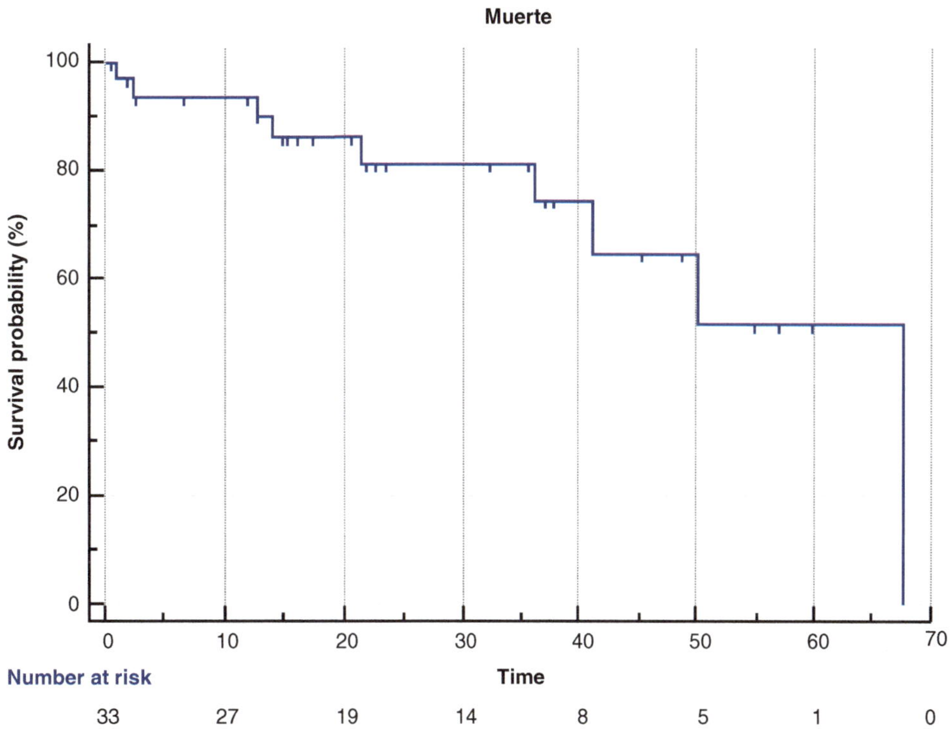


Fig. 9.3 Survival of patients who are on the intermittent peritoneal dialysis program at Hospital Obrero #2, CNS, in Cochabamba, Bolivia

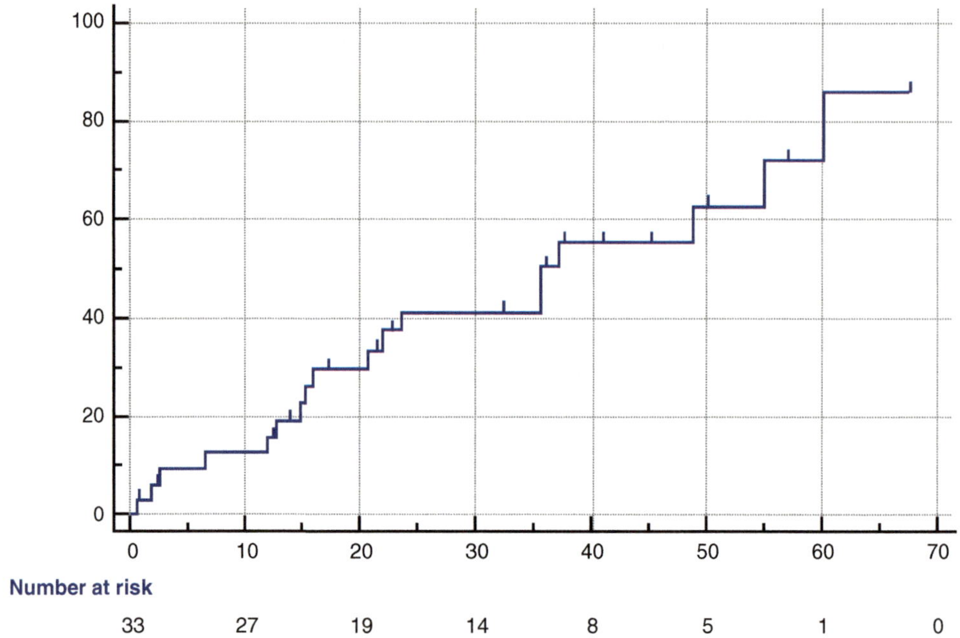


**Fig. 9.4** Cumulative incidence of technique failure and transfer to hemodialysis of patients on the intermittent peritoneal dialysis program

and the patient needs to pay US$ 6 per session (US$ 936 per year). However, not all patients had the capacity to pay this amount, besides the costs of transportation, medication, and monthly laboratory analyses. Since 2014, the municipal governments of each province in Bolivia pay each HD session for all patients who do not have any type of health insurance [18]. Since 2016, municipal governments have started the purchase of HD services from private units due to the saturation of the public units. The reimbursement that each HD center receives should include the cost of medications (i.e., antihypertensive, phosphate binders, vitamins, etc.), erythropoietin, and IV iron. Currently the cost per HD session is US$ 173 in the short-term health insurance system (i.e., CNS) HD centers, and the amount per HD session subject to reimbursement is US$ 103 for patients who benefit from Law no. 475; however, there is no data about the cost per IPD session, given that this modality of dialysis is only done in limited places.

Until March 2019, there were 4400 patients on HD, with a total of 686,400 sessions per year, representing a total cost for the NRHP of US$ 16,050 per patient/year (US$ 103/session) and a total expense of more than 70 million dollars a year [17]. The cost of HD per patients per year in Bolivia is lower as compared with other countries with similar GDP per capita (US$ 16,050 vs. US$ 18,720) [13]. Finally, we want to highlight that current reimbursement policies are focused on intermittent HD, with no peritoneal dialysis (IPD, CAPD, or APD) or home HD reimbursement policies available, except for anecdotal cases.

Reimbursement policies also cover some medications like antihypertensive medications (i.e., B-blockers, ACEIs, ARBs, and calcium channel blockers), ESAs (alpha-EPO), calcium-based phosphate binders, IV iron, and vitamins.

## Acute Kidney Injury in Bolivia

AKI is a global healthcare issue with high morbidity and mortality and caused by multiple and diverse etiologies. It can develop both in the community and in the hospital setting. A recent observational study has shown that the incidence of hospital-acquired AKI in Latin America is 45% and predominately affects a much younger population [19]. While cardiac failure, postoperative AKI, and nephrotoxins are the main etiological risk factors in high- and upper-middle-income countries in the region, in low- and low-middle-income countries (LLMIC), dehydration, infections, animal envenomation, use of herbal medicines, and complicated pregnancy are the most important drivers of AKI. Unfortunately, there is not much published data about the incidence, risk factors, etiology, and outcomes of AKI in Bolivia. Ramirez Torrejon JN and Arze RS published one of the first studies of AKI in Bolivia in 1993; it was a single-center study that described the incidence, etiology, treatment, and outcomes of patients with hospital-acquired AKI (HA-AKI) [20]. During a period of 2 years, they found 41 cases of HA-AKI (defined as a doubling of the baseline serum creatinine) and divided AKI into oliguric and non-oliguric. The first group was defined by a urinary volume <5 ml/kg/h or <400 ml in 24 h in adults and <1 ml/kg/h in children, most of the patients were male (51%), and the mean age was 54 ± 17 years. Common risk factors were hypotensive episodes, most commonly due to cardiogenic shock, sepsis, and hypovolemia, exposure to nephrotoxins (NSAIDs and aminoglycosides), use of contrast media, and rhabdomyolysis. Prerenal AKI was the most common presentation with and incidence of 59%, with oliguria being found in 76% of patients at the time of diagnosis. Ten patients required RRT, PD was used in five of them and intermittent HD in three, and two patients were treated with continuous arteriovenous HF. The mortality rate was 49%, and nine patients died due to sepsis and eight to cardiac failure. In a more recent study, Carpio-Deheza et al. described the incidence of AKI in a single third level center [21]. Using Acute Dialysis Quality Initiative (ADQI) RIFLE criteria and Acute Kidney Injury Network (AKIN) diagnostic criteria, the authors found 65 patients with HA-AKI during 2010; most patients were male (58.3%) and older than 60 years (25%). The three most frequent causes and/or risk factors for HA-AKI described in this study were hypovolemia (41.6%), hypertension (30.5%), and congestive cardiac failure (11.1%). Unfortunately, this study fails to describe what type of medical treatment patients received, RRT requirements, or short-term and long-term outcomes like renal recovery, mortality, and progression to CKD.

In low-income countries like Bolivia, most people who develop AKI continue to die as a consequence of this disorder and are not fortunate to have an early diagnosis or receive adequate treatment [22]. In Bolivia, like in other LLMIC, AKI commonly occurs in the community (CA-AKI) and is a disease of the young, and it is frequently developed as a complication of a single, potentially preventable, treatable, and reversible disease [23]. Community-acquired AKI is often preventable with simple measures like hydration or treatment of an acute infection. In those patients who progress to a stage where RRT is needed, dialysis is usually provided in nephrology units located in third level healthcare centers with ≤5 machines devoted to AKI treatment [24]. Intermittent HD is usually available in 100% of the units and is the most frequent form of RRT employed, while other techniques like prolonged intermittent HD, continuous renal replacement therapies, and PD are less frequently used. In areas with poor infrastructure, most of the patients present to the healthcare system late and often in advance disease stages and where RRT is not available.

Following the example of the 3 by 5 initiative by UNAIDS and WHO to provide three million people with HIV/AIDS living in low-income countries with antiretroviral therapy by 2005, the International Society of Nephrology (ISN) launched the 0by25 initiative with the goal to achieve zero preventable deaths from AKI by 2025 in low-income and low-middle-income countries where lack of early identification and resources for treatment may impact patient outcomes, and Bolivia is one of the three pilot centers of this initiative. Preliminary data from the 0by25 Pilot Feasibility Project, designed to evaluate an education and training program coupled with a point of care (POC) test and teleconsultation to improve detection and management of AKI in low-resource settings, has shown that the incidence of CA-AKI is 30% with a mortality rate at discharge of 3.1% and at 6 months 13.7%; 26% of patients developed CKD at day 90. The 0by25 initiative has shown that the use a POC test could identify a significant number of patients with CA-AKI who might otherwise not be recognized, allowing an early diagnosis and the implementation of an adequate treatment.

## Pediatric Nephrology

The interest on pediatric nephrology as a subspecialty has increased in our country; in the past 10 years the number of pediatric nephrologists has increased from two to ten practitioners. Pediatric nephrologists in Bolivia have helped to increase early diagnosis and improve treatment of glomerular diseases in children, as well as to improve diagnosis and treatment of AKI like improving and expanding the use of PD to patients under 10 kg and especially to critically ill neonates and toddlers [25]. Certain aspects of pediatric nephrology like ongoing patient care needs and its technical aspects (renal biopsy, dialysis, and transplantation) guarantee its continuing future growth as a major pediatric discipline in our country. CKD management by pediatric nephrologists has made us gain a space within pediatric specialties, and our colleagues now refer their patients for treating this condition properly. But if we look to improve outcomes, CKD treatment needs to be provided by a multidisciplinary team. On the other hand, we have an intense work in the diagnosis and routing of the treatment of congenital abnormalities of the kidneys and the urinary tract (CAKUT) since the number of pediatric urologists is insufficient in Bolivia. Pediatric nephrologists have become a fundamental part of the screening and diagnosis of CAKUT. However, some patients have to travel to the main cities of Bolivia or even to border countries like Chile, due to the lack of pediatric urologists.

Nephrocalcinosis and urolithiasis are other important medical conditions in our country. We have been surprised by the amount of kidney stone episodes in children, due to dietary factors, lack of proper fluid intake, increase in sodium load from daily diet (i.e., instant soups, broths, and energy drinks), and from obesity and metabolic syndrome in adolescents. Genetic and/or metabolic disorders are usually involved when the recurrence is the rule in young children [26].

Before the enactment of the Law no. 475 in our country, treatment of CKD in children meant a catastrophic expense for their families [18]. Dialysis and kidney transplantation coverage is now provided to all patients with AKI and ESRD who need acute or chronic RRT. On February 20, 2019, this law was subject to an amendment, which has increased the coverage to children over 5 years of age who had earlier been without health insurance. To benefit from this law, ESRD patients are considered to have a visceral disability (a wrong concept from our point of view). This definition leaves many children with AKI, pre-dialysis CKD, and other kidney diseases without health coverage and treatment. Although these policies are changing and extending health coverage to the pediatric population, it is still not clear how much of the pediatric population this law covers, but these are the first important first taken in order to improve the care of CKD children.

The number of pediatric nephrologists in Bolivia is still low. Currently there are ten distributed in the three main cities of Bolivia (La Paz, Cochabamba, and Santa Cruz de la Sierra) as follows: four in La Paz, four in Cochabamba, and two in Santa Cruz de la Sierra. Pediatric nephrologists do not have their own scientific society, and most of them are affiliated to the Bolivian Society of Nephrology and Hypertension; however, pediatric nephrologists actively communicate among themselves through social media networks and have an active participation in some academic and special events of pediatric nephrology in the region.

Among future perspectives of pediatric nephrologists in Bolivia are to organize an independent scientific society, review the national practice standards of pediatric HD, PD, and renal transplantation, and develop an initiative so that PD could become a sustainable form of RRT in Bolivia.

## Renal Transplantation: Living Donor and Deceased Donor

Even though the dialysis and renal transplantation records in Bolivia are mandatory, compliance with such requirements barely reaches 32% [27], which provides only partial information of living deceased donors transplant in Bolivia. The number of transplants performed in Bolivia the past 3 years has remained above 70 per year according to the information provided by the National Kidney Health Program registry (2016, $n = 89$; 2017, $n = 82$; and 2018, $n = 76$).

In the past 4 years, there has been an increase in the number of nephrologists (5–11 pmp) [28], but we are still below the average as compared to other countries in our region. Moreover, the prevalence of patients living with a functioning transplant totals 31.6 pmp, five times below the average in Latin America (159 pmp) [27]. Some of the causes for this low prevalence are explained on Fig. 9.5. This also explains why our deceased donor transplantation activity is 0.8 pmp, only exceeding the Dominican Republic according to the 2015 registry of the Latin America and the Caribbean Society

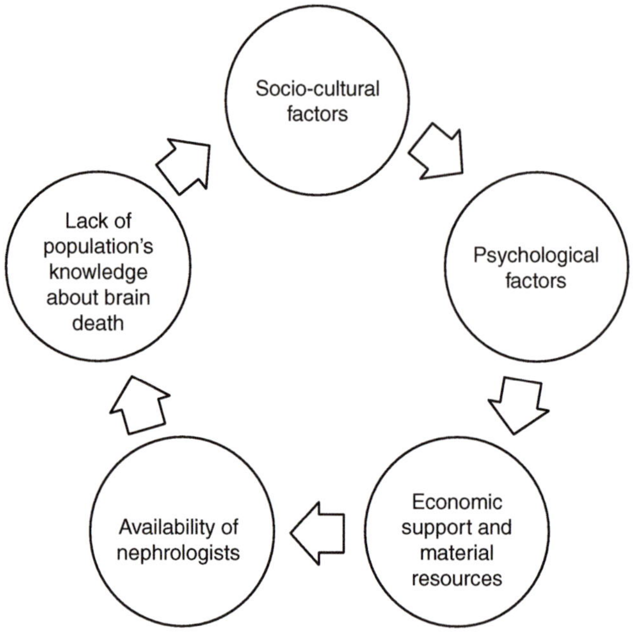


**Fig. 9.5** The interactions of several factors like the lack of population's knowledge about brain death and the low number of nephrologists could explain the low prevalence of living and decease donor transplantation in Bolivia

of Transplantation (STALYC). However, Bolivia is the fourth country with the largest number of living donor renal transplant activity (7.4 pmp) as compared with the rest of the Latin American region that has 7.1 transplants pmp. If we consider both types of transplant donors, we have a total of 9 transplants pmp, with Uruguay, Brazil, and Argentina being the countries with most renal transplantation activity (27–28 pmp). This shows that attitudes toward living donation among the Bolivian population needs to be improved, and we must approach to the attitudes of Bolivians residing in Spain which is favorable and represents a group that may be encouraged to become donors, with only 10% of the population against living donation [29].

To improve CKD prevention and treatment policies, various cooperation agreements were signed among some Latin American countries and STALYC [28, 30]. One of the most important agreements entails the developing and/or improvement of the deceased donor transplantation program. Even though a culture of venerating people who have passed away still exists in our country, a larger number of people are willing to donate organs: 49% are in favor, 21% are against, and 30% are undecided according the study of Rios et al. [31]. Policies on education and information about concepts and definitions of transplantation, xenotransplantation, deceased donation, or brain death are some of the factors that influence donation, as shown by Rios et al. in a survey of Bolivians living in Spain where 73% of the participants were unaware of the different definitions [32]. While lack of knowledge was not statistically significant associated to the decision-making process at the time of organ donation, there are other social, personal, familiar, and educational factors involved and that need to be addressed in our country couple with better health policies in order to improve deceased organ donation [33].

All patients in the dialysis program have the option to get a living or deceased donor kidney transplant. Patients who lack a living donor can access the waiting list for deceased donor transplantation, which is organized and supervised by the Ministry of Health through the National Renal Health Program. Organ allocation is based on standard criteria (UNOS, United Network for Organ Sharing), in addition to the Ministry of Health's Transplantation Manual [1].

The main immunosuppression scheme used in Bolivia is the use of basiliximab 20 mg IV x2 for acute kidney rejection prophylaxis and the use of prednisone, cyclosporine or tacrolimus, and mycophenolate as maintenance immunosuppressive regimen. Since 2014, the cost of immunosuppressant medications for patients without medical insurance is covered by the local governments.

**Table 9.1** Evolution of regulatory acts and laws regulating transplant activity and organ trafficking in Bolivia

| *Enactment dates* | *Transplant Law in Bolivia and the evolution of regulatory acts* |
|---|---|
| November 5, 1996 | First law on transplantation and donation of organs, cells, and tissues (Law no.1716) |
| June 21, 1997 | Act no. 24671 that regulates Law no. 1716, for public and private healthcare and health insurance facilities nationwide |
| December 2011 | Act no. 1115 that repeals Act no. 24671. These are the new regulations for Law no. 1716, which set the scope of application, implementing categories of donors, recipients, and the responsibilities and duties of healthcare facilities and professionals that participate in the donation and transplantation of organs, cells, and tissues |
| January 23, 2014 | Act no.1870 amends and complement Act no. 1115, on paragraph "b," on the definition of brain death. It incorporates that the recipients of organs, cells, and tissues must be Bolivian citizens, with the exception of foreign nationals and their living donors who are in transit. It also provides public support for kidney transplants to patients lacking health insurance |
| *Enactment dates* | *Laws regulating organ trafficking* |
| July 1978 | Article 90 of the health code, sanctioned by Law no. 15629 |
| November 5, 1996 | Articles 17, 18, 19 of Law no. 1716 |
| July 31, 2012 | Article 281 b of the criminal code, amended by Article 34 of Law no. 263 |

## Organ Procurement and Transplantation Network Policies

The Political Constitution of the Plurinational State of Bolivia recognizes that the state shall protect the right to health, promoting public policies that seek to improve the quality of life, collective well-being, and people free access to health services. In addition, it points out that specific laws will regulate the donation and transplantation of cells, tissues, and organs under the principles of humanity, solidarity, opportunity, gratuity, and efficiency. In spite of good intentions and regulations, there is not an organized system to allow a deceased donor procurement activity, representing a limited number of transplants, keeping a long waiting list, and maintaining HD centers overfilled with patients.

The first procurement and cornea transplant was reported in Bolivia in 1948, and the first kidney transplant was performed in 1979, as previously described. Over two decades, the law did not regulate kidney transplants, and only in November 1996, the transplant Law no. 1716 was enacted [34], 17 years after the first kidney transplant [35]. Since then, several amendments have been done by the promulgation of several acts that regulate the transplantation activity in the country (Table 9.1).

In Bolivia information and promotion of organ donation has not had an important impact in the population due to some country's idiosyncratic and religion factors. The programs have not been able to reach the whole territory of the country nor the various social groups; it has not been made any plans for the near future in order to increase the awareness of organ donation in schools, in universities, or to the general population. Another barrier is the lack of a national procurement center and the lack of improvement of current procurement policies. These are major weaknesses of this model, which has failed to increase the number of donors over the years.

In the case of deceased donors, the Regional Transplant Coordinator, working under the Regional Health Service (SEDES), will register the deceased donor in the national waiting list, managed by the Ministry of Health, for the allocation of organs, cells, and tissues among registered recipient patients, using criteria set in standard applicable manuals and protocols [1]. Deceased donation process will be managed by the Regional Transplant Coordinator and overseen by the Regional Transplant Commission, operating under SEDES. Healthcare workers are required to give notice immediately to the Regional Transplant Coordinator of the existence of patients with brain death directly or through the local hospital coordinator (Fig. 9.6).

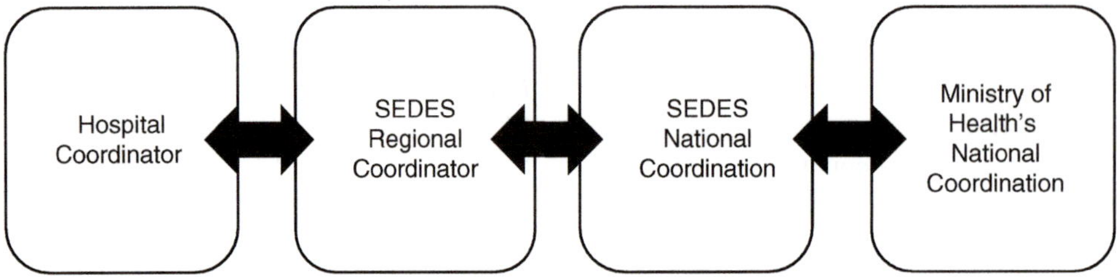


**Fig. 9.6** Deceased donation process of notification. The entire process is overseen by the Regional Transplant Coordinator and overseen by the Regional Transplant Commission, operating under the regional health service (SEDES). Healthcare workers are required to give notice immediately to the Regional Transplant Coordinator of the existence of patients with brain death directly or through the local hospital coordinator

## Nephrology Practice and Job Market

Throughout history, in Bolivia, specialists who have not been incorporated into a hospital which supports and encourages them and offers appropriate, reliable, and high-quality laboratory and imaging technologies, and specialists who have not had a group of colleagues, residents, interns, or students to work with, have tempted to migrate to other countries. However, in recent years more specialist have returned to Bolivia after finishing their training abroad, and they usually are characterized for having devotion to teach, interest in basic or epidemiological clinical research, passion for clinical nephrology, and interest in dialysis in its various forms or toward various aspects of renal transplantation. These specialists have an open and fertile field to develop fully as an outstanding professional in the field of nephrology.

Nephrologists can work in some of the private or public schools of medicine spread over the various regions of Bolivia; they can participate in the training of specialists in one of the five existing fellowship programs in the country; they can contribute to the training of nurses in public or private nursing schools. Finally, they have much to teach to the community in general, about the role of the kidney in health and disease and, above all, about the prevention of CKD and its progression.

Nephrologists with a passion for basic research still have no institution to work, as we lack as a country specialized laboratories. Nevertheless, if they have a passion for clinical and epidemiological research, there is much for them to do. They can organize or participate in courses on research methodology, data analysis, and biostatistics, bibliography search, and writing of medical papers, sponsored by the Scientific Societies of Medical Students of the various schools of medicine, the Bolivian Medical Association, the Bolivian Society of Nephrology, or other scientific societies.

If nephrologists are interested in clinical practice, they can focus on an in-depth study of the main nephropathies, including community- and hospital-acquired AKI, glomerulopathies, tubulointerstitial diseases, hypertension, diabetic nephropathy, renal complications during pregnancy and the various aspects of CKD. Moreover, they can devote themselves to an in-depth analysis and description of infrequent clinical cases and, finally, if they are trained, to the various aspects of interventional nephrology.

If the specialists are interested in RRT, they can actively engage in the startup and development of CAPD and APD units, intermittent HD, and in CRRT.

Finally, if nephrologists are interested in transplantation, they can actively participate in the organization, implementation, and development of the coordination and procurement of organs and in the dissemination of the advantages of renal transplantation and the concept of cerebral death and the importance of organ donation to the community. Furthermore, they can be actively involved in the clinical aspects of transplantation and, above all, in the assessment of recipients and potential donors and in the diagnosis and treatment of the various complications throughout the renal transplantation period.

In conclusion, Bolivia offers the specialist in nephrology great possibilities to work in the different areas of nephrology. However, it must be highlighted that to do so, great motivation and passion for work are required above all, given that contrary to other countries in Latin America, North America, and Europe, the economic incentives are negligible, for example, the average salary for a nephrology in public hospital (run by the Minister of Health) or in hospitals run by the short-term insurances (i.e., Caja Nacional de Salud) ranges from US$ 800 to US$ 1200 per month.

## Conclusion

In Bolivia, CKD prevalence and incidence rates have been growing steadily, probably as a result of the increase in life expectancy, aging of the population, a growing epidemic of type 2 diabetes, and a fast epidemiological transition across the country. Chronic noncommunicable diseases like CKD impose an enormous cost, barely supported at present and unlikely afforded by the government in the future. There is ongoing national CKD detection program in Bolivia, but it needs to be improved. Data about CKD and AKI are scarce, and public health awareness is low. High-risk patients must be studied, using simple determinations such as creatinine and proteinuria. For these programs to succeed, lifestyle changes must be encouraged, and public awareness must be increased through teaching and media-oriented activities. In concert, continuous activities in the area of education, research, and advocacy will be crucial in addressing the challenges of practicing nephrology in Bolivia and will enable the design of effective policies to prevent and control kidney disease in the future.

## References


1. Pacheco-Marquez A, Maury-Fernandez S. Manual de Trasplante Renal. La Paz: Ministerio de Salud y Deportes; 2009. p. 1–151.
2. Asturizaga L, Pacheco-Marquez A, Bocángel D, et al. Manual de Evaluacion y Acreditacion de Establecimientos de Salud y Autorizacion de Profesionales para Trasplantes Renales. La Paz. 2008:1–75.
3. Asturizaga L, Pacheco-Marquez A, Macias D, Murillo L, Valenzuela M. Guia de Evaluacion y Acreditacion de Establecimientos de Salud y Autorizacion de Profesionales para Trasplantes Renales. La Paz. 2008:1–221.
4. Moore LG. Human genetic adaptation to high altitude. High Alt Med Biol. 2001;2(2):257–79.
5. Rennie D, Marticorena E, Monge C, Sirotzky L. Urinary protein excretion in high-altitude residents. J Appl Physiol. 1971;31(2):257–9.
6. Chen W, Liu Q, Wang H, et al. Prevalence and risk factors of chronic kidney disease: a population study in the Tibetan population. Nephrol Dial Transplant. 2011;26(5):1592–9.
7. Jefferson JA, Escudero E, Hurtado ME, et al. Hyperuricemia, hypertension, and proteinuria associated with high-altitude polycythemia. Am J Kidney Dis. 2002;39(6):1135–42.
8. Plata R, Cornejo A, Arratia C, et al. Angiotensin-converting-enzyme inhibition therapy in altitude polycythaemia: a prospective randomised trial. Lancet. 2002;359(9307):663–6.
9. Hurtado-Arestegui A, Plata-Cornejo R, Cornejo A, et al. Higher prevalence of unrecognized kidney disease at high altitude. J Nephrol. 2018;31(2):263–9.
10. Amaru-Lucana R, Vera-Carrasco O. Guia para el Diagnostico y Tratamiento de las Eritrocitosis Patologicas en la Altura. Rev Med. La Paz. 2016;22(2):70–7.
11. Plata R, Silva C, Yahuita J, Perez L, Schieppati A, Remuzzi G. The first clinical and epidemiological programme on renal disease in Bolivia: a model for prevention and early diagnosis of renal diseases in the developing countries. Nephrol Dial Transplant. 1998;13(12):3034–6.
12. Carney EF. Epidemiology: global burden of disease study 2013 reports that disability caused by CKD is increasing worldwide. Nat Rev Nephrol. 2015;11(8):446.
13. van der Tol A, Lameire N, Morton RL, Van Biesen W, Vanholder R. An international analysis of dialysis services reimbursement. Clin J Am Soc Nephrol. 2019;14(1):84–93.
14. Arze R. Historia de la Dialisis en Cochabamba. 2015. http://nefrodial.com.bo/index.php/blog/140-historia-de-la-dialisis-en-cochabamba. Accessed 31 May 2019.
15. Pecoits-Filho R, Abensur H, Cueto-Manzano AM, et al. Overview of peritoneal dialysis in Latin America. Perit Dial Int. 2007;27(3):316–21.
16. D'Achiardi-Rey R, Molano-Triviño A, Echeverri-Sarmiento J, Rivera-Florez A, Sanabria-Arenas M. Educación en diálisis peritoneal crónica en los programs de posgrado de Nefrología en Latinoamérica. Rev Med. 2017;3(39):231–45.
17. "Registro Nacional de Diálisis Peritoneal, Hemodiálisis y Trasplante Renal" 2019. http://www.saludrenal.minsalud.gob.bo/Dialisis/PDF/Situacion_IRCT_06-07.pdf. Accessed 31 May 2019.
18. Bolivia EPd, ed. Ley de Prestaciones de Servicios de Salud Integral del Estado Plurinacional de Bolivia, vol. 475. La Paz: Gaceta Oficial del Estado Plurinacional de Bolivia; 2013. p. 1–8.
19. Mehta RL, Burdmann EA, Cerda J, et al. Recognition and management of acute kidney injury in the International Society of Nephrology 0by25 global snapshot: a multinational cross-sectional study. Lancet. 2016;387(10032):2017–25.
20. Ramirez-Torrejon JN, Arze RS. Fracaso renal agudo en el Centro Medico Quirurgico Boliviano Belga. Nefrologia. 1993;XIII(Supplement 5):146–9.
21. Carpio-Deheza G, Cespedes-Vargas J, Jaillita-Meneses C, et al. Analisis Clinico-Epidemiologico de la Insuficiencia Renal Aguda, en Basa al Empleo de las Clasificaciones RIFLE y AKIN en el Hospital Clinico Viedma. Rev Med-Cient "Luz Vida". 2013;4(1):24–9.
22. Okunola O, Akinsola A, Ayodele O. Kidney diseases in Africa: aetiological considerations, peculiarities and burden. Afr J Med Med Sci. 2012;41(2):119–33.
23. Remuzzi G, Horton R. Acute renal failure: an unacceptable death sentence globally. Lancet. 2013;382(9910):2041–2.
24. Lombardi R, Rosa-Diez G, Ferreiro A, et al. Acute kidney injury in Latin America: a view on renal replacement therapy resources. Nephrol Dial Transplant. 2014;29(7):1369–76.
25. Chesney RW. The development of pediatric nephrology. Pediatr Res. 2002;52(5):770–8.
26. Habbig S, Beck BB, Hoppe B. Nephrocalcinosis and urolithiasis in children. Kidney Int. 2011;80(12):1278–91.
27. Gonzales-Bedat M, Rosa-Diez G, Ferreiro A. El Registro Latinoamericano de Dialisis y Trasplante Renal: la importancia del desarrollo de los registros nacionales en Latinoamaerica. Nefrologia Latinoam. 2017;14(1):12–21.
28. Sola L, Plata-Cornejo R, Fernandez-Cean J. Latin American special project: kidney health cooperation project between Uruguay and Bolivia. Clin Nephrol. 2015;83(7 Suppl 1):21–3.
29. Rios A, Lopez-Navas A, Fernandez-Olivares P, et al. Attitudes toward living donation in the Bolivian population residing in Spain. Transplant Proc. 2015;47(9):2597–9.
30. Perico N, Plata R, Anabaya A, et al. Strategies for national health care systems in emerging countries: the case of screening and prevention of renal disease progression in Bolivia. Kidney Int Suppl. 2005;97:S87–94.
31. Rios A, Lopez-Navas AI, Sanchez A, et al. Factors that affect the attitudes of the Bolivian population in Spain with regard to organ donation for transplant. Transplant Proc. 2018;50(2):319–22.
32. Rios A, Lopez-Navas AI, Flores-Medina J, et al. Knowledge of the concept of brain death: is this an obstacle in the acceptance of donation and transplantation of organs among the Bolivian population residing in Spain? Transplant Proc. 2018;50(8):2257–9.
33. Rios A, Lopez-Navas AI, Flores-Medina J, et al. Level of acceptance of solid organ and tissue xenotransplantation among the Bolivian population residing in Spain. Transplant Proc. 2018;50(8):2300–2.
34. Arze S, Paz Zambrana S. Advances in ethical, social, and economic aspects of chronic renal disease in Bolivia. Transplant Proc. 2016;48(2):559–63.
35. Ley de Donación y Trasplante de órganos, células y tejidos. Bolivia EPd, ed. La Paz: Gaceta Oficial del Estado Plirinacional de Bolivia; 1996. p. 1–2.

# Nephrology in Brazil

# 10

José A. Moura-Neto, Cassiano Augusto Braga Silva, Daniela Ponce, Gianna Mastroianni Kirsztajn, José Osmar Medina Pestana, Renato Demarchi Foresto, Ana Flavia Moura, Carmen Tzanno Branco Martins, Edison Souza, Marcelo Mazza do Nascimento, and José Hermógenes Rocco Suassuna

| | |
|---|---|
| Area[1] | 8,510,820 km$^2$ |
| Population[2] | 210,461,442 (2019) |
| Capital | Brasilia – DF |
| Three most populated cities | 1. São Paulo – SP<br>2. Rio de Janeiro – RJ<br>3. Salvador – BA |
| Official language | Portuguese |
| Gross domestic product (GDP)[3] | 2.054 trillion US dollars (2017)<br>1.869 trillion US dollars (2018) |
| GDP per capita[3] | 9928.56 US dollars (2017)<br>8959.02 US dollars (2018) |
| Human Development Index (HDI)[4] | 0.759 (79° position, 2017) |
| Official currency | Brazilian real (R$) |
| Total number of nephrologists[5] | 4474 |
| National society of nephrology[5] | Brazilian Society of Nephrology<br>www.sbn.org.br |
| Incidence of end-stage renal disease[6] | 2018 – 204 pmp |
| Prevalence of end-stage renal disease[6] (on dialysis) | 2018 – 640 pmp |
| Total number of patients on dialysis (all modalities)[6] | 2017 – 126,583<br>2018 – 133,464 |
| Number of patients on hemodialysis[6] | 2017 – 117,849<br>2018 – 123,187 |
| Number of patients on peritoneal dialysis[6] | 2017 – 8734<br>2018 – 10,277 |
| Number of renal transplantations per year[6] | 2017 – 5929<br>2018 – 5920 |

1. Instituto Brasileiro de Geografia e Estatística (IBGE). Accessed in September 2019. Available in https://www.ibge.gov.br/geociencias/organizacao-do-territorio/estrutura-territorial.html
2. Instituto Brasileiro de Geografia e Estatística (IBGE). Accessed in September 2019. Available in https://www.ibge.gov.br/apps/populacao/projecao/
3. The World Bank. Accessed in August, 2019. Available in https://data.worldbank.org/country/brazil?view=chart
4. United Nations Development Program. Human Development Reports. Accessed in August, 2019. Available in http://hdr.undp.org/sites/default/files/2018_human_development_statistical_update.pdf
5. Brazilian Society of Nephrology (SBN). Accessed in September 2019. Available in https://sbn.org.br/
6. Brazilian Society of Nephrology (SBN). Brazilian Census of Dialysis 2018. Available in http://www.censo-sbn.org.br/censosAnteriores

J. A. Moura-Neto
Brazilian Society of Nephrology (SBN), Salvador, Bahia, Brazil
e-mail: moura@nephrologyworldwide.com

C. A. B. Silva
Grupo CSB, Salvador, BA, Brazil

A. F. Moura
Department of Internal Medicine, Bahiana School of Medicine and Public Health, Salvador, Bahia, Brazil

D. Ponce
Botucatu School of Medicine, University of São Paulo (UNESP), Botucatu, SP, Brazil

G. Mastroianni Kirsztajn
Brazilian Society of Nephrology (SBN), São Paulo, Brazil

Federal University of São Paulo (UNIFESP), São Paulo, SP, Brazil

J. O. Medina Pestana · R. D. Foresto
Hospital do Rim, Oswaldo Ramos Foundation, Federal University of São Paulo (UNIFESP), São Paulo, SP, Brazil

C. T. B. Martins
Brazilian Society of Nephrology (SBN), São Paulo, Brazil

E. Souza
Clinical and Academic Unit of Nephrology, Hospital Universitário Pedro Ernesto, Faculty of Medical Sciences, Universidade do Estado do Rio de Janeiro (UERJ), Rio de Janeiro, RJ, Brazil

M. M. do Nascimento
Brazilian Society of Nephrology (SBN), São Paulo, Brazil

Federal University of Paraná (UFPR), Curitiba, PR, Brazil

J. H. R. Suassuna (✉)
Brazilian Society of Nephrology (SBN), São Paulo, Brazil

Clinical and Academic Unit of Nephrology, Hospital Universitário Pedro Ernesto, Faculty of Medical Sciences, Universidade do Estado do Rio de Janeiro (UERJ), Rio de Janeiro, RJ, Brazil


J. A. Moura-Neto et al. (eds.), *Nephrology Worldwide*, https://doi.org/10.1007/978-3-030-56890-0_10

## Introduction

The Federative Republic of Brazil, globally known as Brazil, is a country of continental dimensions located in South America. It has a long coastline that measures 7491 km along the Atlantic Ocean, and it shares a border with ten countries in South America – almost all of them, except for Chile and Ecuador. The Brazilian population has grown significantly in the past decades. Brazil had 172.3 million inhabitants in 2001. In 2019, the estimated population was 210,461,442 million, which represents an increase of approximately 22% over the last 18 years. The general table summarizes the main information of Brazil [1–6].

The official currency is the Brazilian real, introduced in 1994 and symbolized as R$. In July 2019, R$ 1.00 was worth 0.26 US dollar, 0.23 euro, 28.1 Japanese yen, and 1.79 Chinese yuan renminbi. The Brazilian gross domestic product (GDP) was USD 1.869 trillion in 2018, which makes Brazil the ninth largest economy in the world. Brazil is considered an emerging country and is part of BRICS – a global group formed by the five major emerging national economies [3, 7].

The Brazilian political regime is a democratic republic, ruled by a national president. Brazil has 26 states and a federal district, in which the capital, Brasilia, is located. Each federal entity has administrative, political, and financial autonomy [8]. The country is also divided into five major regions: North, Northeast, Midwest, Southeast, and South (Fig. 10.1). Although the regions have no political or legislative autonomy, there are some cultural, geographical (climate, vegetation), and economic similarities among the states within each region.

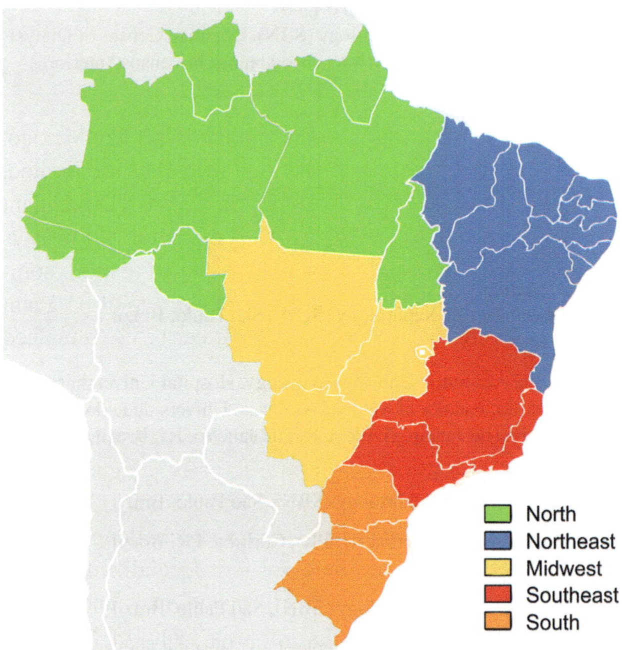


**Fig. 10.1** Regions of Brazil

There are 5570 municipalities, and the five most populated are São Paulo, Rio de Janeiro, Salvador, Brasilia, and Fortaleza. There are 46 municipalities (0.8%) with more than 500,000 inhabitants. The population is concentrated in few cities; 57% of Brazilians reside in 5.7% of the cities [8].

Although previously inhabited by indigenous tribes and settlements for a long time, the Portuguese only arrived on the shores of Bahia in 1500. From that time and until 1815, Brazil was a colony of Portugal. Hence, the official language of Brazil is Portuguese, with slight differences in accent, rhythm, and vocabulary from the language spoken in Portugal. There are also differences in accents within the Brazilian territory, among regions and states, which is more a curiosity than a barrier for communication. Due to the European colonization, the large presence of African slaves descendants, and indigenous Amerindians, Brazil is one of the most ethnically and culturally diverse countries in the world, with diverse regional identities.

Since 1988, health care is a constitutional right in Brazil. It is provided to all Brazilian residents and even foreigners within the national territory through the National Healthcare System, created in 1989 and known by the acronym SUS, which in Portuguese means "the Unified Health System" [9]. Although SUS guarantees universal and "free" access to health care, there are criticisms regarding undercoverage, long wait times, and the quality of healthcare assistance, with a few exceptions. Therefore, many Brazilians (24.2%) – usually the wealthiest – opt to pay for additional private healthcare insurance [10]. However, these patients can freely move to the SUS coverage at any time; this is a common occurrence when patients decide for some reason to stop the monthly payment to the private healthcare insurance.

## Brief History of Nephrology in Brazil

The Brazilian Society of Nephrology (SBN – *Sociedade Brasileira de Nefrologia*) was founded in 1960, by a group of 42 physicians composed of not only nephrologists but also clinicians and cardiologists [11]. Since then, SBN organizes the biannual Brazilian Congress of Nephrology, with around 2000 attendees and the participation of national and international invited speakers. The subspecialty of pediatric nephrology is under the tutelage of both the SBN and the Brazilian Society of Pediatrics, in the form of departments. It has a specific congress, which takes place approximately every 3 years. Below, we highlight milestones that helped to establish the basis of nephrology in the country over the years.

The first hemodialysis (HD) in Brazil was performed in 1949 at the University of São Paulo, on a locally developed artificial kidney, different from the one developed by Willem Kolff [12]. In 1956, acute procedures began to be performed at the Hospital Servidores do Estado (HSE) in Rio de Janeiro with the historic Kolff-Brigham Artificial Kidney [13]. Between 1954 and 1962, Brazil received a total of 4 of the 22 dialysis machines shipped from the USA to centers worldwide [14] – one of them still available for visitation at the museum of the National Academy of Medicine.

A decade later, the first chronic hemodialysis program was officially initiated [15]. The first manual peritoneal dialysis program, for acute and chronic renal failure cases, was started at HSE, in Rio de Janeiro, in the late 1950s [16], but continuous ambulatory peritoneal dialysis (CAPD) was only introduced in 1980, in Curitiba [17].

The first renal transplantation took place in 1964, also at HSE in Rio de Janeiro. The donor was a 9-month-old child with hydrocephalus who sacrificed one of his kidneys for the insertion of a ventriculoureteral shunt. There was immediate graft function, but the clinical course was complicated by acute rejection and death from pneumonia on the eighth postoperative day [18].

The *Brazilian Journal of Nephrology* (BJN) was launched in 1979 as the official scientific publication of the SBN. BJN is a dual language (Portuguese and English), open-access journal, currently published quarterly in online and print versions. Since 2010, the BJN is indexed in Medline/PubMed. Another official publication of the SBN is a widely read magazine (among nephrologists) entitled *SBN Informa*, in circulation since 1994 first as a newsletter and then as a magazine. It is available quarterly in Portuguese – online and in print version.

The Brazilian Organ Transplantation Association (ABTO) was founded in 1986 and has been contributing ever since to the development of renal transplantation in the country [19]. ABTO also issues a scientific publication (*Jornal Brasileiro de Transplantes*), available in Portuguese, as well as the quarterly Brazilian Transplantation Registry, which monitors all the transplantation activity in the country. In 2003, as part of an ABTO campaign to encourage organ donation, transplantation was the main theme of a top samba school, *Mocidade Independente*, in the Brazilian carnival – considered by many to be the world's biggest party. Currently, Brazil has the third largest renal transplantation program in the world [20].

The year of 1996 marks the largest tragedy in the history of Brazilian nephrology. Following a routine session in a dialysis facility in the city of Caruaru, in the state of Pernambuco, 116 out of 131 patients developed nausea, visual disturbances, and muscle weakness. One-hundred patients progressed to acute liver failure, and 52 died over the following days. Subsequently, hepatotoxic cyanotoxins found in the center's water treatment system were identified as the main cause of death [21]. The "Caruaru tragedy" is considered a turning point for health regulation in the country. Its aftermath was critical for the launching of ANVISA – the Brazilian National Health Surveillance Agency. Since then, all dialysis facilities in the country are required by law to follow a set of strict rules and guidelines and are under a stringent policy of inspections by government agencies. As a result, Brazil now has a good overall quality of dialysis in most of its 786 dialysis centers.

## Renal Diseases in Brazil

### Chronic Kidney Disease

Data on the epidemiology of chronic kidney disease (CKD) in Brazil is relatively scarce [22, 23]. In populational screening campaigns in the state of São Paulo, between 2005 and 2010, dipstick proteinuria was found in 7.3% of 38,721 individuals [24], a frequency that is similar to that previously described in other countries [25]. Considering the large sample size of these campaigns, this figure probably approximates the situation for the remainder of the country.

In another study performed a few years earlier in the state of Minas Gerais, the prevalence of CKD stages 3, 4, and 5 combined was 9.6% [26]. This study was based on eGFR calculated from the dataset of a private laboratory, covering the years of 2004 and 2005. The prevalence of CKD was 12.2% in women and 5.8% in men. CKD was detected in 25.2% of individuals over 60 years and in 3.7% in those under 60 years of age.

The prevalence rate of treated ESRD may be estimated from national renal replacement therapy (RRT) registries of dialysis and transplantation. The total number of patients on dialysis in Brazil was estimated at 133,464 in the 2018 SBN's Chronic Dialysis Registry. Based on the same data, the prevalence of dialysis was calculated at 640 patients per million population (pmp), with the lowest rate in the North region (448 pmp) and the highest in the Southeast region (738 pmp). Estimates indicate that 42,546 patients (204 pmp) with CKD started chronic dialysis in the calendar year of 2018. Similarly, the incidence of new patients with CKD on chronic dialysis also varied significantly (75–272 pmp) in the different Brazilian regions. Since 2013, the trend shows average annual increases in incidence (4.5%) and prevalence (6%), as well as in the absolute number of patients on dialysis (6.5%) [6]. According to the latest census, the most prevalent attributed causes of CKD are arterial hypertension (34%), diabetes mellitus (31%), glomerulonephritis (9%), and polycystic kidney disease (4%) [6].

More recently, national public policies aimed at CKD have been enacted with the intention of organizing an integral and comprehensive patient care network, instead of the previous approach, which focused on RRT. Brazilian CKD guidelines now emphasize the need for appropriate primary care for pre-dialysis patients and incentivize specialized outpatient care [27]. However, a significant portion of healthcare resources in Brazil is still spent on RRT, instead of on primary care [28].

## Acute Kidney Injury

Regarding acute kidney injury (AKI), the few available studies show a picture that bears similarities to that of countries with the same socioeconomic profile. As reported worldwide, the etiology of AKI appears to be changing over time, in part due to population aging and associated comorbidity.

Actual incidence rates of AKI are difficult to ascertain due to the variableness of contexts in which it may occur (community, hospital, and intensive care unit –ICU) and the diverse characteristics of affected patients (age, geographical location, social and economic conditions) [29, 30]. There might be a mixed epidemiology pattern in Brazil, with an epidemiologic spectrum typical of developed economies in the largest cities and of low- and middle-income countries in poor and remote areas [31].

Given the huge territorial extension of the country, the choice of the RRT method for AKI varies according to the locality and its different peculiarities, such as the availability of conventional HD, hemodiafiltration (HDF) or continuous renal replacement therapy (CRRT) equipment, and the experience of the nephrology team.

Some centers in Brazil employ PD as the main modality of dialysis for patients with AKI displaying satisfactory results in terms of morbidity and mortality when compared to the traditional HD treatment [32, 33].

An important fact to note is that approximately 75% of the country's RRT centers usually receive AKI patients, depending on the patient's clinical condition and mainly because many HD units are located jointly or inside hospitals [34].

## Renal Disease in Pediatric Population

The 2011 SBN Census recorded 1283 pediatric patients on RRT, ensuing a prevalence rate of 20 ppm and an incidence of 6.6 ppm, with an average age of 12.5 years. Renal diagnosis was unknown or not documented in 32.3% of the cases. Among the main known diagnoses, congenital anomalies of the kidney and the urinary tract (CAKUT) were present in 25.8%, with a predominance in younger patients, while glomerulonephritis was the main cause recorded for children older than 12 years. HD was the main treatment modality, being used in 74.9% of patients [35].

In a 2008 study from the state of São Paulo with 301 patients, the mean age was 9.0 years, and 53.5% of the children were male. The estimated prevalence was 23.4 ppm. CAKUT were also the most common known etiology (24.9%), followed by glomerulopathies (excluding focal segmental glomerulosclerosis) at 18.9%. Once again, HD was the main modality of RRT (71.2%) [36].

Epidemiological information could also be inferred from pediatric kidney transplantation records. Between January 2004 and December 2013, data were collected from 1751 pediatric transplants performed at the main centers in the country. The most common reported etiologies were obstructive uropathy (31%) and glomerular diseases (26%), with focal segmental glomerulosclerosis (FSGS) representing 48% of these. The cause of ESRD was recorded as unknown in 19% of the cases. CAKUT were responsible for the highest proportion of primary diagnoses at all ages [37].

Conclusions drawn from these studies indicate that Brazil has a low prevalence of children on RRT when compared to countries with the same socioeconomic profile. There were substantial differences in prevalence and incidence of pediatric chronic dialysis among the five regions of the country, with higher rates in the richest regions (South and Southeast). Also noteworthy is the high number of patients without a defined renal diagnosis. This may be due to insufficient, inadequate, or late medical care, which can be highly discrepant among different regions of the country.

The 2018 Census of the SBN revealed that 0.4% of dialysis patients in the country are from 0 to 12 years old and another 0.8% from 13 to 18 years old [6].

A recent review article compiled the published Brazilian experience on AKI in the pediatric population. Although most of the studies were single-centered, the available data differ little from those of other countries [30].

In a 2008 retrospective study, among children diagnosed with AKI who underwent PD, the mortality rate was 53.3% in children up to 12 years and 73.9% in the neonatal period [38].

In another study, published in 2009, with children from 1 month to 15 years of age, mortality was 33.6%. This rate was lower compared to other similar studies, probably due to the exclusion of patients younger than 1 month and the inclusion of patients who had not reached the most severe stage of renal dysfunction [39].

More recent studies incorporating pRIFLE for diagnosis and classification of AKI in patients admitted to pediatric ICU have shown that patients with any degree of AKI had higher mortality and hospitalization than those who maintained normal renal function [40, 41]. A prospective epidemiological study showed a high correlation between pRIFLE classification and KDIGO criteria regarding prevalence and mortality among pediatric patients diagnosed with AKI [42].

Another group that studied sepsis-associated AKI showed a 33.7% mortality rate, with length of hospitalization, use of mechanical ventilation, hypoalbuminemia, and need for dialysis as the main risk factors for mortality [43].

A recent dissertation recorded 693 pediatric patients, all with dialysis-requiring AKI, from an administrative database in the state of Rio de Janeiro. The etiology of AKI and mortality changed markedly with each age strata. Sepsis was diagnosed in 58% of the patients, and mortality was 65%, mostly within 24 hours of nephrology consultation, suggesting late referral [44].

## Glomerulopathies

Glomerular diseases constitute the third most prevalent cause of ESRD in Brazil, with a 9% prevalence among dialysis patients, after hypertension and diabetes mellitus [6]. However, in these cases, especially when patients present with advanced renal disease in their initial clinical presentation, diagnosis is often by presumption or exception, based on laboratory presentation often without renal biopsy.

Registries of patients with glomerular disease have helped to establish a better understanding about this group of diseases. The most important registry to date is the Glomerulopathies Registry of São Paulo, created in 1999 and comprising several centers in São Paulo, the most populous Brazilian state. Data from the period of inception until 2005 showed that the most common primary glomerular diseases were FSGS (29.7%), followed by membranous nephropathy (MN) (20.7%), IgA nephropathy (IgAN) (17.8%), minimal change disease (MCD) (9.1%), membranoproliferative glomerulonephritis (MPGN) (7%), and crescentic glomerulonephritis (4.1%). For secondary forms, the most frequent were lupus nephritis (LN) (66.2%), postinfectious glomerulonephritis (PIGN) (12.5%), and diabetic nephropathy (6.2%). The most common indication for renal biopsy was the nephrotic syndrome, followed by asymptomatic hematuria and/or proteinuria, chronic renal failure associated with nephrotic syndrome, rapidly progressive glomerulonephritis, nephritic syndrome, AKI, and macroscopic hematuria [45].

Another registry initiative was established in the state of Pernambuco, located in Northeastern Brazil. Published data are from 1998 to 2016 and comprised 670 native kidney biopsies. Primary etiologies were more frequent (58%) with the predominance of FSGS (43%). Other causes were MN (15%) and MCD (14%), followed by IgAN (9%) and MPGN (9%). Of the secondary glomerulopathies, the main etiologies were LN (67%) and PIGN (10%) [46].

An important study, using data from a reference laboratory in renal pathology, yielded data from 9617 native kidney biopsies from all regions of the country, over the span of 15 years. Again, the most frequent diagnosis was FSGS (24.6%), followed by MN (20.7%), IgAN (20.1%), MCD (15.5%), mesangioproliferative non-IgAN (5.2%), diffuse proliferative GN (4.7%), and MPGN (4.2%). With respect to secondary glomerulopathies, LN was responsible for most cases (45.5%), followed by PIGN (18.9%), and diabetic nephropathy (8.5%). Ninety-three percent (93%) of the biopsies came from adults, 4.3% from children, and 2.2% from elderly patients. Nephrotic syndrome was the main clinical indication for biopsy (39%), followed by asymptomatic urinary abnormalities in children (16%) and adults (20.7%) and acute and chronic renal failures in the elderly (16.8%) [47].

Isolated studies from several centers also consistently showed nephrotic syndrome as the main indication for renal biopsy. With some slight differences, primary glomerulopathies were more prevalent, with FSGS being the most frequent in all studies, followed by either MN or IgAN in second place. Among secondary glomerulopathies, the most frequent was LN, followed by PIGN [48–52].

It is important to note the decrease in the prevalence of schistosomiasis-associated glomerular lesions, Schistosomal glomerulopathy, whose predominant histopathology pattern is MPGN [48, 53]. This coincides with the decreasing incidence of schistosomiasis, particularly in previously endemic regions [54].

In a retrospective study involving renal biopsies of elderly individuals (over 60 years of age), the indications were nephrotic syndrome in 42.1%, proteinuria and hematuria in 27.4%, nephritic syndrome in 18.6%, and AKI in 11.7% of the cases. The most prevalent diagnoses were podocytopathies (FSGS or MCD), in 34.1% of the cases, followed by MN in 25.3% [55].

One study highlighted the patterns of incidence in children and adolescents. The patients were separated into three age groups: 0–6 (group 1), 6–12 (group 2), and 13–18 (group 3) years. In group 1, the findings were MCD/FSGS podocytopathies in 34.7%, hereditary proteinuria in 21.7%, LN in 13%, and IgAN in 8.6%. For group 2, podocytopathies again predominated (44.4%), followed by acute diffuse glomerulonephritis (22.2%), IgAN (11.1%), and Alport syndrome or thin membrane disease (11.1%). In adolescents (group 3), the main diagnoses were LN (22.8%), podocytopathy (20%), IgAN (15.7%), and MN (11.42%) [56].

## Renal Replacement Therapy in Brazil

Renal replacement therapy for ESRD in Brazil encompasses HD and PD modalities, as well as both living and deceased donor transplantation. The majority of prevalent patients are either undergoing HD or already transplanted. Of note, a few dialysis centers offer online HDF for selected ESRD patients. Although there is no official data yet, the number of patients on HDF was probably less than 1% of the total dialysis population in 2019.

**Fig. 10.2** Number of patients on dialysis in Brazil (2000–2018)

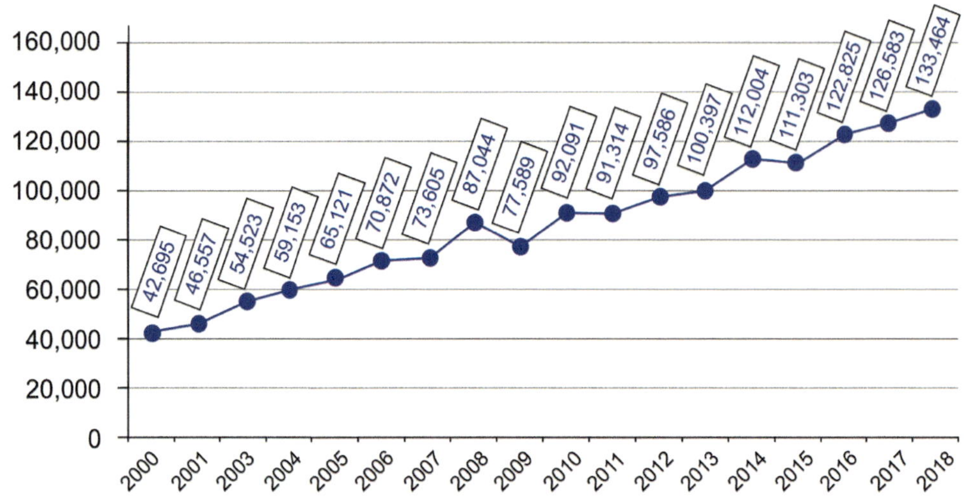


In 2018, there were 133,464 patients on dialysis in Brazil (Fig. 10.2). Most of the data presented herein is from the Brazilian Society of Nephrology's Chronic Dialysis Registry, an annual voluntary online survey. Despite its national scope and informative results, there are potential biases due to its self-reported nature and incomplete coverage – only 36.6% of the total dialysis centers responded to the survey in 2018 [6].

## Hemodialysis

HD is the main modality of RRT in Brazil, currently treating 92% of patients on chronic dialysis. There are 786 dialysis centers in the country. Almost half of them (49%) are concentrated in the Southeast region. The Northeast region and the South region have 20% and 19%, respectively, while only 12% of the centers are in the Midwest and North regions combined [6].

Only about 20% of the total dialysis sessions are funded by private healthcare insurance, while the great majority (80%) is paid for by the federal government, through the SUS. Despite this, most of SUS-funded sessions occur in private facilities (71%). Only 9% of the dialysis centers are in public centers or institutions, and 19% are philanthropic. This indicates that, despite being largely dependent on public funds, the large-scale dialysis enterprise in Brazil is critically influenced by the decisions and the quality of care provided by the private sector.

In recent years, the Brazilian health sector has been opened to foreign capital. Currently, there is a flurry of acquisitions of dialysis facilities by some of the major worldwide dialysis providers. It is still early to evaluate the significance and consequences of this economic move.

As of 2019, reimbursement of HD sessions in Brazil, when compared to other countries, is low and generally insufficient for the high standards required by regulatory agencies. At present, the SUS pays about 50 USD for each HD session. Reimbursement policies by private healthcare insurances are much higher and vary significantly based on several factors, including geographic location, quality of service provided, and the bargaining power of the parties involved. Nevertheless, in general, it ranges from 75 to 150 USD per session. Particularly, in centers located in the major state capitals, with higher costs of renting and enterprising, financial solvency can only be achieved by having a proportion of patients covered by private insurance.

According to the latest estimations, there are about 123,000 patients on chronic HD in Brazil [6]. This figure has grown rapidly over the last few decades. For example, there were only 25,489 patients on chronic HD in 1996 [15].

Regarding vascular access, most patients use arteriovenous fistulas for HD. Nine percent (9.2%) of HD patients have temporary vascular access, 14.4% use tunneled catheters, and 2.6% have grafts. Although most of the patients use arteriovenous fistula, the proportion of venous catheters has grown in the past years: from 15.4% in 2013 to 23.6% in 2018 [6, 57].

The typical HD prescription has a dialysate flow of 500 ml/min and a blood flow rate that varies from 300 to 400 ml/min, depending on the patient and the vascular access. The conventional in-center, 4-hour, thrice-weekly session schedule is the standard in Brazil. Only 2.4% of HD patients dialyze for more than four times per week. Home HD is seldom employed; it is estimated that only 0.1% of the patients are treated with this modality [6].

Kt/V is widely adopted as the main indicator of dialysis adequacy, as required by ANVISA national guidelines.

**Table 10.1** Dialysis adequacy indicators, by ANVISA national guidelines

| Laboratory test | Target |
|---|---|
| Serum phosphorus level | 3.5 – 5.5 mg/dL |
| Serum parathyroid hormone (PTH) level | < 600 pg/mL |
| Hemoglobin level | 10 – 11.5 g/dL |
| Serum calcium level | 8.4 – 10.2 mg/dL |
| Serum albumin level | > 3.5 g/dL |
| Kt/V | > 1.2 |

These also require the provision of other indicators and laboratory tests and their respective targets, as shown in Table 10.1 [58].

Reuse of dialyzers is allowed up to 20 times; however, the dialyzer must be discarded if the priming volume decreases by more than 20% from the nominal value. Reuse is strictly prohibited in patients with hepatitis B, hepatitis C, HIV, or acute kidney injury [59]. The seroprevalence of hepatitis B, hepatitis C, and HIV are, respectively, 0.7%, 3.2%, and 0.9%. Despite still ranking the highest, hepatitis C seroprevalence decreased from 3.8% in 2015 to 3.2% in 2018 [6].

There were 25,986 recorded deaths of patients on either chronic HD or PD in 2018. For 2018, the chronic dialysis census committee of the SBN estimated an annual mortality rate of 19.5% and a monthly hospitalization rate of 5.8% [6].

## Peritoneal Dialysis

PD is another important modality of RRT for patients in ESRD; however, the percentage of patients treated with PD in Brazil is low. According to the 2018 census of the SBN, the proportion of patients on PD is estimated at 7.7% of those on chronic dialysis, down from 10% in 2000 [6]. Despite this, the absolute number of patients on PD more than doubled in two decades, from 4495 in 1996 to 10,277 in 2018.

Although HD predominates, most centers offer both modalities of RRT. Peritoneal dialysis reimbursement is about USD 92 per patient per month, excluding the amount paid for dialysis materials. This might help to explain why PD is largely underused [6].

A similar proportion of patients served by private health insurance and the SUS undergo PD (6.7 vs. 7.6%), but a greater proportion of privately insured patients is under automatic PD (APD): 7.4% vs. 5.4% [60].

In similarity to hemodialysis, Brazilian SUS cover both APD and continuous ambulatory PD (CAPD), with no direct cost for the patient. For those covered by private health insurance, access for both modalities is also available at no additional costs, besides their regular monthly fees.

There are some reasons for the low penetration of PD in Brazil [61]. One aspect might be its low-profit margin in comparison with HD, a phenomenon also observed in other countries [62, 63]. Moreover, there is no coverage for the treatment of peritonitis, the most prominent complication of PD. Other aspects may include lack of training to conduct a PD program. Catheter implantation may also be an issue, even though there is evidence that programs with a nephrologist experienced in catheter implantation recruit more patients while affording the same or better results than when catheters are implanted by surgeons [64–67].

Brazilian centers with higher numbers of patients on PD usually have better outcomes in terms of the method survival [68]. Unfortunately, in many centers PD is used as the last option for patients with no alternative vascular access sites for HD. These patients are not ideal candidates for the PD therapy, largely because they have no residual renal function – which may impact patient survival.

The use of PD in the management of AKI has been embraced by a few centers, in spite of the theoretical classic limitations, such as infectious and mechanical complications and inadequate solute control. To improve these aspects, the use of cycles, flexible catheters, and a high volume of dialysis fluid was proposed. This knowledge has also been used in the case of unplanned onset of chronic PD and has been a tool for increasing the penetration rate of PD among incident patients initiating RRT.

The reasons for targeting more PD patients are several, such as vessel preservation for future vascular access or transplantation – PD presents better results compared to HD in the early years of the program – and also because PD causes fewer changes in patients' lifestyle and is more protective of residual renal function [69–72].

## Renal Transplantation

Brazil's first kidney transplant [73] occurred 10 years after the first successful kidney transplant in Boston [74]. Initial efforts took place within university hospitals, driven primarily by scientific interest. A substantial later surge was fomented through the development of regulatory and legislative initiatives and a very effective state-run policy of financial incentives and provision of universally free immunosuppressive medications [75, 76].

As regards deceased donor transplantation, in the early years, there was no central coordinating structure or financial agreement. It was up to each transplantation center to set up its own program and allocation policy [77]. These were however few in number.

Widening indications for ESRD treatment, the developing of state-sponsored program, and attractive reimbursement policies were met by the preferential expansion of operationally savvy dialysis units in detriment of kidney transplantation.

It was up to 1986 when the Brazilian Association for Organ and Tissue Transplantation (ABTO) was founded and emerged as an important catalyzer for the development of transplantation policies [78]. In 1987, the federal government created a technical council, composed of government and university members, with the aim to support the treatment of patients with ESRD, and establish standards for accreditation, operation and reimbursement of dialysis and transplant centers [79].

The emergence of the SUS in 1988, was followed by government investments in key strategic programs such as National Immunization Program, HIV/AIDS Treatment Program and the Brazilian Transplant Program. Dedicated programs for transplantation, not only for kidney but also for liver, heart, lung, pancreas and bone marrow transplantation, allowed implementation of policies to enhance national organization, logistics, training of professionals and reimbursement [80].

In 1997, the National Transplant System (SNT) was created to coordinate transplant procedures, from waiting lists, organ donation from living and deceased donors, organ allocation and transplantation [78]. In the same year, the Federal Council of Medicine published the resolution defining the criteria for brain death and procedures for the maintenance of the potential donor.

In 1998, the federal government established a fund [81] to replace former reimbursement organizations in financing high complexity procedures such as transplantation, including organ procurement, recovery and allocation, hospital admissions, surgical procedures, diagnostic tests, medical appointments, posttransplantation follow-up, and immunosuppressive medication. Accordingly, all the activities related to organ donation and transplantation were then adequately reimbursed by the SUS. Since then, organ procurement organizations and transplant centers receive bundle reimbursements for each kidney transplant, with up to 60% adjustments based on predefined levels of activity. Yet, reimbursements are not corrected for patient complexity, durations of index hospitalizations, and any other incidental costs.

The result of these government policies, legislations, and investments over the last 30 years is clearly recognized by the analysis of robust data. While in 1988 there were only 920 kidney transplants (5.8 pmp), figures were up to 5920 (28.6 ppm) in 2018, ranking third worldwide in absolute numbers. This drive was primarily due to the increase of effective deceased donors (from 1.8 pmp in 1998 to 17 pmp in 2018) and a corresponding growth in the number of transplants with deceased donors' kidneys (3.8 pmp in 1999 to 23.6 pmp in 2018), which accounted for 83% of all the transplant activity in 2018. The pediatric program followed the same trend, with around 320 annual kidney transplants over the last 5 years, 89% of them with deceased donor kidneys [82]. Living donation is regulated, allowing only living-related donors up to the third degree or spouses.

Currently more than 95% of the kidney transplants are reimbursed by the SUS, including hospital admissions, outpatient visits, laboratory tests, and, importantly, long-term provision of immunosuppressive medication [83]. Despite the apparent success, more is necessary. The impending challenge is to further increase transplantation activities and ensure long-term quality care in order to meet the demands of a growing and aging population. Innovative strategic measures toward improving the care structure and reducing geographic disparities are much too needed.

Regarding the criteria for organ procurement and allocation, management is performed by the SNT of the Ministry of Health. The main feature of the list is that it does not work for arrival order. The determining factor is donor-recipient compatibility, taking into account HLA class I (A and B) and II (DR) typing, crossmatch, and ABO blood typing. The patient can be prioritized in the list according to some severity criteria, which offers the possibility of accelerating the transplantation, but does not guarantee an organ with excellent quality and compatibility. Although the transplantation system is national, organ distribution and waiting list are regionalized. This means that the agency is made available to a recipient in the same state as the federation. This is due to transport logistics, favoring a shorter cold ischemia time [84].

There are currently 22,616 patients on the renal transplant waiting list in Brazil, which is approximately 18% of the total patients on RRT. Admittedly, these figures are still far from ideal and a remaining challenge for the countries' transplant community [85].

## Critical Care Nephrology

In the setting of critical care nephrology, available RRT modality options include conventional HD, prolonged intermittent hemodialysis (PIRRT), PD, and continuous therapies, performed in wards or ICU. Unlike RRT in ESRD, data about RRT in AKI is scarce. By far, the most common modality of RRT for AKI in Brazil is conventional HD, but PIRRT is being increasingly preferred for hemodynamically unstable patients.

The nephrology community is very much interested in intensive care and the provision of care to acute patients. Sessions related to AKI and critical care nephrology are usually the one's with the highest number of attendees in national and regional meetings and have the highest number of views in the SBN online courses and materials.

## Nephrology Practice in Brazil

There are two major pathways to be a nephrologist in Brazil. The more common and traditional is through medical residency. Training institutions are first accredited and then periodically inspected by the Ministry of Education. This pathway requires 4 years of supervised training, 60 hours per week in average. The first 2 years are to be spent in internal medicine and, then, two additional years in nephrology. During these two final years, the training center should provide a complete overview of nephrology, which includes theoretical and practical training at least on HD, PD, ESRD, AKI, critical care nephrology, renal transplantation, and clinical nephrology. Some centers offer additional supervised training in interventional nephrology, although this is still rare. The other pathway is through an approval on the annual test conducted by the SBN. There are some general requirements before the physician is eligible to take this 1-day test and apply for the SBN certification. In particular, the applicant must provide evidence of having worked in an accredited nephrology unit for a number of years. By 2020, 2495 physicians historically have had the SBN certification, since it began in 1972.

Although it is not mandatory, many nephrologists in Brazil choose to have a double degree, being nephrologists by the 4-year medical residency (internal medicine and then nephrology) and certified by the SBN. There is no need to reapply at any time nor other requirements for maintaining the initial certification.

Regarding pediatric nephrology, both pediatricians and nephrologists are required to complete two additional years of medical residency in an accredited training center. Few institutions offer such modality. The exact number of doctors working in nephropediatrics is unknown, but there are 350 qualified nephropediatricians holding SBN's board certification [86].

According to SBN, the average age of nephrologists is 47 years, and 51% are women. More than half of nephrologists (and physicians in general) are concentrated in the Southeast region [87].

According to a 2018 national survey, there are 4474 practicing nephrologists in Brazil. There are around 4000 physician members of SBN by 2020. This is not contradictory, since it is allowed to be a nephrologist without being a SBN member and vice versa. The distribution of nephrologists in Brazil is heterogeneous, with half of them located in only three states: São Paulo (1263), Rio de Janeiro (495), and Minas Gerais (483). The Northern region has the lowest number of nephrologists and nephrology centers. In some remote states, there are less than 20 nephrologists, such as Amapá (7), Roraima (8), Acre (10), Tocantins (13), and Rondônia (16) [87].

Only 7% of the 5570 Brazilian municipalities offer nephrology services and/or have dialysis clinics, precisely those that are most populous, have better hospital, laboratory, and imaging structure, and count on a higher concentration of specialists. Generally, municipalities with dialysis clinics also have hospital-associated ICUs. It is not uncommon for nephrologists to work both in dialysis units and ICUs.

Nephrology as a career is a relatively recent medical specialty in Brazil, having become particularly popular from the 1970 to 1980s, when professionals from other specialties migrated to nephrology attracted by its scientific research and technological advances, including dialysis and transplantation.

The fragmentation of health care in Brazil poses a challenge for nephrology care. In 2005, out of 6384 hospitals, 60% had 50 or fewer beds, and only a handful had more than 400 beds [88]. Most hospitals do not have nephrologists in their staff. Some activities can and are performed by other specialists, most commonly critical care physicians. However, due to expense and the complex infrastructure needed, AKI and inpatient ESRD care is often outsourced to mobile dialysis companies, both in public and private hospitals.

In a recent trend, multinational dialysis providers are developing strategic partnerships with hospital networks to provide inpatient RRT without the participation of the local nephrologist.

Chronic dialysis and transplantation activities still suffer from underfunding, which determines a low rate of expansion of new units. Although there are 786 dialysis outpatient centers currently operational, the country has one of the lowest prevalence rates of dialysis-treated ESRD among Mercosur participants, as well as low reimbursement value for treatment maintenance.

These facts underlie the tendency for lower income and a limited number of posts for certified nephrologists in dialysis clinics. Nephrologists coming to the market have few opportunities in established public and university-based nephrology and kidney transplantation programs and face a great vulnerability in dealing with multinational dialysis providers.

In terms of reimbursement, physicians in general are still one of the best paid professionals in the country. Doctors are still prominent figures, inspiring respect and assuming leadership roles, although a reduction of prestige over the past decades has been observed. The average monthly earning of an ordinary Brazilian nephrologist ranges from USD 4000 to 8000, with the hourly wage at a dialysis center ranging from USD 20 to 40 per hour. This may vary depending on several factors, such as geographic location, number of patients on RRT, proportion of patients with private medical insurance, medical visits to hospitalized patients, among others.

Nephrology practice in Brazil allows a wide range of options, such as basic and clinical research, dialysis, transplantation, public health and epidemiology, management, palliative care, critical care, interventional nephrology, pharmaceutical industry, education, etc. In addition, it requires a multiprofessional team and the interactivity with other specialists for a comprehensive care of the patient. The specialty has a comprehensive theoretical foundation, including physiology, pathophysiology, hydroelectrolytic and basic acid disorders, complex cases, rare diseases, and a plethora of areas that captivate the young physician. However, the technology and therapeutic possibilities often experienced in high-end hospitals or university banks do not reproduce on a day-to-day basis, causing some frustration.

## Highlights of Nephrology in Brazil

### Renal Transplantation in Brazil

As mentioned above, despite all the difficulties involved, Brazil has the largest public transplantation program in the world, with a fair organ allocation system and no social or cultural privileges. The numbers are expressive but still far below the growing demands of the country.

### World Kidney Day in Brazil

In order to disseminate among the population all aspects related to kidney disease through informational and educational materials, SBN locally coordinates the World Kidney Day activities in Brazil, one of the most engaged countries worldwide. Activities take place in all regions of the country, with an average of 500 registered events per year [89]

## Future Perspectives of Nephrology in Brazil

The major current challenge for nephrology in Brazil is to increase the interest among medical graduates. In 2018, only 0.8% of graduating physicians chose nephrology as their medical specialty. This is much lower than other traditional medical specialties, such as obstetrics and gynecology (8.6%), anesthesiology (7.1%), orthopedic surgery (5.2%), dermatology (5.2%), ophthalmology (5.0%), psychiatry (4.8%), and cardiology (3.1%). In 2017, 60.1% of posts for medical residency in nephrology were not occupied [87].

A noteworthy point is the need to increase the general reimbursement for nephrology-related therapies. Payment is outdated for a long time. Greater encouragement is needed, not only for the survival of existing clinics and renewal of the nephrology workforce but also to provide treatment with high quality and with continuous incorporation of state-of-the-art technology, facilitated patient access, and the expansion of expanding dialysis facilities to a larger number of cities.

Another challenging and urgent point, as already mentioned, is the need to increase the use of the PD throughout the country. Specific strategies within the government and the Brazilian Society of Nephrology should be designed to establish the culture of PD, making this modality an option to all patients requiring RRT.

A novel factor to consider results from the approval of the new regulation that allows foreign investment in the healthcare sector. As of 2020, about 100 dialysis centers, of among 550 privately owned centers, have already been acquired by multinational companies or investment funds. This change obliges the country to face this new reality as a great challenge, with positive and negative aspects. Only the future will tell us about its consequences and overall impact on nephrology practice in Brazil.

## Conclusion

Despite its young age, nephrology in Brazil is well-organized as a medical specialty and society, and it has shown advances over the past years. There is much to be proud of. The publicly funded healthcare system promotes universal access to health care for the entire population, which includes primary care and RRT. The renal transplantation program is one of the top three largest in absolute numbers in the world. The country also has shown great engagement year after year through its World Kidney Day celebrations; it stands out globally as one of the countries with the most registered activities, helping to spread the word about the importance of early detection and CKD prevention. Brazilian regulatory agencies set high-quality standards for dialysis, which is positive for the sector and results in dialysis facilities with good overall outcomes. The number of patients on chronic dialysis is steadily rising, but this may be due to better access to treatment, although there is still a "RRT gap" in the poorest regions. Nevertheless, there are challenges and unsolved issues ahead of nephrology in Brazil. Reimbursement policies, especially for HD and PD, need to be further discussed. PD, despite good outcomes, is still underutilized. Multinational companies and foreign industries are now dialysis owners in Brazil; this might change the dynamics within the sector. Finally, attracting the interest of young fellows may be one of the greatest current obstacles of the specialty in the country and needs to be urgently addressed.

**Conflict of Interest** The authors declare that they have no conflict of interest.

## References


1. Instituto Brasileiro de Geografia e Estatística (IBGE) [internet]. Accessed in August, 2019. Available from: https://www.ibge.gov.br/geociencias/organizacao-do-territorio/estrutura-territorial.html.
2. Instituto Brasileiro de Geografia e Estatística (IBGE) [internet]. Accessed in August, 2019. Available from: https://www.ibge.gov.br/apps/populacao/projecao/.
3. The World Bank [internet]. Accessed in August, 2019. Available from: https://data.worldbank.org/country/brazil?view=chart.
4. United Nations Development Programme. Human Development Reports. [internet]. Accessed in August, 2019. Available from: http://hdr.undp.org/sites/default/files/2018_human_development_statistical_update.pdf.
5. Brazilian Society of Nephrology (SBN) [internet]. Accessed in August, 2019. Available from: https://sbn.org.br/.
6. Brazilian Society of Nephrology (SBN) [internet]. Brazilian Census of Dialysis 2018. Available from: http://www.censo-sbn.org.br/censosAnteriores.
7. The World Bank [internet]. Accessed in August, 2019. Available from: https://data.worldbank.org/indicator.
8. Instituto Brasileiro de Geografia e Estatística (IBGE) [internet]. Accessed in August, 2019. Available from: https://www.ibge.gov.br/geociencias/organizacao-do-territorio.html.
9. Brazil. Ministry of Health [internet]. Available from: http://www.saude.gov.br/sistema-unico-de-saude/sistema-unico-de-saude.
10. Brazil. Agência Nacional de Saúde Suplementar [internet]. Accessed in August, 2019. Available in: https://www.ans.gov.br/perfil-do-setor/dados-gerais.
11. Brazilian Society of Nephrology (SBN) [internet]. Accessed in September, 2019. Available from: https://sbn.org.br/institucional/apresentacao/.
12. Junior GBS, Oliveira JGR, Barros E, Martins CTB. A nefrologia e o Sistema de saúde no Brasil. 2019.
13. Mion Junior D, Romão Junior JE. História da Nefrologia Brasileira, Editora Ventura, 1966, Brasil.
14. McBride PT. Dialysis in the United States. In: Genesis of the artificial kidney. Travenol Laboratories Inc, Deerfield; 1979. p. 19–27.
15. Noronha IL, Schor N, Coelho SN, Jorgetti V, Romão Júnior JE, Zatz R, et al. Nephrology, dialysis and transplantation in Brazil. Nephrol Dial Transplant. 1997;12(11):2234–43.
16. Landmann J, Bedran Y, Arduíno E, Godoy M, Francalatti S, Cezimbra JP. The treatment of renal insufficiency with peritoneal dialysis. Med Cir Farm. 1962;298:91–107.
17. Riella MC. História da CAPD no Brasil. J Bras Nefrol. 1994;XCI:117–8.
18. Moura Neto JA, Moura AF, Souza E. *Fifty years* of the first transplant in Brazil. J Bras Transpl. 2016;19(4):26–9.
19. ABTO - Brazilian Association for Organ and Tissue Transplantation [internet]. Available from: http://www.abto.org.br/abtov03/default.aspx?mn=460&c=902&s=0&friendly=historico-da-abto.
20. International Registry in Organ Donation and Transplantation [internet]. Accessed in August, 2019. Available from: http://www.irodat.org/.
21. Azevedo SM, Carmichael WW, Jochimsen EM, Rinehart KL, Lau S, Shaw GR, et al. Human intoxication by microcystins during renal dialysis treatment in Caruaru-Brazil. Toxicology. 2002;181–182:441–6.
22. Perico N, Plata R, Anabaya A, Codreanu I, Schieppati A, Ruggenenti P, et al. Strategies for national health care systems in emerging countries: the case of screening and prevention of renal disease progression in Bolivia. Kidney Int. 2005;97(suppl):S87–94.
23. Cusumano AM, González Bedat MC. Chronic kidney disease in Latin America: time to improve screening and detection. Clin J Am Soc Nephrol. 2008;3:594–600.
24. Lima AO, Kesrouani S, Gomes RA, Cruz J, Mastroianni-Kirsztajn G. Population screening for chronic kidney disease: a survey involving 38,721 Brazilians. Nephrol Dial Transplant. 2012;27 Suppl 3:iii135–8.
25. Dirks JH, de Zeeuw D, Agarwal SK, Atkins RC, Correa-Rotter R, D'Amico G, et al. Prevention of chronic kidney and vascular disease: toward global health equity – the Bellagio 2004 Declaration. Kidney Int Suppl. 2005;98:S1–6.
26. Bastos RMR, Bastos MG, Ribeiro LC, Bastos RV, Teixeira MTB. Prevalence of chronic kidney disease, stages 3, 4 and 5 in adults. Rev Assoc Med Bras. 2009;55(1):40–4.
27. Brazil. Ministry of Health. Portaria GM/MS n° 389. 2014 [internet]. Available from: http://bvsms.saude.gov.br/bvs/saudelegis/gm/2014/prt0389_13_03_2014.html.
28. Santos JRFM, Luz MFS, Silva RRL, Aguiar VF, Moura IH, Silva PS. Estratégias da atenção básica na doença renal crônica: a importância do diagnóstico precoce. Rev Saúde Com. 2017;13(2):863–70.
29. Lombardi R, Rosa-Diez G, Ferreiro A, Greloni G, Yu L, Younes-Ibrahim M, et al., Acute Kidney Injury Committee of the Latin American Society of Nephrology and Hypertension Working Group. Acute kidney injury in Latin America: a view on renal replacement therapy resources. Nephrol Dial Transplant. 2014;29(7):1369–76.
30. Cleto-Yamane TL, Gomes CLR, Suassuna JHR, Nogueira PK. Acute kidney injury epidemiology in pediatrics. J Bras Nefrol. 2019;41(2):275–83.
31. Lombardi R, Yu L, Younes-Ibrahim M, Schor N, Burdmann EA. Epidemiology of acute kidney injury in Latin America. Semin Nephrol. 2008;28(4):320–9.
32. Ponce D, Buffarah MB, Goes C, Balbi A. Peritoneal Dialysis in acute kidney injury: trends in the outcome across time periods. PLoS One. 2015;10(5):e0126436.
33. Ponce D, Berbel MN, Regina de Goes C, Almeida CT, Balbi AL. High-volume peritoneal dialysis in acute kidney injury: indications and limitations. Clin J Am Soc Nephrol. 2012;7(6):887–94.
34. Thomé FS, Sesso RC, Lopes AA, Lugon JR, Martins CT. Brazilian chronic dialysis survey 2017. J Bras Nefrol. 2019;41(2):208–14.
35. Konstantyner T, Sesso R, de Camargo MF, de Santis FL, Koch-Nogueira PC. Pediatric chronic dialysis in Brazil: epidemiology and regional inequalities. PLoS One. 2015;10(8):e0135649.
36. Nogueira PCK, Feltran LS, Camargo MF, Leão ER, Benninghoven JRCS, Gonçalves NZ, et al. Prevalência estimada da doença renal crônica terminal em crianças no Estado de São Paulo. Rev Assoc Med Bras. 2011;57(4):443–9.
37. Garcia C, Pestana JM, Martins S, Nogueira P, Barros V, Rohde R, et al. Collaborative Brazilian Pediatric Renal Transplant Registry (CoBrazPed-RTx): a report from 2004 to 2013. Transplant Proc. 2015;47(4):950–3.
38. Tavares MS. Análise de mortalidade em crianças com insuficiência renal aguda submetidas à diálise peritoneal. J Bras Nefrol. 2008;30:180–433.
39. Bresolin N, Silva C, Halllal A, Toporovski J, Fernandes V, Góes J, et al. Prognosis for children with acute kidney injury in the intensive care unit. Pediatr Nephrol. 2009;24(3):537–44.
40. Bresolin N, Bianchini AP, Haas CA. Pediatric acute kidney injury assessed by pRIFLE as a prognostic factor in the intensive care unit. Pediatr Nephrol. 2013;28(3):485–92.
41. Cabral FC, Ramos Garcia PC, Mattiello R, Dresser D, Fiori HH, Korb C, et al. Influence of acute kidney injury defined by the pediatric risk, injury, failure, loss, end-stage renal disease score on the clinical course of PICU patients. Pediatr Crit Care Med. 2015;16(8):e275–82.

42. Volpon LC, Sugo EK, Consulin JC, Tavares TL, Aragon DC, Carlotti AP. Epidemiology and outcome of acute kidney injury according to pediatric risk, injury, failure, loss, end-stage renal disease and kidney disease: improving global outcomes criteria in critically ill children-a prospective study. Pediatr Crit Care Med. 2016;17(5):e229–38.
43. Riyuzo MC, Silveira LV, Macedo CS, Fioretto JR. Predictive factors of mortality in pediatric patients with acute renal injury associated with sepsis. J Pediatr. 2017;93(1):28–34.
44. Cleto-Yamane TL. Epidemiology of acute kidney injury in children in Rio de Janeiro. Universidade do Estado do Rio de Janeiro, 2019. Master's thesis. Available from: http://www.pgcm.uerj.br.
45. Malafronte P, Mastroianni-Kirsztajn G, Betônico GN, Romão Junior JE, Alves MA, Carvalho MF, et al. Paulista Registry of glomerulonephritis: 5-year data report. Nephrol Dial Transplant. 2006;21(11):3098–105.
46. Costa DM, Valente LM, Gouveia PA, Sarinho FW, Fernandes GV, Cavalcante MA, et al. Comparative analysis of primary and secondary glomerulopathies in the northeast of Brazil: data from the Pernambuco Registry of Glomerulopathies - REPEG. J Bras Nefrol. 2017;39(1):29–35.
47. Polito MG, de Moura LA, Mastroianni-Kirsztajn G. An overview on frequency of renal biopsy diagnosis in Brazil: clinical and pathological patterns based on 9,617 native kidney biopsies. Nephrol Dial Transplant. 2010;25(2):490–6.
48. dos Santos WLC, Sweet GMM, Azevêdo LG, Tavares MB, Soares MFS, Melo CVB, et al. Current distribution pattern of biopsy-proven glomerular disease in Salvador, Brazil, 40 years after an initial assessment. J Bras Nefrol. 2017;39(4):376–83.
49. Crensiglova C, Rehme BB, Kinasz LR, Chula DC, Nascimento MM, Soares MF. Frequency and clinical histological analysis of glomerular diseases in a tertiary hospital in southern Brazil. J Bras Nefrol. 2016;38(1):42–8.
50. Ferraz FH, Martins CG, Cavalcanti JC, Oliveira FL, Quirino RM, Chicon R, et al. Profile of glomerular diseases in a public hospital of Federal District, Brazil. J Bras Nefrol. 2010;32(3):249–56.
51. Cardoso ACD, Mastroianni-Kirsztajn G. Morphological patterns of glomerular diseases in Amazonas (North of Brazil). J Bras Nefrol. 2006;28(1):39–43.
52. Carmo PAV, Carmo WB, Bastos MG, Andrade LCF. Study of glomerular diseases in the Zona da Mata Region of Minas Gerais. J Bras Nefrol. 2008;30/1:15–21.
53. Queiroz FP, Brito E, Martinelli R. Influence of regional factors in the distribution of the histologic patterns of glomerulopathies in the nephrotic syndrome. Nephron. 1975;14:466–70.
54. Brazil. Ministry of Health [internet]. Available from: http://www.saude.gov.br/saude-de-a-z/esquistossomose#epidemiologia.
55. Oliveira LB, Cobo Ede C, Machado JR, Custódio FB, da Silva MV, de Oliveira FA, et al. Clinical and epidemiological prevalence of glomerulopathies elderly in the city of Uberaba - MG. J Bras Nefrol. 2015;37(2):166–70.
56. Rocha LP, Carminati CR, Machado JR, Laterza VL, dos Reis MA, Corrêa RR. Prevalence of nephropathies in children and adolescents and alterations in renal biopsies in Minas Gerais, Brazil, from 1996 to 2010. Ann Diagn Pathol. 2013;17(1):22–7.
57. Sesso RC, Lopes AA, Thomé FS, Lugon JR, Santos DR. Brazilian Chronic Dialysis Survey 2013 – Trend analysis between 2011 and 2013. J Bras Nefrol. 2014;36:476–81.
58. Brazil. Ministry of Health. Portaria n° 1.675, June 7th, 2018 [internet]. Available from: http://bvsms.saude.gov.br/bvs/saudelegis/gm/2018/prt1675_08_06_2018.html.
59. Brazil. Ministry of Health [internet]. Agência Nacional de Vigilância Sanitária – ANVISA. RDC n° 11, March 13th, 2014. Available from: http://portal.anvisa.gov.br/documents/10181/2867923/(1)RDC_11_2014_COMP.pdf/5e552d92-f573-4c54-8cab-b06efa87036e.
60. Sesso RC, Lopes AA, Thomé FS, Lugon JR, Martins CT. Brazilian chronic dialysis survey 2016. J Bras Nefrol. 2017;39(3):261–6.
61. Abensur H. How to explain the low penetration of peritoneal dialysis in Brazil. Braz J Nephrol. 2014;36(3):269–70.
62. Nissenson AR, Prichard SS, Cheng IK, Gokal R, Kubota M, Maiorca R, et al. Non-medical factors that impact on ESRD modality selection. Kidney Int Suppl. 1993;40:S120–7.
63. Pecoits-Filho R, Campos C, Cerdas-Calderon M, Fortes P, Jarpa C, Just P, et al. Policies and health care financing issues for dialysis in Latin America: extracts from the roundtable discussion on the economics of dialysis and chronic kidney disease. Perit Dial Int. 2009;29:S222–6.
64. de Moraes TP, Campos RP, de Alcântara MT, Chula D, Vieira MA, Riella MC, et al. Investigators of BRAZPD. Similar outcomes of catheters implanted by nephrologists and surgeons: analysis of the Brazilian peritoneal dialysis multicentric study. Semin Dial. 2012;25:565–8.
65. Ozener C, Bihorac A, Akoglu E. Technical survival of CAPD catheters: comparison between percutaneous and conventional surgical placement techniques. Nephrol Dial Transplant. 2001;16:1893–9.
66. Wong CM, Ng KP, Keng TC, Lim SK, Tan SY. Impact of interventional nephrology on outcome and penetration rate of a CAPD program. Perit Dial Int. 2011;31:194–6.
67. Asif A, Pflederer TA, Vieira CF, Diego J, Roth D, Agarwal A. Does catheter insertion by nephrologists improve peritoneal dialysis utilization? A multicenter analysis. Semin Dial. 2005;18:157–60.
68. Martin LC, Caramori JC, Fernandes N, Divino-Filho JC, Pecoits-Filho R, Barretti P, et al. Geographic and educational factors and risk of the first peritonitis episode in Brazilian Peritoneal Dialysis study (BRAZPD) patients. Clin J Am Soc Nephrol. 2011;6(8):1944–51.
69. Zhang X, Shou Z, Chen Z, Xu Y, Han F, Yin X, et al. The role of an integrated care model for kidney disease in the development of peritoneal dialysis: a single-center experience in China. Perit Dial Int. 2014;34:S55–8.
70. Ponce D, Berbel MN, Goes CR, Balbi AL. High volume peritoneal dialysis in acute kidney injury: indications and limitations. Clin J Am Soc Nephrol. 2012;7:887–94.
71. Dias DB, Mendes ML, Banin VB, et al. Peritoneal dialysis can be an option for unplanned chronic dialysis: initial results from a developing country. Urol Nephrol Int. 2016;48:901–6.
72. Dias DB, Mendes ML, Banin VB, Barretti P, Ponce D. Urgent-start peritoneal dialysis: the first year of Brazilian experience. Blood Purif. 2017;44:283–7.
73. Vasconcelos MSF, Menezes PA, Menezes JAV, et al. O transplante renal no Hospital dos Servidores do Estado - Rio de Janeiro. Revisão de 380 transplantes. Jornal Brasileiro de Transplantes. 1998;1:71–83.
74. Merril JP, Murray JE, Harrison JH, Guild WR. Successful homotransplantation of human kidney between identical twins. JAMA. 1956;160:277–82.
75. Murray JE, Merril JP, Harrison JH, Wilson RE, Dammin GJ. Prolonged survival of human-kidney homografts by immunosuppressive drug therapy. N Engl J Med. 1963;268:1315–23.
76. Calne RY, Rolles K, White DJ, Thiru S, Evans DB, McMaster P, et al. Cyclosporin A initially as the only immunosuppressant in 34 recipients of cadaveric organs: 32 kidneys, 2 pancreases, and 2 livers. Lancet. 1979;2:1033–6.

77. Pêgo-Fernandes PM, Garcia VD. Current status of transplantation in Brazil. São Paulo Med J. 2010;128(1):3–4.
78. Silva HT Jr, Felipe CR, Abbud-Filho M, Garcia V, Medina-Pestana JO. The emerging role of Brazil in clinical trial conduct for transplantation. Am J Transplant. 2011;11(7):1368–75.
79. Ramos OL. SIRC-TRANS (Editorial). J Bras Nefrol. 1987;9:65.
80. Garcia VD, Abbud-Filho M, Keitel E, Neumann J. Situação atual do processo doação - transplante. In: Garcia VD, editor. Por uma política de transplantes no Brasil. São Paulo: Office Editora e Publicidade Ltda; 2000. p. 19–35.
81. Brasil, Portaria GM/MS n° 531 de 30 de abril de 1999. Diário Oficial da União, Brasília.
82. ABTO - Brazilian Association for Organ and Tissue Transplantation. Brazilian Registry of Transplants. 2018;4:1–104.
83. Medina-Pestana JO. Organization of a high-volume kidney transplant program - the “assembly line” approach. Transplantation. 2006;81(11):1510–20.
84. Brazil. Agência Nacional de Saúde Suplementar [internet]. Available from: http://www.ans.gov.br/images/stories/Legislacao/camara_tecnica/2013_gt_revisao_rol/20130520-doc12_contrib-consnacdesauderegulamentotecnicodosnt.pdf.
85. ABTO - Brazilian Association for Organ and Tissue Transplantation. Brazilian Registry of Transplants. 2019;1:15.
86. Brazilian Society of Nephrology (SBN) [internet]. Accessed in September, 2019. Available from: https://sbn.org.br/nefrologistas-titulados/.
87. Scheffer M. Demografia Médica no Brasil 2018. São Paulo, SP: FMUSP, CFM, Cremesp. 2018. 286 p.
88. Paim J, Travassos C, Almeida C, Bahia L, Macinko J. The Brazilian health system: history, advances, and challenges. Lancet. 2011;377(9779):1778–97.
89. Brazilian Society of Nephrology (SBN) [internet]. Accessed in September, 2019. Available from: https://sbn.org.br/dia-mundial-do-rim/ano-2019/#fndtn-sobre.

# Nephrology in Canada

# 11

Peter G. Blake

| | |
|---|---|
| Area[1] | 9,093,510 km² |
| Population[2] | 37,590,000 (2019) |
| Capital | Ottawa |
| Three most populated cities | 1. Toronto, Ontario<br>2. Montreal, Quebec<br>3. Vancouver, BC |
| Official languages | English and French |
| Gross domestic product (GDP)[3] | 1.709 trillion USD (2018) |
| GDP per capita[3] | 51,358 USD (2018) |
| Human Development Index (HDI)[4] | 0.922 (13° position) |
| Official currency | Canadian dollar (C$) |
| Total number of nephrologists | ~700 |
| National society of nephrology[5] | Canadian Society of Nephrology www.csnscn.ca |
| Incidence of end-stage renal disease[6] | 2016 – 202 pmp |
| Prevalence of end-stage renal disease[6] | 2016 – 1351 pmp |
| Total number of patients on dialysis (all modalities)[6,7] | 2017 – 22,500 (excluding Quebec)<br>2017 – 28,100 (estimate including Quebec) |
| Number of patients on hemodialysis[6,7] | 2017 – 17,936 (excluding Quebec) (includes 1058 on home HD)<br>2017 – 23,600 (estimate including Quebec) (includes 1200 on home HD) |
| Number of patients on peritoneal dialysis[6,7] | 2017 – 4564 (excluding Quebec) (28% CAPD and 72% APD)<br>2017 – 5320 (estimate including Quebec) |
| Number of renal transplantations per year[6,7] | 2017 – 1339 (excluding Quebec)<br>2017 – 1580 (estimate including Quebec) |

1. The World Bank. Accessed in February 2020. https://data.worldbank.org/indicator/AG.LND.TOTL.K2
2. Statistics Canada. Accessed 10 Feb 2020. Available in: https://www.statcan.gc.ca/eng/subjects-start/population_and_demography
3. Trading Economics. Accessed February 2020. https://tradingeconomics.com/canada/
4. United Nations Development Program. Human development reports. Accessed in February 2020. Available in: http://hdr.undp.org/sites/default/files/2018_human_development_statistical_update.pdf
5. Canadian Society of Nephrology/Societe Canadienne de Nephrologie. Accessed February 2020. https://www.csnscn.ca/
6. Canadian Institute for Health Information. Organ replacement in Canada; CORR annual statistics, 2018. Accessed February 2020. https://www.cihi.ca/en/organ-replacement-in-canada-corr-annual-statistics-2018
7. Personal Communication. Dr. Annie Claire Nadeau-Fredette, Universite de Montreal February 2020

## Introduction

Any description of nephrology in Canada needs to begin with a brief review of the geography and demography of the country and of the Canadian health-care system which has some unique and highly relevant features.

Canada has a population of just over 37 million people who live in 10 provinces and 3 territories. Over 60% of the population live in just two central Canadian provinces – Ontario and Quebec. While the area of the country is very large, the overwhelming majority – about 80% – of Canadians live within 150 kilometers of the Canada-United States (US) border, and the population is predominantly urban. Canada is a wealthy country with a gross domestic product of about US$ 50,000 per capita [1, 2].

P. G. Blake (✉)
Western University, London, Ontario, Canada

London Health Sciences Centre, London, Ontario, Canada

Ontario Renal Network, Toronto, Ontario, Canada
e-mail: Peter.Blake@lhsc.on.ca



J. A. Moura-Neto et al. (eds.), *Nephrology Worldwide*, https://doi.org/10.1007/978-3-030-56890-0_11

Politically Canada is a federation which was founded in 1867 and represented a coming together of two colonial peoples – the French based mainly in what is now the province of Quebec and the British based mainly in Ontario and the Maritime provinces and later in Western Canada. The country is very multicultural with over 20% of the population having been born in another country and with over 25% belonging to a so-called visible minority. Particularly important is the approximately 4% of the population whose ancestors lived in the country before it was colonized and who are described as "First Nations" and "Inuit." The "Metis" population are a mix of First Nations and French. These three groups – the First Nations, Inuit, and Metis – are sometimes referred to collectively as "FNIM" and have suffered socioeconomic deprivation and discrimination since colonization [1, 2].

In large part because of the historical importance of ensuring the French population could maintain its culture, language, and other distinct characteristics despite its minority status within the country, Canada is a highly decentralized federation with the individual provinces having substantial power relative to the federal government. Health care, for example, is largely under provincial jurisdiction [3, 4]. The country also has a strong collectivist culture, related to the historical need to protect both French and English rights and perhaps also to its severe climate. This collectivism contrasts sharply with the much more individualistic culture of the United States and is demonstrated by a strong emphasis on government administered social programs [1, 2].

All this is reflected in the Canadian health-care system [3, 4]. The system is administered and funded at a provincial level. However, the federal government provides critical supplemental transfer payments to the individual provinces that are essential to its funding, and, in return, the provinces are required to follow the basic tenets of the federal Canada Health Act passed in 1967. Critically these include a requirement that essential health services have a single public funder only. Internationally, this is uniquely restrictive. There is no other country where essential health care cannot be paid for privately. This means that in Canada government-funded cardiac surgery or cancer chemotherapy or dialysis is available to all and cannot be paid for privately by a Canadian resident unless they leave the country to receive it. Canadian health care is therefore a true single payer system for these services. It does not however cover outpatient medications for all those aged between 18 and 65, a source of recent controversy [5]. Private provision of health care is allowed as long as it is publicly funded, and this is the case for most physician care, for most outpatient laboratory and imaging services, and for many other aspects of health care. However, "private for-profit" hospitals and private dialysis clinics are very uncommon.

For completeness it should be noted that as much as 30% of health care in Canada is paid for privately – through insurance or "out of pocket." This includes medications for most of those aged 18–65, dental care, nonessential medical care such as cosmetic surgery, a high proportion of physiotherapy, optometry, psychology, private rooms in hospitals, medical exams for insurance purposes, and so on [3, 4].

The Canadian health-care system is often criticized internationally and domestically, but it is also widely admired, and the underlying single payer principle is very popular with the general population and often seen by Canadians as a defining feature of national identity that, in particular, distinguishes the country from the neighboring United States [6, 7].

## History of Nephrology in Canada

In 1945, Dr. Gordon Murray, a pioneering and somewhat controversial cardiac surgeon working in Toronto, constructed a hemodialysis (HD) machine with a cellulosic membrane and a venovenous pump as part of his investigation into heparin and extracorporeal circuits [8, 9]. He was apparently unaware of the similar and now famous work done by Dr. Willem Kolff in 1943 in German-occupied Netherlands. In 1946, Murray carried out the first successful HD in Canada for a young woman with acute kidney injury (AKI) [9].

The same Dr. Murray turned his attention in the early 1950s to kidney transplantation and performed four deceased donor transplants on patients with presumed end-stage renal disease (ESRD) using the recipients' iliac vessels, but all were soon rejected and three of the patients died [10]. A fourth survived long term but probably due to recovery of native renal function. Clearly rejection was the unsolved problem here [8].

The first successful kidney transplant in Canada was an identical teenage twin to twin donation carried out in the Royal Victoria Hospital in Montreal in 1958 by a team led by Dr. John Dossetor [11]. Both survived for decades though the recipient required chronic dialysis 16 years posttransplant. In 1963, the first Canadian non-twin transplants occurred in the same center in Montreal and in Saskatoon, and soon the practice became widespread [12, 13].

While acute dialysis was increasingly available in the late 1950s and early 1960s, chronic dialysis programs did not start until the middle to later 1960s. The first reported experience came from McLeod and colleagues in Edmonton, Alberta, in 1965 and later from Morrin and colleagues in Kingston, Ontario, who had four stations operating in 1968 [14, 15]. Chronic dialysis and kidney transplant programs became widespread in the 1970s and 1980s and grew rapidly in the 1990s. Canadian nephrology was quite innovative in these years with, for example, the use of both intermittent and continuous ambulatory peritoneal dialysis (CAPD) in the 1970s and early 1980s being pioneered by Dr. Dimitrios Oreopoulos in Toronto Western Hospital and routine use of subclavian catheter venous access for chronic HD patients being developed by Dr. Robert Uldall at the same time in the same center [16, 17].

In the 1980s, Canada was a world leader in widespread use of CAPD with over 50% of chronic dialysis patients in some provinces being maintained on this therapy [18]. In the 1990s, there was huge growth in the ESRD population and increasing use of chronic HD with units spreading out of teaching hospitals into city suburbs and smaller towns and a consequent relative fall in peritoneal dialysis (PD) use [19, 20]. During the same period, innovative approaches to home HD (HHD) led to growth in that modality. In particular, Canada became a world leader in slow nocturnal and short daily home HD [21, 22].

Kidney transplant also prospered in the 1980s and 1990s with 13 good-sized programs across the country. Dr. Cal Stiller from London, Ontario, led randomized trials confirming that cyclosporine was a major advance in prolonging graft survival [23].

## ESRD Rates

Canada has a Canadian Organ Replacement Register which records transplant and dialysis activity across the country [24]. It is considered relatively complete except for the province of Quebec which has not contributed data for the last decade and which contains about 8.5 million, or 22.5%, of the total Canadian population of 37.6 million people. Incident and prevalent rates of ESRD quoted here therefore are for Canada outside Quebec. Historically they have been somewhat lower in Quebec but this may no longer be so [25].

Canada's incident rate for ESRD varies between provinces but is approximately 200 new cases per million population (pmp) per annum (Table 11.1) [24]. Interprovincial variation is driven in part by differences in the percentage of the population that is FNIM because rates of ESRD are about three times higher in FNIM as compared to Caucasian populations [26]. Accordingly, Manitoba has a higher rate than any other province. Other factors influencing provincial differences are less clearly defined but may include ethnic differences, socioeconomic factors, age distribution, and perhaps the proportion of the population living in rural and remote areas. It is also likely influenced by completeness of reporting. The rate rose steadily during the 1990s but much less so after 2000 when it seemed to plateau at 160–170 pmp. The more recent rise to 200 pmp reflects aging of the population but also better data in Ontario particularly as a consequence of closer linkage between accurate reporting and provision of funding.

**Table 11.1** Incident and prevalent treated ESRD rates per million population by province/region of Canada in 2017

| Province/region | Incident rate pmp | Prevalent rate pmp |
|---|---|---|
| Ontario | 244 | 1430 |
| Quebec | 206[a] | Not available |
| British Columbia (+ Yukon) | 210 | 1326 |
| Alberta (+ Northwest Territory + Nunavut) | 132 | 1109 |
| Saskatchewan | 156 | 1212 |
| Manitoba | 244 | 1704 |
| New Brunswick | 217 | 1262 |
| Nova Scotia (+ Prince Edward Island) | 195 | 1566 |
| Newfoundland | 202 | 1657 |
| Canada (excluding Quebec) | 200 | 1372 |

Adapted from Canadian Organ Replacement Register data in Ref. [24]
[a]Estimate based on personal communication from Dr. A Nadeau-Fredette

**Table 11.2** Comparison of incident and prevalent treated ESRD rates (including transplantation) per million population in 2016 between Canada and selected other countries

| Country | Incidence pmp | Prevalence pmp |
|---|---|---|
| Taiwan | 493 | 3392 |
| USA | 378 | 2198 |
| Japan | 296 | 2599 |
| Portugal | 236 | 1909 |
| **Canada**[a] | **200** | **1346** |
| Brazil | 197 | 865 |
| France | 165 | 1278 |
| Poland | 149 | 806 |
| UK | 120 | 956 |
| Australia | 117 | 988 |
| Iran | 82 | 652 |
| Russia | 58 | 303 |

Adapted from data in Ref. [27]
[a]Canadian rates exclude Quebec

Canada's incident rate places the country in the second highest tier worldwide where incident rates vary between 160 and 250 pmp (Table 11.2). Within this second tier, Canada is just below a small number of countries in Southern and Eastern Europe and parts of Latin America but ahead of most of Western Europe [27]. The rate is much higher than that seen in a third tier of countries which includes Scandinavia, the United Kingdom, and Australia who lie between 100 and 120 pmp. The Canadian rate however is well below that of the first tier of countries, which include the United States, as well as Japan, Taiwan, Korea, and Thailand, all close to or in excess of 300 pmp (Table 11.2).

These international differences may reflect true differences in the incidence of ESRD, driven particularly by differences in rates of diabetic kidney diseases between countries and ethnic groups [27]. They are also influenced by medical and cultural attitudes toward the use of chronic dialysis in older frailer patients, by socioeconomic factors, and by health-care delivery models, particularly the degree to which "private for-profit" providers participate in dialysis delivery, which is of course not a feature in Canada [28].

As in almost all countries, diabetic kidney disease is the largest cause of ESRD in Canada accounting for just under 40% of cases [27]. This is much less than in East Asia, the United States, and Mexico but more than in Western Europe. The proportion of cases attributed to hypertension is much lower than in the United States, perhaps reflecting the relatively small Canadian population with West African origin [29].

The prevalent rate of ESRD, including those alive with transplants, is about 1350 pmp and has risen gradually in the last two decades [24]. Prevalent dialysis rates have slowly risen to 60% of prevalent treated ESRD rates as transplant struggles to grow in proportion to chronic dialysis.

Mean ages for incident and prevalent dialysis patients are about 62 and 65 years, respectively, and have not increased much in the last two decades. Approximately 60% of incident patients are male, and over half have diabetes although in only 40% is it considered the cause of their ESRD [24].

It is important to note that the relatively modest growth in ESRD incident and prevalent rates does not reflect the experience of dialysis providers and funders who continue to see a substantial increase in absolute numbers of patients being treated. There are about 22,500 people on chronic dialysis outside Quebec and about 5700 more in Quebec for a total of over 28,200. About 7300 started chronic dialysis in 2017 including over 1700 in Quebec (personal communication, De Annie Claire Nadeau-Fredette, Universite de Montreal). Absolute numbers of dialysis patients have recently risen at about 2.5–3% per annum [24]. The growth in the Canadian population has recently been rising, largely due to increased immigration, and is now close to 1% per annum, and so even when ESRD rates stand still, the need for dialysis and transplant increases. The aging of the population also contributes approximately a further 1% to this growth in absolute numbers of patients on dialysis.

The relative plateauing in ESRD incidence rate since 2000 likely reflects that most of the unmet need for renal replacement therapy has been dealt with since the marked growth in the 1990s and there is a general opinion that few Canadians who need and wish to receive dialysis are being denied it. The proportion who receive "conservative care" has recently received more attention but has so far not been reliably measured though it is likely substantial [30].

Unadjusted survival rates on dialysis in Canada at 1, 3, 5, and 10 years are 83%, 63%, 45%, and 16%, respectively. Comparable figures a decade ago for 1, 3, and 5 years were 83%, 60%, and 43%, respectively, suggesting gradual improvement in long-term rates [24]. This is reflected in prevalent dialysis rates rising slightly faster than incident rates, 2.8% versus 2.2% annually [24]. Survival rates are, not surprisingly, substantially longer for those whose primary disease is glomerulonephritis compared to diabetes – 93% versus 86% at 1 year, 80% versus 63% at 3 years, and 66% versus 41% at 5 years. Survival is also longer in people starting on PD compared to HD – 92% versus 80% at 1 year and 73% versus 60% at 3 years – but these data are unadjusted and do not reflect the younger age and better baseline health of those doing PD [24].

## Kidney Transplant

Transplant rates have been high by international standards and stable from 2000 to about 2015 at about 35–40 pmp per annum or 50–55 per 1000 dialysis patients per annum with about 40% being accounted for by living donors and the rest by deceased donors [24]. Since 2015, the rate has risen to 45–50 pmp per year or 60 per 1000 dialysis patients. This is because there has been significant growth in deceased donor transplant rates due in part to more liberal donor acceptance criteria. In 2017, there were 1338 adult transplants in Canada of which 803 were deceased donor and 535 living donor. There were about 240 in Quebec for a total of about 1680 nationwide. There are about 40–50 pediatric transplants annually [24]. Internationally, Canadian transplant rates are quite high but below those in the United States, Spain, and the Netherlands and similar to those in Scandinavia and the United Kingdom (Table 11.3). Living donor rates are also high by international standards but have been stagnant for a decade or more and below that of the United States and the Netherlands when expressed pmp or per 1000 dialysis patients [27]. Within Canada, there is significant variation in transplant rates between provinces and between renal programs [31, 32]. There is also variation in wait times and degrees of organ sharing within and between provinces [31].

**Table 11.3** Comparison of kidney transplant rates per million population in 2016 between Canada and selected other countries

| Country | Kidney transplant rate pmp |
|---|---|
| Spain | 64 |
| USA | 62 |
| Netherlands | 59 |
| France | 54 |
| **Canada** | **49** |
| UK | 48 |
| Australia | 45 |
| Brazil | 29 |
| Japan | 13 |
| Taiwan | 13 |
| Russia | 7 |

Adapted from data in Ref. [27]

## Home Dialysis

The proportion of Canadian ESRD patients treated with home dialysis modalities remains relatively high by international standards but is much less than in the 1980s and early 1990s when CAPD was being used in over 35% of prevalent patients [17, 23]. This was due to a combination of enthusiasm for the modality and also to scarcity of HD capacity. Home dialysis use in Canada fell dramatically between 1995 and the early 2000s and then plateaued at under 20%. This was due to a large increase in HD capacity and in particular to the proliferation of HD units in suburbs of larger cities and in smaller towns [19, 20].

There has recently been an increase in home dialysis prevalence back up toward 25%, in part related to efforts by provincial renal agencies [33–36]. This places Canada in the top 12 countries in the world for percent home dialysis use [27]. Increases in home dialysis use have also been attributed to widespread use of assisted PD initiatives, whereby home care nurses visit patients' homes and help them set up their PD cyclers and troubleshoot any problems [37], and also to pre-ESRD clinics, economic incentives, and greater use of urgent start PD [38–40].

Again, there are provincial differences in home dialysis use, and provinces which have had major initiatives to grow home dialysis, such as Ontario and British Columbia, have notably higher rates, while those in Quebec and Newfoundland are lower [24]. About 20% of home dialysis is accounted for by home HD, less than is the case for Australia and New Zealand but much more than in the United States and most of Europe [27].

## HD Practices

There are some specific atypical features with regard to Canadian HD practices. HD patients mainly receive 3–4 h three times weekly with routine monitoring of urea clearances. Only a very small percent of in-center patients receives two treatments a week, but about 5–10% receive four or more treatments weekly, due to fluid overload issues and to a belief in the merits of more frequent HD. Canada has a very high incident and long-term prevalent use of cuffed tunneled jugular venous catheters for dialysis access. In some provinces, prevalent catheter use exceeds 50%. Previously this was attributed to problems with availability of good vascular surgery, but in reality it is more related to a disillusionment with the high complication and failure rates of fistulas on the part of nephrologists and an increasing preference by patients for catheters [41, 42]. In a 2016/2017 survey of prevalent vascular access in Ontario, fistulas were being used in 36% of people on HD, grafts in 5%, and central venous catheters in 59% [34]. Bacteremia rates in the same province are measured continuously and are about 0.2 per 100 catheter days equal to about 1 new episode every 15 years (unpublished data). There has been no evidence that the decline in fistula use has had any adverse effect on mortality in people on HD.

Volumetric machines and high flux dialyzers are now standard with prices for the latter having dropped dramatically in the past 20 years. As a result, dialyzer reuse costs more to do than it saves and so has declined to zero. Online hemodiafiltration is now widely available and is no longer excessively expensive, but it is not widely used due to a lack of convincing evidence of benefit [43]. There are no good data but its use is estimated to be less than 10%.

Hepatitis B and C and human immunodeficiency virus (HIV) are monitored in all people starting dialysis, but there are no recent published data. Estimated prevalence rates in the HD population are under 1% for hepatitis B and HIV and about 5% for hepatitis C. Transmission within dialysis units is considered to be rare because of good adherence to strict infection control practices.

## PD Practices

In 2017, 72% of prevalent PD patients were doing automated PD (APD) using cyclers although many start with CAPD for 4–6 weeks [24]. High APD use is mainly for lifestyle reasons. There are no definitive data published, but icodextrin use is very common and thought to be prescribed to over 60% of people on PD, for metabolic as well as ultrafiltration-related indications. This is not the case for the so called "biocompatible" solutions which are used in less than 10% of patients, probably because of uncertain evidence and extra cost. Incremental PD is widely practiced but often in quite different ways [44]. Some patients are initiated on "day dry" cycler prescriptions or on three CAPD exchanges daily or even on one or two icodextrin dwells daily, especially if fluid removal is the main aim. Government-funded assisted PD is common in some provinces and less available in others. In the most populous province, Ontario, it is used in about 25% of prevalent PD patients at any given time and in about 33% at some stage in a given 12-month period. It typically involves a nurse or a health-care worker doing a patient's cycler setup for them and sometimes also attaching them to the cycler.

Catheters are mainly placed laparoscopically by surgeons, but a significant minority is placed percutaneously by nephrologists or invasive radiologists [45]. Peritonitis rates are routinely monitored. Unpublished data from the Ontario Renal Network indicates that rates in that province are typically 1 every 36–48 months [34].

Technique survival rates have improved with time and, depending on how they are measured, are about 85% at 1 year after censoring for death and transplant [46]. Despite these results there is significant "churn" in the PD population due to the combination of about 10% mortality, 15% technique failure, and 15% transplant rate so that after 1 year 40% of new starts are no longer on the therapy [46]. As mentioned above patient survival rates for PD appear to be good in Canada relative to those for HD though this may partly or wholly reflect positive patient selection with baseline age and comorbidities being generally less in PD patients [47, 48].

## Home HD Practices

HHD is relatively widely used in Canada, at just under 5% of prevalent dialysis patients [24]. Practices are diverse, and at least half receive "frequent" or long duration HHD prescriptions [22, 24, 48, 49]. Slow nocturnal HHD, 5–6 nights weekly for 6–8 h each time, is particularly popular [21, 50]. Others use short daily HHD for about 2 h 5–6 days weekly, and alternative day conventional HD is also used [22, 48, 50]. The "Next Stage" machine which is so popular for HHD in the United States and parts of Europe is used in only about 20% of HHD patients in Canada and is perceived as more expensive and less easily supported outside major cities [51]. Online remote monitoring of HHD patients is now rarely done. Some provinces, notably British Columbia and Ontario, provide specific funding for frequent HHD. A number of provinces reimburse electricity and water costs incurred by patients doing HHD.

Just as is the case with in center HD, central catheters are often the vascular access in HHD, and this has the advantage of avoiding the challenge to patients of learning to needle. For those who do have fistulas, button hole needling has been a source of concern for infection and is less frequently used [52].

Survival rates for people on home HD are very high exceeding those on both center HD and PD [24, 48, 50]. This partly reflects baseline differences in health and perhaps functionality and education, though the benefit persists even when these are adjusted for. However, technique failure rates have risen in recent years and are now similar to those on PD, at least for the first 12 months, likely due to the recruitment of more "marginal" patients to take on the therapy [50].

## Pre-ESRD Care

Specialized multidisciplinary pre-ESRD clinics for patients with advanced chronic kidney disease (CKD) have become standard practice across the country. The purpose of these is to prepare people for dialysis or transplant or conservative care and also to slow progression of advanced CKD and to treat complications [40]. With the increased emphasis on patient-centered care over the past decade, there is a big focus on education, shared decision-making, and patient empowerment in these clinics [40]. Specifically, these clinics are supposed to focus on key decisions around modality selection, access choice, and preemptive transplant where possible.

Eligibility for these clinics varies with some going by estimated glomerular filtration rate (eGFR) levels and others using the Kidney Failure Risk Equation which incorporates proteinuria as well as kidney function [53].

## Transplantation Practices

As stated earlier, Canada has a relatively high rate of kidney transplantation, and about 40% of transplants are from living donors [24]. Despite the high transplant rate when expressed per million population, the lifetime likelihood of a person starting chronic dialysis receiving a transplant is only about 20% [54]. This reflects the high incident rate of ESRD, the relative shortage of donated kidneys, and the fact that the large majority of people on dialysis is not eligible to receive a transplant due to comorbidities and consequent short life expectancy [54].

There are 15 transplant centers, all based in university centers. Organ sharing is largely within provinces or clusters of provinces, rather than nationwide. However, the Canadian Blood Services does facilitate some nationwide organ sharing, such as with highly sensitized patients, kidney paired donors, and living donor recipient "chains" [55].

Rules for organ sharing vary. In Ontario, for example, the region in which a pair of kidneys is retrieved from a deceased donor is allowed to keep one kidney for use by the local transplant center, and the other is shared across the province, with preference given to children and younger adults, to the highly sensitized, and to those with longer time on dialysis [55, 56].

There are significant differences in the likelihood of a person on chronic dialysis receiving a kidney transplant between renal programs that cannot be attributed to organ availability [31, 32]. These are thought to reflect differences in perception by referring nephrologists as to who is eligible for transplant and differences in the efficiency with which candidates are worked up and referred, but there also are patient socioeconomic factors that reduce access for people living further away from transplant centers [31, 32, 54].

Standard immunosuppression involves induction with basiliximab, the chimeric interleukin-2 receptor monoclonal antibody. Thymoglobulin, an antihuman thymocyte globulin polyclonal preparation, is used in induction of patients at higher risk of rejection. Transplant recipients also typically receive a regimen of tacrolimus, mycophenolate, and tapering doses of steroids. Some centers reduce steroids rapidly [56].

Cytomegalovirus mismatching is common and ganciclovir prophylaxis is used. Cellular rejection is usually treated with steroids and thymoglobulin, while antibody-mediated rejection treatment also includes plasma exchange and intravenous immunoglobulin [56].

Recipients with uncomplicated courses are often discharged within 5–7 days posttransplant. Graft survival rates for deceased donor transplants at 1, 3, 5, and 10 years are 93%, 88%, 82%, and 63%, respectively, and the half-life of deceased donor transplants is now at least 12 years. For living donor transplants, graft survival at 1, 3, 5, and 10 years is 97%, 95%, 91%, and 74%, respectively, and half-life is likely at least 18 years [24].

## Funding

As already stated and consistent with Canadian health-care principles, dialysis delivery is completely and only funded by provincial governments, either directly or through provincial renal agencies. Dialysis is almost entirely delivered through hospitals which are either public or, more commonly, not-for-profit independent entities heavily dependent on provincial government funding and therefore answerable to that government. There are almost no private dialysis providers in Canada and a complete absence of the so called 'chains' or large dialysis organizations that are so dominant in the United States and elsewhere. There are also no physician-owned dialysis units [57].

The units themselves are mainly located inside acute care hospitals. Those in hospitals which have multiple nephrologists and a reasonable range of renal services, including facility-based HD, PD, acute dialysis, and general nephrology clinics, are often called "hubs," while those with an HD unit but no nephrologists of their own and very limited ancillary renal services are called "satellites." Typically, "hub" hospitals receive government funding for dialysis and contract with their satellites to deliver HD. Some of the hubs and satellites locate their HD units in leased buildings not on the main hospital site, and some of these are in shopping malls or office blocks, but this is still not very common. In Ontario with over 14 million population, for example, there are 27 renal programs, some very large and some very small. Between them they operate 100 HD units. All 27 of them provide PD, but only 21 of them do home HD, and just 6 do transplant [58].

The method by which government funds the "hub" hospitals providing dialysis varies by province [57, 59]. Some provinces such as Alberta and Manitoba fund dialysis through the hospital's global budget in the same way that they fund surgical operating rooms and medical wards. This approach has become less popular because of the sensitive life sustaining nature of dialysis and because of its tendency to grow from year to year. Accordingly, volume-based funding is becoming more common and is used in Ontario and British Columbia. It is modality specific with different rates for facility-based HD, CAPD, APD, HHD, etc. Recently, "bundled" funding has become popular so that, for example, the rate for facility HD might also include vascular access provision or intradialytic medications or laboratory tests, but no jurisdiction has bundled erythropoiesis-stimulating agents as has occurred in the United States. There is talk of quality-based funding, but, strictly speaking, this has not yet occurred, and there would be little consensus about how "quality" might be measured in such a diverse population as those with ESRD. If the annual bundled funding for center HD is divided by 156, the typical number of HD treatments per year, the rate per dialysis is about US$ 250.

In general, modality-based funding for facility HD is about 50% higher than that for home PD and home HD, consistent with costing studies (Table 11.4) [39, 58, 59]. The higher cost of facility HD is mainly accounted for by nursing salaries. A number of provinces including Ontario and British Columbia have introduced specific "bundled" fees for frequent home HD and even for frequent facility HD, typically defined as five or more treatments a week [9, 58]. It should be noted that provincial modality-based funding formulas do not generally cover outpatient medications, imaging studies, hospital admissions, transport costs, or physician fees. In Ontario, there is a specific annual "bundle" for pre-ESRD multidisciplinary care of patients with a 2-year risk of ESRD greater than 10% or an eGFR of 15 ml/min or less.

Transplantation is generally funded out of the global budget of the hospital where the procedure is performed and often comes from the surgical rather than the renal portion of that budget. In Ontario, there is a one-off payment of

**Table 11.4** Ontario renal network annualized reimbursement bundles by modality, expressed in US$ using exchange rate of C$ 1 = US$ 0.75

| Modality | Annualized payment (US$) | Additions (US$) |
|---|---|---|
| CAPD | 21,822 | Up to 1725 for initial training |
| APD | 28,609 | Up to 1725 for initial training |
| Home HD | 17,348 | 11,400 for initial training |
| Frequent home HD (>4 treatments weekly) | 26,695 | 11,400 for initial training |
| Facility HD[a] | 38,459 | |
| Facility HD (>4 treatments weekly) | 64,056 | |
| Facility slow nocturnal HD | 64,056 | |

[a]Equivalent to US$ 247 per treatment in person receiving 3 treatments weekly

C$25,000 by the Ministry of Health to the hospital performing the transplant and an additional C$5800 if there is a living donor. This funding usually goes to the surgical transplant unit rather than to the nephrology unit. There is no dedicated funding for potential transplant recipient work up. There is funding available in most provinces to cover medical and personal costs of living donors [60, 61].

## Glomerular Diseases

Glomerulonephritis is listed as the primary cause of ESRD in about 11% of incident cases and 21% of prevalent cases receiving renal replacement therapy in Canada [24]. The higher prevalent rate reflects the longer survival of people with glomerulonephritis compared to other causes of ESRD.

Driven by the greater complexity and cost of immunosuppressive medications for glomerular diseases, there has been an increasing trend toward specialized clinics for nondiabetic glomerular diseases, including vasculitis. Provincial renal agencies in British Columbia and Ontario have set up networks of specialist clinics with multidisciplinary teams comprising nephrologists, nurses, pharmacists, and social workers as well as affiliated pathologists to help people navigate renal biopsies, diagnosis, choice and funding of required immunosuppressive agents, and subsequent follow-up [62–64]. Standardized protocols and approval processes for funding of medications such as rituximab and eculizumab have been developed in some provinces.

## Acute Kidney Injury

The incidence of AKI requiring dialysis in Canada is difficult to measure because many of the cases labeled "acute" are actually people with ESRD who are hospitalized [65]. People with AKI severe enough to require dialysis and to be treated in intensive care units may receive conventional acute HD for 3–4 h 3–6 times weekly. However, it is estimated that more than half now receive at least some treatment with either sustained low-efficiency dialysis (SLED) using a conventional HD machine with low blood flows for 6–12 h daily or continuous renal replacement therapy (CRRT), most often delivered using the Baxter "Prisma" machine in either hemofiltration or hemodiafiltration mode [65–67]. SLED and CRRT are about equally popular. In intensive care units where CRRT is used, intensivists are often in charge of initiation and prescription of the therapy. Where conventional HD or SLED is used, it is typically initiated and prescribed by nephrologists.

## First Nations Populations and Kidney Disease

As alluded to earlier, First Nations or FNIM populations in Canada represent about 4% of the country's total population, and with high birth rates, this proportion is likely to increase. FNIM groups have high rates of ESRD, related primarily to high rates of type 2 diabetes mellitus which have rapidly increased over the past 60 years with alteration in diet and lifestyle [26, 68, 69].

The problems associated with CKD and ESRD in FNIM populations are aggravated by the high rates of socioeconomic deprivation, mental health problems, and substance abuse, associated in turn with the legacy of colonialism and displacement that these people have suffered [70].

Incident ESRD rates are estimated to be about three times as high as in the general population, and this raises particular challenges in provinces like Manitoba and Saskatchewan where close to 20% of the population is FNIM. As many as half of FNIM people live on reserves, and in a proportion of these, the reserve location is remote from hospitals and dialysis units. In these scenarios, relocation for HD is required if home dialysis is not feasible or is unsuccessful. In general rates of both home dialysis and transplant are relatively lower in FNIM populations, in part due to social reasons [71, 72].

Initiatives to alleviate the excess load of CKD in FNIM people have included screening and treatment programs for early CKD and use of telemedicine to deliver remote care [73]. Networks of small satellite HD units on or close to reserves have also been developed [74]. However, nothing short of major social change is likely to alleviate this burden of diabetic CKD.

## Medications

There is no universal payment system for medications in Canada, analogous to that for hospital and physician care, and this is frequently criticized by advocates of socialized medicine [5]. The provinces do provide medications free of charge from a broad provincial formulary to all those aged 65 or over and often to those under 18 and also to those on social welfare. Many working Canadians have an employment-related private insurance drug benefit plan that covers a similar or wider range of medications, but there is a significant population between 18 and 65 years of age who have no such insurance. These individuals may receive supplemental provincial funding for medications once their annual costs exceed an income-related deductible. Expensive medications such as erythropoiesis-stimulating agents are often covered completely by special provincial drug programs, and pre-ESRD and dialysis patient have easy access to these in almost all cases. Access to immunosuppressive medications is also rarely an obstacle to kidney transplant patients although income-related deductible payments may be required for those aged under 65.

Relatively newer more expensive medications for dialysis patients such as non-calcium phosphate binders, vitamin D analogues, and cinacalcet are not routinely available free of charge to patients in every province, and typically specific clinical criteria have to be met before the government will fund them [75]. Newer expensive medications such as rituximab or eculizumab, used in the treatment of some types of glomerulonephritis and microangiopathies, are more difficult to access but most provinces have evidence-based criteria in place to fund them for those people who truly need them [62–64].

## Nephrologists

Canada has about 700 practicing adult nephrologists, equal to about 1 per 50,000 population or 1 per 40 chronic dialysis patients [76]. About half have some form of academic appointment, and a large proportion of these have full-time academic positions. The other half are in "community" nephrology, a notable increase from 25 years ago when most chronic dialysis was being delivered through academic centers [19, 20]. The proliferation of new community-based renal programs in the late 1990s led to this increase in non-academic community nephrologists. About a third of nephrologists are women, a notable increase from a decade ago. Over 90% of Canadian nephrologists, both in academic and community nephrology groups, are involved in the care of chronic dialysis patients. Less than 10%, all in academic centers, spend a large part of their clinical time caring for patients with kidney transplants.

Like the majority of Canadian physicians, most nephrologists, including those in full-time academic positions, are paid "fee for service" by provincial government "insurance" plans. These fees are set through negotiations between the provincial health ministries and the provincial medical association. Nephrologists must adhere to this billing arrangement, and "extra billing" of patients is forbidden. Patients do not and may not pay nephrologists. The combination of single government payer and fee for service is unusual in healthcare systems and, to some extent, was a compromise between government and physician groups at the time of the establishment of Canadian Medicare. While it may be seen by some as an imposition on physician independence and on the physician-patient relationship, the reimbursement system does give physicians security of income, the simplicity and time saving of a single payer system, and a proportionality between work done and reimbursement received which is not typically found in salaried systems.

The bulk of nephrologists' income comes from fees for chronic dialysis. Historically these were procedural fees, and those for center-based HD were paid for physician provision/supervision of each treatment, whereas for home dialysis or for satellite HD, there was either no physician fee or a modest specific retainer fee paid per week [77]. This arrangement persists in some provinces, but in others it was perceived as giving physicians a perverse incentive to direct patients to expensive center-based HD and away from home and satellite dialysis. In the late 1990s, Ontario therefore introduced a modality-independent capitation fee, analogous to that in the United States at the time, and other provinces followed suit leading to a fee that is not related to the actual dialysis procedure but rather to the overall care of the patient [78].

Academic nephrologists in most provinces pay a variable percentage of their salary as a "tithe" to their university department of medicine. This can vary from as low as 10% to as much as 30%. However, the same department of medicine typically pays a modest and variable base salary to their nephrologists as reimbursement for teaching, research, and administrative activities and in proportion to their productivity in those areas. The end results of these dollars going in circles are broadly revenue neutral for nephrology groups as a whole. Most academic nephrology groups pool and share their income to some degree so that productive research-focused nephrologists earn similar income to clinical and education-oriented academics who have higher clinical billings. The fee for service system is notably less rewarding for nephrologists who mainly work in kidney transplantation, as distinct from chronic dialysis, but again income pooling in university nephrology groups addresses this. However, the point is often made that chronic dialysis fee for service income is indirectly funding academic nephrology activities. In recognition of this, academic nephrologists in many provinces receive some income from government "alternate funding plans." Transplant nephrologists may also have specific supplemental "alternate funding" government payments allocated to them in recognition of limited billing opportunities. In the province of Alberta, some academic physicians forgo "fee for service" altogether and are reimbursed through a full "alternate funding plan" in order to avoid "fee for service" incentive unduly disrupting or disincentivizing academic activities [79].

There are 15 active nephrology training programs in Canada, though not all consistently have trainees, and only half would consistently have over five trainees at a time [80]. All are affiliated with medical schools, and between them they accept about 25 internal medicine-trained residents annually. Additional trainees come from other countries to do nephrology fellowships in Canada, with or without an eventual plan to return to their home countries, and some eventually stay long term. Training takes a minimum of 2 years though it is typically longer for those interested in acquiring specialized clinical skills or in developing an academic career. Basic training includes teaching in HD and PD, transplant, and general outpatient, inpatient, and intensive care nephrology [81]. Subsequent specialist training fellowships in areas such as transplantation, home dialysis, glomerular disease, clinical research methodology, education, and quality improvement are increasingly popular for those wishing to work in academic centers particularly [81].

The combination of fee for service payment and of the growth that has occurred over the past four decades in the numbers of prevalent dialysis patients has led to relatively high incomes for Canadian nephrologists who typically rate third among internal medical specialists behind cardiologists and gastroenterologists in annual reimbursement received. Incomes in excess of US$ 250,000 annually are not unusual for clinically busy nephrologists who are caring for large numbers of dialysis patients. Partly because of this, nephrology remains a relatively popular specialty among Canadian medical school graduates, and most training positions and staff nephrologist positions are filled. Indeed, there is often keen competition for nephrologist positions in larger Canadian cities [81, 82]. A large majority of nephrologist appointments are now Canadian medical school graduates.

Canada has the Canadian Society of Nephrology (CSN) which meets annually and is very active [83]. The CSN promotes education, research, and debate and develops its own disease management guidelines. Quebec has its own mainly Francophone Societe Quebecoise de Nephrologie [84]. There is also the Canadian Society of Transplantation [85]. At a provincial level, physician groups such as the Ontario Association of Nephrologists promote the economic and professional interests of their members.

## Nurses and Allied Health Professionals

In general dialysis in Canada has been delivered by unionized registered nurses, and this contrasts with the situation in the United States where much less well-reimbursed dialysis technicians provide HD under nursing and physician supervision. However, the ongoing growth in numbers of dialysis patients and the increasing cost constraints in the whole health-care system have led to increased use of less expensive "practical nurses" and dialysis technicians in some provinces. There is a lot of variation across provinces and between centers, but in recent times, this trend has been accentuated because some renal programs have found recruitment of dialysis registered nurses to be a challenge [86, 87].

Registered nurses are increasingly likely to have nursing degrees rather than college diplomas and will have 3–4 years of training. They are typically paid in the range of US$40,0000–70,000 annually, depending on seniority and varying by province. Many academic renal programs employ nurse practitioners who have extra training and who act as physician extenders and often as advocates and practitioners of patient-centered and multidisciplinary care.

Senior nurses have always played a crucial role in administrative, fiscal, and clinical leadership of renal programs in Canada. The director of each program, appointed and employed by the hospital concerned, is typically a senior nurse. In the past nephrologists were often less involved with program administration, but, in recent times, co-management between hospital administrators and nephrologists has become more typical.

Nephrology services in Canada have generally emphasized multidisciplinary patient care, and the roles of allied health professionals such as renal dietitians and social workers have been paramount [88, 89]. Renal pharmacists play a greater role with increasing complexities of medications in many relevant areas including anemia, bone mineral osteodystrophy, glomerular disease, and kidney transplant management [90].

## Pediatric Nephrology

Pediatric nephrology is by its nature much more centralized than its adult counterpart. Canada has about 70 pediatric nephrologists concentrated in 13 major academic centers with chronic pediatric dialysis programs. There are nine pediatric kidney transplant programs of which two only operate on patients aged 12–18 [91] (personal communication Dr. Guido Filler, Western University, London, Canada, July 10, 2019).

Canada has a quite stable incident rate of ESRD in children aged 0–19 year of about 10 per million population (aged 0–19), equivalent to about 75 cases annually. These children have a 10-year survival rate in excess of 80%. This age group is transplanted promptly so that at any given time there are about 400 children alive with ESRD in Canada excluding Quebec, for a prevalent rate of 65 per million, but 330 of them are living with transplants. Of the approximately 70 on chronic dialysis, just over half use PD, and just under half do HD [24].

## Renal Agencies

A feature of Canadian nephrology over the past decade has been the growing popularity of provincial renal "agencies." British Columbia was the pioneer in this regard when it set up the British Columbia Renal Agency in the 1990s [32]. The Ontario Renal Network was established in 2009, and there are similar bodies in Manitoba, Nova Scotia, and Alberta [33, 34, 92, 93]. In general, these are government agencies with a budget provided by their provincial Ministry of Health. They operate at varying degrees of "arm's length" from the ministry and supervise the budget for renal services and act to ensure that patients receive equitable, cost-effective, and good quality renal care.

Generally, these agencies commit to the principles of patient-centered care and, in particular, to that care being better integrated and available closer to home. Accordingly, these agencies promote initiatives such as shared decision-making, growing home dialysis modalities, increasing transplant rates, promoting appropriately deferred start on chronic dialysis, ensuring patients' goals of care are discussed and documented and that palliative options are available when requested, monitoring patient reported outcomes and experience, and developing specialized services for patients with glomerular diseases [62–64, 94].

A particular feature of these agencies is the involvement of nephrologists in policy development and implementation, to a degree that had not occurred in the past. This co-management principle also involves a role for renal program administrators and multidisciplinary groups. Patient involvement is also a strong feature, and in Ontario no policy is now implemented without input from patient and family advisory committees [34].

There is a general impression that these agencies have changed the culture of Canadian nephrology and have had success in growing home dialysis in a number of provinces [33, 34].

It should be noted that, unlike in the United States, these renal agencies do not have specific guidelines for the detailed care of individual people with CKD. Areas, such as dialysis clearances, access and ultrafiltration in people on dialysis, and management of anemia and mineral bone metabolism in CKD and ESRD, are not regulated by these government agencies. Guidelines are provided by the Canadian Society of Nephrology and by other international agencies, but there is no direct governmental policing of these [83, 84]. However renal programs generally self-regulate these practices and outcomes.

## References


1. OECD Data Canada 2019. Accessed at https://data.oecd.org/canada.htm.
2. Fierlebeck K. Political thought in Canada. An intellectual history. 1st ed. Toronto: University of Toronto Press; 2006.
3. Fierlebeck K. Health care in Canada: a citizen's guide to policy and politics. 1st ed. Toronto: University of Toronto Press; 2011.
4. Deber R. Treating health care: how the Canadian system works and how it could work better. 1st ed. Toronto: University of Toronto Press; 2017.
5. Morgan SG, Li W, Yan B, Persaud N. Estimated effects of adding universal public coverage of an essential medicines list to existing public drug plans in Canada. Can Med Assoc J. 2017;189:E295–302.
6. Muzyka D, Hodgson G, Prada G. The inconvenient truths about Canadian health care. Conference Board of Canada. 2012. Accessed at https://www.conferenceboard.ca/CASHC/research/2012/inconvenient_truths.aspx.
7. McGill Health Care in Canada Survey 2018. 2018. Accessed at https://www.mcgill.ca/hcic-sssc/hcic-surveys/2018.
8. McAlister VC. Clinical kidney transplantation: A 50th anniversary review of the first reported series. Am J Surg. 2005;190(3):485–8.
9. Murray G, Delorme E, Thomas N. Development of an artificial kidney. Arch Surg. 1947;55:516–22.
10. Murray G, Holden R. Transplantation of kidneys, experimentally and in human cases. Am J Surg. 1954;87:508–15.
11. McGill Channels. McGill University news and events. McGill University Health Centre celebrates 50th anniversary of Canada's first kidney transplant. https://www.mcgill.ca/channels/news/mcgill-university-health-centre-celebrates-50th-anniversary-canada%E2%80%99s-1st-kidney-transplant-102108. 2008. Accessed July 2019.
12. Dossetor JB, Gault MH, Oliver JA, Inglis FS, Mackinnon KJ, Maclean JD. Cadaver renal homotransplants: initial experience. Can Med Assoc J. 1964;91:733–42.
13. Kidney Foundation of Canada. Saskatchewan. History of transplant in Canada. Accessed at https://www.kidney.ca/sslpage.aspx?pid=645.
14. Virtual Museum of Canada. Athena's heirs: history of medical technology in Canada. The history of hemodialysis: hemodialysis in Canada. 2001. Accessed at website http://www.virtualmuseum.ca/edu/ViewLoitDa.do;jsessionid=AF581B5BC8FB41B28BCF0E164DD82425?method=preview&lang=EN&id=4124.
15. McLeod LE, Mandin H, Davidman M, Ulan R, Lakey WH. Intermittent hemodialysis in terminal chronic renal failure. Can Med Assoc J. 1966;94:318–27.
16. Amair P, Khanna R, Leibel B, Pierratos A, Vas S, Meema E, et al. Continuous ambulatory peritoneal dialysis in diabetics with end-stage renal disease. N Engl J Med. 1982;306:625–30.
17. Uldall PR, Woods F, Bird M, Dyck R. Subclavian cannula for temporary hemodialysis. Proc Clin Dial Transplant Forum. 1979;9:268–72.
18. Fenton SSA, Copleston PF, Desmeules M, Arbus GS, Froment DH, Kjellstrand CM, et al. Renal replacement therapy in Canada 1981–1992. In: Jacobs C, Kjellstrand CM, Koch KM, Winchester JF, editors. Replacement of renal function by dialysis. 4th ed. Dordrecht: Kluwer Academic Publishers; 1996. p. 1406–22.
19. Blake PG, Finkelstein FO. Why is the proportion of patients doing peritoneal dialysis declining in North America? Perit Dial Int. 2001;21:107–14.
20. Blake P. Proliferation of hemodialysis units and declining peritoneal dialysis use: an international trend. Am J Kidney Dis. 2009;54:194–6.
21. Uldall R, Ouwendyk M, Francoeur R, Wallace L, Sit W, Vas S. Slow nocturnal home hemodialysis at the Wellesley Hospital. Adv Ren Replace Ther. 1996;3:133–6.
22. Lindsay RM, Leitch R, Heidenheim AP, Kortas C. London daily/nocturnal hemodialysis study – study design, morbidity and mortality results. Am J Kidney Dis. 2003;42(suppl 1):5–12.
23. Canadian Multicentre Transplant Study Group. A randomized controlled trial of cyclosporine in cadaveric renal transplantation. N Engl J Med. 1983;309:809–15.

24. Canadian Institute for Health Information. Organ replacement in Canada; CORR Annual Statistics, 2018. https://www.cihi.ca/en/organ-replacement-in-canada-corr-annual-statistics-2018. Accessed 21 July 2019.
25. Canadian Institute for Health Information. Organ replacement in Canada; CORR Annual Statistics, 2012.
26. Jiang Y, Osgood N, Lim HJ, Stang MR, Dyck R. Differential mortality and the excess burden of end-stage renal disease among First Nations people with diabetes mellitus: a competing risk analysis. Can Med Assoc J. 2014;186:103–9.
27. United States Renal Data Systems, 2018 Annual data report. Chapter 11. International comparisons. Accessed at https://www.usrds.org/2018/view/v2_11.aspx.
28. Horl WH, de Alvaro F, Williams PF. Healthcare systems and end-stage renal disease (ESRD) therapies – an international review: access to ESRD treatments. Nephrol Dial Transplant. 1999;14(suppl 6):10–5.
29. Limou S, Nelson GW, Kopp JB, Winkler CA. APOL1 kidney risk alleles: population genetics and disease associations. Adv Chronic Kidney Dis. 2014;21:426–33.
30. Hemmelgarn BR, James MT, Manns BJ, O'Hare AM, Muntner P, Ravani P, et al. Rates of treated and untreated kidney failure in older vs younger adults. JAMA. 2012;307:2507–15.
31. Kim SJ, Gill JS, Knoll G, et al. Referral for kidney transplant in Canadian provinces. J Am Soc Nephrol. 2019;30:1708–21.
32. Naylor K, Dixon SN, Garg AX, Kim ST, Blake PG, Nesrallah GE, et al. Variation in access to kidney transplantation across renal programs in Ontario, Canada. Am J Transplant. 2017;17:1585–93.
33. British Columbia Renal Agency. Accessed at http://www.bcrenalagency.ca/kidney-services.
34. Ontario Renal Network. Accessed at https://www.ontariorenalnetwork.ca/en.
35. Alberta Health Services. Renal services. Accessed at https://www.albertahealthservices.ca/info/Page15379.aspx.
36. Oreopoulos DG, Coleman S, Doyle E. Reversing the decreasing peritoneal dialysis (PD) trend in Ontario: a government initiative to increase PD use in Ontario to 30% by 2010. Perit Dial Int. 2007;27:489–95.
37. Oliver MJ, Quinn RR, Richardson AR, Kiss AJ, Lamping DL, Manns BJ. Home care assistance and the utilization of peritoneal dialysis. Kidney Int. 2007;71:673–8.
38. Alkatheeri AM, Blake PG, Gray D, Jain AK. Success of urgent start peritoneal dialysis in a large Canadian renal program. Perit Dial Int. 2016;36:171–6.
39. Manns B, Agar JWM, Biyani M, Blake PG, Cass A, Culleton B, et al. Can economic incentives increase the use of home dialysis? Nephrol Dial Transplant. 2019;34:731–41.
40. Smekal MD, Tam-Tham H, Finlay J, Donald M, Thomas C, Weaver RS, et al. Patient and provider experience and perspectives of a risk-based approach to multidisciplinary care: a mixed methods approach. BMC Nephrol. 2019;20(1):110. https://doi.org/10.1186/s12882-019-1269-2.
41. Blake PG, Quinn RR, Oliver MJ. The risks of vascular access. Kidney Int. 2012;82:623–5.
42. Quinn RR, Oliver MJ, Devoe D, Poinen K, Kabani R, Kamar F, et al. Effect of predialysis fistula attempt on risk of all-cause and access-related death. J Am Soc Nephrol. 2017;28:613–20.
43. Wang AY, Ninomiya T, Al-Kahwa A, et al. Effect on hemodiafiltration and hemofiltration compared with hemodialysis on mortality and cardiovascular disease in chronic kidney failure: a systematic review and meta-analysis of randomized trials. Am J Kidney Dis. 2014;63:968–78.
44. Ankawi GA, Woodcock N, Jain AK, Garg AX, Blake PG. The use of incremental peritoneal dialysis in a large contemporary peritoneal dialysis population. Can J Kidney Health Dis. 2016. https://doi.org/10.1177/2054358116679131. eCollection 2016.
45. Wallace EL, Fisell RB, Golper TA, et al. Catheter insertion and perioperative practices within the ISPD North American Research Consortium. Perit Dial Int. 2016;36:382–6.
46. Schaubel D, Blake PG, Fenton SS. Effect of renal center characteristics on mortality and technique failure on peritoneal dialysis. Kidney Int. 2001;60:1517–24.
47. Yeates K, Zhu N, Vonesh E, Trpski L, Blake P, Fenton S. Peritoneal dialysis and hemodialysis are associated with similar outcomes for end-stage renal disease in Canada. Nephrol Dial Transplant. 2012;27:3568–75.
48. Krahn M, Bremner K, de Oliveira C, Dixon S, McFarlane P, Garg AX, et al. Home dialysis is associated with lower costs and better survival than other modalities: a population-based study in Ontario, Canada. Perit Dial Int. 2019;39:553–61.
49. Pauly RP, Komenda P, Chan CT, et al. Programmatic variation in home hemodialysis in Canada: results from a nationwide survey of practice patterns. Can J Kidney Health DisWW2014;1. https://doi.org/10.1186/2054-3581-1-11.
50. Tennankore KK, Na Y, Wald R, Chan CT, Perl J. Short daily-, nocturnal- and conventional home hemodialysis have similar patient and treatment survival. Kidney Int. 2018;93:188–94.
51. Beaudry A, Ferguson TW, Rigatto C, Tangri N, Dumanski S, Komenda P. Cost of dialysis therapy by modality in Manitoba. Clin J Am Soc Nephrol. 2018;13:1197–203.
52. Grudzinski A, Mendelssohn D, Pierrattos A, Nesrallah G. A systematic review of buttonhole cannulation practices and outcomes. Semin Dial. 2013;26:465–75.
53. Tangri N, Stevens LA, Griffith J, Tighiouart H, Djurdjev O, Naimark D, et al. A predictive model of progression of chronic kidney disease to kidney failure. JAMA. 2011;305:1553–9.
54. Kiberd BD, AlBugami MM, Panek R, Tennankore K. Contraindications to kidney transplantation: uneven grounds? Transplant Res. 2015. https://doi.org/10.1186/s13737-015-0024-x.
55. Ryan J. National organ sharing leads to 500 kidney transplants for highly sensitized patients. 2019. Canadian Blood Services. https://blood.ca/en/research/our-research-stories/research-education-discovery/national-organ-sharing-leads-500-kidney. Accessed 12 Feb 2020.
56. Trillium Gift of Life Network. Clinical handbook for kidney transplantation. June 2017. https://www.giftoflife.on.ca/resources/pdf/transplant/Clinical_Handbook_for_Kidney_Transplantation_FINAL_Web_March_2019.pdf. Accessed 15 Feb 2020.
57. Blake PG, Just P. Economics of Dialysis. In: Horl WH, Koch K-M, Ronco C, Lindsay RM, Winchester JF, editors. Replacement of Renal Function by Dialysis. 5th ed. Dordrecht: Klewer Academic Publishers; 2004.
58. Ontario Renal Network. Local services. https://www.ontariorenalnetwork.ca/en/local-services.
59. Klarenbach SW, Tonelli M, Chui B, Manns BJ. Economic evaluation of dialysis therapies. Nat Rev Nephrol. 2014;10:644–52.
60. Klarenbach S, Gill JS, Knoll G, et al. Economic consequences incurred by living kidney donors: a Canadian multi-center prospective study. Am J Transplant. 2014;14:916–22.
61. Barnieh L, Klarenbach S, Arnold J, et al. Nonreimbursed costs incurred by living kidney donors: a case study from Ontario, Canada. Transplantation. 2019;103:e164–71.
62. Barbour S, Beaulieu M, Gill J, Djurdjev O, Riech H, Levin A. Overview of British Columbia Glomerulonephritis network and registry: integrating knowledge generation and translation within a single framework. BMC Nephrol. 2013;14:236. https://doi.org/10.1186/1471-2369-14-236.
63. Pang J, D'Antonio C, Heale E, et al. Provincial needs assessment to determine the current state of glomerulonephritis

care in Ontario. Can J Kidney Health Dis. 2019. https://doi.org/10.1177/2054358119877405.
64. Barbour S, Lo C, Espino-Hernandez G, Sajjadi S, Feehally J, Klarenbach S, et al. The population-level costs of immunosuppression medications for the treatment of glomerulonephritis are increasing over time due to changing patterns of practice. Nephrol Dial Transplant. 2018;33:626–34.
65. Sawhney S, Fraser SD. Epidemiology of acute kidney injury: utilizing large databases to determine the burden of acute kidney injury. Adv Chronic Kidney Dis. 2017;24:194–204.
66. Nash DM, Przech S, Wald R, O'Reilly D. Systematic review and meta-analysis of renal replacement treatment modalities for acute kidney injury in the intensive care unit. J Crit Care. 2017;41:138–44.
67. Tandukar S, Pavlevsky PM. Continuous renal replacement therapy: who, when, why and how. Chest. 2019;155:626–38.
68. Turin TC, Saad N, Jun M, et al. Lifetime risk of diabetes causing First Nations and non-First Nations people. CMAJ. 2016;188:1147–53.
69. Dyck RF, Jiang Y, Osgood ND, et al. Can J Diabetes. 2014;38:237–43.
70. Tonelli M, Hemmelgarn B, Manns B, et al. Use and outcomes of peritoneal dialysis among Aboriginal hemodialysis people in Canada. J Am Soc Nephrol. 2005;18:482–8.
71. Tonelli M, Chou S, Gourishankar S, Jhangri GS, Bradley J, Hemmelgarn B. Wait-listing for kidney transplant among Aboriginal hemodialysis patients. Am J Kidney Dis. 2005;46:1117–23.
72. Ferguson JW, Tangri N. Zan Screening for chronic kidney disease in Canadian indigenous people is cost-effective. Kidney Int. 2017;92:121–200.
73. Komenda P, Lavallee B, Ferguson TW, et al. Prevalence of chronic kidney disease in rural Canadian Indigenous people: results from the First Nations Community Screening to Improve Kidney Health and Prevent Dialysis (FINISHEDD) screen, triage and treat program. Am J Kidney Dis. 2016;68:582–90.
74. Ferguson TW, Zacahrias J, Walker R, Collister D, Rigatto C, Tangri N, Komenda P. A economic assessment model of rural and remote satellite hemodialysis units. PLoS ONE. 2015. https://doi.org/10.1371/journal.pone.0135587. eCollection 2015.
75. Ministry of Health Ontario. Exceptional access program reimbursement criteria for frequently requested drugs. 21 Sept 2019. http://www.health.gov.on.ca/en/pro/programs/drugs/docs/frequentlyrequested_drugs.pdf. Accessed 29 Dec 2019.
76. Ward DR, Manns B, Gil S, Au F, Kappel JE. Results of 2014–15 Canadian Society of Nephrology workforce survey. Can J Kidney Health Dis. 2016. https://doi.org/10.1186/s40697-016-0117-6. eCollection 2016.
77. Nissenson A, Prichard SS, Cheng IK, Gokal R, Kubota M, Maiorca R, et al. Non-medical factors that impact on ESRD modality selection. Kidney Int Suppl. 1993;40:S120–7.
78. Mendelssohn DC, Langlois N, Blake PG. Peritoneal dialysis in Ontario: a natural experiment in physician reimbursement methodology. Perit Dial Int. 2004;24:531–7.
79. Alberta. Academic Medicine and Health Services Program. 2019. Accessed at https://www.alberta.ca/academic-medicine-health-services-program.aspx.
80. Canadian Residence Matching Service. 2018. www.carms.ca.
81. Blake PG. Supply of nephrologists in Canada remains steady. Nephro News Issues 2018. Accessed at https://www.healio.com/nephrology/kidney-care-community/news/print/nephrology-news-and-issues/%7Be56e17a5-260b-4807-b230-6bae7ef1e7f2%7D/supply-of-nephrologists-in-canada-remains-steady.
82. Bear R. Hiring doctors. Whose interests should come first? Healthy Debate. Nov 15, 2012. Accessed at http://healthydebate.ca/opinions/doctors_and_hospitals_relationship.
83. Canadian Society of Nephrology. Accessed at https://www.csnscn.ca/.
84. Societe Quebecoise de Nephrologie. Accessed at https://sqn.qc.ca/.
85. Canadian Society of Transplant. Accessed at https://www.cst-transplant.ca/.
86. Canadian Association of Nephrology Nurses and Technicians/l'Association Canadienne des infirmieres et infirmiers et des technologies de nephrologie. Accessed at https://cannt-acitn.ca/.
87. Grant K. Supply of nurses falls in Canada for first time in 20 years: report. Globe and Mail. June 23, 2015. Accessed at https://www.theglobeandmail.com/life/health-and-fitness/health/supply-of-nurses-falls-in-canada-for-first-time-in-almost-20-years-report/article25069547/. Accessed 25 July 2019.
88. Canadian Association of Nephrology Social Workers. Accessed at http://www.cansw.org/.
89. Dietitians of Canada/Dietetistes du Canada. Canadian Association of Nephrology Dietitians. Accessed at https://www.dietitians.ca/About-Us/Become-A-Member/Networks/CAND.aspx.
90. Renal Pharmacists Network/Reseau de pharmaciens en nephrology. Accessed at https://renalpharmacists.net/resources/.
91. Bell L, Drummond K, Arbus G, Lirenman D, Wolfish N, Crocker J, et al. History of pediatric nephrology in Canada. Canadian Association of Pediatric Nephrologists/Association des Nephrologies Pediatriques du Canada. 2000. Accessed at https://www.capneph.ca/about-us/history/history-of-pediatric-nephrology-in-canada.html. Accessed 25 July 2019.
92. Kidney Health.ca. Manitoba Renal Program. https://www.kidneyhealth.ca/about-us/manitoba-renal-program/.
93. Woodward GL, Iverson A, Harvey R, Blake PG. Implementation of an agency to improve chronic kidney disease care in Ontario: lessons learned by the Ontario Renal Network. Healthc Q. 2015;17; Spec No 44-7.
94. Nesrallah GE, Dixon SN, MacKinnon M, Jassal SV, Bota SE, et al. Home palliative service utilization and care trajectory among Ontario residents dying on chronic dialysis. Can J Kidney Health Dis. 2018;5:2054358118783761. https://doi.org/10.1177/2054358118783761. eCollection 2018.

# Nephrology in Chile

# 12

Ana Ortiz, Leopoldo Ardiles, Jacqueline Pefaur, Helmuth Goecke, Eric Roessler, Susana Elgueta, and Pía Rosati

| | |
|---|---|
| Area[1] | 756,950 km$^2$ |
| Population[2] | 17,373,831 (2017) |
| Capital | Santiago de Chile |
| Three most populated cities: | 1. Santiago<br>2. Concepción<br>3. Valparaiso |
| Official language | Spanish |
| Gross domestic product (GDP)[3,4] | 277.08 billion USD (2017) |
| GDP per capita[3,4] | 15,346.45 USD (2017) |
| Human Development Index (HDI)[5] | 0.843 (2018) |
| Official currency[3] | Peso |
| Total number of nephrologists | 242 adult nephrologists<br>60 pediatric nephrologists |
| National society of nephrology | Sociedad Chilena de Nefrología<br>www.nefro.cl |
| Incidence of end-stage renal disease | 2018 – 187.4 pmp |
| Prevalence of end-stage renal disease (on dialysis) | 2018 – 1342.2 pmp |
| Total number of patients on dialysis (all modalities) | 2017 – 22,508 patients<br>2018 – 23,739 patients |
| Number of patients on hemodialysis | 2017 – 21,223 patients (1208 pmp)<br>2018 – 22,310 patients (1260 pmp) |
| Number of patients on peritoneal dialysis | 2017 – 1285 patients (74 pmp)<br>2018 – 1429 patients (82.2 pmp) |
| Number of renal transplantations per year | 2017 – 399 (21.7 pmp)<br>2018 – 312 (16 pmp) |

Table References:

1. Geographic Military Institute. (https://www.igm.cl)
2. National Institute of Statistics, Census 2017. (https://www.censo2017.cl)
3. Central bank of Chile 2018. (https://www.bcentral.cl)
4. The World Bank Group. (https://databank.worldbank.org/home.aspx)
5. Human Development Indices and Indicators: 2018 Statistical Update. (http://hdr.undp.org/en/2018-update)

## Introduction

Chile is a country located along the western seaboard of South America, extending over approximately 4329 km within the American continent and including territories in the Antarctica and Oceania. The general information table provides a brief overview of data for the country. Chile is a member of the OECD (Organization for Economic Co-operation and Development) since January 2010.

According to 2017 data from the World Health Organization, life expectancy at birth is 80 years for men and 85 years for women; the birth rate is 13.1 per 1000 inhabitants, and the mortality rate is 6.2 per 1000 inhabitants [1].

Epidemiological indicators obtained in 2010 suggest chronic kidney disease (CKD) prevalence of 2.7%, in presumably healthy people, which increases to 12.1% [2] in

A. Ortiz (✉)
Facultad de Medicina, Pontificia Universidad Católica de Chile, Santiago, Chile
e-mail: mortiz@med.puc.cl

L. Ardiles
Hospital Regional, Facultad de Medicina, Universidad Austral de Chile, Valdivia, Chile

J. Pefaur
Facultad de Medicina, Universidad de Chile Hospital Barros Luco Trudeau, Santiago, Chile

H. Goecke
Hospital Naval Almirante Nef – Universidad de Valparaíso, Viña del Mar, Chile

E. Roessler
Hospital Clínico Pontificia Universidad Católica de Chile, Santiago, Chile

S. Elgueta
Histocompatibility Laboratory, Instituto de Salud Publica, Santiago, Chile

P. Rosati
San Juan de Dios, Santiago, Chile


J. A. Moura-Neto et al. (eds.), *Nephrology Worldwide*, https://doi.org/10.1007/978-3-030-56890-0_12

primary care patients in urban centers. These data have been useful to focus resources in preventive programs in order to delay the progression of renal failure disease as a public policy. The access to diagnosis and therapy of CKD in all its stages is financed and protected by the Explicit Health Guarantees System of universal access (GES) [3].

Prevalence of end-stage renal disease (ESRD) requiring dialysis is 1284 pmp, mainly in hemodialysis (HD), whereas renal transplant rate was 16.6 pmp. Chilean legislation regulates all dialysis centers since 1994. Donation and renal transplant (both living and deceased donors) were legally established in 1996, and efforts are currently being made to establish, by law, a wider policy of presumed donation in people over 18 years of age. Academic nephrologists from the Universidad de Chile, Pontificia Universidad Catolica, Universidad de Valparaiso, and Universidad Austral as well as clinical nephrologists from the metropolitan area or regions, and personnel from state institutions, like the Institute of Public Health (ISP), have participated in the drafting of this chapter.

We present a brief history of Chilean nephrology from its beginning, including the different areas where nephrologists are involved, as well as the present conditions of the specialty in the country.

## Brief History of Nephrology in Chile

In 1962, a course of nephrology was carried out in the Society of Medicine of Santiago directed at that time by Dr. Renato Gazmuri, the first president of the Chilean Society of Nephrology which started its activities on June 24, 1964.

The first unit of pediatric nephrology was created in 1958 in the Arriaran Hospital in Santiago [4], and the university training of pediatric nephrology began in 1988 at the University of Chile.

The first HD was performed, at the San Borja Hospital, in a woman with septic shock in 1957. Six years later, the national health service (FONASA) was founded to deliver necessary financial coverage establishing as a model of public insurance for high-cost diseases in Latin America.

The first dialysis unit was created in 1965 at Jose Joaquin Aguirre Hospital [5].

Acute peritoneal dialysis (PD) started in 1963 at the Navy Hospital of Valparaiso and in the Del Salvador Hospital of Santiago [6] and continued ambulatory peritoneal dialysis (CAPD) in Indisa Clinic and Universidad Católica de Chile in 1994–1995.

In 1974, the Society for Dialysis and Transplanted patients (ASODI) was created, as a nongovernmental nonprofit institution.

The history of transplantation began in the Jose Joaquin Aguirre Hospital, in 1966 [7]. On June 26, Dr. Jorge Kaplan performed the first heart transplant in the Navy Hospital, just a few months after the first heart transplant was performed in the world. The first kidney transplant performed in Chile was in January 1968, with a living related donor [8]. The first liver transplant was performed in 1988; combined kidney/pancreas transplants have been done since 1994 [9], and lung and heart transplant began in 1997.

Organ donation and transplantation have been regulated since 1996 by the Law no. 19451, modified in 2010 (Law no. 20413), establishing a presumed donation policy in people over 18 years [10, 11]. In relation to the extraction of organs from living donors for transplant purposes only, the law allows as capable people only those over 18 years, blood relatives up to fourth degree, or the husband, wife, or stable partner of the receptor. Since 2017, the Law no. 20988 regulates cross kidney transplantation in the cases that living donor is present; however, kidney transplantation cannot be performed from relatives due to blood group incompatibility or the presence of high levels of antibodies, whereas a life gift can be shared via cross transplantation method. The requirements needed for the certification of a nephrologist in Chile include a medical school degree (7 years of undergraduate studies) plus 3 years of training in internal medicine and 2 additional years in nephrology. The training can be done in one of the four public or private university centers (University of Chile, University Catolica of Chile, University Austral in Valdivia, and University of Concepcion). All of these programs have similar core curriculums and are submitted to periodic accreditation in accordance to national regulations. There are 13 training positions available per year, but only 55% of the capacity is occupied. Internist physicians from Latin America can apply for these training positions if they meet the requirements mentioned above.

## Renal Diseases in Chile

### Chronic Kidney Disease in Chile

The epidemiology of CKD in Chile has evolved in association with an improvement in the economic conditions, being dominated today by the effects of the epidemic explosion of the classic cardiovascular risk factors such as diabetes mellitus, arterial hypertension, obesity, sedentary lifestyle, and an extension of the life expectancy. In a survey involving people presumably healthy, the prevalence of CKD in Chile reaches 2.7% [2], but in patients users of primary care, it is 12%, being higher in females (14.5%) and adults over 60 years old (23%), mainly in CKD stage 3 [12].

The law, through the GES, assures the detection, prevention, and treatment of CKD, in any of its stages to all citizens of Chile [3, 13].

## Acute Kidney Injury and Acute Dialysis in Chile

Acute dialysis in Chile was started in a public hospital in 1957. At that time, septic abortion was a major public health problem, and women suffering septic shock used to die because of acute kidney injury (AKI) or hemolysis.

In the 1980s, acute dialysis expanded to many public and private hospitals, covering the epidemiological changes of AKI due to shock, ischemia, or nephrotoxins, which have been treated with intermittent techniques. The first continuous renal replacement therapy (CRRT) in Chile was performed in a teaching hospital in 1990. Acute dialysis has expanded remarkably in the country and is administered fundamentally by intensive care physicians, except in university hospitals, private clinics, and some public hospitals, where the nephrology teams take charge of the procedures.

A recent survey carried out by the Chilean Society of Nephrology in 29 healthcare centers showed that 31% of them had intermittent renal replacement therapy (RRT) only, while 21% had the chance to use CRRT as well. One out of every three centers reported the intensive care physician as responsible for the indication, and 27% of the centers reported the nephrologist to do so; in the rest both of the specialties were involved in the indication of acute RRT [14].

## Renal Replacement Therapy in Chile

The proportion of patients in HD in our country has grown exponentially in the last decade, increasing from 12.7 pmp in 1980 to 1260 pmp in 2018 (22,310 patients). PD is used by a minority (Fig. 12.1), with a low increase throughout the years, with an average annual rise of 8.5%, and 3.5% in 2018.

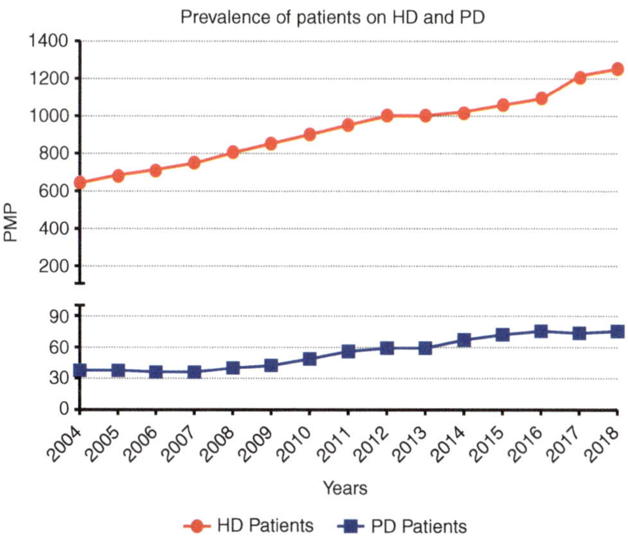


**Fig. 12.1** Prevalence of hemodialysis (HD) and peritoneal dialysis (PD) patients, from 2004 to 2018. Pmp, patients per million of population

The monthly cost of HD is 1024 USD and for PD 1297 USD. In both therapies the national health service (public) reimburses 100% of the cost of treatment and in the cases of private insurance (private), the reimbursement is 80% of the total cost of the therapy.

Convective therapies as chronic RRT has recently begun in the country in the public and private healthcare centers.

## Hemodialysis

HD techniques were established in our country at San Francisco de Borja Hospital, based in Santiago, in 1957. They were initially used for patients with AKI but gradually expanded to patients in CKD stage 5. The first formal dialysis center was created in 1965. Vascular access puncture and Shaldon's catheters in femoral veins were introduced in 1969, following the use of shunts.

The number of patients in chronic HD has increased exponentially. According to the national registry (2018), there are 22,310 patients on chronic HD with a rate of 1264 pmp, treated in 253 centers distributed in 101 cities throughout the country [15].

The most frequent causes of ESRD in dialysis patients are diabetes mellitus (38.9%), nephrosclerosis (10.3%), glomerulopathies (6.3%), and 13% of the cases with unknown causes. The annual mortality rate is 10.7%, and the most frequent causes of death are cardiac (33.4%), infections (16%), stroke (10.4%), and cancer (9.9%) [15].

The prevalence of HD patients with hepatitis B is of 0.11%, hepatitis C 0.64%, and HIV 0.44% (2018).

Vascular access is performed through native arteriovenous fistula in 70.8% of the patients, permanent catheter (24.1%), grafts (2.8%), and temporary dialysis catheters (2.3%) [15].

According to the 2018 national renal data registry report (22,310 patients on HD), 9.9% of these patients have been on HD for 5 years, 8.1% for 10 years, and 0.9% for more than 25 years of treatment [15].

Patients on treatment less than 9 h per week were 2.7%, whereas more than 12 h 15.7%; the ratio of nephrologists to dialysis patients in the country is 1:98.

In HD, each nurse assists a maximum of six adult patients simultaneously and in case of pediatric nurses a total of three patients [16]. These centers reuse blood lines and dialyzers, which is regulated by rules dictated by the Ministry of Health. It is established in Article 25 that the dialyzer residual capacity cannot be less that 80% of its initial volume, and the dialyzer can be reused 26 times, at maximum [16].

HD is financed by the explicit Health Guarantee System that includes treatment and drugs such as erythropoietin, calcitriol, iron, cinacalcet, and phosphate binders. These drugs are included as a package in their private health insurance and free in the case of public health insurance. The private health insurance system covers 80% of the treatment, whereas the patients pay 20% of the total cost. In the case of patients belonging to the public health insurance, the treatment is free.

## Peritoneal Dialysis

Acute PD is rarely performed in our country. Continuous ambulatory peritoneal dialysis (CAPD), automated peritoneal dialysis (APD), continuous cycling peritoneal dialysis (CCPD), and nocturnal intermittent peritoneal dialysis (NIPD) have been used since 1994 as an alternative treatment to HD, and the prevalence throughout the years of patients in PD is shown in Fig. 12.1. Nowadays, there are 1308 adult patients (75.3 pmp), 53% male, average age 49.8 years. Out of the 40 PD centers, 23 are private, 15 are in public hospitals, and 2 are in university clinics [17].

In 2018, most of the adult patients (93%) are in APD and only 3% in CAPD with a peritonitis rate of 0.13 episodes/patient/year and a gross mortality rate of 9.2% per year [17].

PD is financed by the explicit Health Guarantee System including treatment and drugs, such as erythropoietin, calcitriol, iron IV, cinacalcet, and phosphate binders. These drugs are included as a package in their private health insurance and free in the case of public health insurance. The private health insurance system covers 80% of the treatment, whereas the patients pay 20% of the total cost. In the case of patients belonging to the public health insurance, the treatment is free.

In PD, each nurse takes care of 30 adult patients, at maximum, simultaneously and in case of pediatric nurses a total of 15 patients [16].

## Renal Transplantation

The history of transplant in Chile began in 1968. In our days, there are 20 renal transplant centers (18 adult and 2 pediatrics) and 2 histocompatibility laboratories in network. A high proportion (72%) of renal transplants are financed by the state through FONASA (national health fund), 28% by private health institutions (ISAPRES), and 1% by the Armed Forces insurance, all of them under the benefit of GES.

The National Procurement and Transplant Coordination (CNPT) was created by the Ministry of Health in 2010, establishing a sanitary model to assure research and the procurement of encephalic death donors throughout the country. Its activity has been reflected in an increase of the percentage of multi-organ donors in relation to the renal only and promoting the use of expanded cadaver donor (ECD). Indeed, in 2018, 27% of the transplants were performed from ECD donors [18].

The transplant waiting list for cadaver donors is a legal responsibility of the public health institute, with a unique national waiting list for each organ, with priority criteria in accordance to the current legislation and in agreement with the transplant centers. The prioritization of kidney receptors is based mainly on histocompatibility criteria, the waiting time, and PRA percentage.

From 2013 onward, the law for organ allocation considering pediatric patients is a priority in cases of donors less than 45 years. In Chile, by the end of December 2018, a total of 8,646 renal transplants have been performed (32% living and 68% deceased donors) being 9% to pediatric patients. In the last 2 years, 45 pancreas-kidney, 45 liver-kidney, and 2 heart-kidney transplants have been performed [19].

Renal transplant rate in 2017 reached 21.7 pmp and, in 2018, 16.6 pmp (including living and deceased donors). At the end of 2018, the kidney transplant waiting list for cadaver donors included 2057 patients, which represents less than 10% of the patients on dialysis. The number of potential recipients on the waiting list with the highest immunological risk (patients with PRA $\geq$ 80%, re-transplant, or those <18 years) has increased, representing 23% of the waiting list.

The average waiting time for receiving a renal transplant in the last 2 years has been 28 months, but only 9 months for patients <18 years, showing the priority assigned to younger patients [18, 19].

The results show a graft survival of 92% and 85% for living and deceased donors, at 1 year, respectively. At 5 years, 86% for living donors and 75% for deceased and at 10 years 71% and 60% for living and deceased donors, respectively [18].

## Pediatric Nephrology in Chile

Pediatric nephrology was established in 1958, when nephrology units were created in different hospitals. The first specialists were trained under the mentoring of renowned adult nephrologists, including fellowship abroad. Postgraduate university programs started in 1990 [20].

Today, there are 63 active pediatric nephrologists (17 pmp < 15 years), and one-third of them are working in regions away from the capital, Santiago.

In 1980, PD was introduced as a RRT [21]. In 1994, CAPD was included into the services financed by the state [22]. There are ten centers with PD (eight in the public system and two in the private area) and four pediatric HD centers, all of them in the public health system.

According to the national registry, until 2015, the prevalence and incidence of stage 2 and 5 CKD were 50.7 and 10.4 pmp < 15 years, respectively. Eighty-three patients were on PD and 29 in HD. The age of initiation on PD has dropped from 7.8 years to 5.5 years old, being 25% of the children under 6 months.

The average age for initiating HD has been constantly maintained (9 years old). Fifty-three percent of the causes of ESRD are structural abnormalities as reflux, obstruction, and hypoplasia-dysplasia, 15% glomerular, and 10% hereditary.

In addition to the dialytic treatment, children with stages 4 and 5 have access to erythropoietin, calcitriol, iron IV, and growth hormones as they are included in the patients' health insurance.

Pediatric renal transplant started in the 1970s in the Catholic University Clinical Hospital, for patients from the public system, under the support of adult patient transplant teams [8]. Between 1989 and 2012, three public centers [9], corresponding to 95% of the transplanted pediatric patients, performed 462 transplants in children of 10.2 ± 4.2 years old (20% < 6 years of age), 68% of them with deceased donors. Seventy percent of them came from PD, and 9% were transplanted preemptively.

Immunosuppressant therapy considers induction in all patients (20% antithymocyte globulin and 80% receptor inhibitor IL2), tacrolimus, and mycophenolate mofetil, with steroid-free regimen. The results of this program are similar to those described in the international literature. Graft survival rates at 1, 3, and 5 years are 92%, 86%, and 83% for living donors and 87%, 80%, and 71% for deceased donors. The patient survival rate is 99%, 97%, and 96% for living donors and 97%, 97%, and 95% for deceased donors at 1, 3 and 5 years of follow-up, respectively [22].

National statistics show that we have reached up to 575 transplanted patients until 2017 [22].

For that reason, the organ allocation law considers now pediatric patients as a priority, in order to reduce their waiting times. Before prioritization between 2011 and 2012, there were 17 transplants in patients under 18 years of age, while after the prioritization in 2017 and 2018, a total of 35 patients were transplanted.

## Nephrology Practice in Chile

Chile has the unique feature of being a very long country with a few cities concentrating most of the population, social, and medical development. Most of the nephrologists live and work in those cities, leaving smaller cities with few specialists to cope with the nephrology needs.

There are not enough trained nephrologists for the country's demand. Many regions depend on "travelling doctors" going there once a month and working in collaboration with internal medicine or even general practitioner doctors. That is why an enthusiastic effort is being done to create telemedicine programs to solve the problem.

The health system in Chile includes public insurance (Fondo Nacional de Salud, FONASA) which covers most of the population and assures universal access to kidney replacement programs (dialysis and transplantation) all over the country. There is also private health insurance which is responsible for a wealthier population, almost one-third of Chilean inhabitants. The huge prevalence of kidney disease requires a great number of qualified professionals to take care of them.

Most medical doctors work both in public hospitals and private clinics. Some work at dialysis clinics, while some visit hospitalized patients at medical clinics but not being full-time employees of these clinics.

Critical care nephrology needs a lot of development outside of the university or public critical care units, especially because of trained personal shortage (nephrologists, nurses). This is a well-paid work but depends on the number of medical visits made.

According to the time committed to the in public hospitals and private clinics shifts, doctors can get roughly between USD 3000 and 6000 as employees, leaving room for more income from liberal exercise of the profession at their own offices or dialysis clinics as medical director or as attending nephrologists. These extra-hospital jobs can probably double their monthly income.

In case of the nurses of public hospitals and private hospitals, monthly salary is USD 1900–2300; this income can vary depending on the calling shifts.

There is plenty of room for trained nephrologists to work, especially in smaller cities. Foreign professionals, migrating to the country due to different causes, must be certified through passing proficiency tests to perform clinical work in Chile.

Currently, there are 17.4 nephrologists per million populations in Chile.

## Highlight of Nephrology in Chile

### Earthquakes and Nephrology in Chile

Earthquakes have been a constant threat in our country throughout all of its history. Located in the ring of fire of the Pacific, Chile is one of the most seismic regions of the planet. The fearsome and most destructive earthquake occurred in 1960 at 3:11 p.m. in the City of Valdivia situated in the south of Chile. It registered 9.6 on the Richter scale, and more than 2000 people died; this earthquake was followed by a tsunami that washed away the cities along the coast. More than two million people were affected by the disaster.

Saturday, February 27, 2010, local time 3:34 h (6:34 h GMT), the city of Maule was awakened by an earthquake 8.8 on the Richter scale with epicenter at 115 km northeast of the city of Concepcion, one of the largest cities of the country. It was the second most destructive earthquake registered in the country killing a total of 507 people. Most fatalities were attributed to drowning caused by the tsunami and suffocation after the collapse of adobe houses. Many victims were never found, presumably swept by the sea. Although crush injuries were rare, we were aware of two AKI patients requiring dialysis support, who recovered kidney function later. The low prevalence of crush injuries may be largely attributable to the high standards of seismic construction in Chile.

The major problems faced in this hazard were the interruption of communication that were reestablished 3 days post-earthquake only. The local agent for the RDRTF/ISN intervened as a central link between nephrologists and the Chilean Health Ministry. In the affected area, there were more than 2000 chronic dialysis patients, and several dialysis units were immediately out of use due to inadequate water availability.

After 1 week, all chronic patients regained access to dialysis, without increase in the expected mortality for the period. Local and international adequate training may be lifesaving if renal problems occur in earthquake circumstances [23].

Six patients on chronic HD were reported dead immediately post catastrophe, which represents 0.36% of total deaths. In three of these cases, the cause of death was clearly not associated to lack of dialysis treatment but to other medical causes.

The patients with APD, due to lack of electricity in their homes, began doing CAPD; some were transferred to close locations that were supplied with electricity. There were no reports of peritonitis or dead patients [24].

## Future Perspectives of Nephrology in Chile

The following aspects deserve to be included in the planning of strategies oriented to enhance the quality of the nephrology in our country:

1. An increase in the number of specialists: This includes the design of effective strategies to stimulate the interest of young physicians for the specialty.
2. A serious effort in nephroprevention:
   (a) A national network in teleconsultation has to be implemented in primary care facilities in coordination with nephrologists.
   (b) A hard multidisciplinary work needs to be established in order to reduce the epidemic expansion of cardiovascular risk factors in our population and their effects in renal health.
3. Renal replacement therapy (RRT):
   (a) Hemodialysis (HD): An increase in the water quality used in hemodialysis in public and private centers, in order to reach an ultrapure water standard.
   (b) Peritoneal dialysis (PD): The introduction of new dialysis solutions and the use of telemedicine to make an easier and better-assisted therapy.
   (c) Kidney transplant: To improve the strategies to increase the donation of deceased donors, focusing on education and enhancing the confidence in the public transplant network. To start soon with a crossed donation program.
4. Academics, teaching, and research:
   (a) A big effort has to be done to keep and recruit new academic nephrologist into the university teams in order to maintain and increase the capability of human resources training.
   (b) National and private funds need to be raised to improve the research capacities in areas of nephrological clinical impact.

## Conclusive Remarks

Nephrology in Chile has developed rapidly in all its aspects: academics and basic and clinical research with support from universities and scientific societies.

RRT is within reach for all its inhabitants, and the prevention of ESRD progression and renal replacement therapies, HD, PD, and transplantation are protected by law, which guarantees universal access in the private and public health service.

Chile has a high rate of patients undergoing HD treatment (1260 pmp) in 204 HD centers and 49 hospitals that have a HD center.

The increase in the number of renal transplants is limited due to the low number of kidney donations. The number of transplants has not increased despite having the alleged presumed donation policy in people over 18 years of age and multiple advertising campaigns aimed at the general population.

There are a small number of nephrologists to cover the increasing demand and a low interest among young doctors to embrace the specialty.

## References

1. OPS/OMS Chile – New health report of America, 2017. Available from: https://www.paho.org/chi/index.php?option=com_content&view=article&id=956:n.
2. National health survey 2009–2010. MINSAL. Available from: https://www.minsal.cl/portal/url/item/bcb03d7bc28b64dfe040010165012d23.pdf.

3. Explicit Health Guarantees System (GES) health orientation. Available from: http://www.supersalud.gob.cl/difusion/665/w3-article-564.html.
4. Norero C. Historical review of infant nephrology in Chile. Rev Chil Pediatr. 1998;69:236–9.
5. Katz E. Treatment of the terminal chronic kidney failure. Rev Med Chil. 1970;98(3):167–8.
6. Katz E, Acchiardo S, Lomnitz E. Peritoneal dialysis. Rev Med Chil. 1965;93:22–6.
7. Allende J, Diaz H, Kappes J, Lazcano F, Morgado F, Murray G, Oberhauser E, Piwonka G, Roman J, Soto R, Sunkell W, Vukusich A. Renal homologous transplantation. Rev Med Chil. 1967;95:467–4.
8. Orozco R, Vargas R, Rossenblitt M, Hernandez LA, Rubinstein P, Plaza de los Reyes M. Kidney transplant "from life donors" in 3 patients with chronic terminal renal failure. Rev Med Chil. 1969;97:58–68.
9. Buckel E, Morales J, Aguilo J, Rosenfeld R, Pefaur J, Zavala C. Simultaneous pancreas-kidney transplantation. First cases in Chile. Rev Med Chile. 1996;124:83–8.
10. Public law: Establishes rules on transplantation and organ donation. Pub. L. No 19451, April 10, 1996. Available from: https://www.leychile.cl/Navegar?idNorma=30818.
11. Public law: Modifies Law No 19451, in order to determine who can be considered organ donors and how they can express their will. Pub- L. 20413, January 15, 2010. Available from: https://www.leychile.cl/Navegar?idNorma=1010132.
12. Zúñiga C, Múller H, Flores M. Prevalence of chronic kidney disease in subjects consulting in urban primary care clinics. Rev Med Chile. 2011;139:1176–84.
13. Bossert TJ, Leisewitz T. Innovation and change in the chilean health system. N Engl J Med. 2016;374:1–5.
14. Renal replacement therapy in critical ill patients. Autumn course 2017. Available from: https://www.nefro.cl/v2/post.php?id=596.
15. Poblete H XXIV Chilean hemodialysis registry 2018. Chilean Society of Nephrology. Available from: https://www.nefro.cl/v2/biblio/registro/24.pdf.
16. Public law: Regulations on dialysis benefits and the establishments that grant it. Pub. L. No 1107626. Decree No 45. Ministry of Health, September 6, 2017. Available from: https://www.leychile.cl/Navegar?idNorma=1107626&idVersion=2017-09-06.
17. Ortiz A, Peritoneal Dialysis registry 2018. Chilean Society of Nephrology. Available from: https://www.nefro.cl/v2/biblio/registro/24.pdf.
18. Organ and transplant donor data, January – December 2017. Available from: https://www.minsal.cl/wp-content/uploads/2018/01/Datos-P%C3%A1gina-Enero-Diciembre-2017.pdf.
19. Rojas JL. Chilean donation and transplant registration. Santiago, Chile, November 7, 2018.
20. Norero C, Puga F. Pediatric nephrology. In: Albo M, editor. Historia de la Sociedad Chilena de Nefrología. Santiago: Chilean Society of Nephrology; 2004. p. 57–68.
21. Saieh C, Baeza J, Cordero J. Intermittent peritoneal dialysis in pediatrics. Rev Chil Pediatr. 1986;57(2):141–5.
22. Delucchi A, Contreras A, Bidegain A, Quiero X, Barrera P, Pinto V, Lillo A, Martínez A, Villegas R. Pediatric chronic peritoneal dialysis in Chile: Multicentric study. Rev Chil Pediatr. 2002;73:116–26.
23. Vanholder R, Borniche D, Claus S, Correa-Rotter R, Crestani R, Ferir MC, Gibney N, Hurtado A, Luyckx VA, Portilla D, Rodriguez S, Sever MS, Vanmassenhove J, Wainstein R. When the earth trembles in the Americas: the experience of Haiti and Chile 2010. Nephron Clin Pract. 2011;117:184–97.
24. Zuñiga C. Hemodialysis at earthquake time: A report from BioBio region. Chile. Rev Med Clin Condes. 2010;21(4):638–43.

# Nephrology in Cuba

# 13

Raúl Bohorques, Jorge Alfonzo, Miguel Almaguer, Yanet Alvarez, José Florín, Guillermo Guerra, Christian Leyva, Charles Magrans, Jorge Perez-Oliva, and Roberto Rivas

| | |
|---|---|
| Area | 109,884 km$^2$ |
| Population[1] | 11,288,752 (2017) |
| Capital | Havana |
| Three most populated cities: | 1. Havana<br>2. Santiago de Cuba<br>3. Holguin |
| Official language | Spanish |
| Gross domestic product (GDP)[2] | 96.851 billion USD (2017) |
| GDP per capita[2] | 8541.2 USD (2017) |
| Human Development Index (HDI) | 0.777 |
| Official currency | Cuban peso |
| Total number of nephrologists | 433 |
| National society of nephrology | *Sociedad Cubana de Nefrología*<br>www.sld.cu |
| Incidence of end-stage renal disease | 2018 – 107.3 pmp |
| Prevalence of end-stage renal disease (on dialysis) | 2018 – 299.4 pmp |
| Total number of patients on dialysis (all modalities) | 2017 – 3289<br>2018 – 3352 |
| Number of patients on hemodialysis | 2017 – 3224<br>2018 – 3281 |
| Number of patients on peritoneal dialysis | 2017 – 65<br>2018 – 71 |
| Number of renal transplantations per year | 2017 – 203<br>2018 – 178 |

1. Oficina Nacional de Estadística e Información (ONEI). República de Cuba. Anuario Estadístico de Cuba 2017. Edición 2018. Disponible en: www.one.cu/aec2017.htm
2. The World Bank, https://data.worldbank.org/country/cuba

R. Bohorques (✉) · J. Alfonzo · M. Almaguer · Y. Alvarez
G. Guerra C. Leyva · C. Magrans · J. Perez-Oliva · R. Rivas
Instituto de Nefrología, La Habana, Cuba
e-mail: bohorq@infomed.sld.cu; docimef@infomed.sld.cu; nefroprev@infomed.sld.cu; alvarezyanet@infomed.sld.cu; nefrodir@infomed.sld.cu; cleyva@infomed.sld.cu; cmagrans@infomed.sld.cu; scnefro@infomed.sld.cu; rrivas@infomed.sld.cu

J. Florín
Hospital Pediátrico de Centro Habana, La Habana, Cuba
e-mail: florin@infomed.sld.cu

## Introduction

The Republic of Cuba is an archipelago made up of more than 1600 islands, islets, and cays; the capital Havana is located on the island of Cuba, the largest of the archipelago. The surface area of the Cuban archipelago is 109,884.01 km$^2$. The country has a population of 11,288,752 (2017); 20.1% are 60 years or older, and that number is expected to increase to 30.1% by 2030. Life expectancy at birth is, on average, 78.4 years, 76.5 years for men and 80.45 years for women [1].

Cuba is one of the countries with the oldest population in Latin America. The educational level is high, with a literacy rate of 99.7% [2]. Cuba has a high Human Development Index of 0.777 that ranks 73rd out of 188 countries in the world [3]. In respect to the economy, Cuba ranks as an upper middle-income country [4].

In Cuba, there is a unique state-run health system, with universal coverage and access (no exclusions), free of charge for the entire population [5]. The Cuban health system rests on the three key principles of the current strategy for universal health access and coverage as set forth by Pan American Health Organization/World Health Organization (PAHO/WHO): health as a human right, equity, and solidarity [6].

The cornerstone of the national health system (NHS) is primary health care (PHC). Since 1984, the family medicine model has been implemented in the community. Its objective is to contribute to the improvement of the population's health through integrated interventions for individuals, families, communities, and the environment [7]. The NHS has 92,084 physicians (122 inhabitants per physician). The PHC has 450 polyclinics (health-care areas), 13,131 family doctors in community clinics, and 10,869 basic health-care teams. Each team includes an internist, a pediatrician, and an obstetrician-gynecologist, among other specialists, who provide care for 100% of the population [8].

The number of specialized nephrologists amounts to 433 (57.3% of whom are women), a ratio of 38.35 per million population (pmp). A total of 229 general practitioners (GPs)



J. A. Moura-Neto et al. (eds.), *Nephrology Worldwide*, https://doi.org/10.1007/978-3-030-56890-0_13

are enrolled in the 3-year specialty, provided in the 11 provincial medical universities categorized for postgraduate programs [9]. Human resource needs are established by the provincial health divisions, according to the number of centers, incidence of kidney disease, and the age of the practicing nephrologists.

Specialists in nephrology work at the hospital level and also see patients in the polyclinics located in the 168 municipalities. They carry out actions that range from primary prevention, care, consultations, referral to other specialists, rehabilitation through dialysis, and transplantation. In addition, they are involved in academic and research work according to the needs identified at institutional, provincial, or field levels. For this purpose, the analysis of health situations at each level is used as an essential tool, with a comprehensive, interdisciplinary nature, including community participation and inter-sectoral collaboration.

Cuba, a country that has been subject to a financial and economic embargo for approximately 60 years, must incur extremely high expenses every year to respond to the incidence and prevalence of patients with end-stage renal disease (ESRD). Although they are a minority of the population, these patients require medicines, consumables, and technologies for peritoneal dialysis (PD), hemodialysis (HD), and kidney transplantation [10]; all of them are internationally recognized as sources of inequities [11] in a country characterized by an increase in noncommunicable chronic diseases and aging population.

## Brief History of Nephrology in Cuba

Nephrology was recognized as a specialty in Cuba with the creation of the Institute of Nephrology in December 1966. In the past, teaching, medical care, and research activities of this specialty were carried out by urology fellows/residents and pediatricians, the latter with outstanding activity since the decade of the 1950s [12].

In the capital, two pediatric centers stood out for the care of kidney diseases. In 1948, the first kidney biopsies were performed by puncture; a preliminary report was presented at the Congress of Pathology in La Plata, Argentina, in 1950. The report described the technique used in eight patients, and this work was published in the bulletin of the League Against Cancer later in the same year. Kidneys were localized through a pyelogram, and a special type of punch trocar was used which was called a microtome [13].

In the late 1950s and early 1960s, HD was sporadically performed on patients with acute kidney injury (AKI) and exogenous intoxications. With the establishment of the Institute of Nephrology by Professor Abelardo Buch López, whose name this institution bears today, a small program of intermittent dialysis (HD and PD) for patients with ESRD began, which led to the first successful kidney transplant from a cadaveric donor in February 1970. Once the specialty was recognized, the training of nephrologists began and the first graduation occurred in 1970.

The 1970s were marked by the expansion of nephrology care to the center and east of the country, which paved the way for the national coverage of the specialty: the performance of kidney transplants from cadaveric donors and living donors (first-degree relatives), kidney transplants in children [14], as well as the progressive development of care, teaching, and research, as well as the creation of related research laboratories (physiopathology, immunology, and nuclear medicine).

The Cuban Society of Nephrology was constituted in 1974; it is a nongovernmental, civil, scientific organization, linked to similar societies. Since its creation, it has developed ten national congresses with international participation, as well as numerous courses, workshops, and training for both national and foreign nephrologists. The Latin American Society of Nephrology and Hypertension (SLANH) named Professor Abelardo Buch López, founder of the specialty in Cuba, as its honorary president.

In the 1980s, the nephrology national coverage was completed with the establishment of at least one nephrology center with the possibility of providing dialysis treatment in each province. The national coordination center for dialysis and kidney transplantation was created with headquarters in the Institute of Nephrology. Since then, its main mission has been to advise and receive information from all the nephrology centers in the country. This has made it possible to keep a record of all patients treated with RRT.

At the beginning of this century, the Cuban government decided to bring dialysis facilities closer to patients' homes. Today, we have 56 nephrology centers with dialysis possibilities throughout the country spread over 15 provinces and a special municipality, for a population of just over 11 million inhabitants.

## Kidney Diseases in Cuba

Kidney diseases that require specialized care do not differ from that of most countries: hypertension, diabetes mellitus, polycystic kidney disease, glomerular diseases, uropathies, and others. Despite being geographically located in the Caribbean and close to Central America, there are no reports on chronic kidney disease of unknown cause (CKDu), also called Mesoamerican nephropathy.

In Cuba (2014) the main ESRD causes of the incident RRT patients were hypertension (37.1%), diabetes mellitus (32.1%), polycystic kidney (7.3%), and glomerular diseases (5.6%) [15].

A research study comprising 1503 renal biopsies performed in adult patients between 1988 and 2007 at the Institute of Nephrology reported the main histopathological patterns of primary glomerular diseases: focal segmental glomeruloesclerosis (20.6%), mesangioproliferative glomerulonephritis (16.8%), minimal change disease (10.9%), infectious disease-associated glomerulonephritis (6.9%), and membranous glomerulonephritis (5.0%), as well as the main secondary glomerular diseases: lupus nephritis (13.6%), benign nephroangiosclerosis (2.6%), and systemic vasculitis (1.3%) [16].

The epidemiological Cuban study ISYS (Isle of Youth, 2004–2006) reported a chronic kidney disease (CKD) prevalence of 9.63% (stage 1, 3.02%; stage 2, 3.43%; stage 3a, 2.26%; stage 3b, 0.71%; stage 4, 0.15%; and stage 5, 0.03%) in an adult population of 55,646 people [17]. The third National Risk Factors Survey reported a prevalence of CKD (glomerular filtration rate <60 ml/min/1.73 m$^2$) of 5.4% [18].

In Cuba, the mortality rate adjusted for glomerular and kidney diseases (N00-N19, N25-N27) has had a slight increasing trend up to 4.4 per 100,000 inhabitants, and it ranks 13th in the country's overall mortality in 2017 [8]. It is lower than the global adjusted mortality rate of 18.2 per 100,000 inhabitants reported by the Global Burden of Disease Study in 2016 [19]. The third National Risk Factor Survey also measured the risk of having a glomerular filtration rate of <60 ml/min/1.73 m$^2$, given the presence of the following risk factors: obesity 13.6%, diabetes mellitus 13.2%, hypercholesterolemia 10.2%, arterial hypertension 9.2%, smoking 5.9%, and alcohol consumption 3.5% [18].

The intervention strategy for the prevention of CKD has been based on the following pillars:

(a) Integration with the noncommunicable diseases program
(b) Primary health care
(c) Medical care services for CKD patients brought closer to the communities
(d) Interdisciplinary and inter-sectorial interventions
(e) Surveillance
(f) Human resource development and research

The Program for CKD Prevention (1996) is integrated into the noncommunicable diseases program, under the control of the Ministry of Public Health, which has facilitated the implementation and control of interventions [20].

Primary health care has favored the implementation of integrated preventive actions for CKD and noncommunicable diseases. The continuous assessment, risk evaluation, and classification of the population by family physicians are noteworthy. This is an organized, continuous, and dynamic process that permits planned and programmed evaluation of intervention on the health status of individuals and families, under the leadership and coordination of the basic health team.

People are screened and classified into four groups:

- Group I – apparently healthy people
- Group II – people at risk
- Group III – sick people, diagnosed with communicable or noncommunicable diseases
- Group IV – people with disabilities or handicaps

Screening records make it possible to assess the population's health status [7].

Bringing health-care services close to where patients live has been a fundamental principle in the intervention strategy. In addition to care provided by family doctors and basic health teams, nephrologists consult in certain areas of the country. Dialysis facilities have also followed such strategy through a regionalization plan.

The CKD prevention program emphasizes the active participation of the organized community for the identification of risk groups, early diagnosis through the study of renal injury markers, specific treatment of underlying kidney disease, preventing or attempting to delay disease progression and complications, patient rehabilitation, and control of the environment, for which an interdisciplinary and inter-sectorial approach is required.

CKD surveillance is integrated into the systems of the Ministry of Public Health. Passive surveillance is carried out through the registration of deaths (mortality) [8], registration of screened patients by family doctors, and registration of dialysis and kidney transplantation. Active surveillance is carried out through national risk factor surveys and population-based preventive actions, carried out periodically in 1990, 2001, and 2010 [18]. The human resource development plan and research to be carried out are scheduled according to the needs.

The CKD risk factor prevention program has made some progress including an improvement in social determinants, higher educational level in the population, control of environmental pollution with a significant reduction in the use of agrochemicals in agriculture, reduction of low birth weight to 5.1%, smoking reduction to 23.7%, and reduction of overweight to 28.9%, although obesity increased to 14.8%. In primary health care, there has been an increase in the diagnosis of diabetics (699,282), with effective glycemic control (<7 mmol/L) in 67% of them; an increase in diagnosed hypertension (2,531,803), with effective blood pressure control (<140/90 mm/Hg) in 50% of them; and more than 50% using antihypertensive agents with renal protective effect (inhibitors of angiotensin-converting enzyme). There is better control of infectious diseases; 14 infectious diseases have been eliminated, including malaria, and there is a vaccination program against 18 infectious diseases, with coverage for 100% of the population [8, 18].

In primary health care, family doctors have increased the diagnosis of CKD, but it is still not enough based on the number of expected patients.

## Renal Replacement Therapy in Cuba

Our country offers integrated kidney care to patients suffering from advanced CKD who require RRT; however, in the area of dialysis, 97% of patients are on standard HD therapy with polysulfone membranes, the majority of them low flux dialyzers. Most water treatment systems are of reverse osmosis, a few with double pass reverse osmosis systems and heat sterilization. In addition, all provinces in the country have mobile water treatment systems. Convective therapies are only practiced in a small number of patients and are being introduced in two nephrology centers in the capital.

The national pharma and biotechnology industries ensure the sustainability of HD with the production of concentrate for the HD instruments, whereas home-based PD is done by importing the consumables from leading PD companies. Nationally produced recombinant human erythropoietin is provided free of charge to all patients who require it [21].

The RRT methods are kidney transplant, HD, and PD; these three methods are not antagonistic, but rather complementary to each other; a patient can switch from one to another according to clinical, psychological, or social needs, thus extending their life expectancy [22]. The possibility of providing these three therapeutic modalities is known in the world as integrated kidney care.

CKD is a complex phenomenon, a chronic non-transmissible disease, considered to be a modern epidemic in the world, due to the increase in the number of cases each year, partly due to the increase in the life expectancy of the population, allowing more time to the development and/or to the increase in the prevalence of other pathologies such as hypertension, diabetes mellitus, and obesity, which may lead to the development and/or progression of CKD. Its magnitude is a serious medical problem overwhelming the budgets of health-care services in all countries of the world, although with individual differences for each type of RRT; all separately and as a whole are costly techniques [23].

## Peritoneal Dialysis

In our country, both HD and PD have been used since the 1960s. However, for circumstantial reasons, HD has had an adequate technological development, whereas PD began as a technique for hospital intermittent PD, performed mainly by nurses, using dialysis solutions packaged in nationally produced glass flasks. The medical team involved in PD, practically from the beginning, was in charge of recording and publishing their work experiences [24–28].

Continuous ambulatory peritoneal dialysis (CAPD) and automated peritoneal dialysis (APD), was introduced in late 2007 and 2008, respectively, in both adult and pediatric patients, by the Institute of Nephrology, which is the governing center of the specialty in the country for the adults, and months later by the pediatric hospital in Havana that is the national pediatric reference center for kidney diseases.

Since it is a technique-based self-care, home-based PD has, among others, the advantage of being able to treat patients remotely, so from the Institute of Nephrology in the capital, patients are treated for all of the western provinces of the country; two other units are responsible for the care of the central provinces and another in the eastern area, using nephrology centers that are engaged in the performance of kidney transplantation and offer regional care.

After five decades using virtually the same open PD system, often three times a week, for 10 or 12 h each time, HD was, at the same time, incorporating global technological advances that allowed standard HD to be performed. Then it became difficult for nephrologists and health authorities to promote greater numbers of patients treated with PD. It was said that someone in Europe made a remark during an international congress of nephrology that "peritoneal dialysis is a second-class procedure for third-class patients, performed by fourth-class physicians" [12].

Once home-based PD was introduced in a small group of patients, it took some time to obtain results that supported the unavoidable need for changes in the distribution of patients treated with dialysis as an RRT method [29–34]. Since 2014, the Pan American Health Organization (OPAS) and the Latin American Society of Nephrology and Hypertension (SLANH) made a call to increase the rate of RRT in the countries of the region and to reach a 20% utilization of home-based PD.

At the beginning of 2017, taking into account the results obtained up to that time, the public health authorities considered increasing the number of patients treated with home-based PD and decided:

- All pediatric patients who require this procedure may have access to it, with coverage for 100% of these patients.
- To reach an annual increase of 5% of the total number of patients treated with dialysis, until reaching a proportion of 10% of patients on home-based PD and 90% on HD in the next few years, a figure equivalent to the world average at that time. This would slightly represent more than

300 patients treated with home-based PD, as well as gradually phasing out inhospital intermittent PD.
- Home-based PD should provide regional care; this mission will initially be fulfilled by hospitals that currently have kidney transplant services.
- The Institute of Nephrology is responsible for the training of nephrology specialists and nursing staff for the care and follow-up of such patients, as well as maintaining technical and methodological advisory.

Coincidentally, the Central American Association of Nephrology and Hypertension convened a meeting of experts in PD a few months later. This conference was held in the Dominican Republic, with the purpose of evaluating the situation of this therapy in each country and stimulating its use, as it is an efficient method and with a very good cost-effectiveness ratio. After 2 days of work, a consensus document was issued, known as La Romana Declaration: "Peritoneal Dialysis, an Alternative to the Epidemic of Kidney Disease."

Among other aspects, it was recommended to promote the use of home-based PD as an excellent option for RRT, to encourage research on PD in the region, and to stimulate the development and performance of health economics studies, both nationally and among the different countries of the region, as well as to discard programs of intermittent PD, a technique associated with high morbidity/mortality that demotivates and discourages patients from receiving dialysis treatment and is no longer recommended with current clinical and scientific evidence. A summary of that consensus meeting was later published [23].

Cuba has been represented in all Latin American scientific events (except the first one) and in the PD world congresses since 2010, with the presentation of scientific papers. Nephrologists and nurses in charge of home-based PD have received training inside and outside the country. We organize and offer national and international courses accredited by the University of Medical Sciences of Havana.

## Hemodialysis

In 1957, the country's first hemodialysis center for AKI and toxic coma was created [33]. Starting in 1966, with the recognition of the specialty and the creation of the Institute of Nephrology, ESRD care began in an organized manner with IPD and chronic HD. From that moment on, the creation of new nephrology centers with dialysis programs began slowly and progressively, for adult ESRD patients, in hospitals in all provinces and since 1980 in children [34].

International developments in the treatment of CKD in our country showed the magnitude of the problem. In all these years, HD development has been considered in the context of a more comprehensive health policy, which included prevention integrated with other noncommunicable diseases [35–39].

A nephrology center in the eastern part of the country developed a prototype of artificial kidney with proportional pump and single-pass dialysate, which was used in that unit and other centers in that region [40]. This project was later discarded, and the technology used has always been imported.

In 1986, the country's first HD satellite unit was created, which also provided psychological, nutritional, and physical activity support to patients, interacting closely with caregivers [41].

The national medical-pharmaceutical industry produced PD solutions (in glass flasks) and acetate-based HD concentrates, which allowed an initial sustainability for both of them, with emphasis on HD that always predominated vs. proceeding with inhospital IPD.

The history of HD in Cuba is part of the achievements of the national health system and its uninterrupted improvement, in spite of the economic complexities of a poor country without access to international financing sources due to the economic and financial embargo of the United States [42].

The replacement of HD acetate-based concentrate with nationally produced bicarbonate-based one was achieved in 2002. The turning point in the HD development occurred in January 2003, marking the beginning of a stage of accelerated promotion of the specialty and development of its human resources and strategic projection [43]. Fifteen new nephrology centers were inaugurated and another 10 already in operation that went from having 4 or 8 HD stations to up to 18 or 22. The use of cellulose membranes was replaced and the reuse of needles and lines discarded.

But, taking into account the Ministry of Public Health's policy regarding efficient and rational use of resources, reuse of dialyzer in the same patient is permitted. The dialyzer can be reused while the residual volume is higher than 80%. The average dialyzer reuse has been 10–12 times, but reuse is not allowed more than 15 times.

The national dialysis registry allows us to precisely know the number of patients and establish, based on this information, the coverage of the needs of human, logistical, and financial resources for adequate care of these patients.

At present, after 15 years of priority care, despite all economic and financial problems, HD treatment is performed in

**Table 13.1** January 2019 report

| Indicators | 2007 | 2010 | 2011 | 2015 | 2016 | 2017 | 2018 |
|---|---|---|---|---|---|---|---|
| Nephrology-HD centers in operation | 47 | 48 | 49 | 51 | 51 | 55 | 56 |
| Total number of patients on dialysis | 2353 | 2560 | 2724 | 3148 | 3189 | 3289 | 3352 |
| ESRD prevalence (pmp) | 214 | 228.6 | 243.2 | 281.1 | 284.7 | 292 | 299.4 |
| ESRD incidence (pmp) | 100 | 96.1 | 97.8 | 110 | 95 | 97.6 | 107.3 |
| HD prevalence of patients with functional native arteriovenous fistula (%) | 72.5 | 74.1 | 72 | 72 | 73.8 | 83 | 74 |
| HD gross mortality (%) | 28.3 | 27.9 | 23.8 | 26.4 | 23.2 | 24.6 | 25.4 |

Program coordinating center. Kidney disease, dialysis, and transplantation. National Institute of Nephrology

56 nephrology centers, all of them state-owned. More than 3300 prevalent patients are being treated, using nationally produced concentrated solutions for dialysis. Table 13.1 shows the evolution and the current RRT scenario in Cuba. We use imported high-tech equipment such as HD machines and water treatment systems (reverse osmosis); hemodiafiltration (convective therapies) is in the introduction stage. There is a decrease of hepatitis B, with marked stability in recent years, as we use nationally produced vaccines. Moreover, there is a specialty development program which includes the creation of new nephrology centers until 2025.

## Renal Transplantation

The first successful kidney transplant in Cuba was performed in the early 1970s at the Institute of Nephrology. In the following years, this technology extended to the rest of the island, and Cuba currently has nine centers accredited to perform kidney transplantation of cadaveric and living donors [44].

The transplant program covers the entire population as equitably as possible; there are five organizational zones led by a regional coordinator who reports to the National Transplant Organization (NTO). In addition, the major hospitals have local coordinators who are responsible for identifying potential donors and interacting with the family in order to achieve organ and tissue donation. In Cuba, presumptive consent does not apply, i.e., families must approve donations. For now, donors are only used in the case of encephalic death; however, the first steps are being taken to include donors in controlled cardiac arrest. There is a unique selection program that is updated monthly and that takes into account criteria such as ABO and human leukocyte antigen (HLA) compatibility, waiting time in RRT, age, and body weight. Likewise, patients under 19 years of age and patients with vascular capital depletion for HD are prioritized.

Traditionally, only first-degree relatives were accepted as living donors; however, at the end of 2015, in order to stimulate the performance of this type of transplants and in accordance with international practices, the donor selection criteria were broadened to include other types of relatives and patients emotionally related as children or spouses, which was approved in a resolution by the Ministry of Public Health and published in the Official Gazette [45].

During the cadaveric donor transplant operation, HLA typing and flow cytometry crossmatch are performed in most areas of the island; however, lymphocytotoxicity techniques are still applied in the eastern region, since the transplant system is not isolated from the economic impact of the embargo applied by the US government against the Cuban people. The preservation of the organs is done through simple hypothermia with standard preservation liquid. The organs are kept in the Acute Tubular Necrosis (NTA) from where they are distributed to the centers that will perform the grafts. Each transplant center is committed to serving a region that encompasses several provinces or municipalities, with their corresponding HD or PD centers. Such regions are also encouraged to create their pre-dialysis transplant consultations so that patients with advanced kidney disease, who are not yet receiving HD or PD, may choose transplantation as a replacement for kidney function.

Transplant surgical teams include anesthesiologists, surgeons, urologists, and nurses. The selection of patients is made through an automated program with a single database where all patients eligible for transplantation are registered. Nephrologists are in charge of checking patients, selecting the immunosuppression according to the individual immunological risk, and performing postoperative care. Most of the centers apply induction of immunosuppression with biological drugs, especially in cases of higher immune risk. The usual maintenance treatment is cyclosporine A or tacrolimus associated with mycophenolate mofetil or azathioprine and low doses of steroids [46]. Due to financial limitations, there are still very few patients with treatments based on other drugs such as everolimus or sirolimus, and there is no experience in Cuba with the application of belatacept. As with the rest of medical care, kidney transplantation, associated medical care, and the main immunosuppressive drugs, both induction and maintenance, are free for patients.

Clinical follow-up of transplanted patients is usually done in the same transplant center. In fact, nephrologists coordinate the rest of the specialized care required by transplanted patients. The main causes that affect the long-term survival of the graft are cardiovascular disease and chronic rejection and to a lesser extent infections and cancer. The first-year graft survival rate of the first renal transplant was 80.4% (2013) [15].

The staff involved in kidney transplantation is trained in Cuba at the medical university and in different specialized centers, at no cost. Furthermore, there is a rich regional and global exchange through the Transplant Society of Latin America and the Caribbean (STALYC) and centers in Florida and Spain that support the training of specialists. Cuba is usually represented at regional and global congresses on kidney transplantation.

The main challenges facing the Cuban transplant system and nephrology are to increase the number of patients fit for transplant among those undergoing HD and PD, reduce organ waste during operations, and increase graft survival per year, especially by reducing surgical complications. The main achievement is the equitable and free care to all the population of patients requiring kidney transplant on the island.

## Acute Kidney Injury and Critical Care Nephrology

Although the first cases of AKI were described at the beginning of the last century, this disease was "rediscovered" during the last world war in the form of crush syndrome. The concept of AKI as a syndrome was clearly and permanently established in the world medical literature in 1942, when Eric Bywaters and JH Dible studied poly-traumatized patients after the bombings of London in World War II [47]. This syndrome is usually presented as a serious and frequent complication in the clinical evolution of many diverse medical situations: the increase in complex and aggressive surgery, scientific-technical progress applied to very critical patients that allow them to prolong their life long enough to develop AKI, increased use of nephrotoxic substances, population aging, increased frequency and severity of accidents, traumas, catastrophes and natural disasters, as well as regional war conflicts have contributed decisively to the high prevalence of this condition, which offers an interesting paradox. By definition, it is potentially reversible and yet leads to death in more than half of the cases [46]. This persistently high mortality despite recent progress in pathophysiological knowledge, in diagnostic methods, and in the technological development of effective uremia treatments remains a major challenge for current medicine [48–50]. The modern management of AKI should be oriented in a multidisciplinary manner, requiring maximum understanding, intelligence, and effort from qualified personnel [51, 52].

In Cuba, in the prerevolutionary stage, there was no comprehensive health system that would allow us to accurately define the real behavior of the disease we are dealing with in the statistical order, which makes it practically impossible for us to compare current results with previous studies. At the beginning of the 1960s, the first research studies began under the leadership of Professor Abelardo Buch López, showing that the most frequent causes of AKI were incompatible blood transfusion, complicated abortion, and hemodynamic disorders (shock), which determined that health actions were adopted in order to establish preventive and therapeutic measures.

In 1976, the Institute of Nephrology created a department with the function of a nephro-urological intensive care unit (ICU) that still maintains this profile; it is the only one with this characteristic in our country and one of the few in the world, specialized in both assistance, teaching, and research in multidisciplinary care of critical uremic patients. In the rest of the country, these patients are cared for with intensive multipurpose therapies and nephrological support. At present, Cuba has a national health system with an extensive network of polyvalent ICUs with more than 2200 beds, extended throughout the country, equipped with significant human and technological resources, providing specialized care to the entire population.

The number of people in the world who reach or exceed the seventh decade of life has increased, from just over 400 million in 1950 up to 700 million today, with a forecast of over 1 billion in 2025; thus, the total population growth will be characterized in the near future by a growing proportion of elderly people. This process, already in motion, is accompanied by a clear decrease in the birth rate and an ostensible increase in life expectancy, in such a way that demographic trends qualify population aging as a transcendental change in the distribution of population in today's world, turning it into a global phenomenon.

Our country, as a participant in the current world demographic development, is among the four most aged countries in Latin America and the Caribbean. In 1988, elderly Cubans represented 11.7% of the population; today they have increased up to 14%, and according to forecasts, the elderly in 2025 will reach 20.1% of the total population [53]. Population aging does not constitute a health problem; it is rather an achievement of humanity due to technical scientific developments. However, with aging, limitations begin to proliferate as well as a progressive risk of disease and death.

AKI in elderly people, within the framework of 60 years of age according to the classification of the WHO, has a much higher prevalence than in the general population, being considered by some to be a typically geriatric pathology. Volume depletion, hemodynamic alterations, nephrotoxic drugs, and urological obstructions are the main factors responsible for the onset of this syndrome. More and more elderly patients are being admitted to ICUs, leading to a significant increase in the frequency of AKI in such patients, leading to prolonged hospitalization and high mortality, possibly also conditioned by the severity of the same due to underlying diseases [54–57].

At the Congress of Acute Kidney Injury held in the Dominican Republic in April 2016, we presented our 16-year work experience (1999–2015): 223 patients 60 years older or more, in which we concluded that there was a predominance of male patients with parenchymal causes. A high number of patients required dialysis treatment, post-renal or obstructive causes accounting for almost half of the cases. If we take into account the total number of cases treated in that period, regardless of age, 1003 patients were treated in which there was a predominance of men over 50 years of age and parenchymal causes, two thirds of all patients required dialysis treatment, and HD/ultrafiltration was used in most of these cases [57].

## Nephrology Practice in Cuba

The process to become a specialist in nephrology in Cuba is done through the residence in nephrology. First of all, the candidate must have a medical degree. Then, one of these criteria must be met: specialization in internal medicine or in general integral medicine (family medicine) or graduated as medical doctor with an academic index of 4.5 mark or more.

The training is done at institutions which have been accredited by the Ministry of Public Health and the Ministry of High Education. The residence program is given through learning modules at any nephrology center. The pathway requires 3 years of training. The first year should comprise 24 weeks in an area of internal medicine and critical care patients followed by an additional 24 weeks at an internal medicine ward and intensive care unit and another area in basic nephrology at a nephrology ward. The last 2 years in nephrology should be focused on clinical nephrology, HD, PD, renal transplantation, pediatric nephrology, urology, and others. There is a theoretical and practical examination at the end of each year, as well as one thesis and a final theoretical and practical examination at the end of the residency [58].

The second half of the twentieth century was marked by a progressive and permanent development of nephrology practice from the perspective of RRT in ESRD patients, in accordance with the development of technology and pharmaceutical industry linked to dialysis and transplantation. In Cuba, this phenomenon has occurred with a progressive increase in the number of nephrology centers and a response from the national medical-pharmaceutical industry, in terms of dialysis concentrates, solutions, and medicines, but with a strong dependence on imports of technology and expendable resources from very distant countries due to the US embargo, which prevents the use of its powerful and closed market.

The development of nephrology in Cuba: on one hand, the training of specialized personnel – up to more than 400 physicians and more than 1500 nurses specialized in nephrology – in a population of just over 11 million inhabitants and, on the other hand, the development of specialized human resources, which has allowed the progressive increase of nephrology centers, with the aim of bringing them closer to patients' homes and ensuring universal access.

There is a multidisciplinary staff at each of the nephrology centers, integrated by nephrologists, renal care, HD and PD trained nurses, psychologists, dietitians, and social workers.

Although the development of the medical pharmaceutical industry in Cuba has allowed a progressive increase in the coverage of nephrology practice, the conditions of being an underdeveloped country, with a GDP in the range of Latin American countries' average income, dependent on imports and subject to the US strict embargo, have greatly hindered technological development in the medical sector in general and the nephrology sector in particular.

Within this context, convective therapies have been introduced to adapt them to our conditions, to analyze their particularities, and to promote their subsequent implementation and extension to the rest of the country. All activities developed by the national health system are budgeted by the Cuban state, which has an important source in the system of taxes and duties established in the country. All care received by patients is free of charge, and there is no particular reimbursement policy linked to dialysis and transplantation.

## Conclusion

In Cuba, since the official recognition of nephrology as a medical specialty and the foundation of the Institute of Nephrology in 1966, a progressive development has happened, expressed in the performance of scientific work and medical publications, which has allowed at all times the exchange of experiences between Cuban and international nephrologists, mainly from the Latin American area, in national, regional, and global scientific events.

We have a unique health system that ensures universal and free coverage; there are 56 nephrology centers distributed throughout the country, which offer specialized nephrology care, RRT coverage, the possibility of special laboratory tests, imaging, and kidney biopsy. For the care of such patients, the country has more than 400 nephrologists and 1500 specialized nurses who have the possibility of taking periodic refresher courses.

In Cuba, the development of public health in general, and of nephrology in particular, has been hindered by the economic and financial embargo imposed by the United States for about 60 years, which makes the acquisition of equipment and supplies more expensive. In spite of this, we have had achievements and are renown in the international arena.

## References


1. Oficina Nacional de Estadística e Información (ONEI). República de Cuba. Anuario Estadístico de Cuba 2017. Edición 2018 [Internet]. Accessed in Apr 2019. Available from: www.one.cu/aec2017.htm.
2. UNESCO. Cuba 2012. Tasa de alfabetización, total de adultos (% de personas de 15 años o más) [Internet]. Accessed in Apr 2019. Available from: https://datos.bancomundial.org/indicador/SE.ADT.LITR.ZSLOCATIONS=cu.
3. Cuba. Indice de desarrollo humano –IDH- 2017 [Internet]. Accessed in Apr 2019. Available from: https://datosmacro.expansion.com/idh/cuba.
4. The World Bank. Data Cuba 2017 [Internet]. Accessed in Apr 2019. Available from: https://data.worldbank.org/country/cuba; https://data.worldbank.org/indicator/NY.GDP.PCAP.CD locations=CU.
5. Morales R, Mas P, Castell-Florit P, Arocha C, Valdivia N, Druyet D, et al. Transformaciones en el sistema de salud en Cuba y estrategias para su consolidación y sostenibilidad. Rev Panam Salud Publica. 2018;42:6–13.
6. Pan American Health Organization. Directing Council. Strategy for Universal access to health and universal health coverage. Washington, DC: PAHO; 2014. (CD53/5, Rev. 2) [Internet]. Accessed in Apr 2019. Available from: http://www.paho.org/uhexchange/index.php/es/uhhex-change documents/technical-information/26-strategy-for-universal-access-to-health-and-universal-health-coverage/file.
7. Programa del Médico de la Familia. Ministerio de Salud Pública. República de Cuba. Editorial Ciencias Médicas. Ecimed. La Habana. Cuba. 2011 [Internet]. Accessed in Apr 2019. Available from: http://www.sld.cu/sitios/ecimed.
8. Anuario Estadístico de Salud. 2017. Ministerio de Salud Pública. República de Cuba [Internet]. Accessed in Apr 2019. Available from: http://bvscuba.sld.cu/anuario-estadistico-de-cuba/.
9. Anuario Estadístico de Salud 2016 Ministerio de Salud Pública Dirección de Registros Médicos y Estadísticas de Salud. ISSS: versiónelectrónica 1561-4433 [Internet]. Accessed in Apr 2018. Available from: www.sld.cu/sitios/dne/; http://bvscuba.sld.cu/anuario-estadistico-de-cuba/.
10. Online version of ISN Global Kidney Health Atlas 2017 [Internet]. Accessed in Aug 2018. Available from: www.theisn.org/global-atlas.
11. Stanifer JW, Isenburg MV, Chertow GM, Anand S. Chronic kidney disease care models in low- and middle-income countries: a systematic review. BMJ Glob Health. 2018;3(2):e000728.
12. Alfonzo Guerra JP. Historia de la Nefrología en Cuba, vol. 17. La Habana: Editorial Ciencia Médicas; 2013. p. 203–13.
13. Pérez-Ara AMM. La biopsia puntual del riñón no megálico. Consideraciones generales y aportación de un nuevo método. Boletín Liga Contra el cáncer, La Habana. 1950;25:121–47.
14. Buch A, Magrans C, Ferrandis R, Mañalich R, Suarez O, et al. Nuestra experiencia en el transplante renal. Repórter preliminar. Rev Cubana Cir. 1972;11:407–33.
15. Anuario Cuba Nefro-Red 2014. Situación de la Enfermedad Renal Crónica en Cuba. 2014 [Internet]. Accessed Jan 2020. http://www.sld.cu/sitios/nefrologia.
16. Bacallao R, López-Marín L, Llerena B, Heras A, Dávalos JM, Gutiérrez F, Nuñez L, Magrans C. Experiencia de 20 años en biopsia renal percutánea en adultos del Instituto de Nefrología. Rev Cubana Invest Bioméd. 2005;34(3):213–23.
17. Herrera R, Almaguer M, Chipi JA, Pérez-Oliva J, Silva-Aiçaguer LC. Prevalence of chronic kidney disease and associated risk factors in Cuba. In: Garcia G, editor. Chronic kidney disease in disadvantaged population. 1st ed. San Diego: Elsevier, Academic Press; 2017. Section 6.
18. III Encuesta Nacional de Factores de Riesgo y actividades preventivas de enfermedades no transmisibles. Cuba 2010–2011. Editorial Ciencias Médicas (ECIMED). La Habana. Cuba. 2014 [Internet]. Accessed in Apr 2019. Available from: http://www.ecimed.sld.cu.
19. GBD 2016 Causes of Death Collaboration. Global, regional and national age-sex specific mortality for 264 causes of death, 1980–2016, a systematic analysis for the global burden of disease study 2016. Lancet. 2017;390:1151–210.
20. Landrove-Rodríguez O, Morejón-Giraldoni A, Venero-Fernández S, Suárez-Medina R, Almaguer-López M, et al. Enfermedades no Transmisibles: factores de riesgo y acciones para su prevención y control en Cuba. Rev Panam Salud Publica. 2018;42:14–21.
21. Morales R. Las transformaciones del Sistema de Salud Pública cubano. Rev Cub Salud Publica. 2017;43(4):499–500.
22. Otero González A, Iglesias Forneiro A, Camba Caride MJ, Pérez Melón C, Borrajo Prol MP, Novoa Fernández E, et al. Supervivencia en hemodiálisis vs. diálisis peritoneal y por transferencia de técnica. Experiencia en Ourense. 1976–2012. Nefrologia. 2015;35(6):562–6.
23. García-Trabanino R, Arroyo L, Courville K, Chica I, Bohorques R, Rodríguez G, et al. La diálisis peritoneal en Centroamérica y el Caribe: estado actual, necesidades y propuestas. Nefrología Latinoamericana. 2018;15:52–64.
24. Bohorques R, Barranco E, Martínez M. Valoración nutricional de pacientes con insuficiencia renal crónica terminal al iniciar tratamiento dialítico. Rev Cubana Med. 1985;24:871–6.
25. Bohorques R, Rivas R, Nuviola B, Laurencio E. Colocación de catéteres peritoneal fijo por punción. Rev Cub Invest Biom. 1985;4:197–200.
26. Bohorques R, García A. Diálisis Peritoneal intermitente: Tres años de experiencia. Rev Cubana Med. 1986;25:1021–6.
27. Bohorques R, Martínez I, Nuviola B, Rivas R, Martínez A. Diálisis Peritoneal Intermitente en diabéticos. Nefrol Mex. 1988;9(3):97–102.
28. Bohorques R, Rivas R, Fernández O, Martínez I, Martínez A, Rodríguez R. Diálisis peritoneal en urémicos diabéticos y no diabéticos. Nefrol Mex. 1989;10(3):97–102.
29. Bohorques R, Moore A, Martínez A, Bacallao R, Gutiérrez F, Ballard Y. Continuos ambulatory dialysis in Cuba. Experience of the first two years. Perit Dial Int. 2010;30(suppl 30):S 16.
30. Alvarez Y, Bohorques R, Noa L. Sobre el comportamiento de los requerimientos de Eritropoyetina en los pacientes atendidos en un programa de diálisis peritoneal domiciliaria. Rev Cubana Aliment Nutr. 2016;26(2):358–61.
31. Bohorques R, Alvarez Y, Rodas A, Noa L. Influencia del estado nutricional sobre la capacidad funcional del paciente tratado en el hogar mediante Diálisis peritoneal. Rev Cubana Aliment Nutr. 2016;26(1):1–15.
32. Bohorques R, Alvarez Y, Martínez A. Diálisis peritoneal. In: Alfonzo-Guerra JP, editor. Nefrología. La Habana: Ecimed; 2016. p. 383–92.
33. Bohorques R, Alvarez Y, Martínez A. Complicaciones Infecciosas en un programa de Diálisis Peritoneal Domiciliaria, INEF, Cuba. Peritoneal Dialysis International. Agosto, 2011. Volumen 31, suplemento 4, pag 21.
34. Bohorques R, Alvarez Y, Martínez A, Ballard Y, Pérez S, Gutierrez F. Use of home peritoneal dialysis by Cuba Nephrology Institute 2007–2012. Medicc Rev. 2015;17(2):29–32.
35. Buch A, Magrans C, González E, Jirka J. Resumen de nuestra experiencia en el tratamiento de la insuficiencia. renal aguda en Cuba en los últimos 2 años. Rev Cubana Med. La Habana. 1965;5(3):515–26.
36. Valdés-Martín S. Hemodiálisis en niños. Experiencia Cubana. Revista Avances Médicos de Cuba. 2001;VIII, 26:14–5.

37. Herrera R, Magrans C, Buch A, Mañalich R, et al. La insuficiencia renal crónica y la estrategia de Cuba para las enfermedades crónicas no transmisibles hasta el año 2000. Nefrologia. 1993;XIII(Suppl 5):41–5.
38. Pérez-Oliva JF, Portal JA. Enfermedad renal crónica: estrategia nacional para enfrentar este importante problema de salud. Rev Habanciencméd. 2010;9(2):140–2.
39. Almaguer M, Herrera R, Magráns C, Mañalich R, Pérez Oliva JF. Chronic kidney disease in Cuba: epidemiological studies, integral medical care, and strategies for prevention. Ren Fail. 2006;28(8):671–6.
40. Alfonzo JP. Breve historia de la hemodiálisis. In: Magrans C, Barranco E, Ibars E, editors. Hemodialisis y Enfermedad Renal Crónica. La Habana: Ecimed; 2016. p. 1–15.
41. Almaguer M. Desarrollo de la rehabilitación en la enfermedad renal crónica en Cuba. Rev Cubana Med. 1987;26:546–52.
42. Pérez-Oliva JF, Herrera R, Almaguer M, Magráns Ch, Mañalich R, Alfonso JP, et al. Día mundial del riñón y Nefrología en Cuba. Tratar algo más que la enfermedad renal. Revhabanciencméd [Internet]. 2007 Jun [citado 2020 Ene 05];6(2). Available from: http://scielo.sld.cu/scielo.php?script=sci_arttext&pid=S1729519X2007000200019&lng=es.
43. Pérez-Oliva JF, Pérez R, Herrera R, Gutiérrez F, Almaguer M, Magráns C. Current status in ESCKD in Cuba. Nephrology. 2005;25(5):104–6.
44. Mármol A, Pérez A, Pérez de Prado JC, Fernández-Vega S, Gutiérrez F, Arce S. Programa de trasplante renal en Cuba. Rev Cubana Med [Internet]. 2009 Dic [citado 2019 Mayo 06];48(4):238–43 [Internet]. Available from: http://scielo.sld.cu/scielo.php?script=sci_arttext&pid=S003475232009000400012&lng=es.
45. Resolución No. 857 MINSAP. Gaceta Oficial No. 33 Extraordinaria de 17 de septiembre de 2015 [Internet]. Available from: http://www.gacetaoficial.gob.cu/.
46. Leyva C, Hernández LM, Muradas M, Molina S, Fernández-Vega S. Necrosis tubular aguda y rechazo agudo y su impacto en la función del injerto renal. Rev Cubana Urol. 2019;8(1):45–53.
47. Bywaters EGL, Dible JH. The renal lesion in traumatic anuria. J Path Bact. 1942;54:111.
48. Carbonel N. Fracaso Renal Agudo en la unidad de cuidados intensivos. Estudio observacional prospectivo. Nefrologia. 2004;14(1):47–53.
49. Bellomo R, Ronco C, Kellum JA, Mehta RL, Palevsky P. Acute renal failure-definition, outcome measures, animal models, fluids therapy and information technology needs; the second international consensus conference of the acute dialysis quality initiative group. Crit Care. 2008;8:204–12.
50. Alcázar R, Torre M, Santana H. Avances en la insuficiencia renal aguda en el año 2008. Nefrologia. 2009;29(S 5):82–7.
51. Liaño F, Tenorio MT, Rodríguez M. Clasificación, epidemiología y diagnóstico de la insuficiencia renal aguda. In: Roglan A, Net Castel A, editors. Disfunción renal aguda en el paciente crítico. Barcelona: Ars Medica; 2009. p. 1–14.
52. Ronco C. Continuous dialysis is superior to intermittent dialysis in acute renal injury of the critical ill patient. Nat Clin Pract Nephrol. 2007;3(3):118–9.
53. Oficina Nacional de Estadísticae Información de Cuba. El envejecimiento de la población en Cuba y sus territorios. 2009 [Internet]. Accessed in Apr 2019. Available from: http://www.one.cu/envejecimiento2009.htm.
54. Van de Noortgate N, Verbeke F, Dhondt A, et al. The dialytic management of acute renal failure in the elderly. Semin Dial. 2002;15(2):127–32.
55. Silveira Santos CGD, Romani RF, Benvenutti R, Ribas Zahdi JO, Riella MC, Mazza do Nascimento M. Acute kidney injury in elderly population: a prospective observational study. Nephron. 2018;138(2):104–12.
56. Mahesh E, Nallamuthu P, Kumar M, Madhyastha PR, Konanna G. Clinical profile of geriatric acute kidney injury in a tertiary care center from South India. Saudi J Kidney Dis Transpl. 2017;28(4):886–90.
57. Fernández-Vega S, García Y, Alvarez Y, Bohorques R, Rivas R, Leyva C, et al. Estado de la hemodiálisis de urgencia en una institución verticalizada en la atención del nefrópata. Rev Cubana Aliment Nutr. 2014;24(2):50–2.
58. Programa de Residencia de Nefrología. Cuba [Internet]. Accessed Jan 2020. http://www.sld.cu/sitios/nefrología.

# Nephrology in Mexico

# 14

Guillermo Garcia-Garcia, Jonathan Samuel Chavez-Iñiguez, Armando Vazquez-Rangel, Cynthia Gabriela Cervantes-Sanchez, Ramón Paniagua, Rafael Valdez-Ortiz, Rafael Reyes-Acevedo, Mara Medeiros, Maria Alejandra Aguilar-Kitsu, Ricardo Muñoz-Arizpe, Gregorio T. Obrador, and Ximena Rubilar-Araya

| | |
|---|---|
| Area[1] | 1,964,375 km$^2$ |
| Population[2] | 125,929,439 (2019) |
| Capital | Mexico City |
| Three most populated cities | 1. Mexico City – CDMX<br>2. Guadalajara – GDL<br>3. Monterrey – MTY |
| Official language | Spanish |
| Gross domestic product (GDP)[3] | 1.224 trillion USD (2018) |
| GDP per capita[3] | 9180.00 USD (2018) |
| Human Development Index (HDI)[4] | 0.767 (76° position, 2018) |
| Official currency | Mexican peso (MXN) |
| Total number of nephrologists[5] | 1196 |
| National societies of nephrology | Colegio de Nefrologos de Mexico<br>www.cnm.org.mx<br>Instituto Mexicano de Investigaciones Nefrologicas<br>www.imin.org.mx<br>Asociacion Nacional de Nefrologos de Mexico |
| Incidence of end-stage renal disease[6] | 2016 – 355 pmp |
| Prevalence of end-stage renal disease[6] (including patients with a functioning kidney transplant) | 2016 – 1447 pmp |
| Total number of patients on dialysis (all modalities)[6] | 2016 – 100,752 |
| Number of patients on hemodialysis | 2016 – 38,882 |
| Number of patients on peritoneal dialysis | 2016 – 61,870 |
| Number of renal transplantations per year[7] | 2017 – 3180<br>2018 – 3121 |

1. Referencias geográficas y extension territorial de Mexico. Aguascalientes, Mexico: Instituto Nacional de Geografía y Estadística (INEGI); 2018. Accessed in December 2019. Available at https://www.inegi.org.mx/inegi/spc/doc/internet/1-geografiade-mexico/man_refgeog_extterr_vs_enero_30_2088.pdf
2. Proyecciones de la población y conciliación demográfica. Mexico City, Mexico: Consejo Nacional de Población (CONAPO); 2019. Accessed in December 2019. Available at https://www.gob.mx/conapo
3. The World Bank. Mexico Data: The World Bank; 2018. Accessed in December 2019. Available at https://data.worldbank.org/country/mexico
4. Human Development Indicators. Mexico: United Nations Development Programme; 2019. Accessed in December 2019. Available at http://hdr.undp.org/en/countries/profiles/MEX

G. Garcia-Garcia (✉) · J. S. Chavez-Iñiguez
C. G. Cervantes-Sanchez
Nephrology Service, Hospital Civil de Guadalajara Fray Antonio Alcalde, University of Guadalajara Health Sciences Center, Guadalajara, Mexico

A. Vazquez-Rangel
Department of Nephrology, Instituto Nacional de Cardiología Ignacio Chavez, Mexico City, Mexico

R. Paniagua
Unidad de Investigación Médica en Enfermedades Nefrológicas, UMAE Hospital de Especialidades, Centro Médico Nacional Siglo XXI, Instituto Mexicano del Seguro Social, Mexico City, Mexico

R. Valdez-Ortiz
Nephrology Service, Hospital General de Mexico Dr. Eduardo Liceaga, Mexico City, Mexico

R. Reyes-Acevedo
Department of Surgery, Centenario Hospital Miguel Hidalgo de Aguascalientes, Aguascalientes, Mexico

M. Medeiros · R. Muñoz-Arizpe
Unidad de Investigación y Diagnóstico en Nefrologia y Metabolismo Mineral Óseo, Hospital Infantil de México Federico Gómez, Mexico City, Mexico

M. A. Aguilar-Kitsu
Department of Nephrology, Hospital de Pediatría, Centro Medico Nacional Siglo XXI, Instituto Mexicano del Seguro Social, Mexico City, Mexico

G. T. Obrador
Universidad Panamericana School of Medicine, Mexico City, Mexico
e-mail: gobrador@up.edu.mx

X. Rubilar-Araya
Universidad Panamericana School of Nursing, Mexico City, Mexico
e-mail: xrubilar@up.edu.mx



J. A. Moura-Neto et al. (eds.), *Nephrology Worldwide*, https://doi.org/10.1007/978-3-030-56890-0_14

5. Nefrologos con certificación vigente. Mexico City, Mexico: Consejo Mexicano de Nefrología, A.C.; 2019. Accessed in December 2019. Available at http://consejomexicanodenefrologia.org/nefrologos-con-certificacion-vigente/
6. United States Renal Data System. 2019 USRDS annual data report: Epidemiology of kidney disease in the United States. National Institutes of Health, National Institute of Diabetes and Digestive and Kidney Diseases, Bethesda, MD, 2018. Accessed in December 2019. Available at https://usrds.org/2018/view/Default.aspx
7. Boletín Estadístico Informativo del Centro Nacional de Trasplantes. Centro Nacional de Trasplantes (CENATRA); 2018. Accessed in December 2019. Available at https://www.gob.mx/cms/uploads/attachment/file/484466/BEI-CENATRA_Vol._III__No._2_ENE-DIC_2018_WEB.pdf

## Introduction

Mexico is a federal republic composed by 32 states and 2457 municipalities. Its official name is the United Mexican States. It has a land area of 1,923,039 square km and a total area (including the exclusive economic zone) of 5,120,679 square km. To the north it shares a 3145 km common border with the United States of America (USA) and to the southeast with Guatemala and Belize. The west and south are bounded by the Pacific Ocean and to the east by the Gulf of Mexico and the Caribbean Sea. It has a total population of 125,929,439 inhabitants. The three largest agglomerations are the capital Mexico City (21.581 million), Guadalajara (4.980 million), and Monterrey (4.689 million). The general table summarizes the main information of Mexico [1–7]. Governmental powers are divided constitutionally between executive, legislative, and judicial branches. The legislative branch is divided into the senate and the chamber of deputies.

For 300 years, from 1521 to 1821, Mexico was Spain's largest and richest colony in the American continent. After obtaining its independence in 1821, the country became an empire under Agustin de Iturbide. He was deposed in 1823, becoming a federal republic under the name of the United Mexican States. Throughout the nineteenth century, Mexico lived in constant civil unrest. By the end of the nineteenth century, it had had 2 emperors and 49 presidents. In 1836, the vast territory of Texas declared its independence, and after the invasion and defeat by the United States (1846–1848), Mexico lost more than half of its territory, the area that is now California, Nevada, and Utah, most of Arizona and New Mexico, and parts of Wyoming and Colorado [8].

Mexico has a rich cultural history and diversity. In addition to Spanish, the official language, 68 native languages are spoken in the country. Geographically, it can be divided into ten major physiographic regions: Baja California, the Pacific Coastal Lowlands, the Mexican Plateau, the Sierra Madre Oriental, the Sierra Madre Occidental, the Cordillera Neo-Volcánica, the Gulf Coastal Plain, the Southern Highlands, and the Yucatán Peninsula (Fig. 14.1) [1, 9].

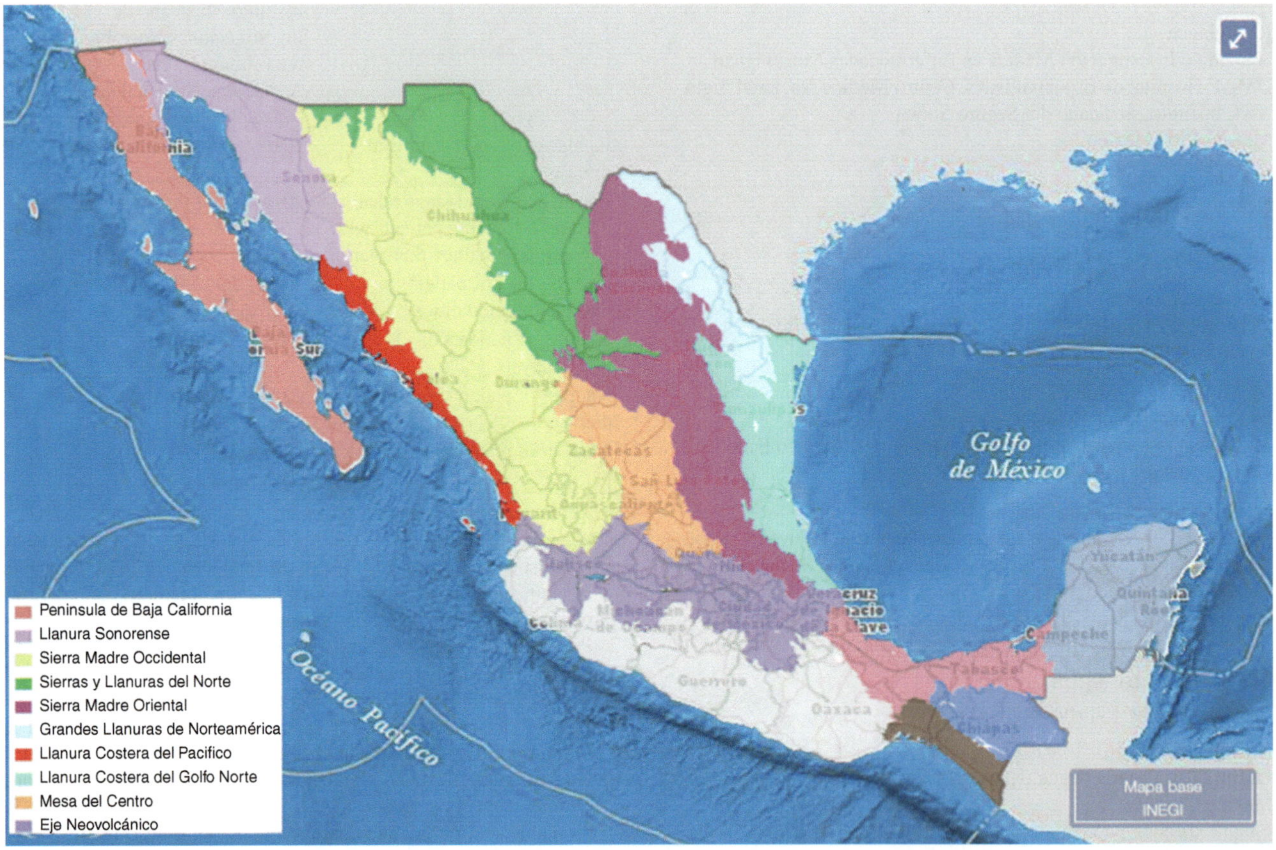


**Fig. 14.1** Political division and physiographic representation of the different provinces and sub-provinces in which Mexico has been divided, according to their geology and topography [1]

Mexico's macroeconomy has supported moderate growth despite several setbacks in recent years. Rising crime and insecurity are negatively affecting economic activity and the population well-being, particularly the underprivileged and women. Tax revenues remain low, and fiscal policy has little redistributive impact resulting in high inequalities. Reducing the high informality (60%) will require actions in enforcement, taxation, business, and labor regulations to drive resources toward a more productive formal market. Increasing the low female labor market participation and expanding high-quality childhood education would improve school outcomes and increase equality of opportunities for higher productivity. It is expected that the economy will gradually grow by 1.6% in 2021. Consumption will be a key driver, together with higher minimum wages and strong remittances. Declining interest rates will increase investment, and monetary policy will appropriately become more flexible due to declining inflation and the prevailing slack in the economy. Boosting productivity will require more competition and continuing efforts to strengthen the rule of law and to reduce crime [10].

Modern Mexican health-care system began in 1943 with the establishment of the Ministry of Health (SSA by its Spanish initials) and the Mexican Institute of Social Security (IMSS by its Spanish initials). In 1959, the Institute of Social Security and Services for Civil Servants (ISSSTE by its Spanish initials) was created to provide social security to federal public sector employees and their families [11]. Although since 1983 health care became a constitutional right, Mexico has a health system characterized by its failure to offer universal protection in health to one-half of its citizens. Access to renal replacement therapy (RRT) is limited or nonexistent for the uninsured population. Social security benefits, including universal access to dialysis and kidney transplantation, are only available to salaried workers employed by the private sector or by the government. However, they represent less than half of the country's population, and only a small percentage can afford private health insurance. As a result, over 50% of the population do not have access to social security benefits and cannot afford private health-care services. This segment of the population seeks care at the facilities of Mexico's Health Ministry, where access to renal replacement therapy (RRT) is limited or nonexistent [12].

The government Popular Insurance Program (Seguro Popular), which was established in 2003, intended to correct these disparities. After 15 years of its implementation, the percentage of the population with some type of public health insurance increased from 41% in 2002 to 81% in 2015, Seguro Popular never covered RRT [12, 13]. In November 2019, the Mexican government replaced Seguro Popular with the Institute of Health for Welfare (INSABI). Although INSABI aims to provide universal access to health care to the population without social security, the fate of access to RRT remains uncertain [14].

## History of Nephrology in Mexico

The start of adult nephrology in Mexico is credited to Dr. Herman Villarreal-Cantu, with the opening of the nephrology department at Mexico's National Heart Institute (INC by its Spanish initials) in 1955, where the practice of hemodialysis (HD) and kidney biopsy began in 1958 [15]. Two years earlier, in 1953, pediatric nephrology care was first offered by Dr. Rafael Soto-Allende and Dr. Gustavo Gordillo Paniagua at Mexico's Federico Gomez Children's Hospital's (HIMFG by its Spanish initials) hematology and nephrology service. This was among the first pediatric nephrology programs in the world [16, 17]. In 1961, the pediatric nephrology section became a separate service under the leadership of Dr. Gordillo- Paniagua.

In 1963, additional adult nephrology programs were established in Mexico City at the IMSS General Hospital by Dr. Emilio Exaire-Murad and at the Instituto Nacional de la Nutrición (INNSZ by its Spanish initials) by Dr. José Carlos Peña-Rodriguez. Additional pediatric nephrology services opened at the IMSS's Children's Hospital in 1963 by Dr. David Santos-Atherton and at the Mexican Pediatrics Institute (INP by its Spanish initials), by Dr. Samuel Zaltzman in 1970 [18].

The first successful kidney transplant in Mexico was performed in 1963 at the IMSS General Hospital, from a living donor, followed 4 years later by the first deceased donor kidney transplant [19]. The first pediatric kidney transplant was performed at the HIMFG in 1967 [17, 20].

Nephrology training began at the INC in 1958, followed by the IMSS General Hospital and the INNSZ in 1963 and by ISSSTE's Hospital 20 de Noviembre in 1976 [15]. Pediatric nephrology training began at the HIMFG in 1963 [15, 20]. The Mexican Board of Nephrology (CMN by its Spanish acronym), a board certifying organization, started its activities in 1985 [21].

Established in 1967, the Sociedad Mexicana de Nefrología was the first nephrology society in the country, being its first president Dr. Herman Villarreal-Cantu [15]. It became the Mexican College of Nephrology (CNM, by its Spanish initials) in 2005 [22]. Since then, two additional nephrology societies have been established: the Instituto Mexicano de Investigaciones Nefrologicas (IMIN), in 1970, and the Asociación Nacional de Nefrólogos de Mexico (ANNMAC) in 2007 [23, 24]. *Nefrologia Mexicana*, the official journal of the Sociedad Mexicana de Nefrología, was established in 1980 [25].

Noteworthy were the organization of the 5th International Society of Nephrology (ISN) International Congress of Nephrology in Mexico City, 1972 [26], and the 1st International Peritoneal Dialysis Symposium, June 1978, in Chapala, Mexico, where continuous ambulatory peritoneal dialysis (CAPD) was the "hot topic" of the conference [27].

## The Mexican Health-Care System

Health services in Mexico are provided through a variety of subsystems. The largest of these is the IMSS, which provides health-care services for formal private workers. The ISSSTE provides similar services for federal government employees. Other key institutions include the network of the Ministry of Health's State Health Services (SHS), for those without employment linked insurance. Only patients and their families with social security have universal access to end-stage renal disease (ESRD) replacement therapies. After the introduction of Seguro Popular (SP) in 2003, publicly funded health insurance extended to 50 million Mexicans who were previously uninsured. Prior to Seguro Popular, these individuals would have had access to the Ministry of Health's SHS but have been liable to a user fee [28]. Unfortunately, Seguro Popular never covered ESRD treatment, except for kidney transplantation in children <18 years of age.

Although the lack of infrastructure and human resources in the Ministry of Health's SHS facilities as well as geographic barriers limits the access to renal replacement therapy (RRT) to patients without social security, the most important factor is that access to dialysis and transplantation in this population is limited only to patients who can afford to pay part or all of the treatment expenses. As a consequence, many uninsured patients refuse dialysis, eventually abandon their treatment, or lose their kidney grafts because sustaining dialysis or immunosuppression becomes unaffordable. This results in marked disparities between the insured and uninsured populations with access to RRT. By 2015, the treated ESRD incidence and prevalence rates in the population with social security were 281 and 1357 per million population, respectively, whereas 130 and 200 per million population were uninsured, respectively (Fig. 14.2) [12].

## Renal Diseases in Mexico

### Chronic Kidney Disease

Chronic kidney disease (CKD) is a public health problem in Mexico with an estimated gross mortality of 40.3 deaths per 100,000 population [29]. Between 1990 and 2013, CKD burden increased, with an age standardized years of life lost and disability-adjusted life year (DALY) rates rising to >130%, the second highest DALY rate due to CKD in the world [30]. It has been estimated that 8.5% of the Mexican population has CKD [31]. Reported CKD prevalence in specific population-targeted screening varied between 16% and 33% [32–34].

Like many other countries, Mexico lacks a national dialysis registry. Reports from the Jalisco Registry estimate an annual incidence rate of 411 per million population and a prevalent rate of 1556 per million population. Over half of new ESRD patients have a primary diagnosis of diabetes [6].

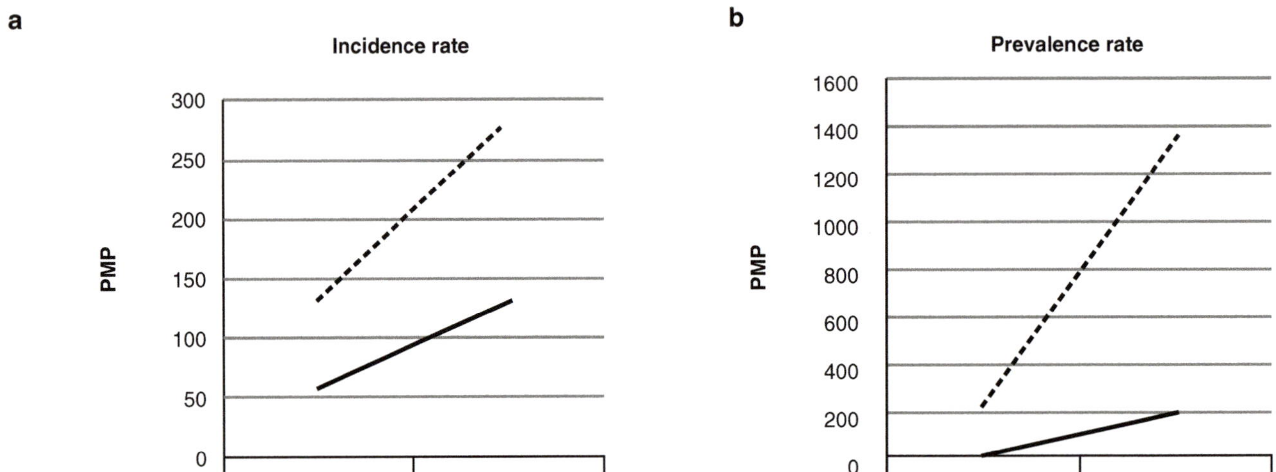


| a | 2000 | 2015 |
|---|---|---|
| Insured pmp | 133 | 281 |
| Uninsured pmp | 58 | 130 |

| b | 2000 | 2015 |
|---|---|---|
| Insured pmp | 243 | 1357 |
| Uninsured pmp | 27 | 200 |

pmp= per million population

**Fig. 14.2** Yearly incidence (**a**) and prevalence (**b**) of treated end-stage renal disease per million population (pmp), 2000–2015, among the insured and uninsured Mexican population. (With permission from Garcia-Garcia et al. [12])

## Acute Kidney Injury

Reports on the epidemiology of acute kidney injury (AKI) in the country are few. In a recent review of reports on AKI in Latin America, published between 1990 and 2016, only nine (14%) articles were from Mexico. Eight of these studies were hospital-acquired AKI cases and one in community-acquired AKI. Reports on the pediatric population were also underrepresented; only one study was on hospital-acquired AKI in children [35].

A new review has increased the number of reports to 15, 2 of them in children, comprising 852 patients. The prevalence on admission to acute care facilities varied between 3.1% and 69%, reflecting the selection criteria and the setting of the study. Over half (53–75%) of the adult cases were males. Sepsis was the main risk factor in the majority of the reports, except in AKI in pregnancy, where preeclampsia represented two-thirds of the cases. Average mortality reported was 38%, being twofold higher in the pediatric population. When reported, progression to ESRD ranged from 1.1% to 75% of the cases (Table 14.1) [36–50].

**Table 14.1** Pooled data published on AKI studies in Mexico

| Author | N | Prevalence | Setting | Males (%) | Etiology n (%) | Pediatric y/n | Mortality n (%) | RRT n (%) | ESRD n (%) |
|---|---|---|---|---|---|---|---|---|---|
| Córdova-Sánchez [36] | 270 | 69% | Oncology ICU | 130 (48) | Sepsis 99 (36.6), congestive heart failure 18 (6.6) | n | 81 (30) | 5 (1.8) | 3 (1.1) |
| Vázquez-Rodríguez [37] | 63 | 5% | Ob/Gyn ICU | | Severe preeclampsia 41 (65); eclampsia 4 (6.3); obstetric hemorrhage with hypovolemic shock 3 (4.7); sepsis 3 (4.7); other 12 (19) | n | 1 (1.5) | 1 (1.5) | 3 (4.7) |
| Valdez-Diaz [38] | 10 | 4.6% | Cardiac angiography | n/a | Contrast media 10 (100) | n | 0 | 0 | n/a |
| Santibáñez-Velázquez [39] | 55 | 11.2% | Tertiary-care facility ICU | 40 (73) | Sepsis 25 (45); postsurgical 19 (34.5); SIRS 5 (9); AMI 3 (5); other 3(5.4) | n | 19 (34.6) | 55 (100) | n/a |
| Alba [40] | 12 | 54% | Tertiary-care facility | n/a | Pneumonia, UTI, infected surgical wound, abdominal abscess | n | 1 (8.3) | n/a | n/a |
| Cruz-Martinez [41] | 78 | n/a | Tertiary-care facility ICU | 53 (67.9) | Sepsis 22 (28.2), trauma 10 (12.8), decompensated DM 11 (17.9), cerebral neoplasia 4 (5.1), AMI 3 (3.8), other 28 (35.8) | n | 22 (28) | 21 (26.9) | n/a |
| Higuera-de la Tijera [42] | 41 | 57% | Tertiary-care facility | n/a | Hepatic encephalopathy 28 (92.6); UGI bleeding 10 (24.3); alcoholic hepatitis 3 (7.3) | n | 37 (90) | n/a | n/a |
| Moguel-González [43] | 28 | 17% | Tertiary-care facility | 15 (53.5) | Cardiac surgery 28 (100) | n | 10 (52.6) | 9 (32%) | n/a |
| Chavez-Iñiguez [44] | 113 | n/a | Tertiary-care facility | 77 (68.1) | Sepsis 35 (31%); CHF 25 (22.8); DKA 15 (12.7) | n | | | 38 (43.6) |
| Meraz-Muñoz [45] | 87 | 54% | Tertiary-care facility | 46 (52.8) | Sepsis 37 (42.5); contrast media 21 (24.1); aminoglycosides 21 (24.1); other 8 (9.1) | n | n/a | n/a | 22 (75) |
| Bautista [46] | 17 | 53.5 | Tertiary-care facility ICU | 13 (76.5) | AH1N1 influenza with ARDS (all) | n | 6 (35.2) | n/a | n/a |
| Vega-Martinez [47] | 20 | 3.1% | Tertiary-care facility ICU | 11 (55) | Sepsis 18 (90) | n | 5 (25) | n/a | n/a |
| Ortega-Hernández [48] | 15 | 19.2% | Tertiary-care facility CCU | 11 (73.3) | Acute coronary syndrome | n | 5 (33) | n/a | n/a |
| Martínez-García [49] | 33 | 36% | Pediatric ICU | n/a | Sepsis 33 (100%) | y | 25 (75.7) | n/a | n/a |
| Cueva-Lepe [50] | 10 | n/a | Pediatric ICU | 3 (30) | Congenital heart disease 8 (80%); sepsis 1 (10%); status epilepticus 1 (10%) | y | 7 (70) | All | 0 |

*RRT* renal replacement therapy, *ESRD* end-stage renal disease, *ICU* intensive care unit, *AMI* acute myocardial infarction, *UTI* urinary tract infection, *DM* diabetes mellitus, *UGI* upper gastrointestinal, *CHF* congestive heart failure, *DKA* diabetic ketoacidosis, *ARDS* acute respiratory distress syndrome

## Renal Replacement Therapy in Mexico

### Peritoneal Dialysis

For many years the treatment of choice for ESRD in Mexico has been peritoneal dialysis (PD). PD began in Mexico shortly after being considered as a viable option for chronic dialysis in the late 1970s. Its dominance as a dialysis modality was not planned. A contributing factor was the 1985 Mexico City's earthquake, when a large number of public hemodialysis (HD) facilities were damaged, which obligated the use of PD on a larger scale. Later events favored the use of PD. First, it did not require special installations; second, it could be prescribed and delivered by non-nephrologists in secondary-care health facilities; and most important, it was found to be less expensive and therefore more affordable than HD, especially in the public health sector.

Most of the information on PD comes from IMSS, the largest dialysis provider in the country. The growth of population on PD has been spectacular over the last two decades. While in 1996 over 6000 patients were on PD [51], a recent study reported that 55,101 patients were on some form of RRT; 59% of them were on PD, 27% on automated PD (APD), and 32% on continuous ambulatory PD (CAPD). The HD population has also grown with respect to the previous years, currently representing 41% of the dialysis population [52].

There are few reports on PD outcomes. In 1997, in a single-center report, catheter failure was found in 68% of the cases, mainly due to mechanical dysfunction. At the end of the first month, only 55% of the catheters were still functioning. The most frequent failure was observed in patients with intermittent PD, a modality often used at the time [53]. Subsequent studies showed an improvement in the 1-year catheter survival at 61% for surgical-inserted catheters and 61–80% 1-year survival for percutaneous-inserted catheters [54, 55].

Similarly, a progressive reduction in the rates of peritonitis has been observed over the years. A report in 1996 showed a rate of 0.8 episodes/year [51], and a controlled clinical trial with a twin-bag disconnect system in CAPD patients reported a rate of 0.06 episodes/year [56]. In 2002, a peritonitis rate of 0.04 episodes/year was found in a study on PD adequacy [57]. In a more recent study, the rate was 0.163 episodes/year. Risk factors were male gender, low income, and low number of hours of patient training. The profile of bacteria detected was similar to that of other countries, with a predominance of *Staphylococcus* species, frequently associated with infection of the exit site [58]; however, in 40% of the cases, PD fluid culture was negative. Similar results have been reported among the uninsured CAPD population [59]. Peritonitis rates on APD have been estimated at 0.33 episodes per year [60].

Reports on quality of care are also scant. In a prospective multicentric study, only 40% of patients had hemoglobin levels within the levels recommended by clinical guidelines [61]. Erythropoietin was used in 13.5% of patients on CAPD and 28.1% on APD patients. The annual frequency of blood transfusions ranged from one to three on CAPD and one to two on APD. In a cohort of prevalent PD and HD patients, calcium and phosphorus metabolism-related variables were analyzed at baseline and followed for more than a year [62]. The percentage of PD patients within target limits was 35% for phosphorous, 32% for calcium, and 12% for PTH. The most frequent pattern was hyperphosphatemia, hypercalcemia, and low PTH. The latter was more frequent in CAPD patients, probably due to the high percentage of diabetic patients. Hypercalcemia was more frequent in PD probably due to high calcium concentration in PD solutions, which is the only type available in Mexico. Other important finding was the high number of CAPD patients with hypophosphatemia (21%), which seems related with malnutrition. The same pattern has been found in other studies in Mexican population. Low level of 25OH-VitD is a frequent finding among Mexican PD patients [63].

Due to the lack of a national registry, the analysis of mortality and technique failure in PD in Mexico comes from single-center reports, clinical studies, and databases generated for administrative ends. In a report from an IMSS tertiary-care facility, estimated CAPD patient survival at 1, 2, and 3 years was 90%, 78%, and 72%, respectively. Reported technique survival at 1, 2, and 3 years was 90%, 61%, and 50% [64]. Outcomes on uninsured PD patients have shown worse results. Reported patient survival at 1, 2, and 5 years was 79%, 55%, and 22%, respectively [65]. Additionally, another study reported a threefold higher mortality in uninsured patients starting dialysis in Mexico in comparison to Hispanic patients in the United States [66]. The high mortality was attributed to the advanced stage of kidney disease at the time of dialysis initiation and to the lack of pre-dialysis nephrology care. In a controlled clinical trial, the reported mortality rate was 15 per 100 patient-year at risk [57]. In another report, 24% of patients died during an 18-month follow-up [62]. Based on databases generated by the system for home delivery of dialysis solutions, between 2009 and 2012, gross mortality was 27.84% (unpublished data). In all the studies, the most frequent cause of death was cardiovascular disease (>40%), and the most frequent cause of technique failure was peritonitis.

APD was introduced in Mexico in 1998. Reported outcomes on APD are superior to CAPD. Patient survival at 1, 2, and 3 years was 82%, 62%, and 52% on APD versus 62%, 49%, and 42% on CAPD. Technique survival at 1, 2, and 3 years was 76%, 56%, and 56% for APD and 67%, 45%, and 42% for CAPD [60].

The cost of RRT has important variations according to the source of information. Data from IMSS indicate expenses of US$ 2562 per patient/year for CAPD and US$ 3842 for APD [52]. However, in a more detailed analysis, direct medical cost was estimated in US$ 16,452, being higher in APD than in CAPD, but the difference was not statistically significant [67]. Annual funding for patients on PD in Mexico has been recently estimated at close to US$ 5000 [68].

## Hemodialysis

HD was introduced in Mexico in the late 1950s at the INC [15, 69]. Initially it was used for the treatment of patients with AKI [70]. The first series of patients with chronic HD was reported at the INNSZ in the early 1960s [71, 72].

Since its introduction, Mexico has experienced a significant increase in the incidence and prevalence of treated ESRD [73]. However, the growth of HD was limited because PD rapidly became the treatment of choice for ESRD, especially in the public sector, for reasons explained before. Nevertheless, over the last decade, the number of HD patients has increased, and currently close to half of ESRD patients on RRT at IMSS are on this modality [52]. This was largely due to the hiring of private dialysis facilities, the majority owned by industry, to provide treatment to the large number of patients in whom PD failed. As the capacity of private HD units increased, a significant number of patients were offered HD as a first option. As a consequence, by 2013, the number of patients on PD had declined close to one-half of the dialysis population (Fig. 14.3) [12].

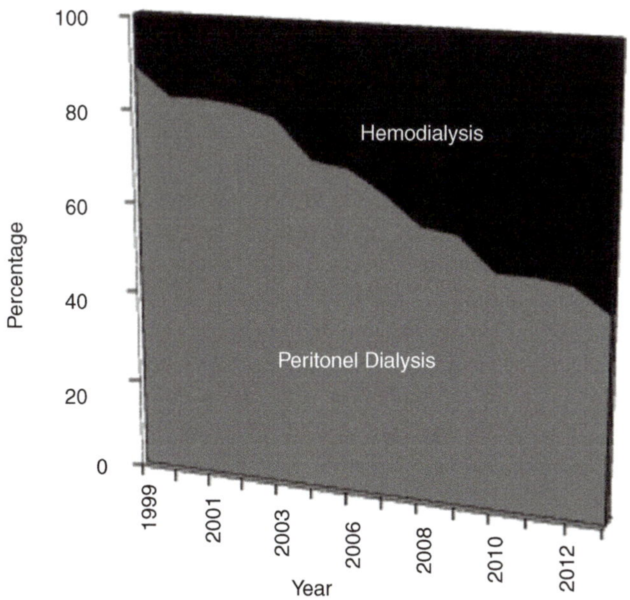


Fig. 14.3 Trends in dialysis prevalence using in-center hemodialysis or peritoneal dialysis, 2000–2013. (With permission from Garcia-Garcia et al. [85])

Similar to PD, reports on outcomes on HD are few and disappointing. A survival analysis on uninsured HD patients showed a three-year mortality rate of 56.7% among patients without a health insurance, compared to 38.2% among those with social security [74]. The higher mortality was attributed to inadequate dialysis because patients without medical insurance must face the financial burden of receiving adequate treatment [75]. A cross-sectional study in 83 public and private HD units from the 32 states in Mexico revealed that over half of them did not meet the standards of care defined by the Ministry of Health [76]. Close to half of the units were classified as delivering poor or very poor quality of care, and over three-fourth scored <70% on infrastructure requirements. Out of 818 patients, only 8% of the patients had an AV fístula. The average number of dialysis sessions was 1.3/week, and only 37% of the patients were receiving 3 sessions per week. Kt/V was not estimated in over half of the patients, and in those who it was measured, 45% had a Kt/V <1.2. The mortality rate ranged from 5.2 per 100 patients in the good quality units to 21 per 100 patients in the poor ones, with an average mortality of 10.7 per 100 patients. The estimated annual funding per patient has been estimated at over US$ 9000 [68, 76].

Although by law hemodialysis units must screen patients for hepatitis B and C every 4 months [77], due to the lack of data collection, reports on the prevalence of hepatitis B and C are scant and outdated. In a cross-sectional study that included 368 patients on maintenance hemodialysis at the IMSS, 7% were positive to hepatitis B, 30 times higher in comparison to the general population [78]. The prevalence of hepatitis C has been reported in 6.7–12.7% of the HD patients [79–81].

The use of hemodiafiltration and continuous renal replacement therapy (CRRT) is minimal and is largely available only in public tertiary-care hospitals and private facilities. A successful hemodiafiltration program has been implemented at the National Heart Institute with good results [82]. However, if access to conventional hemodialysis is limited, the possibility of increasing the use of hemodiafiltration and CRRT seems remote.

There are close to 400 dialysis units in public hospitals and over 3000 private hemodialysis units in Mexico [52, 83]. The size of the units varies between 10 and >100 dialysis stations. By law, the practice of hemodialysis in Mexico requires the presence of one certified nephrologist per dialysis shift (8 h) and one registered nurse for every four patients. Only nephrologists are allowed to prescribe the treatment. The dialysis nurse must approve a 6-month course on the technique of dialysis in an authorized training center. The law requires that presence of a renal dietitian and a psychologist for at least 2 days a week. However, it has been reported that only 52% of the units met these requirements [76]. Dialysis technician as a profession does not exist in Mexico [77, 84].

Dializer reuse is allowed, and it is widely used in both public and private dialysis units. It requires informed consent by the patient, and the dializer can be reused up to 12 times. Reuse is forbidden in patients positive for HIV and hepatitis B and C. The reuse of dialysis tubing is strictly forbidden [77].

## Renal Transplantation

The first successful kidney transplant in Mexico was performed in 1963. In 1984 legislation on organ and tissue transplantation was introduced resulting in a significant increase in kidney transplantation activity in Mexico. Between 1984 and 2015, the kidney transplant rate increased from 1.57 to 22.8 pmp, and the percentage of deceased donor kidney transplantation increased from 12% to 33%; organ-donation rate increased from 6.4 pmp in 2006 to 16 pmp in 2015 [85]. By 2018, over 50,000 kidney transplants had been done in Mexico [86]. Overall kidney transplant rates are similar to those reported in high-income countries and are among the highest in Latin America [87, 88]. However, this success has not been shared equally by the uninsured population. Because Seguro Popular does not pay for the cost of kidney transplantation and immunosuppressive therapy, transplantation rates are significantly lower (130 per million population vs 13 per million population) among patients without social security (Fig. 14.4) [12]. Consequently, the largest percentage of kidney transplants are performed at social security transplant facilities (56%), followed by the private sector (25%), and lastly by the Ministry of Health (19%). At present there are 389 licensed centers to practice transplantation, and over 15,000 ESRD patients are on the waiting list [86].

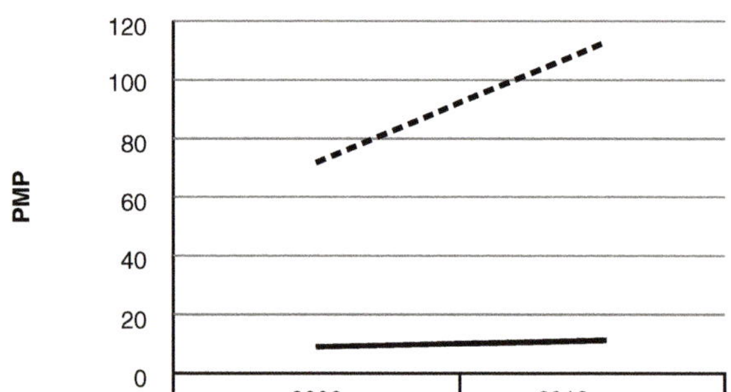


| | 2000 | 2013 |
|---|---|---|
| Insured pmp | 72 | 112 |
| Uninsured pmp | 9 | 11 |

pmp= per million population

**Fig. 14.4** Kidney transplantation rates among the insured and uninsured patients, 2000–2013, pmp (per million population). (With permission from Garcia-Garcia et al. [85])

Organ donation and kidney transplantation rates are unequally distributed in Mexico. A recent analysis of deceased donor (DD) kidney transplantation, between 2007 and 2018, revealed that half of the organs were retrieved from only 5 out of 32 Mexican states (Mexico City, Jalisco, Nuevo Leon, Guanajuato, Estado de Mexico); 43% were obtained in 14 states; and only 6% came from the remaining 23 states of the country. As a result, over half of DD kidney transplants were done in four states (Mexico City, Jalisco, Nuevo Leon, and Guanajuato). Overall, the largest percentage (45.8%) of DD kidney transplants was done in social security facilities, 42.7% in the Ministry of Health hospitals, and 11.7% in private institutions [86, 89].

The National Transplantation Center (CENATRA by its Spanish initials), an agency of the Ministry of Health, oversees organ donation and transplantation in Mexico. CENATRA promotes organ donation and education of transplant professionals, while documenting all donation and transplant activities through the National Transplant Registry. CENATRA is directly involved neither with organ procurement or transplantation nor with the distribution and allocation of DD organs; Mexican law delegates those decisions to each hospital transplant committee. CENATRA, however, oversees all transplant activities in collaboration with the Federal Commission for Protection against Sanitary Risk (COFEPRIS), the regulatory agency that license all transplant centers [90]. Although there are no relevant legal, social, or religious obstacles for deceased donation, Mexico has an organ donation rate of 3.9 per million population (pmp), significantly lower than other Latin American countries like Colombia (8.9 pmp), Argentina (13.4 pmp), and Uruguay (18.9 pmp) [91]. Low DD rates are at least partly explained by a fragmented and poorly coordinated organ procurement system. Although there is a national coordinating center, every state independently coordinates the logistics of organ procurement and allocation. There is national waiting list, but in practice each transplant facility manages its own waiting list. Procured organs are first offered to patients listed in the hospital where the donation has occurred. If there are no suitable receptors in that center, organs are offered first to other centers belonging to the same health system (IMSS, ISSSTE, Ministry of Health, or private sector). Finally, if no candidate is eligible within the same sector, the organs are offered to any institution with a suitable receptor [92]. Organ distribution is prioritized by time spent on the waiting list, not by HLA matching, which is rarely performed. As a result, patients listed in public hospitals, with larger waiting lists, must wait longer for an organ than patients listed in private facilities, where the list is normally smaller. In addition, health professionals in public hospitals work for a fixed salary. The lack of additional reimbursement for transplant procedures results in lower organ retrieval and transplantation, especially on weekends and holidays at the public transplant facilities [85].

With certain restrictions, unrelated living donation is allowed in the Mexican legislation. A recent analysis of LD transplant activity between 2015 and 2017 revealed that 730 non-related donors were accepted, representing 11.3% of total LD transplants and 8% of total kidney transplants done in that period. Interestingly, unrelated donor transplant represented 7% of total LD transplants in public institutions as compared with 27.4% in private institutions [86, 89]. Although the benefits of living donor kidney transplantation are recognized, the poorly organized deceased donor organ system in Mexico results on the utilization of LD as the main source of organs for kidney transplantation, with the risk of coercion and commercialization.

Currently, over 15,000 patients are registered on the waiting list for deceased donor kidney transplantation [89]. However, this number underestimates the total number of patients in need for kidney transplantation, since uninsured ESRD patients are underrepresented in the list.

## Pediatric Nephrology

### Epidemiology of Pediatric CKD in Mexico

Data analysis from the Latin American Registry of Transplantation and from the HIMFG showed that in close to 60% of ESRD patients the etiology is unknown, followed by congenital abnormalities of kidney and urinary tract (CAKUT) and glomerular disease [93, 94].

CKD risk factors in children, like prematurity, overweight, and obesity, are highly prevalent in Mexico. It is estimated that 6.6% of deliveries are preterm [95]. Results from the Halfway National Health and Nutrition Survey 2016 reported that 21.4% of girls and 16.2% of boys were overweight, while 10.2% and 13.2%, respectively, were obese [96].

Reports on the prevalence of CKD in children are few. Koshi et al. detected proteinuria in 16.1% in children screened on World Kidney Day; 15% had BMI > 95th percentile for age [97]. In apparently healthy children in Calvillo, Mexico, a region with allegedly high prevalence of CKD, 8.3% had proteinuria, 2.9% had proteinuria and hematuria, and 0.25% had eGFR <60 ml/min/1.73 $m^2$ [98]. Having a first- or second-degree family with kidney disease has been reported a risk factor for CKD [99, 100]. In a report on asymptomatic Mexican children with family history of RRT, 24% had urinary tract abnormalities, and 63.6% had CKD stage 2 [101]. When screening children with known risk factors, 33% presented abnormal urinary findings, and 2.2% had an eGFR <60 ml/min/1.73 $m^2$ [102, 103].

### Renal Replacement Therapy

Kidney transplantation is the best option for children with ESRD. The results of graft and patient survival in Mexican children are similar to those reported by other registries. Data from the Latin American Pediatric Kidney Transplantation Registry (RELATREP) reported a 4-year patient survival of 92.6%; LD and DD 4-year graft survival were 87% and 79%, respectively. Graft loss was due mainly to chronic allograft rejection (18%), vascular thrombosis (18%), and acute rejection (14%); 17% of the patients died with a functioning kidney graft; main causes of death were infectious diseases (63%) and cardiovascular complications (25%) [94, 104, 105].

The most common RRT used in Mexican children is PD. In a report from IMSS, out of 1342 children on RRT in 2009, 94% were on PD and 6% on HD [106]. Reported incidence of peritonitis varies from 0.25 to 0.63 episodes/patient-year [107, 108]. In a small single-center study, nosocomial peritonitis in children on PD occurred in 22% of the patients [109].

Outcomes on HD in the pediatric population are missing. Due to its high cost, few public hospitals offer CRRT for children; this option is offered mainly in private facilities. Programs to assist in the transition from pediatric to adult care are inexistent.

Similar to the adult population, uninsured children have limited access to dialysis and kidney transplantation. ESRD children without social security must pay for their treatment.

Many abandon their treatment or lose their kidney graft when dialysis or immunosuppression therapy becomes unaffordable. In 2012, Seguro Popular began a pilot program to pay for kidney transplantation (including a fixed period of pretransplant hemodialysis) in children ≤17 years without social security. Despite its success, the future of the program is uncertain due to drastic cuts in the national health budget made by the new federal administration [110].

There some are important issues regarding immunosuppressive therapy for children in Mexico. First, there are no pediatric formulations for most of the drugs commonly used in organ transplantation (tacrolimus and mofetil mycophenolate); it has been reported that the manipulation of adult formulations introduces a source of error [111]. Generic immunosuppressive drugs are widely available; however, there is a growing concern about the quality of some of the drugs provided [112]. In a population study of tacrolimus pharmacokinetics in Mexican pediatric transplant patients, the drug formulation and the CYP3A5 genotype were the most important covariates affecting tacrolimus concentration. A calculator has been developed to facilitate dose individualization in children [113].

Finally, despite the shortage of pediatric nephrologists in Mexico, the lack of opportunities to work in public and private institutions forced many to work as general pediatricians or as nephrologists in charge of adult hemodialysis facilities.

## Nephrology Practice in Mexico

### Nephrology Workforce

Based on an analysis of the Mexican Board of Nephrology (CMN for its initials in Spanish) database and the results of a recent online survey of all Mexican nephrology training programs, by February 2019, there were 1196 board-certified nephrologists practicing in Mexico (976 adult and 220 pediatric) [114]. The national rate of nephrologists was 9.1 per million population (pmp), but there were marked differences among states. Mexico City had the highest rate (45 pmp), followed by Jalisco (16–20 pmp) and Nuevo Leon (11–15 pmp). Incidentally, these three states have the highest GDP in the country. Most of the remaining northern and central states had rates between 6 and 10 pmp, and with few exceptions, the less developed southern states had rates between 0 and 5 pmp (Fig. 14.5).

Regarding nephrology training capacity, currently, there are 24 adult and 6 pediatric nephrology training programs. Prior training requirements for adult and pediatric nephrology are at least 2 years of internal medicine and 3 years of pediatrics, respectively; the length of adult and pediatric nephrology fellowships is 3 and 2 years, respectively [115]. A total of 166 annual positions (132 adult and 34 pediatric) are offered to Mexican and foreign candidates, and the ratio of applicants to offered positions is 2:1 for adult and 1:1 for pediatric nephrology. Considering an annual output of new Mexican nephrologists of 114 and no losses due to death, retirement, or other reasons, the projection is that it will take about two decades to achieve the rate of 20 nephrologists pmp that has been recommended by the Latin American Society of Nephrology and Hypertension (SLANH) by 2020. Doubling of the current annual output of new Mexican nephrologists could reduce this time to only a decade.

The majority of nephrologists works in the public sector, with monthly salaries ranging between US$ 500 and 1500

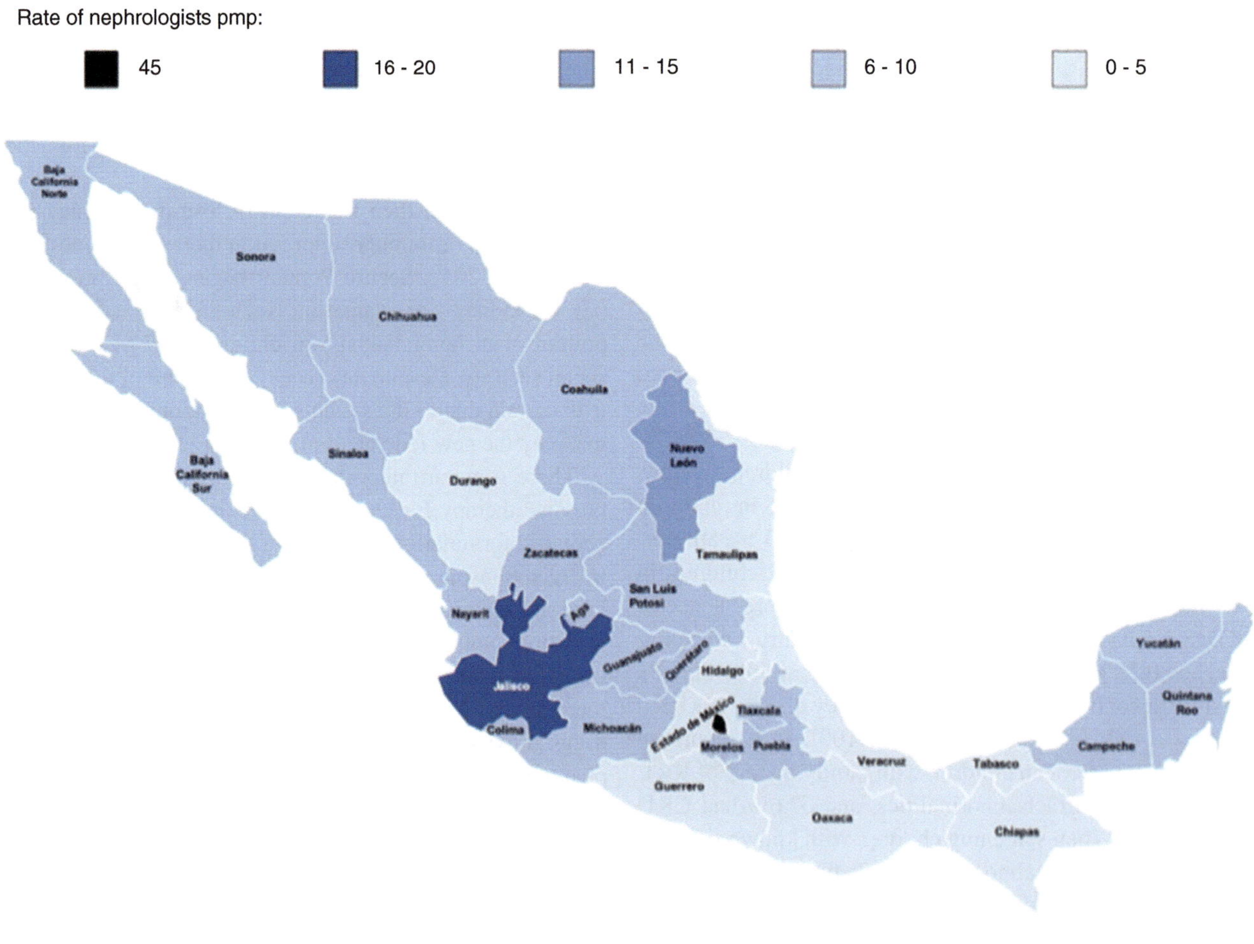


Fig. 14.5 Geographical distribution of nephrologists in Mexico, pmp (per million population)

depending on the type of position. Consequently, most nephrologists do private practice to supplement their income and, for a small proportion of nephrologists, is their only source of income.

Available information on other health professionals, such as renal nurses and dietitians, is inexistent or scant. Neither actual or estimated figures nor a formal certification process to practice renal nursing or nutrition exists. However, there is the Mexican Association of Nephrology Nurses (AMENAC for its initials in Spanish), which provides continuing education and training. Nurses may qualify to provide renal care through short diploma courses or by enrolling in a 1-year renal nurse specialty. Regarding renal dieticians, there is the Mexican College of Renal Dieticians (COMENUR for its initials in Spanish), which was founded in 2016 after the closing of the Mexican Association of Renal Dietitians (AMENUR for its initials in Spanish), which began in 2008. Currently, there are close to 100 members, albeit not all are renal dieticians (Angeles Espinoza, PhD, personal communication). Several online and on-site diploma courses on renal nutrition are available with variable duration, as well as an annual congress organized by COMENUR.

## Emerging Issues

### CKD of Unknown Origin

It has been suggested that Mexico may have newly identified CKD of unknown origin (CKDu) hotspots. Studies from Tierra Blanca, a rural region in Mexico, have shown that the prevalence of probable CKD is high (25%) among the population, of which almost half of the cases had no known traditional risks factors, such as diabetes or hypertension [116, 117]. Lozano-Kasten et al. screened 394 children residing in a community with high incidence of CKD of unknown origin in Jalisco; he reported that 45.7% of children had persistent albuminuria [118]. In the same community, in a cross-sectional study comparing CKD prevalence in Poncitlan residents to those residing in other Jalisco municipalities, a twofold and threefold increase in the prevalence of CKD and proteinuria, respectively, was found in adults residing in Poncitlan. In children the prevalence of CKD was similar (3.4% vs 0.7%) in the two populations; however, the prevalence of proteinuria was tenfold higher in children residing in Poncitlan in comparison to other municipalities [119].

### Pregnancy and CKD

Pregnancy in CKD patients is being frequently recognized in Mexico and is linked to adverse outcomes [120–123]. More than half of Mexican women are in childbearing age [124]. The high prevalence of CKD (6%) in women of childbearing age [125] is of particular relevance in countries like Mexico, where CKD prevalence is higher and resources are limited. In a prospective observational study in poor CKD pregnant women, preeclampsia (32% vs 4%), prematurity (48% vs 15%), and low birth weight (48% vs 12%) were more common in CKD patients in comparison to a group of pregnant women with normal kidney function. Fifteen (75%) remained dialysis dependent [123].

There are a number of problems faced by uninsured CKD pregnant women. First, the lack of CKD surveillance in Mexico limits the potential for early diagnosis and timely referral of CKD pregnancies. Diagnosing CKD during pregnancy represents an additional challenge in the care of this population. There are few specialized centers for the care of CKD pregnancy in the country, and access to dialysis is limited or unavailable in many of Mexico's Health Ministry facilities. When dialysis is available, providing treatment in overcrowded facilities, even at the standard prescription rate, is difficult. A particular issue is the fact that a large percentage of patients remained dialysis dependent. Since pregnancy-related coverage by Seguro Popular is limited to 42 days after delivery, patients with established ESRD must continue on dialysis at their own expense, with the risk of abandoning treatment when dialysis becomes unaffordable, leaving their children motherless [122, 123].

## Conclusion

After 65 years of the beginning of nephrology in Mexico, CKD care remains unjust, unequal, and below the quality of international standards. The current infrastructure and resources are insufficient to satisfy the demand of renal care in our society. Therefore, it is important to consider CKD a public health priority and to implement a comprehensive program for the prevention and control of this illness.

The establishment of a national public policy for the prevention and treatment of CKD is urgently needed. The policy must include:

(a) The implementation of community CKD screening programs tied to the ongoing strategies to prevent obesity, diabetes, and hypertension in our society
(b) Improvement of the current infrastructure and human resources, increasing the number of offered positions and training centers to match the high demand of nephrologists and allied health professionals
(c) The establishment of a national dialysis registry
(d) The extension of INSABI to cover treatment to retard CKD progression and universal access to RRT in patients without social security
(e) The promotion of a PD-first policy and kidney transplantation as the treatments of choice

(f) The use of generic immunosuppressive drugs to make this therapy more affordable
(g) To develop a more equitable organ allocation system to ensure that all patients have an equal chance of receiving a suitable organ

Pregnant CKD Mexican women have a high rate of adverse maternal-fetal outcomes. Even in a context of limited resources, the results of providing good care on maternal-fetal mortality are encouraging; an integrated approach and follow-up for pregnant patients with all stages of CKD should include preconception counseling and information on birth control. There is a need to increase the programs of CKD surveillance during pregnancy and to allow Mexican women who start dialysis during pregnancy to continue on RRT after delivery and raise their children. The emerging of newly identified CKDu hotspots suggests that CKD surveillance coupled with interventional treatment programs focusing on methods to slow or prevent progressive kidney function loss is urgently needed in these high-risk populations.

## Future Perspectives of Nephrology in Mexico

With the reforms in the health system introduced by the new federal administration, the future of health care, particularly renal care, in Mexico looks uncertain. As part of the austerity measures announced by the new president, the government has made substantial cuts in the health budget that have resulted in shortage of human resources and drug supplies [126]. Research has also faced cuts. The role of board certification, as a requisite to be licensed to practice nephrology and other specialties, has been questioned [127]. Seguro Popular has been dismantled and replaced by the newly created Institute of Health for Welfare [128]. Although Mexico's Health National Plan 2019–2024 includes universal access to health care, including free access to high-complexity services for patients without social security, details on how this will be implemented are yet to be seen [129].

## References


1. Referencias geográficas y extension territorial de Mexico. Aguascalientes: Instituto Nacional de Geografía y Estadística (INEGI); 2018. Available from: https://www.inegi.org.mx/inegi/spc/doc/internet/1-geografiademexico/man_refgeog_extterr_vs_enero_30_2088.pdf.
2. Proyecciones de la población y conciliación demográfica. Mexico City: Consejo Nacional de Población (CONAPO); 2019. Available from: https://www.gob.mx/conapo.
3. The World Bank. Mexico data. The World Bank; 2018. Available from: https://data.worldbank.org/country/mexico.
4. Human Development Indicators. Mexico: United Nations Development Programme; 2019. Available from: http://hdr.undp.org/en/countries/profiles/MEX.
5. Nefrologos con certificación vigente. Mexico City: Consejo Mexicano de Nefrología, A.C.; 2019. Available from: http://consejo-mexicanodenefrologia.org/nefrologos-con-certificacion-vigente/.
6. United States Renal Data System. 2018 USRDS annual data report: epidemiology of kidney disease in the United States Bethesda: National Institutes of Health, National Institute of Diabetes and Digestive and Kidney Diseases; 2018. Available from: https://www.usrds.org/2018/view/Default.aspx.
7. Boletín Estadístico Informativo del Centro Nacional de Trasplantes: Centro Nacional de Trasplantes (CENATRA); 2018. Available from: https://www.gob.mx/cms/uploads/attachment/file/484466/BEI-CENATRA_Vol._III__No._2_ENE-DIC_2018_WEB.pdf.
8. Mexico. Facts, history and news: info please; 2012. Available from: https://www.infoplease.com/world/countries/mexico.
9. Catalogo de las lenguas indígenas nacionales: Variantes lingüisticas de México con sus autodenominaciones y referencias geostadísticas. Mexico City: Instituto Nacional de Lenguas Indígenas (INALI); 2008. Available from: https://www.inali.gob.mx/clin-inali/.
10. Mexico Economic Snapshot: Organization for Economic Co-operation and Development (OECD); 2019. Available from: http://www.oecd.org/economy/mexico-economic-snapshot/.
11. Frenk J, González-Pier E, Gómez-Dantés O, Lezana MA, Knaul FM. Comprehensive reform to improve health system performance in Mexico. Lancet. 2006;368(9546):1524–34.
12. Garcia-Garcia G, Chavez-Iñiguez JS. The tragedy of having ESRD in Mexico. Kidney Int Rep. 2018;3(5):1027–9.
13. Frenk J, Knaul FM, Gomez-Dantes O, Arreola-Ornelas H. La brecha de la salud. Mexico City: Nexos; 2018. Available from: https://www.nexos.com.mx/?p=35971.
14. Instituto De Salud para el Bienestar. Mexico City: Secretaria de Salud; 2020. Available from: https://www.gob.mx/insabi.
15. Torres-Zamora M. History of the Mexican Society of Nephrology, currently Colegio de Nefrologos de Mexico. Nefrologia Mexicana. 2011;32(4):107–8.
16. Mota-Hernandez F, Velazquez-Jone L. Homenaje a Dr. Gustavo Gordillo Paniagua (1923–2012). Arch Latin Nefr Ped. 2013;13:3–28.
17. Garcia-Aranda JA, Madeiros M. Hospital Infantil de Mexico Federico Gomez. historical brief. Rev Investig Clin. 2009;61(5):351–3.
18. Santos-Atherton D. Antecedentes. In: Treviño-Becerra A, editor. Relatos: 50 años de la nefrología en Mexico: de Sociedad a Colegio. Mexico City: Editorial Prado; 2017. p. 23–6.
19. Teran-Ortiz LA, Diaz-Muñoz I, Alvarez-Balbas L, Silvia O-E. Los trasplantes de organos y tejidos en Mexico. Medicina Universitaria. 2001;3(12):191–4.
20. Garcia-Alvarez R, Fernandez de Castro J. Remembranzas de un pediatra: origen y breve historia de la nefrologia pediatrica en Mexico. Rev Med Pediatr. 2013;80(5):211–2.
21. Treviño-Becerra A. Consejo Mexicano de Nefrología. In: Treviño-Becerra A, editor. Relatos: 50 años de la nefrologia en Mexico: de Sociedad a Colegio. Mexico City: Editorial Prado; 2017. p. 281–8.
22. Trinidad-Ramos P. Transición de la Sociedad Mexicana de Nefrologia, A.C., a Colegio de Nefrologos de Mexico, A.C. In: Treviño-Becerra A, editor. Relatos: 50 años de la nefrologia en Mexico: de Sociedad a Colegio. Mexico City: Editorial Prado; 2017. p. 257–64.
23. Abraham-Bermudez J. Instituto Mexicano de Investigaciones Nefrologicas. In: Treviño-Becerra A, editor. Relatos: 50 años de la nefrologia en Mexico: de Sociedad a Colegio. Mexico City: Editorial Prado; 2017. p. 265–72.

24. Garcia-Garcia G. Asociacion Nacional de Nefrologos de Mexico. In: Treviño-Becerra A, editor. Relatos: 50 años de la nefrologia en Mexico: de Sociedad a Colegio. Mexico City: Editorial Prado; 2017. p. 273–4.
25. Torres-Zamora MI. Revista Nefrologia Mexicana. In: Treviño-Becerra A, editor. Relatos: 50 años de la nefrologia en Mexico: de Sociedad a Colegio. Mexico City: Editorial Prado; 2017. p. 241–4.
26. Robinson RR, Richet G. International society of nephrology: a forty year history. 1960–2000. Kidney Int Suppl. 2001;79:S1–100.
27. Nolph KD. 1975 to 1984—an important decade for peritoneal dialysis: memories with personal anecdotes. Perit Dial Int. 2002;22(5):608–13.
28. OECD Reviews of Health Systems. Mexico 2016. 2016. Available from: https://www.oecd-ilibrary.org/social-issues-migration-health/oecd-reviews-of-health-systems-mexico-2016_9789264230491-en.
29. Aldrete-Velasco J, Chiquete E, Rodriguez-Garcia J, Rincon-Pedrero R, Correa-Rotter R, Garcia-Peña R, et al. Chronic kidney disease mortality and its relation to diabetes in Mexico. Med Int Mex. 2018;34(4):536–50.
30. Gómez-Dantés H, Fullman N, Lamadrid-Figueroa H, Cahuana-Hurtado L, Darney B, Avila-Burgos L, et al. Dissonant health transition in the states of Mexico, 1990–2013: a systematic analysis for the global burden of disease study 2013. Lancet. 2016;388(10058):2386–402.
31. Amato D, Alvarez-Aguilar C, Castañeda-Limones R, Rodriguez E, Avila-Diaz M, Arreola F, et al. Prevalence of chronic kidney disease in an urban Mexican population. Kidney Int Suppl. 2005;97:S11–7.
32. Gutierrez-Padilla JA, Mendoza-Garcia M, Plascencia-Perez S, Renoirte-Lopez K, Garcia-Garcia G, Lloyd A, et al. Screening for CKD and cardiovascular disease risk factors using mobile clinics in Jalisco, Mexico. Am J Kidney Dis. 2010;55(3):474–84.
33. Garcia-Garcia G, Gutierrez-Padilla AJ, Chavez-Iniguez J, Perez-Gomez HR, Mendoza-Garcia M, Gonzalez-De la Pena MD, et al. Identifying undetected cases of chronic kidney disease in Mexico. Targeting high-risk populations. Arch Med Res. 2013;44(8):623–7.
34. Obrador GT, Garcia-Garcia G, Villa AR, Rubilar X, Olvera N, Ferreira E, et al. Prevalence of chronic kidney disease in the kidney early evaluation program (KEEP) Mexico and comparison with KEEP US. Kidney Int. 2010;77:S2–8.
35. Chávez-Iñiguez JS, García-García G, Lombardi R. Epidemiología y desenlaces de la lesión renal aguda en Latinoamérica. Gac Med Mex. 2018;154(Suppl 1):S6–S14.
36. Córdova-Sánchez BM, Herrera-Gómez Á, Ñamendys-Silva SA. Acute kidney injury classified by serum creatinine and urine output in critically ill cancer patients. Biomed Res Int. 2016;2016:6805169.
37. Vázquez-Rodríguez JG, Solís-Castillo LA, Cruz-Martínez FJ. Frequency and clinical evolution of acute renal failure in obstetric patients treated in the intensive care unit of a high-specialty hospital in Mexico City. Med Intensiva. 2017;41(4):255–7.
38. Valdez-Diaz R, Wong-Estrello R, Flores-Ydrack E, Basoni-Ruiz AE, Esquivel-Molina CG, Gonzalez-Ortiz LA, et al. Nefropatia por medio de contraste en angiografia cardiaca. Med Int Mex. 2010;26(3):226–36.
39. Santibáñez-Velázquez M, Sánchez-Montoya F, Alvirde-Gutiérrez L. Survival in acute renal failure with conventional therapy or continuous replacement therapy. Rev Med Inst Mex Seguro Soc. 2014;52(3):254–7.
40. Alba L, Espinosa R, Castro L, Reyes E. Incidence of nephrotoxicity in patients infected, treated with colistimethate. Enf Inf Microbiol. 2013;33(3):109–12.
41. Cruz-Martinez E, Hernandez-Rojas ME, Molinar-Ramos F. Funcion renal del paciente critico con falla renal aguda en relacion a niveles de depuracion de creatinina. Rev Asoc Mex Med Crit. 1999;13(5):155–9.
42. Higuera-de la Tijera MF, Pérez-Hernández JL, Servín-Caamaño AL, Serralde-Zúñiga AE, Cruz-Palacios A. The amount of alcohol intake, upper gastrointestinal bleeding, acute renal failure and hepatic encephalopathy as the risk factors implied in the increase of patients with alcoholic hepatitis. Rev Gastroenterol Mex. 2009;74(4):306–13.
43. Moguel-González B, Wasung-de-Lay M, Tella-Vega P, Riquelme-Mc-Loughlin C, Villa AR, Madero M, et al. Acute kidney injury in cardiac surgery. Rev Investig Clin. 2013;65(6):467–75.
44. Chavez-Iñiguez JS, Garcia-Garcia G, Briseño-Ramirez J, Medina-Gonzalez R, Jimenez-Cornejo M. The effect of resolution time of acute kidney injury on clinical outcomes. Indian J Nephrol. 2017;27(2):99–103.
45. Meraz-Muñoz A, Gomez-Ruiz I, Correa-Rotter R, Ramirez-Sandoval JC. Chronic kidney disease after acute kidney injury associated with intravenous colistin use in survivors of severe infections: a comparative cohort study. J Crit Care. 2018;44:244–8.
46. Bautista E, Arcos M, Jimenez-Alvarez L, García-Sancho MC, Vázquez ME, Peña E, et al. Angiogenic and inflammatory markers in acute respiratory distress syndrome and renal injury associated to A/H1N1 virus infection. Exp Mol Pathol. 2013;94(3):486–92.
47. Vega-Martinez D, Aguirre-Avalos G, Chavez-Iñiguez JS, Colunga-Lozano LE, Estrada-Gil FC. Precision diagnostica de prueba de estres con furosemida para prediccion de daño renal agudo severo. Rev Asoc Mex Med Crit Ter Int. 2016;30(4):230–4.
48. Ortega-Hernández J, Springall R, Sánchez-Muñoz F, Arana-Martinez JC, González-Pacheco H, Bojalil R. Acute coronary syndrome and acute kidney injury: role of inflammation in worsening renal function. BMC Cardiovasc Disord. 2017;17(1):202.
49. Martínez-García JJ, León-Sicairos NM, Canizalez-Román A, García-Arellano BA. Fluid balance and acute kidney injury in septic shock. Bol Med Hosp Infant Mex. 2017;74(4):282–8.
50. Cueva-Lepe AR, Risco-Cortes RE, Caballero-de AC. Estudio comparativo de hemodiafiltracion y dialisis peritoneal en niños con insuficiencia renal aguda oligurica en estado critico. Rev Asoc Mex Med Crit Ter Int. 2001;15(1):11–7.
51. Su-Hernández L, Abascal-Macías A, Méndez-Bueno FJ, Paniagua R, Amato D. Epidemiologic and demographic aspects of peritoneal dialysis in Mexico. Perit Dial Int. 1996;16(4):362–5.
52. Méndez-Durán A, Ignorosa-Luna MH, Pérez-Aguilar G, Rivera-Rodríguez FJ, González-Izquierdo JJ, Dávila-Torres J. Current status of alternative therapies renal function at the Instituto Mexicano del Seguro Social. Rev Med Inst Mex Seguro Soc. 2016;54(5):588–93.
53. Leaños-Miranda A, Garduño-Espinosa J, Martínez-García MC. Factors associated with peritoneal dialysis catheter failure in chronic renal insufficiency. Rev Investig Clin. 1997;49(3):189–95.
54. Padilla-Ochoa R, Garcia-Garcia G, Torres-Muñoz A, Lepe-Murillo L, Briseño-Renteria G, Luquin-Arellano VH, et al. Peritoneal dialysis catheter survival. A comparison between surgical and percutaneous catheter insertion techniques. Perit Dial Int. 2007;27:S7.
55. Murillo-Lepe L, Padilla-Ochoa R, Marquez-Magaña I, Renoirte-Lopez K, Garcia-Garcia G. PD catheter survival. A comparison between two percutaneous catheter insertion techniques. J Am Soc Nephrol. 2007;18:476A.
56. Monteón F, Correa-Rotter R, Paniagua R, Amato D, Hurtado ME, Medina JL, et al. Prevention of peritonitis with disconnect systems in CAPD: a randomized controlled trial. The Mexican Nephrology collaborative study group. Kidney Int. 1998;54(6):2123–8.
57. Paniagua R, Amato D, Vonesh E, Correa-Rotter R, Ramos A, Moran J, et al. Effects of increased peritoneal clearances on mortality rates in peritoneal dialysis: ADEMEX, a prospective, randomized, controlled trial. J Am Soc Nephrol. 2002;13(5):1307–20.

58. Amato D, de Jesús VM, Miranda G, Leaños B, Alcántara G, Hurtado ME, et al. Staphylococcal peritonitis in continuous ambulatory peritoneal dialysis: colonization with identical strains at exit site, nose, and hands. Am J Kidney Dis. 2001;37(1):43–8.
59. Garcia-Garcia G, Tachiquín-Bautista N, Luquin-Arellano VH, Ibarra-Hernandez M, Aviles-Gomez R, Briseño-Renteria G, et al. Risk of peritonitis among disadvantaged CAPD patients in Mexico. Contrib Nephrol. 2007;154:145–52.
60. Sanchez AR, Madonia C, Rascon-Pacheco RA. Improved patient/technique survival and peritonitis rates in patients treated with automated peritoneal dialysis when compared to continuous ambulatory peritoneal dialysis in a Mexican PD center. Kidney Int Suppl. 2008;108:S76–80.
61. Murguía-Miranda C, Ventura MJ, Ávila-Díaz M, Prado-Uribe MC, Mora-Villalpando C, Ilabaca B, et al. Adherence to clinical practice guidelines for anemia among Mexican chronic dialysis patients. Int J Urol Nephrol. 2016;4(4):120–7.
62. Paniagua R, Ventura MD, Ávila-Díaz M, Hinojosa-Heredia H, Méndez-Duran A, Cisneros A, et al. Reaching targets for mineral metabolism clinical practice guidelines and its impact on outcomes among Mexican chronic dialysis patients. Arch Med Res. 2013;44(3):229–34.
63. Ramirez-Sandoval JC, Arvizu-Hernandez M, Cruz C, Vazquez-Cantu B, Rojas-Concha LJ, Tamez L, et al. Cholecalciferol supplementation increases FGF23 in peritoneal dialysis patients with hypovitaminosis D: a randomized clinical trial. J Nephrol. 2019;32(4):645–59.
64. Rojas-Campos E, Alcántar-Medina M, Cortés-Sanabria L, Martínez-Ramírez HR, Camarena JL, Chávez S, et al. Patient and technique survival in continuous ambulatory peritoneal dialysis in a single center of the west of Mexico. Rev Investig Clin. 2007;59(3):184–91.
65. Aviles-Gomez R, Luquin-Arellano VH, Garcia-Garcia G, Ibarra-Hernandez M, Briseno-Renteria G. Is renal replacement therapy for all possible in developing countries? Ethn Dis. 2006;16(2):70–2.
66. Garcia-Garcia G, Briseño-Rentería G, Luquín-Arellan VH, Gao Z, Gill J, Tonelli M. Survival among patients with kidney failure in Jalisco, Mexico. J Am Soc Nephrol. 2007;18(6):1922–7.
67. Cortés-Sanabria L, Rodríguez-Arreola BE, Ortiz-Juárez VR, Soto-Molina H, Pazarín-Villaseñor L, Martínez-Ramírez HR, et al. Comparison of direct medical costs between automated and continuous ambulatory peritoneal dialysis. Perit Dial Int. 2013;33(6):679–86.
68. van der Tol A, Lameire N, Morton RL, Van Biesen W, Vanholder R. An international analysis of dialysis services reimbursement. Clin J Am Soc Nephrol. 2019;14(1):84–93.
69. Villarreal H. The artificial kidney and its applications. Rev Investig Clin. 1961;13:103–9.
70. Villarreal H, Flores C, Torres J, Ocando V, Colmenares P. The use of the artificial kidney in acute renal insufficiency. Arch Inst Cardiol Mex. 1962;32:569–80.
71. Peña JC, Duhalt R, Navarrette R, García Zozaya JL. Periodic hemodialysis in the treatment of chronic renal insufficiency. Gac Med Mex. 1968;98(2):150–67.
72. Peña JC. [The renal transplant history in the Instituto Nacional de Ciencias Médicas y de la Nutrición "Salvador Zubirán" (1966)]. Rev Investig Clin. 2005;57(2):120–123.
73. Saran R, Robinson B, Abbott KC, Agodoa LY, Albertus P, Ayanian J, et al. US renal data system 2016 annual data report: epidemiology of kidney disease in the United States. Am J Kidney Dis. 2017;69(3 Suppl 1):A7–8.
74. Valdez-Ortiz R, Navarro-Reynoso F, Olvera-Soto MG, Martin-Alemañy G. Mortality in patients with chronic renal disease without health insurance in Mexico: opportunities for a national renal health policy. Kidney Int Rep. 2018;3:1171–82.
75. Mercado-Martínez FJ, Correa-Mauricio ME. Living in hemodialysis without social insurance: the voices of renal sick people and their families. Salud Publica Mex. 2015;57(2):155–60.
76. Tirado-Gómez LL, Durán-Arenas JL, Rojas-Russell ME, Venado-Estrada A, Pacheco-Domínguez RL, López-Cervantes M. An evaluation of the characteristics, processes and outcomes of hemodialysis units in Mexico. Salud Publica Mex. 2011;53 Suppl 4:491–8.
77. Norma Oficial Mexicana NOM-003-SSA3-2010 para la practica de hemodiálisis Mexico City: Secretaria de Salud; 2010. Available from: https://www.gob.mx/cms/uploads/attachment/file/35874/NOM-003-SSA3-2010.pdf.
78. Paniagua R, Villasís-Keever A, MeC P-U, Ventura-García MD, Alcántara-Ortega G, Ponce de Leon SR, et al. Elevated prevalence of hepatitis B in Mexican hemodialysis patients. A multicentric survey. Arch Med Res. 2010;41(4):251–4.
79. González-Michaca L. Hepatitis C virus infection in patients with end stage renal disease. Rev Investig Clin. 2000;52(5):546–56.
80. Méndez-Sánchez N, Motola-Kuba D, Chavez-Tapia NC, Bahena J, Correa-Rotter R, Uribe M. Prevalence of hepatitis C virus infection among hemodialysis patients at a tertiary-care hospital in Mexico City, Mexico. J Clin Microbiol. 2004;42(9):4321–2.
81. Gómez-Gutiérrez C, Chávez-Tapia NC, Ponciano-Rodríguez G, Uribe M, Méndez-Sánchez N. Prevalence of hepatitis C virus infection among patients undergoing haemodialysis in Latin America. Ann Hepatol. 2015;14(6):807–14.
82. Mora-Bravo FG, De-La-Cruz G, Rivera S, Ramírez AM, Raimann JG, Pérez-Grovas H. Association of intradialytic hypotension and convective volume in hemodiafiltration: results from a retrospective cohort study. BMC Nephrol. 2012;13:106.
83. Estaciones (unidades) de Hemodiálisis: Instituto Nacional de Geografía y Estadística (INEGI); 2016. Available from: http://www3.inegi.org.mx/rnm/index.php/catalog/291/variable/V567.
84. Guía Tecnológica No. 15. Sistema de Hemodiálisis. Mexico City: Secretaria de Salud. Centro Nacional de Excelencia Técnica en Salud; 2004. Available from: http://www.cenetec.salud.gob.mx/descargas/biomedica/guias_tecnologicas/15gt_hemodialisis.pdf.
85. Garcia-Garcia G, Garcia-Bejarano H, Breien-Coronado H, Perez-Cortes G, Pazarin-Villaseñor L, De la Torre-Campos L, et al. End-stage renal disease in Mexico. In: Garcia-Garcia G, Agodoa L, Norris K, editors. Chronic kidney disease in disadvantaged populations. New York: Elsevier; 2017. p. 77–82.
86. Centro Nacional de Trasplantes. Reporte Anual 2017 de donación y trasplantes en Mexico. Mexico City: Secretaria de Salud; 2017. Available from: https://www.gob.mx/cms/uploads/attachment/file/289636/Presentaci_n_anual_2017.pdf.
87. Obrador GT, Rubilar X, Agazzi E, Estefan J. The challenge of providing renal replacement therapy in developing countries: the Latin American perspective. Am J Kidney Dis. 2016;67(3):499–506.
88. Rosa-Diez G, Gonzalez-Bedat M, Ferreiro A, García-García G, Fernandez-Cean J, Douthat W. Burden of end-stage renal disease (ESRD) in Latin America. Clin Nephrol. 2016;86:29–33.
89. Centro Nacional de Trasplantes. Estado actual de receptores, donación y trasplantes en Mexico. 2do trimestre 2018. Mexico City: Secretaria de Salud; 2018. Available from: https://www.gob.mx/cms/uploads/attachment/file/343098/SegundoTrimestre2018.pdf.
90. Reyes-Acevedo R, Obrador GT, Alberú-Gómez J, Gracida-Juárez C, André Madrigal J, Aburto-Morales S. Current state and challenges for organ donation and transplantation in Mexico. Transplantation. 2019;103(4):648–50.
91. Organizacion Nacional de Trasplantes. Newsletter Transplant 2018. International figures on donation and transplantation 2017. Spain: Organización Nacional de Trasplantes; 2018. Available from: http://www.ont.es/publicaciones/Documents/NewsleTTER2018finalCE.pdf.

92. Centro Nacional de Trasplantes. Distribución y asignación de órganos y tejidos. Mexico City: Centro Nacional de Trasplantes; 2016. Available from: https://www.gob.mx/cenatra/acciones-y-programas/distribucion-y-asignacion-de-organos-y-tejidos.
93. Medeiros-Domingo M, Romero-Navarro B, Valverde-Rosas S, Delgadillo R, Varela-Fascinetto G, Munoz-Arizpe R. Renal transplantation in children. Rev Investig Clin. 2005;57(2):230–6.
94. Latin American Pediatric Nephrology A, Latin American Pediatric Renal Transplant Cooperative S. Latin American registry of pediatric renal transplantation 2004–2008. Pediatr Transplant. 2010;14(6):701–8.
95. McDonald JA, Mojarro O, Sutton PD, Ventura SJ. A binational overview of reproductive health outcomes among US Hispanic and Mexican women in the border region. Prev Chronic Dis. 2013;10:E137.
96. Shamah-Levy T, Cuevas-Nasu L, Gaona-Pineda EB, Gómez-Acosta LM, Morales-Rúan MDC, Hernández-Ávila M, et al. Overweight and obesity in children and adolescents, 2016 Halfway National Health and Nutrition Survey update. Salud Publica Mex. 2018;60(3):244–53.
97. Koshy SM, Garcia-Garcia G, Pamplona JS, Renoirte-Lopez K, Perez-Cortes G, Gutierrez MLS, et al. Screening for kidney disease in children on world kidney day in Jalisco, Mexico. Pediatr Nephrol. 2009;24(6):1219–25.
98. Góngora-Ortega J, Serna-Vela Francisco J, Gutiérrez-Mendoza I, Pérez-Guzmán C, Hernández-Garduño E, Ron-Torres O. Prevalence of chronic kidney disease in children in Aguascalientes, Mexico. Salud Publica Mex. 2008;50(6):436–7.
99. McClellan WM, Satko SG, Gladstone E, Krisher JO, Narva AS, Freedman BI. Individuals with a family history of ESRD are a high-risk population for CKD: implications for targeted surveillance and intervention activities. Am J Kidney Dis. 2009;53(3 Suppl 3):S100–6.
100. Bulum B, Ozçakar ZB, Ustüner E, Düşünceli E, Kavaz A, Duman D, et al. High frequency of kidney and urinary tract anomalies in asymptomatic first-degree relatives of patients with CAKUT. Pediatr Nephrol. 2013;28(11):2143–7.
101. Medeiros M, Andrade Veneros GD, Toussaint Martinez de Castro G, Ortiz Vasquez L, Hernandez Sanchez AM, Olvera N, et al. Prevalence of kidney disease in asymptomatic children with family history of renal replacement therapy. Bol Med Hosp Infant Mex. 2015;72(4):257–61.
102. Medeiros M, Olvera N, Reyes R, Velasquez Jones L, Toussaint G, Obrador Vera GT. Early detection of kidney disease in children and adolescents in Mexico: a pilot study [Abstract]. J Am Soc Nephrol. 2013;24(Renal Week suppl):174A–5A.
103. Ortega-Romero M, Méndez-Hernández P, Cruz-Angulo MDC, Hernández-Sánchez AM, Álvarez-Elías AC, Muñoz-Arizpe R, et al. Chronic kidney disease in children aged 6–15 years and associated risk factors in Apizaco, Tlaxcala, Mexico, a pilot study. Nephron. 2019;143(4):264–73.
104. Medeiros-Domingo M, Romero-Navarro B, Valverde-Rosas S, Delgadillo R, Varela-Fascinetto G, Muñoz-Arizpe R. Renal transplantation in children. Rev Investig Clin. 2005;57(2):230–6.
105. Orta N, García C, Delucchi A, Medeiros M. Registro Latinoamericano de Trasplante Renal Pediatrico (RELATREP) 2004–2014. Arch Latin Nefr Ped. 2016;16:22–34.
106. Mendez-Duran A, Mendez-Bueno JF, Tapia-Yañez T, Muñoz-Montes A, Aguilar-Sanchez L. Epidemiology of chronic kidney failure in Mexico. Dial Traspl. 2010;31(1):7–11.
107. Fabian Velasco R, Lagunas Munoz J, Sanchez Saavedra V, Mena Brito Trejo JE, Qureshi AR, Garcia-Lopez E, et al. Automated peritoneal dialysis as the modality of choice: a single-center, 3-year experience with 458 children in Mexico. Pediatr Nephrol. 2008;23(3):465–71.
108. Robles-Vásquez N, Aguilar-Kitsu MA, Mendoza-Guevara L, Miranda-Novales MG. Complicaciones infecciosas en niños con enfermedad renal enterapia sustitutiva. Rev Med Inst Mex Seguro Soc. 2015;53(Suppl 3):S246–52.
109. Lopez-Gonzalez D, Garduno J, Reyes-Lopez A, Partida-Gaytan A, Medeiros M. Risk factors associated with nosocomial peritonitis in children on peritoneal dialysis. Rev Investig Clin. 2015;67(3):170–6.
110. Agren D. AMLO's Mexico leads to drastic cuts to health system. Lancet. 2019;393(10188):2289–90.
111. Medeiros M, Castaneda-Hernandez G, Ross CJ, Carleton BC. Use of pharmacogenomics in pediatric renal transplant recipients. Front Genet. 2015;6:41.
112. Jacobo-Cabral CO, Garcia-Roca P, Reyes H, Lozada-Rojas L, Cruz-Antonio L, Medeiros M, et al. Limustin(R), a non-innovator tacrolimus formulation, yields reduced drug exposure in pediatric renal transplant recipients. Pediatr Transplant. 2014;18(7):706–13.
113. Jacobo-Cabral CO, Garcia-Roca P, Romero-Tejeda EM, Reyes H, Medeiros M, Castaneda-Hernandez G, et al. Population pharmacokinetic analysis of tacrolimus in Mexican paediatric renal transplant patients: role of CYP3A5 genotype and formulation. Br J Clin Pharmacol. 2015;80(4):630–41.
114. Consejo Mexicano de Nefrologia, A.C.: nefrologos con certificacion vigente: Consejo Mexicano de Nefrologia, A.C.; 2019. Available from: http://consejomexicanodenefrologia.org/nefrologos-con-certificacion-vigente/.
115. Consejo Mexicano de Nefrologia, A.C.: Sedes de entrenamiento. Mexico City: Consejo Mexicano de Nefrologia, A.C.; 2019. Available from: http://consejomexicanodenefrologia.org/quienes-somos/.
116. Aguilar DJ, Madero M. Other potential CKD hotspots in the world: the cases of Mexico and the United States. Semin Nephrol. 2019;39(3):300–7.
117. Obrador GT, Levin A. CKD hotspots: challenges and areas of opportunity. Semin Nephrol. 2019;39(3):308–14.
118. Lozano-Kasten F, Sierra-Diaz E, de Jesus Celis-de la Rosa A, Margarita Soto Gutiérrez M, Aarón Peregrina Lucano A, Childhood RGoSaEDi. Prevalence of albuminuria in children living in a rural agricultural and fishing subsistence community in Lake Chapala, Mexico. Int J Environ Res Public Health. 2017;14(12):1577.
119. Garcia-Garcia G, Gutiérrez-Padilla A, Perez-Gomez HR, Chavez-Iñiguez JS, Morraz-Mejia EF, Amador-Jimenez MJ, Romero-Muñoz AC, Gonzalez-De la Peña MDM, Klarenbach S, Tonelli M. Chronic kidney disease of unknown cause in Mexico: the case of Poncitlan, Jalisco. Clin Nephrol. 2020;93(1):42–8.
120. Vázquez-Rodríguez JG, Rivera-Hernández M. Perinatal complications in patients with chronic renal failure. Ginecol Obstet Mex. 2011;79(5):261–8.
121. Vazquez JAG, Calva IEM, Fernandez RM, Leon VE, Cardona M, Noyola H. Pregnancy in end-stage renal disease patients and treatment with peritoneal dialysis: report of two cases. Perit Dial Int. 2007;27(3):353–8.
122. Ibarra-Hernandez M, Orozco-Guillen OA, de la Alcantar-Vallin ML, Garrido-Roldan R, Jimenez-Alvarado MP, Castro KB, et al. Acute kidney injury in pregnancy and the role of underlying CKD: a point of view from Mexico. J Nephrol. 2017;30(6):773–80.
123. Ibarra-Hernandez M, Alcantar-Vallin ML, Soto-Cruz A, Jimenez-Alvarado PM, Villa-Villagran F, Diaz-Avila JJ, et al. Challenges in managing pregnancy in underserved women with chronic kidney disease. Am J Nephrol. 2019;49(5):386–96.
124. Consejo Nacional de Población. Situación de la Salud Sexual y Reproductiva. República Mexicana. Panorama demográfico y principales características de las mujeres en edad reproductiva. Mexico City: Consejo Nacional de Poblacion; 2016. Available

from: https://www.gob.mx/cms/uploads/attachment/file/237216/Cuadernillo_SSR_RM.pdf.
125. Webster P, Lightstone L, McKay DB, Josephson MA. Pregnancy in chronic kidney disease and kidney transplantation. Kidney Int. 2017;91(5):1047–56.
126. Agren D. AMLO's Mexico leads to drastic cuts to health budget. Lancet. 2019;393(10118):2289–90.
127. Senado de la República. Gaceta de la Comisión Permanente. Iniciativa con proyecto de decreto por el que se reforma el Artículo 81 de la Ley General de Salud. Mexico City: Senado de la República. Gaceta de la Comisión Permamente; 2019. Available from: http://www.senado.gob.mx/64/gaceta_comision_permanente/documento/97421.
128. Muñoz AE. Se crea el Instituto de Salud para el Bienestar. Mexico City: La Jornada; 2019. Available from: https://www.jornada.com.mx/ultimas/politica/2019/07/13/se-crea-el-instituto-de-salud-para-el-bienestar-8896.html.
129. Secretaria de Salud. Proyecto Plan Nacional de Salud 2019–2024. Mexico City: Secretaria de Salud; 2019. Available from: http://www.hgm.salud.gob.mx/descargas/pdf/dirgral/Plan_Nacional_Salud_2019_2024.pdf.

# Nephrology in the United States of America

# 15

Samaya J. Anumudu and Stephen Z. Fadem

| | |
|---|---|
| Area | 9.834 million km$^2$ |
| Population | 327.2 million (2018) |
| Capital | Washington, DC |
| Three most populated cities[1] | 1. New York (8,398,748)<br>2. Los Angeles (3,990,456)<br>3. Chicago (2,705,994) |
| Official language | English |
| Gross domestic product (GDP)[2] | 19.39 trillion USD |
| GDP per capita[2] | 59,531.66 USD |
| Human Development Index (HDI)[3] | 0.920 |
| Official currency | US dollar (USD) |
| Total number of nephrologists[4] | 10,883 |
| National society of nephrology | American Society of Nephrology (ASN)<br>www.asn-online.org |
| Incidence of end-stage renal disease | 2016 – 373.4 pmp<br>2017 – 380.5 pmp |
| Prevalence of end-stage renal disease[5] | 2016 – 2160.7 pmp<br>2017 – 2282 pmp |
| Total number of patients on dialysis (all modalities) | 2016 – 511,270<br>2017 – 520,769 |
| Number of patients on hemodialysis | 2016 – 457,957<br>2017 – 468,139 |
| Number of patients on peritoneal dialysis | 2016 – 51,005<br>2017 – 52,630 |
| Number of kidney transplants per year[6] | 2017 – 21,167 |
| Prevalence of transplant patients[5] | 2016 – 215,061<br>2017 – 222,848 |

Table references:
1. US Census Bureau
2. World Bank
3. United Nations
4. ASN
5. USRDS ADR 2019
6. UNOS

## Introduction

The specialty of nephrology includes the management of patients with acute and chronic kidney injury, the deciphering of complex acid-base disorders, or the identification and management of patients with glomerular diseases. For many nephrologists, the specialty centers around the diagnosis and treatment of patients who have various stages of kidney disease. What was once a disease that was 100% lethal can now be treated and well managed. Challenges exist, but the field is far more gratifying given this population of patients can enjoy a decent quality of life and be active members of society. This chapter will examine the beginnings of the field and how United States (US) nephrologists are approaching modalities of care as well as various specific issues such as hospitalization rates, arteriovenous access barriers, hospitalizations, volume and cardiovascular disease, the mineral and bone disorder, potassium, and transplantation. It will discuss various opportunities for young physicians and conclude with what lies in the future for nephrologists and, more importantly, for patients.

## About the USA

The United States of America (USA) evolved between the 1600s and 1700s to become first British colonies and then to win freedom. In 1789, after a bitter revolutionary war with Great Britain, it created a constitution that set up an infrastructure that would "secure the blessings of liberty to ourselves and our posterity." The US Constitution created three branches of government, a legislative, an executive, and a judicial branch, each designed with checks and balances. The legislative branch is composed of two individuals from each state elected to the senate and a varying number of representatives elected from census determined congressional districts to the house of representatives. There is a president, elected by representatives from each state for a 4-year term who presides over an executive branch that

S. J. Anumudu · S. Z. Fadem (✉)
Baylor College of Medicine, Houston, TX, USA
e-mail: samaya.qureshi@bcm.edu; fadem@bcm.edu


J. A. Moura-Neto et al. (eds.), *Nephrology Worldwide*, https://doi.org/10.1007/978-3-030-56890-0_15

includes among its administrative bureaus the Department of Health and Human Services headed by a secretary of HHS and the Department of Justice headed by an attorney general. The state department is under the executive branch and presides over international affairs, and the secretary of defense heads the vast Defense Department that oversees the military. And a third branch, the judicial branch, is composed of nine Supreme Court justices who are appointed by the president but approved by congress and hold their office for life. Under the constitutional democracy, the USA grew through the doctrine of manifest destiny to expand across the North American continent and now includes 50 states including Hawaii and Alaska. A highly contentious two-party system stimulates heated debate among those who classify themselves as Democrats or Republicans. The purpose of this division is to engender productive discussion between those with differing ideas, but productivity in the USA is at its best when a cooperative spirit exists between party members.

The USA is a global superpower and among the wealthiest nations. The Brookings Institution reports that American households hold over US$ 98 trillion dollars of wealth (2018) and US$ 113 trillion dollars in assets. The households in the USA also hold US$ 15 trillion dollars in debt. A college-educated American has 4–5 times the wealth as one without such an education, and education through high school in the USA is compulsory. Those with a graduate or professional degree enjoy an eightfold increase in wealth over a high school graduate. Entrepreneurism in the USA, a capitalistic environment, has been historically very richly rewarded with 80% of the wealth distributed among 20% of the people [1]. The wealthy include inventors and creators. The USA is the founding home for Google, ExxonMobil, Walmart, Apple computer, Microsoft, IBM, ATT, and several other major entities known throughout the world.

Despite being established in 1630 by English refugees seeking religious freedom as the "city upon the hill," the USA was stained by slavery which denied justice and freedom to slaves of African descendancy until 1865. Although a vicious civil war led to the emancipation of blacks, the wealth and prosperity gap remained huge. In the years between 2013 and 2016, the net worth of Hispanic and black families has risen between 30% and 50% [2].

The USA has multiple problems yet to resolve – high crime is often committed with lethal firearms and the weaponization of America. The accessibility of weapons to those with severe mental health issues has created the problem of mass shootings that has yet to resolve. America is in the midst of an opioid crisis. The CDC reports that 4.8% of persons fail to obtain medical care due to costs. Although health care for medical emergencies is guaranteed by federal statute, 27.5 million US residents lack insurance coverage [3].

## Brief History of Nephrology in the USA

Kidney disease is a worldwide and universal problem. It is impossible to speak about its history without referencing the contributions of scientists or physicians from many nations. The concept of dialysis was discovered in Scotland by Thomas Graham (1805–1869) who, in 1861, noticed a semipermeable membrane could separate colloids from crystalloids. He described that this method, which he termed dialysis, could separate salt and urea from the blood. However, this process would not be possible for 100 more years. Parallel to his observation was the discovery of the explosive, gun cotton, in 1846, and a tamer agent known as collodion. This substance was also a cellulose nitrate that was used for wound dressings and in the new field of photography. The film was also attempted in a dialysis experiment. In 1913, John Jacob Abel (1859–1938) and two assistants, Leonard George Roundtree (1883–1959) and Benjamin Turner (1871–1945), successfully completed a dialysis procedure in dogs using hirudin prepared from leeches with collodion membranes. A journalist for *The Times* of London coined the term "artificial kidney" to describe this event, and it was later mentioned in the January 12, 1914, edition of *The New York Times*. When the procedure was attempted in a human patient, it failed, and the concept was abandoned.

Dialysis would never have been possible without an anticoagulant. In 1916, Jay Maclean, a medical student volunteering in the Johns Hopkins laboratory of William Henry Howell, described an anticoagulant that was called heparin. Although it was first discovered in liver tissues, its main site of production is in the intestines and lung [4]. Collodion was replaced as a potential dialysis membrane by regenerated cellulose. Cellophane was not commercially profitable for DuPont until 1927 when a process was implemented that would make it waterproof. Meanwhile, in 1925, Erwin Freund founded the Visking company and used regenerated cellulose to wrap sausage. It was this product that found its way into the dialysis world [4, 5].

The news of heparin and Visking's sausage wrapping as potential products in the artificial kidney reached Willem Kolff of the Netherlands, who between 1939 and 1943 created a wooden rotating drum dialysis machine wrapped with 20 meters of sausage casing. His dialysis efforts were not met with success until 1945. After World War II, he sent prototype machines around the world. When speaking at Grand Rounds, he met George Thorn and John Merrill of the Peter Bent Brigham Hospital (The Brigham), who teamed with him to create a stainless steel version of the machine – the Kolff-Brigham kidney. By 1948, 40 stainless steel Kolff-Brigham kidneys were manufactured and shipped around the world [6].

By the 1950s, dialysis became more commonplace but was mainly used to treat acute renal failure – now termed acute kidney injury (AKI). Often, as a consequence of nephrotoxic medications, trauma, or surgery, dialysis would sustain the patient through a critical period and give the kidneys a chance to recover. While first considered a deluxe toy, dialysis proved itself a useful lifesaving procedure during the Korean War as a major tool to treat AKI related to battle field injuries.

Belding Scribner, a physician in Seattle, identified that the reason dialysis could only be performed temporarily was because of the access used. Along with engineer Wayne Quinton, he developed a U-shaped detachable Teflon shunt that could be placed in the artery and vein and connected to dialysis tubing for each treatment. In March 1960, he dialyzed Clyde Shields, a 39-year-old machinist. Shields lived an additional 11 years, initially dialyzing for 24 h every fifth day. His fifth patient, Tim Albers, survived an additional 36 years. Scribner and his patients demonstrated that dialysis could be useful not just for AKI but for patients with end-stage renal disease (ESRD). By January 1962, there were not enough dialysis beds to accommodate all of the chronic patients who needed therapy. Stringent criteria were established to determine who could qualify for lifesaving treatment. In November 1962, a journalist, Shana Alexander, published an article in *Life Magazine* titled "They Decide Who Lives, Who Dies: Medical Miracle and a Moral Burden of a Small Committee." This article was a wake-up call for the public that there was a therapy that would reverse an otherwise terminal disease yet a lack of resources available to provide for the need.

Scribner, as part of the Washington sector of dialysis innovation, played key roles in the development of home dialysis, the dialysis machine we use today, and, along with colleagues such as Joseph Eschbach, Henry Tenckhoff, and Wayne Quinton, made sentinel advances in the management of anemia, home peritoneal, and chronic dialysis care [7, 8].

John Putnam Merrill, an internist and cardiologist, initially scoffed at the "chore" of dialysis that he felt should be assigned to surgeons. But in accepting this chore, he created the subspecialty of nephrology. In the past several years, there has been a doubling in the number of nephrologists in the USA. In 1999, there were 4718 nephrologists, and in 2013, the last reporting period, there were 9007 nephrologists [9].

Merrill relegated the "chore" to fellows, namely, Eugene Schupak, Constantine "Gus" Hampers, and Ted Hagar. As fellows, their task was to purchase sausage casing from Oscar Meyer and wrap it around the drum and as well mix the chemicals for each dialysis procedure. The camaraderie between the trio survived their fellowship days. In 1965, the six dialysis stations at The Brigham could not provide for the burgeoning dialysis needs of the entire New England area, and additional programs were established by Hampers and Hagar at Normandy House, an extended care facility in 1966, and the Babcock Center in 1970. Care was provided at a fraction of the cost of hospital care. In 1968, National Medical Care (NMC) was established with approval of George Thorn, John Merrill, and Joseph E. Murray. It developed into a profitable business, and by 1970, NMC had four centers and generated profits of US$ 265,546 on 2 million dollars revenue. In 1984, NMC was purchased by WR Grace, and in 1996 it was sold to Fresenius Medical Care (FMC). It currently has a nearly US$ 23 billion market cap and owns or operates 3971 dialysis centers worldwide with its global headquarters in Bad Homburg, Germany [10].

Today, there are over 400,000 patients who dialyze in one of the 7749 dialysis centers in the USA. A majority dialyze within two major large dialysis organizations (LDOs), Fresenius or DaVita, which have 70% of the market share [11].

DaVita was started as Medical Ambulatory Care, Inc. in 1979 but was purchased by Donaldson Lufkin Jenrette in 1994. They recruited Victor Chaltiel (1941–2014), an ambitious businessman who was later a candidate for the mayor of Las Vegas. In 1994, the name changed to Total Renal Care (TRC) and became a public company the following year. It continued to expand, purchasing another dialysis company, Renal Treatment Centers in 1998. The integration was fraught with problems and TRC nearly went bankrupt. In recruiting a new CEO, Kent Thiry, the company reinvented itself and in 2000 emerged as DaVita. In July 2004, DaVita acquired Gambro Dialysis for 3.05 billion dollars and under Thiry became the second largest LDO. It currently has a market cap of US$ 9.3 billion [12]. It now has 2664 outpatient dialysis centers in the USA and 241 in other countries [13].

In 1997, the National Kidney Foundation (NKF), one of the largest national nephrology associations in the USA, published the first two in a series of clinical practice guidelines – the Dialysis Outcomes Quality Initiative – under the leadership of Garabed Eknoyan and Nathan Levin in an effort to standardize clinical and dialysis practices, improve outcomes and survival, and improve patient care efficiency by establishing a set of guidelines based on rigorous structured review and evidence-based medicine. The first guidelines centered around hemodialysis (HD) and peritoneal dialysis (PD) adequacy, anemia management, and vascular access. By 2000 the scope was broadened to encompass kidney disease, not just dialysis, and is presently referred to as the Kidney Disease Outcomes Quality Initiatives – KDOQI. In 2004, a worldwide guidelines project was established – Kidney Disease Improving Global Outcomes – KDIGO.

## Renal Diseases in the USA

According to the Centers for Disease Control and Prevention (CDC), approximately 15% of US adults or 37 million people are estimated to have CKD. Most adults with CKD do not know they have it and should be referred for nephrology care when diagnosed. CKD is most prevalent in people aged 65 years or older (~38%), slightly more common in women (15%) than men (12%), and more common in non-Hispanic blacks than non-Hispanic Asians and whites. In regard to ESRD, African Americans are about three times more likely than whites to develop ESRD. Approximately 125,000 people in the USA started treatment for ESRD, and more than 726,000 individuals were on dialysis or living with a kidney transplant in 2016. Unfortunately, more than 240 individuals die on dialysis daily [14].

The leading causes of chronic kidney disease (CKD) in adults are diabetes and hypertension. A major risk factor for the development of CKD is the development of AKI. Among patients with AKI, 31% will develop CKD within a year [15]. Other risk factors also include obesity, heart disease, glomerulonephritis, cystic kidney disease, chronic interstitial nephritis, family history of kidney disease, congenital conditions, and medications. Among children and adolescents less than 18 years of age in the USA, glomerulonephritis and polycystic kidney disease are the main causes of ESRD (https://www.usrds.org/2018/download/v2_c07_ESRD_Pediatric_18_usrds.pdf) [15].

Kidney disease is the tenth leading cause of premature death in the USA. In the last period for which data is available, 2016, there were 124,675 newly reported cases of ESRD. This constitutes a plateau over the past 5 years. The lifetime risk of being diagnosed with ESRD is 4% in males and 2.9% in females and ranges from a low of 2.3% in white females to 8.1% in black males. There were 726,331 prevalent cases of ESRD in 2016, the number increasing by 20,000 per year. The prevalence is 9.5 times greater in Hawaiians and Pacific islanders and 3.7 times greater in blacks than in whites [15].

Over the past 15 years, the ESRD population unadjusted death rate has decreased by 27% and is now down to 134 per 1000 patient-years for ESRD. Forty percent to 50% of patients die during the first 3 years. Of the 30 million people in the USA with CKD, only 1.56% will ever reach dialysis [15].

## Renal Replacement Therapy in the USA

Renal replacement therapy in the USA is done in centers via HD or at home with either PD or HD. When a patient with CKD has an estimated glomerular filtration rate (eGFR) less than 20 ml/min/1.73m$^2$, he or she is able to be listed and become eligible for a kidney transplant.

Sadly, in 2017, 35.4% of ESRD patients received minimal or no care from a nephrologist prior to starting dialysis. The mean eGFR at the initiation point of dialysis was 9.7 ml/min/1.73m$^2$ – down from 10.4 in 2010. Among incident patients, 87.3% began renal replacement therapy with HD and 9.7% with PD, and only 2.8% received a preemptive kidney transplant. Among prevalent dialysis patients, 29.6% have a functioning kidney transplant, 7.5% are treated with PD, and 63.15% of prevalent patients receive HD. Only 2.5% of patients do home HD [15].

## Hemodialysis

Staff assisted in center is the most common therapy in the USA – comprising 86.9% of all starting patients. A third (33.4%) of incident patients received no pre-ESRD or little pre-ESRD nephrology care, and 80% of HD patients start dialysis using an indwelling catheter. Dialysis times are generally 4 h three times a week with a blood flow of 450 ml/min if a successful fistula is in place. While reuse of dialyzers was once popular (in 1997, 82% of dialysis facilities participated in a reuse program), it is rarely if ever in use today [16]. Hemodiafiltration is not generally offered in the outpatient dialysis setting. The typical patient dialyzes three times a week in a large dialysis center. Mortality in the dialysis population has been steadily declining in the past 15 years. The adjusted death rate has decreased by 29% with patients over the age of 65 years old comprising 44% of the population. The mortality rate is 166 per 1000 patient-years for the HD population [15].

Governance of the dialysis facility is typically represented by the facility administrator, the medical director, and for the 70% of patients dialyzing in one of the two largest dialysis facilities, Fresenius North America and DaVita Kidney Care, a corporate representative – generally the regional operations director. On a monthly basis, the interdisciplinary team comprised of a nephrologist, the social worker, dietitian, and renal nurse meets to discuss individual patient care. A facility health meeting made up of the medical director, the clinical coordinator, the facility administrator, social worker, and dietitian meets to discuss trends and the processes in place to advance facility quality and continually improve outcomes.

## Home Hemodialysis

In 1963, John Merrill was able to demonstrate that patient's families could be trained to operate a dialysis machine and dialyze patients at home. The following year, Stanley Shaldon, while in London, was able to demonstrate that patients could not only successfully learn to manage their own dialysis but to dialyze overnight.

In Seattle, initial dialysis machines made use of a 380 liter stainless steel tank. The water and solutes were mixed and then stirred with canoe paddles. Albert "Les" Babb, a professor of nuclear and chemical engineering at the University of Washington, worked with Scribner to develop a machine that would mix fluid in a set ratio and recirculate it until it passed through the dialysis filter and could be discarded. The proportioning machine was born.

In 1964, Caroline Helm, a 16-year-old girl with lupus nephritis, developed the need for dialysis but did not qualify for in-center care because she fell below the minimum age of 18. But Caroline's father and Babb were friends, and for her, Babb developed a single patient machine with monitors and fail-safe devices. It even included a laminated front that would blend with the family furniture. This single patient proportioning machine became the prototype for nearly every dialysis unit now in existence. Two years later home dialysis was adopted in Seattle as a means of providing more dialysis to patients. Eventually 90% of Seattle patients were undergoing dialysis at home [17].

Despite its prominence in early dialysis care, home HD has not been utilized well in the USA. This may be due to multiple factors including lack of patients receiving pre-ESRD education. In a survey conducted by the American Association of Kidney Patients (AAKP), 32% responded that they were not educated about home dialysis. In the past 5 years, the percentage of patients who undergo home HD has been relatively flat, ranging from 1.6% in 2011 to 1.8% in 2016 [15].

## Peritoneal Dialysis

Of the home modalities in the USA, PD is most often chosen by patients. Although it was in use for the management of AKI in the 1940s, PD catheters were stiff, and without a suitable access, it could not be considered for chronic therapy. In 1968, Henry Tenckhoff developed the silastic implantable catheter, which was later modified by adding Dacron cuffs, which is in use today [17].

In Austin, Texas, during the 1970s, Robert Popovich and Jack Moncrieff pioneered the chronic ambulatory peritoneal dialysis (CAPD) procedures in use today. A further advancement was the development of plastic dialysis bags instead of glass bottles by Dimitri Oreopoulos in Toronto. Another pioneer, Zbylut Twardowski, developed a means to measure PD equilibrium and use it in patient management and a grading system for exit sites [18]. Automated peritoneal dialysis (APD) is possible because of the HomeChoice machine, created through the clever ingenuity of Dean Kamen in collaboration with Baxter.

PD has lower mortality rates than HD (153.5 vs 166.3 all cause prevalent mortality per 1000 patient-years). In 2017, 10.1% of incident ESRD patients started with PD. The prevalence of PD is only 7.1%. Most current figures demonstrate that in 2017 52,630 were undergoing either APD (the vast majority) or CAPD. In the years between 2001 and 2016, the adjusted mortality rate fell by 28% in HD but 43% in PD patients. The 3-year survival odds at 3 years are 70% for PD and 57% for HD. The lower mortality for PD may be explained by patient selection; those who select PD must have the dexterity and cognitive skills to manage it by themselves on a more or less constant basis. PD is more economical, and based on US Renal Data System (USRDS) data, a year of HD costs approximately US$ 72,000, while PD costs US$ 53,000 [15].

## Government Involvement in Dialysis

By 1961, Belding Scribner had established the first outpatient dialysis unit in the world, a three-station outpatient center in the nursing residence basement of the Swedish Hospital. Soon, the center was at capacity, and the Seattle Artificial Kidney Center (now Northwest Kidney Center) was built. Of 30 candidates, only 10 could be accepted, and the rest would die. The *Life Magazine* feature by Shana Alexander highlighted the problem in 1962, and the veterans administration established 30 dialysis centers. Edwin Newman's 1965 NBC television documentary, "Who Shall Live?," sparked further interest in the program, and the Public Health Service set up a 5-year grant program, creating 12 more dialysis centers and 14 home programs the following year. When this program ended, it became regional. A government committee headed by Carl Gottschalk recommended government support for dialysis and kidney transplantation.

The National Association of Patients on Hemodialysis (NAPH) was created in October 1969 by Samuel Orenstein and William Blackton. They dialyzed together for 18 h a day in Brooklyn's Kings County Hospital dialysis unit and played a key role in persuading congress that dialysis could be feasible and safely done. In 1966, after undergoing dialysis training in Seattle, a young premed Stanford student, Andrew Peter Lundin, applied to medical schools across the country. Eli Friedman, Professor at SUNY Downstate Health Sciences University in Brooklyn and a pioneer in American dialysis, persuaded his admissions committee to accept Lundin, who while dialyzing alongside Orenstein and Blackton became a practicing academic nephrologist. He had been active in the NAPH from its beginnings and died in 2001. Simultaneously, George Schreiner, also a major pioneer in American dialysis and a member of the Gottschalk Committee, was involved in the National Kidney Foundation (NKF). He invited his neighbor Charles Plante to become their lobbyist, and together they crafted the legislative policies that would place dialysis as a Medicare benefit. Schreiner testified before congress 30 times. To demonstrate to the Wilbur Mills Ways and Means Committee that it was safe and feasible, a dialysis patient, Shep Glazer, daringly dialyzed before them in the committee room in 1971. The result of the Gottschalk Committee, AAKP, NKF, and several others was that in October 30, 1972, congress amended the Social Security Act to include dialysis benefits (Public Law 92-603). The law became effective in July 1973 and is now the highest source of support for kidney patients.

It was projected that annual dialysis costs would never top 250 million dollars. In 2016, 35.4 billion dollars was spent on all ESRD care and 7.2% of all Medicare claims. Of this portion, 28 billion dollars is spent on dialysis alone. It is the most important revenue source for large dialysis organizations like DaVita, which receives 69% of its revenue from Medicare.

The Medicare program is under the auspices of the Centers for Medicare and Medicaid Services (CMS) and tasked with both certifying ESRD facilities and monitoring and recertifying those that meet basic conditions for coverage. The original conditions were adopted in 1976, and the updated version was published April 15, 2008.

These conditions stress flexibility with respect to implementing facility-specific outcome measures. The goals are to ensure protection of patients' rights and physical safety, patient satisfaction and engagement in care, and the elimination of unnecessary administrative policies. The focus is on the "continuous, interdisciplinary, integrated care system that a dialysis patient experiences, centered around patient assessment, care planning, service delivery and quality assessment, and performance improvement." The burden of responsibility for implementing and continuing policies that meet these objections is tasked to the facility governing body and medical director. As outlined in §494.150, the medical director must participate in staff training and performance assessments, in the development, review, and approval of and adherence to patient care policies and procedures. These procedures pertain to safety, infection control, as well as patient admissions, transfers, and discharges. It is estimated that 87% of approximately 9000 nephrologists in clinical practice serve as a medical director (http://dialysisunits.com).

## Dialysis Adequacy

Dialysis adequacy is determined in part by dialyzer membrane characteristics. Dialyzer technology rapidly moved from the large rotating drum to smaller and more compact devices. When in 1960 Clyde Shields was dialyzed, the device used was a parallel plate dialyzer that had been invented by Leonard Skeggs and Jack Leonards working in Cleveland. Frederic Kiil in Norway modified this dialyzer and made it popular for use when Scribner started the home dialysis program in 1964. Skeggs went on to invent the serial multiple analyzer (SMA), automating the chemistry analysis of serum samples and revolutionizing the way kidney disease could be identified. The coil dialyzer was developed by Kolff in 1956 after he moved to the USA and consisted of orange juice cans fitted to a Maytag washing machine. When Maytag forbad its commercial use, Travenol designed a machine of its own, the RSP (recirculating single pass) [4].

Although the hollow fiber technique was developed in the 1940s, it was never commercialized until Dow Chemical Company began to manufacture it for reverse osmosis. The hollow fiber technology was first used to manufacture cuprophane dialyzers by Cordis-Dow, in a joint venture with the Dow Chemical Company. However, biocompatibility was a problem as the cellulose-based dialyzers made of cuprophane or cellulose acetate led to amyloidosis. Union Carbide introduced polysulfones in 1965, and Fresenius capitalized on their superiority for clearing the beta microglobulins associated with amyloidosis. Hollow fiber membranes have now replaced all earlier dialyzers, and are highly efficient, biocompatible, and more compact.

In 1967, Frank Gotch, nephew of a legendary professional wrestler of the same name, along with John Sargent evaluated the characteristics of the Dow hollow fiber dialyzer and by 1974 had developed a kinetic modeling equation. Ten years after the introduction of chronic dialysis, there was no agreement as to what adequacy was. The National Cooperative Dialysis Study (NCDS) that began the following year was a prospective randomized trial performed to study the adequacy of dialysis. Patients were randomized to two different time-averaged urea concentrations, 50–90 mg/dL and 90–130 mg/dL. They were also randomized to shorter and longer treatment periods, 3 ± 0.5 and 5 ± 0.5 h. NCDS emphasized that the time on dialysis, the characteristics inherent in the dialyzer membrane, and the volume of distribution of total body water were functions of dialyzer clearance and time on treatment. Gotch concluded that Kt/V depended upon protein catabolism and was a predictor of dialysis failure. In 1985, the model suggested that the minimum adequate dose of three times weekly dialysis was single pool (sp) $spKt/V_{urea}$ of 1.0. For years nephrologists attempted to follow the NCDS strategy, a mistake falsely based on the age-old premise that urea was the major toxin of uremia. As dialysis treatments were shortened, the mortality rates rose.

In 1989, the Dallas Conference on Morbidity and Mortality in Hemodialysis was held and demonstrated that mortality rates decreased when dialysis times increased. The results resulted in the creation of a randomized control trial to determine the appropriate time for dialysis. The HEMO study looked at spKt/V groups of 1.71 and 1.32 and in 2001 concluded that a high dose offered no advantage; the NKF KDOQI guidelines have since established the minimum delivered $spKt/V_{urea}$ to be 1.2 and the target spKt/V to be 1.4 per HD session in patients treated three times a week. In the USA, these goals are being met. Only 3.5% of prevalent dialysis patients have a spKt/V less than 1.2. Nearly half of the patients (49%) have a spKt/V between 1.2 and 1.59, and 47.4% have a spKt/V greater than 1.6.

The frequency and duration of dialysis have been quantified and studied by Dialysis Outcomes and Practice Patterns Study (DOPPS). In the USA, 96.6% of patients currently dialyze three times a week. There has been no trend. It has also been shown that shortening the length of dialysis sessions is associated with a higher mortality rate. DOPPS has looked at 5203 prevalent dialysis patients and found that 30.8% dialyze less than 210 min, 39.6% dialyze between 210 and 240 min, and 29.7% dialyze over 4 h. In 2010, 22.4% of patients dialyzed over 240 min, representing an upward trend.

## The Arteriovenous Access

In 1966, Michael Brescia and James Cimino along with Kenneth Appel and Baruch Hurwich reported a technique to create a fistula between the artery and vein in the arm and successfully cannulate it with a #14 needle. Cimino later reported he got the idea from a surgical procedure developed at the Mayo Clinic in the 1930s to increase blood flow in the limbs of polio victims (Oct 1, 2006, Renal and Urology News). The procedure has been a success and continues to be the gold standard for access. In the USA, 73.2% of accesses are arteriovenous (AV) fistulas.

Synthetic vascular grafts created from a stretched form of polytetrafluoroethylene (Gore-Tex) has been in use since around 1969 and substituted for the Brescia-Cimino fistula 16.6% of the time in the USA [15]. They do not last as long or permit as high a blood flow and have a higher rate of infection when compared to AV fistulae.

Patients are recommended to have AV fistulas in place for their access as part of a national vascular access improvement initiative – the Fistula First Initiative (FFI) – established in 2003 by CMS. Through education and support, the rate of fistula placement has steadily improved. However, still many fistulas that are placed fail [19], and as a result, 12.1% of US patients require dialysis through a catheter [20]. The continued use of a catheter is the result of either patient preference, exhaustion of sites, or lack of stability to undergo access surgery. Some patients have extensive peripheral vascular disease by the time they reach the point of requiring dialysis; thus it becomes difficult to place permanent access.

Catheter disadvantages include an increased incidence of infection and a lower maximum blood flow than other forms of access. They also have higher hospitalization rates and are costlier, mainly because a nurse is required to initiate treatment in catheter patients. In addition to complications, the presence of a dialysis catheter is associated with a higher mortality rate in dialysis patients.

The ideal scenario is for patients to be closely followed and carefully managed by the nephrologist for several years, receive extensive education regarding dialysis modalities, and after making a selection, transition to dialysis with a permanent access in place. Unfortunately, this is not always the case. Patients who have not been adequately educated on dialysis modalities during the earlier stages of disease often present to a hospital acutely ill but only rarely have a fistula placed during the initial admission because of financial payment disincentives. Patients with ESRD secondary to hypertension are less likely than diabetic patients to receive pre-ESRD education. Furthermore only 13.3% of patients who received pre-ESRD education received dietary instruction. Patients without education were less prepared for dialysis and more likely to start with an indwelling catheter rather than the preferred AV fistula. USRDS reports data from 2016 that 80% of newly diagnosed patients initiate HD with a catheter and that at 90 days 69% are still using the catheter. Only 17% of patients initiate dialysis with an AV fistula in the USA. It is a relief to know that at the end of 2 years 71% of HD patients have a working AV fistula in place. Around 50% of incident patients start dialysis with an eGFR between 5 and <10 ml/min/1.73$m^2$, while around 29% initiate treatment when the eGFR is between 10 and <15 [15].

Poor access planning and surgical technique are both barriers to higher fistula rates, and 39% of fistulas fail to sufficiently mature for use. Of those that do mature, the median time to first use is 108 days. AV access accounts for 9.2% hospitalizations, 8.5% readmissions within 30 days, and 7.6% of emergency room admissions [15]. Although, historically, the emphasis has been to place an AV fistula, elderly patients have a slower maturation time and a higher degree of access failures and require more careful planning. Additionally, some patients may not have adequate arterial blood flow because of peripheral vascular disease [15].

## Hospitalizations

Despite the conditions for coverage and their requirement that continuous quality improvement processes be put into place, some indicators that reflect both increased expenses to the Medicare system and quality of life for patients are not improving rapidly and signify that an ongoing challenge exists. According to the July 2014 DOPPS data, the mean percentage of ESRD facilities with hospitalization claims over a 6-month period was 38.4%. The percentage of ESRD beneficiaries with at least one hospitalization claim was 12.9% [8].

In 2016, Medicare was the primary spender for US – 10.2 *billion of in patient care. That was nearly as much as it spent as the US* – 11.1 billion as primary payer for outpatient services. The USRDS reports that adjusted hospital admission rates have declined 15% over the past 9 years, from 2.0 to 1.7 per patient-year. Reasons for hospitalizations often relate to the complexity of comorbidities attendant in a population that reaches the most advanced stages of disease. The serum albumin is an index of chronic illness [21]. The USRDS reported that in a sample of HD patients from May 2017, 18.9% had serum albumin levels less than 3.5 g/dL.

The most likely cause for a hospital encounter in ESRD patients is infection [15]. The number of hospital days per patient-year for infection is 3.6. Septicemia is the most frequent cause of admission, readmission, and emergency visit – 9.3%, 8.6%, and 9.2%, respectively [15]. The risk of having bacteremia in a patient on HD is 26 times higher than in the general population, and the dialysis catheter is the most common site of infection [22]. Newer therapies are emerging to reduce the incidence of catheter-related infections. The ClearGuard HD antimicrobial barrier cap was compared with the Tego connector plus Curos disinfecting cap and demonstrated a significantly lower incidence of blood stream infection (0.28 vs 0.75 positive blood cultures/1000 central venous catheter days $p = 0.001$) [23].

Hospitalizations are highest in the first year of dialysis, suggesting that CKD education and preparation for either a preemptive transplant or the desired modality may lessen transition costs even further [15].

Even more daunting is the frequency of 30-day readmissions for hospital patients. Roughly 37% of patients who were admitted to the hospital were readmitted within 30 days between the periods of 2014 and 2016. This percentage is relatively steady; between 2007 and 2011 39% were readmitted. The USRDS demonstrates that readmissions for cardiovascular disease are 39.2%. Many (45.8%) of the readmissions are to treat cardiovascular in contrast to a new condition, a reflection of the chronicity of this disorder. Although constituting only 2.6% of the reasons for hospitalization, 41.9% of those sustaining an acute myocardial infarction account are readmitted following discharge. Stroke patients are also frequently readmitted, 40.9%. Stroke patients also have a 30-day post-discharge mortality of 7.8% [15].

The expense of end of life treatment practices in the USA for patients with ESRD is increasing. Despite that 23.3% of ESRD patients withdraw from dialysis, and 26% enroll in hospice care before death, and 39% of ESRD patients die in the hospital. Fifty-five percent are seen by at least 10 physicians and 62% by at least 5 specialties during their final 90 days. Most recently, the median number of days these ESRD patients spend in the hospital is 15 days. Sixty-three percent of patients with ESRD are admitted to a critical care unit during the final 90 days of life. The median cost in the year of death per person of ESRD patient was $103,932 in 2015, with $7687 being in the final week of life [15].

## Heart Disease and Volume

In 2009, a 20th anniversary meeting of Dallas Conference on Morbidity and Mortality was held on April 23, at the Sheraton Boston Hotel to look at factors that were determining patient care. At the time the meeting was held, dialysis mortality was 20% per year with hospital costs exceeding $20,000 per patient. Less than 20% of patients were rehabilitated. Myocardial fibrosis emerged as a major culprit in the high mortality and was felt as the result of poor blood pressure control and a failure to achieve euvolemia. It was acknowledged that normalization of blood pressure and intravascular volume was difficult with conventional dialysis and that in addition to modifying dialysis schedules, reducing sodium and repeated dietary counseling would be necessary [24].

In the USA, angiotensin-converting enzyme (ACE) inhibitors or angiotensin-receptor blocker (ARB) therapy is prescribed in 59.9% of patients with heart failure. Cardiovascular disease occurs in 64.5% of patients with CKD who are ≥66 years old. It is associated with a shortened survival; only 59% of patients ≥66 years old with stage 4–5 CKD who sustain an acute myocardial infarction survive 2 years. When it is present, congestive heart failure is an independent mortality risk factor in CKD and is associated with a 2-year survival probability of 77.8%. 23.8% of CKD patients have atrial fibrillation, but around 50% of patients with heart failure and CKD have atrial fibrillation. In the USA, 30.9% of patients with atrial fibrillation and CKD are treated with anticoagulants. Peripheral vascular disease occurs in 25.2% of CKD patients, and a stroke or transient ischemic attack is also more common, occurring in 16.1% of CKD patients in contrast to 6.7% of patients ≥66 years old without CKD [20].

Using DOPPS data and looking at treatment times and ultrafiltration rates in 22,000 HD patients, Saran et al. published in 2006 that every 30-min longer period on HD was associated with a 7% lower relative risk of mortality (RR = 0.93 $p < 0.0001$). Ultrafiltration removal of over 10 ml/kg per hour was associated with a higher relative risk of mortality (RR = 1.09 $p = 0.02$) and an odds ratio for intradialytic hypotension of 1.30 ($p = 0.045$) [20]. In 2015, Flythe et al. published that post-dialysis weights that exceeded the target by 2 kg in at least 30% of treatments were associated with an adjusted hazard ratio of 1.28 (95% CI 1.15–1.43) and completing dialysis treatments with a weight below the target weight by 2 kg resulted in an adjusted hazard ratio of 1.22 (95% CI 1.05–1.4) for all-cause mortality [25]. It is well established that removing volume at high ultrafiltration rates is associated with a higher mortality [26]. Greater than 13 ml/kg/hour is associated with a relative risk of mortality of 1.59 (95% CI 1.29–

1.96) [27]. In the Feb 2019 DOPPS study, of 5145 patients, the intradialytic weight loss was 2.68% per treatment. For a 70 kg patient, this would compute to 1.88 kg, which if removed over a 4-hour treatment would be 470 ml/hour or 6.7 ml/kg/hour [20]. Regrettably, many hospital visits are for volume overload. The hospitalization rate for cardiovascular disease is 2.6 per patient-year and represents a continued challenge for nephrologists [15].

## CKD Mineral and Bone Disorder (CKD-MBD)

Among complex disorders associated with advancing kidney disease are those that surround the metabolism of the tightly regulated divalent cation, calcium. As kidney disease advances, the renal tubular cell production of 1-alpha hydroxylase decreases, resulting in a marked decrease in the hydroxylation of 25-hydroxyvitamin D (3) to its active form. Active vitamin D is essential for cell differentiation, the modulation of immune responses, and both the transcellular and paracellular absorption of calcium from the gastrointestinal tract [28]. It participates in a feedback loop that controls the synthesis of parathyroid hormone (PTH), an 84 amino acid that regulates calcium absorption from bone through an indirect stimulation of osteoclasts. In CKD, the elevated serum phosphorus stimulates FGF23 to rise and modulate phosphorus excretion, but as the disease progresses, the serum phosphorus also rises. The high serum phosphorus turns on transcription factors that deposit calcium into the media of vascular smooth muscle cells. In the patient with abnormal kidneys, bone calcium falls, and calcium abnormally deposits in the blood vessel media. This pathology results in vascular calcification, aortic valve disease, vascular stiffness, and increased bone fractures [29]. Management strategies are to reduce serum phosphorus and prevent or treat the rise in PTH. Popular therapies are the use of phosphate binders, vitamin D analogs, and a calcimimetic.

In the USA, the most popular vitamin D receptor analog is doxercalciferol, being used 84.2% of the time in the DOPPS dialysis sample, as compared with 15.8% use for paricalcitol. At the time of reporting, calcitriol use was zero. Twenty-nine percent of dialysis patients are on a calcimimetic, although in its oral form, cinacalcet, it was sometimes poorly tolerated. A newer parenteral calcimimetic, etelcalcetide, is in use 6.1% of the time [20].

Serum phosphorus remains a challenge to control. 23.5% of dialysis patients are in the 3.5–4.5 mg/dL range, while 26.3% are between 4.6 and 5.5 mg/dL. 42.7% have serum phosphorus values greater than 5.5 mg/dL and in 22.4% are between 5.0% and 5.4% [20].

## Serum Potassium

In 61.0% of ESRD patients the serum potassium is between 3.5 and 4.9 mEq/L, and in 23%, it is between 5.0 and 5.4 mEq/L. 11% have a serum potassium greater than 5.5 mEq/L. An elevated potassium greater than 5.5 mEq/L indicates for the most part either dietary indiscretion or inadequate dialysis, and for years the standard has been to supplement selected patient with persistent hyperkalemia with sodium polystyrene sulfate [20]. Now, there are now two newer medications that have been successfully tested in the ESRD population. In patients with multiple episodes of hyperkalemia, patiromer on a daily basis statistically reduces the serum potassium by −0.5 mEq/L over a follow-up period, the median of which was 141 days [30]. Sodium zirconium cyclosilicate was studied in an ESRD population on a once daily basis on non-dialysis days. Forty one percent (41.2%) in the zirconium responded compared to 1.0% of placebo. Serious adverse events were roughly the same 7% vs 8% in the zirconium and placebo groups. Both groups had comparable interdialytic weight gains, and the drug was well tolerated [31].

## Renal Transplantation

Valley Forge General Hospital was a major casualty center for battlefield injuries near Philadelphia during World War II. It was here that the noted plastic surgeon, Joseph E. Murray, working as an Army surgeon, developed a keen interest in immunology and the skin. On December 23, 1954, Murray, now a surgeon at the Peter Bent Brigham Hospital, performed the first kidney transplant. It was between 24-year-old identical twins, and the recipient lived an additional 9 years without immunosuppression. He also pioneered cadaveric transplantation and the use of immunosuppressants in organ transplantation. In 1990, he was awarded the Nobel Prize in Physiology or Medicine.

Today, there are 231 transplant centers in the USA. As of December 31, 2016, there were 81,418 dialysis patients waiting for a transplant. 20,161 transplants were performed in 2016, 28% from living donors. There were 215,061 patients who have a functioning kidney transplant as of that date. The probability of 1-year survival with a living related donor is 99% and 96% for a deceased donor [15].

Kidney transplantation consists of either living or deceased donors. Advances have been made in both, yet there is a wide gap between those persons who are on a waiting list and the numbers of available kidneys. With respect to living donors, kidney-paired donations have enabled families and friends to indirectly donate to an individual when the kidney is not a biocompatible match. They can thus donate to a second individual who is a compatible recipient provided a prospective donor for that individual can donate back. While even more complex pairing systems can be arranged, the net result is that each recipient receives a biocompatible living donor kidney, even if from a stranger.

Kidneys that have been harvested from decedents are allocated to recipients by computer matching, managed through the Organ Procurement and Transplantation Network (OPTN) under strict policies. OPTN is government based and managed by the United Network for Organ Sharing (UNOS). Recipients are active candidates on a registered waiting list. To fairly allocate how deceased donor kidneys are appropriated, they are first indexed. The computer instruction set compares the data on the deceased organ donor with data on the waiting list and ranks candidate recipients according to OPTN policies. Since the time spent on the waiting list is counted toward the appropriation priority, early referral is advised. The Kidney Donor Profile Index (KDPI) established in 2014 combines a variety of donor factors into an index that helps establish how long the donor kidney is expected to function. The lower the score the better the predicted function. In general, 65% of deceased donor kidneys have KDPI between 21% and 85% and can be expected to function around 9 years, while a KDPI greater than 85% may be predicted to function only greater than 5½ years. The Estimated Post-Transplant Survival (EPTS) score is assigned to all active patients on the waiting list. It is based on the patient's time on dialysis, whether or not they are diabetic, whether or not they have had a previous kidney transplant, and their age. The score ranges from 0% to 100%. The ETPS score is used in tandem with the KDPI to match kidneys that have a longer predicted survival with appropriate candidates. Thus, an EPTS score of 20% or less will receive a higher priority of kidneys with a KDPI of 20% or less. In 2017 there were 92,685 patients on the waiting list for a kidney transplant [32].

Age in and of itself is not an exclusion for transplantation. In 2017, 23% of all US transplants were performed in persons over 65 years old. In 2018, there were 21,157 transplants recorded in the OPTN registry. Of these, 4419 were over 65 years old. 8259 transplants (38%) were performed in persons between the ages of 50 and 64. The trend toward transplanting older patients has increased. In 1988, only 212 of the 8878 transplants in the registry were in persons above age 65 [32].

The waiting time for a kidney transplant is a concerning long-term trend, as the time continues to increase. In 2017, 37.8% waited on the list over 3 years. 16.6% of patients have been on the list greater than 5 years [32]. The 2014 kidney allocation system (KAS) allows patients to start their waiting list time from the date of first dialysis.

There are racial disparities among prevalent transplant patients. When related to the number of prevalent African American patients on HD (141,383), only 44,002 have a functioning transplant (31%). This compares to 60% of white, 40% of Hispanic, and 59% of Asians. The reasons for these disparities are complex and may in part relate to provider awareness. The UNOS kidney allocation system changes that were implemented in December 2014 were designed to increase fairness in allocating kidneys and to also reduce the racial disparities. Disparities are being further addressed by the establishment of a clinical trial that involves educational materials for the staff and patients in 600 US dialysis facilities with low wait-listing [33]. However, all-cause graft loss in deceased donor kidney transplants has decreased from 51.4% to 30.6% [34].

Immunosuppression related to kidney transplantation is generally driven by the center's protocol. Most commonly, in high-risk patients – African Americans, panel-reactive antibody tests greater than 20%, or who lost a previous transplant because of immunologic reasons – thymoglobulin is initiated intraoperatively. Tacrolimus is given as initial therapy when the fall in serum creatinine is 30% from baseline or when function delayed is started at the completion of thymoglobulin to a target of 50–75% of goal level until a recovery in kidney function. Our center also uses mycophenolate mofetil (MMF) and corticosteroids. In non-high-risk patients, daclizumab or basiliximab is used instead of thymoglobulin. A steroid sparing can be used with thymoglobulin induction in non-high-risk patients. Our center uses tacrolimus with a goal of 8–10 ng/mL for the first 30 days and 7–9 ng/mL for the next 60 days. From the 90th day to the completion of 1 year, our goal is 6–8 ng/mL and 4–8 ng/mL after 1 year. We also use MMF and prednisone – 30 mg daily for the first 2 weeks and tapering by 5 mg every 2 weeks until 10 mg daily. At the 180th day, patients with good graft function who are not on a steroid-sparing regimen are placed on 5 mg daily of prednisone. Our protocol also addresses anti-infectious, gastrointestinal, cardiac, and osteoporosis prophylaxis.

## Pediatric Nephrology

The pediatric nephrologist encounters a different spectrum of disease than adult counterparts, as they must diagnose and treat a variety of congenital disorders as well. Congenital anomalies of the kidney and the urinary tract (CAKUT) occur as a disruptive process of urologic development and account for the majority of cases of CKD and ESRD in children. The malformations vary from renal agenesis to horseshoe kidneys and duplication of the ureter [35]. The number of children with ESRD has decreased from 17.5 per million to 12.9 per million by 2017. The total number of incident ESRD patients under 21 years old was 1319 for 2017. Of those 51.3%

received HD, 27.8% PD, and 20.8% a renal transplant. There are currently 9667 prevalent ESRD patients, 16.6% of whom are on HD and 10.1% on PD. 73.3% have received a kidney transplant. 44.7% of patients under 21 years old receive pre-ESRD for greater than 12 months, but there are still 19.1% of pediatric patients who receive no care at all. In contrast to adults, the mean eGFR for pediatrics is 14.0 ml/min/1.73m$^2$. 41.5% receive dietary care.

The North American Pediatric Renal Trials and Collaborative Studies (NAPRTCS) registry of dialysis patients demonstrates that focal segmental glomerulosclerosis occurs in 14.3% of patients, while a dysplastic or hypodysplastic kidneys occur 13.9% of the time. The third most common cause of renal abnormalities in children is obstructive uropathy, which occurs 12.6% of the time. Reflux nephropathy occurs in 3.5% of patients, hemolytic uremic syndrome in 3.0%, while chronic glomerulonephritis and congenital nephrotic syndrome occur in 2.9 and 2.6 percent of dialysis patients. The NAPRTCS database reveals that pediatric dialysis patients initiating dialysis have a height $z$-score < 2 standard deviations less than average and are hypertensive. The most common cause of death was cardiopulmonary disease with young age, growth deficits, and black race predicting a poorer prognosis for survival. Survival increased significantly between the 2002–2011 and the earlier 1992–2001 cohorts [36].

## Other Renal Diseases

The nephrologist follows a variety of kidney disorders as part of his or her daily routine. These include glomerular disorders, inherited disease, interstitial nephritis secondary to medications, and acid-base/electrolyte abnormalities. Hospital-based nephrologists deal with fluid management and a variety of critical care issues, acute acid-base disorders and AKI. These next few paragraphs will highlight a few of these conditions.

The incidence of glomerular disorders was examined in 2016 in a Medicare and an employer health plan. It was found that the incidence of secondary glomerular disease – that related to a primary non-renal systemic disorder – was 134 per 100,000 in the Medicare cohort and 10 per 100,000 in the employer health plan. Primary glomerular disorders occurred in 57 per 100,000 in the Medicare and 20 per 100,000 in the health plan cohorts. Primary glomerulonephritis patients are more likely to progress to ESRD than secondary glomerulonephritis patients in both the health plan 46.2 vs 19.5 and Medicare 72.9 vs 24.1. Data for Medicare demonstrated that the death rate was higher in secondary glomerulonephritis patient 186.1 vs 127.2 in the Medicare population. It was also noted that hospitalization rates were substantially higher in glomerulonephritis patient [37].

The prevalence of kidney stones in the USA is 10.6% for men and 7.1% for women. The incidences of kidney stones rise with age, peaking in 60–69-year-old men at 19.1% and women 9.4%. Kidney stones are more common in a southern latitude with a higher sunlight index. It is not clear whether oxalate in vegetables is associated with a higher kidney stone incidence. However, the incidence rises with sugar-sweetened sodas, animal protein intake and supplemental calcium (in men), and decreased fluid intake. It decreases with increased fluid intake, increased dietary calcium intake, coffee and tea consumption, and fresh fruit intake. Kidney stones are associated with cardiovascular disease, the metabolic syndrome, hypertension, and diabetes. They are associated with CKD. As expected, kidney stone patients have a higher hospitalization rate, especially emergency department visits [38].

Polycystic kidney disease is a single gene disorder that is autosomal dominant, reportedly prevalent in 1 in 400 to 1 in 1000 live births, and has been calculated to affect greater than 10 million persons worldwide. In the USA, the incidence has been studied in Olmstead County and is 2.06/100,000 person-years. In a rare variant, the prevalence is estimated to be 1 in 26,500 live births in North, Central and South America [39].

Alport syndrome is a rare X-linked disease that in 805 of patients is caused by mutations in the COL4A5 gene, affecting type 4 collagen in glomeruli. It leads to progressive renal failure, is associated with hearing loss, and occurs mainly in men [40]. Clinical trials for therapy related to Alport syndrome are underway.

Diseases such as Bartter syndrome (prevalence 1/1,000,000) and Gitelman syndrome (prevalence 1/40,000) are uncommonly encountered by the nephrologist. They are each caused by gene mutations that affect tubular transport in either the thick ascending limb, as in Bartter syndrome, or the distal convoluted tubule [41]. Other disorders such as Fabry disease are uncommon. Nephrologists in both an inpatient and an outpatient setting must deal with hemo-mediated kidney injury, acute kidney injury, and interstitial nephritis that are related to drug-induced nephrotoxicity. Treatments vary, but acute kidney disorders are usually reversible by removing their underlying cause [42].

## Nephrology Practice in the USA

In the USA, after completing 2–3 years of nephrology fellowship, individuals start clinical practice in either private or academic sectors. Some graduates may pursue an extra year of fellowship to specialize in transplant and then pursue one of the above two models for transplant practice.

In the private practice spectrum, physicians either go in to solo practice or join smaller- to medium-sized groups ranging from 2 to 4 partners or larger groups with 5+ individuals. Each practice consists of physicians and physician extenders that see patients in the clinic, dialysis centers, hospitals, and often in interventional access centers. Private practice is more likely to be associated with business opportunities that include ownership or joint ventures into dialysis clinics (15.7% vs 4.1%), ambulatory surgery centers, and interventional access centers (5% vs 2.5%) than academic practices. Private practice physicians also participate in medical directorships (33.9% vs 15.6%) but conduct clinical research trials less commonly (8.3% vs 57.4%). Some private practice physicians elect to assume teaching responsibilities in local medical schools and may opt for non-tenured clinical tract with respect to academic appointments. Almost half (47.1%) of the physicians elect to join either a group practice nephrology or multispecialty clinic. 52.9% of men and 38.7% of women elect to go into private practice. 60.6% of group practice nephrologists have weekend call 13 times or more each year, in contrast to only 24.1% academic nephrologists. 39.1% of group and 18.1% of academic nephrologists have night call greater than 26 or more weeks per year. The average annual salary for the private practice nephrologist is US$ 207,176 vs US$ 176,438 for academia [43].

In the academic model, individuals join nephrology departments at large academic centers and balance duties between clinical practice, research, and training. Naturally, in the academic setting, direct involvement with trainees exists, providing excellent opportunities for teaching and for shaping future nephrologists. With respect to research, academic nephrologists conduct either clinical research or basic science investigations, and some combine both along with clinical practice. A tenured appointment for an academic position offers much greater security than a clinical appointment. About half (47.1%) of nephrologists completing their renal fellowship training enter academic medicine, the same as for private practice. 53.8% are women and 42.4% are men. 5.8% of fellows align with neither tract. Academic physicians receive more support for career development opportunities (37.3% vs 16.9%) and Visa sponsorships (18.6% vs 13.6%). Sign-on bonuses (28% vs 5.1%) and income guarantees (33.2% vs 16.9%) are more likely to accompany private group practice in contrast to academia. Academic physicians are less likely to be dissatisfied with work hours (23.5% vs 35%) and work life balance (26.1% vs 33.6%). Academic nephrologists are more likely to recommend nephrology to medical students and residents (81% vs 69.7%) [43].

Regardless, unfortunately women are currently paid less than men in both settings $206,043 vs $175,152. According to an ASN survey, 25% of all nephrologists are unhappy with their salaries but find the intellectual challenges and relationships with patients highly rewarding [43].

Salaries for dialysis nurses in the USA vary but are generally between US$ 72,000 per year and US$ 95,000 per year. Nurse practitioners are compensated at a higher rate, around US$ 107,000 per year [44].

## Future Perspectives of Nephrology in the USA

We have come a long way from 1961 when Belding Scribner established the first outpatient dialysis unit in the world. It was not until 12 years later, during Richard Nixon's reelection campaign, that Congress passed Public Law 92-603 extending Medicare coverage to individuals with ESRD requiring HD or transplantation.

What followed PL 92-603 was various policy and payment models over the years to improve patient care and physician reimbursement. Since then, dialysis has become the most expensive item that Medicare reimburses, and there are challenges for the program to add value as well as improve the quality of life and well-being for ESRD patients. Recently, there has been more movement and encouragement for increasing preventative care and education in CKD and improving access and rates of kidney transplantation. What is being evaluated is incorporating various incentives to help build this framework and improve access to care for this vulnerable population. A major impetus is on home dialysis. Thus, we have come full circle, as the original models of dialysis therapy envisioned strong home programs.

However, despite that patients are starting dialysis at an older age, the trends toward mortality in dialysis are improving as we discover better ways to care for patients. As our population ages, renal replacement therapy must adapt to accommodate the need for quality life and a minimized burden of care.

As we advance care, we will discover several innovations along the way. An innovation initiative known as KidneyX (https://www.kidneyx.org) is a public-private partnership between the US Department of Health and Human Services and the American Society of Nephrology. It recently awarded a $75,000 prize to a team of collaborators, Shuvo Roy and William Frissell, to accelerate their development of an implantable dialysis device. Victor Gura, a nephrologist in Los Angeles, has developed an ergonomic miniature dialysis machine that is wearable. His machine weighs less than 10 pounds, is operated by 9-volt batteries, and uses less than 400 ml of fluid. A clinical trial was conducted between 2014 and 2016 [45].

The innovative concepts to manage patients with ESRD lie in the field of bioengineering, where steps in developing bioengineered organs and tissues for clinical use are being investigated [46]. Teams are investigating how to harvest stem cells from a prospective kidney transplant and implant them into the blastocyst of an animal made deficient of kidney genes. As the animal develops, a phenotypic human kidney is generated that is immunologically compatible with the recipient and can be transplanted back. A proof of concept has been demonstrated by implanting pluripotential stem cells from a mouse into a Sall1-targeted anephric rat [47]. Other tissues and organs are being studied by other groups, and technical challenges are slowly being hurdled [48].

## Conclusion

Nephrologists in the USA provide dialysis care to over 450,000 patients and manage over 200,000 functioning transplants. The fascinating development of technologies makes the care of patients with ESRD gratifying. Despite our advances, we face major challenges – the burdensome cost of care, the lack of patients being started with a fistula, the fact that many patients are not being started on the modality they would choose if they were educated on their choices and managed earlier in the course of their disease, and the association of cardiovascular disease with CKD and the lack of transplantable kidneys. Efforts to increase home dialysis and education of CKD patients are underway. While it may sound like science fiction, there are several initiatives to develop more innovative ways to provide wearable and implantable dialysis machines and even to grow human kidneys for transplantation in another animal. Overall, the future to improve kidney disease is promising.

## References

1. Brookings Institute. 15 December 2019. Available from: https://www.brookings.edu/.
2. Changes in U.S. family finances from 2013 to 2016: evidence from the survey of consumer finances: The Federal Reserve System. Available from: https://www.federalreserve.gov/publications/files/scf17.pdf.
3. National Center for Health Statistics. 15 December 2019. Available from: https://www.cdc.gov/nchs/fastats/access-to-health-care.htm.
4. Fadem SZ. Issues in dialysis. 1st ed. New York: Nova Science Publishers; 2012. 361 p.
5. Cameron JS. The prehistory of haemodialysis as a treatment for uraemia. G Ital Nefrol. 2016;33(Suppl 66):33.S66.2.
6. Murphy WP Jr, Swan RC Jr, Walter CW, Weller JM, Merrill JP. Use of an artificial kidney. III. Current procedures in clinical hemodialysis. J Lab Clin Med. 1952;40(3):436–44.
7. Blagg CR. Belding Hibbard Scribner—better known as Scrib. Clin J Am Soc Nephrol. 2010;5(12):2146.
8. Blagg CR. The 50th anniversary of long-term hemodialysis: University of Washington Hospital, March 9th, 1960. J Nephrol. 2011;24(Suppl 17):S84–8.
9. Chronic Kidney Disease (CKD) Surveillance System – Centers for Disease Control and Prevention (CDC). 12 December 2019. Available from: https://nccd.cdc.gov/ckd/Default.aspx.
10. Fresenius Medical Care AG & Co. KGaA (FMS). Available from: https://finance.yahoo.com/quote/FMS/.
11. Shinkman R. The big business of dialysis care. NEJM Catalyst. 2016 https://catalyst.nejm.org/doi/full/10.1056/CAT.16.0826.
12. DaVita Inc. (DVA). Available from: https://finance.yahoo.com/quote/DVA/.
13. DaVita Inc 2018 Form 10-K Annual Report. 2018.
14. Chronic Kidney Disease in the United States – 2019. Atlanta: Centers for Disease Control and Prevention; 2019. Available from: https://www.cdc.gov/kidneydisease/pdf/2019_National-Chronic-Kidney-Disease-Fact-Sheet.pdf.
15. U.S. Renal Data System. USRDS 2018 annual data report volume 2: end-stage renal disease in the United States. Bethesda: National Institute of Health; 2018.
16. Denny GB, Golper TA. Does hemodialyzer reuse have a place in current ESRD care: "to be or not to be?". Semin Dial. 2014;27(3):256–8.
17. Fadem SZ. Milestones in dialysis in issues in dialysis. New York: Nova Science Publishers; 2012.
18. Prowant BF, Schmidt LM, Twardowski ZJ, Griebel CK, Burrows LK, Ryan LP, et al. Peritoneal dialysis catheter exit site care. ANNA J. 1988;15(4):219–23.
19. Ackad A, Simonian GT, Steel K, Parisi C, Mancini S, Douglas C, et al. A journey in reversing practice patterns: a multidisciplinary experience in implementing DOQI guidelines for vascular access. Nephrol Dial Transplant. 2005;20(7):1450–5.
20. DOPPS practice monitor: reporting contemporary trends in US dialysis practice. Ann Arbor: Arbor Research Collaborative for Health; 2019 [updated 2019, May]. Available from: https://www.dopps.org/dpm/.
21. Friedman AN, Fadem SZ. Reassessment of albumin as a nutritional marker in kidney disease. J Am Soc Nephrol. 2010;21(2):223–30.
22. Suzuki M, Satoh N, Nakamura M, Horita S, Seki G, Moriya K. Bacteremia in hemodialysis patients. World J Nephrol. 2016;5(6):489–96.
23. Brunelli SM, Van Wyck DB, Njord L, Ziebol RJ, Lynch LE, Killion DP. Cluster-randomized trial of devices to prevent catheter-related bloodstream infection. J Am Soc Nephrol. 2018;29(4):1336–43.
24. Parker TF 3rd, Glassock RJ, Steinman TI. Conclusions, consensus, and directions for the future. Clin J Am Soc Nephrol. 2009;4(Suppl 1):S139–44.
25. Flythe JE, Kshirsagar AV, Falk RJ, Brunelli SM. Associations of posthemodialysis weights above and below target weight with all-cause and cardiovascular mortality. Clin J Am Soc Nephrol. 2015;10(5):808–16.
26. Flythe JE, Brunelli SM. The risks of high ultrafiltration rate in chronic hemodialysis: implications for patient care. Semin Dial. 2011;24(3):259–65.
27. Flythe JE, Kimmel SE, Brunelli SM. Rapid fluid removal during dialysis is associated with cardiovascular morbidity and mortality. Kidney Int. 2011;79(2):250–7.
28. Christakos S, Dhawan P, Porta A, Mady LJ, Seth T. Vitamin D and intestinal calcium absorption. Mol Cell Endocrinol. 2011;347(1–2):25–9.
29. Chistiakov DA, Sobenin IA, Orekhov AN, Bobryshev YV. Mechanisms of medial arterial calcification in diabetes. Curr Pharm Des. 2014;20(37):5870–83.
30. Kovesdy CP, Rowan CG, Conrad A, Spiegel DM, Fogli J, Oestreicher N, et al. Real-world evaluation of patiromer for the treatment of hyperkalemia in hemodialysis patients. Kidney Int Rep. 2019;4(2):301–9.
31. Fishbane S, Ford M, Fukagawa M, McCafferty K, Rastogi A, Spinowitz B, et al. A phase 3b, randomized, double-blind, placebo-controlled study of sodium zirconium cyclosilicate for reducing the incidence of predialysis hyperkalemia. J Am Soc Nephrol. 2019;30:1723–33.
32. National Data – Organ Procurement and Transplantation Network. Richmond: UNOS; 2019.

33. Patzer RE, Smith K, Basu M, Gander J, Mohan S, Escoffery C, et al. The ASCENT (allocation system changes for equity in kidney transplantation) study: a randomized effectiveness-implementation study to improve kidney transplant waitlisting and reduce racial disparity. Kidney Int Rep. 2017;2(3):433–41.
34. Purnell TS, Luo X, Kucirka LM, Cooper LA, Crews DC, Massie AB, et al. Reduced racial disparity in kidney transplant outcomes in the United States from 1990 to 2012. J Am Soc Nephrol. 2016;27(8):2511–8.
35. Nicolaou N, Renkema KY, Bongers EMHF, Giles RH, Knoers NVAM. Genetic, environmental, and epigenetic factors involved in CAKUT. Nat Rev Nephrol. 2015;11(12):720–31.
36. Weaver DJ Jr, Somers MJG, Martz K, Mitsnefes MM. Clinical outcomes and survival in pediatric patients initiating chronic dialysis: a report of the NAPRTCS registry. Pediatr Nephrol. 2017;32(12):2319–30.
37. Wetmore JB, Guo H, Liu J, Collins AJ, Gilbertson DT. The incidence, prevalence, and outcomes of glomerulonephritis derived from a large retrospective analysis. Kidney Int. 2016;90(4):853–60.
38. Ziemba JB, Matlaga BR. Epidemiology and economics of nephrolithiasis. Investig Clin Urol. 2017;58(5):299–306.
39. Bergmann C, Guay-Woodford LM, Harris PC, Horie S, Peters DJM, Torres VE. Polycystic kidney disease. Nat Rev Dis Primers. 2018;4(1):50.
40. Kashtan CE, Ding J, Gregory M, Gross O, Heidet L, Knebelmann B, et al. Clinical practice recommendations for the treatment of Alport syndrome: a statement of the Alport syndrome research collaborative. Pediatr Nephrol. 2013;28(1):5–11.
41. Caberto S, Fadem S. In: Fadem S, editor. Genetic renal tubular disorders in essentials of chronic kidney disease. New York: Nova Science Publishers; 2015.
42. Rastogi A, Arman F, Asaturyan A, Ameen K, Singhal R. Other causes of chronic kidney disease. In: Fadem S, editor. Essentials of chronic kidney disease. New York: Nova Science Publishers; 2015.
43. Quigley L. E S. report on a survey of nephrologists in early years of practice. Washington, DC: George Washington Health Workforce Institute; 2018.
44. Salaries.com. Available from: https://www.salary.com/research/salary/benchmark/staff-nurse-rn-renal-dialysis-salary/.
45. Gura V, Rivara MB, Bieber S, Munshi R, Smith NC, Linke L, et al. A wearable artificial kidney for patients with end-stage renal disease. JCI Insight. 2016;1(8):e86397.
46. Nichols JE, La Francesca S, Vega SP, Niles JA, Argueta LB, Riddle M, et al. Giving new life to old lungs: methods to produce and assess whole human paediatric bioengineered lungs. J Tissue Eng Regen Med. 2017;11(7):2136–52.
47. Goto T, Hara H, Sanbo M, Masaki H, Sato H, Yamaguchi T, et al. Generation of pluripotent stem cell-derived mouse kidneys in Sall1-targeted anephric rats. Nat Commun. 2019;10(1):451.
48. Roelen BAJ. Regenerative medicine: taming the chimaera. Stem Cell Rep. 2018;11(4):849–51.

# Nephrology in Uruguay

16

Liliana Gadola, Oscar Noboa, Pablo Rios, Alejandro Ferreiro, María Carlota Gonzalez-Bedat, Liliana Chifflet, Milka Bengochea, Sergio Orihuela, Anabella Rebori, Laura Sola, Raúl Mizraji, Raúl Lombardi, Margarita Halty, and Francisco Gonzalez-Martinez

| | |
|---|---|
| Area | 176,215 km$^2$ |
| Population[1,2] | 3,505,985 (2018) |
| Capital | Montevideo |
| Three most populated cities | 1. Montevideo<br>2. Canelones<br>3. Salto |
| Official language | Spanish |
| Gross domestic product (GDP)[2] | 56,156.97 million USD (2017) |
| GDP per capita[3] | 16,245.60 USD (2017) |
| Human Development Index (HDI)[4] | 0.818 (2017) |
| Official currency | Uruguayan *peso* |
| Total number of nephrologists | 175 |
| National society of nephrology | *Sociedad Uruguaya de Nefrología*<br>www.nefrouruguay.org.uy |
| Incidence of end-stage renal disease | 2018 – 165 pmp |
| Prevalence of end-stage renal disease | 2018 – 771 pmp (on dialysis)<br>461 pmp (renal transplantation) |
| Total number of patients on dialysis (all modalities)[5] | 2017 – 3322<br>2018 – 3365 |
| Number of patients on hemodialysis[5] | 2017 – 3024<br>2018 – 3069 |
| Number of patients on peritoneal dialysis [5] | 2017 – 298<br>2018 – 296 (58% on CAPD) |
| Number of renal transplantations per year | 2017 – 134<br>2018 – 152 |

References:
1. https://www.worldometers.info/world-population/uruguay-population/
2. http://www.ine.gub.uy/web/guest/estimaciones-y-proyecciones
3. https://datos.bancomundial.org/
4. http://hdr.undp.org/en/data
5. https://www.fnr.gub.uy/sites/default/files/estadisticas/ia2018/ia_dial_2018.pdf

## Introduction

Uruguay (*República Oriental del Uruguay*) is a South American country (3,505,985 inhabitants, area of 176,215 Km$^2$). Uruguay is a democratic unitary state, of a presidential nature. The government is divided into three independent powers: executive, legislative, and judicial. It has a consolidated political party system and is characterized for its secularism, advanced social laws, and the social security, health, and educational systems. The entire population has access to clean water from a state provider and free access to education (from elementary to university), so it has high levels of literacy. Life expectancy at birth is 77.6 years for total population (male 74.4 years and female 80.8 years in 2018).

L. Gadola (✉) · O. Noboa · A. Ferreiro · R. Lombardi
Centro de Nefrología, Hospital de Clínicas, Facultad de Medicina, Universidad de la República, Montevideo, Uruguay

P. Rios
Programa de Salud Renal. Fondo Nacional de Recursos, Montevideo, Uruguay

M. C. Gonzalez-Bedat
Registro Uruguayo de Diálisis. Sociedad Uruguaya de Nefrología, Montevideo, Uruguay

L. Chifflet
Fondo Nacional de Recursos, Montevideo, Uruguay

M. Bengochea · R. Mizraji
Instituto Nacional de Donación y Trasplantes. Hospital de Clínicas, Facultad de Medicina, Universidad de la República, Montevideo, Uruguay

S. Orihuela
Instituto de Nefrología y Urología - Trasplante Renal, Hospital Italiano, Montevideo, Uruguay

A. Rebori
Unidad de Nefrología pediátrica de ASSE, Hospital Pereira Rossell, Montevideo, Uruguay

L. Sola
Comisión Asesora del Programa de Salud Renal, Montevideo, Uruguay

M. Halty
Clínica Pediátrica, Centro Hospitalario Pereira Rossell, Facultad de Medicina, Universidad de la República, Montevideo, Uruguay

F. Gonzalez-Martinez
Facultad de Medicina, Universidad de la República, Montevideo, Uruguay



J. A. Moura-Neto et al. (eds.), *Nephrology Worldwide*, https://doi.org/10.1007/978-3-030-56890-0_16

Nephrology is an internal medicine subspecialty practiced in the country since 1940. It was recognized as a specialty, and a postgraduate course began at the School of Medicine (*Facultad de Medicina, Universidad de la República*) in 1979, with a complete syllabus. Since then, 250 nephrologists have graduated. Nowadays, there are 175 practicing nephrologists (50.6 per million population) distributed throughout the country but mainly within the capital city, Montevideo, where half of the total population lives. Renal replacement treatment (RRT) for chronic kidney disease (CKD) stage 5 has been universally available since 1980. The country also has a National Integrated Health System (SNIS) that provides medical care for the entire population since 2007.

## Brief History of Nephrology in Uruguay

In 1942, Franchi-Padé ("the father" of Uruguayan nephrology) published the book *Enfermedades Médicas de los Riñones* [1] and an original article about renal glomerular and tubular function evaluation in an international publication [2]. Since then, kidney biopsies have been performed in the country, and the glomerulopathies registry was initially coordinated at the university hospital, albeit it is now a national registry [3].

In April 1957, the first acute peritoneal dialysis (PD) was performed [4], and, in January 1958, the first acute hemodialysis (HD) [5] was performed. In May 1967, the first chronic kidney disease patient (with a polycystic kidney disease) was chronically hemodialyzed through a Scribner's shunt [6]. In June 1969, the first kidney transplantation was performed from a deceased donor, although with very short survival. A better outcome was obtained with the first living donor kidney transplantation performed in January 1973 (sister to brother) [7, 8]. In September 1969, the Act on Tissue and Solid Organ Transplantation began to be discussed, and this act was passed into law in August 1971 (Law no. 14005, subsequently no. 17668) and was later regulated in 1977. The National Institute of Tissue and Organ Donation was then created, becoming responsible for histocompatibility evaluation and for the regulation of universal procurement and distribution of tissue and solid organs for transplantation. Since then, kidney transplantation has expanded.

Law no. 14897 (subsequently no. 16343) was passed in 1979, and as result, the National Resources Fund was created, and the economic and administrative bases for CKD treatment were established (simultaneously with those for other high-cost treatments). Since then, dialysis and transplantation have been available for the entire Uruguayan population.

The fact that Uruguayan fellows attend regional (Argentina, Brazil, and Chile) and international (France, Spain, Italy, Japan, the USA) reference centers has been of the utmost importance for the education of Uruguayan nephrologists and the development of the clinical and research activities in the field of nephrology. International cooperation agreements with France and Spain supported by the ISN in the last few years have been especially instrumental in having a fluid bilateral exchange that strongly contributed to the pursuit of excellence within the field of national nephrology.

The Uruguayan Society of Nephrology (*SUN* by its Spanish acronym) and, afterwards, the National Resources Fund held the Uruguayan Registry of Dialysis (*RUD* by its Spanish acronym) and the Registry of Transplantations (*RUT* by its Spanish acronym), a mandatory registry that included all dialyzed patients, their clinical and biochemical data and outcomes [9, 10], as well as all kidney transplantations performed in the country. Kidney transplantation teams also registered detailed clinical data, treatments, and outcomes [11]. Since 2004, a National Renal Healthcare Program (NRHP) was created to improve CKD patients' diagnoses and treatments, and a CKD registry was established, which nowadays includes over 20,000 patients with non-dialysis CKD [12, 13].

## Renal Diseases in Uruguay

Uruguayan nephrologists provide secondary and tertiary care to patients depending on their clinical condition, using a referral and counter-referral system with primary care physicians (PCP) or other specialists at the primary level. Every institution linked to the National Integrated Health System (*SNIS)* provides outpatient nephrological care, dialysis equipment, and healthcare to hospitalized patients at the standard or intensive care sector.

## National Renal Healthcare Program

In April 2004, the NRHP was created by the Uruguayan Society of Nephrology (*SUN*) and the School of Medicine (*Universidad de la República).* Its goal was to improve renal healthcare and, more specifically, (a) to promote renal healthcare education and a healthy lifestyle among the general population in order to reduce cardiovascular and renal risk factors; (b) to increase accessibility to renal healthcare at the primary level; (c) to promote early diagnosis of CKD among at-risk population; (d) to improve the care given to patients at all stages of CKD, and (e) to prevent cardiovascular morbidity and mortality, which are high within the targeted population [14]. An Advisory Committee for Renal Health (ACRH), composed of representatives from the National Resources Fund (FNR), the SUN, the School of Medicine (*Universidad de la República*), and a delegate from the Ministry of Health [14, 15], was committed to its implementation and evaluation. Simultaneously, an online CKD registry was created and held by the *FNR*. Patients were registered whenever eGFR was lower than 60 ml/min/1.73 $m^2$ (initially by MDRD 4 equation and later by CKD-EPI) or when persistent proteinuria higher than 300 mg/day (or microalbuminuria, higher than 30 mg/day in diabetic patients) was present. In order to minimize failure to follow-up, this CKD registry had a centralized "alarm system" that is activated whenever patients failed to keep an appointment. These patients were called by an *FNR* social worker or by the nurse from each nephrology team and scheduled for another appointment.

CKD screening has been incorporated into health checkups. In Uruguay, since 1936, it is mandatory for students, individuals with a stable job, and people who practice sports to have a regular health checkup once every 2 years. In 2009, the Department of Health passed a decree providing for serum creatinine tests to be included in diabetic and hypertensive individuals' health checkups. Patients who were positive for urine abnormalities or high serum creatinine levels in these checkups would be referred to PCPs or nephrologists to complete their evaluation. Between January 1, 2009, and December 12, 2012, 11,161 people were tested for serum creatinine levels at health checkups. CKD prevalence was higher in people with diabetes and hypertension (16.9%) followed by those with diabetes and without hypertension (11.9%) [15–18].

## The CKD Registry

The registry and variables included have already been reported [17]. Between October 1, 2004, and December 31, 2018, 21,399 patients were registered. The patients' median age was 70 years (IQT 60–77), and 43.7% of them were female. The follow-up was 4.5 years, and the most frequent diagnoses were vascular nephropathy (40.8%), diabetic nephropathy (19.1%), obstructive nephropathy (7.9%), and primary glomerulonephritis (4.8%). The most frequent risk factors for kidney disease were hypertension (86.9%), dyslipidemia (54.2%), diabetes (37.3%), and obesity (37.7%). Most patients were referred to a nephrologist at CKD stage 3 (58.2%), followed by stage 1–2 (17%) and stage 4–5 (24.8%). The latter were considered late referrals. 17.7% of patients had proteinuria >0.3 g/d. Every year, the ACRH carries out an annual evaluation and invites all nephrology groups included in the NRHP. Group coordinators meet to discuss the progress of clinical indicators, and each group is given performance results for each indicator, as well as the median and percentiles 25–75 for the program. This meeting is important to address each group's strengths and weaknesses, as well as to holistically assess the program.

After 4.5 years of average follow-up, 4614 (22%) patients died, and 1275 (6%) had ESRD, 7890 patients (36%) had stabilized renal function (loss of eGFR <1 ml/min/year), 1909 (12.3%) patients had rapid progression (>5 ml/min/year), and 3641 patients (16%) had slow progression (1–5 ml/min/year). The remaining 14.5% were not followed up. The survival of patients controlled at 10 years was significantly ($p < 0.05$) higher (71%) when compared to those not controlled (43%). Patients from the NRHP were 7 years older at admission to dialysis than patients without nephrological assistance before beginning dialysis, adjusted for nephropathy [14]. The mortality rate was 6.20/100 patients/year. The main cause of death was cardiovascular: 2.03/100 patients/year. Proteinuria and glomerular filtration rates were independent risk factors for new cardiovascular events [18].

## Registry of Glomerulopathies and Kidney Biopsies

Glomerulopathies have a national incidence of 58 cases per million population (pmp) [3]. The Glomerulopathies Prevention and Treatment Program (*PPTG* by its Spanish acronym) was created in 1989 by the Glomerulopathies Study Group from the Nephrology Department at the School of Medicine and by the Uruguayan Society of Nephrology. The Uruguayan Registry of Glomerulopathies has been running since 1970 by the Nephrology Department, and since 1985, it is sponsored by the Uruguayan Society of Nephrology and includes patients from every institution nationwide. In 2000, a ministerial ordinance made the *PPTG* official, granting the Nephrology Department at the School of Medicine power to develop that program, and made it mandatory to notify the registry of all clinically diagnosed cases of glomerulopathy and of their evolution (Uruguayan Registry of Glomerulopathies/Kidney Biopsies). Since 2001, the Managing Commission for the National Resources Fund sponsors the *PPTG* and collaborates with data collection. Some of the goals of the *PPTG* are to analyze epidemiology and to update the diagnosis and treatment of glomerulopathies in Uruguay.

The main activities carried out by the coordinating commission of the *PPTG* are (1) epidemiological surveillance through the Uruguayan Registry of Glomerulopathies (*RUG* for its Spanish acronym) to make relevant national health recommendations; (2) weekly meetings (glomerulopathies grand round) to discuss clinical cases and their kidney biopsies, streamed live to enable the participation of nephrologists nationwide; (3) peer review of international-related publications; and (4) periodically updating of clinical practice guides for the diagnosis and treatment of glomerulopathies (www.nefrologia.hc.edu.uy/images/Guias_de_Practica_clinica_para_tratamiento_de_las_Glomerulopatias._Version_2018.pdf). Nephrologists, internists, pathologists, laboratory technicians, hematologists, and gynecologists collaborate with the guides, verifying preexisting guides using the *AGREE* tool, conducting an updated bibliographical search, and, finally, attending the national consensus that completes the draft for the documents [19]. Having widely disseminated and regularly updated treatment guidelines has led to a more homogeneous treatment of glomerulopathies in the country.

The Registry of Glomerulopathies has shown that the incidence of multiple glomerulopathies has varied throughout the years [3, 20]. From 1990 to 2014, 3390 biopsies on native kidneys corresponding to glomerular disease were performed in patients older than 14. The average biopsy rate was 58 per pmp/year. The glomerular disease incidence rate progressively increased over that period ($p < 0.05$). Trends analysis over 5-year periods demonstrated a progressive increase of IgA nephropathy (3.08 pmp/year 1990–1994 to 12.53 pmp/year 2010–2014 $p < 0.05$), membranous nephropathy (2.38 pmp/year 1990–1994 to 8.04 pmp/year 2010–2014 $p < 0.05$), and lupus nephritis (4.23 pmp/year 1990–1994 to 7.81 pmp/year 2010–2014 $p < 0.05$). Focal segmental glomerulosclerosis increased until 1996 and decreased afterwards [20].

Tubulointerstitial nephritis (TIN) study was performed with data from both registries (NRHP and *RUG*). This study showed that the female gender had a higher risk of TIN caused mainly by medications. The most common clinical presentation for the biopsied group was as rapidly progressive renal failure (RPRF). A better evolution of the estimated glomerular filtration (eGF) was associated to a lower tubule-interstitial fibrosis score at biopsy in patients who received steroid treatment, exclusive or associated to other immunosuppressive agents (OR 0.143; 95% CI, 0.028–0.720; $p < 0.05$) [21].

The diagnosis and treatment of hypertension warrant special attention by Uruguayan nephrologists, and a group of them actively participates in national and international epidemiology research, having produced numerous publications [22]. Information campaigns on vascular risk factors and on limiting the use of salt in the diet of the population have been performed.

## Acute Kidney Injury and Critical Care Nephrology

There is no information on the epidemiology of acute kidney injury (AKI) in the community. Nevertheless, multiple reports exist providing information on specific situations or contexts (leptospirosis, sepsis, cardiac surgery, pregnancy, nephrotoxins, etc.). During an observational study of 40 intensive care units (ICU) in the country spanning over 2 weeks, a 9.1% frequency of AKI (AKIN criteria) was observed [23]. The main causes were ischemic acute tubular necrosis and sepsis, 52% in the context of multiple organ failure and 13.6% of which required RRT. Other studies report a frequency of 2.3% [24, 25] for severe AKI with RRT in cardiac surgery, of 5.6% [26] at ICU, and 0.3 pmp/year in the case of severe leptospirosis [27].

AKI has been identified as a public health issue and has been included in the events report for patient check-ups from the Renal Health Program Registry. Several interdisciplinary educational activities have been carried out to disseminate reno-protective strategies in the community and hospital areas, and both scientific societies and academia have participated in such activities [28]. More specifically, in 2014, the Ministry of Health made it mandatory to diagnose, report, and apply a prevention protocol for AKI caused by administration of iodinated contrast agents [29].

The treatment of AKI, regardless of its severity, is universally covered, can be equally accessed by the entire population, and is under charge and responsibility of both public and private integral healthcare providers. The regulatory ordinance authorizing the installation of critical care facilities requires having RRT techniques. Historically, due to availability and funding, the main form of RRT for AKI was intermittent HD, with anecdotal reports of peritoneal dialysis (PD) administration. Continuous RRT have not been habitually incorporated in the country. Consequently, in the past 10 years, sustained low-efficiency dialysis (SLED) was used, and, more recently, online hemodiafiltration for AKI in critical patients has been introduced. Nowadays, most hospitals offer RRT managed by their own professional teams organized into AKI treatment units equipped with HD machines with bicarbonate and controlled ultrafiltration (UF). Most units use treated water obtained through portable osmosis systems, and only two units have a water treatment system that obtains ultrapure water.

There is no national registry for AKI episodes or their results. Nevertheless, hospital and long-term mortality for AKI, treated with RRT and reported in studies, resembles the mortality reported from observational studies in developed countries [23, 26, 30].

## Renal Replacement Therapy in Uruguay

### Epidemiology

As from 1980, RRT started to be developed in Uruguay when the National Resources Fund Act became alive. The Fund is funded by every inhabitant of the country (with the exception of members from the armed forces and of police officers), and it finances several high-cost treatments, such as the chronic dialysis and renal transplantation programs.

The Uruguayan Society of Nephrology created the Uruguayan Registry of Dialysis (*RUD*), and the Uruguayan Society of Transplantations created the Uruguayan Registry of Transplantations (*RUT)* in 1981. Presently, the *RUD* is a mandatory registry of patients, and it collaborates with the National Resources Fund, annually providing reports on data it shares with the *RUT* [9–11]. As from its creation, both the *RUD* and the *RUT* have accumulated data on the entire population that underwent different forms of RRT in the country. By means of different studies conducted, this has made it possible to know the epidemiology of CKD in RRT in the country [31–34], as well as to compare treatment results with results from other countries and regions [35–37].

The incidence of CKD in dialysis treatment has increased from 32 (in 1981) to 165 pmp (in 2017) [36, 38], with certain stability since 2008, and a constant predominance of male vs. female gender (215 vs. 118 pmp, respectively) and of patients from Montevideo (the capital city) vs. those from other parts of the country (187 vs. 151 pmp) in 2018. The average age of incident RRT patients progressively increased and reached 61.6 years in 2018. The etiology of CKD was diabetes at 28%, cardiovascular at 25%, chronic glomerulonephritis at 11%, obstructive tubule-interstitial nephropathy at 11%, nonobstructive TIN at 2%, and other causes at 23% in 2018. In 2018, the most frequent prescribed dialysis therapy was HD in 89.6% of the cases, whereas PD was prescribed in 10.4% of the cases.

The prevalence of dialysis therapy increased from 38 in 1981 to 771 ppm in 2018, also moving toward stability since 2008, with a rate of 706 ppm in HD and 64 pmp in PD.

Only 14% of dialysis patients were waitlisted to receive kidney transplant in 2018 (13% from HD and 26% from PD).

Gross mortality was 24.9% in 1987, decreasing to 17.4% in 2018 (17,5% in HD and 15,8% in PD patients, stable between 15% and 17% in the last 10 years). The most frequent causes of death in 2018 were cardiovascular (35%), infectious (19%), suspended treatment (7%), neoplasm (6%), and others (34%).

The incidence of kidney transplant increased from 3 pmp in 1981 to 44 pmp in 2018, and the prevalence of successful kidney transplant was 3 pmp in 1981 but increased to 461 pmp in 2018 [9–11]. At present, 2689 kidney transplants have been performed in the country.

## Reimbursement Policies

### Chronic Kidney Disease Treatment: Legal Framework and Financial Coverage

In Uruguay, the right of healthcare to each inhabitant is regulated by Law no. 18211 from 2007, which created the National Integrated Healthcare System (*SNIS)* and the National Health Insurance (*SNS* by its Spanish acronym), which compose the National Health Fund (*FONASA* by its Spanish acronym) [39].

Services are provided through comprehensive public and private healthcare providers and are defined within a Holistic Healthcare Plan, a benefits plan that ensures universal coverage through an explicit list of healthcare and medication services [40].

In order to provide healthcare for people without insurance and to cover out-of-pocket expenses, the *SNIS* is financed by public sources, by the *SNS* (employer, worker, and retired workers taxes), and by general revenue. Throughout the years, the contribution from the *SNS* has increased, and the out-of-pocket expenses have progressively decreased, with Uruguay becoming the second Latin American country with the lowest percentage of out-of-pocket expenses for healthcare [41].

*FONASA* makes a per capita payment to integral healthcare providers according to age and gender and a variable payment based on performance and goal achievements. Additionally, public healthcare providers are financed using general revenue, as defined in the national budget. In the case of more complex, high-cost services and medications, the National Resources Fund (*FNR)* provides financing pursuant to Law no. 16343 of 1993 and acts as additional healthcare public insurance along with *FONASA*, thus reinsuring integral healthcare providers. Thereby, Uruguay reaches universal healthcare coverage, with equity and without exposing people to financial hardship [39, 40].

The *FNR* has been in place since 1980, financing the High Care Specialized Institutes (*IMAE* by their Spanish acronym). The public and private dialysis and transplantation Institutes are among these IMAE. When the *SNIS* was created, the *FNR* also began providing coverage for high-cost medications. Currently, it is a nongovernmental public entity governed by an Honorary Managing Committee comprised of nine members: five representing the government and four representing healthcare providers and the *IMAE* [42–44]. It is funded by *FONASA* (82%), general revenue (10%), and out-of-pocket expenses (6%). Two percent of the funds stem from gambling taxes. In 2018, the *FNR* spent 250 million dollars [45].

In Uruguay, public and private healthcare providers and dialysis and renal transplant institutes are responsible for RRT in ESRD. These institutes are funded by the *FNR* through tariffs agreed upon by the executive branch and the Association of *IMAE* centers [46]. Moreover, the *FNR* funds treatments with immunosuppressive agents (tacrolimus and everolimus) for transplanted patients [47, 48]. Both living and deceased donor renal transplantations are funded, as well as combined organ transplantations (heart-kidney, pancreas-kidney, liver-kidney), covering the transplantation procedure and all complications that may arise [47, 48].

In the case of HD, the *FNR* pays the *Institutes* a tariff for each dialysis session performed. (At 2019, $5324 = US dollars 38). Regarding PD, the *IMAE* receives a fixed amount per patient treated (At 2019, US dollars 1547/patient-month). Furthermore, the *FNR* acquires PD materials and provides them to patients through suppliers. The FNR also covers all the PD complications costs [47].

Additionally, the *FNR* has prevention programs, targeting the treatment of risk factors for the most prevalent noncommunicable chronic diseases in the country as a risk management strategy for new procedures.

The Renal Health Program [49] and the Glomerulopathies Prevention and Treatment Program developed by the National Resources Fund, the Ministry of Health, the Nephrology Department from the School of Medicine (*Universidad de la República)*, and the Uruguayan Society of Nephrology aim to prevent and screen for kidney disease and stop/slow down its progression in cases in which it has already begun. These programs provide easy access to nephrological attention and have partial financial cover by the FNR.

The *FNR* develops quality and results assessment and follow-ups for services funded [50] and publishes results indicators differentiated by dialysis and transplant institutes (*IMAE)* [51]. Multidisciplinary teams from the *FNR* periodically audit facilities, equipment, and processes, boosting risk evaluation policies, medical error prevention, and epidemiology surveillance. These teams control compliance with legal regulations and protocols, estimate staff training and strengthening, and seek to ensure that every treatment the population has access to is of equal quality [52].

## Hemodialysis

Chronic HD is broadly developed throughout the country and can be accessed universally, as earlier mentioned, in hospital centers and clinics. In 2018, 3069 patients received chronic HD. There are 37 chronic HD centers, 17 located in Montevideo and 20 in the rest of the country, most of which (92%) treat between 30 and 90 patients, and 5% of them treat over 90 patients [11]. All centers have been authorized by sanitary authorities (Ministry of Health) and funded by the National Resources Fund. Operational rules have been well defined [53–55], are the same for all centers, and are annually audited by sanitary authorities [56].

Water treatment for HD complies with the best international standards [57, 58]; reverse osmosis is used in every center (most centers using double pass reverse osmosis system), and aluminum, endotoxins, and microbiology levels are periodically controlled. Online hemodiafiltration (HDF) with "ultrapure" water is also carried out in one center (at the University Nephrology Department) for 28 patients. Until 2018, all centers reused dialyzers (reuse median of 15 reuses), which were stored in peracetic acid. Since 2019, some centers have decided not to reuse; however, dialyzer reuse is allowed if the priming volume is at least 80% of the initial, and they are handled and stored as defined [53]. High-flux dialyzers from international suppliers are used. Dialysis solutions used are produced by the pharmaceutical industry under strict quality control (composition and microbiology) by sanitary authorities. Bicarbonate and controlled ultrafiltration HD/HDF machines are used.

Most patients receive 3 weekly sessions of HD, lasting 231 ± 18 min/session [11, 38] on average, blood flow at least 350 ml/min. Vascular access is achieved through native arteriovenous fistula in 53% of patients, prosthetic fistula in 24% of patients, double-lumen tunneled central venous catheter in 14% in patients, and temporary central venous catheter in the remaining cases [11, 38]. When completing HD/HDF, all data for the procedures, prescribed treatments, and eventual complications are reported online at the computerized control system of the *FNR* (known as *María* system).

Pursuant to the regulations of the *FNR*, multidisciplinary teams provide care under the technical supervision of a nephrologist with proven experience [53–55]. A nephrologist (1 to every 16 patients) is always present during the dialysis sessions, and there is a nurse to every 16 patients and a hemodialysis technician to every 3–4 patients. Nutritionists and psychologists periodically check up on patients, and a social worker collaborates with them.

When beginning RRT, and semiannually, viral markers for hepatitis A, B, and C and HIV are controlled. AgHBs (0.7% positive) and susceptible patients received hepatitis B vaccination. In 2016, 65% of patients developed HB antibodies after vaccination. The prevalence of antibodies to hepatitis C was 2.2% and to HIV was below 1% [11]. Between 82% and 100% of patients on HD receive treatment with subcutaneous erythropoietin.

Compliance goals and objectives for monthly clinical and biochemical parameters (blood pressure, weight, azotemia, electrolytes, hemoglobin, phosphate, calcium, etc.) have been recorded for each session and are audited annually by sanitary authorities and included in the Uruguayan Registry of Dialysis, which allows for an annually published [11, 38] healthcare quality control [55, 58]. Mortality rate was 15.2/100 patient-year in 2016 and adjusted to age, sex, and diabetes 9.2/100 patient-year [11, 38]. At present 346 patients (13.2% of prevalent patients) have been on HD for more than 10 years.

## Peritoneal Dialysis

PD is prescribed almost exclusively for the treatment of ESRD in adult patients and almost never for the treatment of AKI, except in pediatric population, as it will be described later. PD is used less often than HD, and only 10% of dialyzed patients use this treatment, although it is universally available and all patients on RRT may use it [30]. In 2018, there were eight PD centers authorized by the Ministry of Health and funded by the *FNR* as is HD. Every inhabitant has access to these centers, being free to choose one for treatment. Half of the centers provide care for 30–60 patients, and the remaining centers serve less than 30 patients each. In 2018, 296 patients were dialyzed using this treatment method. Seven centers are in Montevideo (albeit they serve patients from other areas of the country), and one is in the city of San José. The *FNR* supplies these centers by calling for public tenders for suppliers (who then distribute supplies to the patients' home), and nephrologists are free to choose a supplier and PD plan for each patient.

Based on preference of the PD team and on the clinical situation of each patient, peritoneal catheters (Tenckhoff, double cuff, straight, or coil catheters) are placed by puncture by nephrologists, by surgical technique with enhanced local anesthesia, or by video laparoscopy.

Standard dextrose (or glucose) and icodextrin PD solutions are used, albeit icodextrin is only limited to people under the age of 14, diabetic patients, or patients with very rapid peritoneal transport. Cyclers are obtained from only one supplier, which limits their use in clinical practice. Approximately 48% of patients use automated PD [11, 38]. By 2018, there were no bicarbonate or amino acid solutions available.

Pursuant to regulations by the *FNR* [53, 55], PD teams for each center are made up of a nephrologist with proven experience in the field acting as technical director, nephrologists, nurses, dietitians, social workers, and a psychologist/psychiatrist, all of which provide multidisciplinary care focused on the patient and his/her family and social circle.

Clinical and biochemical checkups are conducted at least once a month on all patients treated, and all data are collected. Medications, PD prescriptions, and complications/hospitalizations are reported online at the computerized control system of the *FNR* (*María* system). Ninety-six percent of patients on PD receive treatment with subcutaneous erythropoietin.

As on HD centers, these centers have quality control criteria, goals, and objectives based on the best scientific evidence available and annual auditing for all centers conducted by national sanitary authorities (National Resources Fund and Ministry of Health) [24].

Since 2004, the Peritoneal Dialysis Group from the *SUN* steers the National Registry of Peritonitis in PD in order to determine the most common bacteria and their antibiotic sensitivity and to define the initial empiric peritonitis therapy for this population [58–60]. The national peritonitis rate has decreased (from 0.49 in 2004 to 0.33 peritonitis/patient-year in 2017), mainly cases caused by gram-positive bacteria [58].

Patient survival for patients treated with PD is similar to that of patients treated with HD, as well as clinical and biochemical controls [11, 38]. The Uruguayan Registry of Dialysis and the National Resources Fund annually publish results on morbidity and survival indicators [11, 38]. Mortality rate was 16.2/100 patient-year in 2016 and adjusted to age, sex, and diabetes 11.4/100 patient-year [11, 38]. At present 36 patients (13.8% of prevalent patients) have been on PD for more than 10 years.

In the last few years, several young nephrologists from South America have come to Uruguay to complete their PD training with scholarships from Sociedad Latinoamericana de Nefrología e Hipertensión (*SLANH)* and International Society for Peritoneal Dialysis (ISPD).

## Renal Transplantation: Living and Deceased Donor

The first renal transplantation in Uruguay was performed in 1969 [61]. Currently, there are three transplantation centers in Uruguay authorized to conduct kidney transplantations and one authorized to conduct hepatorenal transplantations, although the process of procuring and assigning deceased donor organs is centralized and regulated by law as described in the following paragraph. The teams providing care are multidisciplinary, directed by a nephrologist with proven experience [53], surgeons, urologists, anesthesiologists, nephrologists, nurses, nutritionists, psychologists, and social workers. Since 1979, 2689 kidney transplants have been performed.

In 2018, 44 kidney transplants pmp were performed, the highest figure in Latin America, as it has been the case for the past two decades [62, 63]. Ninety-three percent of these kidney transplants were performed with a deceased donor, and 7% with a living related donor [64], ratio that has remained historically stable with clear predominance of deceased donors. For 5.4% of patients, kidney transplant was the first treatment for CKD (preemptive). The age of donors and recipients has increased, with current ages at 39 ± 16 and 46 ± 15 years, respectively. The pretransplant time on dialysis has decreased and is currently 56.7 ± 47.0 months [65]. In 2018, the prevalence of kidney transplant was 461 pmp.

Immunosuppression usually includes tacrolimus, mycophenolate, and corticosteroids and, in 81% of cases, induction with mono- and polyclonal antibodies. The survival rate for kidney transplants performed during this century is of 96%, 90%, and 81% at 1, 5, and 10 years, respectively, and the survival rate for death-censored graft survival is of 92%, 80%, and 68%, respectively. By 2018, the prevalence of patients living with successful kidney transplant was 461 pmp, making up 31.5% of the total number of patients with RRT (dialysis and transplantation).

## Simultaneous Transplantation of Kidney and Other Organs

**Cardiorenal** The first kidney transplant simultaneous to a heart transplant was performed in 1995. Only two transplantations of this nature have been performed so far.

**Renal-pancreatic** The first simultaneous kidney and pancreas transplantation was performed in 2002, within the framework of a national program developed by the School of Medicine. Since then, 57 transplantations of this nature have been performed. There were no cases of pancreatic transplantations followed by kidney transplantations (PAK) or of isolated pancreatic transplantation. This program is now suspended.

**Hepatorenal** The first simultaneous kidney and liver transplantation was performed in 2014 at the bi-institutional unit from the School of Medicine-Military Hospital where the National Liver Transplant Program operated. To this date, ten transplantations of this nature have been performed.

**Professional Training** The study of kidney transplants is part of the syllabi for nephrologists, urologists, surgeons, and other specialists, and there is also available a "Diploma in Organ Procurement and Histocompatibility." Given the excellent results obtained, professionals from several Latin American countries such as Chile, Paraguay, Bolivia, Peru, and Ecuador complete their transplantation training in Uruguay.

## Organ Procurement and Transplantation Network Policies

The National Institute for Organ, Tissue and Cell Donation and Transplantation and for Regenerative Medicine (*INDT* by its Spanish acronym), a public entity reporting to the Ministry of Health and the *Universidad de la República*, has been around for over 40 years and has legal authority over all programs and therapeutic or scientific activities using human organs, tissues, or cells.

The institute has healthcare, regulation, teaching, research, and extension goals.

Within the area of healthcare, the institute is responsible for donations, procurement, immunogenetic studying of donors and recipients, managing single waitlists, assigning each organ transplant, and ablating, processing, and assigning tissue, as well as for studying and looking for donors for hematopoietic transplantation.

Through various legal frameworks, Uruguay has managed to maintain deceased donation rates above the Latin American average; in 2018, the rates per million population (pmp) were of 23.8 for organs and 15.8 for tissue.

Regulations have fostered changes that allowed for developing different types of organ, tissue, and cell transplantations. Organ transplantations with living donors are allowed among collateral relatives or up to four degrees of consanguinity, and, in the case of hematopoietic transplantation, it is also possible to make a nondirected donation through a registry for unrelated persons.

For over three decades, INDT operated based on the legal form of donation of explicit consent granted by an individual or by his/her relatives, form established by Law no. 14005 approved in 1971, a groundbreaking law for Latin America establishing a broad criteria for death that remains functional and in force, when performing transplantation activities. As from 2003, an amendment introduced the figure of presumed donors in the case of death that required forensic examination, and, as from 2013, Law no. 18968 came into force, establishing the status of presumed donor for all cases in which an individual has not stated otherwise while alive. This amendment made it necessary to notify families about donations rather than to consult them on the matter.

Kidney transplants and corneal grafts are the oldest and more active transplantations, with transplantation rates per million population of 48.9 and 44.2, respectively. Even so, the rate of waitlisted patients per million population is of 140 and 170, respectively.

The institute is organized into five technical areas: transplant coordination, immunogenetics laboratory assignment unit, multi-tissue bank, registry and statistics, and cellular transplantation (search and registration of HSC (hematopoietic stem cells) donors).

Regarding the kidney transplantation program, we must highlight the active work conducted by the Transplantation Coordination whose operation is based on joint coordination, especially on coordinating with clinics. A legally approved National Network for Donations and Transplantations is currently being implemented by appointing institutional key agents for donation and transplantation activities. The Donation and Transplantation Coordination is made up of intensivists and psychologists in charge of choosing and keeping donors and of interviewing their relatives, respectively.

Within the field of education, the *INDT* is responsible for three postgraduate diplomas: transplant coordination, immunogenetic basis of transplantation, and multi-tissue bank. Thus, ours is one of the first countries to offer university diplomas for these disciplines.

## Nephrology Practice in Uruguay

The Postgraduate Degree in Nephrology from the School of Medicine, *Universidad de la República*, was approved by the university authorities on May 8, 1979 [6]. The fact that this postgraduate degree is the only training program available (Nephrology Department from the *Hospital de Clínicas)* contributes to homogenize nephrology practices all over the country. This development was boosted in 1990 with the creation of the residency program that, since 1993, includes a nephrology residency; initially, it was carried out during the last year of the internal medicine residency, but, afterwards, a specific nephrology residency was created.

Afterwards, associated public and private teaching centers were accredited by the Graduate Department of the School of Medicine, allowing the nephrology residencies program to expand.

Nowadays, the postgraduate degree takes 3 years with additional time to write a thesis. Two final evaluation tests are performed. Many nephrologists have trained further through scholarships abroad and, in some cases, have been able to homologate degrees obtained abroad (Spain).

The training for nephrology nurses initially developed as a specialization within the practical work and, more recently, has been developed in specialized courses in the School of Nursing.

In 2018, there were 158 practicing nephrologists in Uruguay, corresponding to a rate of 50.6 nephrologists pmp.

Nephrological activity has diversified throughout the years. This, along with the expansion of the national integrated healthcare system, has led to full employment in the area of nephrology for doctors and nurses alike.

The field of development for nephrological activity includes:

1. Outpatient healthcare activities are carried out across the country. The renal health program indicates the need to provide 2 h of outpatient nephrological care to every 10,000 users (20 years or older). Depending on the complexity of the care system, nephrologists are organized into practice groups that establish a fluid relationship with other healthcare professionals. Normally, this outpatient care is associated with a hospital care group. Patients may also be directed to certain healthcare centers for specialized consults for glomerular diseases, lithiasis, and advanced chronic disease.
2. Hospital care oversees RRT with nephrologists who care for hospitalized patients or patients in emergency facilities, either when covering an in-hospital shift in high complexity healthcare centers or when being on call. In every case, these services are overseen by nephrologists.
3. Nephrology departments in public and private hospitals develop general nephrological follow-up, outpatients care, and acute dialysis units, always under the supervision of an experienced nephrologist. These programs, along with the growing Renal Health Program, have progressively engaged more nephrologists providing hospital care, including the RRT for hospitalized patients, and the diagnosis and follow-up of patients with CKD at different stages of kidney disease.
4. Activity at outpatient and in-hospital chronic HD centers, with on-site supervision during dialysis shifts and clinical follow-up for patients on chronic dialysis. This activity is complemented with multidisciplinary regular clinical meetings. Nephrologists with over 5 years of experience are technical directors at these centers (pursuant to regulations by *FNR*). It can be estimated that 40% of the workload for nephrologists comes from this area.
5. PD centers employ one nephrologist to every 20–30 patients. Since PD is less developed, only 10% of the workload comes from this area. Once again, nephrologists with proven experience act as technical directors for these centers.
6. Kidney transplantation centers employ about 20 nephrologists for direct care who deal with waitlists, monitoring the pre-transplantation period and doing post-transplantation follow-up. Once again, nephrologists with proven experience at renal transplantation act as technical directors for these centers.
7. Academic activity is centralized at the Center of Nephrology from the *Universidad de la República* and the Associated Nephrology Units. The University Nephrology Department, with a staff of almost 20 nephrologists, conducts nephrology courses for trainees and continuous medical education.

Nephrological research in Uruguay is conducted by different research groups [3, 9, 12, 21, 22, 25, 33, 38, 58, 61, 64–67] from the Uruguayan Society of Nephrology and the School of Medicine (*Universidad de la República)* who have produced about 233 scientific papers published in peer-reviewed journals (search in PubMed: KIDNEY and URUGUAY).

Given how medicine works in the country, nephrologists normally have more than one paid job, for example, working at a hospital and then working at an outpatient chronic dialysis center. Nephrologist monthly salary is on average US dollars 2800 per 30 h/week, and renal nurse monthly salary is on average US dollars 2100 per 36 h/week.

## Pediatric Nephrology

Until 1960 in Uruguay, general pediatricians dealt with nephrological pathologies. The first renal biopsy was performed in 1959. During the 1960s, pediatric nephrology polyclinics were created at *Hospital Pedro Visca* and *Hospital Pereira Rosell*. In 1983, both units merged and settled at *Hospital Pereira Rosell* [66]. That year, two pediatric chronic dialysis centers were created: HD and PD [67]. Between 1979 and 1989, the Pediatric Uro-nephrology Department was based at *Hospital de Clínicas* and directed by urology professors. Practicing pediatricians would get the degree of adult nephrologist or would train abroad with pediatric nephrologists (France, Japan).

The Pediatric Nephrology Postgraduate course was approved by the Postgraduate School of the *Universidad de la República* on April 12, 2013, and by the Central Board of Directors on July 1, 2014 [67]. The first generation of postgraduate students started school in 2015. Nowadays, there are six pediatric nephrologists who hold this degree, and five professionals have retired in the last 5 years.

The incidence of pediatric patients with CKD in our country is unknown. The Pediatric Renal Health Program will begin operations at the Congenital Defects and Rare Diseases Center. There are 121 patients <16 year with CKD receiving care at that center and have been referred by public and private care providers. Forty-two percent of the patients present with nephro-urological malformations, 27.8% present with malformations at the neural tube, 17.4% present with CKD due to genetic causes, 11.3% present with acquired CKD, and, for 0.9%, the causes are unknown. 67.8%, 13%, 7%, 4.3%, and 6.1% are at CKD stages 1, 2, 3, 4, and 5 respectively. The last group is comprised of seven patients: one has received a transplant, one is on HD, and five are on PD. Five of the patients from stages 4 and 5 are currently being studied for transplantation (Data from Reference Center).

Since 1983, 203 children <15 years have been dialyzed: 108 on HD and 95 on PD (Data from the Uruguayan Registry of Dialysis). In December 2018, there were 16 children on PD and 5 on HD (3 on temporary HD) between the ages of 2 and 17. Two of these patients started on PD within the first month of life, and another patient started on PD at 6 months (Data from the Pediatric Dialysis Center, *SENNIAD*). All children receive nightly cyclic dialysis and, when prescribed, daily icodextrin PD solution.

PD and HD teams are multidisciplinary and made up of pediatric nephrologists, pediatricians studying nephrology, nurses, dietitians, psychologists, and social workers. Given the importance of nutrition and growth in pediatrics, dietitians are present when routine checkups on pediatric PD patients are performed. For HD, it is fundamental for teachers to participate as they coordinate activities based on the status of the patient. All teams comply with national regulations for dialyzed patients [53–55]. The team in charge of pediatric dialysis for chronic patients also dialyzes acute patients, with PD being the preferable technique chosen for young children, both chronic and acute.

The first pediatric transplantation was performed on a 14-year-old girl in 1978 at the Nephrology and Urology Institute (*INU* by its Spanish acronym); to this date, 61 transplantations in <15 years old have been performed there, with 12 of those patients not having been dialyzed prior to that (preemptive transplant) [10].

In 2018, five patients between the ages of 9 and 16 received renal transplants: two are recipient from living and three from deceased donors (one of them received a re-transplantation). There was one case of arterial thrombosis primary failure, but the other grafts were successful.

## Highlights of Nephrology in Uruguay

Nephrology in Uruguay has been characterized by multidisciplinary teamwork focused on patients and by having nationwide registries for main activities such as renal biopsies, CKD, dialysis, kidney transplantations, their complications, and results. Cross-referencing data with that of the national registry of deaths has allowed for certainty about the survival rate of treated patients. Having universal access to RRT since the 1980s has made care homogenous, and having centralized funding has fostered the creation of mandatory registries. Consensual rules and guidelines for clinical practice that favor homogenous nephrological care nationwide and epidemiology research have come to exist thanks to specific research groups, university professors, and/or to the Uruguayan Society of Nephrology (glomerulopathies, anemia in CKD, bone mineral metabolism, PD, AKI, etc.). The Renal Health Program has fostered the development of prevention activities and has shown that patients monitored are at lower risk to start RRT and present lower mortality rates.

## Future Perspectives of Nephrology in Uruguay

Looking toward the future, it would be beneficial to extend the Renal Health Program to every institution of the *SNIS* in order to prevent or slow the progression of CKD. Additionally, the rational incorporation of new drugs and diagnostic methods for nephropathies is expected, with the idea of granting everyone access to them. Regarding the population in RRT, the objective is to expand the use of online HDF, make the use of icodextrin in PD available to all patients, make it easy to enter kidney transplant waitlists (improving the rate of waitlisted patients/patients on chronic dialysis), improve the transplantation rate (children and adults) through the optimization of the organ procurement program and the implementation of donation upon cardiac arrest programs, and promote safe organ donations for and from living related donors.

Uruguay has modestly contributed to scientific data in this field, periodically publishing original articles at peer-reviewed journals on the specialty and collaborating, on multiple occasions, with other international groups. One area of interest is to integrate international research networks, in order to participate in multicenter clinical trials.

## Conclusion

Nephrology has gradually developed in Uruguay and yet has allowed for providing full, universal nephrological care to all inhabitants, both children and adults, across the nation. Looking toward improvement, the national nephrology registries activities have further assured a continuous quality control of the care provided, control carried out by both nephrologists and health authorities.

## References


1. Franchi-Padé H. Enfermedades médicas de los riñones. Montevideo: Ed Científica del SMU, 1942. 2 vols. Available from: https://www.smu.org.uy/publicaciones/libros/historicos/emr-1/ and https://www.smu.org.uy/publicaciones/libros/historicos/emr-2/.
2. Franchi-Padé H. La multi-instantanée fonctionnelle du rein. La Semaine des Hopitaux de Paris. 1954;30(3):E172–81.
3. Mazzuchi N, Acosta N, Caorsi H, Schwedt E, Di Martino LA, Mautone M, Gadola L, Petraglia A, Noboa O. Programa de Prevención y Tratamiento de las Glomerulopatías. Frequency of diagnosis and clinic presentation of glomerulopathies in Uruguay. Nefrologia. 2005;25(2):113–20.
4. Lombardi R, et al. Diálisis peritoneal. El Día Médico Uruguayo. 1973;XI(476):262–6.
5. Fernández A, Espasandín W, Petruccelli D. Tratamiento de la insuficiencia renal aguda. Montevideo: Facultad de Medicina; 1962.
6. Petruccelli D, Llopart T, Corio E, Turnes A. Recuerdos de los comienzos de la Nefrología en Uruguay. Montevideo: Ed Tradinco; 2009.
7. Petruccelli D. Informe sobre trasplantes. Arch Med Intern. 1985;VII(1–4):45–8.
8. Ambrosoni P. Uruguay (Nefrología). Nefrologia. 1992;XII(Supl 3):52–61.
9. González-Bedat MC, Ferreiro Fuentes A, Chifflet Bide L, Ceretta ML. Registro Uruguayo de Diálisis: Informe anual 2016. Montevideo: RUD. 2018. http://nefrouruguay.org.uy/wp-content/uploads/2014/01/informeRUD2016.pdf. Accessed 2 June 2019.
10. Fondo Nacional de Recursos. Unidad de Registros Médicos. Informe anual de diálisis crónica: año. 2018. Montevideo. https://www.fnr.gub.uy/sites/default/files/estadisticas/ia2018/ia_dial_2018.pdf. Accessed 2 June 2019.
11. Orihuela S, Curi L, Nin M, Manzo L, Gonzalez G, Nuñez N, Kurdian M, Cuñeti L, Larre-Borges P, González-Martínez F. First 1500 kidney transplants at the Institute of Nephrology and Urology in Uruguay: analysis of the results. Transplant Proc. 2016;48(2):616–9.
12. Schwedt E, Solá L, Ríos PG, Mazzuchi N, National Renal Healthcare Program. Improving the management of chronic kidney disease in Uruguay: a National Renal Healthcare Program. Nephron Clin Pract. 2010;114(1):c47–59. https://doi.org/10.1159/000245069.
13. Mazzuchi N, Schwedt E, Solá L, González C, Ferreiro A. Risk factors and prevention of end stage renal disease in Uruguay. Ren Fail. 2006;28:617–25.
14. Mazzuchi N, Rios P, Canzani O, De Souza N, Gadola L, Lamadrid V, Sola L. Impacto del control clínico en el Programa de Salud Renal en la supervivencia de pacientes. Fondo Nacional de Recursos. Publicaciones científicas. Accessed 2 June 2019. http://www.fnr.gub.uy/trabajos_cientificos_psr.
15. Ríos P, Schwedt E, Solá L, Gadola L, De Souza N, Lamadrid V. Importance of preventive medical examination for early diagnosis of renal disease in Uruguay - the National Renal Health Program. Arch Med Interna. 2015;37(3):114–21.
16. Schwedt E, Solá L, Ríos PG, Mazzuchi N. Improving the management of chronic kidney disease in Uruguay: a National Renal Healthcare Program. Nephron Clin Pract. 2010;114:c47–59.
17. Ríos-Sarro P, Sola L, Gadola L. Prevalence of CKD in Uruguay. In: García-García G, Agodoa LY, Norris KC, editors. Chronic kidney disease in disadvantaged populations. London: Academic Press; 2017. p. 35–44. https://doi.org/10.1016/B978-0-12-804311-0.00005-4.
18. Subiza AK, Odriozola M, Ríos P, Lamadrid V, Mazzuchi N, Gadola L. Riesgo cardiovascular en enfermedad renal crónica. Rev Urug Cardiol. 2016;31:206–18.
19. Guía de Práctica clínica en el tratamiento de las glomerulopatías. Gadola L, Noboa O, Otatti G, Cabrera MJ, González-Martinez F, Caorsi H. Ed Cuadrado, 2018, Uruguay. ISBN 978-9974-8564-2-4.
20. Garau M, Cabrera J, Ottati G, Caorsi H, Gonzalez Martinez F, Acosta N, Aunchayna MH, Gadola L, Noboa O. PLoS One. 2018;13(10):e0206637. https://doi.org/10.1371/journal.pone.0206637.
21. Urrestarazu A, Figueroa S, Coitiño R, Coria V, Acosta N, Aunchayna MH, Garau M, Gadola L. Nefropatías tubulointersticiales no obstructivas biopsiadas en Uruguay. Nefrología Latinoamericana. 2017;14(4):144–52. https://doi.org/10.1016/j.nefrol.2017.06.001.
22. Boggia J, Luzardo L, Lujambio I, Sottolano M, Robaina S, Thijs L, Olascoaga A, Noboa O, Struijker-Boudier HA, Safar ME, Staessen JA. The diurnal profile of central hemodynamics in a general Uruguayan population. Am J Hypertens. 2016;29(6):737–46. https://doi.org/10.1093/ajh/hpv169.
23. Tenzi J, Ferreiro A, Lombardi L, Schwedt E, Nin N, Cancela M, González F. Injuria renal aguda en medicina intensiva. Encuesta multicéntrica nacional. Paciente crítico. 2009;19:9–16.
24. Llopart T, Lombardi R, Forselledo M, et al. Acute renal failure in open heart surgery. Ren Fail. 1997;19:319–23.
25. Lombardi R, Ferreiro A. Risk factor profile for acute kidney injury after cardiac surgery is different according to the level of baseline renal function. Ren Fail. 2008;30:155–60.

26. Masquil D, Ferreiro A. Epidemiología, curso e indicadores pronósticos de la injuria renal aguda en la unidad de cuidados intensivos. Abstract in XIII Congreso Latinoamericano de Nefrología. Sociedad Latinoamericana de Nefrología. Lima. Setiembre 2019. https://slanh.net/congreso-slanh-2019-lima-peru/. Accessed 18 Dec 2019.
27. Lombardi R. Acute renal failure in leptospirosis in Uruguay. Ren Fail. 1997;19(2):315–8.
28. Lombardi R, Ferreiro A, Rosa-Diez G. Raising awareness of acute kidney injury: a Latin American experience. Kidney Int Rep. 2018;3(6):1416–23. https://doi.org/10.1016/j.ekir.2018.08.003.
29. Uruguay. Ministerio de Salud. Ordenanza número 89/2014 del Ministerio de Salud: Protocolo de preparación de pacientes que recibirán medios de contraste. Montevideo. 2014. https://www.gub.uy/ministerio-salud-publica/sites/ministerio-salud-publica/files/2019-02/Ord.%20Min.%20N°%2089%20y%20Anexos.pdf. Accessed 9 June 2019.
30. Ferreiro A, Lombardi R. Acute kidney injury after cardiac surgery is associated with mid-term but not long-term mortality: a cohort-based study. PLoS One. 2017;12(7):e0181158. https://doi.org/10.1371/journal.pone.0181158.
31. Llopart T, González F, Alvarez A, Alvarez I, Fernández JM, Nin J, Schwedt E, Ambrosoni P, Mazzuchi N. Situación de la hemodiálisis crónica en el Uruguay. Rev Med Urug. 1986;2:90–4.
32. Schwedt E, Fernández J, González F, Ambrosoni P, Mazzuchi N. Diez años de hemodiálisis en Uruguay. Condiciones de ingreso, características del tratamiento y resultados. Nefrologia. 1993;13(Suppl 4):20–9.
33. Fernández J, Schwedt E, Ambrosoni P, González F, Mazzuchi N. Eleven years of chronic hemodialysis in Uruguay: mortality time course. Kidney Int. 1995;47:1721–75.
34. Mazzuchi N, Fernández-Cean JM, Schwedt E, González-Martínez F, et al. Registro Latinoamericano de Diálisis y Trasplante. Informe 1998. Nefrología latinoamericana. 1998;5:105–59.
35. González-Bedat MC, Rosa-Diez G. Registro Latinoamericano de Diálisis y Trasplante Renal: Informe 2015–2016. http://test1.slanh.net/wp-content/uploads/2018/10/INFORME-2015-2016.pdf. Accessed 2 June 2019.
36. González C, coord. Registro Uruguayo de Diálisis. Incidencia anual de diálisis 1981–2018. http://nefrouruguay.org.uy/wp-content/uploads/2019/03/INCIDENCIA-PREVALENCIA-1981-2018.pdf. Accessed 2 June 2019.
37. United States Renal Data System. 2018 USRDS annual data report: epidemiology of kidney disease in the United States. Bethesda: National Institutes of Health, National Institute of Diabetes and Digestive and Kidney Diseases; 2018.
38. González C, Fernández-Cean J, González-Martínez F, Schwedt E, Mazzuchi N. Chronic dialysis in Uruguay: mortality trends from 1981 to 1998. Nefrologia. 2001;21(4):342–8.
39. Uruguay. Ministerio de Salud Pública. Sistema Nacional Integrado de Salud. Montevideo, s.d. https://www.gub.uy/ministerio-salud-publica/politica-y-gestion/sistema-nacional-integrado-salud. Accessed 2 June 2019.
40. Molins S, Alonso L, Fernández J. Uruguay: El plan integral de atención a la salud. In: Gideon U, Biltrán R, Ignez T, editors. Planes de beneficios en salud en América Latina: una comparación regional. Washington, DC: BID; 2014. p. 115–43.
41. World Health Organization. Global health expenditure database. Geneva. 2019. https://data.worldbank.org/indicator/SH.XPD.OOPC.CH.ZS. Accessed 2 June 2019.
42. Uruguay. Fondo Nacional de Recursos ¿Qué es el Fondo Nacional de Recursos? Montevideo. n.d. http://www.fnr.gub.uy/que_es_fnr. Accessed 2 June 2019.
43. Uruguay. Fondo Nacional de Recursos. Misión, visión, valores y principios. Montevideo. n.d. http://www.fnr.gub.uy/mision. Accessed 2 June 2019.
44. Uruguay. Fondo Nacional de Recursos. Organización institucional. Montevideo. n.d. http://www.fnr.gub.uy/organizacion_institucional. Accessed 2 June 2019.
45. Uruguay. Fondo Nacional de Recursos. Información económica y financiera. Montevideo. n.d. http://www.fnr.gub.uy/info_economico_financiera. Accessed 2 June 2019.
46. Uruguay. Fondo Nacional de Recursos. Aranceles 2019. Montevideo. n.d. http://www.fnr.gub.uy/sites/default/files/finanzas/aranceles/aranceles_2019.pdf. Accessed 2 June 2019.
47. Uruguay. Fondo Nacional de Recursos. Técnicas. Montevideo. n.d. http://www.fnr.gub.uy/tecnicas. Accessed 2 June 2019.
48. Uruguay. Fondo Nacional de Recursos. Tratamiento con Medicamentos. Montevideo. n.d. http://www.fnr.gub.uy/tratamientos_con_medicamentos. Accessed 2 June 2019.
49. Uruguay. Fondo Nacional de Recursos. Programa de Salud Renal. Montevideo. n.d. http://www.fnr.gub.uy/home_psaludrenal. Accessed 2 June 2019.
50. Uruguay. Fondo Nacional de Recursos. Resultados. Montevideo. n.d. http://www.fnr.gub.uy/resultados. Accessed 2 June 2019.
51. Uruguay. Fondo Nacional de Recursos. Resultados Hemodiálisis: Año 2017. Montevideo. n.d. http://www.fnr.gub.uy/resultados_hemodialisis_2017. Accessed 2 June 2019.
52. Uruguay. Fondo Nacional de Recursos. Estándares de evaluación y seguimiento para la mejora de calidad de los IMAE. 2nd ed. Montevideo: FNR. Publicación Técnica N° 20. 2012. http://www.fnr.gub.uy/sites/default/files/libro_mejora_calidad_139_web.pdf. Accessed 2 June 2019.
53. Uruguay. Fondo Nacional de Recursos. Tratamiento dialítico. Normativa de cobertura FNR. Montevideo: julio 2006. http://www.fnr.gub.uy/sites/default/files/normativas/tecnicas/n_dialisis.pdf. Accessed 2 June 2019.
54. Uruguay. Fondo Nacional de Recursos. Guías para el diseño de la Unidad de Hemodiálisis. Montevideo: nov. 2007. http://www.fnr.gub.uy/sites/default/files/publicaciones/FNR_GuiaDeHemodialisis.pdf. Accessed 2 June 2019.
55. Aguirrezábal X, Bazet C, Beltrán L, Blanco J, Castillo T, Díaz L, et al. Guías de gestión de calidad del agua para diálisis. Montevideo: FNR. n.d. http://www.fnr.gub.uy/sites/default/files/publicaciones/FNR_guia_dialisis.pdf. Accessed 2 June 2019.
56. Blanco JC, Leiva G, Castillo T, Nin M, Chifflet L, Opertti A, et al. Guías de gestión de calidad del agua para diálisis. 2° ed. Montevideo: FNR, 2014. http://fnr.gub.uy/sites/default/files/publicaciones/FNR_guia_dialisis_2014.pdf. Accessed 2 June 2019.
57. Mazzuchi N, Carbonell E, Fernández-Cean J. Importance of blood pressure control in hemodialysis patient survival. Kidney Int. 2000;58(5):2147–54.
58. Gadola L, Gomez T, Saez L, et al. Diez años del registro uruguayo de peritonitis en diálisis peritoneal. Rev Med Urug. 2016;32(3):87–98.
59. Gadola L, Poggi C, Poggio M, Sáez L, Ferrari A, Romero J, Fumero S, Ghelfi G, Chifflet L, Borges PL. Using a multidisciplinary training program to reduce peritonitis in peritoneal dialysis patients. Perit Dial Int. 2013;33(1):38–45. https://doi.org/10.3747/pdi.2011.00109.
60. Gadola L, Poggi C, Dominguez P, Poggio MV, Lungo E, Cardozo C. Risk factors and prevention of peritoneal dialysis-related peritonitis. Perit Dial Int. 2019;39(2):119–25. https://doi.org/10.3747/pdi.2017.00287.
61. González-Martínez F, Orihuela S, Alvarez I, Dibello N, Curi L, Nin M, Wimber E, Mizraji R, Bengochea M, González G, Manzo

L, Toledo R, Silva W, Chopitea A, Lopez D, Balboa O, Porto D, Noboa O. Development of the national kidney transplantation program in Uruguay. Transplant Proc. 2015;47(8):2336–9.
62. Duro García V, Santiago-Delpín E, Tanus R. Latin America transplantation registry report 2015–2016. Np: STALYC. n.d. https://www.stalyc.net/registros/file/74-latin-america-transplantation-registry-report-2015-2016.html. Accessed 2 June 2019.
63. Uruguay. Fondo Nacional de Recursos. Visualizador de actos médicos realizados. 2018. Montevideo. n.d. http://www.fnr.gub.uy/visualizador_realizaciones_2018 Accessed 2 June 2019.
64. Olaizola I, Aznarez A, Jorgetti V, Petraglia A, Caorsi H, Acuña G, Fajardo L, Ambrosoni P, Mazzuchi N. Are there any differences in the parathyroid response in the different types of renal osteodystrophy? Nephrol Dial Transplant. 1998;13(3):15–8.
65. Ambrosoni P, Olaizola I, Heuguerot C, Parodi MN, Caorsi H, Caputti S, López J, Di Trápani N, Petraglia A. The role of imaging techniques in the study of renal osteodystrophy. Am J Med Sci. 2000;320(2):90–5.
66. Grunberg J. Historia de la nefrología pediátrica uruguaya. 1904–2007. Arch Med Int. 2007;XXIX(4):110–2.
67. Universidad de la República. Escuela de Graduados de la Facultad de Medicina. Montevideo: sd. http://www.egradu.fmed.edu.uy/sites/www.egradu.fmed.edu.uy/files//Programa_de_postgrados/Especialidades/NEFROLOGÍA%20PEDIÁTRICA.pdf. Accessed 2 June 2019.

# Nephrology in Venezuela

17

Ezequiel Bellorin-Font, Raul G. Carlini, Carmen Luisa Milanés, Pablo Amair, Douglas Urbina, Nelson Orta Sibu, Marcos Ariza, Jose R. Weisinger, and Evelyn Alonzo

| | |
|---|---|
| Area[1] | 916,445 km$^2$ |
| Population[2] | 32,219,521 (2019) |
| Capital | Caracas, DC |
| Three most populated cities | 1. Caracas<br>2. Maracaibo<br>3. Valencia |
| Official language | Spanish |
| Gross domestic product (GDP)[3] | 276.30 billion US Dollar (2018, PPP) |
| GDP per capita[3] | 8652 US Dollar (2018, PPP) |
| Human development index (HDI)[4] | 0.726 (96° position out of 189 countries) |
| Official currency | Bolívar (Bs.) |
| Total number of nephrologists[5] | 2009 – 614 nephrologists<br>2014 – 545 nephrologists |
| National society of nephrology[5] | Sociedad Venezolana de Nefrología (Venezuelan Society of Nephrology) www.svnefrologia.com |
| Incidence of end-stage renal disease | Not available |
| Prevalence of end-stage renal disease (on dialysis) | 2019 – 321 pmp |
| Total number of patients on dialysis (all modalities) | 2019 – 10,680 patients |
| Number of patients on hemodialysis | 2019 – 10,360 patients |
| Number of patients on peritoneal dialysis | 2019 – 320 patients |
| Number of renal transplantations per year[6] | 2012 – 339 patients<br>2018 – 43 patients<br>2019 – No patients |

1. Venezuela. Accessed in January 2020. Available in https://www.worldatlas.com/webimage/countrys/samerica/ve.htm
2. Instituto Nacional de Estadística, INE. Accessed in January 2020. Available in http://www.redatam.ine.gob.ve/Censo2011/index.html
3. The World Bank. Venezuela Data. Accessed in January 2020. Available in https://www.worldbank.org/en/country/venezuela
4. Human Development Report 2019. United Nations Development Program. Accessed in January 2020. Available in http://hdr.undp.org/sites/all/themes/hdr_theme/country-notes/VEN.pdf.
5. Sociedad Venezolana de Nefrologia Accessed in January 2020. Available in https://www.svnefrologia.com/
6. Unidad de Registros. Organización Nacional de Trasplante de Venezuela. Accessed in October 2019. Available in http://www.ontv-venezuela.org/

## Introduction

The Bolivarian Republic of Venezuela (Venezuela) is located in northern South America. The country is bound on the north by the Caribbean Sea and the Atlantic Ocean, on the east by Guyana, on the South by Brazil, and on the west by Colombia. It has a territory of 916,445 km$^2$, divided in 23 federal states and a federal district (Fig. 17.1) [1, 2]. States are divided in a total of 355 municipalities. Venezuelan official language is Spanish. The general table summarizes the main information of Venezuela [1–6].

There are no official statistics about the ethnicity of the Venezuelan population, but it is estimated that there is a large Mestizo and European descendent population comprising more than 90%, whereas African descendent and indigenous may comprise around 3.5% and 2.5%, respectively. Other groups comprise about 1.5% [1].

Freedom of religion in Venezuela is guaranteed by the national constitution. However, the majority of the population is mostly Christian, with predominance of Catholic

E. Bellorin-Font (✉)
Saint Louis University, St. Louis, MO, USA
e-mail: ezequiel.bellorinfont@health.slu.edu

R. G. Carlini · P. Amair
Venezuelan Society of Nephrology, Caracas, Venezuela

D. Urbina
Hospital Universitario de Caracas, Caracas, Venezuela

C. L. Milanés · E. Alonzo
National Organization of Transplant of Venezuela, Valencia, Venezuela

N. O. Sibu
Universidad de Carabobo, Valencia, Venezuela

M. Ariza
Hospital de Niños, Caracas, Venezuela

J. R. Weisinger
International University of Florida, Gainesville, FL, USA


J. A. Moura-Neto et al. (eds.), *Nephrology Worldwide*, https://doi.org/10.1007/978-3-030-56890-0_17

Roman and in lesser degree, Protestant groups. Other smaller groups are constituted by Muslims, Jews, and Indian to a lesser extent. Religious tolerance for minority groups is generally observed. After the last census of 2011, the estimated population of Venezuela for 2019 was 32,219,521 habitants with a density of 32.3 per $km^2$ (data.UN.org). Approximately 34% of the population is under 19 years of age. Caracas, the capital city, is the largest city in Venezuela with a population of roughly 5,576,000, Maracaibo with a population of 2,450,599 and Valencia with 2,299,026 habitants are the second and third largest cities, respectively [1, 2]. However, at the present time, these numbers might be misleading as current estimates indicate that as a consequence of the national political and socioeconomic crisis, at least 4,000,000 Venezuelans have fled the country representing over 13% of the country's total population [7].

Venezuela was the first South American country to proclaim its independence from Spain in 1811. Over the years, Venezuelan political evolution has cursed between military governments, dictatorships, and democracy. Democracy has been the form of government since 1958. The current political situation of the country is complex. After a period of 40 years of stable democratic representative governments that followed the last recognized dictatorship in 1958, the new constitution adopted in 1999, declared the end of the representative democracy and proclaimed the Bolivarian Republic of Venezuela with a form of direct democracy that has lasted until the present time. The bicameral National Congress was abolished and a unicameral National Assembly was instituted. The current political situation in Venezuela is highly volatile and is accompanied of social unrest as well as economic instability leading to a marked decrease in the internal growth domestic product.

The economy of Venezuela is based mainly on oil and to a lesser extent on manufacturing sectors. During the last years, the capability of the Venezuelan oil industry has decreased progressively in terms of both production and refining. Thus, the oil production has decreased from

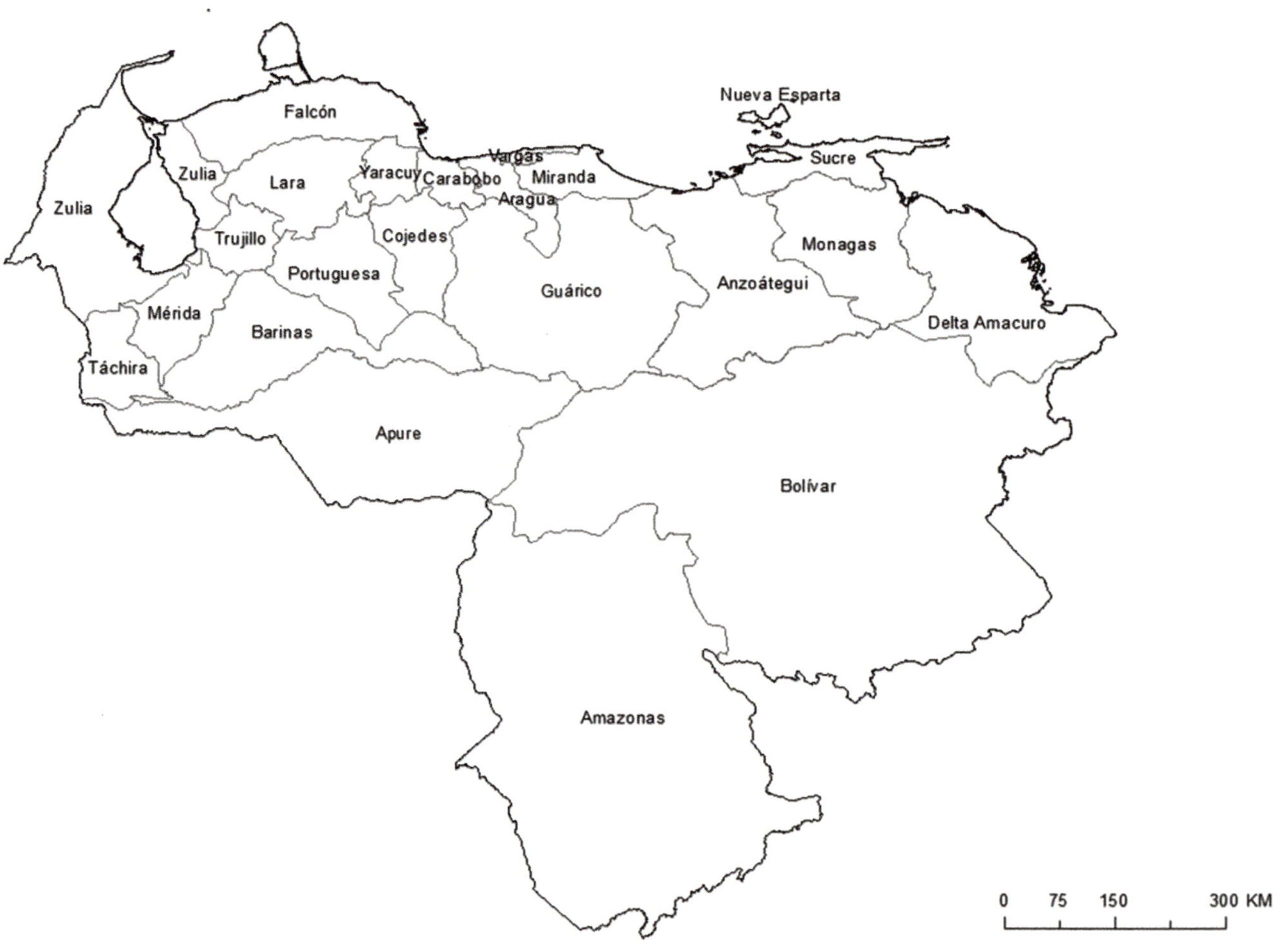


Fig. 17.1 Venezuela political map

3,155,000 barrels per day in 2000 to around 700,000 in 2019. This has resulted in a marked decrease in the economy of the country.

The currency of Venezuela is the Bolivar. The official exchange rate by November 2019 was 30,435.05 per USD. However, given the high inflation rate, estimated in 13,475.8% in November 2019, the exchange rate is highly fluctuating. The 2018 report of the "Economic Commission for Latin America and the Caribbean (ECLAC)" stated that the Bolivarian Republic of Venezuela was going through what could be the highest inflationary episode in the history of Latin America and the Caribbean, with an inflation that in 2018 would have reached 130,060.2% and a hyperinflation whose start dates back to November 2017 [3, 4, 8]. In 2018, the Survey on Living Conditions in Venezuela (ENCOVI) conducted by the main universities of the country revealed that extreme poverty increased from 23.6% to 61.2% in four years (2014–2018) and almost ten points between 2016 and 2017 [9].

Health is guaranteed as a constitutional right in Venezuela. The Ministry of Health (Ministerio del Poder Popular para la Salud) is responsible for the design, control, and execution of health policies, whereas the Social Security (Instituto Venezolano de los Seguros Sociales-IVSS) provides attention to employees based on their contributions and the funds provided by employers and the national government. However, since 2000, the Social Security is also involved in providing health services free of charge to the general population. It is also responsible for the national program of dialysis and the supply of immunosuppressive therapy for transplant patients. In addition to these two public systems, private health insurance companies and self-payed medicine are available for people and private companies with resources to cover such costs. Even though all these options are available, at the present time, an adequate coverage of health needs in the country is far from being satisfactory. Indeed, most health centers from primary to tertiary level are working well below than expected due to insufficient budget to cover costs of medication, personnel, equipment, and infrastructure.

## Brief History of Nephrology in Venezuela

Much of the early history of nephrology in Venezuela has been obtained from oral interviews over many years from some of Venezuela's most distinguished and celebrated nephrologists, many of whom have been recognized over many years, both nationally and internationally. While some of this early history has not been in published form yet, its value and importance serve as a significant reference to the development and advances of nephrology in Venezuela.

In the very early 1960s, as it has been told, it was common practice for many Venezuelan physicians to seek advanced specialized training from diverse and prestigious universities abroad, particularly in the USA, Europe, and Mexico. It is important to remember that nephrology, as a multifaceted specialty as we know currently, did not exist before the 1950s. Thus, the birth of nephrology is internationally recognized to have its initiation in 1960 [10] and the early years that followed. As there were no fellowships or advanced training programs in nephrology available in Venezuela in those times, many physicians traveled outside the country to continue their studies and research. Upon their return to Venezuela, they began their work in the largest cities of several states throughout the country. These nephrology pioneers worked almost independently from each other. Some had to begin their activity attending patients in cardiology or internal medicine departments in order to later achieve, with much effort, perseverance, and passion for their work, the creation of the first Venezuelan nephrology centers.

Over the years, university postgraduate training and degree in nephrology were established, and new specialists were incorporated into the renal care of patients. At the same time, a considerable number of physicians continued to be trained outside the country, mainly in the USA, France, and Mexico. Upon their return to Venezuela, some of these physicians were incorporated in to national universities and laboratories in order to continue the research they had learned and developed during their stay abroad, while others devoted themselves to daily clinical practice and teaching. All of them, collectively, contributed to the growth and strengthening of nephrology in the country.

The number of nephrologists over the years is not well known. According to the archives of the Venezuelan Society of Nephrology, in 1972 the society had 17 members. By 2008, the maximum number of 618 members (24 nephrologist/pmp) was reached; however, the membership had decreased considerably by 2018 [11]. It is important to mention that these figures may not reflect the exact number of nephrologists in the country, as there is an undetermined number of specialists who are not enrolled in the Society. In addition, more recently, an increasing number of nephrologists, as in other specialties, have left the country as a consequence of the deteriorating political and economic conditions that Venezuela has been facing during the last years.

The certification process in nephrology and other medical specialties in Venezuela is done by the College of Physicians (Colegio Médico) and universities. There are two ways to obtain it: perform a university graduate training in nephrology through a programmed residence of 2–3 years or by carrying out a non-university residency program for 2 years with recognition by the College of Physicians. In both cases, a residency in internal medicine for 2 years in an accredited hospital is required as a pre-requisite. In recent years, due to the scarcity of human resources, some of the nephrology graduate programs request at least 1 year of residence in internal medicine. The graduate program includes a practical-theoretical program in clinical nephrology, dialysis in its two modalities (peritoneal and hemodialysis), and renal transplantation. As part of the evaluation of proficiency, graduate students must take periodic written and oral exams on nephrology.

Similarly, in order to obtain the pediatric nephrology specialty certification, it is required the completion of a 3-year residence in pediatrics at an accredited hospital, followed by a 2-year graduate residency in pediatric nephrology undertaken at one of the five organized graduate programs in the country. All programs have a defined theoretical content with an overview of general and pediatric nephrology, as well as practical training in specific topics including pediatric hemodialysis and both acute and chronic peritoneal dialysis. Three of these programs also include training in pediatric renal transplantation.

Programs are under the supervision of Ministry of Health directly and the local authorities and required the complexion of a thesis to obtain the university degree in the specialty of nephrology.

The salary for physicians and nurses working in hospitals of the Hospital of the Ministry of Health depends on their years of service and the number of hours of work. As an example, in 2019, the monthly salaries of a physician during his nephrology fellowship was equivalent to 8.00 USD (262,206 Bs), 12.00 USD (391,498 Bs) for an attending physician with 8 hours daily hiring, and 13.00 USD (416,240 Bs) for a head-of-service.

**Table 17.1** Patterns, organizations, and programs of renal health policies in Venezuela

| Pattern | Institution | Program | Year |
|---|---|---|---|
| Patient survival | National Center for Dialysis and Transplantation, the Ministry of Health | Program of attention to renal disease, focused on RRT<br>Development of a national network for renal disease | 1977 |
| Limitation of damage | National Center for Renal Disease, the Ministry of Health | Program of attention to renal disease<br>Integration of three levels of health | 1995 |
| Education to general population for healthy habits and life<br>Improvement of quality of life<br>Prevention of risk factors for renal disease<br>Early detection and treatment<br>Guarantee RRT for ESKD and AKI | Program of renal health. The Ministry of Health<br>Ministry of the Popular Power for Health (MPPS) | Program of Renal Health | 2001<br>Updated 2006<br>2009 |

## Evolution of Nephrology Programs

In general, the development of nephrological care in Venezuela followed the general principles of health: (1) patient survival, (2) damage control of chronic kidney disease (CKD), and (3) improvement of health quality. In Venezuela, these principles have had an historical correlation with the change of denomination of the institutions and health programs. As shown in Table 17.1, along the years, these principles have evolved with changes in the name and scope of the Ministry of Health: from the "Ministry of Health and Social Assistance" (1936) to the "Ministry of Health and Social Development" (1999) and finally, in 2009, the "Ministry of the Popular Power for Health (MPPS)" to changes in the conception of renal diseases as a public health problem. Thus, the programs for renal disease control, initially centered in the control of the disease, have evolved to the promotion of renal health.

In fact, as time went on, and based on a better knowledge of the epidemiology of kidney disease and new developments in the pathophysiology and treatment of kidney disease, the Ministry of Health redesigned its policy based on four elements:

1. Prevention by means of early detection and referral to multidisciplinary health teams, as well as promotion of health habits in the community.
2. Prevention of progression of renal disease by pharmacologic and non-pharmacologic means.
3. An increase in the rate of coverage and reduction of disparities in the access to dialysis.
4. An increase in the rates of renal transplantation [12] through better organ procurement programs and reinforcement of transplant centers.

**Table 17.2** Public policies and actions that have influenced the development of nephrology in Venezuela

| Policy | Institution | Year |
|---|---|---|
| Creation of the National Center for Dialysis and Transplantation [13] | Ministry of Health | 1977 |
| Creation of the Direction of Nephrology, Dialysis and Transplantation. (http://www.ivss.gov.ve/contenido/Nefrologia,-dialisis-y-trasplante-renal) | Venezuelan Institute of the Social Security (IVSS) | 1992 |
| The National Coordinated Program of kidney transplant in Venezuela [14] | Ministry of Health | 1986 |
| Law of organ transplantation and anatomy materials in human being [15] | Ministry of Health | 1992 |
| Creation of the National Organization of Transplant of Venezuela (ONTV) [16] | NGO | 1997 |
| Norms for the authorization, regulation, and control of medical health establishments as transplant centers [17] | Ministry of Health | 2000 |
| Creation of the Organ and Procurement Program (SPOT) (D. Urbina, personal communication; [18]) | ONTV (NGO) Ministry of Health | 2001 2003 |
| Regulations and guidelines for the architectonic requirements and functioning of dialysis units in public and private institutions in the Venezuela [19] | Ministry of Health | 2004 |
| Law of donation and organ transplant, tissue and cells and in human beings [20] | Ministry of Health | 2011 |

Unfortunately, part of these achievements has been lost in the last years due to the national political crisis that has affected directly the health programs for the population [13]. Table 17.2 summarizes several public policies and actions that have influenced the development of nephrology in the country. Some of these aspects will be addressed in the following sections of this chapter.

## Kidney Diseases

### Epidemiology of Kidney Disease

Very few studies address the epidemiology of kidney disease in Venezuela. However, several papers have been published about specific diseases, some of them endemic and others, over the course of epidemic bursts.

From 1985 to 1989, the most frequent causes of nephrology consultation were arterial hypertension (35.5%) and glomerulonephritis (16%) followed by chronic renal failure (14.2%) and urinary tract infection (13.5%) [21]. Interestingly, however, the prevalence of diseases leading to end stage renal disease (ESRD) has changed considerably during the last 20 years. In 1999, diabetes, hypertension, and glomerular diseases accounted for more than 60% of the patient on chronic dialysis, followed by tubulointerstitial nephritis (9%) and obstructive nephropathies (5%); other diseases such as adult polycystic kidney disease and lupus nephritis were relatively less frequent in the dialysis population [22]. More recently (2010), diabetes and hypertension have become the first causes of admission to dialysis. It should be taking into account that a high percentage of the ESRD population reaches specialized medical care at very advanced stages and without a clear history of renal disease, thus making an etiologic diagnosis almost impossible. Furthermore, because hypertension is an almost constant finding of ESRD, its place as one of the leading causes of admission to dialysis may represent an overestimation.

Regarding the etiology of biopsy-proven kidney disease, a retrospective analysis of 3541 native kidney biopsies performed between 1998 and 2008, and originated mainly from the nephrology services of university hospitals, showed focal segmental glomerulosclerosis (FSGS) as the most frequent renal disease, accounting for 54% of primary nephropathies, whereas lupus nephropathy accounted for 46% of the causes of secondary glomerulopathies [23].

Acute post-streptococcal glomerulonephritis (AGN) has been recognized as an endemic disease in the city of Maracaibo (Zulia State) and perhaps also in other parts of the country. In 1968 an outbreak of 348 cases of AGN was described in Maracaibo [24] by Rodriguez-Iturbe et al. Between 1973 and 1974, 120 of those patients were reexamined; all but one had been completely asymptomatic. Out of the 120 patients, 16 (13.3%) had one or more of the following abnormalities (AGN, group A): decreased creatinine clearance, microscopic hematuria, proteinuria of 1 g/day or more and hypertension, whereas 104 patients (86.7%) were normal by all clinical and laboratory parameters tested (AGN, group B). These findings led to the conclusion that uremia is rare in the first decade after epidemic post-streptococcal glomerulonephritis [20].

### Kidney Disease in the General Population

The prevalence of CKD in the general adult population in Venezuela is not well known. Only three studies have been carried out in small, non-urban population groups. In 2003, a study conducted from 1991 to 1998 estimated that the incidence of CKD stage 5 in Goajiro Indians was 220 pmp/year [25]. Another investigation in 300 individuals from four aboriginal groups conducted in the Bolívar state showed that the two ethnic groups that are in contact with urban areas had a significantly higher blood pressure than the other two who lived distant from these zones. To assess the prevalence of ESRD among indigenous populations, we retrospectively examined the records from two University hospitals in the area. Type 2 diabetes was the cause of ESRD in 66.6% of persons from four different ethnic groups. These data suggest that the incidence of diabetes in this ESRD population is more than twice that of the country as a whole [19]. In another study carried out in 2000 in Choroni, a seashore town in the Aragua state with a total population of 2539 inhabitants, of which 1665 were ≥15 years old and 1436 of them (86.2%) were included in the analysis, the prevalence of CKD in any of its evolutionary stages, was equivalent to 4178 pmp. The main causes of CKD were hypertensive vascular nephropathy, polycystic kidney disease, diabetic nephropathy, and primary glomerulopathy [26]. However, it is important to consider that this sample represents a cluster with special demographic and geographic characteristics and did not represent the prevalence of kidney disease in the whole country. In fact, an analysis in the whole Aragua state based on 40,083 death certificates in people ≥15 years old from 1986 to 1995, a diagnosis of CKD was reported in 1679 cases, equivalent to an estimated prevalence of 134 pmp. The most frequent associated diagnosis in these cases were diabetes mellitus and arterial hypertension [27].

## Prevention of Kidney Disease

As an additional mean to look for possible solutions to the increasing demand in nephrological care, since 1977 the program of attention to renal disease of the Ministry of Health proposed actions to develop prevention programs in nephrology, focusing efforts and resources through the incorporation of the primary and secondary levels into the tertiary level of the health-care system. The purpose of this integration of the three levels of health care was to create a broad coverage system to optimize the care of the CKD population.

Unfortunately, at that time the effectiveness of this program to attain specific objectives was limited, due in part to the relatively scarce medical resources available to apply preventive measures to control the progression of kidney disease and limited resources to approach early detection of kidney disease on a national scale.

Since 2001, with new developments and tendencies in the world focusing on renal health, the Ministry of Health reformulated its objectives creating the program of renal health with a wider conception emphasizing the promotion of education on primary prevention and control of risk factors for renal disease in the population, particularly oriented to those most frequently associated to CKD, such as diabetes and hypertension, among others. In this sense, the program hired and trained renal health coordinators for 19 of the 22 states of the country. These coordinators were involved in specific actions related to education, particularly to the disadvantaged population, schools, and patient associations. Of note, these coordinators joined efforts with other coordinators from related programs such as cardiovascular disease and diabetes. As an example, it can be mentioned that in 2008 these coordinators (renal, cardiovascular, and diabetes) working together delivered 50,763 educational talks among the three programs national wide, on prevention and risk factors for these diseases. In addition, the renal health program carried out CKD investigations in 80,886 persons, of which 4504 had risk factors for kidney disease [28]. Unfortunately, as occurred with other programs, most of these activities have been halted by the deteriorating political and economic conditions.

## Renal Replacement Therapy Scenario

### Hemodialysis

Hemodialysis is the most prevalent form of RRT in Venezuela. As will be described in the following paragraphs, the program has evolved to a progressive coverage of the needs of RRT based on public policies designed and executed by the Ministry of Health and the Social Security. The majority of dialysis centers provide hemodialysis three times a week with a duration of approximately 4 hours for treatment. Patients receive chronic RRT at no cost.

In Venezuela, the public health system is constituted by all institutions financed by the state. As mentioned above, the Ministry of Health is in charge of the development and execution of the country health policies, including those related to renal replacement therapy, whereas the Social Security is in charge of providing health care to workers from the public and private sectors, as well as their family. All RRT supplies and the payment to private dialysis units for dialysis service are also covered by the Social Security. Very few patients on chronic RRT are covered by the private sector. During the initial years of nephrology in Venezuela, renal replacement therapy (RRT) was performed mainly in Ministry of Health, Social Security, and military hospitals. In 1976, only three hospitals in the country had human and technical resources for the specialized care of renal disease, including hemodialysis (HD), peritoneal dialysis (PD), and kidney transplant. In addition, six regional hospitals had nephrologists for the management of clinical nephrology, but not RRT. The absolute number of HD stations was 57, being 75% of them located in Caracas, the country's capital, and Maracaibo, the second largest city of the country. The absolute number of patients was 72 for a country with an estimated population of 13.7 million inhabitants in 1976, equivalent to a prevalence of treatment of 5 pmp (Fig. 17.2) [21]. That year the Ministry of Health acknowledged for the first time CKD as a public health problem and created the National Center for Dialysis and Transplantation (CNDT) ascribed to the Division of

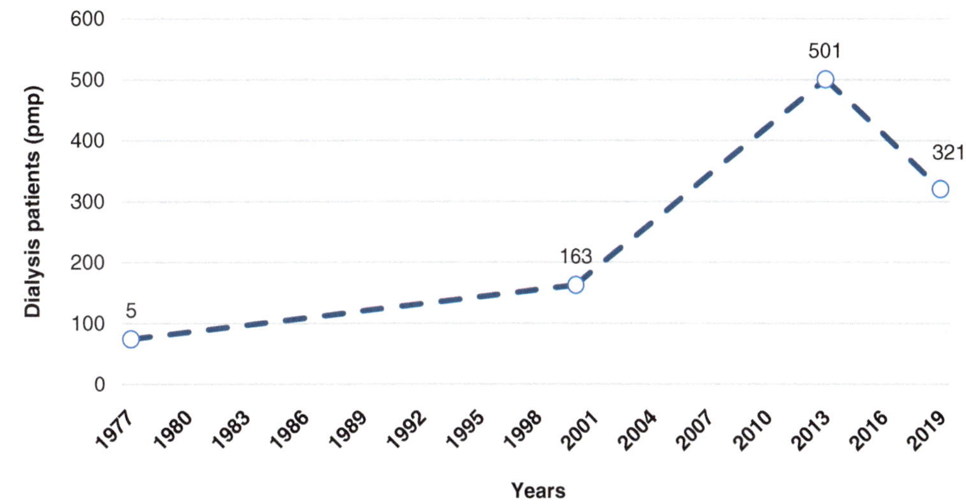


**Fig. 17.2** Prevalence of patients on dialysis in Venezuela (1977–2019). Numbers above points represent the rate of patient per million population (pmp)

Chronic Diseases [29]. The objectives of the center were the definition, planning, and execution of a national program to fight kidney disease through the creation of norms, guidelines, and procedures for the prevention, clinical care, education, and research in all nephrology areas, dialysis, and transplant centers in hospitals of the public health system, as well as professional advice to other centers and institutions of the private and non-governmental sectors. The CNDT had an advisory committee formed by recognized national nephrology leaders, the Venezuelan Society of Nephrology, and representatives of other institutions involved in patient care [29].

These advances in public policy brought about significant relief to the RRT demand. Thus, RRT had been in use in Venezuela since the early years of nephrology, only a relatively low number of patients had access to this type of therapy due to economic constraints, as well as to geographical, technical, and human resources limitations. The development of national ESRD policies by the national government through the Ministry of Health and the Social Security in the late 1970s and early 1980s helped increasing the rate of RRT coverage, progressively [29]. Thus, according to the Venezuelan registry of dialysis and transplantation, between 1990 and 1999 the coverage increased to 197/pmp, a rate still well below (48.7%) the minimum standard expected at that time by the SLANH for our region [30, 31]. However, it was evident a clear trend towards increasing the rates of coverage. The creation of the National Direction of Nephrology, Dialysis and Transplantation (by the Social Security), with the aim of standardizing and regulating the treatment of ESRD for patients covered by the social security system, was an important factor in the progressive increase in coverage rates in subsequent years [32]. The Direction participated in the authorization and supervision of private outpatient dialysis units, providing RRT to the population, the purchase of dialysis supplies, and the RRT reimbursement (J. Domínguez, personal communication, 2019). In 1979, the first national private HD unit was created (L. Troconis, personal communication, 2019), followed by the establishment of other outpatient private units in several cities of the country and, later, to the creation of an association representing private outpatient dialysis facilities under regulation and control by the Social Security (the Venezuelan Association of Non-Hospital Dialysis Units – AVUDE). These events resulted in a faster growth in the number of patients receiving RRT as well as in the number of outpatient centers authorized to provide dialysis treatment. In the ensuing years, the Social Security assumed progressively the full cost of dialysis supplies in the country and the reimbursement for treatment in private units authorized by the institution.

As part of the new actions of the program, in 2004 the Ministry of Health published the regulations and guidelines for the architectonic and operational requirements of dialysis units in public and private institutions in Venezuela [33], which helped not only to the development of dialysis centers according with national and international regulations but also to provide a better environment for patients, quality improvement of the treatment, and prevention of complications. In 2006, 122 dialysis units were in operation in the country, 29 of the Ministry of Health, 10 of the Social Security, and 83 outpatient private units under contract with the Social Security, all of them adapted to the regulations mentioned above. Five years later (2011), there were a total of 136 dialysis units in the country, of which 33 were in Ministry of Health hospitals, 12 in Social Security hospitals, and 91 in outpatient facilities under contract with the Social Security [15].

Unfortunately, these achievements have been progressively lost in the last 5 years. In this period, a complex social, economic, and political situation has led not only to the arrest of the CKD treatment programs growth, but also to a severe deterioration of almost the entire structure of the RRT program. This can be appreciated in the following

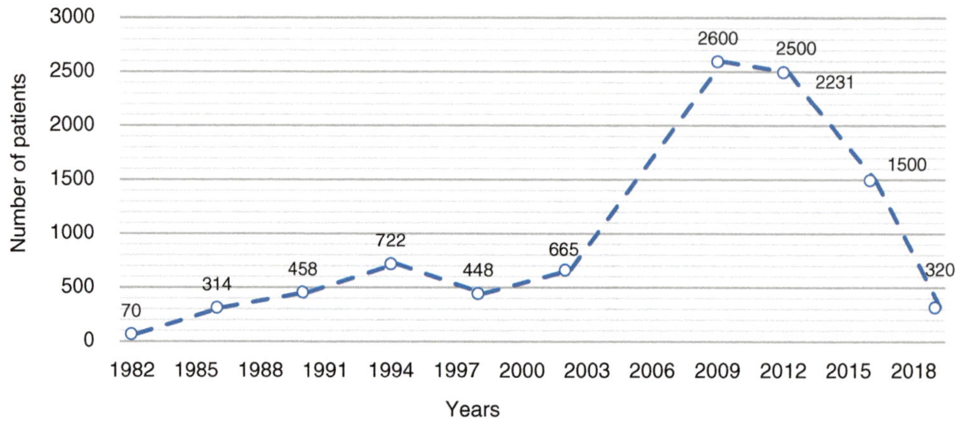


**Fig. 17.3** Evolution of peritoneal dialysis in Venezuela (1982–2019). Number above points represent absolute number of patients

unofficial numbers. By 2013, there were 15,130 patients on dialysis in Venezuela (12,899 on HD and 2231 on PD). At the estimated population of 30.3 million inhabitants, this corresponds to a prevalence of 500 pmp, equivalent to 71.5% of the current goal for Latin America according to the SLANH [34]. However, it should be mentioned that while this figure may give the impression of relatively high dialysis coverage for the Latin American standard, actually the coverage is not uniform in the country, and an important proportion of it is at the expense of units located in large cities. Unofficial estimates indicate that currently (2019) there are a total of 10,680 dialysis patients, of which 10,360 are in HD and 320 in PD. This represents a decrease of 29% of the total number of dialysis patients, corresponding to a decline of 19.6% in HD and 85.6% in PD patients as compared with 2013. As for population coverage concerns, it has decreased to 321 pmp assuming a decrease in the total country's population of about four million people due to migration to other countries as a consequence of the worsening social, political and economic conditions [35]. At the present time, throughout the country, there are 141 dialysis units, which represent a scant growth of 5 dialysis units in the last 7 years.

The reuse of hemodialysis filters and lines was investigated in 1987 and 1988 at the NCDT of the Ministry of Health, and a prototype device for filter reuse (IRMA-I) was built. After a cost/benefit analysis under the prevailing economic conditions in the country as well as an analysis of environmental impact studies, the decision of the Ministry of Health was not to initiate a reuse program of hollow fiber dialyzers in Venezuela.

## Peritoneal Dialysis in the Country

Peritoneal dialysis began in Venezuela in the early 1960s mainly for the treatment of acute kidney injury (AKI) and for some ESRD patients. However, with the increasing availability of HD, the use of acute PD decreased notoriously. In addition, unsatisfactory results associated to the use of PD fluid in glass bottles and rigid catheters rendered PD for the treatment of CKD short lived.

A new perspective arose with the introduction of continuous ambulatory PD (CAPD) as a method for treatment of CKD in large scale. Three university hospitals started CAPD programs simultaneously at the end of 1979 and early 1980, using commercial plastic bags and permanent PD catheters. This development led to a rapid increase in the number of ESRD patients under this modality of RRT. Thus, approximately 16% of all dialysis patients were under this type of treatment in 1983 and by 1987, this percentage reached approximately 50% due to a shortage of HD machines in the country [14]. Figure 17.3 displays the evolution of the PD program over time. In 1982, there were approximately 70 ESRD patients on PD, increasing to 665 patients by 2002 [36]. That was the equivalent to 10% of the whole dialysis population. Of these, 78% used CAPD, 20% automated PD (APD), and 2% intermittent PD (IPD). In the following years, the PD program had an important expansion at the national level, not only with the opening of new units but also in education through guidelines, meetings, and workshops for nephrologists, paramedical personnel, and patients. In 2012 there were 2500 patients using this method, representing 19% of the dialysis population, with 92 PD units throughout the country. The PD program growth was suddenly interrupted in 2016 when the Social Security released a statement informing the suspension of the delivery of PD supplies to the PD units/centers. The distribution of PD supplies continued only to active patients. This resulted in an impossibility to admit new patients into the program. But the most complex situation was that the home delivery of PD materials was inadequate. Consequently, many patients were re-allocated to HD. Table 17.3 shows the national impact of the interruption of the PD program. The goals of RRT for Latin America according to the SLANH, Pan American Health Organization (OPAS), and World Health Organization (WHO) for the period 2015–2019 included an increase of total RRT to 700 pmp and an increase in the proportion of patients assigned to PD with a goal of 20% of the total patients on RRT [34].

Table 17.3 Decline of the peritoneal dialysis program in Venezuela (2009–2019)

| Years | 2009 | 2012 | 2013 | 2016 | 2019 |
|---|---|---|---|---|---|
| Patients on PD (*n*) | 2600 | 2500 | 2231 | 1500 | 320 |
| Patients on PD (%) | 30 | 19 | 14.7 | 10 | 3 |
| Active PD units (*n*) | NA | 92 | NA | 54 | NA |

Number and percentage of patients on PD (peritoneal dialysis) in Venezuela from 2009 to 2019. *NA* Not available

## Continuous Renal Replacement Therapies (CRRT)

Continuous renal replacement therapies (CRRT) are uncommonly used in Venezuela, mostly due to high costs; equipment and supplies are available only in a few private centers. Nephrologists perform the procedures in most cases. To our knowledge, the only study published comprises 66 patients in an intensive care unit (ICU) treated with continuous venovenous hemofiltration (CVVH) using a three pump system. The results were comparable to other published studies [37].

## Dialysis Reimbursement Policies

In Venezuela, health is a fundamental social right established in the national Constitution [16]. According to this, all Venezuelan citizens are entitled to all health services, which include dialysis. In this regard, the nephrology centers of the Ministry of Health offer unrestricted dialysis care (HD, PD, and medications) to all patients with such requirements. The Social Security system likewise provides RRT to their affiliated patients and family, whether in their own hospitals or centers or in outpatient private dialysis units under contract with the institution through an agreement for materials supply and reimbursement for services. This also includes some medicines directly related to the CKD treatment, such as erythropoietin, vitamin D analogs, and intravenous iron. Therefore, RRT is, at least theoretically, covered by the public health system at no cost for the patient. The coverage does not include acute RRT for inpatients in private hospitals.

Although access to health care is theoretically universal, there is a deficit in total coverage of the population as well as disparity in the access to RRT. Thus, while the urban population in middle size to large cities may approach the expected coverage for the region, many small cities, towns, and rural areas are clearly ill covered. This disparity has increased with the reduction by 30% in the total number of dialysis patients in the last years. With current rising trends in the incidence of ESRD and costs of medical technology, the long-term goal of complete RRT coverage will become increasingly out of reach. In fact, with the ongoing economic and political crisis in the country, not only the expected coverage has not been attained but in fact has decreased considerably.

## Acute Kidney Injury and Critical Care Nephrology

In Venezuela, the epidemiology of AKI is not completely defined, but sepsis, shock, nephrotoxicity, obstructive uropathy, and acute CKD decompensation are among the most frequent causes identified of AKI requiring RRT. It can also be noted that most of the nephrology centers in public and private hospitals have the capability for the diagnosis and treatment of this complication. At the beginning of the dialysis practice, in the 1960s, PD was the most used therapy modality for AKI. This procedure continued to be performed for many years, until HD became the method of choice. Currently, conventional intermittent HD, mainly performed by nephrologists, is the RRT of choice for AKI patients requiring dialysis (D. Urbina, personal communication).

While it is true that there is no epidemiologic information on AKI, it is important to mention what is occurring in Venezuela with the increasing number of malaria cases and AKI. In a review conducted between 1982 and 2001, there were 76 cases of AKI due to malaria treated in the nephrology center of the one of the teaching hospitals that covers a broad endemic area. Sixty-two of them (82%) required dialysis (50% HD and 13% PD) [18]. More recently, only in the year 2018, there were 54 cases of AKI associated to malaria, 13 of which required HD (M. Grace, personal communication). Therefore, with the increasing trend of malaria it is possible that the requirements of RRT will increase.

## Renal Transplantation

### Living Donor and Deceased Donor

Kidney transplant in Venezuela has been an important part of the nephrology armamentarium since 1967 when the first renal transplant was performed at the University Hospital of Maracaibo, followed a year later for a second transplant at the University Hospital of Caracas. Along the ensuing 52 years, the implementation and execution of the Venezuelan renal transplant program can be differentiated in at least three periods (Fig. 17.4).

**Period A: 1967–1997:** This period was characterized by the development of national nephrology, dialysis, renal transplant centers, human resource training, the development of a solution for organ preservation [38] that was used in Venezuela for more than 25 years, a national histocompatibility laboratory, the establishment of the regulatory and legal framework for transplants [17], and a progressive growth of the number of successful kidney transplants, mainly in three hospitals: University Hospital of Maracaibo, University Hospital of Caracas, and Hospital Miguel Perez Carreño, as reference centers. Along the following years, the

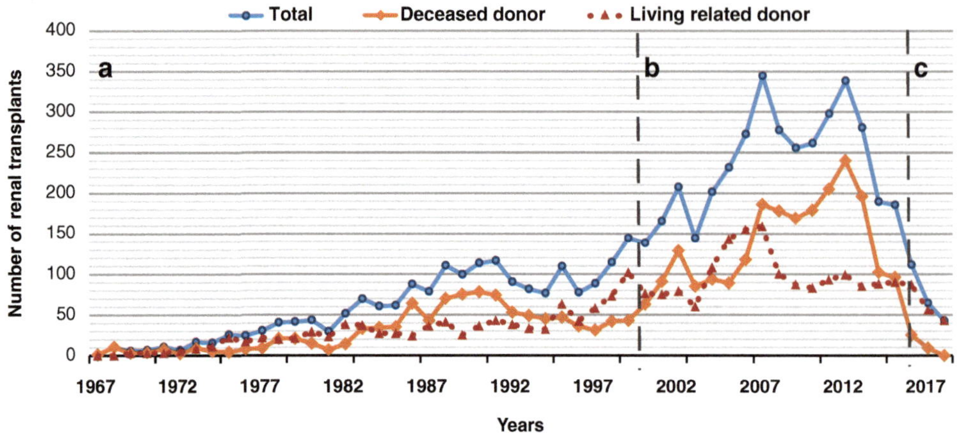


**Fig. 17.4** Renal transplant in Venezuela 1967–2018. (**a**) Period from 1967 to 1997. (**b**) Period from 1997 to 2014. (**c**) Period from 2015 to 2019

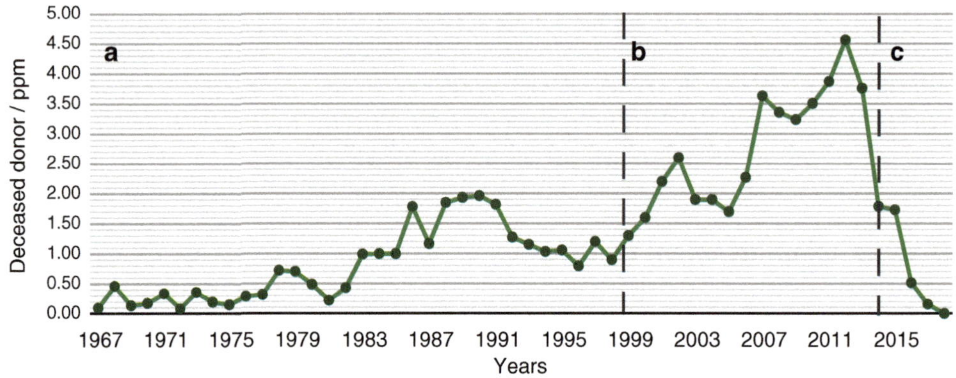


**Fig. 17.5** Procurement of kidneys obtained from deceased donors in Venezuela 1967–2018. (**a**) Period from 1967 to 1997. (**b**) Period from 1997 to 2014. (**c**) Period from 2015 to 2019

program increased with the creation of five additional transplant centers. The total number of transplants during this period was 1606; 54% of them from deceased donors (Figs. 17.4a and 17.5a) [39, 40].

Renal transplant activities of both donation and transplantation were highly variable, mainly due to scarce financial resources to develop the area and the insufficient professional expertise in the procedure. In order to increase the number of kidneys from deceased donors, the Ministry of Health created the Coordinated National Program for Kidney Transplantation in 1986 and obtained the approval of a resolution by the National Congress whereby it was mandatory for emergency rooms and ICUs the admission notification of patients with extensive cerebral damage to the transplant program [41].

By the end of the 1990s, despite policies and strategies developed by the CNDT of the Ministry of Health, and the Social Security, organ donation continued to be deficient or not concurring with the expected figures, mainly due to insufficient source from deceased renal donors (Fig. 17.5a). Furthermore, a relatively small number of potential candidates for deceased and living donor kidney transplant attended the transplant centers to perform the pre-transplant evaluation required for the surgery. In addition, there were limitations of resources in transplant centers to perform such evaluation. All these factors determined a low coverage of transplants in the country. This is how in 1997 a group of transplant experts from the active centers, interested in promoting the development of a robust national program oriented towards an increase in the waiting list of patient for transplant and the number of transplants, proposed, as an alternative to respond to this need, the creation of a non-governmental organization, the National Organization of Transplant of Venezuela (ONTV) [42, 43].

**Period B: 1997–2014:** The transplant community gathered in the newly created ONTV developed specific plans and actions to improve the transplant activity, taking as the primary objective to obtaining quality organs and tissues from deceased donors and guarantee the sustainability of the transplant process [44]. Therefore, the organization developed and submitted for consideration to the Ministry of Health, the project of the Organ and Tissue Procurement System (SPOT). This proposal was approved in January 2001 [45] and ratified in September 2003 [46] to be applied in the whole country with force of law. These resolutions were the public policies that ruled the national transplant program [47] until its repeal in November 2014 [48].

As a result of this intense and increasingly demanding activity of donation and transplantation, in 2006 the Ministry of Health, in its concern to guarantee and comply with the constitutional principle of the right to life and the right to health, promoted the implementation of the National Organ and Tissue Donation and Transplantation Program (PNDTOT), separating it from the renal health program.

## Organ Procurement and Transplantation Network Policies

Built on the resolutions of 2001 and 2003, the SPOT program was directed by ONTV and both of them were under the supervision of the Ministry of Health. Several strategies were put into action to increase procurement, optimization of organ sharing, and improvement of the performance of transplant centers nationwide in order to meet the demand of patients that requiring a life-saving transplant. As a result, there was a progressive increase in the number of deceased donor transplants that outweighed the number of living donor transplants. The average of transplants increased about 4 times, (220 transplants per year) to a total of 3963 during the period, 56% of them from deceased donors. This growth in the number of transplants was accompanied by new norms [49], an increase in transplant centers from 8 to 13, and an improvement in the supply of immunosuppressive drugs under the coverage of the Ministry of Health and the Social Security at no charge to the patient.

At the end of this period (2014), the following objectives were accomplished:

- A predominance of deceased donor (56%) over living donor transplants performed during the period.
- An increase in the national coverage of attention, control, and registration of patients on the waiting list for organ and tissue transplantation. Patients on the waiting list increased about 3 times, from 400 patients in 2004 to 1220 in 2014.
- Achievements of record figures in the kidney transplant activity (Fig. 17.4b).
- Strengthening of transplant centers through the hiring of trained staff, provision of supplies, and financing of clinical procedures required for pre-transplant evaluation of patients to be admitted in the waiting list, as well as their post-transplant follow-up.
- The Ministry of Health assigned a special fund to cover, by mean of inter-institutional agreements, the cost of transplant in other countries for patients with specific needs not able to be accomplished in the country.
- Coverage of post-transplant immunosuppressive treatment by the Social Security.
- Design and putting into practice the policies, plans, and norms to consolidate the donation, procurement, and distribution of organs for renal transplantation, as well as the surveillance and control of the transplant activity.
- Promulgation of the new law of Organ Donation and Transplantation in 2011 [50], which includes a presumed consent or opting-out law. Notwithstanding, the relatives of the potential donors continued to be approached when possible as a mean to understanding the wishes of the deceased about donation, or as a way to getting the permission to proceed with donation when the wishes of the deceased were unknown.

Unfortunately, as showed in Fig. 17.4b, there was a progressive decrease in the number of transplants between 2008 and 2011 partly due to the increase in unmet financial requirements as a consequence of a fixed budget, which represented only 31% of the estimated ideal needs. In addition, despite the previous improvement in the program, the number of patients enrolled in waiting lists for kidney transplant was only 8–12% during that period, although at least 30–40% of dialysis patients were expected to be on the list. The percentage of patients in the waiting list that received a transplant ranged between 15% and 30%.

The second period ends with the transfer of the power of execution of the SPOT by the ONTV to a public foundation attached to the Ministry of Health, the Venezuelan Foundation for Donations and Transplantation of Organs and Tissues (FUNDAVENE). In July 2014 this organization [51] assumed the stewardship and execution of all the aspects of the donation and transplant activity at the national level.

**Period C: 2015–2018:** As shown in Figs. 17.4c and 17.5c, during this period, the average of transplants per year decreased to 102. The total number of transplants during the period was 406 (32% from deceased donors). Since May 2017, the deceased donor transplant procurement activities were discontinued, and there is no active waiting list since then. At the same time, transplants from living donors also decreased markedly due to deficiencies in public transplant centers. Only a somehow residual activity has remained in some private centers until the present time.

Among the factors behind the virtual closure of the transplant program in Venezuela, we can mention the following:

1. Staff without technical competence in donation and transplantation ruling the official foundation in charge of the transplant program.
2. A progressive decrease until cessation of financial support to execute the activities of organ and tissue procurement.

3. Deterioration of hospital infrastructure and support services.
4. Decrease in the availability of specialized human resources trained in transplant activities due to a high migration rate (according to the Venezuelan Medical Federation, it is estimated that more than 30,000 physicians have emigrated from Venezuela during the last 5 years).
5. Irregular supply of immunosuppressive agents used to prevent or control transplant rejection.

In conclusion, after a progressive improvement in transplant activity in Venezuela based on the development of public policies, plans, and programs, in recent years, we have witnessed difficulties to meet the demand of transplants of the Venezuelan population due to the progressive deterioration in various areas such as security, food, and timely access to the health system in general. These factors have led to a detriment in the quality of life of the population with emphasis on vulnerable sectors such as children, older adults, and patients with chronic diseases, including CKD.

In the health sector, the progressive deterioration of institutions is evident in the constant deficit of medicines, material resources, and surgical and professional staff, the latter due in part to the flight and the decrease of contestants in our universities [52].

The situation of patients with kidney disease in its different expressions and their treatment with dialysis and kidney transplantation are severely compromised. The limitation and even the lack of resources for the care of these patients have been documented by various professional and non-governmental organizations [53–56]. In this context, it is particularly noteworthy the continuous shortage of immunosuppressive agent to prevent rejection in patients already transplanted.

For the next few years, a series of priority issues must be addressed to restore donation and transplantation in the country. These include, but are not restricted to:

1. Guarantee the integration of the components of the donation and transplant system to the National Health System.
2. Guarantee optimal working conditions for professional personnel linked to the activity.
3. Resume the training of the human resources necessary to expand the activities of donation and transplantation.
4. Provide organs and tissues from deceased donors for transplantation to meet patient's needs.
5. Optimize the quality and safety of the deceased donor organ and tissue donation process.
6. Establish information systems for donation and transplantation of organs, integrated, robust, and safe.
7. Promote the sustainability of a national system of donation and organ and tissue transplantation.
8. Assure the delivery of immunosuppressive drugs to transplant recipients.
9. Strengthen compliance with regulations against transplant tourism and organ trafficking.
10. Address new ethical dilemmas in the field of transplantation that the current crisis in the sector in the country may trigger.

## Pediatric Nephrology

The development of pediatric nephrology in Venezuela can be traced back to the 1960s, with the creation of the pediatric nephrology service at the Children's Hospital of Caracas. Subsequently the specialty began to develop in other cities in the country. Currently, there are five services with four programs of chronic dialysis and transplantation, which constitute referral centers in the country. Additionally, there are many services of pediatrics with at least one pediatric nephrologist.

During the 1960s and 1970s, about ten pediatric nephrologists were trained abroad, mainly in Mexico, the USA, and Europe. These pioneers progressively developed five training centers in Caracas, Valencia, Maracaibo, Merida, and Barcelona, respectively. The Venezuelan Pediatric Nephrology Chapter of the Venezuelan Society of Pediatrics, created in 1993, has more than 120 members, 80% of them working at public hospitals and well-integrated to the Latin American Association for Pediatrics Nephrology (ALANEPE) and other international scientific societies of nephrology. This structure and organization have allowed reasonable and good attention of nephro-urological pathologies in children and adolescents in the country for decades. However, this has been dramatically affected during the last years due to the complex political and negative economic situation of the country.

## Epidemiological Aspects of Pediatric Nephrology

The current population of the country has decreased about 15% during the last decade because of emigration; more than 85% of the population live in urban areas and about 33% is younger than 15 years of age.

Data from a regional analysis promoted by ALANEPE, which included Venezuela, showed that most of the pediatric nephrologists have undergone formal training in pediatric nephrology, 80% of them work in public hospitals and outpatient clinics, 75% were involved with teaching activities, 50% of them at university hospitals. Ninety percent were actively involved with acute dialysis methods, 80% with chronic dialysis modalities, 50% with continuous hemofiltration, and 50% with kidney transplantation. The most important professional obstacles faced by the responders were economic issues, especially related to inadequate government support for pediatric ESRD, general care and facilities, and the paucity of pediatric urologists, pathologists, and radiologists [57].

The Pediatric Nephrology Chapter of the Venezuelan Society of Pediatrics and the Venezuelan Society of Nephrology reported some years ago epidemiologic data on renal diseases in children. The Information was obtained from 14 hospital centers with at least one pediatric nephrologist. Over 3624 patients were evaluated during a period of 1 year, either through a first outpatient consultation or at a first hospital admission [58, 59].

The patients were grouped into the following categories: (a) urinary tract infection (32%), with detection of abnormalities of urinary tract in 25% of them; (b) tubular and metabolic disorders (28%) mainly idiopathic hypercalciuria and hyperuricosuria; (c) "glomerulonephritis" (9.5%); (d) urolithiasis (7%); (e) acute nephritic syndrome (4.5%); (f) "primary" hematuria (4.2%); (g) AKI (2.8%); (h) ESRD (1.6%); and (i) miscellaneous diseases (4.8%) [57, 58].

## Hypercalciuria and Nephrolithiasis in Children

The epidemiology of nephrolithiasis was studied in a multicenter study, which included 13 centers in Latin America, 2 of them in Venezuela. Eight hundred and seventy children, 63% boys and 37% girls of 2 months to 17 years of age, were evaluated. The initial symptoms reported most frequently were hematuria and abdominal or lumbar pain in 39% of patients. Interestingly, kidney malformations were found in 8.9% of cases [59–61]. With the epidemiological demonstration of the frequency of hypercalciuria and urolithiasis in several areas of Latin America, a Latin American Registry on Urolithiasis is under organization.

## Epidemiological Aspects of Chronic Kidney Disease in Children

A study on the epidemiology of CKD in children and adolescents in several Latin American countries (Argentina, Brazil, Colombia, Mexico, Uruguay, Chile, and Venezuela) showed that the incidence of CKD has a wide variability in the region, ranging between 2.8 and 15.8 new cases pmp. The incidence in Venezuela was about nine cases/year/pmp. The etiology of ESRD was glomerulopathies in 36% of the cases, obstructive uropathies and reflux nephropathy in 31%, systemic diseases in 9%, and other disorders in 15%. The histopathologic entity most frequently associated with ESRD was focal segmental glomerulosclerosis [62, 63].

## Continuous Ambulatory Peritoneal Dialysis in Children

Data concerning clinical practice and long-term outcome of PD in Latin America are scarce, although regional registries are increasing in number and quality.

Pediatric patients possibly represent 20–30% of the total PD population in Latin America. In Venezuela, 31/500 PD patients were in the pediatric age range in 2007. The main underlying renal disorders, in different proportions according to centers, for starting PD included renal dysplasia, reflux nephropathy, hemolytic uremic syndrome, obstructive uropathy, and chronic glomerulonephritis. In Venezuela, at least one half of the PD patients are on CAPD [64].

A recent report on chronic PD in Venezuela in one of the two largest pediatric nephrology centers showed that during a 33 years' period (1984–2017), 164 patients under 18 years of age (age range 18 months to 18 years) were included in the program. Primary glomerulopathies accounted for 36% of the cases, followed by uropathies (33%); other causes included heredofamilial diseases (13%), lupus nephritis and others systemic diseases.

Of the 164 patients, 31% underwent renal transplantation, 33% were either loss to follow-up or died, and 37% were maintained in the program or referred to adult nephrology units [65].

## Renal Transplantation in Children

Data on the experience in pediatric renal transplantation has been published in the Registry of Pediatric Renal Transplantation in Latin America. Report 2018 [66]. This registry, initiated in 2004, analyzes demographic, epidemiological, clinical data and global results of renal transplantation in children and adolescents in Latin America in the period 2004–2017. Eighteen countries sent information including Venezuela (about 400 kidney transplants) corresponding to a total of 4753 pediatric renal transplants in 4578 patients. The mean age of the patients was 11.5 ± 7.5 years. The main causes of kidney disease in these patients were glomerulopathies (24%) (44% FSGS), hereditary diseases (13%), and renal hypoplasia/dysplasia (6%). Other causes included vascular diseases, and in more than 20% of cases, an etiology was not determined, unknown diseases 14%. Sixty percent of the transplants were from deceased donors and 40% from living donors.

Actuarial patient survival at 1, 2, 3, and 4 years were 95, 94, 92, and 91%, respectively, whereas graft survival were 92, 90, 87 y 83%, respectively [67, 68].

## Science and Research in Nephrology in Venezuela

Since the appearance of nephrology as a specialty, there was a growth in number and quality of academic and clinical nephrology activities in Venezuela that started to take downturn at the beginning of this century.

This initial growth started when multiple physicians and scientists went overseas in the late 1960s, basically to the USA and Europe, to be trained in the top academic centers and with the leaders of the specialty at that time. Even though many were offered positions at their training centers, the vast majority returned to Venezuela creating centers of excellence where they continued to train young physicians and incorporated many master's degrees and PhD into kidney disease scientific research. During the last several decades, around ten programs of nephrology training, most of them attached to universities, have been developed, providing many nephrologists involved in clinical activities, research, and education around the country.

Initially there were three centers, one of them at a basic research institute (Instituto Venezolano de Investigaciones Científicas (IVIC)) and two major university affiliated hospitals (Hospital Universitario de Maracaibo and Hospital Universitario de Caracas). The main research areas in these centers have been renal and transport physiology, glomerulonephritis, and immunology factors involved in hypertension, renal transplant, and bone and mineral research in renal disease, all together with more than 500 publications over the last four decades. Other research areas in these and other centers include clinical nephrology and epidemiology.

Different government administrations in the last three decades of the twentieth century, during a time of economic prosperity, provided significant research resources and postgraduate training economic aid in the formation of new investigators through a commission of the Presidency of the Republic (The National Council for Scientific and Technologic Research-CONICIT), the Ministry of Health through the National Center for Dialysis and Transplantation (CNDT), and universities. Monetary resources were an important component in research production, not only through direct project funding but also by financing specialty training and exposing young faculty members and scientists to research.

This led to a significant growth in academic production and research publications in nephrology. Simultaneously, many young residents and fellows took with them this inclination for academic medicine and scientific research to other centers and universities around the country.

This was demonstrated in a study that examined the number and impact of peer-reviewed publications from Latin America included in the Institute of Scientific Information (ISI) and MEDLINE databases from 1981 to 1997. In addition, it was analyzed the number of abstracts submitted to the congresses of the International Society of Nephrology (ISN), American Society of Nephrology (ASN), and SLANH during that time. The results showed that the number of peer-reviewed publications in nephrology from authors in Latin America represented less than 1% of the world's total. Only 13 out of the 22 Latin American countries accounted for these publications, being one Venezuela. At the same time, the citation impact (3.52) was below the world average (7.82). However, this index showed a tendency towards growth in the five most productive countries. Likewise, the number of abstracts submitted to international nephrology meetings by Latin American authors has shown a steady growth but remained proportionately low compared with the rest of the world.

Similarly, it was examined the average impact of the uro-nephrological publications from Latin American countries between 1981 and 1997. In that period, only Brazil, Chile, Mexico, and Venezuela had an impact factor above the Latin American average, and only Venezuela exceeded the world average, a finding that could be partially explained by the total low number of articles and the fact that they have been generated in a few highly qualified research centers.

In that article, it was also demonstrated the importance of research funding on scientific productivity as there was a highly significant correlation between the nephrological publications included in the ISI and MEDLINE databases as a function of the gross national product (GNP). Unfortunately, the situation progressively deteriorated at the turn of this century when a socioeconomic and political crisis with massive emigration from the country has occurred. This is the worst economic crisis in Venezuela's history and the worst facing a country that is not experiencing war since the mid-twentieth century.

This crisis has affected the life of the average Venezuelan on all levels, with a United Nation report estimating in March 2019 that 94% of Venezuelans live in poverty, and more than 10% (3.4 million) have left their country.

Many of the emigrants have been well-trained physicians, scientists, and academicians, including of course, many nephrologists that have been welcomed in many countries around the world. All the clinical and academic programs as well as scientific research have progressively declined and, practically at the present time, have come to a halt.

We think that it could take up to a generation, once this crisis vanishes away, in order to get back in track of what this country once was in academic, research, and clinical nephrology.

## Conclusions

Several years have elapsed since the initiation of nephrology in Venezuela. As in many other countries, it started in the 1960s and developed progressively into a mature specialty with well-designed plans and programs in the areas of epidemiology, diagnosis, and treatment of renal diseases, as well as a progressive growth of RRT for the ESRD population. Education and research in renal diseases and physiology also grew particularly associated to universities and research institutions. These developments were in the majority of cases based on evolving public policies adapted not only to the requirements of the population but also to the advances in the specialty. As a result, in terms of population coverage, RRT approached the goal set by the OPAS and SLANH for the region. However, deficiencies, most of the time related to budget constraints, geographical difficulties for effective access of people to treatment centers, and human resources, did not allow a homogeneous coverage. Thus, although access to treatment, including RRT, is theoretically a fundamental social right established in the national constitution, it must be recognized that coverage has been considerably higher in middle to large cities as compared to small cities and rural areas and that coverage figures expressed by pmp are somehow misleading. This disparity has increased more recently due, among other reasons, to a political, social, and economic crisis that has disturbed the whole country. Health in all its expressions has been one of the most affected and visible areas. Thus, in terms of RRT, there has been a reduction in about 30% of the total number of patients on dialysis in the last years that affects equally adults and children. With the rising trends in the incidence of ESRD and costs of medical technology, adequate coverage of RRT will become increasingly out of reach.

The situation of the national transplant program is perhaps more striking. After a progressive improvement in the number of kidney transplants based on a robust legal structure and the building of capacity to ruling the program, the erroneous substitution of an organization with expertise in the management of the program by another with no competence in the area, together with a marked budget reduction led to a complete stagnation of the deceased donor transplants and a reduction of living transplant to a minimum. This situation is aggravated by a marked shortage of immunosuppressive agents to prevent rejection.

It should be pointed out that these limitations are just a part of a general crisis of the health system in Venezuela, which includes limitations for early detection of diseases, prevention, specialized diagnosis, and basic treatment of acute and chronic diseases. These problems are aggravated by a progressive migration of the human resources required to attend the community and a reduction in the number of health science students and teachers in our universities as a consequence of the crisis. These problems have been addressed in a number of publications and alerts from several organizations (ISN, SLANH, SVN).

With all these difficulties, there is no doubt that the health system and particularly the attention of renal diseases in Venezuela need to be rethought. It is evident that the excessive interference of national politics into the system is in the center of the crisis. Regarding RRT, it is necessary to retake the road of development to stabilize the different programs of attention and patient care. Budgets require to be balanced between the basic programs of attention to the population and those oriented to the treatment of costly diseases. Decreasing costs of RRT is without doubt a way to maintain or increase population coverage in an era of restrictive budgets. In this regard, it is curious that costs of in-center therapies such as HD, which requires equipment, space adapted to regulations, and specialized human resources, among others, are similar to that of PD which in most of the cases does not require such investments. A global tendency to improve coverage is to increase PD. This approach would also serve to reach many patients living in rural areas or far from larger cities with established dialysis units and to reduce disparity in attention at the same times.

Optimal working conditions for professional personnel involved in RRT is necessary to make this activity more attractive and guarantee a better and continued attention to the patient. In this regard, assuring the continuity or the re-initiation of training programs for technical personnel is an important ingredient to expand the activities of both dialysis and transplantation.

With regard to transplant, it is necessary to rebuild a strong program of organ procurement from deceased donor and to incentive living organ donation. Assuring the delivery of immunosuppressive drugs to transplant recipients is a very important part of this component of the program.

Within this context, it is necessary to strengthen compliance with regulations against transplant tourism and organ trafficking as well addressing possible ethical dilemmas in the field of transplantation that the current crisis in the sector in the country may trigger.

We know that the multifaceted crisis Venezuela is suffering is difficult to control and even more, to solve. The damage to the nation has been immense at all levels. Actions to retake a path towards stabilization or growth of the attention to kidney disease in all expressions have to be rethought within policies to rebuild the national health system; no simple or individual remedies seem possible at this time. But we are also certain that the country will at some point start retaking the route towards political stability, economic growth, and social development.

**Acknowledgments**

- **The Pioneers of Nephrology in Venezuela**

Alberto Guinand Baldó, Hugo Dávila, Gastón Vargas, José Chesnau, Alberto Bercowsky, Renato Acosta, Harry Acquatella, Guillermo Whittembury, León Lapco, Vicente Ocando, Ana Recagno, Nahem Seguías, Marcos Boissiere, Waldemar Kiechle, José Padrino, Bernardo Rodríguez-Iturbe, Abdón Alayón, José Luis García Zozaya, Dídimo Rubio, Alberto Bercowsky, Gustavo Sandoval, Virgilio Paz-Martínez, Bruno Burger, Manuel E Pérez Rojas, Valentín Ramírez, Jorge Domínguez, Dietrich Schaeck, Lionel Agostini, Norman Cordero, Raúl Goyo, José A. Pinto, Lirimo Rubio, Rafael García, Pedro Garroni. Luis Troconis.
The authors recognize the invaluable contribution of all nephrologist to the development of nephrology in Venezuela, particularly those who have had a pioneering role in the initiation of nephrology services and units around the country, and that with exemplary actions have contributed to the growth of a strong national program for the attention of renal diseases, education, and research in nephrology. We also would like to recognize the dedication of all nephrology residents who, with extraordinary compromise, have help to maintain the attention to those patients in need of nephrological care, even under the precarious conditions imposed by the critical situation that the country in general is facing.

## References

1. Venezuela. WorldAtlas.com. Accessed in January 2020. Available in https://www.worldatlas.com/webimage/countrys/samerica/ve.htm.
2. Instituto Nacional de Estadística, INE. Accessed in January 2020. Available in http://www.redatam.ine.gob.ve/Censo2011/index.html.
3. The World Bank. Venezuela Data. Accessed in January 2020. Available in https://www.worldbank.org/en/country/venezuela.
4. Human Development Report 2019. United Nations Development Program. Accessed in January 2020. Available in http://hdr.undp.org/sites/all/themes/hdr_theme/country-notes/VEN.pdf.
5. Sociedad Venezolana de Nefrología. Accessed in January 2020. Available in https://www.svnefrologia.com/.
6. Unidad de Registros. Organización Nacional de Trasplante de Venezuela. Accessed in October 2019. Available in http://www.ontv-venezuela.org/.
7. OAS Working Group to Address the Regional Crisis Caused by Venezuela's Migrant and Refugee Flows Accessed in January 2020. Available in http://shapersforvenezuela.com/wp-content/uploads/2019/07/OAS-Working-Group-to-Address-the-Regional-Crisis-Caused-by-Venezuelas-Migrant-and-Refugee-Flows.pdf.
8. Economic Survey of Latin America and the Caribbean. 2019 Bolivarian Republic Venezuela. Accessed in January 2020. Available in https://repositorio.cepal.org/bitstream/handle/11362/44675/144/EEI2019_Venezuela_en.pdf.
9. Encuesta Nacional de Condiciones de Vida de la Población Venezolana (ENCOVI) https://encovi.ucab.edu.ve/ediciones/encovi-2017/.
10. Hamburger J. Naissance et essor de la néphrologie. Nephrologie. 1980;1:1):1–2.
11. Libro de Actas Sociedad Venezolana de Nefrología SVN.pdf. pag 11-13.Google Docs. 2019. [online] Available at: https://bit.ly/2LRzpoh. Accessed 14 July 2019.
12. International Registry In Organ Donation And Transplantation – Venezuela. Accessed in January 2020. Available in http://www.irodat.org/?p=database&c=VE#data.
13. Bellorín-Font E, Milanés C, Carlini R, Rojas E. El Problema de las Enfermedades Renales en Venezuela y Estrategias de Control. 2001. pdf. Ministerio de Salud y Desarrollo Social. Dirección de Salud Poblacional. Dirección Técnica de Programas. Programa de Enfermedad Renal. [online] Google Docs. Available at: https://bit.ly/2XPIfJR. Accessed 10 July 2019.
14. Riella M, Locatelli A. History of peritoneal Dialysis in Latin America. Perit Dial Int. 2007;27:322–7.
15. Carlini R, González H. Situación actual del Programa de Salud Renal. Dirección General de Programas. Ministerio del Poder Popular para la Salud. Google Docs. 2011 [cited 17 July 2019]. Available from: http://cort.as/-LNHe.
16. Constitution of the Bolivarian Republic of Venezuela. 1999. http-://www.asambleanacional.gob.ve/documentos_archivos/constitucion-nacional-7.pdf.
17. Gaceta Oficial 4.497 Extraordinario. Ley de Trasplante 1992. Google Docs. 1992 [cited 12 July 2019]. Available from: https://bit.ly/32qwkSi.
18. Tilac CA. Falla Renal Aguda. Paludismo. Leptospirosis. Caracas. Ed. Corporación Minerva C.A. 2007. pp. 1–158.
19. Bellorin-Font E, Pernalete N, Meza J, Milanes CL, Carlini RG. Access to and coverage of renal replacement therapy in minority and ethnic in Venezuela. Kidney Int Suppl. 2005;97:S18–22.
20. García R, Rubio L, Rodríguez-Iturbe B. Long-term prognosis of epidemic poststreptococcal glomerulonephritis in Maracaibo: follow-up studies 11-12 years after the acute episode. Clin Nephrol. 1981;15(6):291–8.
21. Centro Nacional de Diálisis y Trasplante. División de Enfermedades Crónicas. Ministerio de Sanidad y Asistencia Social. Evolución del Programa de Lucha Contra las Enfermedades Renales en Venezuela Oct 1986. pdf [Internet]. Google Docs. 2019 [cited 15 July 2019]. Available from: https://bit.ly/2LR1oo6.
22. Bellorin-Font E, Milanés C, Rodríguez-Iturbe B. End-stage Renal disease and its treatment in Venezuela. Artif Organs. 2002;26(9):747–9.
23. Allende V, Planchart A, Pinto J. Registro de Biopsias Renales. IAPUCV Presentation presented at; 2014; XII Congreso Venezolano de Nefrología, Valencia. Edo Carabobo.
24. Rodriguez-Iturbe B, García R, Rubio L, Cuenca L, Treser G, Lange K. Epidemic glomerulonephritis in Maracaibo. Evidence for progression to chronicity. Clin Nephrol. 1976;5(5):197–206.
25. Herrera J, Rodriguez-Iturbe B. End stage renal diseases and acute glomerulonephritis in Goajiro Indians. Kidney Int. 2003;63:822–6.
26. Santa Cruz PL. La insuficiencia renal crónica como problema de salud: una reflexión en el tiempo. Nefrologia. 2000;20(5):465–6.
27. Santa Cruz PL, León M E, Urbina D, Paz-Martínez V, Hernández A, Agüero F. Insuficiencia renal crónica (IRC) mortalidad en el estado Aragua durante el decenio 1986–1995. (Abstract). V Congreso Venezolano de Nefrología. 1996. [Internet]. Google Docs. 1986 [cited 14 July 2019]. Available from: https://bit.ly/32ooBUN.

28. Carlini R. González H. IV Reunión Consenso Nacional de Nefrología Hotel Ávila Caracas 29 y 30 de Julio de 2009.Programa de Salud Renal. Google Docs. [cited 17 July 2019]. Available from: http://cort.as/-LO_b.
29. Gaceta Oficial N° 31.149 Enero 10 1977 de la República de Venezuela. Resolución por la cual se crea el Centro Nacional de Diálisis y Trasplante en Diciembre, 29,1976. Ministerio de Sanidad y Asistencia Social. Google Docs. 1977 [cited 12 July 2019]. Available from: https://bit.ly/2Lh5436.
30. Milanes C, Infante M, Ariza M, Mamblona R. Registro Venezolano de Dialisis y Trasplante 1998–1999 [Internet]. Google Docs. 2000 [cited 29 July 2019]. Available from: http://cort.as/-M5en.
31. Goeree R, Manalich J, Grootendorst P, Beecroft ML, Churchill DN. Cost analysis of dialysis treatments for end-stage renal disease. Clin Invest Med. 1996;18:455–64.
32. Creation of the Direction of Nephrology, Dialysis and Transplantation. [Internet]. Caracas: [cited 2019 Jul 2]; [about 2 screens]. Available from: http://www.ivss.gov.ve/contenido/Nefrologia,-dialisis-y-trasplante-renal.
33. Gaceta Oficial N° 37.976 Julio 9 2004.Requisitos Funcionamiento y Arquitectónicos Unidad de Hemodiálisis. Google Docs. 2019 [cited 15 July 2019]. Available from: https://bit.ly/2YUU3HY.
34. Gonzalez-Bedat MC, Rosa-Diez G, Ferreira A. El Registro Latinoamericano de Diálisis y Trasplante Renal: la importancia del desarrollo de los registros nacionales en Latinoamérica. Nefrología Latinoam. 2017;14(1):12–21.
35. The UN Refugee Agency UNHCR. Situation in Venezuela. 2019. [online] Available at: https://www.acnur.org/situacion-en-venezuela.html. Accessed 15 July 2019.
36. Barile M. Situación actual de la Diálisis Peritoneal en Venezuela 2002. Jornada "XXV años de Diálisis Peritoneal Ambulatoria Continua" Caracas 2 julio 2005 Google Docs. [cited 17 July 2019]. Available from: http://cort.as/-M2C3.
37. Prú C, Besso J, Padrón J, Jiménez CC, Martinelli A, Acosta T, et al. Hemofiltración veno-venosa continua (HFVVC) en una Unidad de Ciudades Intensivos (UCI). Experiencia de 60 casos. Nefrología Venez. 2006;8(1):6–11.
38. Acquatella H, Pérez-González M, Morales JM, Whittembury G. Ionic and histological changes in the kidney after perfusion and storage for transplantation: use of high Na- versus high K-containing solutions. Transplantation. 1972;14(4):480–9.
39. Milanés C, Bellorin-Font E, Weisinger J, Pernalete N, Urbina D, Paz-Martinez V. Necesidades y demandas de riñones para trasplante en Venezuela. Invest Clín. 1993;34(1):15–27.
40. Milanés C, Almao R, Leal J, Martínez E, Martínez L, Salgado O, et al. Importancia del Programa de Coordinadores Hospitalarios (PCH) en la obtención de riñones para trasplante. Nefrología Latinoam. 1995;2:122.
41. Resolución G-624 del Ministerio de Sanidad y Asistencia Social. Creación del PCNTR y establecimiento de la obligatoriedad de notificación sobre la presencia de donantes potenciales de órganos en los hospitales adscritos al programa Gaceta Oficial No. 33468 (13 de mayo de 1986).
42. Registro mercantil ONTV.1997 Google docs. 2019 [cited 12 July 2019]. Available from: https://bit.ly/32nyAtj.
43. Estatutos ONTV. 1997. Google Docs. 2019 [cited 12 July 2019]. Available from: https://bit.ly/30tYWIj.
44. Milanés C, Hernández E, Clesca P, Becerra J, Serrano L, Mamblona R, et al. Organización Nacional de Trasplante de Venezuela: a new iniciative to approach donation an transplantation in our country. Transplant Proc. 2001;33:2047–8.
45. Resolución N°. 027 del 29 de enero de 2001. Autorización a la Organización Nacional de Trasplante de Venezuela (ONTV), para desarrollar el Proyecto "Sistema de Procura de Órganos y Tejidos" (SPOT). Gaceta Oficial N° 37.135 Febrero 06 2001. Google Docs. 2001 [cited 12 July 2019]. Available from: https://bit.ly/2XEv0re.
46. Resolución N° 578 del 15 de septiembre de 2003. Resolución por la cual se autoriza a la Organización Nacional de Trasplante de Venezuela (ONTV), para desarrollar el Proyecto "Sistema de Procura de Órganos y Tejidos" (SPOT). Gaceta Oficial N° 37.778 Septiembre 18 2003. Google Docs. 2003 [cited 12 July 2019]. Available from: https://bit.ly/32kqe5G.
47. Milanés C, Hernández E, González L, Sivira H, Mamblona R, Clesca P, et al. Organ and tissue procurement system (Otps). A novel intervention to increase organ donation rates in Venezuela. Prog Transplant. 2003;13(1):65–8.
48. Resolución N° 473 del 17 de noviembre 2014. Resolución mediante la cual se deja sin efecto la Resolución Número 578, de fecha 15 de septiembre de 2003, en los términos que en ella se señalan. (G.O N° 37.778 de fecha 18/09/2003, mediante la cual se autorizó a la Organización Nacional de Trasplante de Venezuela, para desarrollar el Proyecto "Sistema de Procura de Órganos de Tejidos"). Gaceta Oficial de la República Bolivariana 40.550 (27 de noviembre de 2014). Google Docs. 2014 [cited 12 July 2019]. Available from: http://cort.as/-M2P2.
49. Resolución N° 525 del 11 de Octubre de 2000. Normas para la autorización, regulación y control de establecimientos de salud como Centro de Trasplante Gaceta Oficial No. 37061 (20 de Octubre de 2000), Google Docs. 2000 [cited 16 July 2019]. Available from: http://cort.as/-M2PK.
50. Ley sobre donación y trasplante de órganos, tejidos y células en seres humanos. Gaceta Oficial de la República Bolivariana de Venezuela N° 39.808 (25 de noviembre de 2011) Google Docs. 2019 [cited 12 July 2019]. Available from: https://bit.ly/2NOi2rh.
51. Acta Constitutiva y Estatutos Sociales de la Fundación Venezolanas de Donaciones y Trasplantes de Órganos, Tejidos y Células (FUNDAVENE). Gaceta Oficial de la República Bolivariana de Venezuela N° 40.449 (08 de Julio de 2014). Google Docs. 2019. [online] Available at: http://cort.as/-M2Qm. Accessed 29 July 2019.
52. Page KR, Doocy S, Reyna Ganteaume F, Castro JS, Spiegel P, Beyrer C. Venezuela's public health crisis: a regional emergency. Lancet. 2019;393(10177):1254–60. https://doi.org/10.1016/S0140-6736(19)30344-7.
53. Comunicados ONTV.pdf [Internet]. Google Docs. 2019 [cited 12 July 2019]. Available from: https://bit.ly/2JHa8uh.
54. Comunicado Sociedad Venezolana de Nefrología 29–05-2017.pdf [Internet]. Google Docs. 2017 [cited 12 July 2019]. Available from: https://bit.ly/2ScIycm.
55. Sociedad Latinoamericana de Nefrología e Hipertensión SLANH. Comunicado ante la Crisis de la Nefrología Venezolana. Feb 2018. Available from: https://slanh.net/comunicado-ante-la-crisis-de-la-nefrologia-venezolana/.
56. Statement of The International Society Of Nephrology and The Latin American Society Of Nephrology and Hypertension About The Nephrology Crisis In Venezuela. March 26, 2018. Available from: https://www.theisn.org/news/item/3286-isn-and-slanh-stand-united-on-venezuela-s-kidney-health-crisis.
57. Orta N, Lopez M. Report to the International Pediatric Nephrology Association 2016. Available from: https://mailing.europa-organisation.com/2016/IPNA-ASSO/newsletter/161124/pediatric_nephrology_in_venezuela.pdf.
58. Orta Sibu N, Moriyon JC, Ariza M, et al. Epidemiología de las enfermedades renales en niños en Venezuela. Arch Venez Pediatr. 2001;64:76–86.
59. Orta-Sibu N, López M, Moriyon J, et al. Renal diseases in children in Venezuela (South America). Pediatr Nephrol. 2002;17:566–70.

60. Cattini Perrone H. Epidemiology of nephrolithiasis. Pediatr Nephrol. 1998; 12: 10 Supp. C46.
61. López MM, Castillo LA, Chávez JB, Ramones C. Hypercalciuria and recurrent urinary tract infection in Venezuelan children. Pediatr Nephrol. 1999;13:433–7.
62. Penido MG, Diniz JS, Moreira ML, et al. Idiopathic hypercalciuria: presentation of 471 cases. J Pediatr. 2001;77:101–4.
63. Orta-Sibú N. Epidemiological aspects of chronic renal failure in Latin American countries. Arch Venez Pediatr. 1999;62(suppl2):83.
64. Koch V, Orta N, Exeni R. Pediatric nephrology in Latin America. ALANEPE. In: Avner E, editor. Pediatric nephrology. Berlin, Heidelberg: Springer; 2016. https://doi.org/10.1007/978-3-662-43596-0_70.
65. Cano F, Orta N. Pediatric peritoneal dialysis in Latin America looking at for common answers over diversity. Pediatr Nephrol. 2007;22:1413.
66. Orta N, Lara E, Dominguez L, et al. Congress of the Spanish Association of Ped Nef. Valencia, Spain; 2018.
67. Garcia CD, Delucchi A, Orta N, et al. Latin American pediatric renal transplant registry: 2004–2012 report. Am J Transplant. 2014;14(53):359: 502.
68. Ariza M, Orta N, López M, Bosque M, et al. Trasplante Renal en Niños en Venezuela: Resultados 1982-2006. Rev Nefrología Venez. 2008;9(3):47–55.

# Part III

# Asia

# Nephrology in Bangladesh

# 18

Harun Ur Rashid, Mohammad Rafiqul Alam, Asia Khanam, M. Muhibur Rahman, Shamim Ahmed, Mamun Mostafi, Shakib Uz Zaman Arefin, Tasnuva Sarah Kashem, Nura Afza Salma Begum, Kazi Shahnoor Alam, and Nazrul Islam

## Abbreviations

| | |
|---|---|
| AAMI | Advancement of Medical Instrumentation |
| ABO | ABO blood group |
| ACEI | Angiotensin-converting enzyme inhibitors |
| AKI | Acute kidney injury |
| APD | Automated peritoneal *dialysis* |
| ARBs | Angiotensin II receptor blockers |
| AVF | Arteriovenous fistula |
| BIRDEM | Bangladesh Institute of Research and Rehabilitation in Diabetes, Endocrine and Metabolic Disorders |
| BMRC | Bangladesh Medical Research Council |
| BRA | Bangladesh Renal Association |
| BRJ | Bangladesh Renal Journal |
| BSMMU | Bangabandhu Sheikh Mujib Medical University |
| BSPD | Bangladesh Society for Peritoneal Dialysis |
| c-ANCA | Cytoplasmic anti-neutrophil cytoplasmic antibodies |
| CAPD | Continuous ambulatory peritoneal dialysis |
| CGN | Chronic glomerulonephritis |
| CIA | Central Intelligence Agency |
| CKD | Chronic kidney disease |
| CKD-EPI | Chronic Kidney Disease Epidemiology Collaboration |
| CMV | Cytomegalovirus |
| CRRT | Continuous renal replacement therapies |
| CT | Computed tomography |
| CVD | Cardiovascular diseases |
| CVVH | Continuous veno-venous haemofiltration |
| DKD | Diabetic kidney disease |
| DM | Diabetes mellitus |
| eGFR | Estimated glomerular filtration rate |
| ESRD | End-stage renal disease |
| FSGS | Focal segmental glomerulosclerosis |
| GDP | Gross domestic product |
| GFR | Glomerular filtration rate |
| GN | Glomerulonephritis |
| GoB | Government of Bangladesh |
| GP | General practitioners |
| HD | Haemodialysis |
| HDI | Human Development Index |
| HIV | Human immunodeficiency virus |
| HLA | Human leukocyte antigen |
| HTN | Hypertension |
| ICUs | Intensive care unit |
| IFKF | International Federation of Kidney Foundation |
| IgAN | IgA nephropathy |
| IHD | Ischaemic heart disease |
| IPD | Intermittent peritoneal dialysis |
| IPGMR | Institute of Postgraduate Medicine and Research |
| ISN | International Society of Nephrology |
| K/DOQI | Kidney Disease Outcomes Quality Initiative |
| KAMPS | Kidney Awareness Monitoring and Prevention Society |
| KDIGO | Kidney Disease Improving Global Outcomes |
| KFB | Kidney Foundation, Bangladesh |
| *KYAMC* | Khaja Yunus Ali Medical College |

H. U. Rashid (✉) · S. Ahmed · S. U. Z. Arefin · T. S. Kashem
N. A. S. Begum
Department of Nephrology, Kidney Foundation Hospital and Research Institute, Dhaka, Bangladesh
e-mail: rashid@bol-online.com

M. R. Alam · A. Khanam
Department of Nephrology, BSMMU-Bangabandhu Sheikh Mujib Medical University, Dhaka, Bangladesh

M. M. Rahman
Department of Nephrology, Popular Medical College Hospital, Dhaka, Bangladesh

M. Mostafi
Department of Nephrology, Gonoshathaya Nagar Hospital Dhanmondi, Dhaka, Bangladesh

K. S. Alam
Department of Nephrology, National Institute of Kidney Diseases & Urology, Dhaka, Bangladesh

N. Islam
Department of Nephrology, Dhaka Medical College and Hospital, Dhaka, Bangladesh


J. A. Moura-Neto et al. (eds.), *Nephrology Worldwide*, https://doi.org/10.1007/978-3-030-56890-0_18

| | |
|---|---|
| MCD | Minimal change disease |
| McPGN | Mesangioproliferative glomerulonephritis |
| MD | Doctor of medicine |
| MN | Membranous nephropathy |
| MPGN | Membranoproliferative glomerulonephritis |
| NGO | Non-government organization |
| NS | Nephrotic syndrome |
| NSAIDS | Non-steroidal anti-inflammatory drugs |
| p-ANCA | Perinuclear anti-neutrophil cytoplasmic antibodies |
| PD | Peritoneal dialysis |
| PhD | Doctor of philosophy |
| PMP | Per million population |
| PNSB | Pediatric Nephrology Society of Bangladesh |
| PPP | Public-private partnership |
| PSGN | Post-streptococcal glomerulonephritis |
| RO | Reverse osmosis |
| RRT | Renal replacement therapy |
| SLED | Sustained low efficiency dialysis |
| SOT | Society of Organ Transplantation |
| T2DM | Type 2 diabetes mellitus |
| UFF | Ultrafiltration failure |
| UGC | University Grants Commission |
| UK | United Kingdom |
| USA | United States of America |
| USD | United States dollar |
| USRDS | United States Renal Data System |
| WHO | World Health Organization |

## General Information Table

| | |
|---|---|
| Area | 147.57 $km^2$ |
| Population[1] | 163.65 million |
| Capital | Dhaka |
| Three most populated cities: | 1. Dhaka (36,054,418)<br>2. Chattogram (28,423,019)<br>3. Rajshahi (18,484,858) |
| Official language | Bangla |
| Gross domestic product (GDP)[1] | 274.1 billion USD (2017–2018) |
| GDP per capita[1] | 1675 USD (2017–2018) |
| Human Development Index (HDI)[2] | 0.608 (2017) |
| Official currency | Taka |
| Total number of nephrologists* | 205 |
| National society of nephrology | 1. Bangladesh Renal Association (BRA)<br>2. Kidney Foundation, Bangladesh (KFB)<br>3. Kidney Awareness Monitoring and Prevention Society (KAMPS)<br>4. Society of Organ Transplantation (SOT), Bangladesh.<br>5. Bangladesh Society for Peritoneal Dialysis (BSPD)<br>6. Pediatric Nephrology Society of Bangladesh (PNSB) |
| Incidence of end-stage renal disease[3] | 2018 – 244.4 pmp |
| Prevalence of end-stage renal disease[3] (including patients with a functioning kidney transplant) | 2018 – 305.5 pmp |
| Total number of patients on dialysis (all modalities)[3] | 2017 – ~18,579 (113.52 pmp)<br>2018 – ~19,123 (116.8 pmp) |
| Number of patients on haemodialysis[3] | 2017 – ~18,000 (110 pmp)<br>2018 – ~18,500 (113 pmp) |
| Number of patients on peritoneal dialysis[3] | 2017 – 579 (3.5 pmp)<br>2018 – 623 (3.8 pmp) |
| Number of renal transplantations per year[3] | 2017 – 159 (1.0 pmp)<br>2018 – 187 (1.1 pmp) |

Table References:

1. Bangladesh Bureau of Statistics. Gross Domestic Product (GDP) of Bangladesh (Final) 2017–18; 8. Available from http://bbs.portal.gov.bd/site/page/dc2bc6ce-7080-48b3-9a04-73cec782d0df/-. Accessed on 23.06.2019.
2. United Nations Development Programme. Human Development Indices and Indicators: 2018 Statistical Update, Bangladesh. Available fromhttp://hdr.undp.org/sites/all/themes/hdr_theme/country-notes/BGD.pdf. Accessed on 23.06.2019.
3. Rashid HU. Year book of Kidney Foundation, Bangladesh, 2019 (in Press).

## Introduction

Bangladesh is one of the most densely populated areas in the world and is bordered by India and Myanmar. The total population is 163.65 million, of whom 65% live in rural areas. The World Bank classifies Bangladesh as a low-middle-income country.

According to the Global Burden of Disease Study, Bangladesh is in the bottom half of the list of 191 countries in terms of their socio-demographic index. However, the economic and health indicators of Bangladesh have remarkably improved from 2010 to 2016 as compared to Nepal, India and Pakistan. Unfortunately, the maternal, infant and under 5 mortality rates are still high (Table 18.1) [1].

The national policies for non-communicable disease control are still in the early stages of development. These policies are targeted towards management of diabetes mellitus (DM), hypertension (HTN), cardiovascular diseases (CVD) and cancer. The government has started to include kidney diseases among the non-communicable diseases. At present, the priority of healthcare budget is population control, sanitation, safe water supply, mother and child care and prevention of communicable disease.

There is a rising trend in the incidence and prevalence of kidney diseases in Bangladesh. Most of this increase is driven by population growth. The incidence of chronic kidney diseases (CKD) is increasing due to the increased incidence of DM and HTN in the last decades. The burden of acute kidney injury (AKI) has not been accurately estimated in Bangladesh. Most cases of AKI seen in public hospitals are acquired in the community and are related to suboptimal sanitation and water quality, tropical infections, inadvertent

**Table 18.1** General demographic, economic and health indicators of Bangladesh

| Indicator | Bangladesh |
|---|---|
| Percentage of rural population (%) | 65 |
| Life expectancy at birth, total (yr) | 72.5 |
| Population growth (annual %) | 1.1 |
| Mortality rate, infant (per 1000 live births) | 28.2 |
| Birth rate, crude (per 1000 people) | 18.9 |
| Cause of death, by non-communicable diseases (% of total) | 66.9 |
| Current health expenditure (% of GDP) | 2.6 |
| Domestic general government health expenditure per capita (current international dollars) | 12.9 |
| Out-of-pocket expenditure (% of current health expenditure) | 71.8 |
| Number of physicians (per 1000 people) | 0.5 |
| Maternal mortality ratio (modelled estimate, per 100,000 live births) | 176 |
| Mortality rate, under 5 (per 1000 live births) | 34.2 |
| Health Access and Quality[a] | 47.6 |
| Social Development Index[b] | 0.51 |

Data from The World Development Report 2016 (https://data.worldbank.org/products/wdi), the Global Burden of Disease Study 2016 (http://www.healthdata.org/gbd), the World Health Organization Global Health Observatory (http://www.who.int/gho/countries/en/) and CIA World Fact book (https://www.cia.gov/library/publications/resources/the-world-factbook/) [1]

*GDP* gross domestic product, *PPP* purchasing power parity

[a]Health Access and Quality (0–100): measures personal access to healthcare and its quality, derived from the outcomes of 32 diseases that can be avoided or effectively treated with proper medical care

[b]Social Development Index (0–1): measures development status of countries based on average income per person, educational attainment and total fertility rate

use of drugs like antibiotics and analgesics and poor obstetric care [2, 3].

There is no policy for determining eligibility to renal replacement therapy (RRT) or choice of dialysis modality in our country. More than 95% of patients are receiving haemodialysis (HD) [4]. In recent years, peritoneal dialysis (PD) patients are increasing in some hospitals. The availability of kidney transplantation is even more limited.

Renal services, however, are gradually expanding in Bangladesh with the support from the government, nonprofit hospitals like Kidney Foundation Bangladesh (KFB) and other charitable organizations.

## Brief History of Nephrology in Bangladesh

There has been phenomenal improvement of nephrology in Bangladesh since its independence in 1971. In 1973, there was only one nephrologist in the country named Professor Dr. Matiur Rahman. He was trained in Glasgow (UK) and joined as associate professor of urology at the, then, Institute of Postgraduate Medicine and Research (IPGMR), now called Bangabandhu Sheikh Mujib Medical University

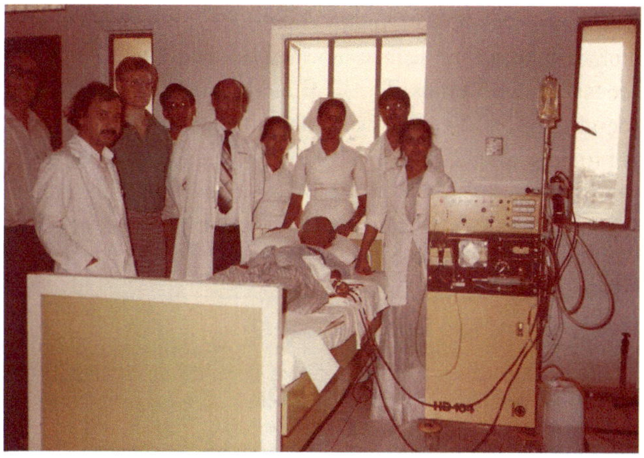

**Fig. 18.1** First HD at IPGMR, 1986 with Professor Dr. Matiur Rahman, Professor Dr. Harun Ur Rashid and nephrology team members

(BSMMU), in the name of the father of the nation. He launched a nine-bed nephrology ward. In 1977 another postgraduate doctor in internal medicine Dr. Harun Ur Rashid (corresponding author of this book) went to the University of Newcastle Upon Tyne (UK) for higher training in nephrology. He returned home in 1981 after completing his PhD degree and joined as associate professor at that nephrology unit. Both the specialists worked together and expanded nephrology in Bangladesh from grass root level of clinical nephrology up to kidney transplantation.

The first renal biopsy was performed in 1973. In 1974 the treatment of end-stage renal disease (ESRD) with intermittent peritoneal dialysis (IPD) made nephrology a distinct specialty. Although the first haemodialysis (HD) was attempted in 1965, it could not be continued because of the lack of specialists to implant Scribner shunts. Since 1986, HD has been considered as a regular form of therapy (Fig. 18.1). The first live related kidney transplantation (KT) performed in 1982 was the start of a new era of modern nephrology practice in Bangladesh [5]. Continuous ambulatory peritoneal dialysis (CAPD) was also started in 1982 [6]. However, due to non-availability of PD fluids, CAPD was stopped for a few years and restarted in 1992.

The formation of the Bangladesh Renal Association in 1977 was a major breakthrough in the growth of nephrology in Bangladesh. The First National Convention and Scientific Seminar in nephrology was held in 1981 soon after Dr. Harun Ur Rashid joined in nephrology unit in IPGMR. Since then, scientific seminars in nephrology have been held every year. Nephrologists from foreign countries including Asia, Europe, and the USA attend the seminars as guest speakers. The only nephrology journal of the country named *Bangladesh Renal Journal (BRJ)* started its journey in 1982 [7]. Postgraduate courses in nephrology were started in 1986 at IPGMR, and the first physician obtained MD in nephrology in 1991.

Research in the field of kidney disease has progressed slowly during the last four decades and has been confined largely to the teaching hospitals. The KFB has set up a voluntary renal registry for ESRD since 2002, and since then KFB has been publishing the ESRD registry every year. It has also been sending data regarding ESRD, dialysis and transplantation to United States Renal Data System (USRDS) since 2003.

## Renal Diseases in Bangladesh

### Chronic Kidney Disease (CKD)

The number of patients with CKD is increasing in Bangladesh. Unfortunately, it is not yet possible to define the incidence, prevalence and pattern of kidney diseases in the country to its full extent. However, study from disadvantaged urban and rural population suggested that the prevalence of CKD was 16–18%; of them 11% were in stage III–V. Hospital-based survey revealed that about 200–250 patients per million population (pmp) are reaching ESRD each year in Bangladesh [8].

The pattern of kidney disease in Bangladesh has been changing over the last three decades. Acute post-streptococcal glomerulonephritis (PSGN) and nephrotic syndrome (NS) were the two predominant kidney diseases in the past. Chronic pyelonephritis, urinary tract infection, renal stone disease, obstructive uropathy, AKI and CKD were also part of the renal disease spectrum [9]. At that time, diabetic nephropathy (DKD) and hypertension (HTN) were not considered to be important causes of renal disease. At present, the principal causes of CKD have shifted from PSGN and NS to chronic glomerulonephritis (CGN) (37%), followed by DKD (33%) and hypertension 16% (Table 18.2) [8].

### Glomerulonephritis/Nephrotic Syndrome

In a study from 1990 to 2004, the histological diagnosis of GN/NS in 1238 patients was evaluated. The study showed that the primary causes were mesangioproliferative glomerulonephritis (McPGN) 30%, membranous nephropathy(MGN) 18%, membranoproliferative glomerulonephritis (MPGN) 14%, proliferative glomerulonephritis (PGN) 12.6%, focal segmental glomerulosclerosis (FSGS) 9%, minimal change disease (MCD) 8% and IgA nephropathy 8%, whereas renal lupus (74%), post-streptococcal GN (PSGN) (21%) and secondary MGN (1%) were the most common causes of secondary GN. It is notable that McPGN was the commonest cause, followed by MGN, whereas IgA nephropathy contributed least among the causes of GN. Clinical presentations of those patients were also studied (Table 18.3) [10].

#### Management

In large hospitals, renal biopsies are performed to obtain a diagnosis before initiating GN treatment, whereas at districts and sub-centres (upazilas), GN is treated symptomatically and then referred to a specialist. KDIGO guideline is usually followed by most of the nephrologists. However, nephrologists use various textbooks as a reference to treat GN. For example, idiopathic MGN is treated with oral prednisolone and cyclophosphamide by the majority of nephrologists; Ponticelli regimen is rarely followed. Cyclosporine, tacrolimus and rituximab are gold dust in Bangladesh due to its high cost. For FSGS, prednisolone is the first choice; as second-line treatment tacrolimus or cyclosporine is used mainly in tertiary hospitals by a limited number of nephrologists.

### Diabetes and Kidney Disease

#### Incidence and Prevalence

Diabetes mellitus (DM) is a leading cause of death and disability worldwide. In Bangladesh, the prevalence of diabetes among adults has escalated substantially from 4% in 1995–

**Table 18.2** Aetiology of ESRD in CKD and RRT patients [4, 8]

| Disease | CKD | HD | | CAPD | Transplant |
|---|---|---|---|---|---|
| | | 1998 ($n = 994$) | 2012–2014 ($n = 954$) | | |
| CGN | 37% | 40% | 25% | 20% | 63% |
| DM | 33% | 31% | 41% | 75% | 8% |
| HTN | 16% | 15% | 33% | 4% | 7% |

*CGN* chronic glomerulonephritis, *DM* diabetes mellitus, *HTN* hypertension

**Table 18.3** Histology and clinical presentation of glomerulonephritis ($n$ = 1187) [10]

| Histology | Number (percentage) | Proteinuria >3.5gm/24 hours | HTN BP > 140/90 mmHg | Creatinine S/Cr > 140 μmol/L |
|---|---|---|---|---|
| MGN | 214 (18%) | 51% | 41% | 17% |
| PGN | 150 (12.6%) | 26% | 32% | 49 |
| IgAN | 95 (8%) | 46% | 28% | 21% |
| MPGN | 166 (14%) | 45% | 25% | 37% |
| FSGS | 107 (9%) | 53% | 24% | 29% |
| McPGN | 356 (30%) | 32% | 17% | 30% |
| MCD | 95 (8%) | 61% | 3% | 4% |

Abbreviations: *MCD* minimal change disease, *FSGS* focal segmental glomerulosclerosis, *IgAN* IgA nephropathy, *MPGN* membranoproliferative glomerulonephritis, *PGN* proliferative glomerulonephritis, *McPGN* mesangioproliferative glomerulonephritis, *MGN* membranous nephropathy

2000 to 9% in 2006–2010 [11]. Diabetes is the second most common cause of CKD in Bangladesh. A study with 400 type 2 diabetes mellitus (T2DM) patients in a tertiary diabetes hospital (BIRDEM) in 2014 showed that the prevalence of nephropathy was 24.0% (male 27.1% and female 21.8%) [12]. Another study at the same institute in 2015 demonstrated that more than half (54.5%) of T2DM patients had CKD stages 3–5 according to CKD-EPI equations (male 42% and female 63.6%) [13].

#### Prevention and Treatment

The prevention and treatment of DK is based on the management of hypertension, hyperglycaemia, microalbuminuria and other co-morbidities. The treatment goal is fasting blood sugar ≤6.5 mmol and HbA1c <7.0. In practice, this is very difficult to achieve, and only 34% of the patients have an effective control of blood sugar in Bangladesh. Poor compliance of patients to medications and to preventive measures such as lifestyle modification is the main obstacle to achieve treatment goals. In a study by Mumu et al., non-adherence to diabetic diet was 90%, to foot care 70%, to physical exercise 25% and to self-blood glucose monitoring 32% [14].

#### Healthcare Expenditure

Healthcare expenditure for DM and DKD is increasing at an alarming rate. A study revealed that the annual cost of diabetes care per person in an outpatient department of a tertiary care facility was USD 314. Based on this information, it has been estimated a total annual burden of 1.5 billion USD to treat 5.1 million diabetic patients in the whole country, which is a large burden for a low-middle-income country like Bangladesh [15].

The Bangladesh Diabetic Association, established in 1958, is the largest non-governmental organization, which offers treatment to diabetic patients and provides free insulin to limited number of underprivileged population through its 60 branches in the country.

## Hypertension and Kidney Disease

#### Incidence and Prevalence

HTN is an important worldwide public health challenge because of the concomitant risks of cardiovascular and kidney disease. High blood pressure can be either a cause or a consequence of CKD. Patients with CKD have a high prevalence of high blood pressure even when GFR is only mildly reduced. The appropriate evaluation and management of high blood pressure remains a major component of the management of patients with CKD.

HTN is the third most common cause of CKD in Bangladesh. Although HTN is quite common, most people are unaware of its presence and consequences. In a study among 1000 urban disadvantaged and 1265 rural people, the prevalence of HTN was 11.6–19%, respectively. Strikingly, less than half of these people (only 35%) were aware of their HTN, and the other 65% were identified during the survey. More strikingly, less than half (43%) of the self-reported hypertensive patients were on medication, and among them only 25% had optimum blood pressure control [16, 17]. Another community-based study from two sites in Bangladesh and three sites in India revealed that the prevalence of HTN was 65%, and among them, only 45% were aware of their condition, 40% were taking antihypertensive medications, but only 10% achieved the target level. The prevalence was higher in urban than rural areas [18].

Pre-hypertension also elevates the risks of cardiovascular disease and CKD. In a study by Khanam et al., the prevalence of pre-hypertension and hypertension was 31.9% and 16.0%, respectively. Men had a higher prevalence (33.6%) of pre-hypertension compared to women (30.3%) [19].

#### Management

Hypertension is managed by both general practitioners (GP) and different specialists. The majority of the antihypertensive medications are locally manufactured at affordable prices when compared to other South Asian countries. There is a national guideline, for management of hypertension and hypertensive kidney disease, prepared by specialists from Bangladesh in cooperation with the World Health Organization (WHO) in 2013 [20]. However, there is a lack of awareness among the population about the complications and effects of HTN. Moreover, there is poor compliance with lifestyle modification and medications among the patients.

## Acute Kidney Injury and Critical Care Nephrology

#### Epidemiology

AKI is associated with high morbidity and mortality throughout the world. The epidemiology of AKI in Bangladesh differs from that in the developed world in many ways. In developed countries, AKI is predominantly seen in hospitalized patients, in intensive care units (ICUs) and in elderly patients. However, in Bangladesh it is noted among young patients, and most patients present after developing AKI in the community.

#### Incidence and Causes

The incidence of AKI in hospitalized patients varies from 5% to 25% in Bangladesh. The predominant causes of AKI are acute gastroenteritis (related to suboptimal sanitation and water quality), inadvertent use of drugs, tropical infections, sepsis, poor obstetric care, insufficient monitoring after major surgeries, contrast use, burns, trauma, etc. [2, 3]. However, renal and postrenal causes are also common.

There are several reports of AKI published from different hospitals. In a study of 236 cases of AKI detected among admitted patients over a 9-year period, the causes of AKI were categorized as medical 65.3%, surgical 23.7% and obstetrics 11% [3]. One hundred and five cases of AKI were reported in a military hospital from 2007 to 2011, with 23% developing AKI from gastroenteritis, 9.5% rhabdomyolysis, 7.6% septicaemia, 8.5% GN and 6.6% falciparum malaria [21]. Another study demonstrated a 38% diagnosis of AKI in ICU patients [22]. Contrast-induced AKI was also reported (11%) by Alam et al. [22].

The incidence of AKI increases by 18–24% during monsoon season secondary to an increase in new cases of acute gastroenteritis, dengue, leptospirosis and bacillary dysentery. Malaria is prevalent in South Asian region, particularly in India and Bangladesh. Falciparum malaria is an important cause of AKI in Bangladesh in hill tract districts. It is estimated that 1% of malaria cases develop severe malaria, jaundice and AKI, a complication associated with 45% mortality.

In Bangladesh drug-induced nephrotoxicity was noted in about 15–26.3% of AKI cases [21, 23]. Common causative agents are NSAIDS (naproxen, diclofenac), ciprofloxacin, aminoglycosides (gentamicin, amikacin), ACEI, ARBs, contrast dye, cyclosporine and tacrolimus. In rural areas, herbal and homeopathic remedies are the major contributors to AKI, whereas AKI due to star fruit and snake bite is also common in Bangladesh.

#### Diagnosis, Treatment and Prognosis

In Bangladesh, AKI is generally diagnosed on the basis of serum creatinine and eGFR. There are substantial variations in diagnostic and therapeutic capabilities between the hospitals, community clinics and medical colleges across the country.

Oral rehydration solutions are available everywhere including villages and community clinics. However, intravenous fluids, antimalarial drugs and common antibiotics are only available in district hospitals and sub-centres. After initial management, patients are usually referred to tertiary care centres. At tertiary centres, critically ill patients are managed at ICUs. Inotrope drugs like dopamine, dobutamine and noradrenalin are only available at tertiary centres. However, for the prevention or treatment of AKI, low-dose dopamine or diuretics are not recommended across the country. For the management of hyperkalaemia, calcium gluconate, 7.5% sodium bicarbonate, calcium resonium, insulin and salbutamol inhalation are usually used. If medical treatment fails and the AKI patients require dialysis, they normally receive HD or SLED in most centres and CRRT in a few centres and IPD in district medical college. In some places, especially in a resource-limited setting, IPD is the only dialysis method available to manage AKI patients.

The prognosis of AKI patients has improved significantly over the years. A study in 1997 showed that the survival rate in medical, surgical and obstetric cases were 67.5%, 82.1% and 92.3%, respectively [3]. A more recent study in 2011, including 105 AKI patients, demonstrated that HD was required in 49 cases (46%), CRRT in 6 (5.7%) and PD in 5 (4.7%); complete recovery was recorded in 88 patients (83%), 8 progressed to CKD (8%), 6 developed ESRD (6%), and 3 died (3%) [21].

The management of AKI is still limited by inadequate resources, lack of laboratory facility, insufficient medical and nursing personal and unorganized medical infrastructure. Delay in recognition and inappropriate treatment result in significant morbidity and mortality from AKI in remote places of Bangladesh.

## Paediatric Nephrology

#### History

Paediatric nephrology started its journey as a wing of paediatrics in the year 1982 in the IPGMR. In 1986, paediatric nephrology was established as a separate unit. First PD was performed in 1982, first paediatric HD in 2004 and first KT in January 2006. The Pediatric Nephrology Society of Bangladesh (PNSB) was established in 2004.

#### Incidence, Prevalence and Renal Disease Pattern

The prevalence of paediatric renal patients in Bangladesh is quite high. About 4–5 million children are suffering from different renal diseases. The incidence of paediatric renal patients is increasing day by day [24].

There is no epidemiological study to report the pattern of renal diseases in children of our country. One study was carried out in four tertiary care centres in order to observe the pattern of renal diseases in children in 2015. A total of 6453 patients were studied, 1123 were inpatient and 5330 were outpatient. Mean age was 5.8 ± 3.5 years for inpatients and 6.90 ± 1.37 years for outpatients. Of the inpatients, 64.1% were male and 35.8% female, whereas of the outpatients, 62.59% were male and 37.4% female. Nephrotic syndrome (76% in inpatient) was the most common disease followed by CKD (6%) in inpatient and urinary tract infections (9.4%) in outpatients. Common presentations were proteinuria (27.6%), oliguria or anuria (26.2%) and oedema (25.7%) [25].

The incidence of AKI in children has declined due to better management of infections, diarrhoea, dehydration, and prevention of toxin-associated renal injury. Ignorance and lack of awareness among parents and physicians and limited opportunities for management have continued to result in considerable morbidity and mortality in children with CKD.

## Renal Replacement Therapy in Bangladesh

**Introduction**

Worldwide, over two million people are being kept alive by RRT, the majority of which are from the developed high-income countries. In Bangladesh, according to hospital statistics, 35,000–40,000 patients reach ESRD every year. The existing facilities can hardly accommodate 9000–10,000 new patients, which means RRT is not available for 70–75% of ESRD patients [8].

**Incidence and Prevalence**

The number of new patients reaching ESRD and starting on RRT is increasing dramatically in Bangladesh. In 2017, about 9364 (57.2 pmp) new patients were started on RRT, and in 2018 the incidence increased to 10,421 (63.6 pmp). Majority of these patients started HD (96%) followed by CAPD and renal transplantation [26] (Fig. 18.2). In 1996, only 2048 (17 pmp) patients were on different forms of RRT which rose to around 16,068 (107 pmp) in 2009, 19,546 (122 pmp) in 2017 and 20,260 (123.8 ppm) in 2018 [26].

**Age and Sex**

On December 31, 2013, the mean age of the patients on RRT was 46 years (range 12–76 years). The mean age of patients on HD, CAPD and renal transplant was 41 years, 52 years and 34 years, respectively [8].

### Haemodialysis (HD)

RRT has evolved over the years, and Bangladesh can now offer various techniques of RRT such as maintenance HD (MHD), continuous RRT (CVVH), sustained low efficiency dialysis (SLED) and peritoneal dialysis (CAPD) [14]. However, HD has been the major modality of RRT in Bangladesh.

**Incidence and Prevalence**

In 2017, the number of new patients starting HD was 9000 (55 pmp), and in 2018 it was 10,000 (61.1 pmp). Among the 19,546 patients on RRT in 2017, 18,000 (110 pmp) were on HD, and in 2018 out of 20,260 RRT patients, 18,500 (113 pmp) were on HD (Fig. 18.3) [26].

**Haemodialysis Service in Bangladesh**

There are now 170 HD centres across the country. Not all dialysis centres have a designated nephrologist, as most of them are based in the capital. In 84% of the dialysis centres, there are on-site doctors, and 16% centres are visited by doctors when needed. The doctors in these centres are mainly medical officers trained in management of hypertension and other co-morbid conditions that are common in dialysis patients, but they do not receive any formal nephrology training. There are 750–1000 dialysis nurses operating these centres. There are only 40 dialysis engineers responsible for the preventive and corrective maintenance of the dialysis machines [4]. The majority of the HD centres are based in Dhaka catering to the 15 million population of Dhaka division. The rest is scattered across the country, mainly in other six divisions Barisal, Chittagong, Dhaka, Khulna, Sylhet and Rajshahi. More than 80% of dialysis centres are profit-oriented, and only 20% are non-profit hospitals, including public and NGOs [8].

**Typical HD Prescription**

The frequency of HD is mainly twice a week. About 69% of the patients are dialyzed twice weekly compared to 22% who are on thrice weekly dialysis, 2.5% once weekly and 1.5% on four times a week dialysis. Depending on the financial situa-

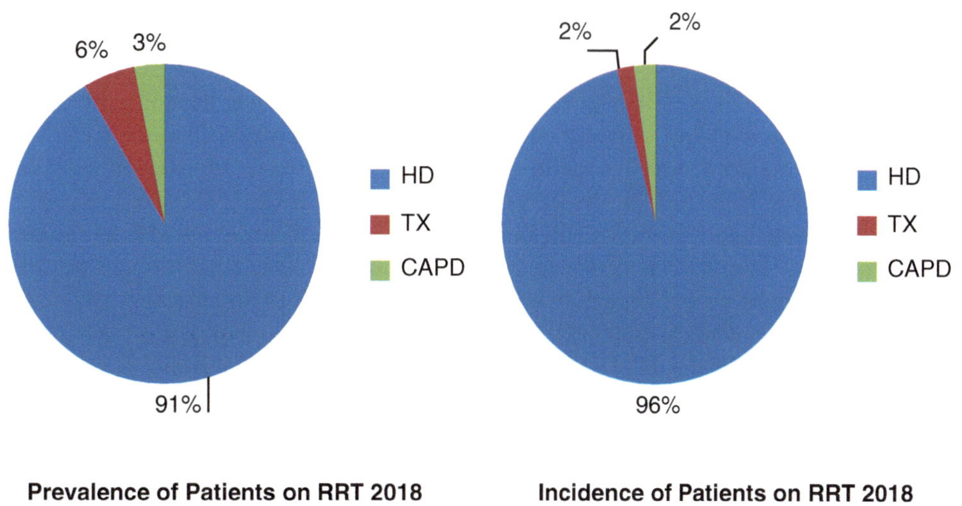


**Fig. 18.2** Incidence and prevalence of renal replacement therapy (RRT)

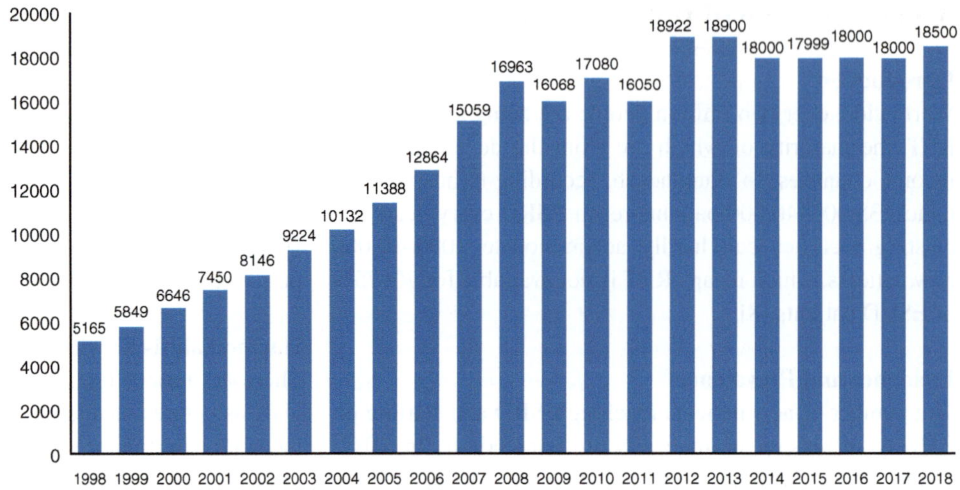


**Fig. 18.3** Prevalence of haemodialysis in Bangladesh (1998–2018) [26]

tion of the patient, 15% of them have a variable frequency of dialysis each week. The average blood flow is 250–300 [27]. In 1988, most of the dialyzate used were acetate buffer until bicarbonate buffer was introduced in South Asia in the 1990s. Acetate buffer is still used in about 5% of the HD patients in Dhaka and in more than 80% of the dialysis units in rural areas due to low cost [28]. Most of the HD sessions are performed mainly at centres located in district and divisions, and only 20% of total HD patients in Bangladesh are based in rural areas. In the early 1990s, cuprophane, cellulose acetate and polysulfone hollow fibre dialyzers were used. The sizes of the dialyzer membranes used then were 1 $m^2$, 1.1 $m^2$ and 0.9 $m^2$. Now the dialyzer membrane used is mainly polysulfone with size range from 1.5 $m^2$, 1.7 $m^2$ to 1.9 $m^2$ [28]. The dialyzer reuse is an integral part of HD in Bangladesh. Previously, the dialyzer membrane was cleaned manually by first rinsing with filtered water until it was blood free and then cleaned using 4% formalin [29]. Nowadays there are machines available in HD units to clean the dialyzers properly. The dialysers are checked mainly manually. Few centres in the capital use reprocessor machines. The frequency of reuse is recommended between five and ten times.

**Water Quality**

In HD, more than 90% of the dialyzate delivered to the dialyzer is water. Water quality is extremely important for standard HD. A standard water treatment system in the Bangladesh dialysis centres involves pre-treatment stages (softener, activated carbon, downsizing micro-filter). The reverse osmosis (RO) unit and deionizer are generally used to obtain ultrapure water. Ultrapure water must present <0.1 cfu/ml and endotoxin <0.03 IU/ml as per European standards. Water quality should be maintained by most HD units across the country as per environmental laws of Bangladesh. There is very few data on how the centres are maintaining the standards across the country. Shaha et al. conducted a survey at six different dialysis centres and found that 67% of the tap water and 80% of treated water used in dialysis centres in Bangladesh complied bacteriologically with Advancement of Medical Instrumentation (AAMI) standards [30].

**HD Vascular Access**

Most patients present as a crash-lander, requiring temporary catheter to initiate urgent dialysis. Those who can afford to continue dialysis have the fistula done at a later stage. In a single-centre study of 2409 patients, 82% initiated HD with non-cuffed catheter and 8% with AV fistula. Among the fistulas 51% had brachial fistula, and 38% had radial fistula [31].

**Causes of ESRD in HD Patients**

A study demonstrated the causes of ESRD in HD patients from 2012 to 2014 as CGN (25.5%), DKD (41%) and HTN (33%). Another study in 1998 showed that, then, the causes were CGN (40%), DKD (31%), HTN (15%), obstructive uropathy (8%) and undetermined (10%) (Table 18.2).The number of patients with diabetic nephropathy reaching ESRD has increased dramatically from 24% in 1994 to 31% in 1998 and 41% in 2014 [4].

**Outcome of HD Patients**

A study including 1000 HD patients of twenty centres demonstrated that the mean age of patients was 40 ± 15 years (range 16–68); 546 were males, and 454 were females. Mean haemoglobin was 8–10 gm/dl, and erythropoietin was received by 39% of the patients [8]. Another single-centre study demonstrated that the average KT/V in patients was 1.03 (range 0.9–1.4), calcium 2.09 mmol/L, phosphate 1.5 mmol/L, uric acid 285.5 μmol/L, total protein 70 g/l and serum albumin 38 g/l [27].

**Complications, Mortality and Morbidity**

Infection is very common in patients on dialysis. The most common is infection of the temporary venous catheter followed by respiratory tract infection, tuberculosis, hepatitis C, hepatitis B, acute pancreatitis, acute hepatitis and skin infection. Other than infections, HD patients also suffer from co-morbid conditions. In a study by Alam et al., the prevalence of co-morbid conditions in patients with HD ($n = 328$) was noted as hypertension 81%, heart failure 27%, coronary artery disease 18%, cardiovascular disease 16%, peripheral vascular disease 2%, diabetes 7%, cancer 3%, lipid abnormality 17%, chronic liver disease 9% and other 25% [32]. Notably HTN, diabetes and heart diseases associated with ESRD are more prevalent among urban HD patients than rural HD patients. Anaemia, anorexia, pruritus, respiratory tract infection, chronic uraemia and malnutrition were more prevalent among rural residents than urban HD patient [33]. This could be due to low quality of HD in the rural sector where the cost of dialysis is less. HD patients are hospitalized more frequently than general people. In a study by Jishu et al., the mean hospital admission was 2.8 times per patient during the study period [34].

HD patient survival rates were estimated to be at 1, 3 and 5 years of 90%, 75% and 55%, respectively, in 1993 and of 90%, 70% and 40% in 2016 [35, 36] (Fig. 18.4).The decrease of survival in recent years could be due to increase number of DKD and older patients in HD as compared to earlier studies. The causes of death were left ventricular failure (LVF) (50%), congestive cardiac failure (CCF) (20%), cerebrovascular disease (CVD) (20%) and coronary artery disease (CAD) (10%). The longest surviving HD patient has been dialysed for 21 years at one public centre [37].

### Cost of HD

The costs of HD are dependent on several factors. The corporate hospitals are more expensive than other HD centres. Acetate dialyzate is cheaper than bicarbonate by USD 1.00.

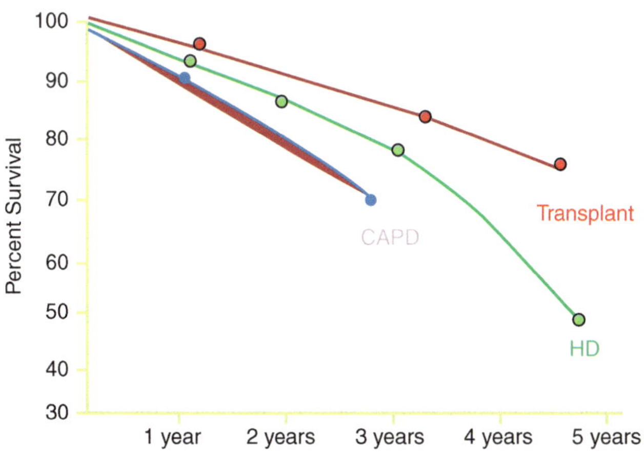


**Fig. 18.4** Survival of ESRD patients on HD, CAPD and transplantation [36]

The total cost of dialysis also depends on the dialyzer membrane type and size; for example, 1.9 $m^2$ dialyzers are more expensive than 1.5 $m^2$ dialyzers, and polysulfone filter is more expensive than cellulose. The cost of HD in profit hospitals ranges from USD 44.00 to 60.00 per HD session, whereas in non-profit hospitals it ranges from USD 10.00 to 30.00 per HD session. The government of Bangladesh (GoB) offers dialysis at a subsidized cost to ESRD patients, but the availability of these services is limited. About 80% of the cost comes from out-of-pocket expenditure.

Bangladesh is trying to keep up in the race of advancement with the entire world. There have been some major advances in the field, but, unfortunately, due to the cost, there are certain orthodox practices that still prevail in the rural areas. Awareness and prevention are the keys to reduce the number of ESRD patients in Bangladesh.

## Continuous Ambulatory Peritoneal Dialysis (CAPD)

### History

CAPD was first introduced in the world by Popovich and Moncrief in 1976. IPD was started in 1973 and CAPD in 1981 in Bangladesh. PD was performed in a total of seven patients until December 1982. Unfortunately, it could not be continued due to non-availability of PD catheters and PD fluid; then, in 1993 CAPD was restarted.

### Incidence and Prevalence

Over the last 10 years, effort is being made to popularize CAPD in Bangladesh. Acceptance rate is now gradually increasing among the patients, peritonitis rate is decreasing, and survival rate has been prolonged. In 2017 the number of new patients started CAPD was 205 (1.3 pmp), and in 2018 it was 234 (1.4 pmp). The prevalence of CAPD patients was 579 (3.5 pmp) in 2017 and 623 (3.8 pmp) in 2018 [26].

### Cause of ESRD in CAPD Patients

The causes of ESRD among CAPD patients are DKD (75%), CGN (20%), HTN (4%) and others (1%) (Table 18.2).The mean age of these patients is 56 years (range 6–85 years; male 450, female 377) [4].

### Indication of CAPD

The main indications of CAPD are haemodynamic instability (40%), poor vascular access (22%), poor general condition (20%) and remote residence (8%). In earlier periods, many patients were selected for PD, not as a matter of choice but because they were not fit for other modalities of RRT. Less than 20% of PD patients are initiated on PD directly; the rest have been transferred from HD after a period of time on HD [4].

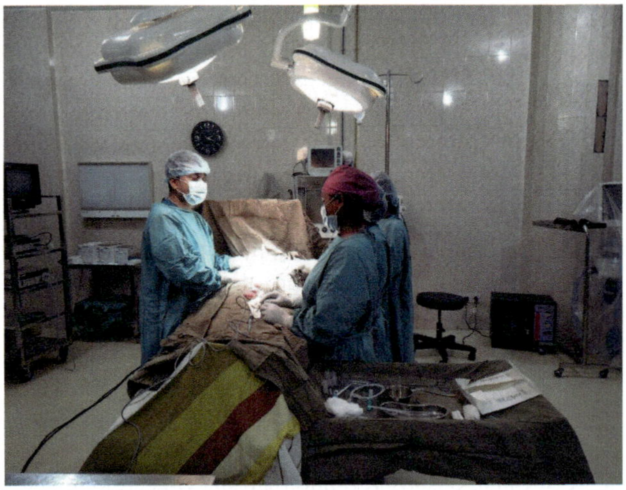

Fig. 18.5 Nephrologists performing PD catheter insertion by percutaneous technique in Bangladesh

**CAPD Technique**

In Bangladesh, PD catheters are inserted either percutaneously (Seldinger technique) or surgically (open dissection method). However, percutaneous puncture technique performed by nephrologist is preferred by the patients (Fig. 18.5). The coiled and straight-tip Tenckhoff catheters are used. It was noted that the outcome of percutaneously placed catheters is comparable to the surgically placed catheters. However, percutaneously placed catheters have the advantage of lower costs, avoidance of operation theatre scheduling issues, smaller incisions and shorter period between catheter insertion and initiation of dialysis. Flushing of the catheter is usually done on third, fourth and fifth days, and manual exchange is started from seventh day using twin bag system. During the first 1 week, treating nephrologists and PD nurses give education and training to patients and their attendants [38].

**PD Bags**

CAPD fluids are imported from Singapore and supplied by Baxter. The solutions are packaged in clear flexible plastic bags, typically made from polyvinyl chloride. Only 2 L bags of 1.5%, 2.5% or 4.25% dextrose solutions (Dianeal) are available. Very recently Extraneal (icodextrin) from Baxter is available in Bangladesh.

**Cost of PD**

The cost of PD is equal or lower than HD, if HD is performed at for-profit dialysis centres. There are few CAPD facilities in public hospitals. In Bangladesh, most of the patients do three exchanges per day; very few perform two exchanges per day due to financial constrain. If three exchanges per day are performed, then the cost for 1 day is around USD 12.00 and for 1 year USD 4380 [8].

**Complications of PD**

Infections (exit site infection, tunnel infection and peritonitis) are the most common complication of CAPD in Bangladesh. However, the incidence of peritonitis has decreased from 1 in 14 patient months in 2003 to 1 in 34 patient months in 2010 [8]. A more recent study revealed that a peritonitis rate of 1 episode in 30 patient months, technique failure due to omental wrap, tip migration and fluid leak were reported in about 1% patients, and 5% patients required catheter removal [39]. In a study by Iqbal et al., organisms responsible for peritonitis and their sensitivity to antibiotics were evaluated and found that 77% samples were culture-positive; the organisms isolated were gram-positive bacteria (*Staphylococcus* and *Streptococcus* species) in 41% of cases, gram-negative bacteria (*Escherichia coli*, *Pseudomonas*, *Klebsiella* species) in 52% and fungus in 7% [40]. Patients with suspected peritonitis are usually advised to come to hospital for treatment. However, those who are unable to come to hospital immediately are advised to start the empirical antibiotics at home.

Non-infectious complications of CAPD are classified in two groups on the basis of onset from the time of insertion of catheter: early onset (1–4 months) and late onset (12–24 months). Early onset complications include exit site leakage, catheter malposition, haemoperitoneum, right-sided hydrothorax and ultrafiltration failure (UFF). The late-onset complications include abdominal hernia, scrotal swelling, encapsulated peritonitis and catheter cuff protrusion. A study found that pain was the most common non-infectious complication (30.8%), followed by ultrafiltration failure (4.7%), hydrothorax (1.9%), fluid leakage (0.9%) and others (27.1%) [38].

Malnutrition is a common problem in CKD patients especially those on PD. While mild to moderate malnutrition is present in 30–70% of PD patients, severe malnutrition develops in 2–9% of patients. The cause is multifactorial and includes delayed dialysis initiation, extreme protein restriction in the pre-dialysis period which often continues even after starting dialysis because of inadequate dietary advice, uremic toxicity, catabolic factors and intercurrent infections.

**Survival of CAPD Patients**

A number of recent studies have shown that survival rates of HD and PD are similar, and PD patients have better cardiovascular stability over HD patients. Patient survival at 1, 2, 3 and 5 years was found to be 68%, 48%, 38% and 22%, respectively. The cause of death is usually acute myocardial infarctions, cerebrovascular disease, pneumonia, malnutrition, peritonitis and others [39]. Another single-centre study has shown that 1- and 3-year survival is 90% and 68%, respectively (Fig. 18.4) [36].

**Challenges and Obstacles of PD**

The major challenge of CAPD in Bangladesh is peritonitis either alone or in association with exit site and tunnel infections. Unfortunately, culture-negative peritonitis rates are high, which hinder the selection of appropriate antibiotics, and, therefore, resolution of infection is sometimes not achieved. This contributes to technique failure and shift from PD to HD. Inadequate sampling, lack of trained and dedicated manpower, lack of automated PD effluent culture system and poor culture technique are the possible reasons for high culture-negative infections. Other major challenges faced are high gram-negative peritonitis rates, infection from multidrug-resistant pathogens, shift from *Candida albicans* to non-*C. albicans* and mycelial infections [41, 42].

Proper training of patients and their relatives about aseptic exchange technique, good exit site care, improvement in catheter insertion technique, strengthening microbiology laboratory and rational use of antibiotics based on local susceptibility data are likely to reduce the peritonitis rate and preserve the peritoneal membrane function, thereby improving clinical outcome of peritonitis and helping in PD growth of Bangladesh.

Other obstacles in CAPD are lack of awareness among general people and physicians, lack of confidence and uncertainty among patients and relatives and even in nephrologists, high cost of treatment, etc. [41].

**Future**

There are tremendous opportunities to expand CAPD in Bangladesh. Most of the dialysis centres are in the capital and in large cities. Due to lack of facility, a vast number of rural and semi-urban population are unable to travel long distances to avail HD. Hence, CAPD can be an available and effective form of therapy in this group of population.

Financing is the major barrier for CAPD. HD in public hospitals is partly reimbursed by the government, whereas CAPD patients pay out of pocket. As a result, most patients prefer HD as the first choice. To expand CAPD we need to manufacture PD fluids and accessories locally and need some reimbursement by the government and NGOs.

Peritoneal Dialysis Society of Bangladesh was established in 2017 to expand CAPD in the country. The KFB is also working to enhance knowledge and awareness about PD among nephrologists, physicians and general people through educational programs, posters and electronic media and providing training to doctors and nurses. PD needs to be positioned as part integrated of the ESRD care, complementing HD, by improving awareness, patient training, care of PD-related infections and management of malnutrition.

## Renal Transplantation

**Introduction**

Organ transplantation is one of the best achievements in the medical history of twentieth century, and in Bangladesh KT is a well-established form of RRT.

**History**

The first living-related KT was performed in December 1982 at IPGMR, Dhaka, Bangladesh, almost 30 years after successful twin transplantation in the USA in 1954. The patient was 29 years old, and the cause of ESRD was CGN. His sister who was 42 years old donated her kidney. He was well post-transplant. Unfortunately, he developed pneumonia and passed away 4 weeks after transplantation with a functioning graft [5]. From 1982 to 1986, only six patients were transplanted at that centre, and survival rate was less than 12 months. Successful KT started in 1988. Until 2003 there was only one centre in the country which performed KTs. From 2004 on, other centres started to perform KT in Bangladesh, and currently ten centres in the country are recognized by the government for performing KT. However, only four centres are performing KT regularly. The other six centres were not regular but are now gathering more interest in transplant [43]. There are now 1791 KTs successfully performed in Bangladesh [44].

**Incidence and Prevalence**

In 2017, the incidence of KT was 1.0 pmp (168 new patients) and 1.14 pmp in 2018 (187 new patients); each year about 120–190 KT surgeries are being performed. The prevalence of renal transplant patients in 2017 was 967 (6 pmp), and in 2018 it was 1137 (6.9 pmp) [26].

**Workforce**

The total number of urologists in Bangladesh is 160, out of which the number of transplant surgeons is only 25. However, few surgeons are interested in transplantation, and, as a result, the number of transplantation is not increasing as expected.

**Organ Act Law**

Bangladesh Organ Act Law was passed in the parliament in 1999. According to the law, parents to child, siblings to siblings, spouse to spouse and blood-related close relatives like uncle and aunt were eligible to donate solid organs [45]. To expand the living donor pool, the Organ Act Law was revised in January 2018, and grandfather, grandmother and blood-related cousins were included in the eligible donor list. However, live unrelated organ donation is completely prohibited, whereas deceased transplantation is supported by the Organ Act Law. Donors should be between 18 and 65 years of age and free from hepatitis B, hepatitis C and HIV. Recipients should be between 2 and 70 years of age [46]. Selling and buying solid organs are completely prohibited. This law has a provision of 2–3 years of rigorous imprisonment or USD 5882 to USD 11,674 fine, or both for violation of the law, aiming to check the illegal trade of human organs [46].

#### Cause of ESRD in Transplant Patients

CGN (63%) was by far the commonest cause of ESRD in transplanted patients in Bangladesh. Other causes include DKD, HTN, polycystic kidney disease, renal lupus, Alport syndrome and unknown in one-tenth of the cases (Table 18.2) [4].

#### Preparation and Immunosuppression

Preparation for transplantation starts either in the clinic or during inpatient stay in hospital. Once patients reach ESRD, they are informed about KT in details. Then, patients discuss with their families, friends and close relatives. Once they wish to go ahead with transplantation, appropriate investigations are carried out, and they are reviewed by ethical and medical board. Transplant team reviews the patients only before surgery. During preparation, patients are usually recommended to take hepatitis B, pneumococcal and meningococcal vaccination. Usually patients undergo MHD for 3–6 months before transplantation. However, in few cases pre-emptive transplantation does take place.

The immunosuppression protocol from 1988 to 2005 was triple therapy including cyclosporine, azathioprine and prednisolone for initial 6 months followed by withdrawal of cyclosporine in majority of cases and continuation of azathioprine and prednisolone at appropriate dose. From 2006 cyclosporine was replaced by tacrolimus in majority of centres, and azathioprine was replaced by mycophenolate mofetil in some centres.

For induction, generally methylprednisolone is used, and basiliximab is avoided because of its high cost. However, basiliximab is recommended specially if the donor is spouse and the HLA tissue match is poor.

Post-operatively, the patient stays in the hospital for a minimum of 14 days, and the donor stays for 7 days. In most centres, patients are followed up by their nephrologists. After discharge, patients are followed up weekly for first 3 months, thereafter fortnightly for next 3 months, then monthly up to 1 year and then 2–3 monthly. Immunosuppression dose is gradually reduced after 6 months depending on cyclosporine or tacrolimus level. Tacrolimus trough level is usually 8–10 for first 3 months and reduced to 6–8 after 3–6 months thereafter 5–6. Mycophenolate dose is adjusted as per body weight. Patients weighing >60 kg are given 1500–2000 g/day, whereas patients <60 kg are usually prescribed 1000 g. Prednisolone is given as 0.5 mg/kg body weight at start and reduced to 5 mg after 6 months.

#### Transplant Outcome

Studies performed in Bangladesh to see the outcome of renal transplant patients are not many. However, studies concluded that the survival of transplant patients in Bangladesh is comparable to that in developed countries [47, 48].

In an earlier study (1993) including 94 patients, the graft survival was 96% at 1 year and 81% at 3 years [48]. A study including 262 patients who were followed up for 16 years (1988–2004) demonstrated that the 1-, 3-, 5-, 7- and 10-year survival rates of patients were 93%, 90%, 83%, 80% and 70%, respectively [49]. More recent studies showed that the 1-, 3-, and 5-year survival rates of transplant patients were 94%, 86% and 77%, respectively, in one centre and 92%, 85% and 80% in another centre (Fig. 18.4) [36, 47]. The longest surviving renal graft has been functioning for 33 years.

Female transplant patients are not usually encouraged to get pregnant because of the high risk of graft failure and risk of maternal and foetal morbidity and mortality. However, few patients become pregnant 14–28 months post-transplant and have successful pregnancy outcome with good graft function after delivery.

## Complication of Renal Transplantation

### Immediate Complications

Infections remain the major concern in renal transplant patients in Bangladesh. The infections are usually respiratory (40%), followed by urinary tract infections and tuberculosis (10%) [8]. Acute rejection is the second most important complication comprising 20–25%. The other complications are acute tubular necrosis, CMV infection, superficial fungal infections and post-transplant diabetes mellitus. The surgical complications are urinoma, abscess and pelvic lymphocele [50].

### Late Complications

The chronic complications are allograft nephropathy, transplant glomerulopathy, drug toxicity, cancer and graft failure.

## Mortality and Morbidity

The main cause of death in Bangladeshi transplanted patients is infection, but cardiovascular disease also accounts for a significant number of deaths [49]. Biopsy of transplanted kidney is limited and only performed in few centres of Bangladesh. Unfortunately, we lack the capacity to perform C4D staining, staining for BK virus or CMV, electron microscopy and other specialized stains in our biopsy samples.

### Outcome of Kidney Donors

In Bangladesh, females are the main bulk of donors. In a study, 76% of donors were females (mothers 40%, wives 24% and sisters 12%), and only 24% were male. Donors are usually 21–55 years old. Outcome of donors is always a big concern for patients and their relatives as no one wants any harm to the donors. A study revealed that 5 years post nephrectomy, there was no significant rise of blood pressure, blood urea, serum creatinine or urinary protein in the donors. However, a small statistically non-significant fall in creatinine clearance from 75 ± 11.6 ml/min to 65 ± 5.7 ml/min was noted after 5 years. The study concluded that kidney donors did not suffer from any immediate or long-term complications after kidney donation [51].

### Transplant Tourism and Organ Trafficking

Because of the significant shortage of organs, organ trafficking and transplant tourism have become a global problem accounting for about 10% of organ transplants that are performed annually around the world. In Bangladesh, organ trafficking is one of the reasons behind the low number of transplantations performed each year. Even though organ trafficking is completely prohibited in Bangladeshi law and outlawed in almost every country in the world, each year nearly 250 Bangladeshi patients are transplanted outside Bangladesh [52].

### Cost of Transplantation

The cost for pre-transplant donor investigations is around USD 500, and that of the recipient is around USD 350. The cost of transplantation surgery with ICU and post-ICU stay for 14 days in public hospitals is around USD 1200.00. In non-profit centres, it is around USD 2200.00–3200.00 and in for-profit hospitals around USD 6000.00–10,000.00. After discharge from the hospital, patients bear the cost of medications, lab investigations and doctor's fee which is around USD 2900.00–3500.00 for the first 6 months and thereafter, it reduces to around USD 3000.00 per year [4]. Patients usually pay the cost of transplantation and post-operative medications in the private sectors. In the public hospitals, out-of-pocket expenditure comprises about 80% of total costs, whereas only 20% comes from government funding.

### Barriers for Transplantation

Despite being the most costly RRT, the number of transplant remains low in Bangladesh. Potential barriers for living related donors include scarcity of donors mainly due to lack of awareness among people and fear of donation, high cost of immunosuppressive drugs, lack of trained workforce both medical and paramedical, frequent post-transplant infections and lack of necessary laboratory facilities [46].

Though deceased transplantation is the main form of transplantation in developed countries and is permitted by the law in Bangladesh, it is yet to be performed. Obstacles for deceased transplantation are (a) lack of proper ICU infrastructure for early identification and management of brain death donors; (b) lack of proper knowledge about deceased transplantation in the public and even physicians; (c) certain sociocultural beliefs of people such as 'dead body should be buried whole' and 'donation after death is against religious convictions'; (d) high cost with lack of certainty; and (e) lack of workforce and laboratory facilities.

## Nephrology Practice in Bangladesh

### Health System

The healthcare service in Bangladesh is divided into primary healthcare in rural areas, secondary health care in unions and sub-centres (upazila), district hospitals in each district and tertiary care hospitals in divisional cities (Fig. 18.6).

The primary centres in villages provide basic health services like family planning, vaccination, etc. through 16,400 community clinics run by health workers. The union health and sub-centres in 450 upazilas are run by graduate doctors. Each upazila has 30–50-bed hospital and limited lab facility. The 64 district hospitals provide secondary care, while tertiary care in all specialties including nephrology is provided by 112 medical college hospitals and 8 postgraduate institutes (Fig. 18.6).

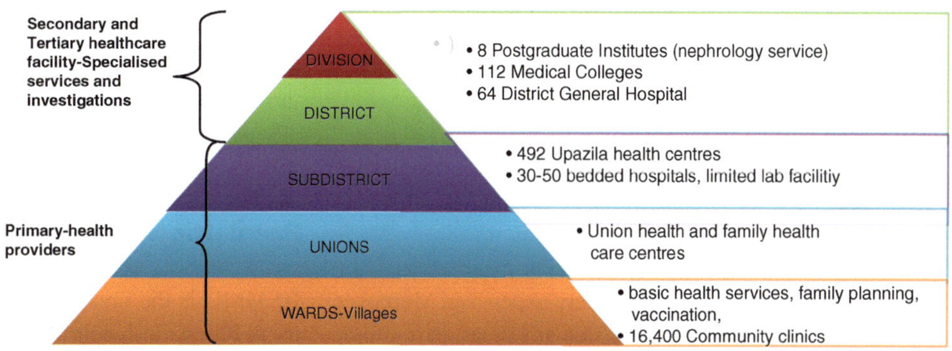


**Fig. 18.6** Health system of Bangladesh

There are many NGOs that provide renal services, namely, KFB and 'Center for Kidney Disease and Urology', which are the prime non-profit hospitals for KT and dialysis. Seventy-five per cent of KTs are performed in these two centres, whereas 50% of PD services is provided by KFB alone. Another NGO, Gonoshasthaya Hospital, has been providing HD at an affordable price for poor patients for the last 2 years.

## Workforce and Job Market

In Bangladesh, there is insufficient number and uneven distribution of trained medical and paramedical professionals. There is a huge gap between the number of renal patients and the number of nephrologists available in Bangladesh. There are about 205 nephrologists across the country, which means that for about 0.8 million people, only one nephrologist is available. Moreover, the majority of the nephrologists (about 70%) work in the capital, which has a population of 15 million, only whereas districts and sub-centres comprise 70% of the total population and have few or no nephrologists to serve the renal patients. As a result, people from villages and districts have to travel a long distance to reach the city in order to consult with a nephrologist. There are also gaps in allied health professionals working in renal wards and dialysis units. There is no national training programme for renal nurses, technicians and renal nutritionists. Normally general nurses and nutritionists get supervised training in renal wards and dialysis units for 1–3 months and thereafter provide service for renal patients. The government, however, is launching a 1-year renal nursing training programme in the Kidney Foundation of Bangladesh.

Due to this huge shortage, there is a high demand of nephrologists and allied health professionals. Although there are limited nephrology posts in government medical college hospitals, they still have vacancies. In private hospitals of large cities, ample job opportunities are available. Because of the huge load of kidney patients, nephrologists are usually busy seeing patients and are unable to perform regular research works. The salary scale in public sectors for assistant professor ranges from USD 400.00 to 900.00, for associate professors from USD 600.00 to 1200.00 and for professors from USD 1000.00 to 3000.00. In for-profit hospitals, the salary scale is three times higher than the government sector. In addition to the salary, doctors earn from private practice and from nephrology interventions.

## Facilities

The kidney care facilities in government hospitals are limited, whereas private hospitals are very expensive. Moreover, there is lack of laboratory facility in many areas, particularly in rural setup. Basic laboratory services like urine test, estimation of serum creatinine, ultrasonography and X-rays are available in upazilas and in districts, but not in villages. CT scans are available in large cities. Albumin creatinine ratio, protein creatinine ratio, complement assay, antinuclear factor, anti-double stranded antibody, c-ANCA and p-ANCA and other specialized services are only available in a few centres in large cities. However, assay methodologies of different laboratories are not uniformly standardized.

Renal biopsies are performed in eight medical college hospitals and in four private hospitals. Immunofluorescence of the sample is available in limited centres only. Electron microscopy is unavailable across the country. There are 150 histopathologists in Bangladesh; but only 10 (5%) of them report renal histology.

## Training and Research

Nephrology training programmes and kidney diseases research have progressed slowly over the last five decades and are largely confined to the teaching hospitals. There are now six centres offering higher training in nephrology. Both MD nephrology and FCPS nephrology are 5-year training programmes in nephrology. There are masters and PhD programmes available for nutritionists in collaboration with both local and foreign universities. Short training programme on deceased kidney transplantation is also available in collaboration with Korea University Anam Hospital.

The Bangladesh Renal Association (BRA), KFB and Kidney Awareness Monitoring and Prevention Society (KAMPS) all are working on awareness, prevention, treatment and research. BRA is affiliated with the International Society of Nephrology (ISN). KFB is a sister renal centre of ISN and is affiliated with the International Federation of Kidney Foundation (IFKF). KFB in addition to providing services at affordable price is conducting various researches in collaboration with Royal London Hospital (UK) and Wayne State University (Michigan, USA).

Postgraduate doctors usually perform epidemiological and clinical studies as a part of their MD nephrology course. Besides that, some nephrologists pursue research by personal interest. Funding for research is available from Bangladesh Medical Research Council (BMRC), University Grants Commission (UGC) and the government funding scheme. ISN also supports capacity building and research in Bangladesh through partnership with ISN. *Bangladesh Renal Journal* usually publishes local and foreign researches twice a year.

## Paediatric Nephrology Practice

BSMMU is the first and leading paediatric nephrology centre in Bangladesh with 30 inpatient beds and 4 haemodialysis beds. This is the only paediatric renal transplant centre in

Bangladesh. To date 11 paediatric KTs have been performed. There are two postgraduate programmes on paediatric nephrology: MD residency and FCPS. In 2018, there were 35 paediatric nephrologists across the country with a ratio of paediatric nephrologists to paediatric population (>19 years or less) to be approximately 1:1.1 million. The Pediatric Nephrology Society of Bangladesh (PNSB) arranges programmes to enhance public awareness about paediatric renal disease every year in the eve of world kidney day, and it arranges international conferences every biannually, national seminar every year and regional seminars in every 2–3 months.

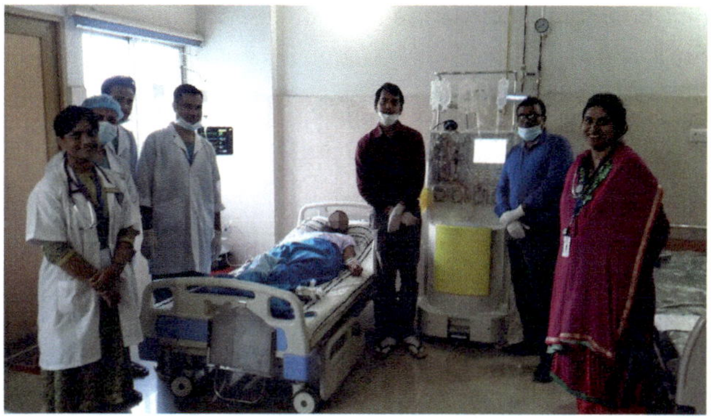

Fig. 18.7 Plasma exchange for ABO-incompatible kidney transplantation, 2018

## Limitations of Renal Services in Bangladesh

The hurdles yet to be addressed are inability of general people to bear the cost of renal treatment (though the cost is less than in neighbouring countries), lack of government subsidy and lack of adequate facilities. The insufficient number and uneven distribution of trained medical and allied health professionals, lack of proper referral system, follow-up and concise national guidelines are other factors that need attention to ensure good sustainable renal care across the country.

## Highlights of Nephrology in Bangladesh

### Interventional Nephrology

Nephrologists in Bangladesh are now increasingly using their hands-on ultrasound guiding temporary and permanent HD catheters and renal biopsies. PD catheter implantation and some AVF are also performed by nephrologists. The job of vascular surgeon is reserved mainly for complicated AVF.

### Transplant

ABO-incompatible kidney transplantation has started in one centre in 2018 in Bangladesh, and there are now five patients successfully transplanted (Fig. 18.7).

### Awareness Programmes

The use of electronic and print media is playing an important role to improve awareness about DM, HTN and kidney diseases among common people, general physicians and allied health professionals. Articles are now published in print media in local language demonstrating different aspects of kidney diseases. Doctors are also appearing in talk shows and radio programmes to discuss health issues. Some private hospitals and clinics are using Skype and telephone to communicate with patients living in remote places free of cost. To create awareness, 'World Kidney Day', 'World Health Day' and most of the days from the 'health awareness calendar' are celebrated throughout the country.

### Pioneer Award

The International Society of Nephrology (ISN), a leading organization of nephrologists of 152 countries, has selected Professor Harun Ur Rashid, an eminent nephrologist of Bangladesh and the founding president of Kidney Foundation, for the South Asian region ISN Pioneer Award 2017. The award was given in recognition to his remarkable leadership in initiating and developing nephrology and KT in Bangladesh.

## Future Perspectives of Nephrology in Bangladesh

There has been enormous development in all sectors of nephrology including diagnosis, treatment availability, prognosis of patients, workforce, etc., since its inaugural year in 1973. It is expected that by 2030 there will be further improvements in the management of AKI, CKD and ESRD care.

### Prevention

The government is also giving more importance to the prevention of DM, HTN and CKD by involving the community clinics. Community clinics in Bangladesh currently offer primary healthcare mainly vaccination, mother and child healthcare and population control to about 6000 people in every village. The government of Bangladesh is now prepar-

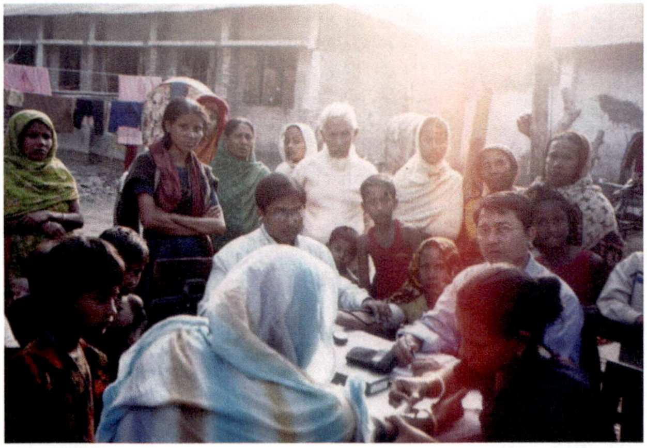

**Fig. 18.8** Screening camp for CKD, hypertension and diabetes for disadvantaged population, 2005

ing to include detection of non-communicable diseases in each community clinic so that DM, HTN and CKD could be diagnosed at a very early stage and treatment could be initiated at the earliest stage of the disease. The community clinics will be entitled to check height, weight, blood pressure, blood sugar and urine for albumin and sugar of all people attending the clinics every day (Fig. 18.8). If any of the above parameters are found abnormal, patients will be referred to sub-centres and district hospitals, and they will be further screened, estimating serum creatinine and eGFR. District hospitals and sub-centres will refer the case to a nephrologist if serum creatinine is greater than 176 μmol/l. In a 10-year period, we are expecting that if DM, HTN and CKD can be detected at an early stage, 40–50% of prevention will be possible in Bangladesh.

## HD

Our government is now targeting 50% access to ESRD treatment. The government is now setting up ten-bed dialysis units in all 64 districts of Bangladesh. The government has just started public-private partnership (PPP) as a pilot scheme to offer affordable dialysis at a mere cost of USD 5.0 per session [4]. New methods of RRT therapy such as haemofiltration and haemodiafiltration are being piloted at some of the ICUs across the country and are expected to expand.

## CAPD

CAPD is gradually establishing as a popular modality of dialysis. KFB is providing training on CAPD in collaboration with international organizations, which will promote CAPD further in Bangladesh. Automated peritoneal dialysis (APD) is expected to become available in near future. The government is also taking measures to manufacture PD fluid in the country.

## Transplantation

In the near future, we are hoping to see a lot more transplantations to happen. To increase the number of live related transplantations, the 'Organ Act Law' was revised in 2018, extending the list of eligible living donors and permitting deceased transplantation.

Several round table discussions, conferences and seminars have been arranged to disseminate the idea of deceased donation and to discuss about practicalities of deceased donation. The Society of Organ Transplantation in Bangladesh is trying to organize the deceased transplantation program. Steps are underway to improve brain death committees in designated ICUs, to form an organ procurement committee and provide training for transplant coordinator and grief counsellors. Each dialysis unit is now also encouraged to keep a registry of their patients' blood group and tissue type. In order to train transplant coordinators, ICU specialists and transplant surgeons, a bilateral agreement with other Asian countries has also established.

ABO-incompatible KT has recently started, which will further increase the donor pool. Strategies also need to be developed to perform HLA-incompatible transplantations and 'paired kidney exchange' in the future. With all these efforts and enforcement of law, it is expected that the number of KTs performed each year in our country will hike in the near future, and, thereby, transplant tourism and organ trafficking will reduce.

## Healthcare System

Healthcare delivery system in Bangladesh is anticipated to change in near future. KFB has taken initiative to formulate and implement local guidelines for the management of kidney diseases. Communication with patients will improve remarkably with the use of digital technology (electronic and print media, Skype, telephone calls). The government is also taking measures to increase renal nursing and renal nutrition training in different government and private non-profit hospitals.

Along with the government, KFB is also working to enhance all aspects of kidney care including HD, CAPD, transplantation, DM screening, HTN, proteinuria and prevention of kidney disease. It has already established four dialysis units in peripheries and is planning to establish dialysis units in large cities and in districts. KFB and other organizations are training doctors, nurses and nutritionists, trying to disseminate knowledge and enhance awareness through electronic and print media. Regular national and international seminars and conferences are being held. We hope that with the increasing support from the government and other organizations, kidney care will be accessible and affordable to the whole population in the near future.

## Conclusion

Kidney disease is emerging as an important public health issue due to its rising incidence and prevalence, high morbidity, mortality and high healthcare cost. Although there has been phenomenal improvement in nephrology care in Bangladesh, renal services are still not accessible and affordable to the majority of the population. Lack of workforce, facilities, national guideline, lack of insurance and government subsidy make difficulties in the proper care of renal patients. Moreover, inequality between organizations and lack of national policy complicate things further. The expanding private sector is providing secondary and tertiary care, but it does not have a comprehensive health policy to strengthen the entire health system. The government of Bangladesh is beginning to recognize the economic and health impact of kidney diseases and is initiating strategies for prevention of AKI and CKD and to provide accessible and affordable renal care. Few NGOs are working alongside the government and delivering significant contribution to the ongoing improvement. However, research on nephrology and training for nephrologists and for allied health professionals are still in the early stages and hence need special concentration. In the future, with the support of the government, NGOs and other charitable organizations, kidney care in Bangladesh is expected to improve further and meet international standards of renal care.

**We Thank the Following Doctors for Their Suggestion in Writing This Chapter**

1. Golam Moinuddin, MD, Professor of Pediatric Nephrology, Bangabandhu Sheikh Mujib Medical University, Dhaka
2. Nizam Uddin Chowdhury, FCPS, MD, Professor and Chairman, Dept. of Nephrology, Dhaka Medical College
3. MA Samad, FCPS, MD, Professor of Nephrology, BRB Hospital, Dhaka
4. AKM Monowarul Islam, MD, Professor and Head, Dept. of Nephrology, Rajshahi Medical College, Rajshahi
5. Shahidul Islam Selim, MCPS, MD, Professor of Nephrology, Bangabandhu Sheikh Mujib Medical University, Dhaka
6. Sarwar Iqbal, MD, Professor of Nephrology, BIRDEM Medical College, Dhaka
7. Probir Kumar Dutta, FCPS, MD, Professor of Nephrology, Chittagong Medical College, Chittagong
8. Muhammad Nazrul Islam, FCPS, MD, Associate Professor of Nephrology, Bangabandhu Sheikh Mujib Medical University
9. Babrul Alam, MD, Associate Professor of Nephrology, National Institute of Kidney Disease and Urology, Dhaka
10. A H Hamid, MD, Associate Professor of Nephrology, Bangabandhu Sheikh Mujib Medical University
11. KM Hadiuzzaman, MD, Associate Professor of Nephrology, Bangabandhu Sheikh Mujib Medical University
12. Syed Fazlul Islam, Assistant Professor of Nephrology, Bangabandhu Sheikh Mujib Medical University
13. Nurul Huda, FCPS, MD, Associate Professor of Nephrology, Chittagong Medical College, Chittagong
14. Mobasher Alam, MD, Associate Professor and Head, Rangpur Medical College
15. A.H.M Ahsan, MD, Associate Professor, Bogra Medical College
16. Enamul Kabir, MD, Assistant Professor, Shaheed Abu Naser Specialized Hospital, Khulna
17. Alamgir Chowdhury, MD, Associate Professor, Sylhet M.A.G Osmani Medical College
18. Abdul Aziz, MD, Consultant Paediatric Medicine, CMH, Dhaka

## References

1. Jha V, Rashid HU, Agarwal SK, Akhtar SF, Kafle RK, Sheriff R. The state of nephrology in South Asia. Kidney Int. 2019;95:31–7.
2. Rashid HU, Hossain M, Khanam A. Outcome of acute renal failure in adults in a teaching hospital in Bangladesh. Ren Fail. 1993;15(5):603–7.
3. Rashid HU, Ahmed S, Hossain R, Khanam A. Acute renal failure in adult in a teaching hospital. Bangladesh Renal Journal. 1997;16(2):41–4.
4. Rashid HU. Bangladesh renal registry-2002–2013. Kidney Foundation, Bangladesh: 2013. p. 10–16.
5. Alam S, Chowdhury D, Rashid HU. A case of living donor transplant in IPGMR. Bangladesh Renal Journal. 1982;1(1):12–4.
6. Rahman M, Haq SA, Haq A. Preliminary experience with continuous ambulatory peritoneal dialysis. Bangladesh Med Res Counc Bull. 1982;8(2):52–8.
7. Rashid HU. Articles of special interest-birth of specialist journal. Bangladesh Renal Journal. 1982;1(1):1.
8. Rashid HU. Management of end stage renal disease-Bangladesh perspective. Open Urol Nephrol J. 2014;7:108–12.
9. Rashid HU. Health delivery system for renal disease care in Bangladesh. Saudi J Kidney Dis Transpl. 2004;15(2):185–9.
10. Khanam A, Alam MR, Islam S, Rashid HU, Rahman H. Histological pattern of glomerulonephritis in a teaching hospital. Bangladesh Renal Journal. 2004;23(1):14–7.

11. Saqib N, Saquib J, Ahamed T, Khanam MA, Culler MR. Cardio vascular diseases and type II diabetic in Bangladesh. A systematic review and nephropathy of studies between 1995 and 2010. BMC Public Health. 2012;12:434.
12. Sayama H, Muttalib MA, Islam MI. Prevalence of nephropathy with evaluation of HbA1c level and other associated risk factors in type 2 diabetic patients in is tertiary level hospital. KYAMC J. 2017;8(1):21–6.
13. Rahman MA, Mitra P, Haque HA, Samadoni TS, Zaman S, Nizamuddin K. Prevalence of chronic kidney disease stages 3–5 among patients with type 2 diabetes mellitus in Bangladesh. IMC J Med Sci. 2017;11(1):19–24.
14. Mumu SJ, Saleh F, Ara F, Ali L. Non-adherence to lifestyle modification and its determinants among Bangladeshi type 2 diabetic patients. Int J Epidemiol. 2015;44:148–9.
15. Afroz A, Habib SH, Chowdhury HA, Paul D, Shahjahan M, Hafez MA, et al. Healthcare cost of type 2 diabetes mellitus in Bangladesh: a hospital-based study. Int J Diabetes Dev Ctries. 2016;30(2):235–41.
16. Alam KS, Huda MN, Rashid HU, Saha M. Prevalence of diabetes mellitus, hypertension, proteinuria and association of these risk factors with estimated glomerular filtration rate (eGFR) in adult disadvantaged population. Bangladesh Renal Journal. 2010;29(1):1–6.
17. Faroque MO, Rashid HU, Rahman MH, Alam MR, Islam S, Khan F, et al. Prevalence of diabetes mellitus, hypertension and proteinuria in rural area of Bangladesh. Bangladesh Renal Journal. 2010;29(1):7–11.
18. Hypertension Study Group. Prevalence, awareness, treatment and control of hypertension among the elderly in Bangladesh and India: a multicentre study. Bull World Health Organ. 2001;79(6):490–500.
19. Khanam MA, Lindeboom W, Razzaque A, Niessen L, Milton AH. Prevalence and determinants of pre-hypertension and hypertension among the adults in rural Bangladesh: findings from a community-based study. BMC Public Health. 2015;15:203.
20. Malik A, Khandaker RK, Zaman M, Choudhury SR. National guidelines for management of hypertension in Bangladesh. Dhaka: World Health Organization; 2013. p. 1–66.
21. Mostafi M, Nessa MA, Fakir MAH, Bhuiyan MAQ, Rahman AM. Presentation and outcome of acute kidney injury in a Tertiary Military Hospital of Bangladesh. Bangladesh J Med. 2011;22(2):35–40.
22. Alam B, Islam N, Khatun F, Moniruzzaman M, Alam M, Faraji AH, et al. Co-morbidity and acute kidney injury among critically ill patients. Bangladesh Renal Journal. 2011;30(2):29–36.
23. Arefin MSZ, Rashid HU, Ahamed PI, Rubel RA. Improving outcomes from acute kidney injury. Proceedings of World Congress of Nephrology 2015. Cape Town; 2015.
24. Afroz S, Hossain D, Huque S, et al. Editorial. Paediatr Nephrol J Bangladesh. 2016;1(1):1.
25. Qader A, MuinUddin G, Rahman R, et al. Renal diseases in children attending pediatric nephrology centers of Dhaka City. J Pediatr Nephrol. 2016;4(3):86–91.
26. Rashid HU. Year book of Kidney Foundation, Bangladesh. Kidney Foundation, Bangladesh; 2019 (in Press).
27. Arefin SU, Rashid HU. Experience of haemodialysis in a tertiary care hospital of Bangladesh. Proceeding of 9th International Congress of the International Society for Hemodialysis (ISHD) 2015. Kuala Lumpur, Malaysia; 2015.
28. Chowdhury NS, Islam FM, Zafreen F, Begum BA, Sultana N, et al. Effect of surface area of dialyzer membrane on the adequacy of haemodialysis. J Armed Forces Med Coll Bangladesh. 2011;7(2):9–11.
29. Kashem MDA, Dutta PK, Huda N, Das S, Yunus IB. Dialyzer reuse. A logical practice in hemodialysis. J Chittagong Med Coll Teach Assoc. 2011;22(1):11–4.
30. ShahaAK. Analysis of water quality in different Haemodialysis centers in Bangladesh. BSMMU Project. 2008;1(1):11–4.
31. Rashid HU. Year book of Kidney Foundation, Bangladesh. Kidney Foundation, Bangladesh; 2016.
32. Alam MR, Khanam A, Alam KS, Muqueet MA, Ahmed T. Prevalence of co-morbidity in hemodialysis patients. Bangladesh Renal Journal. 2004;23(2):56–60.
33. Reza HM, Ahmed AS, Rahman MA, Shuvo SD, Ahmed T. Comparison of nutritional status between patients from urban area with rural area undergoing hemodialysis in Kushtia district, Bangladesh: a cross-sectional study. Asian J Med Biol Res. 2016;2(4):603–10.
34. Jishu DN, Kashem A. Etiology and frequency of hospital admissions in maintenance hemodialysis patients in chronic kidney disease. Saudi J Kidney Dis Transpl. 2019;30(2):508–12.
35. Rashid HU, Khan F, Ahmad S, Rahman M. Experience of haemodialysis in Bangladesh. Bangladesh Renal Journal. 1993;1291(17):19.
36. Rashid HU, Arefin S, Hasan S, Alam K. The role of the Kidney Foundation of Bangladesh in promoting kidney care in a resource-limited environment. Clin Nephrol. 2016;86(1):64–8.
37. Rana AS, Hossain K, Islam S. 21 years of haemodialysis with healthy life: a case report. Bangladesh Renal Journal. 2012;31(1):22.
38. Arefin MSU. A 2-year follow-up study of patients oncontinuous ambulatory peritoneal dialysis (CAPD) in specialized hospital in Dhaka, Bangladesh. J Dhaka Med Coll. 2015;24(2):132–5.
39. Iqbal S, Iqbal MM, Chowdhury TA, Rahim MA, Bhuiyan ASMMM, Ananna MA, et al. Experience managing adult patients on continuous ambulatory peritoneal dialysis in Bangladesh. Adv Perit Dial. 2018;34:38–41.
40. Iqbal MM, Sattar H, Islam MN, Ahmed AH, Rahman MH, Rashid HU, et al. Spectrum of organisms causing peritonitis in peritoneal dialysis patients--experience from Bangladesh. Adv Perit Dial. 2008;24:40–3.
41. Savla D, Ahmed S, Yeates K, Matthew A, Anand S. Barriers to increasing use of peritoneal dialysis in Bangladesh: a survey of patients and providers. Perit Dial Int. 2017;37:234–7.
42. Prasad KN. PD fluid cell count, biochemical analysis and culture in diagnosis of peritonitis. Proceeding of 2nd Annual convention and scientific seminar on CAPD. 2014;18.
43. Rashid HU. Proceeding of 4th national convention and scientific seminar on "organ transplantation". Society of Organ Transplantation (SOT), Bangladesh. 2018;2–3.
44. Rashid HU. Year book of Kidney Foundation, Bangladesh. Kidney Foundation, Bangladesh; 2018.
45. The Bangladesh Gazette. Organ Transplantation act (Bangladesh) 1999. Registration No – D A-1; Tuesday 13 Apr 1999.
46. The Bangladesh Gazette. Transplantation of human organs (amendment) bill, 2018. Registration No – D A-1; Sunday 28 Jan 2018.
47. Mitra P, Hossain MG, Hossan ME, Khoda MME, Rahim MA, Hossain MJ, et al. A decade of live related donor kidney transplant. Experience in a tertiary care hospital of Bangladesh. BIRDEM Med J. 2018;8:198–202.
48. Rashid H, Rasul G, Rahman M, Jinnat S, Wahab M. Experience of kidney transplantation in Bangladesh. Transplant Proc. 1992;24:1831.
49. Rashid HU, Rahman M, Sharmin S, Selim S, Alam M, Khanam A, et al. Single center experience of renal transplantation in Bangladesh with short term use of cyclosporine. Bangladesh Ren J. 2005;24:12.
50. Iqbal M, Islam Z, Salam A, Rashid H. Ipsilateral leg swelling and graft dysfunction-A sequel of post transplant pelvic lymphocele. Bangladesh Ren J. 2000;19:67–71.
51. Islam MS. Evaluation of living related kidney transplant donor: study of 50 donors. Pulse. 2011;5:16–21.
52. Moniruzzaman M. "Living Cadavers" in Bangladesh: ethics of the human organ bazaar. Doctoral dissertation; 2010.

# Nephrology in Cambodia

# 19

Chanseila Hy, Pichthida Thim, Kea Keng, Elin Phon, Vadhana Lim, and Toru Hyodo

| | |
|---|---|
| Area[1] | 181,035 Km$^2$ |
| Population[1] | 15,288,489 (2020) |
| Capital | Phnom Penh – PP |
| Three most populated cities[2] | 1. Phnom Penh – PP<br>2. Takeo – T<br>3. Kampong Saom – PS |
| Official language | Khmer |
| Gross Domestic Product (GDP)[1] | 76,635 billion USD (PPP, 2019)<br>26,628 billion USD (nominal, 2019) |
| GDP per capita[1] | 4645 USD (PPP, 2019)<br>1614 USD (nominal, 2019) |
| Human Development Index (HDI)[1] | 0.581 (146° position, 2018) |
| Official currency | Riel (KHR) |
| Total number of nephrologists | 10 |
| National Society of Nephrology | Cambodian Association of Nephrology<br>http://cambodia-nephrology.org |
| Incidence of end-stage renal disease | 2018 – unknown |
| Prevalence of end-stage renal disease (on dialysis) | 2018 – ~40 pmp |
| Total number of patients on dialysis (all modalities) | 2017 – 407 (Phnom Penh)<br>2018 – 600 (Phnom Penh, Battambang, and Siem Reap) |
| Number of patients on hemodialysis[5] | 2017 – 407 (Phnom Penh)<br>2018 – 600 (Phnom Penh, Battambang, and Siem Reap) |
| Number of patients on peritoneal dialysis | 2017 – 0<br>2018 – 0 |
| Number of renal transplantations per year | 2017 – 0<br>2018 – 0 |

[1]Wikipedia the Free Encyclopedia. Accessed in Mar 2020. Available in: https://en.wikipedia.org/wiki/Cambodia [1]

[2]Cambodia – 10 Largest Cities. Accessed in Mar 2020. Available in; https://www.geonames.org/KH/largest-cities-in-cambodia.html [2]

[5]Pichthida T, Hyodo T, Elin P, Tan S, Kim S, Yim S, Chanseila H, Tith C, Sokhom P, Sochun L, Svay K, Chan S, Vadhana L. Cambodian renal registry 2017 and 2018 (Limited to Phnom Penh). Cambodian J Nephrol. 2019;4:14–21. https://www.cambodia-nephrology.org/ [5]

## Introduction

Cambodia is located in Southeast Asia. It shares borders with Vietnam, Laos, and Thailand. There are 25 provinces. The capital city is Phnom Penh. In 2018, total life expectancy is 69.4 years with male 67.3 and female 71.2. Annual household income per capita is US$ 1376 in 2017. Khmer language is the official language and is spoken by most of the population of Cambodia. Regarding religious practices, 97.9% of the population is Theravada Buddhist, 1.1% Islam, 0.5% Christian, and the majority of the remaining population follows, animism, or atheism [1, 2].

After World War II (1939–1945), there was modernization in the medical system. During the Songkum Reasniyum regime (1953–1970), there was a huge accomplishment in the medical sector since main public hospitals were built. Unfortunately, the medical system disintegrated when the Khmer Rouge came to power, where only natural and herbal medications were used for treatment. The Khmer Rouge was a brutal regime that ruled Cambodia, under the leadership of Marxist dictator Pol Pot, from 1975 to 1979. Nowadays, with a multiparty democracy under a constitutional monarchy, our medical field has been improving gradually. However, it hasn't reached the standard yet due to poverty, corruption, and lack of education. The lack of accurate statistics and surveys makes planning for the development of the healthcare system difficult [1].

## Brief History of Nephrology in Cambodia

Cambodia suffered through a genocidal regime and dozens of years of civil war, leaving the country decimated. During the Pol Pot regime between 1975 and 1979, most of the educated population were killed. All hospitals were closed and the national healthcare system essentially ceased to function. When the regime fell in 1979, the new Cambodian government started to rebuild the country from the scratch. However, development proceeded haltingly, as the civil war continued for another decade until 1998. Fortunately, many

C. Hy · P. Thim · K. Keng · E. Phon · V. Lim
Cambodian Association of Nephrology, Phnom Penh, Cambodia

T. Hyodo (✉)
Cambodian Association of Nephrology, Phnom Penh, Cambodia

NGO Ubiquitous Blood Purification International, Yokohama, Japan



J. A. Moura-Neto et al. (eds.), *Nephrology Worldwide*, https://doi.org/10.1007/978-3-030-56890-0_19

of our public hospitals started being reopened in 1979, but we have had to confront many obstacles along the way, such as a lack or shortage of equipment and healthcare workers. In the field of nephrology, particularly, general practitioners had to manage patients with kidney disease because there were no nephrologists or hemodialysis (HD) facilities until 1997, when the first HD center opened in Calmette Hospital in Phnom Penh. Initially, there were only four machines, which served approximately ten patients. More HD centers were opened as the incidence of end-stage renal disease (ESRD) increased. Now, we have 12 such centers nationwide. According to unofficial (non-governmental) data collected by members of the Cambodian Association of Nephrology (CAN), there are currently about 600 HD patients in Cambodia (500 in Phnom Penh, 50 in Battambang, and 50 in Siem Reap) [3–5].

We have only ten nephrologists working in the country, all of whom trained in developed countries like France, Japan, and China. Supported by the Japanese nongovernmental organization Ubiquitous Blood Purification International (NGO UBPI; President, Hideki Kawanishi, MD), CAN was established in 2016 to rebuild the workforce in nephrology and HD. *The Cambodian Journal of Nephrology* (ISSN 2518-0381), CAN's official journal, was established with support from Reiseikai Media (Cambodia and Japan) Co., Ltd. (CEO, Haruki Wakai, MD) (Fig. 19.1) [6]. The NGO UBPI membership is made up of members from the Japanese Society for Dialysis Therapy (JSDT) and the International Society of Nephrology (ISN), Japanese Society for Technology of Blood Purification (JSTB), Japan Association for Clinical Engineers (JACE), and the Japanese Society of Renal Nutrition and Metabolism (JSRNM). As a result, CAN maintains close relationships with JSDT and ISN, with CAN becoming an Affiliated Society of ISN in 2017. CAN's goal is to improve the quality of care and provide standardized treatments to patients with chronic kidney disease (CKD) in Cambodia through its close relationships with overseas organizations.

Nowadays, although the healthcare system has improved dramatically in terms of both medical equipment and personnel, nephrologists still have limited capabilities – we cannot perform renal biopsy, kidney transplantation (KT), or hemodiafiltration – and the lack of dietitians limits our management of CKD over the long term.

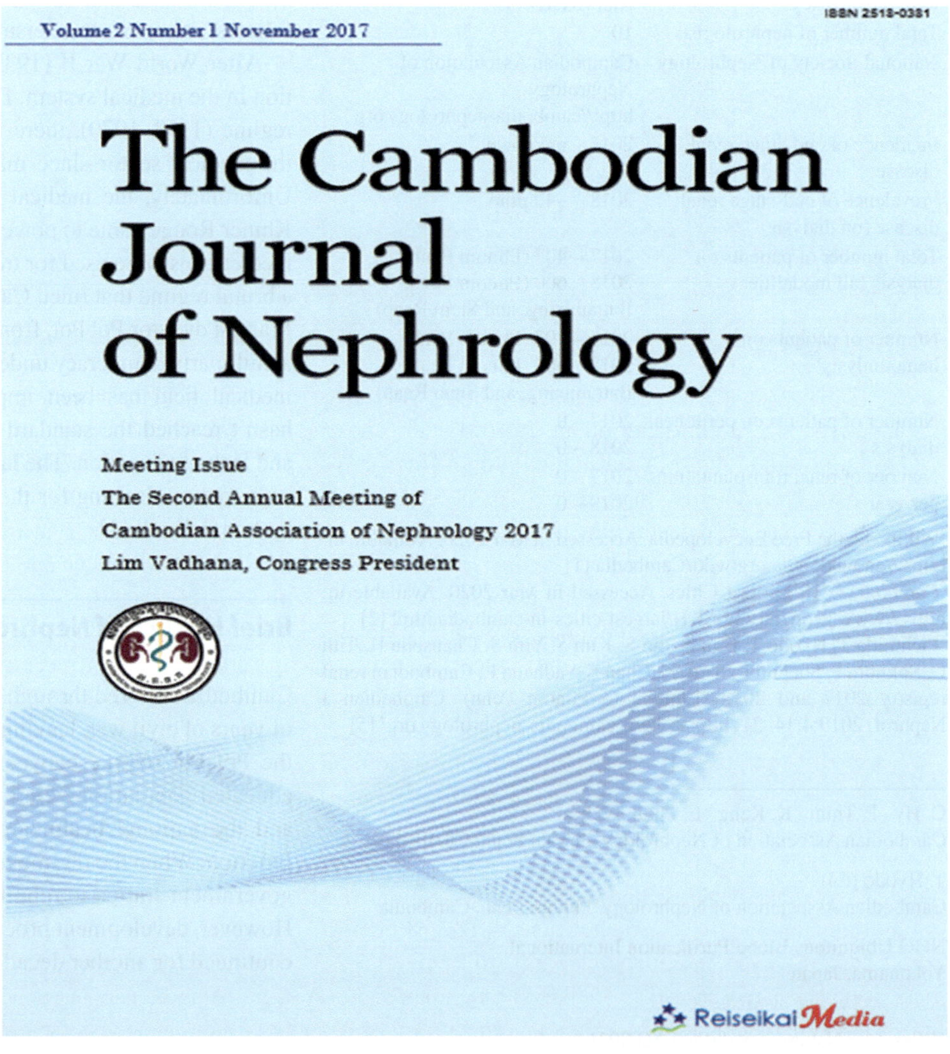


**Fig. 19.1** The Cambodian Association of Nephrology official journal *The Cambodian Journal of Nephrology*. ISSN 2518-0381

## Renal Diseases in Cambodia

### ESRD Epidemiological Study by CAN

Common renal diseases in Cambodia that may lead to ESRD are hypertensive nephropathy, diabetic nephropathy, bilateral renal stones, and glomerulopathies. The true incidence and prevalence of ESRD and HD are not known because we do not have an official governmental system that tracks renal diseases, but estimates suggest that the prevalence may be rising year after year. In 2017, CAN members began collecting unofficial data as part of preparations for an official renal registry. The 2017 data was presented at the Non-Western World Symposium held at the 63rd Annual Meeting of the Japanese Society for Dialysis Therapy (JSDT) [4].

In August 2017 and 2018, in efforts to collect further data, we conducted a cross-sectional study at the six main HD centers in Phnom Penh [5]. We compared the follow-up data from 407 patients in 2017 with data from 499 patients in 2018: age, sex, geographic location, underlying diseases, HD frequency per month, and HD session duration. Data were analyzed using SPSS, with numerical and categorical data given as means, medians, and percentages. Of the patients surveyed, 90.7% in 2017 and 91.0% in 2018 had been receiving HD until the previous year; thus, 9.3% in 2017 and 9.0% in 2018 were new HD patients. In 2017, 55.0% were living in Phnom Penh and 45.0% were living in the provinces; in 2018 the numbers were slightly different, at 57.5% and 42.5%, respectively. Men accounted for 57.2% of the total in 2017 and 51.3% in 2018. Age distribution, HD frequency per month, and underlying diseases are shown in Figs. 19.2, 19.3, and 19.4 [5]. HD duration per session was 4 hours at all HD centers. The peak age distribution was between 51 and 60 years. Mean HD frequency per month was 7.8 ± 2.4 in 2017 and slightly lower at 7.2 ± 2.5 (mean ± SD) in 2018. As for the underlying disease, diabetes mellitus is also as serious as in the advanced countries.

As for the dialysis vintage, we do not have the precise data. However, we can estimate it from the report by Chan Sovandy [7]. The patients' HD histories in four HD centers of Phnom Penh were analyzed. In Calmette Hospital, they have around 150 patients. Ninety (60%) patients have been on HD for more than 10 years, 23 (15%) 7 years, 23 (15%) 5 years, and 15 (10%) less than 1 year. In Preah Ketomela Hospital, they have 60 patients. Six patients (10%) have been on HD more than 10 years, 30 patients (50%) 5–6 years, and 24 patients (40%) less than 1 year. In Preah Kossamak Hospital, they have 40 patients. Twenty-four patients (60%) have been on HD for 3–4 years, 12 (20%) less than 2 years, and 4 patients (10%) less than 6 months. In Sen Sok

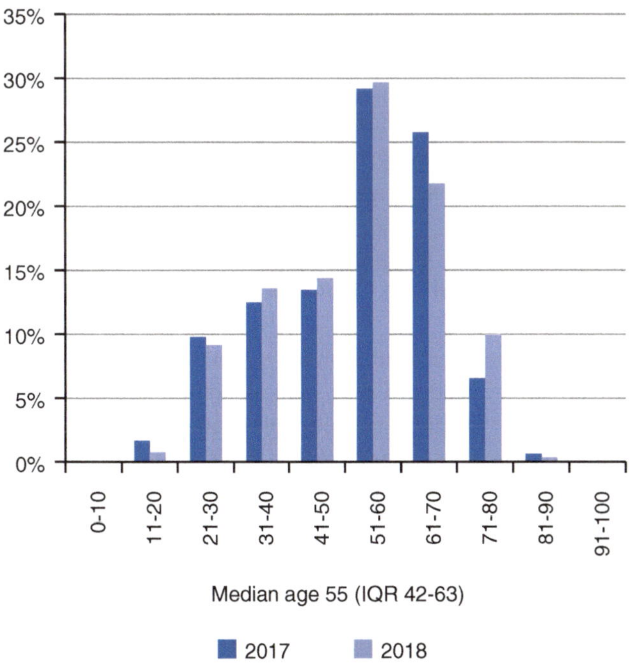


Fig. 19.2 The age distribution of hemodialysis patients in 2017 ($n = 407$) and 2018 ($n = 499$). The peak age distribution was between 51 and 60 years

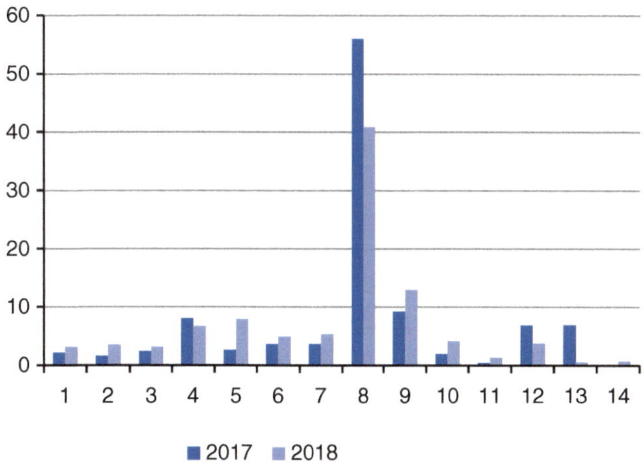


Fig. 19.3 Frequency of hemodialysis per month in 2017 ($n = 407$) and 2018 ($n = 499$). Mean HD frequency per month was 7.8 ± 2.4 in 2017 and slightly lower at 7.2 ± 2.5 (mean ± SD) in 2018

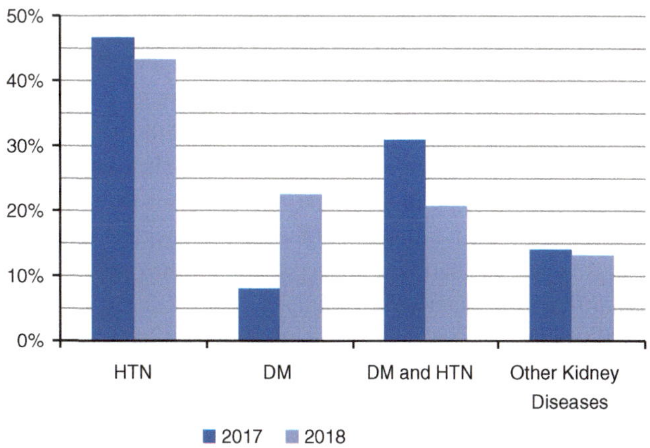


Fig. 19.4 Underlying diseases of hemodialysis patients in 2017 ($n = 407$) and 2018 ($n = 499$). HTN, hypertension; DM, diabetes mellitus; diabetes is also serious as in the advanced countries

International University Hospital, they have eight patients. Three patients have been on HD for 2–5 years.

As for the incidence of hepatitis B, hepatitis C, and HIV population, there are no data even in Calmette Hospital. We did not investigate the percentage of temporary catheters, AV fistula, grafts, or long-term catheter in the surveys of 2017 and 2018. However, we estimate around 98% of HD patients using AV fistula (AVF) for dialysis. Only around 2% of the HD patients use tunnel catheter at first, because AVF are rarely created before dialysis therapy start. The mortality rate could not be surveyed in the above study. However, the annual mortality rate of dialysis patients in Calmette Hospital is around 15% per year.

The results of our study indicate that the prevalence of ESRD and HD is increasing in Cambodia. Among the issues we identified was poor adherence to HD treatment, which needs to be tackled. State and private health insurance subsidies would help with this, and a focus on primary, secondary, and tertiary prevention of hypertension and diabetes mellitus would also be crucial.

## Hypertension

In Cambodia, hypertension is the leading cause of cardiovascular diseases such as myocardial infarction and stroke. Hypertensive patients, especially those with essential hypertension, have been poorly managed with an unattainable targeted blood pressure due to incorrect treatment and follow-up among the general population. Even after doctors explaining the importance of taking medications regularly, patients still think they need to take antihypertensives only when their blood pressure is high (e.g., >160/100 mmHg). Also, many traditional Cambodian foods, which are commonly eaten in rural areas, are very salty, and inevitably renal function deterioration occurs fast.

## Diabetes Mellitus

Maintaining blood sugar or HbA1c at the target level in diabetic patients is quite a challenge for doctors in Cambodia. Patients tend to have a poor understanding of the disease and the importance of their diet in its treatment. They need close monitoring of their blood sugar levels to ensure that they receive adequate treatment, but they tend to neglect to attend follow-ups and maintain dietary therapy. As a result, their renal functions deteriorate rapidly.

Recently, the easy diabetic diet therapy "the basic carbohydrate counting" [8] has become rapidly popular among young doctors and medical students due to the seminars by NGO UBPI since 2015 and the education provided by the Annual CAN Congress [9, 10]. This will certainly result in educational benefit for the Cambodian people of the diabetic diet therapy.

## Glomerulonephritis

Determining the exact cause of glomerulonephritis in Cambodia is a major challenge due to the fact that renal biopsy cannot be performed. This is because we lack not only the equipment for acquiring and staining renal biopsy specimens but also pathologists who can interpret the images. When a renal biopsy is needed, we usually recommend that patients visit a neighboring country like Vietnam or Thailand. If they cannot afford the trip and the cost of hospital care abroad, in practice, we have to decide how to proceed. For patients that we suspect have glomerulonephritis (proteinuria >1 g/24 h, excluding hypertension or diabetic nephropathy), we start them on glucocorticoids (Cortancyl®). Occasionally, we may encounter cases of glomerulonephritis secondary to, for example, disseminated lupus erythematosus or multiple myeloma. When we suspect glomerulonephritis with nephrotic syndrome (proteinuria >3 g/24 h, excluding diabetic nephropathy and hypertensive nephropathy), we normally start patients on methylprednisolone 1 g/day by bolus for 3 days followed by prednisolone 1 mg/kg (body weight)/day. We can normally control proteinuria over 24 h after about 3–4 weeks of treatment. If 24-h proteinuria decreases, we can start to taper the prednisolone over a total treatment duration time of about 6–9 months. But if the amount of proteinuria remains fairly constant or increases, we will switch to one of the immunosuppressive drugs available in Cambodia, namely, such as mycophenolate mofetil (Cellcept®), azathioprine (Imurel®), or cyclophosphamide (Endoxan®).

## Bilateral Renal Stones

In rural areas, people recognize that they might have kidney stones when symptoms such as renal colicky pain appear. Patients sometimes visit a doctor when they have symptoms of obstructive renal failure. The number of cases with bilateral kidney stones progressing to ESRD is estimated to be about 3% of all CKD patients.

## Other Renal Failure Etiologies

We also encounter a substantial amount of different etiologies that may lead to CKD, such as polycystic kidney disease, contrast medium-induced nephropathy, and nonsteroidal anti-inflammatory drug (NSAID) abuse. The data collected by members of CAN about the underlying diseases in HD patients in 2017 and 2018 are shown in Fig. 19.4. Acute kidney injury (AKI) accounts for around 5% of renal diseases and is usually caused by rhabdomyolysis following a traffic accident, methanol intoxication, improper NSAID use, or toxicity after consuming fish gallbladder (we return to describing all causes in detail in the section entitled AKI).

## The Renal Replacement Therapy Setting

### Hemodialysis Protocol

Normally we tell all patients that three sessions per week are needed for adequate HD, but the cost prohibits many patients from receiving this prescription; most patients cannot afford and choose to do only two sessions per week while following a strict diet. Some patients even decide to do only one session per week despite fully understanding the consequences of inadequate dialysis. The standard blood flow rate is 250 mL/min, but we increase this to 280 or 300 mL/min in some patients if their fistula is good. The standard dialysate flow rate is 500 mL/min.

**Standard HD protocol:**

- HD machine: Surdial (Nipro Corp.)
- Dialyzer type: FB170 Tga (diacetate membrane)
- Surface area: 1.7 $m^2$
- Blood flow rate: 250 mL/min
- Standard heparin: loading dose of 3000 IU and midterm dose of 1500 IU of unfractionated heparin
- Dialysate type: bicarbonate
- Dialysate flow rate: 500 mL/min

## Dialysis Access

For patients on long-term dialysis, we prefer a distal radial-cephalic AVF for vascular access. We create a middle-arm radial-cephalic or proximal brachial-cephalic AVF when it is not possible to make a distal radial-cephalic AVF. Central dialysis catheters (CDC) are temporarily placed in patients with AKI or in urgent start chronic dialysis patients with no established vascular access. The preferred central venous sites are the jugular vein and femoral vein. Sometimes, establishing AVF access is a challenge because of diffuse atherosclerosis or AVF failure that cannot be repaired; in such cases, we place a tunneled CDC. An AVF costs around 250 US dollars to create and the cost of a tunneled CDC is around 1000 US dollars. The cost of a normal CDC for temporary use in dialysis is around 100 US dollars.

## Dialyzers and HD Machines

### Dialyzer

The two most commonly used dialyzers in Cambodia are the FB170 Tga and Polyflux. High-flux dialyzers are not available, so to save costs, dialyzer reuse is basically universally practiced. Dialyzers are reused three to five times. The average cost of a dialyzer is 30 US dollars, and patients have an additional fee whenever they change to a new dialyzer. For example, for a normal dialysis session costing 50 US dollars, they will have to pay 80 US dollars to use a new dialyzer. From time to time, dialyzers are manually cleaned and reprocessed by nonmedical staffs. The efficiency of reuse is not appropriately evaluated against standard measurements, with resultant negative effects on dialysis adequacy and outcomes. The formal process is described here below.

### Dialyzer Reprocessing

A dialysis reprocessing system is a medical device that automates the dialyzer cleaning and reprocessing activities in a dialysis center or hospital. The reprocessing procedure involves cleaning, testing, filling the dialyzer with a sterilant (Renalin® Cold Sterilant), inspecting, labeling, storing, and rinsing the dialyzer before it is used for the next renal replacement therapy (RRT) session. The most frequently used dialyzer reprocessing system in Cambodia is the Renatron II 100 series®. Nurses who work at dialysis centers are normally responsible for dialyzer reprocessing.

### HD Machine Console

The HD machine used in most HD centers is a single patient dialysis machine (Nipro Corp.) and the Surdial® console (imported by Dynamic Pharma Co.). Recently, a few HD centers started using a newer HD machine, the 4008s NG® (Fresenius Ltd.).

## Treatment of Anemia

Erythropoietin is commonly used for dialysis patients and patients with long-term renal failure. The following erythropoiesis-stimulating agents (ESA) are available in Cambodia: epoetin alfa (Hemapo® 3000 IU and 10,000 IU), epoetin beta (Recormon® 2000 IU, 4000 IU, and 10,000 IU), darbepoetin alfa (DERISE® 50 μg, 100 μg, and 200 μg), and methoxy polyethylene glycol-epoetin beta (Mircera® 50 μg and 100 μg). For ESA alfa and beta dosages, the loading dose is 50 IU/kg thrice weekly, while the maintenance dose is 75–300 IU/kg once weekly. ESA alfa and beta are the most prescribed ones in Cambodia because they are cheaper than other agents and are easy to find. For our HD patients, we start with 3000 IU twice weekly and monitor hemoglobin 4 weeks later. We increase the dose until reaching the maximum dose (10,000 IU, thrice weekly) until hemoglobin is between 100 and 120 g/L.

Blood iron and ferritin are controlled monthly. In the case of iron deficiency, we add iron orally or intravenously when oral iron intake is not adequate. The brands of intravenous iron currently available in Cambodia are Ferofer® and Venofer®. Unfortunately, because some patients can't afford ESA, they decide to have a transfusion of one or two bags of blood each month. A standard blood bag in Cambodia is 350 mL blood, collected in 49 mL sodium citrate, phosphate-dextrose-adenine (CPDA-1) anticoagulant/preservation

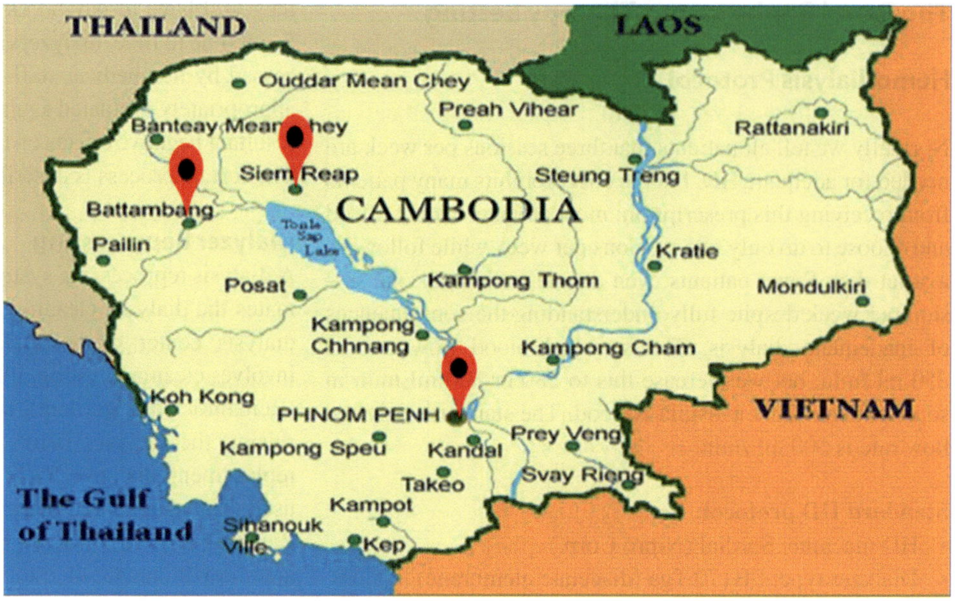

**Fig. 19.5** The location in the country where hemodialysis centers exist. Phnom Penh, Siem Reap, and Battambang

solution. Patients need to find a donor to donate one bag of blood, if they want a transfusion.

## Mineral and Bone Disorders

Like hemoglobin, calcium and phosphorus levels are controlled monthly. Unfortunately, it is difficult to measure parathyroid hormone (PTH) levels. PTH can be measured at any private laboratory, such as the Pasteur Institute of Cambodia (blood samples are sent to France for testing at a cost of around 120 US dollars), Biomed Laboratory, or Paramed Laboratory (samples are sent to a neighboring countries like Vietnam or Thailand). For prevention and treatment of osteitis fibrosa in CKD patients, we usually manage with dietary phosphate restriction and administration of an oral phosphate binder (Sevelamer®) and calcitriol (Rocaltrol®). Calcimimetic agents are not yet available in Cambodia.

## HD Centers

In Cambodia, only HD is available. There were initially only four HD machines when the Chea Sim Center was opened at Calmette Hospital in 1997. In 2007, three HD centers were established; two of them were government dialysis centers at Preah Ket Mealea Hospital and the Health Science Institute Hospital. The latter stopped HD due to lack of funding in 2014. Another center is the La Santé Hemodialysis Center (a private clinic). In 2010, the Cambodia-Japan Friendship Blood Purification Center was established at Sen Sok International University Hospital with support from the NGO UBPI (the secretary general in 2010: Dr. Hideo Hidai). In 2012, the first provincial HD center was opened at Siem Reap Referral Hospital with the support of the Takatsuki Rotary Club in Japan and Dr. Nobuhisa Shibahara of NGO UBPI. Then in 2013, a private center, the Yi Kouk Hemodialysis Center, was established in Battambang province, and another HD center was established in Preah Kossamak Hospital. To date, a few private HD centers have been established, but they do not treat large numbers of patients. There are presently 12 HD centers in three regions only: Phnom Penh, Siem Reap, and Battambang (Fig. 19.5) [11].

## Maintenance HD Systems

The HD machine maintenance system in Cambodia is quite similar among the dialysis centers. Service engineers from the dialysis machine manufacturers come regularly to do a thorough checkup and perform maintenance on the machine every month as follows:

- Check the control panel.
- Test the function of each part of the machine (pump, drain valve, water refill valve, drain ball valve, used ball valve), and then flush and drain out the machine in clean mode.
- Check the function of each machine in clean mode and disinfect mode, and check the spray nozzle rod and clean float sensor.
- Check the bacterial and endotoxin levels in the dialysate, and perform reverse osmosis of the water at the console site every 3 months.
- Sterilize the console and the waterline from the tank every month.

## Peritoneal Dialysis

Recently, we have been able to introduce peritoneal dialysis (PD) in Cambodia. Nephrologists have been trained to perform the procedure, specialized nurses can explain and take care of PD patients, and urologists can implant a peritoneal catheter into the peritoneal cavity. However, most patients seem reluctant to choose PD because it is a complicated procedure and requires a high degree of understanding. Those who do choose PD face problems such as hygienic control and going through the daily dialysate input/output procedure. It is very difficult to find facilities or pharmacies in Cambodia where patients can buy the necessary PD solutions and ancillaries. Therefore, it isn't such a practical method in Cambodia at present. In 2010, one of the authors (TH) asked a PD company to introduce continuous ambulatory peritoneal dialysis (CAPD) to the Cambodian market, but it was impossible because the market was not mature enough and the situation has not changed as of 2019. So, we have no experience on CAPD in Cambodia. Acute PD was applied to only three cases of AKI at the Calmette Hospital, with PD solution donated from an organization.

## Dialysis Reimbursement Policies

CKD and RRT have been a significant financial burden to patients and their families, yet the government has not given it high priority when creating healthcare policies. That is why the cost of RRT continues to be a major issue in Cambodia. Excluding the costs involved with the dialyzer and blood lines, the average cost of HD is 50 US dollars per session. This explains why many patients demand their dialyzer to be reused, at least, 3 or 4 times before changing to a new one. The costs of medicines such as antidiabetic, antihypertensive agents, and ESA are also borne by the patient. If a patient receives HD twice weekly, they have to pay around 800–900 US dollars per month. For the context, the annual household income per capita is estimated to be 1614 US dollars in 2019 [1]. Patients are totally responsible for their treatment costs, which include the additional costs of transportation and accommodation for patients who must travel to the city for treatment from the provinces. This heavy financial burden forces some patients to abandon dialysis therapy and die; others sell their properties, such as their house or piece of land, to pay for treatment; some have to live a lower quality of life because of inadequate dialysis and resulting anemia. This situation is similar to that in Japan before 1972 (the year the Japanese national health insurance system was established and HD patients started receiving HD for free).

## Acute Kidney Injury

AKI, formerly known as acute renal failure, is a syndrome characterized by rapid loss of the kidney's excretory function, and it is typically diagnosed based on accumulation of the end products of nitrogen metabolism (urea and creatinine), decreased urine output, or both. Patients are given RRT if AKI is present with severe biochemical or volume-related disturbances or if other uremia-related complications are of concern. The effects of AKI on in-hospital mortality, length of stay, and healthcare costs have not been well investigated in Cambodia. However, the leading causes of AKI in Cambodia are well established and include fish gallbladder toxicity, rhabdomyolysis following a traffic accident, and NSAID abuse.

### Fish Gallbladder Toxicity

People in rural areas believe that fish gallbladders can cure acne, improve poor vision, lighten the complexion, and are generally good for health. The gallbladders of the freshwater fishes grass carp (*Ctenopharyngodon idellus*) and black sharkminnow (*Morulius chrysophekadion*) are most commonly consumed. After a few days of eating it, the symptoms of AKI appear, and the patients come to the hospital with abdominal pain, repeated vomiting, oliguria, dyspnea, generalized edema, and pulmonary edema. A diagnosis of AKI secondary to fish gallbladder poisoning is made based on history taking and biochemical investigations showing high levels of urea and creatinine in the blood. The main treatment is HD via a CDC inserted in the femoral or jugular vein. Renal function improves and normalizes over a period of 5 weeks. We always ask the patients to explain the risk of fish gallbladder toxicity to their communities when they leave the hospital. The Cambodian Ministry of Health has developed a health education program to educate people in rural areas about the dangers of this toxicity, but the information has not yet been widely disseminated [12].

### Rhabdomyolysis Following a Traffic Accident

Traffic accidents continue to be a problem in Cambodia. People ride or drive carelessly and mostly do not respect the traffic laws. This means that the number of traffic accidents remains very high, so high that they are a leading cause of death. Sometimes muscle injuries sustained in traffic accidents cause rhabdomyolysis-induced AKI. Rhabdomyolysis, a clinical syndrome caused by damage to skeletal muscle and the release of its breakdown products into the blood, can be followed by renal dysfunction in the form of AKI as a severe complication. The clinical symptoms of rhabdomyolysis are myalgia and weakness and swelling of the damaged muscles, which is usually associated with myoglobinuria. When we see patients with multiple muscle injuries sustained in a traffic accident, we diagnose rhabdomyolysis-induced AKI when patients have any symptoms of rhabdomyolysis and oligo-anuria or generalized edema, elevated blood urea and creatinine, and extremely high creatine phosphokinase in the blood. In the case of preserved diuresis, we start with conservative management usually involving massive hydration with crystalloid solution, mannitol administration, urine alkalization, and forced diuresis. The initiation of RRT is decided based on the status of renal impairment and complications such as life-threatening hyperkalemia, hypercalcemia, hyperazotemia, anuria, or significant fluid overload with no response to diuretic therapy. Vascular access for temporary dialysis is a CDC inserted in the femoral or jugular vein. After RRT, renal function usually improves in 3–4 weeks.

### Improper Use of NSAIDs

Due to inadequate public healthcare services and low income, people tend to buy medicines from the pharmacy when they get sick rather than visit a doctor. They often buy painkillers (paracetamol and *NSAIDs*) and steroids. When not prescribed by a doctor, NSAIDs are often taken improperly, leading to serious complications such as gastric hemorrhage and AKI (due to elevated creatinine levels). Fortunately, the improper use of NSAIDs rarely causes severe AKI and need of HD. In these cases, we advise patients to stop taking the NSAIDs and follow them up regularly, monitoring their blood creatinine levels and explaining to them the possible complications of NSAIDs and kidney diseases. There have also been some cases of AKI caused by snake bites or wasp stings.

## Critical Care in Nephrology

When life-threatening complications of renal failure occur, such as severe pulmonary edema, severe metabolic disorders (metabolic acidosis), hyperkalemia with EKG changes, and uremic syndrome with loss of consciousness, we normally admit patients to the intensive care unit (ICU). Generally, when HD is needed, a doctor in the ICU places the CDC, and ICU staff then perform HD following the advice of a nephrologist. We do this routinely in all of the major hospitals in the city. When the patients improve, we transfer them to a general medicine ward or nephrology ward for follow-up. After receiving critical care, they will need to start dialysis at an HD center nearby or at the hospital. For patients with ESRD who need long-term RRT, we explain about the need to create an AVF, and we set up their schedules with the HD center.

### CDC Infections

A CDC is normally used for 3–4 weeks before we remove it. Sometimes, we might remove it earlier, especially when there are signs and symptoms of a catheter infection (redness, pain, or swelling at or near the catheter site, pain or tenderness along the path of the catheter, or drainage from the skin around the catheter) in order to avoid severe sepsis and septic shock, as well as malfunctioning CDC, or when it causes too much pain. Lack of hygiene is a major cause of CDC-related infection.

## Pediatric Nephrology

In Cambodia, pediatric nephrology is underdeveloped; prevalence and incidence of pediatric renal disease are not known. There are no pediatric nephrologists practicing in the country. Diseases that are commonly observed in this population are urinary tract infection, nephrotic syndrome, acute glomerulonephritis, lupus nephritis, polycystic kidney disease, vesicoureteral reflux, and neurogenic bladder. We also encounter cases of AKI caused by snake bites, wasp stings, and most commonly severe sepsis that result in multiple organ failure. Some investigative procedures such as KUB (kidneys, ureters, and bladder) ultrasound, intravenous pyelogram, and voiding cysto-ureterogram are available. Renal biopsy and renal pathology are not available. Recently, intermittent PD was performed successfully in two pediatric cases of AKI caused by snake bite and wasp sting at a children's hospital, Angkor Hospital for Children, in Siem Reap. Because PD solution cannot be imported, ICU doctors prepared the PD solution themselves. HD and KT are not performed for children in Cambodia, and therefore children with ESRD only receive conservative therapy.

## Kidney Transplantation

This treatment modality is not available in Cambodia. Patients who need a KT have to travel to a neighboring country where it is undertaken with living donors. In our experience, most patients go to India because the procedure is widely available and is affordable compared with other countries in the region. According to patients who underwent KT in India, the procedure costs around 40,000 US dollars. To develop this treatment modality in Cambodia, we need to overcome several major challenges. These include the lack of specialized personnel in KT (both a urologist for the operation and a nephrologist for posttransplantation follow-up), the lack of qualified laboratories that can run essential tests (e.g., checking the trough levels for immunosuppressive drugs), the lack of important training in renal biopsy (we do not have any pathologists who can assess renal biopsy specimens), and inadequate laws regarding transplantation. Recently, nephrologists and urologists met to discuss how to introduce KT in Cambodia with the help of specialists from France. The journey will be long, but the first steps have been taken. A law to regulate organ transplantation was recently proposed, and it is hoped that KT will soon become available in Cambodia.

## Highlights of Nephrology in Cambodia

The practice of nephrology in Cambodia is quite complicated. There are many issues that must be addressed.

### Human Resource Problems

The quality of doctors who treat CKD patients depends on their knowledge and work location. For example, in rural areas (i.e., in provinces far from the cities), there are no nephrologists, it is difficult to find trusted laboratories, and local doctors often have limited knowledge of nephrology. Many patients come to general hospitals with ESRD and its complications (pulmonary edema, metabolic acidosis, hyperkalemia, or severe anemia). In addition to HD, the development of other nephrological procedures is still proceeding haltingly. Increasing numbers of patients are reaching ESRD without a biopsy-proven diagnosis as renal biopsy remains unavailable. This is mainly due to the lack of pathologists to assess the biopsy specimens. Also, there are not enough nephrologists in the country to manage the large number of CKD patients. There are only 11 qualified nephrologists in the country and all work in the capital. One or two new nephrologists graduate each year, but this is too few to address the shortage. Generally, the nurses working at HD centers have attended some short training courses on HD and how to operate the HD machines, but only one or two specialized nurses are employed at each center. There are no dietitians, nurses, or doctors responsible for explaining dialysis diets to patients.

### General Population's Knowledge

The knowledge gap between healthcare personnel and the general population is sometimes marked. Some patients do not sufficiently understand their doctors' explanations and have difficulty grasping the step-by-step plan for managing their health. In rural areas, people often choose traditional treatments first, when they have mild symptoms like edema. As a result, they often come to the hospital at a very late stage (of when they are already at the terminal stage of renal failure), and there is no option but dialysis. An intensive public health campaign, especially targeting those living far from the city, could help to address this issue.

### Financial Burden

A number of procedures need to be developed in our country to improve quality of care and for effective diagnostic workups and treatments. However, such services are expensive, and because Cambodia remains a lower-middle-income country and because patients must pay for healthcare services themselves, medical care is unaffordable for most of the population. To move forward, proper business plans must be created before investment in advanced medical equipment can take place. Most Cambodians do not purchase health insurance, so healthcare expenses are generally paid out of pocket. In case of chronic diseases such as CKD that require long-term dialysis, this can be often catastrophic and impoverishing.

### Availability of Dialysis

All 12 HD centers in Cambodia are in big cities like Battambang, Siem Reap, and Phnom Penh. HD patients who do not live near these cities have to regularly travel long distances (sometimes 200–300 km) for HD, which imposes a heavy burden on them. The location of all HD centers in Cambodia is shown in Fig. 19.5.

## Nephrology Practice and the Job Market

In Cambodia, nephrology practice is focused on HD therapy. Other kidney diseases are usually managed by nephrologists, generalists, or other specialists. In fact, some doctors working at HD centers are actually generalists. This is a result of the lack of a standard policy for HD centers and means that the efficacy of treatment in nephrology is not well standardized. As for the dialysis facility setting, there are no psychologist, social workers, renal dietitians, and dialysis clinical engineers in Cambodia. And we have no national rules for the setting.

Nurses providing dialysis nursing care do not have specialist training in HD. HD centers hire nurses based on their nursing experience. The average salary depends on whether the position is part-time or full-time and is around 300–400 US dollars per month for working full-time at a HD center. The number of nurses at each center depends on the number of dialysis machines in use. As for the average salary for nephrologists in Cambodia, it is around 500–800 US$ per month.

## Certificated Nephrologists in Cambodia

There is no official process to train nephrologist in Cambodia. The doctor who went to study nephrology in France is recognized as a nephrologist. Currently, there are ten doctors who went to study nephrology in France.

Here is a brief process to become a recognized nephrologist in Cambodia: First you need to get medical certificate (study in medical university from year 1 to year 6). After finishing year 6, students need to pass a competition exam to start a specialist training to become a nephrologist. Total years of specialist training is 4 years. The first 2 years are to be spent in internal medicine, and then, two additional years in nephrology. During the final year, the training must be in France through cooperation between medical university in Cambodia and medical university in France. When they come back, they become recognized as nephrologist in Cambodia.

## The Nursing Care System at Chea Sim Hemodialysis Center at Calmette Hospital

The center has 26 machines and 13 nurses that serve around 150 patients each month. The center offers a morning session starting from 7 am and an afternoon session starting from 12 pm. Two nurses are on call for 24 h every 4 days. When not on call, they either work the morning session or the afternoon session. One nurse is responsible for three patients at a time, and there are three stages in HD-related patient care as follows:

- Stage 1: Before starting HD, nurses check the patient's name on the schedule and complete documentation including the patient's name, date of dialysis, dry weight, weight gain, fluid to be removed, type of dialysate solution (acetate or bicarbonate), and type of dialyzer. We reuse a dialyzer 3–4 times and blood lines 4–5 times. We do not reuse syringes and fistula needles. The nurses must always verify that the dialyzer and blood lines attached to the machine are matched to the correct patient before initiating dialysis. We store the reuse equipment with formaldehyde solution 40% in a small tank which has the name of the patient on it. Finally, nurses rinse the dialyzer and blood lines which we store with formaldehyde solution with 1 liter of normal saline. The process of rinsing dialyzer and blood line takes about 15 minutes to ensure that all the parts are safe for use before they connect to the patient. The nurses prepare the syringes, needles, and antiseptic solutions ready for needling into the AVF.
- Stage 2: During dialysis, the patient's vital signs are constantly monitored. Nurses monitor the machine, keep an eye out for patient movements that could affect the functioning of the dialysis machine, and make sure that the patient is comfortable. The most frequent complications during dialysis are hypotension and hypoglycemia. From time to time, severe complications occur, such as hemorrhage, stroke, and cardiac arrest. In such cases, we stop the dialysis immediately and transfer the patient to the emergency ward.
- Stage 3: A routine session takes 4 hours. When dialysis finishes, the nurse infuses all blood back into the patient's circulation and measures their vital signs and consciousness before letting them leave the bed. Finally, the patient's post-dialysis weights are recorded, and the equipment is collected from the machine and cleaned.

## Cambodian Association of Nephrology

As the demand for dialysis grows with the number of ESRD patients increasing, more than 10 HD centers have been opened to serve the 600 or so HD patients around the country. The Cambodian Association of Nephrology (CAN) was established in 2016 to train the next generation of nephrologists, nurses, and doctors who will work in the fields of nephrology and HD.

### The Association's Goals

- Provide better care for patients with kidney diseases and on dialysis by training doctors and nurses who will work in the fields of nephrology and dialysis. Such training has been conducted at the annual meeting since CAN was established.
- Raise awareness about ESRD and dialysis. In Cambodia, especially in rural areas, doctors' knowledge of CKD remains limited. A program is being planned to educate Cambodian doctors about nephrology and the symptoms of renal diseases.
- Find solutions to lower the cost of dialysis. Around 80% of patients can barely afford HD and the medicines they need to take.
- Establish an exchange program with developed countries to improve the knowledge of Cambodian doctors.

### Recent CAN Activities

- CAN held its first annual meeting in 2016. The principal topics at each annual meeting are CKD management and HD procedures. CAN works closely with a team made of JSDT, JSTB, JSCE, JSRNM, and NGO UBPI members with one or two of their representatives attending and giv-

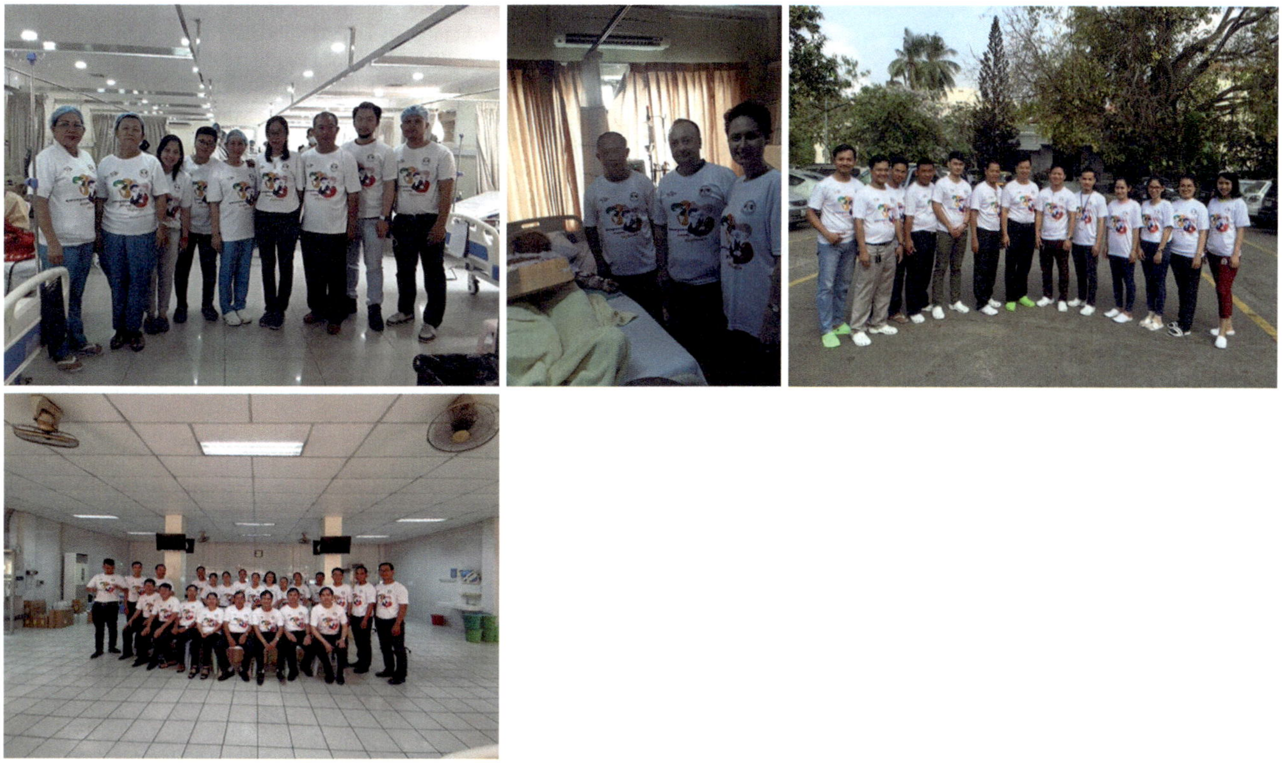

**Fig. 19.6** World Kidney Day events in Cambodia 2019

ing the lectures in our annual CAN meetings. JSDT establishes the Human Resource Development Program Committee for Dialysis Specialists in Developing Countries and since 2016 has accepted several young doctors and students from CAN and Cambodian medical colleges for short-term dialysis and CKD training courses (around 8 days). Speakers from other countries such as Vietnam, Germany, and France have also attended our annual meetings. The goal of the meetings is for experienced nephrologists to provide new information to Cambodian healthcare professionals working in nephrology.

- CAN officially became an affiliate of the International Society of Nephrology in June 2017.
- The preparation for renal transplantation has begun at Calmette Hospital with assistance of French nephrologists.
- CAN began holding "World Kidney Day" events in 2018. Figure 19.6 shows "World Kidney Day 2019" events in Cambodia.
- CAN established its own official journal, *The Cambodian Journal of Nephrology* (ISSN 2518-0381), in conjunction with Reiseikai Media (Cambodia) Co., Ltd. (Fig. 19.1).

## The Future of Nephrology in Cambodia

As mentioned above, nephrology practice in Cambodia lags behind that of neighboring countries. To overcome this, we focus our efforts on achieving our goals. CAN was established not only to train the next generation of Cambodian nephrologists but also to share experiences and information and to promote nephrology through annual meetings, journal articles, and collaboration with international organizations (ISN and APSN). To provide effective medical care to patients, it is clear that new procedures are required. Our nephrologists need opportunities to train in developed countries to further hone their skills. Some nephrologists have already trained in France, Australia, Japan, and Thailand, but this just scratches the surface. Recently, a team of nephrologists from France came to help our nephrologists develop procedures for KT. We hope that this medical procedure will become available in Cambodia in the near future. CAN's next aim is to secure funding to lower the cost of dialysis and to organize educational programs for doctors practicing in rural areas (i.e., to teach them about renal symptoms that are cause for concern) and to raise public awareness of kidney diseases.

## Conclusion

Innovative improvements in dialysis practice are being made to optimize outcomes in Cambodia. In the aftermath of the Khmer Rouge genocide and years of civil war, Cambodia has made many efforts to rebuild and develop the healthcare sector. These efforts have brought us the current healthcare system, which still has many challenges and obstacles to overcome but is making progress toward providing universal and adequate nephrology care to all patients in need. Nevertheless, outcomes would be improved substantially by having more well-trained personnel and more opportunities for better follow-up.

## References

1. Wikipedia the Free Encyclopedia. Accessed in Mar 2020. Available in: https://en.wikipedia.org/wiki/Cambodia.
2. Cambodia – 10 largest cities. Accessed in Mar 2020. Available in; https://www.geonames.org/KH/largest-cities-in-cambodia.html.
3. Kanitha S. Cambodia country status. Blood Purif. 2017;44(Suppl 1):5–6.
4. Pichthida T, Elin P, Chanseila H, Sovandy C. The history and current status of hemodialysis in Cambodia: from registry 2017. J Jpn Soc Dial Ther. 2018;51(Suppl 1):413.
5. Pichthida T, Hyodo T, Elin P, Tan S, Kim S, Yim S, Chanseila H, Tith C, Sokhom P, Sochun L, Svay K, Chan S, Vadhana L. Cambodian renal registry 2017 and 2018 (Limited to Phnom Penh). Cambodian J Nephrol. 2019;4:14–21. https://www.cambodia-nephrology.org/.
6. Website of the Cambodian Association of Nephrology. https://www.cambodia-nephrology.org/
7. Sovandy C. Long term hemodialysis in Cambodia. Cambodian J Nephrol. 2019;4:7. https://www.cambodia-nephrology.org/.
8. Kitajima Y, Mikami N, Hyodo T, Hida M, Kawakami J. Carbohydrate counting: a simple method of dietary management for glycemic control in Japanese diabetic hemodialysis patients. Contrib Nephrol. Basel, Karger. 2017;189:262–9.
9. Hyodo T. A simple method of dietary management for glycemic control in diabetic hemodialysis patients: the usefulness of basic carbohydrate counting. Cambodian J Nephrol. 2015;1:10. https://www.cambodia-nephrology.org/.
10. Hyodo T, Kitajima Y. Basic carbohydrate counting for glycemic control in diabetic hemodialysis patients. Cambodian J Nephrol. 2017;2:18–29. https://www.cambodia-nephrology.org/.
11. Google Map of Cambodia.
12. Kanitha S. Acute kidney injury due to fish gallbladder ingestion: a case report from Cambodia. Blood Purif. 2017;44(suppl 1):22–5.

# Nephrology in China

# 20

Angela Yee-Moon Wang, Yu An, Guang-Yan Cai, Jiang-Hua Chen, Wei Chen, Xiang-Mei Chen, Zhao Cui, Chuan-Ming Hao, Fan-Fan Hou, Bi-Cheng Liu, Zhi-Hong Liu, Qing-Yu Niu, Qi-Quan Sun, Ren-Ding Wang, Damin Xu, Chao Yang, Li Yang, Luxia Zhang, Ming-Hui Zhao, Li Zuo, and Xue-Qing Yu

| | |
|---|---|
| Area | 9,597,000 km$^2$ |
| Population | 1.428 billion (2018) |
| Capital | Beijing |
| Three most populated cities | 1. Guangzhou<br>2. Shanghai<br>3. Chongqing |
| Official language | Chinese[‡‡] |
| Gross Domestic Product (GDP) | 99,086.5 billion RMB (2019); represent 21.95% of the world economy[‡] |
| GDP per capita | 70,892 RMB (2019) |
| Human Development Index | 0.758 (2018) |
| Official currency | Renminbi (RMB) |
| Total number of nephrologists | ~15,000 |
| National Society of Nephrology | Chinese Society of Nephrology<br>www.csnchina.org |
| Incidence of kidney failure[1] | 2015 – 122.19 pmp (age-adjusted) |
| Prevalence of kidney failure[1] (on dialysis) | 2015 – 402.18 pmp on HD, 39.95 pmp on PD (data in 2015) |
| Total number of patients on dialysis[2] (all modalities) | 2017 – 610,811 |
| Number of patients on hemodialysis[2] | 2017 – 524,467 |
| Number of patients on peritoneal dialysis[2] | 2017 – 86,344<br>2018 – 99,145 (20% of total dialysis population) |
| Number of renal transplantations per year | 7087 per year (between 2008 and 2018) |

[1]Wang F, Yang C, Long J, Zhao X, Tang W, Zhang D, et al. Executive summary for the 2015 Annual Data Report of the China Kidney Disease Network (CK-NET). Kidney Int. 2019;95(3):501–5
[2]Data from Chinese National Renal Data Registry
[‡]Sources: National Bureau of Statistics of People's Republic of China. http://www.stats.gov.cn/tjsj/zxfb/202002/t20200228_1728913.html

A. Y.-M. Wang (✉)
Department of Medicine, Queen Mary Hospital, The University of Hong Kong, Hong Kong Special Administrative Region, China
e-mail: angela_wang@connect.hku.hk

Y. An · Z.-H. Liu
National Clinical Research Center of Kidney Diseases, Jinling Hospital, Nanjing University School of Medicine, Nanjing, China

G.-Y. Cai · X.-M. Chen
Department of Nephrology, Chinese PLA General Hospital, State Key Laboratory of Kidney Diseases, National Clinical Research Center for Kidney Diseases, Beijing, China

J.-H. Chen · R.-D. Wang
Kidney Disease Center, The First Affiliated Hospital, College of Medicine, Zhejiang University, Hangzhou, China

National Key Clinical Department of Kidney Diseases, Institute of Nephrology, Zhejiang University, Hangzhou, China

W. Chen · X.-Q. Yu
Department of Nephrology, The First Affiliated Hospital, Sun Yat-sen University, Guangzhou, Guangdong, China

Key Laboratory of Nephrology, National Health Commission and Guangdong Province, Guangzhou, Guangdong, China

Z. Cui · D. Xu · C. Yang · L. Yang
Renal Division, Peking University First Hospital, Beijing, China

C.-M. Hao
Huashan Hospital Fudan University, Shanghai, China

F.-F. Hou
Division of Nephrology, Nanfang Hospital, Southern Medical University, State Key Laboratory of Organ Failure Research, National Clinical Research Center for Kidney Disease, Guangzhou, China

B.-C. Liu
Institute of Nephrology, Zhong Da Hospital, Southeast University School of Medicine, Nanjing, China

Q.-Y. Niu · L. Zuo
Department of Nephrology, Peking University People's Hospital, Beijing, China

Q.-Q. Sun
Third Affiliated Hospital of Sun Yat-sen University, Guangzhou, China

L. Zhang
Renal Division, Peking University First Hospital, Beijing, China

National Institute of Health Data Science at Peking University, Beijing, China

M.-H. Zhao
Renal Division, Peking University First Hospital, Beijing, China

Peking Tsinghua Center for Life Sciences, Beijing, China


J. A. Moura-Neto et al. (eds.), *Nephrology Worldwide*, https://doi.org/10.1007/978-3-030-56890-0_20

## Introduction

People's Republic of China (PRC) is a big country with an area of 9.6 million $km^2$ and over 1.4 billion population. It has 34 provincial-level administrative units: 23 provinces, 4 municipalities (Beijing, Tianjin, Shanghai, Chongqing), 5 autonomous regions (Guangxi, Inner Mongolia, Tibet, Ningxia, Xinjiang), and 2 special administrative regions (Hong Kong, Macau) with a total of 686 cities (Fig. 20.1). To the Han Chinese population, the territory of the country is defined by the regions of Tibet, Inner Mongolia, and Manchuria and the Xinjiang Province which is the most western land of China. China is the fourth largest country in the world after the United States of America, Russia, and Canada. China has great physical diversity. The eastern plains and southern coasts of the country consist of fertile lowlands and foothills and represent most of China's agricultural output and human population. The southern areas of the country (South of the Yangtze River) consist of hilly and mountainous terrain. The west and north of the country are dominated by sunken basins, rolling plateaus, and towering massifs and contain part of the highest tableland on earth, the Tibetan Plateau, and have much lower agricultural potential and population.

The people of China have gradually moved from rural farming areas to business-centered cities. The annual rate of increase in urbanization from 2015 to 2018 was 2.42%. Currently, China has an urban population of 59.3%. The most populated urban areas are Shanghai 25.582 million, Tianjin 13.215 million, Guangdong 12.683 million, Beijing (capital) 19.618 million, Shenzhen 11.908 million, and Chongqing 14.838 million. The life expectancy for the total population stands at 75.7 years in 2016 with men averaged out at 73.6 years and women 78 years [1].

The Chinese Mainland has a three-tiered system for healthcare delivery that remains today, consisting of large hospitals (first tier), intermediary hospitals (second tier), and community-based services/facilities (third tier). The public health sector is the main healthcare provider. In 2017, 82% of inpatient care was provided by public hospitals [2].

The central government is responsible for overall national health legislation, policy, and administration and is guided by the working principle of universal health coverage. However, benefits remain low, and quality and extent of care and coverage vary widely. Co-pays are often very high, certain drugs are excluded from coverage, and out-of-pocket expenses are insufficiently reimbursed. The out-of-pocket cost issue is the most pressing, especially in rural areas. In 2013, out-of-pocket spending per capita accounted approximately 34% of total healthcare expenditures [3].

The 2009 reform (the 12th 5-year plan) of the Chinese government was set out to establish a more affordable system to supply essential drugs for all levels of medical facilities and achieve national comprehensive universal health insurance coverage by 2020, by shifting resources into primary care. It included measures to strengthen a nationwide network of community health clinics and also train primary care physicians in order to divert resources away from the expensive acute hospital system. A key initiative involved the development of "medical alliances" which consists of group of hospitals including a tertiary hospital and primary care facilities that work together in a more coordinated fashion. It was hoped that this type of care coordination would meet the demand for chronic disease care and help to better contain rising costs and improve healthcare quality [4, 5].

In 2014, the Chinese Mainland spent approximately 5.6% of its gross domestic product (GDP) (3531 billion Renminbi) on healthcare, lower than most developed nations in the Organization for Economic Cooperation and Development (OECD), with 30% funded by central government and local government and 38% by publicly financed health insurance, private health insurance, or social health donations [4]. In 2018, the total healthcare expenditure was around 6.39% of its GDP (data from Bloomberg 2019 Nov). Trends in total healthcare expenditure by the government and social health insurance system showed bigger increases than out-of-pocket payments between 2000 and 2017 [5]. The Chinese Mainland has three main basic health insurance schemes – rural and urban resident-based health insurance, which are funded mainly by government subsidies (about 70% of the total funds), and employee-based health insurance funded by employer and employee contributions. Publicly financed insurance consisted of urban employment-based basic medical insurance launched in 1988, urban resident basic medical insurance launched in 2009 (which provides coverage for urban residents without formal employment), and the new cooperative medical scheme for rural residents launched in 2003 which covered more than 90% of all rural residents in 2010. A brief overview of the three main insurance schemes is outlined in Table 20.1 [6].

The health system reform in the Chinese Mainland in the past decade covered five main areas: social health security, essential medicines, primary healthcare, basic public health service package, and public hospitals. The reform policies were designed to tackle access to healthcare and financial protection. Some key progress made in health reform policies included the following: (a) 95% of the population covered by the social health insurance schemes by the end of 2017; (b) catastrophic illness insurance systems were established in all provinces; (c) the Chinese government has invested ¥ 965 billion in primary

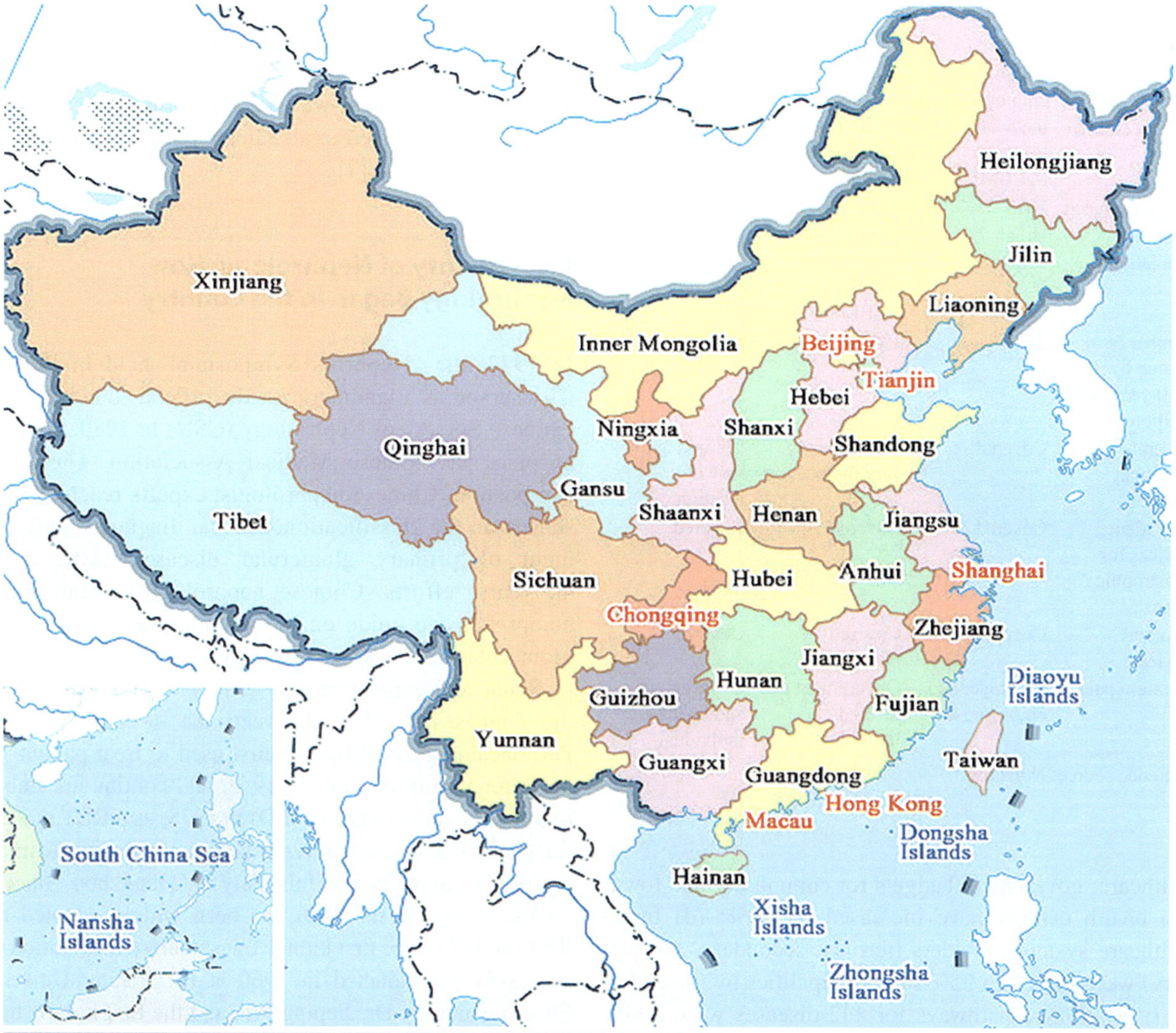


| Provinces (省) | | | | | Claimed Province |
|---|---|---|---|---|---|
| • Anhui (安徽省)<br>• Fujian (福建省)<br>• Gansu (甘肃省)<br>• Guangdong (广东省)<br>• Guizhou (贵州省) | • Hainan (海南省)<br>• Hebei (河北省)<br>• Heilongjiang (黑龙江省)<br>• Henan (河南省)<br>• Hubei (湖北省) | • Hunan (湖南省)<br>• Jiangsu (江苏省)<br>• Jiangxi (江西省)<br>• Jilin (吉林省)<br>• Liaoning (辽宁省) | • Qinghai (青海省)<br>• Shaanxi (陕西省)<br>• Shandong (山东省)<br>• Shanxi (山西省)<br>• Sichuan (四川省) | • Yunnan (云南省)<br>• Zhejiang (浙江省) | • *Taiwan* (台湾省) *governed by R.O.China* |

| Autonomous regions (自治区) | Municipalities (直辖市) | Special administrative regions (特别行政区) |
|---|---|---|
| • Guangxi (广西壮族自治区)<br>• Inner Mongolia / *Nei Menggu* (内蒙古自治区)<br>• Ningxia (宁夏回族自治区)<br>• Xinjiang (新疆维吾尔自治区)<br>• Tibet / *Xizang* (西藏自治区) | • Beijing (北京市)<br>• Chongqing (重庆市)<br>• Shanghai (上海市)<br>• Tianjin (天津市) | • Hong Kong / *Xianggang* (香港特别行政区)<br>• Macau / *Aomen* (澳门特别行政区) |

**Fig. 20.1** Map of China, provinces, municipalities, special administrative regions, and autonomous regions

**Table 20.1** An overview of major health insurance schemes in the Chinese Mainland

| | Urban employee basic medical insurance (UEBMI) | Urban resident basic medical insurance | New rural cooperative medical insurance |
|---|---|---|---|
| Year introduced | 1998 | 2007 | 2003 |
| Insured population | Urban employees | Urban residents who are not covered by UEBMI | Rural residents |
| Number of insured by 2010 year-end (million) | 237 | 195 | 836 |
| General outpatient services | Covered | Limited and vary by location | Limited and vary by location |
| Outpatient services for catastrophic illnesses | Covered | Covered | Covered |
| Inpatient services | Covered | Covered | Covered |
| Premium paid by | Employer and employee | Government and insured individual | Government and insured individual |

Reference source: Nofri [6]

healthcare; government budgets for community and township health centers have increased by 20%; (d) tiered healthcare system providers (tertiary, secondary, and primary) were started in 95% of municipalities by the end of 2017; (e) clinical pathways for 442 diseases were developed by the end of 2015 and 65% of secondary and tertiary hospitals implemented case-based payment reform by the end of 2017; (f) pricing policies also improved with removal of price mark-ups of drugs as a source of finance for public hospitals or primary healthcare providers; and (g) integration of rural and urban basic health insurance systems is also currently underway [5].

In 2016, Mr. Xi released the country's first long-term blueprint to improve healthcare since the nation's founding in 1949, called Healthy China 2030, which pledged to bolster health innovation and make access to medical care more equal and achieve health targets aligned with the United Nation's sustainable development goals. Healthy China 2030 was built on four core principles, namely, health priority, innovation, scientific development, and justice and equity (Fig. 20.2). The blueprint emphasized the importance of both prevention and cure, focusing on prevention and control, Chinese and Western medicine, and changes in service mode to reduce gaps in basic health services. The rural areas of the country are given special attention to promote equal access to basic public health services and to maintain public welfare. Furthermore, healthcare is prioritized and placed in a strategic position in public policy implementation [7].

## Brief History of Nephrology: How Nephrology Began in the Country

In 1977, the "Nephritis Symposium" held in Beidaihe City served as a landmark for the official founding of the Chinese Society of Nephrology (CSN) in 1980, under the auspices of Chinese Medical Association. During the symposium, Chinese nephrologist experts reached a consensus on the classification, clinical diagnosis, and treatment of primary glomerular diseases. After nearly 40 years' efforts, Chinese nephrologists established a comprehensive guide on the diagnosis and treatment of glomerular diseases.

Renal replacement therapy (RRT) was first available in the Chinese Mainland between the 1960s and 1970s. Peritoneal dialysis (PD) was first used to treat patient with acute renal failure (AKI) in 1963, and continuous ambulatory peritoneal dialysis (CAPD) in 1978, as a RRT modality for patients with chronic renal failure at the First Affiliated Hospital of Sun Yat-sen University in Guangzhou. Since the 1970s, hemodialysis (HD) has been widely adopted as a RRT modality. The first kidney transplantation operation was successfully conducted in 1960 at the Peking University First Hospital by Dr. Jieping Wu, and the first kidney transplantation with long-term patient survival was done by Dr. Huamei of the First Affiliated Hospital of Sun Yat-sen University and Dr. Huijuan Yu of Beijing Friendship Hospital in 1972 in Guangzhou.

Over the years, CSN working in close partnerships with the Chinese government has made significant progress in improving the standard and quality of the healthcare system and care delivery models for patients with kidney disease in the Chinese Mainland. At the same time, CSN has provided continuous medical education for health professionals and nephrology specialist training. CSN launched the National Dialysis Registry in 1999 with the first electronic registry established in 2009. A total of 14,000 HD patients and 6000 PD patients' data has been captured in the registry since 2009. CSN has been working closely with the Chinese government to update the Dialysis Registry. In 2010, the Chinese National Renal Data System (CNRDS) was launched [8]. There is also significant development and progress made in

| 13 Core Indicators under 5 health themes | | | | |
|---|---|---|---|---|
| Health level | Healthy life | Health services and security | Environmental health | Health industry |
| 1. Average life expectancy | 1. Number of people doing physical exercise | 1. Proportion of personal health spending in the total health expenditure | 1. Rate of good air quality of all cities at prefecture level or above | 1. Total investment scale of health services |
| 2. Mortality rate of infants | 2. Level of health literacy among residents | 2. Number of registered doctors and registered nurses per 1000 residents | 2. Rate of surface water quality better than III | |
| 3. Mortality rate of children <5years age | | 3. Premature mortality as a result of major non-communicable diseases | | |
| 4. Mortality rate of pregnant women | | | | |
| 5. Proportion of those meeting the national physical determination standard among urban and rural residents | | | | |

**Fig. 20.2** Framework of Healthy China 2030 vision with 4 key principles, namely, health priority, reform and innovation, scientific development, and justice and equity, and 13 core indicators under 5 main themes in health

kidney research from basic science to epidemiology and clinical trials in the Chinese Mainland in the last 40 years. Professional nephrology associations were established at both provincial and city level across the entire country. The number of participants at the CSN annual meeting has increased dramatically in the last 40 years from having only a dozen of participants in the initial years to now over 10,000 participants in 2018.

To tackle the growing burden of chronic kidney disease (CKD), CSN has continued to advocate efforts on CKD prevention, screening, early detection, and treatment with an aim to delay the progression of CKD, reduce the need for RRT, improve patients' quality of life and survival, reduce complications and hospitalizations, and reduce healthcare expenditure. CSN has partnered with several other key international nephrology societies and organizations to facilitate further development of kidney care and research and to reduce the burden of kidney diseases in the Chinese Mainland.

## Highlights of Nephrology in the Chinese Mainland

Nephrologists in the Chinese Mainland have conducted nationally representative studies to examine the burden of different kidney diseases. These data form an important basis to guide the government's decision-making on healthcare policies and financing on kidney disease care in the Chinese Mainland. CKD is a public health issue. A cross-sectional survey conducted in a nationally representative sample of adults in China in 2012 showed that the overall prevalence of CKD was 10.8% (95% CI [confidence intervals] 10.2–11.3) and was higher in the northern (16.9% [95%CI 15.1–18.7]) and southwestern (18.3% [95% CI 16.4–20.4]) regions compared with other regions. The degree of kidney damage was associated with the socioeconomic status of each region, in that patients from regions with lower socioeconomic status had more kidney damage [9]. Subsequent to this national cross-sectional survey, the prevalence of CKD in China was reported from two other sources. First is the Hospital Quality Monitoring System (HQMS), a mandatory national, hospitalized patients' database set up by the National Health Commission of China that tracks all hospitalized patients' discharge records from tertiary hospitals in the Chinese Mainland between 2010 and 2015. In contrast to tertiary hospitals in developed countries, tertiary hospitals in the Chinese Mainland provide primary, secondary, and tertiary care and have a nationwide catchment of a nonselective patient population. The database contains data of 35.3 million patients hospitalized between 2010 and 2015. Second, there was a general population-based study with a nationally representative sample of 47,204 subjects recruited between 2009 and 2010. Data from these two additional sources have shown that CKD related to diabetic kidney disease (DKD) is now more common than CKD related to glomerular disease (GD) in both the general population cohort and in the hospitalized patients' database since 2011 [10].

A nationwide, cross-sectional survey of adult hospitalized patients in 2013 showed that AKI also incurred enormous financial burden to the healthcare system in the Chinese Mainland. In addition, AKI was substantially underdiagnosed and undertreated, reflecting a huge service gap and unmet need in early detection and early initiation of treatment for hospitalized patients with AKI and lack of accessibility to acute dialysis support for AKI in rural parts of China. Many other developing countries in the world also face similar problems. The findings urged nephrologists in China to take up the lead and responsibility to improve AKI detection and improve accessibility to acute dialysis support for AKI [11].

The CNRDS, a nationwide kidney failure (ESRD) data collection system, is a landmark development of nephrology for the Chinese Mainland in 2010. It contains the largest and most comprehensive national ESRD patients' registration. By the end of 2017, the CNRDS included data of 524,467 HD patients and 86,344 PD patients from 5479 HD centers and 981 PD centers, respectively, covering 31 provinces, autonomous regions, and municipalities. The registry provides information on the national burden of ESRD as well as the prevalence, incidence, and severity of CKD in the Chinese Mainland and helps to raise the government's awareness of the importance and burden of ESRD. Most important of all, it prompts national coverage of ESRD in the country's Critical Illness Insurance Program. The CNRDS Annual Data Report (ADR) provides the annual number of prevalent and incident dialysis patients and their mortality rates, enabling quality assurance of kidney care delivered. The CNRDS also enables monitoring of various ESRD-related complications including anemia and mineral and bone disorder so to assure quality of care for various ESRD-related complications.

Academic nephrologists in the Chinese Mainland also play an increasingly important role in conducting global clinical trials that made an impact to the global clinical practice guidelines (CPGs) development. Some examples are the Therapeutic Evaluation of Steroids in IgA Nephropathy Global (TESTING) study [12], the Study of Diabetic Nephropathy with Atrasentan (SONAR) [13], and the Canagliflozin and Renal Endpoints in Diabetes with Established Nephropathy Clinical Evaluation (CREDENCE) [14].

Chinese nephrologists also contributed to the development of many international CPGs, including those of Kidney Disease: Improving Global Outcomes (KDIGO), International Society for Peritoneal Dialysis (ISPD), International IgA Nephropathy Network (IIgANN), and Renal Pathology Society (RPS). Chinese nephrologists also involved in steering clinical trials on roxadustat treatment for anemia in patients with kidney disease undergoing long-term dialysis and in non-dialysis CKD patients [15, 16]. Based on the results of these trials, roxadustat was recently approved as a new drug treatment for renal anemia in patients with kidney disease in the Chinese Mainland. These landmark trials marked the emerging role of Chinese nephrologists in leading global clinical trials in kidney diseases.

Chinese nephrologists also performed significant groundbreaking work in basic research in kidney diseases. Mutations in two genes, polycystic kidney disease-1 (PKD1) and PKD2, accounted for most cases of autosomal dominant polycystic kidney disease (ADPKD). A research group from China reported the 3.6-angstrom cryo-electron microscopic structure of truncated human PKD1-PKD2 complex assembled in a 1:3 ratio and established a framework for dissecting the function and disease mechanisms of the PKD proteins [17]. The study, for the first time, identified the structure of transient receptor potential channel family hetero-complex for further study to understand the pathogenesis of PKD.

A two-stage genome-wide association study (GWAS) of IgAN in the Han Chinese showed that IgAN was associated with variants near genes involved in innate immunity and inflammation [18]. This work from China contributed significantly to the understanding of genetic factors in the pathogenesis of complex kidney diseases and provided important evidence that genetic factors play an important role in the pathogenesis of IgAN.

## Prevalence and Awareness of CKD

The Chinese Mainland has not had a national surveillance system for kidney disease until recently. This constitutes an important barrier to understand the exact scope of the problem and develop effective preventive and therapeutic strategies. In a cross-sectional nationwide survey of a representative adult population in the Chinese Mainland between 2009 and 2010, the overall prevalence of CKD was estimated around 10.8% [9], being comparable to that of developed countries such as the United States (US) (13.0%) [19] and Norway (10.2%) [20]. It also implies that the Chinese Mainland has nearly 119.5 million adults with kidney disease. However, the prevalence and severity of CKD vary according to the economic development of the region, defined by the National Bureau of Statistics

Table 20.2 Prevalence of CKD (%) in the Chinese Mainland stratified by geographical region and urban or rural residency (%)

| | eGFR <60 mL/min/1.73 m$^2$ | Albuminuria | CKD |
|---|---|---|---|
| *Region* | | | |
| East | 1.1 | 7.5 | 8.4 |
| South | 1.3 | 6.0 | 6.7 |
| Middle | 1.4 | 13.1 | 14.2 |
| North | 2.5 | 15.4 | 16.9 |
| Northwest | 1.5 | 5.6 | 6.7 |
| Southwest | 3.8 | 15.1 | 18.3 |
| *Residency* | | | |
| Urban | 2.3 | 7.0 | 8.9 |
| Rural | 1.6 | 10.1 | 11.3 |
| *Total* | 1.7 | 9.4 | 10.8 |

Note: Data were age- and gender-adjusted prevalence (%). Albuminuria was defined as a urinary albumin-to-creatinine ratio > 30 mg/g creatinine. CKD was defined as eGFR <60 mL/min/1.73 m$^2$ or albuminuria
Abbreviations: *CKD* chronic kidney disease, *eGFR* estimated glomerular filtration rate

(Table 20.2). As an example, the prevalence of CKD was higher in the north (16.9%) and southwest (18.3%) regions compared to other regions (Table 20.2) [9]. Rural areas showed lower prevalence of estimated glomerular filtration rate (eGFR) <60 mL/min/1.73 m$^2$, but higher prevalence of albuminuria, compared with urban areas [1]. Furthermore, the prevalence of albuminuria was positively associated with economic status (evaluated by GDP) in rural areas but negatively associated with economic status in urban areas [1].

Most subjects (84%) presented in early stages of CKD with albuminuria and well-preserved kidney function [9]. This indicates the potential to institute early CKD screening, detection, and prevention programs as well as education campaigns to raise more awareness of the importance of kidney health. In a more recent comparative study between China and the USA, the prevalence of eGFR <60 mL/min/1.73 m$^2$ was higher in the USA than in China (6.5% vs. 2.7%) [21]. Nearly two-thirds of this difference was accounted for by the higher prevalence of various CKD risk factors, including increasing age, male gender, diabetes, hypertension, central obesity, cardiovascular disease (CVD), and hyperuricemia in the USA [21].

The Chinese Center for Disease Control and Prevention included both eGFR and urine albumin-creatinine ratio, in the China Chronic Disease and Nutrition Surveillance in 2018, a nationally representative adult population from 302 monitoring sites, in order to estimate the latest prevalence of CKD in the Chinese Mainland. Despite a high prevalence of CKD, the awareness of CKD diagnosis was low (10.04%) [22]. Subjects with advanced CKD were more aware of their diagnosis (15.6% for normoalbuminuria and 61.8% for albuminuria group) than those with early CKD or with normoalbuminuria (7.7–16.7%) [22]. The National Health and Nutrition Examination Survey (NHANES) 1999–2004 showed that 6.0% of CKD subjects in the USA were aware of their diagnosis [23], an awareness rate lower than that reported in China. Compared with those unaware of their CKD diagnosis, subjects aware of their CKD diagnosis were more likely to be educated, have free medical insurance, received health examination during the previous 2 years, and have hypertension, family history of kidney disease, and self-report concern about kidney disease [22].

## Burden of Kidney Failure

The growing burden of CKD in China implies an increasing population requiring RRT [24]. The China Kidney Disease Network (CK-NET) developed a national surveillance system for kidney diseases by integrating national administrative and claims data that covers millions of CKD subjects from all regions of China. According to the CK-NET 2015 ADR, the estimated prevalence of HD and PD was 402.18 and 39.95 per million population (pmp), respectively, and the age-adjusted incidence rate for dialysis was 122.19 pmp [25]. The prevalence rates of dialysis population were higher than that reported previously for the Chinese Mainland [26]. Although HD and PD patients in total constituted only a small percentage (0.16% and 0.02%, respectively) of the entire insured population in the Chinese Mainland, they incurred a disproportionately high percentage of healthcare expenditures (2.08% and 0.34%, respectively) [25].

The Beijing Regional HD Registry and Shanghai Renal Registry reported that the prevalence and incidence of maintenance HD in 2011 were 524.6 pmp and 107.3 pmp in Beijing [27] and 544.7 pmp and 82.9 pmp in Shanghai [28], respectively. The prevalence of ESRD was still lower in the Chinese Mainland than in most other parts of Asia such as Taiwan (2285 pmp in 2007) and Japan (2233 pmp in 2007) [29]. Factors contributing to the very different prevalence rates of ESRD in the Chinese Mainland versus other Asian countries may be related to limited affordability and poor accessibility to RRT in less developed regions [30]. With government support, the number of HD centers has grown to more than 4000 in 2015 [31]. New HD facilities were set up at both county level and township level to improve accessibility and provision of HD service in less developed regions of the Chinese Mainland.

## Evolving Spectrum of Causes of CKD/ESRD

The relative proportion of various causes of ESRD varies according to the race and geographical regions of China [32]. Diabetes is a leading cause, accounting for one-third of all incident ESRD patients worldwide [33]. However, this differs from the Chinese Mainland, where GD is the predominant cause of ESRD. Data from the CNRDS 2015 showed that GD was the most common cause of ESRD (54.2%), followed by diabetes (17.0%) and hypertension (9.9%) [31].

The rapid urbanization of the Chinese Mainland in the last three decades with dramatic changes in lifestyle and dietary habits of native Chinese resulted in a very considerable increase in the burden of various metabolic and noncommunicable diseases such as obesity, diabetes, and hypertension [34]. The prevalence of obesity has increased from 0.6% in 1982 to 2.9% in 2002 [35], and that of diabetes has increased from 0.7% in 1980 [36] to 10.9% in 2013 [37]. The substantial burden of noncommunicable diseases has increased the incidence and prevalence of CKD and changed the relative proportion of causes of CKD/ESRD in the Chinese Mainland over the years.

Data from HQMS showed that CKD patients constituted 4.8% of all hospitalized patients in the Chinese Mainland. The most common causes of CKD in hospitalized patients were DKD (27.0%), hypertensive nephropathy (HTN) (20.8%), obstructive nephropathy (ON) (15.6%), and GD (15.1%) (Fig. 20.3). An increasing number of hospitalizations were observed in patients with CKD due to diabetes [10]. The relative proportion of different causes of CKD varies according to the socioeconomic status and geographic areas (Fig. 20.4). For example, DKD (32.7%) and HTN (23.0%) were the leading causes of CKD in hospitalized patients in urban areas. However, in rural areas, the top 3 leading causes of CKD were ON (21.4%), GD (18.5%), and DKD (17.4%) in hospitalized patients (Fig. 20.2) [38]. In North China, the percentage of hospitalized patients with CKD due to diabetes was higher among residents from urban than rural areas, while more hospitalized CKD patients in rural areas had GD than urban areas [38]. On the other hand, South China had higher prevalence of CKD due to ON than North China [38] (Fig. 20.3) [10]. In 2017, 1.14% of all hospitalized patients had CKD due to DKD and 0.68% of all hospitalized patients had CKD due to GD (unpublished data). The HQMS also showed an increasing proportion of hypertensive kidney disease and ON (mostly associated with kidney stones) as causes of CKD between 2010 and 2015 [38].

In the last decade, GD was a principal cause of CKD in the Chinese Mainland [10, 39], accounting for nearly half of the causes of ESRD in dialysis patients in 1999 [40]. However, its prevalence has decreased since 2013 [10]. The percentage of hospitalized patients with CKD due to IgAN decreased from 19.0% in 2010 to 10.6% in 2015 [41]. In a nationwide survey conducted in 938 hospitals (both tertiary and community hospitals) between 2004 and 2014 [42] including 71,151 biopsy-proven GD, IgAN (36.3%) was the most common primary GD, followed by

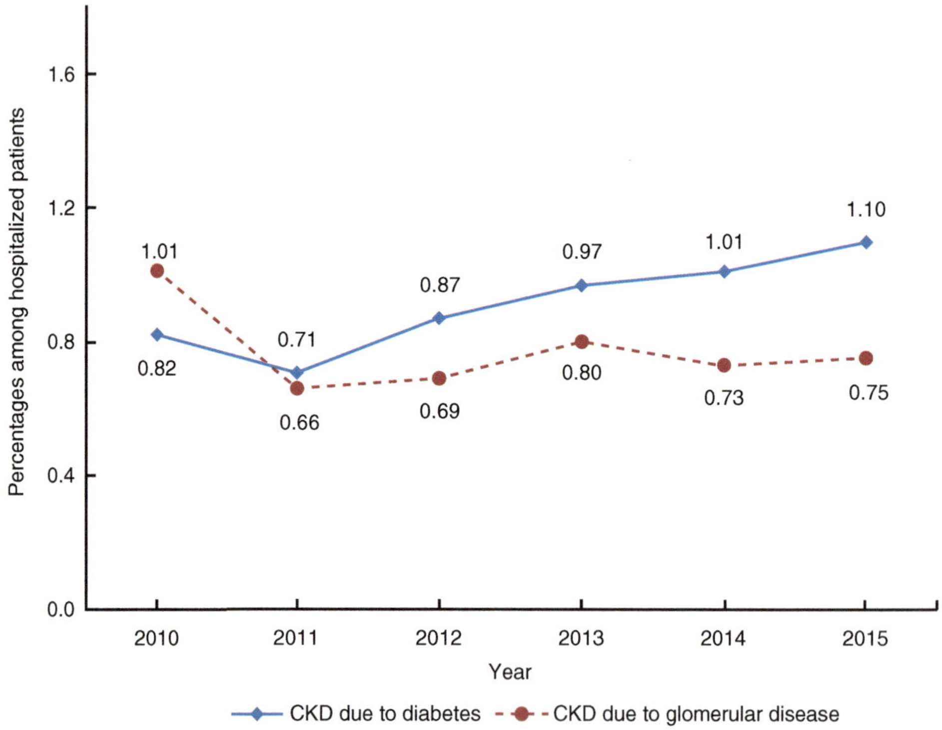


**Fig. 20.3** Trends in CKD due to diabetes or GD among hospitalized patients in the Chinese Mainland from 2010 to 2015. Percentages were calculated based on the overall numbers of hospitalized patients for each year, obtained from the Hospital Quality Monitoring System. Abbreviations: CKD, chronic kidney disease; GD, glomerular disease

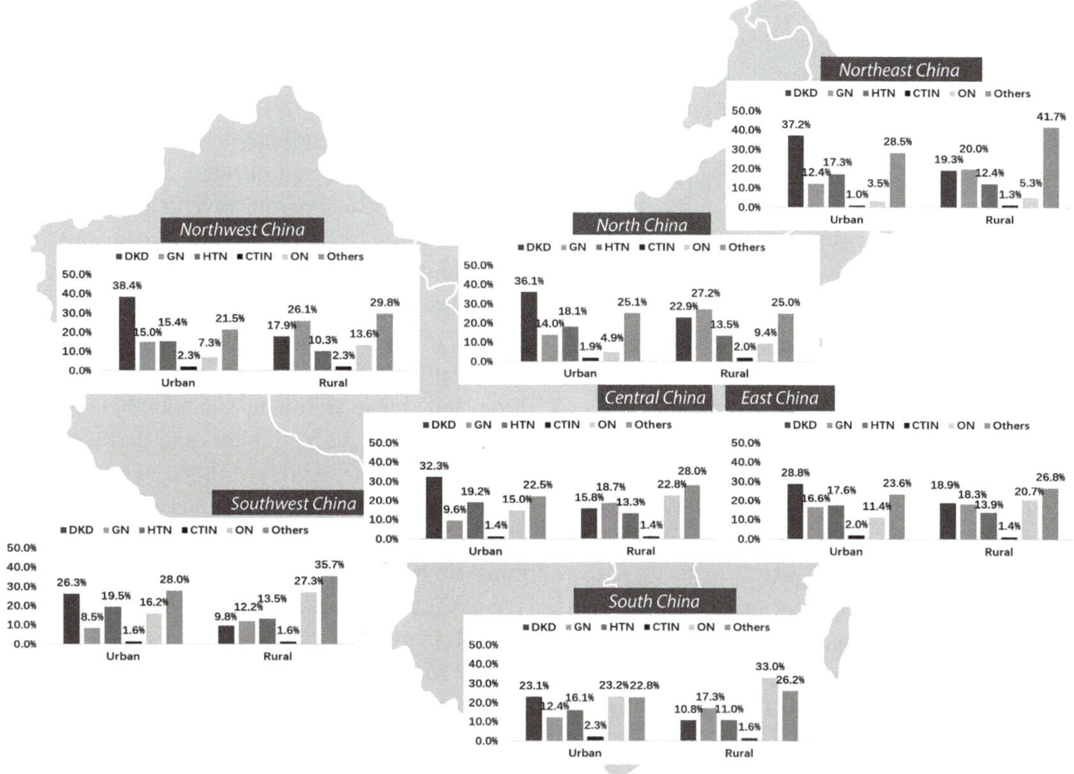


**Fig. 20.4** Proportion of various causes of CKD stratified by geographic regions among hospitalized population with CKD in 2015. Note: numbers represented percentages among patients with CKD. Reproduced from Huang et al. [38]. (With permission from John Wiley and Sons, Inc). Abbreviations: DKD diabetic kidney disease, GN glomerulonephritis, HTN hypertensive nephropathy, CTIN chronic tubulointerstitial nephritis, ON obstructive nephropathy

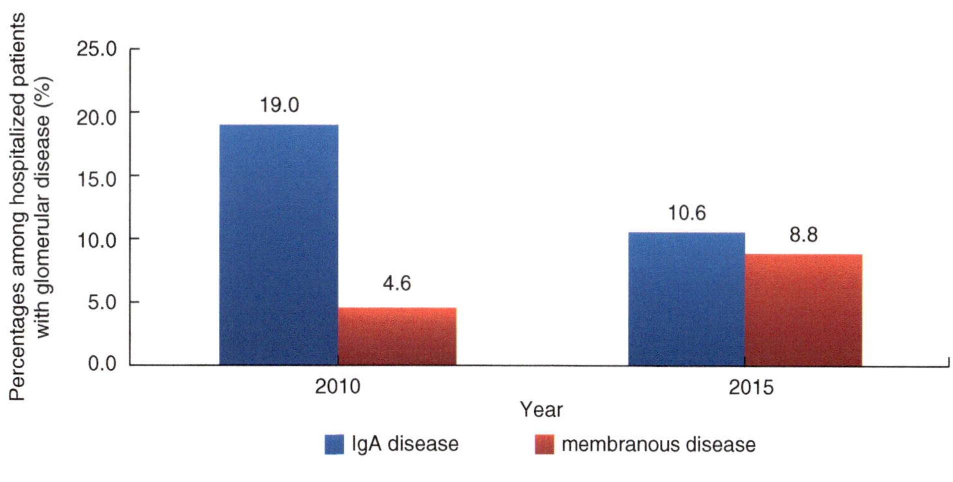


**Fig. 20.5** Proportion of IgA disease and membranous disease among hospitalized patients with primary glomerular nephropathy in 2010 and 2015. Note: numbers represented percentages among hospitalized patients with primary glomerular nephropathy

membranous nephropathy (MN) (30.2%) with age and region standardization. In adults aged <45 years, IgAN was a leading cause of primary GD. However, in adults aged >45 years, MN was the most frequent primary GD. Lupus nephritis and vasculitis-related nephritis were the most common secondary GD [41]. The proportion of hospitalized patients with CKD due to MN almost doubled, from 4.6% in 2010 to 8.8% in 2015 (Fig. 20.5), possibly partly attributed to long-term exposure to air particulate matter (PM) that posed a serious environmental hazard in some parts, especially in the northern region. Each 10 μg/m$^3$ increase in $PM_{2.5}$ was associated with a 14% higher odds of MN in regions with $PM_{2.5} > 70$ μg/m$^3$ compared to regions with $PM_{2.5} < 70$ μg/m$^3$ [42].

## IgA Nephropathy (IgAN)

Three genome-wide association studies (GWAS) in the Chinese population [18, 43, 44] identified five genetic loci associated with IgAN [43]. Besides three independent loci in human leukocyte antigen (HLA) regions, variants in the complement factor H (CFH) and the related CFHR3 and CFHR1 genes on chromosome 1q32 that affected complement activation through their influence on CFH levels and genetic variants of oncostatin M (OSM) and interleukin 6 family (LIF) on chromosome 22q12 may predispose individuals to develop IgAN [45]. A subsequent GWAS in the Chinese population identified two additional loci: 17p13 containing TNF superfamily member 13 (TNFSF13) and 8p23 containing defensin alpha (DEFA) [18]. Polymorphisms within the DEFA genes were involved in gene transcription regulation, and associated with clinical phenotype of gross hematuria, suggesting mucosal immunity may involve in the pathogenesis of IgAN [46, 47]. Another GWAS [44] in 20,612 individuals of European and East Asian origin identified six new loci that increased susceptibility to IgAN, namely, four in integrin subunit alpha M-X (ITGAM-ITGAX), vav guanine nucleotide exchange factor 3 (VAV3), and caspase recruitment domain family member 9 (CARD9) and two at HLA-DQB1 and DEFA. This suggests interaction between the host and intestinal pathogens may play a possible role in shaping genetic predisposition to IgAN [44].

Glycosyltransferases are involved in the synthesis of the O-glycan of IgA1 molecules, and abnormal O-glycosylation of IgA1 molecules is involved in the pathogenesis of IgAN [48, 49]. One protective (YATIG) and two risk (YAGDA, YATDG) regulatory haplotypes in key glycosyltransferase genes for IgA1 O-glycosylation (C1GALT1) gene were associated with IgAN [50]. ADG haplotype in the promoter region of ST6GALNAC2, a key glycosyltransferase gene, has functional significance in increasing predisposition to IgAN [51]. Association has been demonstrated between C1GALT1 and ST6GALNAC2 gene with IgA1 glycosylation, as well as with the severity of IgAN [52].

The TESTING study [12] was a multicenter, double-blind, randomized controlled trial (RCT) that evaluated the efficacy and safety of corticosteroids in IgAN patients with proteinuria >1 g/day and eGFR between 20 and 120 mL/min/1.73 m$^2$, after at least 3 months of blood pressure control with renin-angiotensin-aldosterone system (RAAS) blockade. Study recruitment was discontinued after 262 subjects entered study and followed for a median of 2.1 years, because of significantly more serious adverse events in the methylprednisolone group (14.7%) than placebo group (3.2%) ($p$ = 0.001; risk difference 11.5%), mostly due to serious infections (8.1% vs. 0; risk difference 8.1%; $p < 0.001$), including two deaths. However, methylprednisolone group showed significant benefits in reducing the incidence of primary renal endpoint (5.9%) than placebo (15.9%) with a risk reduction of 63% ($p = 0.02$). The study protocol was amended using a reduced dose of methylprednisolone with septrin as prophylaxis and is currently ongoing.

Another recent multicenter RCT from the Chinese Mainland [53], comparing mycophenolate mofetil (MMF) plus prednisone versus full-dose prednisone in IgAN with active proliferative lesions, failed to show renal benefits with MMF, but combining MMF with prednisolone showed fewer adverse events compared to full-dose prednisolone.

In a prospective follow-up study of IgAN in the Chinese Mainland (mean follow-up, 45 months) of which subjects received mainly RAS inhibitors and steroids added, if persistent proteinuria ($n$ = 703) [54], the mean eGFR decline was −3.1 ml/min/1.73 m$^2$ per year, and annual rate of ESRD was 2.3%. Baseline eGFR (hazard ratio, 0.76 per 10 ml/min/1.73 m$^2$), proteinuria at 6 months (hazard ratio, 1.53 per 1 g/day), and systolic blood pressure at 6 months (hazard ratio, 1.36 per 10 mmHg) were associated with an increased risk of composite kidney failure events using multivariable Cox regression analysis. Baseline eGFR (regression coefficient, 20.1), time-averaged proteinuria (regression coefficient, 20.2), and time-averaged mean arterial pressure (regression coefficient, 20.15) were independent predictors of eGFR slope by linear regression.

## Membranous Nephropathy (MN)

The prevalence of MN has increased quite substantially in the Chinese Mainland in the last 10 years. A nationwide survey of biopsy-proven GD showed that MN accounted for 12.2% of all GD in 2004 but doubled to 24.9% in 2014 (24.9%). The proportion of other major GD has remained similar [42]. This meant that the percentage of MN has increased by an average of 13% per year. Among hospitalized patients with primary GD, MN increased from 4.5% in 2010 to 8.8% in 2015 [55] (Fig. 20.5). Notably, the proportion of MN exceeded that of IgAN in the northern and northeastern China since 2014 and is now the leading cause of GD in these regions.

Air pollution has become a serious public health problem in some cities in the Chinese Mainland and may account for the rising prevalence of MN. Between 2004 and 2014 [56], the 3-year average levels of aerosol optical depth (AOD)-derived $PM_{2.5}$ have increased and plateaued in 2008, with a mean ambient level of 55.6 μg/m$^3$ (range, 8.1–110.5 μg/m$^3$). The aerosol level of $PM_{2.5}$ was much higher than that reported in many developed countries. Indeed, a nationwide survey [42] showed that long-term exposure to high levels of $PM_{2.5}$ was associated with an increased risk of MN. Every 10 μg/

$m^3$ increase in $PM_{2.5}$ concentration was associated with a 14% higher odds of MN in the regions with a $PM_{2.5} > 70$ μg/$m^3$. Assuming a causal relationship, 15.2% of MN in the Chinese Mainland may be attributed to $PM_{2.5}$ exposure. HQMS data showed that these patients were clustered in the Hebei Province and Guangxi Province [55]. The association between $PM_{2.5}$ exposure and an increased risk of MN was confirmed in the Northern region demarcated by the Yangtze River. On the other hand, in Southern China, the Zhuang population, the largest minority population in China, showed a high preponderance of MN, but MN in this population was not associated with $PM_{2.5}$ exposure [55]. These data showed how genes and environmental factors may both contribute to an increased risk of MN in the Chinese Mainland.

In a cross-sectional study ($n$ = 578) in the Chinese Mainland [57], 89% of patients with MN were phospholipase A2 receptor (PLA2R)-associated, including 68% with circulating anti-PLA2R antibodies and 21% negative for the antibody but showing granular expression of PLA2R in glomeruli. Eleven percent had no detectable anti-PLA2R antibody or PLA2R antigen in immune deposits. Two percent had thrombospondin type I domain-containing 7A (THSD7A)-associated MN, which accounted for 16% of the PLA2R-negative patients. These percentages were similar to those reported in the Western population.

A GWAS of primary MN identified two significant genetic loci: chromosome 2q24 containing the PLA2R1 gene (SNP rs4664308) and chromosome 6p21 containing the HLA complex class II HLA-DQα1 chain (HLA-DQA1) (SNP rs2187668), with strong gene-gene interactions between the two risk alleles [58]. Validation studies in China showed that individuals carrying these risk alleles were strongly associated with positive serum anti-PLA2R antibodies (73%) and glomerular expression of PLA2R (75%) [59]. In contrast, among individuals who did not carry these genotypes, none had anti-PLA2R antibodies and glomerular expression of PLA2R was weak or absent. This suggested that individuals carrying these risk alleles were predisposed to the generation of circulating anti-PLA2R autoantibodies that contribute to the pathogenesis of MN.

Three other studies from the Chinese Mainland also provided novel insights into the contribution of specific HLA alleles in primary MN [60–62]. A case-control association analysis identified DRB1*1501 and DRB1*0301 as increasing the risk of primary MN among Han Chinese. Both HLA alleles exhibited interactions with PLA2R1 variant rs4664308 and were associated with circulating anti-PLA2R antibodies [60]. Another study demonstrated the association of DRB1*1501 with anti-PLA2R-positive MN and suggested DRB3*0202 as the second independent risk factor for MN. DRB3*0202 resides on the same haplotype as DRB1*0301 [61]. Extending these findings, another study showed that DRB1*0301 was associated with higher level of anti-PLA2R antibodies and DRB1*1502 was associated with lower eGFR at baseline, a worse renal outcome, and a higher risk of ESRD [62].

In a follow-up study ($n$ = 371) in the Chinese Mainland [63], 68.5% of patients were treated with immunosuppressive agents with or without corticosteroids, and the others by RAS blockade alone. During a median follow-up of 27 months, 87.6% achieved remission (of which 45.3% had complete remission and 42.3% had partial remission). Relapse occurred in 27.7% and 2.2% progressed to ESRD, while 18.1% experienced worsening kidney function with eGFR decline over 50%. Multivariable Cox regression analysis identified the positivity of anti-PLA2R antibodies (HR = 2.5, $p$ = 0.009) and failure to remit (HR = 3.2, $p$ = 0.004) as independent risk factors for worsening kidney function in the Chinese population. The severity of chronic tubule-interstitial injury (HR = 25.8, $p$ = 0.035) and failure to remit (HR = 10.2, $p$ = 0.010) were independent risk factors for ESRD in Chinese.

As in the western population, rituximab induced remission in 41.7% of primary MN not responding to other immunosuppressive therapy (with 36.1% being partial and 5.6% being complete remission) [64]. Those who responded to rituximab had lower baseline levels of anti-PLA2R antibodies and all subjects had antibody depletion or reduction with rituximab.

## Minimal Change Disease (MCD)

A nationwide survey of kidney biopsies done in 7962 children <18 years in the Chinese Mainland [65] showed that nephrotic syndrome was the most frequent (50%) presentation and MCD was the most common primary GD (29%) followed by IgAN (17%). Henoch-Schönlein purpura nephritis (13%) and lupus nephritis (9%) were the most common secondary GD. The proportion of MCD was significantly higher in boys (38%) than in girls (13%), whereas lupus nephritis was more prevalent in girls (20%) than in boys (3%). Purpura nephritis (23%) was the major pathological diagnosis in younger children (0–12 years old). MCD (33%) was the most common glomerular disease in adolescents (13–18 years old). The proportions of MCD, purpura nephritis, and MN increased between 2004 and 2014, while the proportion of FSGS declined.

A RCT was conducted in 8 kidney centers in the Chinese Mainland, of which 119 adults with nephrotic syndrome due to MCD ($n$ = 119) were randomized to receive either glucocorticoid or tacrolimus after 10-day treatment of intravenous methylprednisolone (0.8 mg/kg/day). The study showed non-inferiority of tacrolimus monotherapy to glucocorticoid. Remission occurred in 96.2% of glucocorticoid-treated subjects and 98.3% of tacrolimus-treated subjects with no significant difference between them. Relapse rate was similar (49.0% and 45.5%, respectively) for glucocorticoid- and tacrolimus-treated subjects. However, adverse events occurred more frequently in glucocorticoid group [66].

## Focal Segmental Glomerulosclerosis (FSGS)

FSGS accounts for 3–4% of primary GD in the Chinese Mainland. Mutations of type IV collagen α3–5 (COL4A3–5) [67], inverted formin 2 (INF2) [68], transient receptor potential cation channel 6 (TRPC6) [69], and α-actinin-4 (ACTN4) [69] may contribute to FSGS development under dominant forms. NPHS1 gene mutations were quite common in sporadic Chinese FSGS patients [70]. Mutations in nuclear pore complex nucleoporin160 kD (NUP160) were implicated in steroid-resistant nephrotic syndrome [71].

Chronic tubulointerstitial injury predicted a worse prognosis of FSGS. Han et al. found that C3a and suPAR drive versican V1 expression in tubular cells by promoting transcription and splicing, respectively, and increases in tubular cell-derived versican V1 induced interstitial fibrosis by activating fibroblasts in FSGS [72].

The efficacy of glucocorticoids in ameliorating FSGS depends on the capacity to expand myeloid-derived suppressor cells (MDSCs). Rapid elevation of MDSCs in peripheral blood may predict the efficacy of glucocorticoids in FSGS [73]. miR-30s protected podocytes by targeting Notch1 and p53 and loss of miR-30s may facilitate podocyte injury. Sustained miR-30 expression may be a novel mechanism underlying the therapeutic effectiveness of corticosteroids in treating podocytopathy [74].

Adult-onset FSGS is often associated with poor response to corticosteroid and immunosuppressive treatment and poor kidney survival. In a cohort ($n = 98$) of Chinese patients with biopsy-proven primary FSGS using treatment recommended by KDIGO guidelines 2012, 84.7% achieved remission during a median follow-up of 58.9 months, 60.2% had relapse, 11.2% progressed to ESRD, and 19.4% had worsening kidney function with serum creatinine increased >30% from baseline or >1.5 mg/dL. Multivariable Cox regression analysis showed that baseline eGFR, combined IgM and C3 deposition, and IgM deposition alone were independent factors predicting worsening kidney function [75].

## Lupus Nephritis (LN)

Lupus nephritis is the most common secondary GD in Chinese. Chinese lupus patients showed a higher incidence of kidney involvement (50–60%) compared with Caucasians (30–40%) and had more severe kidney disease with worse long-term outcomes [76, 77]. A large number of genetic variants were associated with systemic lupus erythematosus (SLE) in Chinese. One GWAS in a Chinese Han population identified nine new susceptibility loci (ETS1, IKZF1, RASGRP3, SLC15A4, TNIP1, 7q11.23, 10q11.22, 11q23.3, and 16p11.2) and confirmed seven previously reported susceptibility loci (BLK, IRF5, STAT4, TNFAIP3, TNFSF4, 6q21, and 22q11.21) for SLE [78]. Another GWAS involving a total of 3300 Asian SLE patients from Hong Kong, Mainland China, and Thailand [79] found genetic variants in ETS1 (rs1128334) and WDFY4 (rs7097397) associated with SLE. In a meta-analysis of GWAS in the Chinese Han population with replication in four additional Asian cohorts in a total of 5365 SLE subjects and 10,054 controls [80], genetic variants in or near CDKN1B, TET3, CD80, DRAM1, and ARID5B were associated with SLE. These findings suggest potential roles of cell-cycle regulation, autophagy, and DNA demethylation in the pathogenesis of SLE. Genetic biomarkers that correlated with LN are however limited and require further exploration [81–86].

The first RCT using mycophenolate mofetil (MMF) was conducted in Chinese patients with diffuse proliferative LN [87] and showed a renal remission rate of >80% with 12-month treatment of corticosteroids and MMF, comparable to a sequential regimen of 6-month oral cyclophosphamide induction followed by 6-month maintenance azathioprine. MMF was associated with fewer adverse events including infections as compared with cyclophosphamide. The subsequent Aspreva Lupus Management Study (ALMS) confirmed that Chinese LN patients had similar renal response rates to MMF or intravenous cyclophosphamide induction therapy [88]. Low-dose corticosteroids combined with azathioprine or MMF are now two commonly used maintenance immunosuppressive regimens for LN in China.

In Chinese patients with class IV LN, corticosteroids and cyclosporine also led to significant reduction in proteinuria after 1 month and histological improvement at 1 year with no significant deterioration in serum creatinine or creatinine clearance after a follow-up of 48 months [89]. Dual immunosuppressive treatment with corticosteroids and tacrolimus achieved a response rate similar to that with corticosteroids plus either cyclophosphamide or MMF in the treatment of class III/IV LN [90, 91].

Previous study from the Chinese Mainland showed that triple immunosuppression comprising corticosteroids, tacrolimus, and reduced-dose of MMF was more effective than corticosteroids plus cyclophosphamide in patients with class IV+V LN [92]. More recently [93], this "multi-targeted therapy" was shown to achieve a higher complete remission rate (45.9 vs. 25.6%; $p < 0.001$) and overall response rate (83.5 vs. 63.0%; $p < 0.001$) at 6 months with similar adverse events when compared with corticosteroids and intravenous cyclophosphamide in patients with class III/IV +/− V LN. This multi-targeted therapy, when used as a maintenance treatment in patients who initially responded, showed similar cumulative renal relapse rates and similar eGFR but with fewer adverse events and lower withdrawal rate than maintenance azathioprine [94]. Another study comparing leflunomide with intravenous cyclophosphamide in treating type IV LN in the Chinese Mainland showed comparable complete remission and partial remission rates with the two treatments [95].

## Anti-neutrophil Cytoplasmic Antibody (ANCA)-Associated Vasculitis (AAV)

AAV nephritis is a common form of secondary GD in elderly Chinese. Data from the HQMS between 2010 and 2015 showed that 0.25% of the hospitalized patients had AAV. The prevalence of AAV was stable throughout the 5-year period, and increased with latitude, and was associated with exposure to carbon monoxide. In Yunnan Province, the prevalence of AAV increased by 1.37-fold after the Zhaotong earthquake in 2014. The Dong population, an ethnic minority of Chinese, showed the highest prevalence of AAV (0.67%). The mean age of diagnosis of AAV was 60.0 ± 15.6 years and 46.4% were men [96].

In Chinese, microscopic polyarteritis (MPA) constituted about 80% of AAV [97, 98]. Even among patients with granulomatosis polyangiitis (GPA), 60% had ANCA specificity for MPO [98]. DQA1*0302 and DQB1*0303 are risk alleles, predisposing to the development of MPO-ANCA AAV in Chinese. HLA-DPB1 variant rs3117242 was also associated with GPA in Han Chinese population [99, 100]. Positive ANCA was also reported in 15–64% of patients receiving propylthiouracil but only a quarter developed clinical vasculitis [101, 102]. Their ANCA was against multiple antigens. Patients with propylthiouracil-induced AAV had less organ involvement and milder kidney lesions, compared to those with primary AAV.

Rituximab is a recent adopted induction and maintenance treatment regimen for AAV. Recent data showed the importance of alternative complement pathway activation in the pathogenesis of human AAV [103–105]. In particular, C5a plays a critical role in ANCA-mediated neutrophil activation. Inhibition of C5a has emerged as a potential therapeutic approach for AAV. Treatment resistance however occurred in 10.7% of patients and around one-third relapsed [106]. Relapses were likely to develop in the same organ as with the disease onset [107].

One center from the Chinese Mainland reported that 33.9% of AAV patients died during follow-up, including 20.9% within the first 12 months after diagnosis. This was before the availability of rituximab [108]. Secondary infection was the leading cause of death in the first year. Other independent predictors included older age, pulmonary involvement of AAV, and initial kidney function. Cardiovascular events became the leading cause of death for those who survived the first year.

## Hepatitis B Virus (HBV)-Associated GD

China's HBV prevention program that targeted toward interrupting perinatal transmission has been highly effective. Compared with the survey done before vaccination was available in 1992, the prevalence of HBV surface antigen (HBsAg) positivity has declined 46% in 2006 and 52% in 2014. Among children aged less than 5 years, HBsAg positivity has declined by 97% [109]. Work is ongoing to completely eradicate hepatitis B infection in the Chinese Mainland by 2030.

The China Kadoorie Biobank followed 469,459 participants for a median of 9.1 years (4.2 million person-years) of which 4555 were incident CKD cases. HBsAg-positive subjects showed a 1.37 higher adjusted hazard for incident CKD compared with HBsAg-negative subjects [110].

A single-center review of 11,618 kidney biopsies showed that among the biopsies with a diagnosis of secondary GD, LN accounted for 26.5%, Henoch-Schönlein purpura GD accounted for 25.8%, HBV-associated GD accounted for 14.6%, and DKD accounted for 10.7%. The detection rate of HBV-related GD between 2008 and 2012 (with age adjustment) has declined significantly compared to the period between 1987 and 1992 ($p < 0.001$) [111].

## Diabetic Kidney Disease and Obesity-Related Kidney Disease

### Prevalence of Diabetes and Obesity in China

China faces a huge burden of diabetes with rapid societal modernization and adoption of a "westernized diet" by many local Chinese. The International Diabetes Federation (IDF) estimated that the burden of diabetes will increase from 90 million population in 2011 to nearly 130 million by 2030 in China [112]. According to the most recent national survey, the overall estimated prevalence of diabetes and prediabetes were 10.9% and 35.7%, respectively, indicating that an estimated 110 million people currently suffer from diabetes in China. Of this population, only 36.5% were aware of the diagnosis of diabetes and 32.2% received antidiabetic medications [37]. The increase in the prevalence of diabetes is attributed mostly to an increase in type II diabetes, which accounts for approximately 95% of

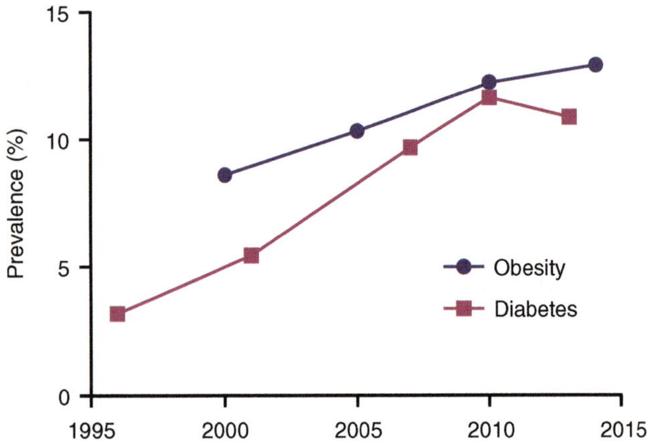


**Fig. 20.6** Prevalence of diabetes and obesity in the Chinese Mainland in the last decades. (Date referred to Ma et al. [114] and Tian et al. [115])

all diabetes in the Chinese Mainland. Chinese patients generally have type II diabetes diagnosed at a relatively younger age and with a lower body mass index than the Western population [113].

Similarly, the prevalence of obesity (defined as having a body mass index ≥27.5 kg/m$^2$ in Chinese) showed a significant increase from 8.6% in 2000 to 10.3% in 2005 and 12.9% in 2014 (Fig. 20.6). The prevalence of central obesity (defined as a waist circumference greater than 90 cm in men and greater than 85 cm in women) has dramatically increased from 13.9% in 2000 to 18.3% in 2005, and 24.9% in 2014, reflecting an enormous public health issue for the Chinese Mainland [115].

## Prevalence of Diabetic Kidney Disease (DKD) and Obesity-Related Kidney Disease in China

The dramatic increase in the prevalence of diabetes and obesity in recent years changed the epidemiology of CKD in the Chinese Mainland. The CRDS 2011 showed that DKD accounted for 16.4% of the ESRD, second to GD (57.4%) [30]. In the CRDS 2015, GD was still the leading cause of ESRD in HD patients (45.8%) but the proportion of DKD had increased to 21.2% [116]. The prevalence of diabetes in the overall dialysis population was 27.1% with no significant difference between HD (26.7%) and PD (28.5%) [25].

DKD has become more prevalent than GD in hospitalized patients in the Chinese Mainland since 2011. The percentage of hospitalized patients with CKD due to diabetes was lower than that due to GD in 2010 (0.82% vs. 1.01%). However, in 2015, more hospitalized CKD patients had diabetes than GD as their causes of CKD (1.10% and 0.75%, respectively) [10]. According to the ADR of the CK-NET in 2015, DKD was the most common cause of CKD among hospitalized patients in the Chinese Mainland (27.0%), followed by hypertensive nephropathy (HTN) (20.8%) and GD (15.1%) [25]. Notably, the prevalence of DKD was higher in developed areas than in rural areas. Among CKD population in developed areas, 32.7% had DKD. In rural areas, DKD accounted for 17.4% of all hospitalized patients with CKD [25].

Cross-sectional surveys from Shanghai and Hong Kong estimated the frequency of DKD ranged between 10% and ~ 40% in patients with diabetes [114]. A new national CPG of DKD was recently published to standardize the screening, diagnosis, and treatment of DKD in China [117]. In keeping with the guidelines from the American Diabetes Association, the Chinese CPG recommended annual screening of urinary albumin-to-creatinine ratio (UACR) and eGFR in patients with type I diabetes with disease duration of ≥5 years and in those with type II diabetes immediately after diagnosis. DKD is diagnosed based on the presence of diabetes with increased UACR (≥30 mg/g) and/or eGFR (<60 ml/min/1.73 m$^2$) after excluding other CKD due to nondiabetic kidney disease [117, 118]. Renal biopsy may be considered if the diagnosis is uncertain, for example, in patients with sudden onset of overt proteinuria, obvious or microscopic hematuria, or rapid progressive decline in kidney function.

Although kidney biopsy is not routinely performed in all patients with DKD, there is a rising trend of biopsy-proven kidney damage due to diabetes in the past two decades [119]. Based on the Renal Biopsy Registry of the National Clinical Research Center of Kidney Disease that included 40,749 renal biopsies, the frequency of DKD nearly doubled from 2003 to 2014. DKD accounted for 13% of all secondary GD between 2003 and 2006 but increased to 24% between 2011 and 2014. Among patients with age between 45 and 70 years, DKD was the predominant cause of secondary GD, accounting nearly 40% [119]. Reports from other centers in the Chinese Mainland indicated that the prevalence of DKD ranged between 25% and 74% among patients with type II diabetes [120].

Obesity contributed significantly to CKD across all age groups and in both gender. A cross-sectional survey from the Chinese Mainland showed that among men aged ≥45 years, the prevalence of impaired kidney function in nonobese, peripherally obese, and centrally obese subjects was 5.1%, 5.1%, and 10.1%, respectively. Among women aged 45 years or older, the prevalence of impaired kidney function was 4.9%, 7.9%, and 20.3%, respectively [121]. The incidence of biopsy-proven obesity-related glomerulopathy (histologically manifested as obesity-associated FSGS with glomerulomegaly or obesity-associated glomerulomegaly alone) showed progressive increase over the years, from 0.63% of all secondary GD in 1992–2002 to 4.94% in 2003–2014 [119, 122].

## Current Treatment and Prognosis of DKD in the Chinese Mainland

The Chinese CPG of DKD recommends lifestyle interventions, glycosylated hemoglobin target <7% and blood pressure <130/80 mmHg as well as low-density lipoprotein cholesterol <2.6 mmol/l for the general DKD population and <1.8 mmol/l for those with previous history of atherosclerotic cardiovascular disease or eGFR <60 ml/min/1.73 $m^2$. Less stringent glycosylated hemoglobin targets are recommended for patients with impaired kidney function (≤8%) and older adults (8.5%). Sodium-glucose cotransporter-2 (SGLT2) inhibitors are currently recommended for DKD patients who fail to meet their glycemic target after metformin in the Chinese Mainland. Glucagon-like peptide-1 receptor agonists are recommended when SGLT2 inhibitors are not tolerated or contraindicated [117]. Referral to nephrologists is recommended for subjects with an eGFR <30 ml/min/1.73 $m^2$, or eGFR <60 ml/min/1.73 $m^2$ and accompanied by metabolic disorders, or uncertainty about the etiology of kidney disease [117].

Recent prospective study including 8811 subjects with DKD in Tangshan, China, followed for a median of 6.9 years [123] showed that the incidence of cardiovascular events, ESRD requiring dialysis, and all-cause mortality were 1227.3, 93.7, and 1626.4 per 100,000 person-years in subjects with DKD having isolated kidney function decline. The incidence of cardiovascular events, ESRD requiring dialysis, and all-cause mortality increased to 1976.6, 602.2, and 3886.5 per 100,000 person-years, respectively, in subjects with DKD having overt proteinuria combined with kidney function decline compared with 951.8, 2.4, and 354 per 100,000 person-years, respectively, for diabetic subjects without DKD [123].

The huge growing burden of DKD has prompted Chinese government and clinicians to focus on early screening, prevention, and evidence-based intervention for diabetes and DKD in China. Since the late 1980s, a series of primary prevention programs for diabetes and obesity were implemented in different parts of the Chinese Mainland. For example, the Da Qing Diabetes Prevention Study demonstrated positive benefits of lifestyle intervention in reducing the risk of cardiovascular and all-cause mortality among subjects with impaired glucose tolerance during a 23-year follow-up [124].

## Reimbursement Policies for DKD

In 2009, the Chinese government announced a healthcare reform plan to provide affordable and equitable basic universal healthcare by 2020. The basic national medical insurance scheme now covers over 95% of the residents in both developed and rural areas [125]. As CKD and diabetes are major chronic diseases, the basic medical insurance scheme provides insurance cover, most of which are partial cover, for all patients with DKD, including those with ESRD receiving HD or PD treatment. However, the reimbursement rates may vary from 70% to 90% of the expenses across regions with different socioeconomic status. New antidiabetic drugs such as SGLT-2 inhibitors and GLP-1 agonists are reimbursed by the national medical insurance scheme and available for use in DKD.

## Hypertension and Hypertension-Related Kidney Disease

The 2012–2015 national hypertension survey showed that the overall crude prevalence of hypertension was 27.9% (weighted rate 23.2%) in Chinese residents aged 18 and over and has increased compared to previously [126]. The prevalence of CKD in hypertensive subjects was 10.9–11.29% in the Chinese Mainland [127, 128]. On the other hand, CKD subjects showed a very high prevalence of hypertension. In one of the largest cross-sectional surveys that enrolled 6079 CKD participants (mean age, 51.0 ± 16.37 years) with or without hypertension from 22 centers across the Chinese Mainland, the prevalence, awareness, and treatment rates of hypertension were 71.2%, 95.4%, and 93.7%, respectively. However, blood pressure control rates (<140/90 and <130/80 mmHg) were only 41.1% and 15.0%, respectively. The prevalence of hypertension increased with increasing age, smoking, body mass index, low physical exercise, family history of hypertension, hyperuricemia, and increasing CKD severity.

Among patients with stage 1–5 CKD, 31% had hypertension. In patients with stage 3–5 CKD, 68–71% had hypertension. Blood pressure control rate was associated with CKD stage, blood pressure monitoring at home, and use of drug combinations [129]. Among patients receiving dialysis treatment, hypertension-related kidney disease (17%) was second to GD as the most common causes of ESRD [130].

Given the poor control rates of high blood pressure in the Chinese Mainland, the Intelligent Hypertension Center (IHEC) was set up by the China High Blood Pressure Alliance and Shanghai Hypertension Research Institute in recent years (http://www.ihec.org.cn), with the aim to standardize blood pressure management and improve blood pressure control rates in China using Internet platform and mobile technology. The China National Health and Food Safety Standard recommended that salt intake for healthy adult do not exceed 6 g salt (with 1 g salt equals to 400 mg sodium). However, it was noted that the daily salt intake for healthy adult in China averaged about 10.5 g (Chinese reference source).

The 2018 Chinese Guidelines for Prevention and Treatment of Hypertension recommended that the blood pressure goal for general hypertensive patients should be <140/90 mmHg (I, A) and further lower to <130/80 mmHg as tolerated or if patients belong to high-risk category (I, A).

In patients with CKD and urine albumin excretion <30 mg/24 h (or equivalence), blood pressure goal should be <140/90 mmHg (I, A), and with albuminuria ≥30 mg/24 h (or equivalence) <130/80 mmHg (IIA, B).

The initial antihypertensive therapy in CKD patients should include one ACEI (IIa) or ARB (IIb) alone or in combination with other antihypertensive drugs. Combination of ACEI and ARB is not recommended (A).

The recommended target blood pressure in patients with diabetes mellitus should be <130/80 mmHg (II a, B).

In the general elderly population aged 65–79 years with BPs ≥150 mmHg systolic and 90 mmHg diastolic, drug therapy is recommended (IA), and when BPs are ≥140 mmHg systolic and 90 mmHg diastolic, pharmacologic treatment should be considered (IIa, B); for elderly aged ≥80 years, pharmacologic treatment should be initiated if SBP ≥160 mmHg (IIa, B).

In elderly aged 65–79 years, pharmacologic treatment should be initiated if SBP ≥150 mmHg and DBP ≥90 mmHg. If the treatment is well tolerated, BP can be lowered to <140 mmHg systolic and 90 mmHg diastolic (IIa, B), and for elderly aged ≥80 years, BP should be lowered to <150 mmHg systolic and <90 mmHg diastolic (IIa, B) [131].

## Aging and Kidney Disease Burden

The Chinese Mainland has been an aging society since 1999 [132]. China's one-child policy, together with improvement in healthcare, has contributed to increased life expectancy and decreased China's birth rate. This demographic shift presents considerable social and economic challenges. According to the 6th China National Census, populations over the age of 60 years accounted for 13.26% of the total population in the Chinese Mainland [133].

An aging kidney is vulnerable to various stressors due to its structural and functional alterations. Aging is one of the major risk factors for the development of CKD [134]. Acute injury in aged kidney tends not to recover, leading to a higher risk of CKD and greater progression to ESRD in elderly [135]. The incidence and prevalence of CKD increased with increasing age. According to a population study from Beijing, the prevalence of CKD in the elderly aged between 60–69 years, 70–79 years, and older than 80 years was 20.8%, 30.5%, and 37.8%, respectively, and was much higher than that reported in the general population in the Chinese Mainland (10.8%) [9, 136] (Fig. 20.7).

The CK-NET ADR 2015 reported that 4.8% of the 18.5 million hospitalized patients had CKD [25]. The prevalence of CKD increased with age, reaching 6.2% and 9.69% for those patients aged 60 years and 85 years or older, respectively. Nearly half of the CKD patients were aged 60 years or older. Diabetes and hypertension were common among these patients (13.9% and 11.3%, respectively) and were common causes of CKD in the Chinese Mainland (27.0% for DKD and 20.8% for HTN).

The in-hospital mortality rate of CKD patients also increased with increasing age. The in-hospital mortality rate was 2.47% for subjects aged between 65 and 69 years but increased to 7.63% for those aged 80 years or over and was much higher than subjects with diabetes and non-CKD in the same age group (Table 20.3) [137]. Data from the CNRDS also observed an increase in the mean age of prevalent dialysis patients, from 53.1 years in 2011 to 55.7 years in 2015. Patients' aged ≥60 years accounted for 33.42% of incident dialysis population in 2011 and rose to 39.87% in 2015. In economically developed areas of China, nearly half of the incident dialysis patients had age ≥60 years [138].

Death was a more likely event than progression to ESRD in CKD subjects aged ≥60 years due to complications and comorbidities. CK-NET data showed that the mortality rates among Chinese CKD subjects aged 18–44 years, 45–64 years, and > 65 years were 11.80, 31.57, and 91.69 per 1000 patient-years, respectively. The all-cause mortality risk was nearly sevenfold higher in CKD subjects aged ≥65 years than in

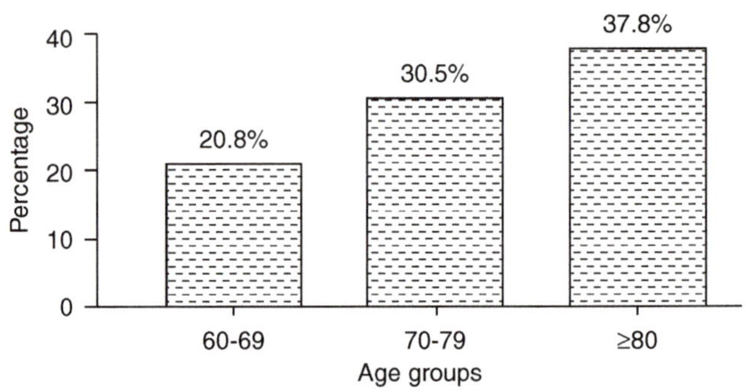


Fig. 20.7 The prevalence of CKD in elderly

Table 20.3 In-hospital mortality rate (%). Mortality rate is in % stratified by age group

| Age group | CKD | DM | Non-CKD |
|---|---|---|---|
| 65–69 | 2.47 | 1.27 | 0.95 |
| 70–74 | 3.43 | 1.83 | 1.30 |
| 75–79 | 5.12 | 2.79 | 1.96 |
| 80–84 | 7.63 | 4.32 | 2.94 |

*Note*: *CKD* chronic kidney disease, *DM* diabetes mellitus subjects aged 18–44 years [138]. However, mortality rate from CK-NET registry may be underestimated because patients covered by commercial insurance scheme in the CK-NET registry may generally have higher socioeconomic status and better health awareness than those without insurance coverage.

Elderly CKD subjects also suffered more depression, cognitive impairment, and protein-energy wasting [139]. The C-OPTION was a prospective observational study in 1079 elderly CKD subjects recruited from 32 clinic centers from 24 provinces in the Chinese Mainland [140]. The estimated prevalence of depression was around 23.0% in elderly Chinese CKD subjects and the severity of depression correlated with the degree of kidney dysfunction. Furthermore, depression had a major negative impact on health-related quality of life (HRQOL) [141]. Further studies will need to examine risk factors for CKD progression among elderly population and develop models to identify elderly who are at high risk for CKD progression.

## Renal Replacement Therapy

In keeping with a global increase in the incidence and prevalence of ESRD [142], the burden of ESRD is on the rise in the Chinese Mainland. According to the CNRDS, the number of ESRD patients receiving dialysis treatment has increased from 261,877 in 2011 to 610,811 by the end of 2017 (Fig. 20.8) [143]. This poses a huge burden on healthcare resources and manpower need. Among the registered dialysis population, HD accounted for 86%, while PD accounted for 14% (Fig. 20.8).

The reasons for limited access to PD in the Chinese Mainland include geographical variations in socioeconomic status, differences in access to healthcare between rural and urban areas, lack of training and education for healthcare professionals, and quality control in most parts of China. To facilitate and increase PD utilization, the Chinese government adjusted the reimbursement policies, introduced new insurance systems (especially in rural areas), and initiated and supported the local production of PD solutions. Currently, 90% of the PD solutions consumed in the Chinese Mainland were imported, and international trade agreements were in place to reduce overall costs.

Kidney transplantation program began in the 1960s and the number of kidney transplants showed steady increase since 1985, with 1-year transplant graft survival above 80% between 1985 and 1993. There were two landmark developments for kidney transplantation policy in the Chinese Mainland in the last 10 years. First, it has become mandatory to allocate kidney organs for kidney transplantation through the China Organ Transplant Response System (COTRS) which is a national, open, and transparent computerized organ allocation system set up since September 1, 2013 [137]. Second, since January 1, 2015, organs from death row prisoners were banned and civil donation has become the only legal source of organ donation. The number of kidney transplantations has grown from 1009 cases in 2010 to

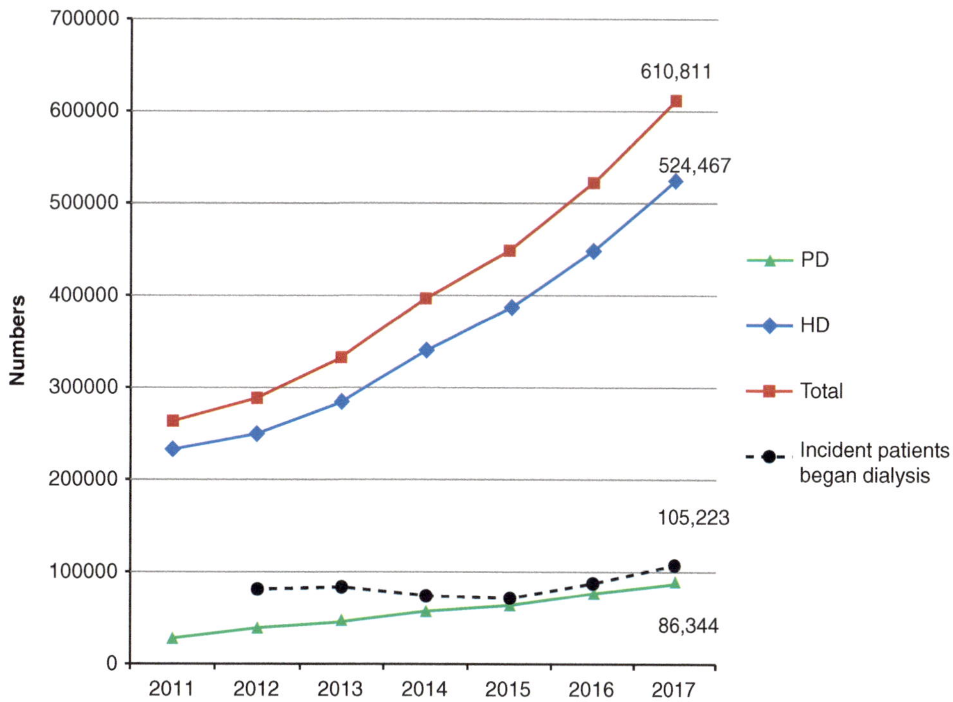


**Fig. 20.8** The increasing number of hemodialysis, peritoneal dialysis, and total dialysis patients in the Chinese Mainland between 2011 and 2017. Data was from the Chinese National Renal Data System. Solid line indicated prevalent dialysis patients at each year and dashed line indicated incident patients began dialysis at each year

13,029 cases in 2018 [144] (Fig. 20.9). The estimated 1-year and 5-year kidney graft survival rate ranged between 91% and 98.3% and 73.2% and 88.6% in different centers, respectively [144].

## Hemodialysis

### Prevalence of HD

HD is the predominant dialysis modality, accounting for 90.96% of all dialysis in the Chinese Mainland [127]. According to a nationwide registration in 1999, the prevalence of dialysis was 33.2 pmp [145] and increased rapidly to 237.3 pmp in 2012 [26] and 442.13 pmp in 2015 [127]. The 2018 National Report on the Services, Quality and Safety in Medical Care System issued by the National Health Commission of the PRC showed that HD patients have continued to grow from 174.1 pmp in 2011 to 379.1 pmp in 2017 in the Chinese Mainland (Fig. 20.10). The prevalence of HD showed a significant increase in the last 10 years as government-operated medical insurance scheme reimburses a large proportion of the RRT since 2010. Patients only need to contribute a small amount for their RRT. However, the prevalence of RRT in the Chinese Mainland remains much lower compared with other developed regions/countries including Hong Kong Special Administrative Region (HKSAR) [146], Taiwan Province [147], Singapore, Japan, and the USA.

It is anticipated that the prevalence of RRT will continue to increase in the Chinese Mainland and there will be a rapid growth in the number of dialysis centers in the near future. The physician- and nurse-to-patient ratios in HD centers are currently much lower when compared with other countries.

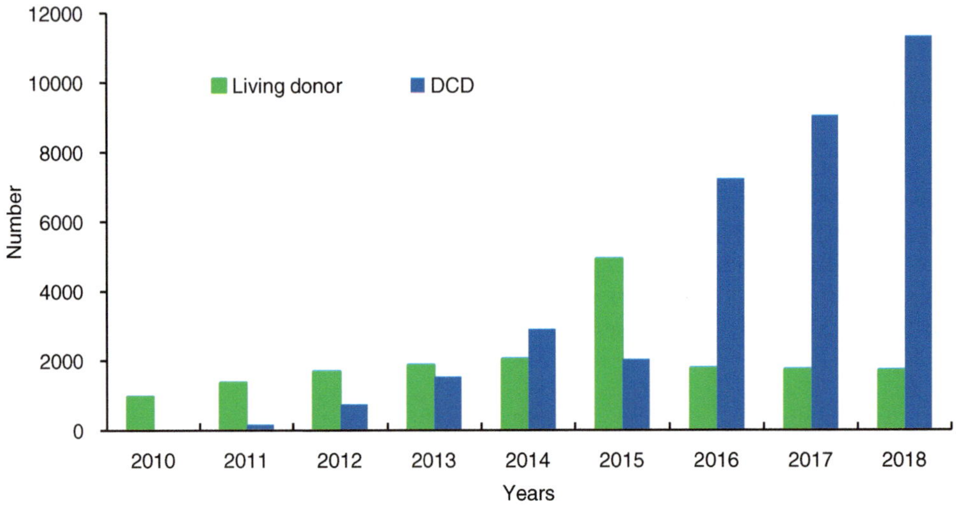


**Fig. 20.9** Number of kidney transplantations in the Chinese Mainland between 2009 and 2018. Abbreviation: DCD, donation after circulatory death

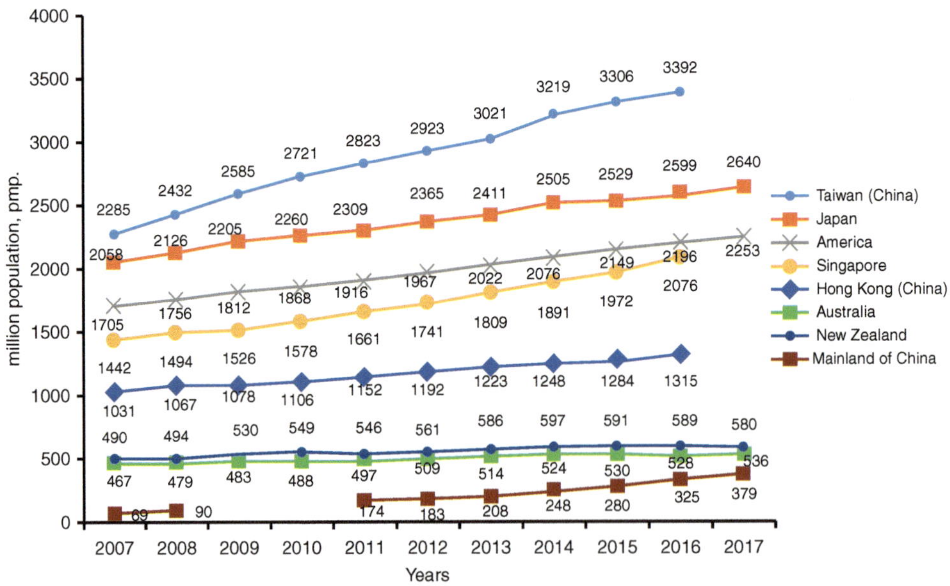


**Fig. 20.10** Number of prevalent dialysis patients per million population by year in different countries and cities

In Chinese Mainland, the average number of dialysis stations in each dialysis center is around 25–30, but larger ones may have more than 100 stations. The average number of patients per center is around 100. As an example, in Beijing and Shanghai, the smallest center has only 4 dialysis stations with 12 patients, but the largest HD center has 150 dialysis stations with 600 patients (unpublished data). The standard operating procedures (SOP) formulated by the Chinese National Health Commission require that there should be at least two physicians in each HD center and one nurse taking care of no more than five patients during one HD session. Meanwhile, each HD center should have one dialysis technician taking care of machines and water and dialysate quality. For PD centers, there should be one physician and one nurse taking care of 20–30 PD patients. Every 50 or 80 PD patients increase in the center should be accompanied by one nurse and one physician increase. On average, each nurse takes care of around 100 PD patients in most PD centers. Currently there are around 2000 PD physicians and 900 PD nurses in the Chinese Mainland. The number of patients per PD center may range between 20 and 1000. Most centers in the Chinese Mainland do not have psychologist, social worker, or renal dietitian.

## Current Status of HD

From the CK-NET 2015 ADR, arteriovenous fistula (AVF) and arteriovenous graft (AVG) were the predominant vascular access used, accounting for 80.48% of all vascular accesses used in prevalent HD patients [127]. Fewer diabetics used AVF and/or AVG than nondiabetics (57.73% versus 84.80%). On the other hand, incident HD patients used more catheters as vascular access than prevalent patients. From the Shanghai 2015 ADR, 31.38% of incident HD patients used short-term catheter, and 13.67% used long-term catheter (Fig. 20.11). The mean HD session length adopted in HD facilities was 243 min, and the mean blood flow rate was 235 mL/min [148]. Nearly a quarter of the HD population receives twice-weekly HD [148, 149]. According to observational data from the China Dialysis Outcomes and Practice Patterns Study (DOPPS), 19% of patients received twice-weekly HD, and 78% received thrice-weekly HD. Patients who received twice-weekly HD had similar survival and hospitalization rates compared with patients who received thrice-weekly HD [150].

Hemodiafiltration (HDF) use increased from 7% in 2007 to 42% in 2014 [151] and majority of patients received HDF once a week. Usually online HDF is done. Most centers use post-dilution method and the convective volume commonly used is around 15 L per session. According to China DOPPS5 (2012–2015), 15.6% of HD patients had hepatitis B and 8.5% had hepatitis C (unpublished data). Dialyzer reuse is allowed but no centers in China currently reuse dialyzers.

## Survival Rate of Patients Receiving Hemodialysis

A study from Beijing that followed 11,175 HD patients for 8 years showed that patients who initiated dialysis with an eGFR ≥15 ml/min per 1.73 $m^2$ and between 10 and 15 ml/min per 1.73 $m^2$ had higher mortality rate than those that started dialysis with eGFR between 5 and 10 or <5 ml/min per 1.73 $m^2$ (unpublished data). In Beijing, patients who initiated dialysis "early" (eGFR>10 ml/min per 1.73 $m^2$) accounted for 15% of new dialysis start [152], and thus, there is a potential to delay the start of dialysis in the ESRD population in the Chinese Mainland.

Notably, the mortality rate in the first 2 months after dialysis initiation was high in the Chinese Mainland; thereafter mortality rate reduced to a lower level and stabilized at 90 days after dialysis initiation [152]. The mortality rate was nearly 30 per 100 patient-years for diabetic patients in the first month after dialysis initiation but was much higher in nondiabetic patients (50 per 100 patient-years) [152]. The

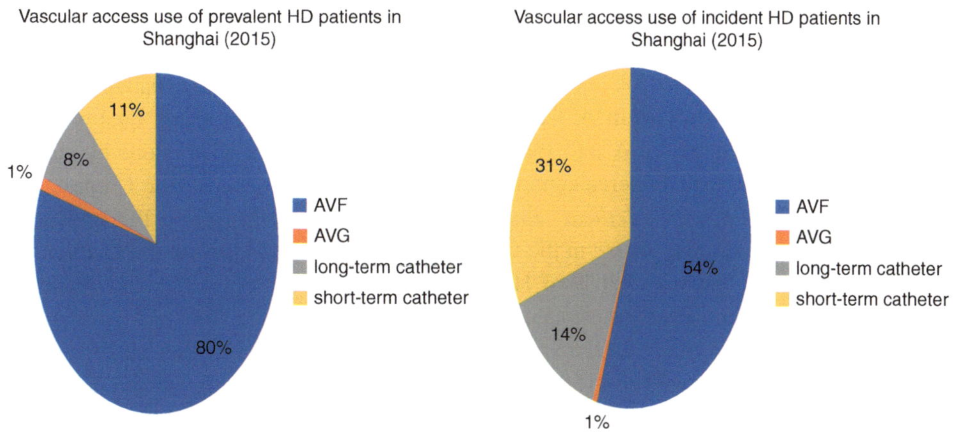


**Fig. 20.11** Vascular access use of prevalent/incident HD patients in Shanghai, China (2015)

exact explanation for this finding is uncertain. One speculation may be that better pre-dialysis care in diabetic patients may contribute to survival benefits 90 days after dialysis initiation than nondiabetics.

The raw annual maintenance HD (MHD) mortality in Beijing has increased from 47.8 per 1000 patient-years in 2007 to 76.8 in 2010 [153] but was still lower when compared with the US Renal Data System (USRDS) results (236.3 in 2009). In Shanghai, the annual MHD patients mortality rate was 7.5% in 2005 [154] and was lower than the mortality reported in Europe (15.6%) and the USA (21.7%) in 2003 but similar to that reported in Japan (6.6%). The observed survival advantage for HD patients in China/Asia compared to the western counterparts could be in part explained by differences in race and practice patterns among different countries.

## Management of Anemia and Mineral and Bone Disorder

Anemia management in dialysis patients is a challenge in the Chinese Mainland. Data from China DOPPS4 showed that 21% of MHD patients had hemoglobin (Hgb) level <9 g/dl, compared with ≤10% in Japan and the USA [155]. Possible reasons for more anemia in Chinese HD patients could be the following: First, more patients from China received twice-weekly HD than other DOPPS countries. Second, erythropoietin-stimulating agent (ESA) dose used in China was lower than in the USA. Third, there was low insurance coverage for ESA treatment in China. In 2018, roxadustat, an oral hypoxia-inducible factor stabilizer and propyl hydroxylase inhibitor, was approved for treatment of anemia in dialysis patients in the Chinese Mainland. A 26-week, phase 3 trial showed that oral roxadustat was non-inferior to parenteral epoetin alfa in treating anemia in Chinese dialysis patients [15], providing a novel treatment for renal anemia.

According to the questionnaires distributed to the dialysis facility director in DOPPS5, the Chinese translated KDIGO guideline was the reference guide for mineral and bone disorder (BMD) management in the Chinese Mainland. However, serum calcium, phosphorus, and parathyroid hormone (PTH) control were not optimal. DOPPS5 showed that more HD patients in the Chinese Mainland had hypocalcemia than in the USA and Europe, and the percentage of subjects with hypercalcemia was higher than other countries (*Chinese Medical Journal*, in press). Phosphate control was also worse in the Chinese Mainland than other DOPPS countries (26% of HD patients in the Chinese Mainland had serum phosphate >7.0 mg/dL compared with 7–10% in other DOPPS countries). Twenty-seven percent had serum PTH <150 pg/ml, and 21% had PTH >600 pg/ml.

## HD Quality Control

In 1998, Shanghai took the lead to set up the Hemodialysis Quality Control Center. The Beijing Health Bureau also established the Hemodialysis Quality Control and Improvement Center (BJHDQCIC) in 2002. Since then, dialysis quality control centers were established in various provinces and regions to promote the standardization of HD and strengthen the quality control of HD service.

This coincided with the setup of CNRDS in 2010, of which comprehensive epidemiological data of all dialysis patients were collected nationwide. It enables the government to work out healthcare financing and formulate health policies. The CNRDS also published the Blood Purification SOP in 2010 that provided detailed guidelines recommendations on safe and quality HD service delivery.

In 2017, China national standardization management committee published a consortium on standard management regulations. Some organizations published their consortium standard for HD facility configuration (to be published by ZGC Nephrology Blood Purification Innovation Alliance) and service (published by Chinese Hospital Association) [156] to assure safe and quality HD service provision by all HD facilities.

## Peritoneal Dialysis

Similar to some developing countries in Asia [157], the Chinese Mainland is home to a large number of low-income people who live in rural and remote areas where HD facility may not be available or not accessible [158]. PD serves as a more feasible and cost-effective alternative dialysis modality than HD and has been in use in the Chinese Mainland for over 30 years [158]. Most patients do CAPD with four bags (2L/bag) per day, while only 0.9% of patients receive automated peritoneal dialysis (APD) [158]. Primary GD accounted for about 50% of background kidney disease in PD patients, while DKD accounted only for 15%~16% [143]. Table 20.4 shows the background causes of kidney disease in incident PD patients. Observational studies showed that patients receiving PD had comparable clinical outcomes and quality of life as those receiving HD [159]. Since PD is done by patients/caregivers at home and incurs lower cost, the Chinese government has been actively promoting more PD utilization nationwide. This explains the rapid growth in PD utilization in the Chinese Mainland in the last 10 years [158]. The provision of PD education programs for health professionals by high-quality PD centers and nephrologists and health professionals trained in PD also contribute to increased PD utilization in the Chinese Mainland [160]. A representative model is the satellite center

**Table 20.4** The composition of primary kidney diseases for incident PD patients at each year

| Year | Primary glomerular disease (%) | Diabetic kidney disease (%) | Hypertensive nephropathy (%) | Polycystic kidney disease (%) | Tubulointerstitial disease (%) | Others (%) |
|---|---|---|---|---|---|---|
| 2013 | 52.6 | 15.6 | 14.9 | 1.5 | 1.4 | 14.0 |
| 2014 | 54.1 | 16.2 | 14.4 | 1.5 | 1.5 | 12.3 |
| 2015 | 50.8 | 16.1 | 15.1 | 1.4 | 1.7 | 14.9 |
| 2016 | 50.0 | 16.2 | 16.6 | 1.4 | 1.6 | 14.2 |
| 2017 | 51.1 | 13.0 | 14.3 | 1.3 | 1.6 | 18.8 |

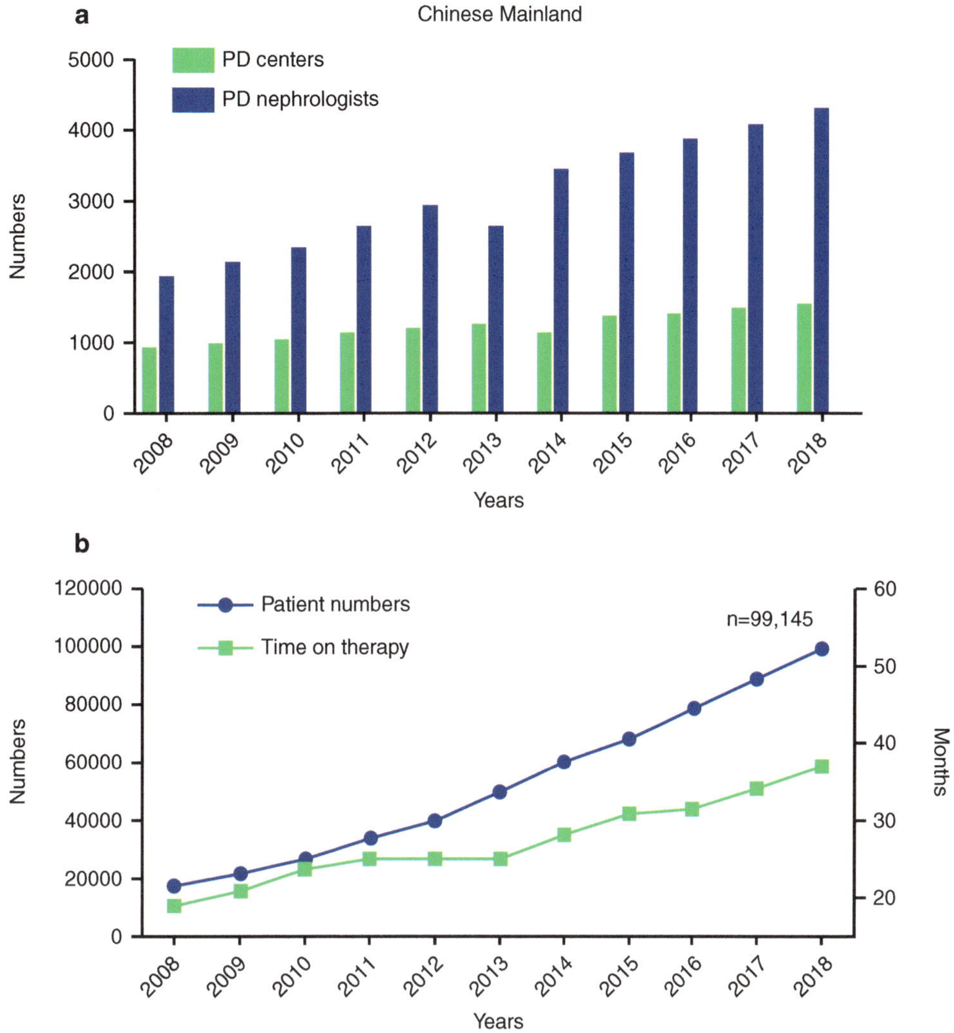


**Fig. 20.12** (**a**) An increasing number of PD centers and nephrologists working in PD treatment in the Chinese Mainland in the last 10 years. (**b**) An increasing number of PD patients along with increasing duration of PD therapy over in the Chinese Mainland the last 10 years

program established at the Sun Yat-sen University PD center in Guangzhou, China. The center has trained dozens of centers, and over hundreds of nephrologists and nurses have become very experienced with PD practices and procedures across the Guangdong Province [161]. As depicted in Fig. 20.10, PD centers have increased from 930 in 2008 to 1560 in 2018 in the Chinese Mainland, reflecting an average increase of 63 new PD centers per annum [143]. Accordingly, the number of nephrologists who practice PD has more than doubled in 10 years' time (Fig. 20.12a) [143]. The number of ESRD patients receiving PD treatment has also grown remarkably from 17,897 in 2008 to the latest 99,145 in 2018, and the number is still on the rise (Fig. 20.12b) [143]. Figure 20.13 shows the distribution of PD utilization on a provincial level by 2018, the top ranked provinces being Guangdong and Zhejiang, with over 9000 PD patients in total [143]. Government's active promotion, national medical insurance coverage, improvement in PD technology, PD being a home-based therapy, and lower overall cost than HD are all important elements that drive the growth in PD utilization [162]. Currently, PD accounts for only about 20% of the dialysis modality in ESRD [158]. Since less developed cities and more remote areas have resource constraints in expanding HD facility and service, it adds incentives for

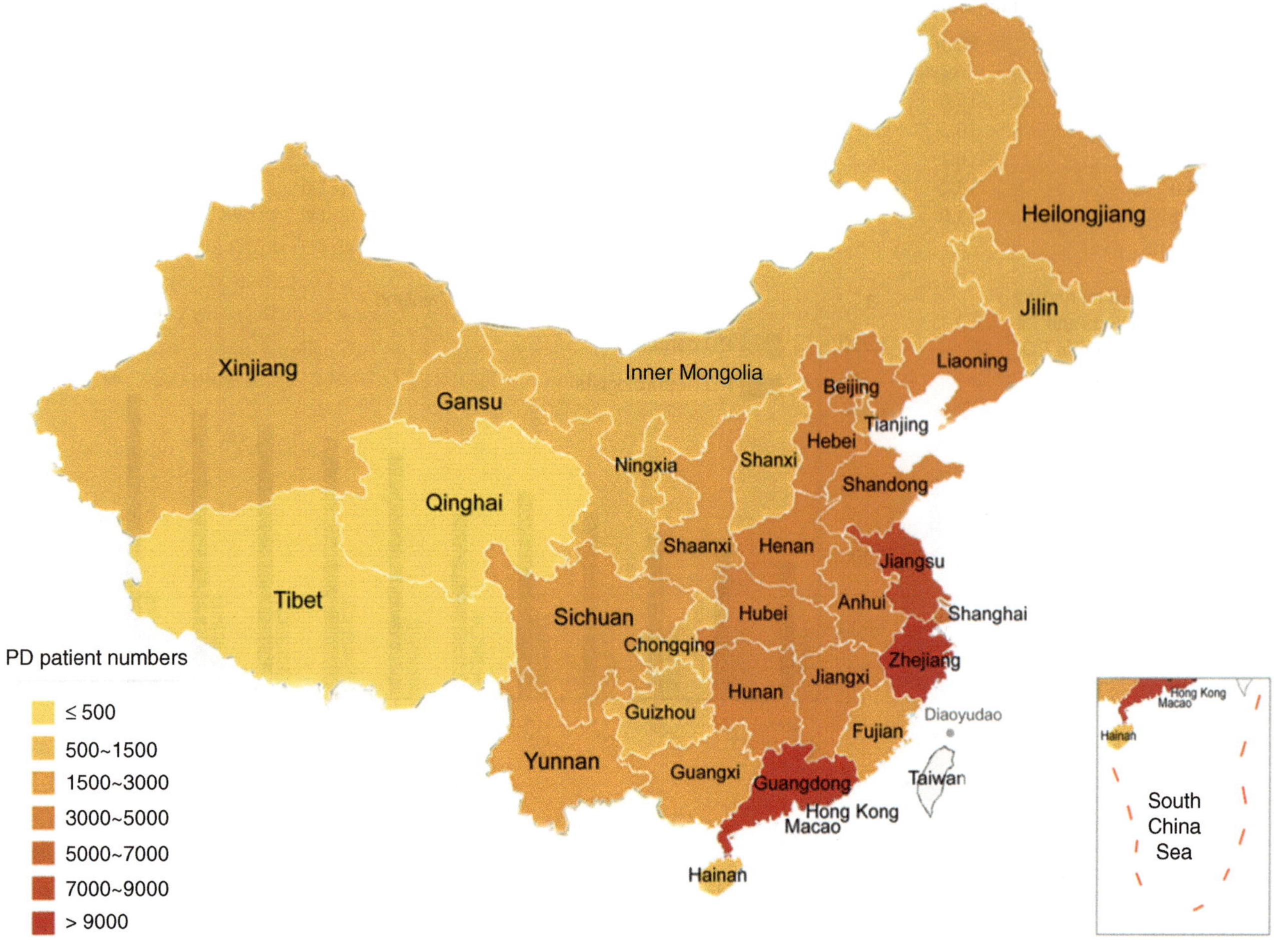


**Fig. 20.13** The distribution of PD utilization in a provincial level in the Chinese Mainland. Note: PD, peritoneal dialysis. Data calculated from CNRDS [1], while Hong Kong, Macao, and Taiwan were not included in the statistical map

more PD utilization as the therapy is home-based and overall less costly than HD. Furthermore, patients are more engaged and empowered in managing their own dialysis treatment [160], and the average time on PD therapy (technique survival) has increased from a mean of 19.2 to 37.1 months in the last decade [144] (Table 20.5).

Nephrologists in the Chinese Mainland have put tremendous efforts in developing high-quality PD programs in the last 10 years [158, 160, 170]. Table 20.5 listed the published reports of clinical outcomes of PD patients from large university-affiliated PD centers in the Chinese Mainland between 2008 and 2018, showing high patient survival rates and technique survival rates as well as low peritonitis rates [163–165, 168, 171, 172] compared to international reports. A recent observational study from the Chinese Mainland reported that patients who initiated PD during 2011–2015 had better survival than those that initiated PD between 2005 and 2010 [163]. Cardiovascular disease and infection are the two leading causes of death in PD patients. The key elements of a successful PD program include a multidisciplinary, collaborative team with nephrologists, nurses, and patients/carers together with a comprehensive social support system [160]. Nephrologists in the Chinese Mainland have dedicated tremendous efforts in developing PD research programs in basic, translational, and clinical science with an aim to identify evidence-based interventions to advance PD care quality. Between 2008 and 2018, the numbers of PD-related publications from the Chinese Mainland in local and international journals have increased substantially [173]. Of note, the number of PD-related publications in internationally indexed journals has increased from 34 in 2008 to 92 in 2016, with an average annual growth rate of 13% [173]. This reflects strong interests and engagement of nephrologists in the Chinese Mainland in PD research, growing impact of Chinese Mainland's PD research on the global PD community, and China gradually taking the lead as one of the major countries that contribute to advances in PD technology and practices.

Table 20.5 A review of the clinical outcomes of PD patients in major PD centers of the Chinese Mainland

| District | Reference | Number of cases | Time of review | Peritonitis rate (patients' month per episode) | Technique survival | Patient survival |
|---|---|---|---|---|---|---|
| Guangzhou | Yang et al. [163, 164] | 2021 | 2006–2014 | 75[170] | 1 year: 97%<br>3 years: 90%<br>5 years: 83%<br>10 years: 57% | 1 year: 97%<br>3 years: 87%<br>5 years: 74% |
| Beijing | Xu et al. [165] | 307 | 2002–2007 | 50.1~76.7 | – | 1 year: 97%<br>3 years: 71%<br>5 years: 51% |
| Beijing | Li et al. [166] | 577 | 1996–2015 | 77 | 1 year: 96.5%<br>3 years:89.1%<br>5 years: 81.7% | 1 year: 91.3%<br>3 years: 70.9%<br>5 years: 49.7% |
| Shanghai | Fang et al. [167] | 339 | 2005–2009 | 62.5 | 1 year: 96%<br>3 years: 92%<br>5 years: 82% | 1 year: 93%<br>3 years: 82%<br>5 years: 71% |
| Zhejiang | Chen et al. [168] | 712 | 2004–2011 | 75 | 1 year: 95%<br>3 years: 88%<br>5 years: 80% | 1 year: 96%<br>3 years: 85%<br>5 years: 76% |
| Nanjing | Liu et al. [169] | 619 | 2005–2011 | 22.86~77.25 | 1 year: 90%~96%<br>2 years: 79%~93%<br>3 years: 77%~93% | 1 year: 93%~97%<br>2 years: 82%~96%<br>3 years: 67%~96% |

## Dialysis Reimbursement Policies

The median annual overall cost for PD was lower than that of HD (73,266 RMB vs. 87,125 RMB per patient per year) [137]. With China Healthcare Reform, basic medical insurance now provides coverage for over 95% of its residents. The National Social Medical Insurance reimburses around 70% of the total medical expenditures with PD. In urban areas, for example, HD and PD patients had, on average, around 70.5% and 68.4% of the medical expenditures reimbursed, respectively [137, 158]. The National Development and Reform Commission has recently increased government insurance coverage for dialysis-related expenses [158]. This will facilitate and improve accessibility to dialysis treatment for ESRD patients in the Chinese Mainland.

## Organ Procurement and Transplant Policies

In 2007, the Chinese Mainland promulgated the Regulations on Human Organ Transplantation with a new national program for deceased organ donation, procurement, allocation, and transplantation implemented in 2013 [174]. Organs harvest from executed prisoners has been banned since January 2015 [175]. Three categories of deceased donors issued by the Organ Transplantation Committee under the Ministry of Health in China were summarized as follows: Category I, donation after brain death (DBD); Category II, donation after cardiac death (DCD), the same as the Maastricht categories (started in the Chinese Mainland in 2010) [176]; and Category III, DBCD, organ donation after brain death followed by circulatory death [177].

According to China's Human Organs Acquisition and Distribution Management Regulations, organ donation is to be coordinated and processed by organ procurement organizations (OPOs), which are composed of organ transplant surgeons, neurologists, neurosurgeons, nurses, critical care medicine experts, and transplant coordinators.

## The Process of Organ Donation

After a potential deceased donor is identified in a hospital, the doctors will inform patient's relatives of his/her illness status. The transplant coordinator will be involved in offering the potential donor's immediate family the option of being a DCD donor. The potential donor could have his/her organs donated if (1) the deceased has expressed willingness to donate organs in either a living will or other written form; (2) their immediate family provides written consent for organ donation if the deceased has not expressed opposition to donating his/her organs prior to death; or (3) the deceased has verbally expressed a wish to donate while in a conscious state in the presence of two doctors, who are not part of the organ procurement or transplantation team, and the deceased' s immediate family does not object [176]. The attending physicians will contact the OPO, and the OPO will be responsible for overall evaluation of the potential organ donor. The neurologists/neurosurgeons need to make sure that the deceased fulfills the Harvard definition of brain death. The transplant surgeons will be involved in organ evaluation but the transplant team is not allowed to contact relatives of the donor. The transplant coordinators are responsible for all the liaisons work. They need to confirm that the deceased individual meets all the abovementioned criteria as an organ donor and all the required written consents have been signed by the deceased donor's immediate family with witness from an independent observer from the Red Cross. In Guangdong Province, the package of clinical and ethical data will be presented to the ethical committee for approval before organ donation. To avoid organ trafficking, direct financial compensation to the deceased donor's family is forbidden. However, medical aid and funeral allowance is permissible.

DBDs will be procured after declaration of brain death according to the diagnostic criteria of brain death [178]. Following declaration of brain death in DBCD or DCDs, written consent for deceased organ donation and withdrawal of life support will be obtained from the donor's immediate family. The obtained consent for organ donation will then be reported to the Organ Donation Committee, who will supervise the DBCD or DCD process. Deceased donors are monitored with invasive blood pressure sensors in the operating room. Following condolences, mechanical ventilation and vasopressors will be withdrawn and vital signs will continue to be monitored. The definition of cardiac death is determined according to the aforementioned criteria, and death is declared after 5 minutes of observation following cardiac arrest and then the organ procurement will initiate. The protocols for DBD, DBCD, and DCD in the Chinese Mainland are detailed in the national guidelines for organ donation [174, 177].

## Organ Allocation and Transplant Waitlist Registry

The legal framework for organ donation is in place in accordance with the WHO guidelines on organ transplantation. A third-party nonprofit organization is involved in implementing organ donation policy according to the law [179]. Deceased organ allocation in the Chinese Mainland is now done via China's Organ Transplant Response System (COTRS), an electronic distribution system maintained by the independent China Transplant Response System Research Center that is affiliated with the University of Hong Kong. The principles in the State Council Regulation call for "fairness, justice, and transparency" in assessing the medical need of waitlisted patients. This State Council directive is designed to ensure fairness and public trust in the organ allocation system [174].

Before harvesting the deceased organs, information of the deceased donor will be uploaded to the organ allocation system. Organ allocation takes into consideration medical urgency, waiting time for patients on the waitlist, HLA compatibility, and patients' clinical need. The organ allocation is conducted electronically to ensure transparency and fairness of the process. In principle, the hospital where the OPO is located has the highest priority to receive the organs. If no eligible recipients are identified from that hospital, the donated organs will be allocated to another hospital that is out of region from the primary OPO. After kidney transplant, data of the recipients will be uploaded to the registry system within 72 hours. The China Health Authority will verify the recipients' identity to avoid illegal change of recipients.

A national registry of transplant recipients has been established [174] and is integrated with the COTRS and other regulatory databases. This enables a national surveillance network for organ procurement and transplantation in the Chinese Mainland and prevents possible illegal organ trafficking, procurement, and transplant activities.

## Future Perspectives of Organ Donation

The Chinese Mainland needs to set up a national registration for volunteers of organ donation and actively promote both living-related and deceased donor's organ donation. Other issues to be addressed include setting up an independent foundation managed by an independent third party to provide some medical aid and funeral service allowances to donor's immediate family [180].

## Kidney Transplantation in the New Era

Organ Transplantation began in the Chinese Mainland in the 1960s and is one of the largest organ transplant programs in the world, reaching over 13,000 transplants per year in 2004. The first living-related kidney transplant was done in 1972. The number of organ donors and organ transplants has steadily increased since the use of DCD in 2010 (Fig. 20.14). According to the Chinese Scientific Registry of Kidney Transplantation (CSRKT), 37,873 kidney transplants from DCD and 15,309 from living donor were performed between 2010 and 2018 [181]. However, this number remained far from meeting the demand for organ transplants in ESRD patients in the Chinese Mainland. It was estimated that 1–1.5 million people in the Chinese Mainland require organ transplantation every year. However, data from the China Organ Donation Administration Center showed that the estimated deceased organ donation rate increased gradually to 3.71 per million Chinese population in 2017 (Fig. 20.15) and only around 10,000 patients received organ transplantation per year.

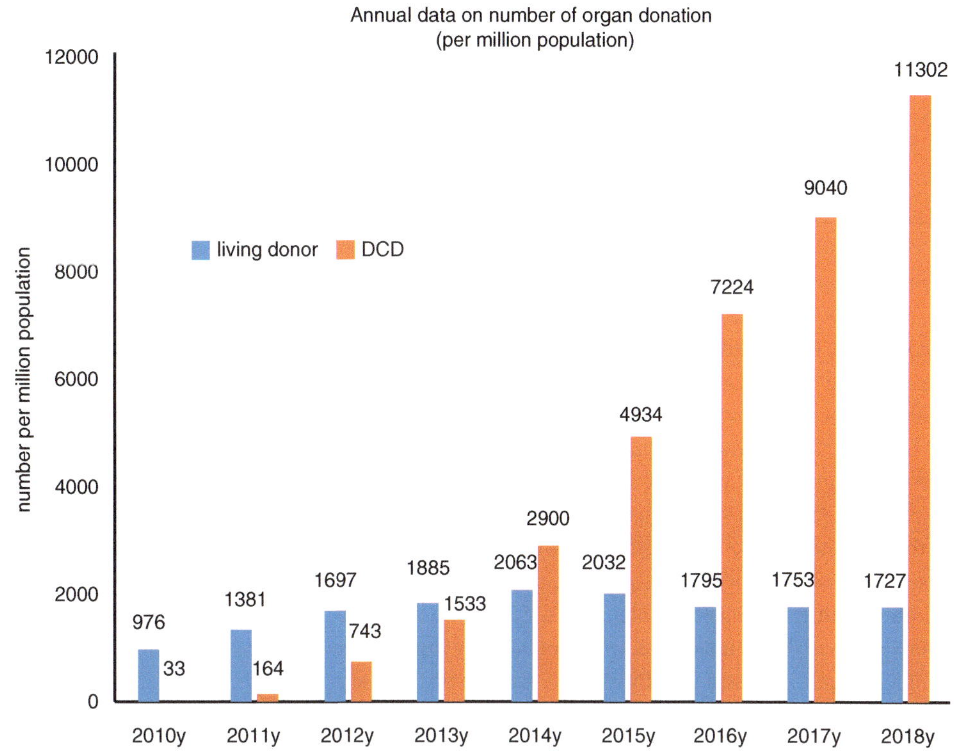


**Fig. 20.14** China annual kidney transplantation from different donor sources between 2010 and 2018. (Data from Chinese Scientific Registry of Kidney Transplantation)

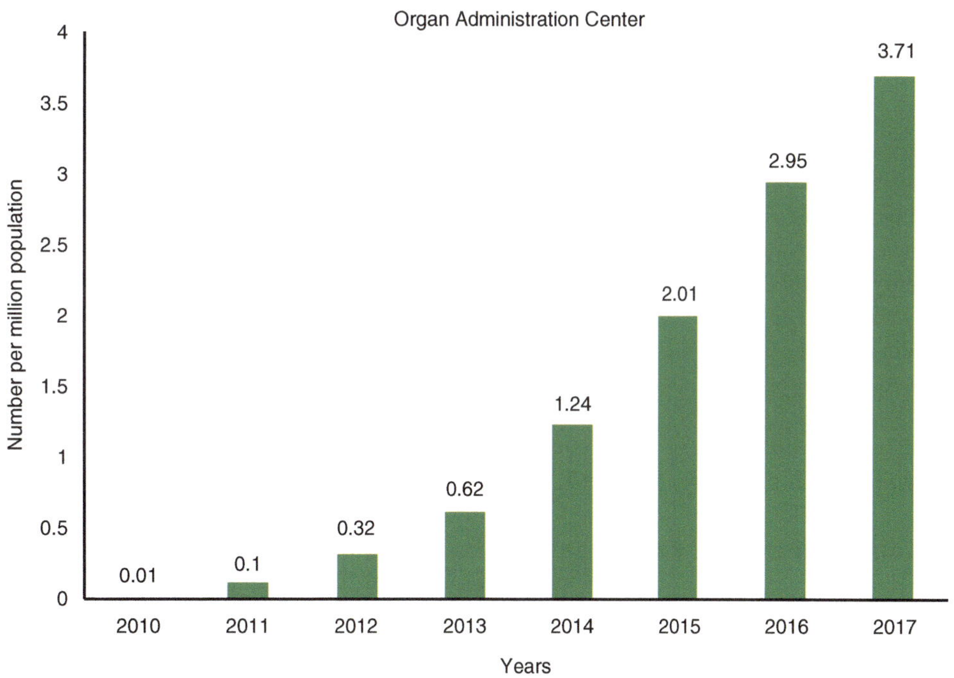


**Fig. 20.15** Annual data on organ donation (per million population). (Data from Chinese Organ Administration Center)

A questionnaire survey conducted among holders of driving license in the Chinese Mainland showed that although 74.4% of survey respondents supported voluntary organ donation and 64.0% advocated organ donation after death, only 48.4% expressed willingness to be organ donors themselves [182]. In another recent survey of organ donation among healthcare professionals in eight hospitals in 2013/2014, only 19.6% of the surveyed healthcare professionals knew where organ procurement and donations were conducted, and only 13.7% knew how the procedure of organ donation happens [183]. Thus, more active promotion campaigns and education are required to promote voluntary organ donations among healthcare professionals, other than the public in China.

In 2014, the Chinese Mainland launched its official organ donation registration websites www.savelife.org.cn or www.rcsccod.cn. All Chinese citizens can register as organ donors in the two sites. Since then, organ donation from community-based deceased donor has become one of the two legitimate primary sources of transplantable organs. Allocation of organs from deceased donor are conducted automatically through the China Organ Transplant Response Electronic System (COTRS, http://www.cot.org.cn) since September 1, 2013, as mandated by the Chinese government to ensure fairness and transparency in the donor organ allocation process [184].

The Red Cross Society has played an important role in registering organ donations in the Chinese Mainland in the past two decades since its establishment. From 2008 to 2009, the Red Cross Society received 10,423 registrations of donations [185]. Furthermore, the organization of organ donation and transplantation in the Chinese Mainland was restructured. According to the COTRS and scientific registries (as of February 3, 2016), between January 1, 2015, and December 31, 2015, there were 2766 community-based deceased organ donations, resulting in 2150 liver transplants, 4931 kidney transplants, 279 heart transplants, and 118 lung transplants.

Figure 20.16 presents the annual number of kidney transplants performed between 2010 and 2018 from different donor sources in the Chinese Mainland (data from CSRKT). DCD is now the dominant source of organ donation and transplantation since 2014. The total number of cases has increased from 2900 in 2014 to 11,302 in 2018. Despite some initial fluctuations, there was a steady increase of kidney transplants in the Chinese Mainland since 2015, especially donations after cardiac death, which is anticipated to continue to increase. Some kidney transplant-related data from 2018 are shown in Figs. 20.17, 20.18, and 20.19.

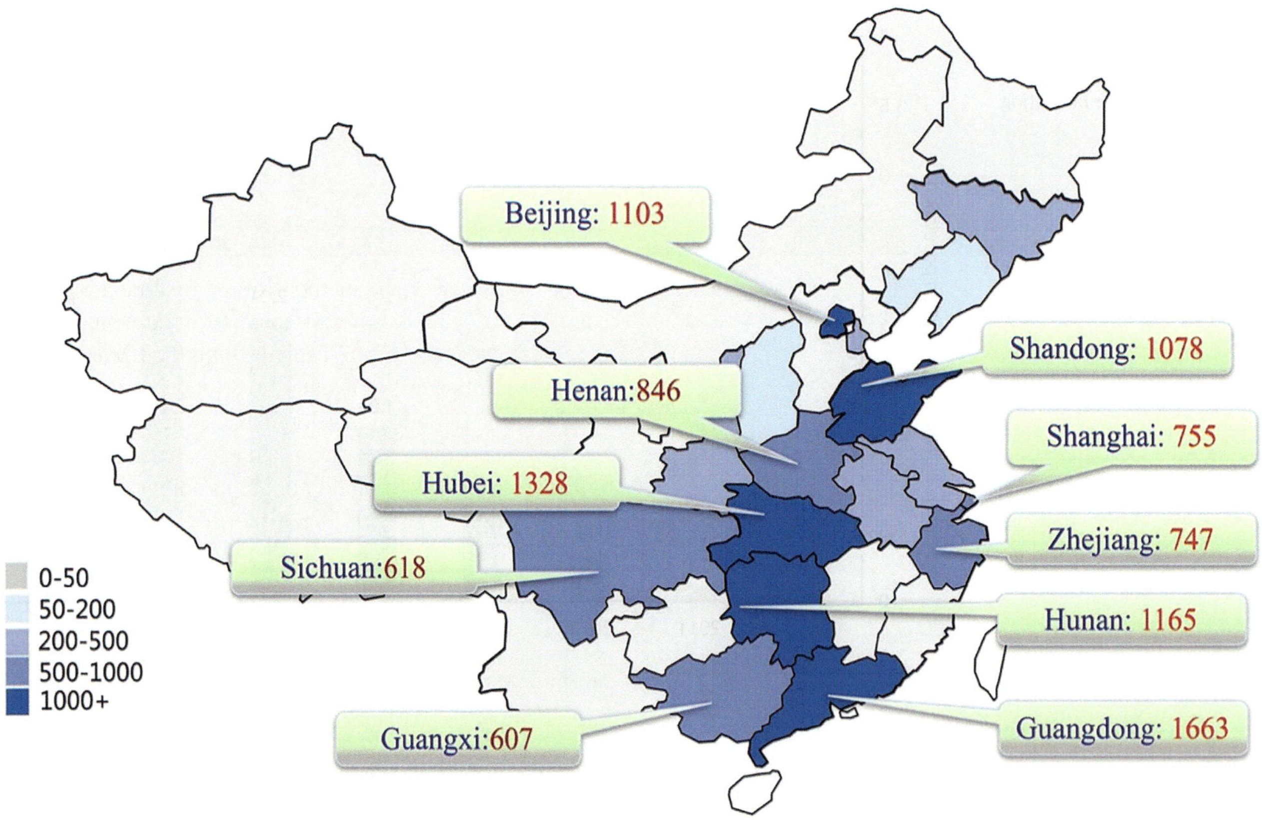


Fig. 20.16 An overview of kidney transplant in 2018. (Data from CSRKT)

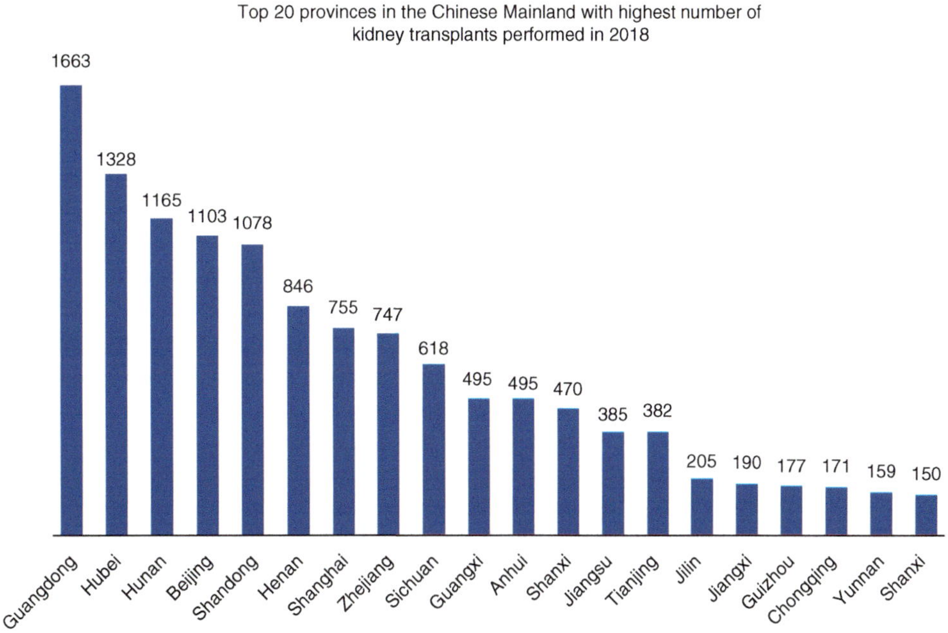


**Fig. 20.17** Top 20 provinces in the Chinese Mainland with highest number of kidney transplants performed in 2018. (Data from CSRKT)

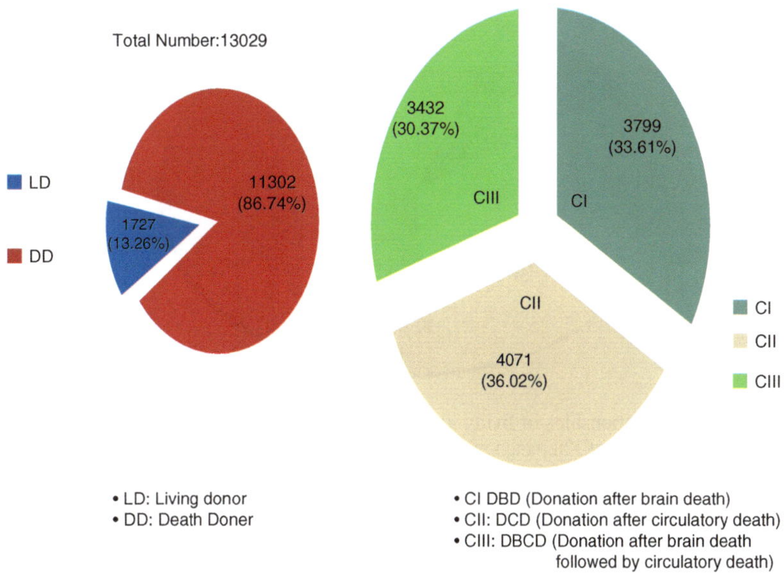


**Fig. 20.18** Deceased donor organ donations in the Chinese Mainland in 2018. abbreviations; DBD, donation after brain death; DCD, donation after circulatory death; DBCD donation after brain death followed by circulatory death

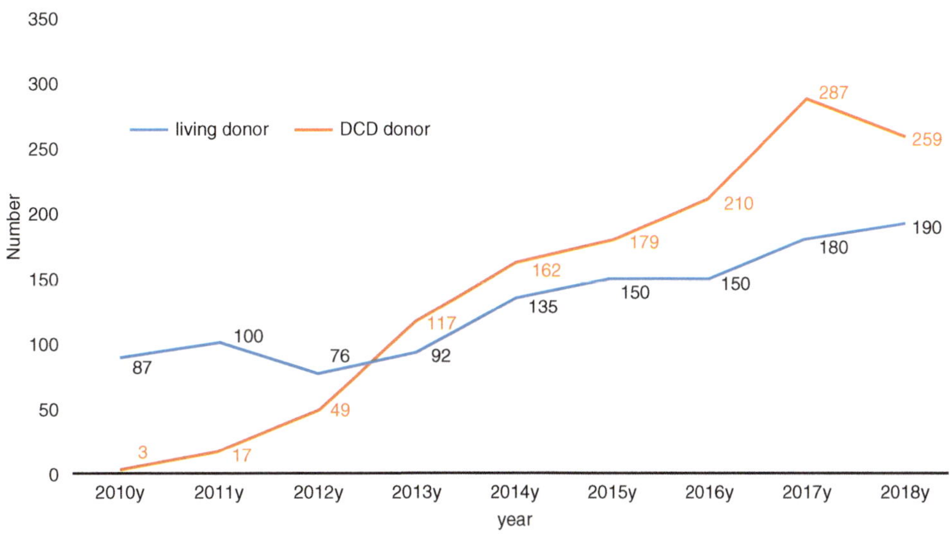


**Fig. 20.19** Annual number of kidney transplantation from DCD donor and living donor in the First Affiliated Hospital of Zhejiang University

Kidney transplantation from DCD also increased steadily from near zero case in 2011 to 1283 cases in 2018 in the First Affiliated Hospital of Zhejiang University (Fig. 20.20), one of the major kidney transplant centers in China. This steady increase is expected to continue to the next decade. The number of living donor kidney transplantations in our center has also grown steadily since 2007 (Fig. 20.20). Figure 20.21 presents a snapshot of percentages of eight different donor-recipient relationships in living-related kidney transplantation performed in the First Affiliated Hospital of Zhejiang University. The percentages of donation from mother to son were the highest, reaching 33% among all living-related donations, while donation from mother to daughter and father to son was 21% and 18%, respectively (Fig. 20.21). Kidney transplantation from DCD showed a high rate of delayed graft function (DGF) and infections. Of the 1283 kidney transplantations from DCD performed without machine perfusion up to end of 2018, the rate of delayed graft function (DGF) was 17.2%, but 93.2% recovered from the DGF. Patients with DGF achieved similar eGFR at 1 year posttransplant when compared to patients without DGF (unpublished data).

Infection was an important complication posttransplant, accounting for 70% of all peri-transplantation deaths. Acute rejection is another important complication. According to unpublished data from the First Affiliated Hospital of Zhejiang University, 3.57% of kidney transplants from living donor and 3.99% from DCD had biopsy-proven acute rejection within the first 6 months posttransplant. Biopsy-proven acute rejection was diagnosed in 5.45% and 6.65% of living donor and DCD kidney transplant at 12 months posttransplant; and 9.02% of living donor and 8.11% of DCD until the end of 2018, respectively.

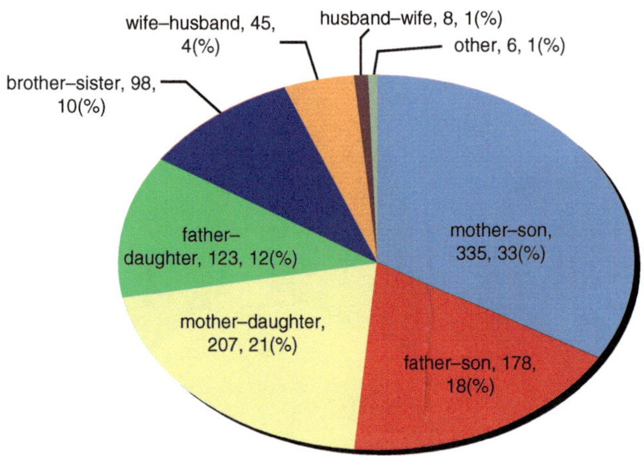


**Fig. 20.20** Relationships of living kidney transplantation in the First Affiliated Hospital of Zhejiang University

## Acute Kidney Injury (AKI) and Critical Care Nephrology

### AKI Disease Burden

A nationwide cross-sectional AKI survey conducted by the *International Society of Nephrology (ISN) 0 by 25 China Consortium* screened 2.2 million adult hospitalized patients from 44 academic or local hospitals in 22 provinces from the Chinese Mainland, based on changes in serum creatinine by the Laboratory Information System [11]. The overall detection rate of AKI was 1.0% by KDIGO criteria (and varied between 0.8% and 1.2% among different geographic regions) and 2.0% by expanded criteria (i.e., ≥50% rise in serum creatinine during hospital stay). The in-hospital mortality rate for AKI was around 12.4% and was lower than that reported from US nationwide inpatient data in 2002 (20.3%) [186]. Over half of the patients with AKI were >60 years old, and

**Fig. 20.21** Percentage of biopsy-proven acute rejection in the First Affiliated Hospital of Zhejiang University

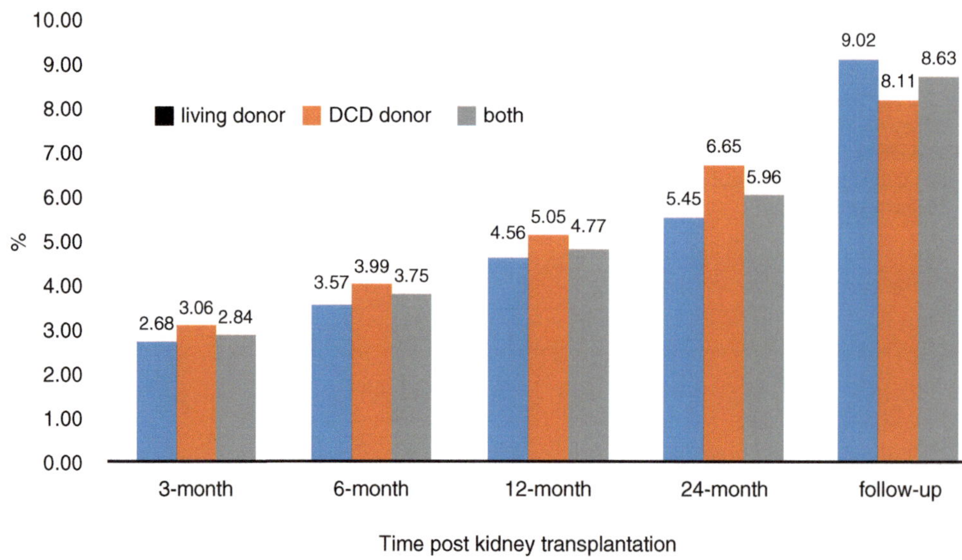

half of the AKI were prerenal in nature, with renal hypoperfusion, nephrotoxic drugs, or environmental toxins being the most common causes. A striking feature of AKI in the Chinese Mainland is a high proportion of nephrotoxic drug exposure (71.6%) before or at the time of AKI compared with those reported in other developed countries (average between 20% and 50%) [187–189]. Nearly half of the AKI occurred in patients with severe critical illness and over a quarter of the AKI were of stage 3 or worse. Furthermore, increasing age, presence of cardiovascular disease, delayed AKI recognition, critical illness, higher peak AKI stage, and need for RRT were all independent risk factors predicting mortality from AKI. Notably, around 74.2% of the AKI that developed during hospitalization was not recognized by physicians. Of the 25.8% of AKI that were recognized, diagnosis was delayed in 17.6%. Regions of lower socioeconomic status were independently associated with more under-recognition or delayed diagnosis of AKI. On the other hand, patients with preexisting CKD, more severe AKI, and early referral to nephrologists were less likely to be under-recognized for their AKI. Since only 25% of the hospitalized patients had serum creatinine measurement repeated during hospitalization, the prevalence of AKI was likely vastly underestimated. Having a timely diagnosis of AKI with early referral to nephrologists may be an important strategy to lower mortality rates from AKI in the Chinese Mainland.

In another multicenter retrospective cohort study conducted in 9 regional central hospitals in the Chinese Mainland in 659,945 adults hospitalized with a wide variety of clinical settings, the estimated incidence of community-acquired (CA)-AKI was 2.5%, and hospital-acquired (HA)-AKI was 9.1%, giving rise to an overall incidence of AKI of 11.6%. Preexisting CKD was identified as a major risk factor of AKI, contributing 20% for the risk of CA-AKI and 12% for the risk of HA-AKI. The three most common clinical settings associated with CA-AKI were sepsis (15.2%), urinary tract obstruction (12.3%), and CKD (11.8%). On the other hand, cardiac surgery (43.7%), sepsis (32%), and intensive care (30.3%) were the three most common clinical settings associated with HA-AKI. Nephrotoxic drugs were important causes of AKI, accounting for 39.2% of CA-AKI and 42.9% of HA-AKI. Chinese traditional medicines/remedies were also important causes of AKI, accounting for 15.3% of CA-AKI and 16.2% of HA-AKI, while contrast agents contributed to 9.1% of the HA-AKI [190]. The estimated in-hospital mortality of AKI in this study was 8.8% and increased in a stepwise fashion with increasing severity of AKI. The risk of mortality with AKI further increased among subjects with preexisting CKD and subjects who need intensive care [190].

Treatment of AKI poses significant financial burden to the hospital systems in the Chinese Mainland. According to an analysis by Xu et al., HA-AKI increased healthcare expenditure by more than 66% compared to patients without AKI. Average length of stay for patients complicated with AKI increased by a median of 5 days compared to those with no AKI. According to a report from National Health and Family Planning Commission of PRC, an estimated 1.4 million people with AKI by KDIGO criteria (2.9 million by the expanded criteria) were hospitalized in 2013 and consumed about US$13 billion, accounting for 10% of total healthcare expenditure in the Chinese Mainland. If patients with severe AKI were discharged without further treatment, an estimated 700,000 patients would have died from AKI during 2013. However, only 16.7% of the AKI were presented to the healthcare system. Thus, the real clinical significance and financial impact of AKI may be grossly underestimated in the Chinese Mainland.

CA-AKI accounted for nearly 50% of all AKI in the Chinese Mainland [11]. Patients in Northern China were more likely to develop AKI due to renal hypoperfusion, whereas more AKI in Southern China were due to exposure to nephrotoxins or urinary tract obstructions [191]. Rates of timely diagnosis of AKI and appropriate initiation of RRT were higher in more developed regions of China [191].

Based on a pediatric AKI survey from 25 regional, central, general, and children hospitals in the Chinese Mainland, the estimated incidence of AKI in pediatric population was 20%, of which 7% were community-acquired and 13% were hospital-acquired. The three most common settings with AKI were heart failure (25%), respiratory failure (24%), and congenital heart disease/cardiac surgery (24%) [192]. The incidence of AKI in pediatric intensive care unit (PICU) was very high (46% on admission and 56% during the PICU stay) in one report from HKSAR [193].

## Critical Care Nephrology

AKI in the ICU settings was very often more complicated than AKI outside ICU and associated with more postoperative complications, sepsis, advanced invasive procedures such as extracorporeal membrane oxygenation (ECMO), and vasoactive support. According to a nationwide survey, 21.6% and 28.5% of the AKI occurred in surgical departments and ICUs, respectively [11]. ICU had the highest detection rate of AKI (22.46%) and had more severe AKI (nearly a third of the AKI were stage 3) and higher mortality rate (50%) than AKI outside ICU [194]. The most common risk factors for AKI in the ICU settings in the Chinese Mainland were renal hypoperfusion, use of nephrotoxic drugs, sepsis, and other critical illnesses. Data from a prospective, multicenter, observational study conducted in 22 ICUs in the Chinese Mainland showed that around 31.6% of the ICU patients developed AKI, with 30% being stage 3 AKI, and 27% of patients with AKI died during hospitalization [195]. Tables 20.6 and 20.7 summarize the recent epidemiologic studies of AKI in the adult and pediatric intensive care units in the Chinese Mainland, respectively.

## Access to RRT for AKI

A nationwide survey in the Chinese Mainland showed that only 59.3% of patients with AKI requiring RRT received the required treatment. This meant nearly 41% of patients with AKI did not receive RRT as required. Extrapolating this data to the whole of China, this meant that an estimated 139,000 patients who should receive RRT for their AKI did not receive the required treatment. Patients who were elderly, men, from lower socioeconomic areas, from local hospitals, and complicated with malignancies or other severe comorbidities were less likely to receive RRT. Subjects who received RRT had lower mortality than those not receiving RRT despite requiring the treatment. In terms of the RRT modality for AKI, continuous renal replacement therapy (CRRT) was used in 53.9% of AKI cases, intermittent HD in 38%, and PD in 1.1% [203]. On the other hand, over a third of the patients who received CRRT did not require the treatment, suggesting that CRRT may be overutilized in some AKIs. The medical costs incurred in providing CRRT for those not requiring this modality [median (interquartile range), USD 7944 [4248, 16,055] vs. 5100 [2948, 9396], $p < 0.001$] and the mortality rate were higher (10.6% vs. 4.4%, $p = 0.047$) compared to those receiving other RRT modalities [203].

Two hundred ICU physicians were surveyed about their clinical practice in sepsis-induced AKI. Forty percent of ICU patients with sepsis had AKI and 25% required extracorporeal therapy. CRRT was the most commonly used modality and the median duration of CRRT was 12 hours per day for 5 days. Heparin-based anticoagulation rather than regional citrate

**Table 20.6** Recent epidemiology studies of AKI in the adult intensive care unit in the Chinese Mainland

| No. | Study | ICU admissions | Incidence of AKI | Mortality rate | RRT rates | Risk factors | Ref |
|---|---|---|---|---|---|---|---|
| 1 | 2013 nationwide retrospective survey of AKI | 9657 | 22% | 21.8% | 17.4% | Renal hypoperfusion, nephrotoxic drugs, other critical illness | [194] |
| 2 | Prospective survey of AKI from 30 ICUs at 28 large tertiary hospitals | 2526 (1731 postoperative, 917 sepsis) | 46.3 (44.8% for postoperative, 11.6% for septic AKI) | 25.7% (9.3% and 5.1% for postoperative and sepsis, respectively) | 18.9% (35.5% for septic AKI) | Emergency surgery, CKD, nephrotoxic drugs, cardiovascular surgery, APACHE II, SOFA score, fluid overload, use of diuretics, and sepsis | [196–198] |
| 3 | Retrospective review of stroke patients from neurology department | 647 | 20.9% | 36.3% | – | Higher NIHSS score, lower baseline eGFR, the presence of hypertension, and infectious complications | [199] |
| 4 | Prospective cohort study of 3063 patients in 22 tertiary ICUs in 2009 | 1058 for KDIGO study and 1255 enrolled for RIFLE study | 55.4% for KDIGO study and 31.6% for RIFLE study | 25.8% for KDIGO study and 35.9% for RIFLE study | 26.5% for RIFLE study | A higher burden of comorbidities and higher overall severity of illness scores | [195, 200] |

Abbreviation: *ICU* intensive care unit, *CKD* chronic kidney disease, *APACHE* Acute Physiology and Chronic Health Evaluation, *SOFA* sepsis-related organ failure assessment, *NIHSS* National Institute of Health Stroke Scale, *eGFR* estimated glomerular filtration rate, *RIFLE* risk, injury, failure, loss, and end stage, *RRT*, renal replacement therapy

**Table 20.7** Recent epidemiology studies of AKI in the pediatric intensive care units in the Chinese Mainland

| No. | Study | ICU admissions | Incidence of AKI | Mortality rate | RRT, rates | Risk factors | Ref |
|---|---|---|---|---|---|---|---|
| 1 | Observational study from PICU of Children's Hospital of Soochow University | 370 | 6.8% | – | – | Fluid overload | [201] |
| 2 | Multicentric retrospective cohort study of 25 medical centers comprising 9 of the 15 children's hospitals and 16 of the 17 general hospitals | 14,866 | 34.6% | – | – | – | [192] |
| 3 | Critically ill children admitted to PICU with confirmed influenza A (H1N1) or enterovirus 71 infection (EV71 group) from Oct. 2009 to Oct. 2010 | 28 | 25% | 71.4% | – | – | [202] |
| 4 | A local pediatric intensive care unit in Hong Kong between 2005 and 2007 | 140 | 56% | 21% | 6% | – | [193] |

Abbreviation: *PICU* pediatric intensive care unit, *RRT*, Renal Replacement Therapy.

anticoagulation method was preferred. Femoral vein was the predominant vascular access for CRRT. However, there was a lack of evaluation of treatment efficiency and no systematic follow-up. The mismatch between high cost of CRRT and lack of insurance cover and social support created difficulty in deciding the initiation of CRRT [204]. A retrospective study from a tertiary hospital in Ningbo, China, showed that lack of insurance coverage was one of the independent predictors of AKI-associated mortality in the ICU [205]. PD may serve as a useful alternative modality for AKI treatment in neonates. This was supported by a retrospective analysis in children that received PD as the RRT modality for AKI in a teaching hospital in Northwest China between 2003 and 2013 [206]. However, the lack of PD equipment for use in very young infants and neonates may pose a major barrier to adopt PD as the RRT modality in very young patients [207].

In order to improve AKI management and outcomes, an AKI electronic alert based on electronic monitoring of serial changes in serum creatinine levels in the medical laboratory system has been set up in several academic hospitals in China, such as Peking University First Hospital and Guangdong General Hospital. This enabled early detection and diagnosis of AKI [208]. Pilot studies (Chinese Clinical Trial Registry No. ChiCTR900021115, http://www.chictr.org.cn/index.aspx) were initiated to evaluate AKI care bundle which included screening of high-risk subjects, optimizing kidney perfusion in at-risk subjects, adjustment of drug dosages, etc. A multicenter clinical trial is currently underway to evaluate PD as a RRT modality for AKI. Preventive strategies for AKI in high-risk clinical settings such as cardiac surgery and nephrotoxin exposure are also under evaluation. There are also studies examining factors or biomarkers that may be useful for risk stratification in AKI.

In conclusion, AKI poses a huge financial burden to China healthcare and hospital system. There are major challenges in making early AKI diagnosis and initiation of treatment. More collaborative efforts are required not only from the healthcare professionals but also from the Chinese government in order to optimize the social-economic support and management of AKI, thereby improving the outcomes of patients complicated with AKI.

## Nephrology Practice and Job Market in the Chinese Mainland

The nephrology workforce is essential in tackling the increasing burden of kidney disease and providing kidney care in the Chinese Mainland. With the growing burden of CKD and an enormous demand of providing RRT for CKD patients approaching ESRD, current kidney care system in the Chinese Mainland faces an unprecedented challenge. However, the exact number of the nephrology workforce and its distribution in the Chinese Mainland are currently not known due to limited studies and lack of a central medical registration office that captures clinical manpower data. In this section, we provide a brief review of nephrology workforce and nephrologists specialist training structure in the Chinese Mainland.

Most nephrology divisions are based in tertiary comprehensive hospitals, while some are in secondary referral hospitals. In 2017, there were 2340 tertiary hospitals in mainland China (with 593 in North China, 538 in East China, 455 in South China, 323 in Southwest China, 269 in Northeast China, and 162 in Northwest China) (Fig. 20.22) [209]. The distribution of tertiary hospitals reflects the distribution of nephrology divisions in the Chinese Mainland. Overall, the density of nephrology divisions in the Chinese Mainland averaged around 1.69 pmp. There are about 8.46–33.84 nephrologists pmp in the Chinese Mainland, assuming that each nephrology division had at least 5–20 nephrologists. The estimated density of nephrologists for the Chinese Mainland was higher than that reported (5.18 pmp) in the Global Kidney Health Atlas (GKHA) project of the ISN and

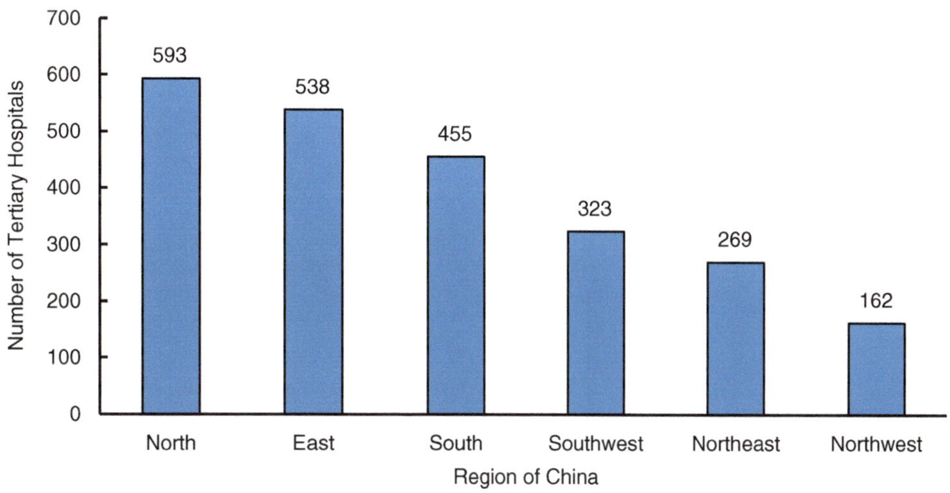


**Fig. 20.22** Number of tertiary hospitals in different regions of the Chinese Mainland

surpassed the density of nephrologists in upper-middle-income countries (7.23 pmp) [210]. However, nephrologists' densities vary widely across different regions. The number of nephrologists is much lower in many county hospitals in underdeveloped and rural areas, while in many developed cities such as Beijing, Shanghai, Guangzhou, and Nanjing where large research centers of kidney disease are located, nephrologists' densities are comparable to that reported in high-income countries (28.52 pmp) [210]. The variations in nephrologists' densities across the country may impact the quality of kidney care delivery in different regions. According to the Science and Technology Evaluation Metrics report of China nephrology divisions from the Chinese Academy of Medical Science, more than 30% of the 100 top-tier nephrology divisions in the Chinese Mainland are located in three major cities (14 divisions in Shanghai, 12 in Beijing, and 8 in Guangzhou). However, in the rural or underdeveloped areas, such as Southwest and Northwest Region that accounted for more than 20% of the total population, the number of top-tier nephrology divisions is disproportionately low with only 13 divisions being among the 100 top-tier nephrology divisions in the country [211].

Apart from inpatient department of nephrology, the outpatient dialysis center constitutes another important working area for nephrologists. According to the unpublished data from CNRDS, the numbers of HD centers and PD centers in the Chinese Mainland were 5419 and 1211, respectively, in 2017. Most dialysis centers were based in tertiary and secondary referral hospitals and managed by nephrologists. In recent years, dialysis corporations, such as Fresenius and Wego, have started to set up dialysis chains in the Chinese Mainland. However, the number of these community-based dialysis centers remains very limited and serves no more than 5% of the total dialysis patients. This was different from the situation in developed countries like the USA, where community-based centers are very prevalent and operated by large dialysis organizations such as DaVita and Fresenius. The "tertiary hospital-based" structure has in part resulted in an imbalance distribution of dialysis centers in the Chinese Mainland. The Chinese government currently encourages investment and setting up of private or independent dialysis centers in order to meet the increasing market need and demand for dialysis in the country. It is foreseen that there will be a rapid growth in the number of dialysis centers in the near future. The ratios of physician to patient and nurse to patient in HD or PD centers is currently much lower in the Chinese Mainland compared with other countries.

The training program for nephrologists in the Chinese Mainland is divided into three phases: Phase 1 involves a standardized training program for residents for general internal medicine. Phase 2 involves standardized training program for specialists (nephrologists) and phase 3 involves continuous medical education of specialists (nephrologists) (Fig. 20.23). Unlike the resident training program, specialist training (or fellowship training) program for nephrologists

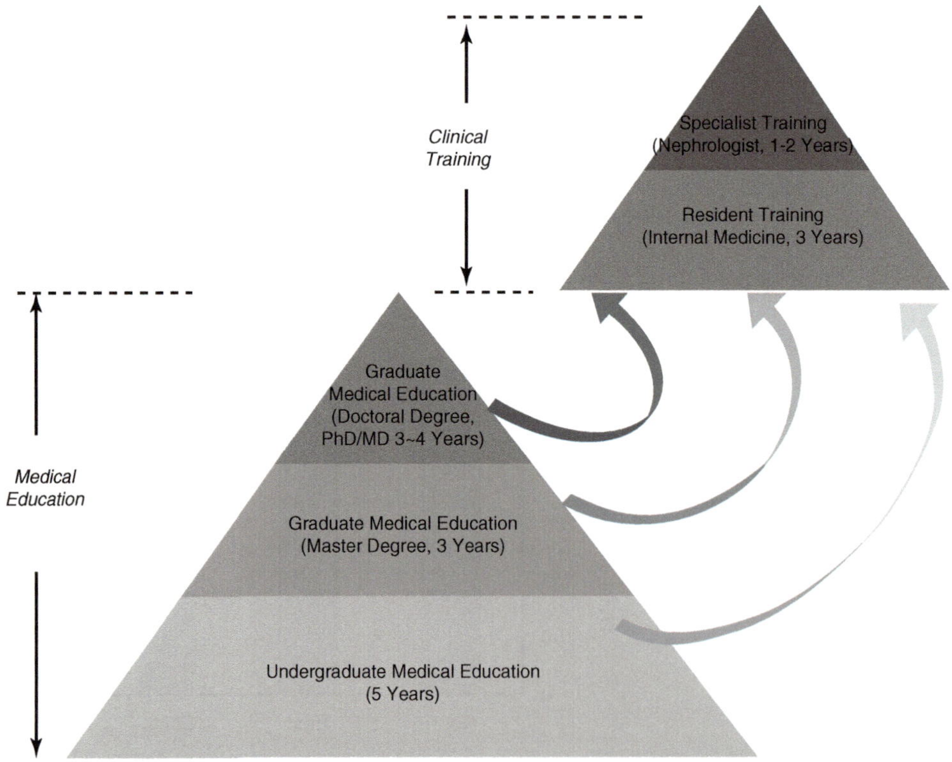


**Fig. 20.23** The medical education and clinical training of nephrologists in the Chinese Mainland

(or other specialties) has not been implemented nationwide. Only a small proportion of nephrologists in developed regions of China receive specialist training in tertiary hospitals/medical centers in the country or receive fellowship training abroad. In the GKHA project, the Chinese Mainland reported a nephrology trainee density of 1.46 pmp, a little lower than the global average level of 1.87 pmp and much lower than that of high-income countries (6.03 pmp) [210]. There is great disparity in the highest degree attained by nephrologists working in tertiary and secondary referral hospitals. A master's degree is usually an essential prerequisite for practicing nephrologists in first- or second-tier cities of the Chinese Mainland, and a large proportion of them (specifically for those age below 45 years) also hold a doctoral degree (MD or PhD). However, a bachelor degree is usually the highest degree attained by most nephrologists working in the third- or fourth-tier cities or underdeveloped areas. The salaries of nephrologists vary among different parts of the Chinese Mainland but are comparable to those of other physicians.

Apart from the nephrologists' workforce, the Chinese Mainland faces significant gaps and deficiencies in specialized nephrology nursing manpower, especially nurses with skills and experience in providing dialysis service. The Chinese Mainland is in need of more renal pathologists. There are also significant gaps in other nephrology-related workforce or allied health professionals' manpower such as renal dietitians [210].

Apart from clinical service provision, academic research is an integral part in many teaching hospitals. However, there are very few full-time academic positions in the Chinese Mainland. Research is mostly done by graduate students of Doctor of Philosophy (PhD) or master's degree (MD). In general, research grants in the Chinese Mainland do not include the salary of research staff. This is very different from research grants funded in most other countries. This may possibly explain why the country has very low number of full-time researchers. Nevertheless, many young nephrologists are still interested in and enthusiastic with academic and research work as academic achievement adds merit for their career development and job promotion in most university-affiliated hospitals. Research grants are mostly supported by the National Natural Scientific Foundation, which provides 300–400 grant programs annually with each grant fund around USD 35,000–80,000. Chinese nephrologists have increasing academic contributions and publications in world leading, high impact kidney and medical journals in the recent years. There are also an increasing number of Chinese nephrologists involved in the leadership of global nephrology societies such as ISN, KDIGO, and ISPD. Chinese nephrologists are very open in establishing connections with global or regional nephrology organizations in order to contribute to kidney research and advances in kidney care.

## RRT in HK Special Administrative Region (SAR)

The hospital system in HKSAR is independent and entirely different from that in the Chinese Mainland. The Hospital Authority (HA) of HKSAR was set up in Hong Kong in 1990 and is responsible for providing RRT and kidney care in over 80% of the ESRD patients in Hong Kong. The remaining 20% of ESRD patients are managed in private settings/hospitals. The RRT public services in Hong Kong are delivered through 7 clusters with 15 renal units under the HA. There are four kidney transplant centers in Hong Kong, including Princess Margaret Hospital, Prince of Wales Hospital, Queen Elizabeth Hospital, and Queen Mary Hospital. The Hong Kong Renal Registry (HKRR) was set up by the HA in 1995 and is an online computerized registry developed by the Central Renal Committee of HA of Hong Kong to capture data of all patients receiving RRT in the public healthcare system under HA of Hong Kong. Each individual renal center can access patients' data from their own center online, and each center is responsible for inputting data of all patients receiving RRT in their center. The system provides important data for the unit as a whole and for the HA Head Office to produce an up-to-date registry data for the RRT situation in the whole HA. The information is useful for audit and monitoring purpose as well as healthcare financing and planning of future renal service development in Hong Kong. The HKRR also comprises the Organ Registry and Transplant System (ORTS) that includes the Organ Procurement System and Transplant Immunogenetics System. The Organ Procurement System collects demographic details, immunological and virology results of all cadaveric donors. Transplant and Immunogenetics System centralizes all the transplant immunogenetics and tissue typing data of deceased donor and patients on transplant waiting list. The HKRR also serves the function of deceased donor kidney allocation. A scoring system was developed, based on the years on RRT, HLA matching, and age of patients, so to assign the priority of the patients on the transplant waiting list. When a deceased donor is confirmed, tissue typing of the deceased donor will be performed by the Tissue Typing Laboratory centralized in the Queen Mary Hospital, Hong Kong, and inputted in the system so to generate the final scoring for deceased donor kidney allocation [212].

RRT service development in Hong Kong has undergone the following milestones over the years. The first acute HD was done in HK in 1962 followed by the development of chronic HD. In 1969, the first cadaveric kidney transplant was performed and in 1980 the first living-related kidney transplant was performed. In the 1980s, CAPD was introduced in Hong Kong. In 1985, PD-first policy was adopted by the HA of Hong Kong of which PD was reimbursed by the government as a first-line dialysis modality in patients with ESRD. Automated PD (APD) was introduced in 1989. PD patients may face technique failure either due to PD-related complications such as peritonitis, peritoneal sclerosis/adhesions, or inadequate PD due to peritoneal membrane failure, requiring permanent switch to HD. Thus, there is an increasing demand for long-term HD support. HA of Hong Kong introduced the nocturnal home HD program in 2006 and the public-private partnership HD program since 2010 to cope with an increasing demand of HD services [212].

Data first captured by the HKRR in 1996 showed that the number of incident ESRD patients in Hong Kong was 615. This number showed steady increase to 1147 in 2013, equivalent to an incidence rate of 159 pmp. By 2013, there were 8510 patients receiving RRT in Hong Kong with 3501 kidney transplants, 1192 HD, and 3817 PD. The ratio of PD:HD was 76.2:23.8. Over 90% of the HD is provided by hospital HD centers. Eighty-six percent of all PD patients received CAPD, while the remaining 14% received automated PD. The use of APD showed a gradual increase in Hong Kong over the years. In 1997, only 3.14% of PD patients used APD but APD use was slowly increased to 5.52% in 2007 and 13.89% in 2013. Data from the HKRR 2016 showed that the annual mortality rate per 100 patient-years was 1.88 for patients who received a renal transplant, 17.89 for patients on PD, and 18.89 for those on HD in Hong Kong [213].

Data from the HKRR showed a trend of increasing age in incident PD patients over the last 17 years from 1996 to 2013. The median age of incident patients into the RRT program was 59.1 years in 2013 with the biggest increase in the age group 45–64 years and age group over 75 years. There was a male preponderance in both incident (male-to-female ratio, 1.54) and prevalent (male-to-female ratio, 1.29) dialysis population. Over the years, the demographics of background causes of kidney disease also changed. In 1995, GD accounted for 29% of the causes of kidney disease in incident dialysis patients but dropped to 17% in 2013. On the other hand, DKD increased from 26.2% in 1996 to 49.6% in 2013 as the cause of incident ESRD cases requiring RRT and is the leading cause of ESRD followed by GD and unknown causes [212].

Hong Kong faces a serious shortage of organ donations that did not seem to improve much over the years. In 2013, there were 1991 ESRD patients on the kidney transplant waiting list. However, only 69 deceased donor kidney transplants and 12 living-related kidney transplants were conducted in Hong Kong. In fact, the number of living-related kidney transplants has not shown much increase in the last 15 years (from 297 cases in 1996 to 415 cases in 2013). However, prevalent kidney transplant patients showed a steady rise from 956 in 1996 to 3498 in 2013, mainly because of an increase in deceased donor kidney transplants (from 659 cases in 1996 to 3085 cases in 2013). Data from the HKRR showed that a living-related kidney transplant had higher 10-year graft survival rate (81%) compared with deceased donor kidney transplant (70%). The 20-year graft survival rate was 44% for deceased donor and 61% for living donor kidney transplant. However, the average waiting time could be approximately 6 years but may also be as long as 28 years [213, 214]. Public education is therefore essential to raise general awareness of the need for deceased organ donation. In the second half of 2018, HA of Hong Kong introduced a pair exchange scheme for kidney transplants that enables two pairs of donor-recipients to exchange kidney donors so that each recipient can receive a better-matched organ.

In terms of anemia treatment, there was a big increase in the proportion of dialysis patients receiving ESA treatment from 29.3% in 1996 to 65% in 2013 as the Hong Kong government has provided additional funding to support ESA treatment in dialysis patients. Currently, HKRR did not include data on patients with CKD or AKI. Thus, representative territory-wide data in these regards were not available.

**Declaration of Conflict of Interest** Angela Yee-Moon Wang, MD, PhD, has received speaker honorarium from Fresenius Kabi and Sanofi Renal and research funds from Baxter Corporation and Sanofi Renal.

Yu An, MD, declares no conflict of interest.

Guang-Yan Cai, MD, PhD, declares no conflict of interest.

Jiang-Hua Chen, MD, declares no conflict of interest.

Xiang-Mei Chen, MD, PhD, declares no conflict of interest.

Wei Chen, MD, PhD, declares no conflict of interest.

Zhao Cui, MD, declares no conflict of interest.

Chuan-Ming Hao, MD, PhD, declares no conflict of interest.

Fan-Fan Hou, MD, PhD, is a study investigator and a consultant for and received honoraria from AstraZeneca.

Bi Cheng Liu, MD, PhD, declares no conflict of interest.

Zhi-Hong Liu, MD, declares no conflict of interest.

Qing-Yu Niu, PhD, declares no conflict of interest.

Qi-Quan Sun, MD, declares no conflict of interest.

Ren-Ding Wang, MD, declares no conflict of interest.

Damin Xu, MD, declares no conflict of interest.

Chao Yang, MD, declares no conflict of interest.

Li Yang, MD, declares no conflict of interest.

Luxia Zhang, MD, PhD, received research funding from AstraZeneca.

Ming-Hui Zhao, PhD, declares no conflict of interest.

Li Zuo, MD, PhD, declares no conflict of interest.

Xue-Qing Yu, MD, PhD, Disclosure: China Q study sponsored by Baxter Healthcare Corporation; Lowering uric acid in PD patients by Wanbang company, China; Orchestra Study by Kyowa-Kirin, China; ROXADUSTAT Study by AstraZeneca; Lupus Nephritis Study by GSK. Consultant for Fresenius Kabi, Baxter Healthcare Corporation, and AstraZeneca.

## References


1. East Asia/Southeast Asia: China The World Factbook – Central Intelligence Agency. www.cia.gov. Archived from the original on 2016-10-13. Retrieved 25 Nov 2018. 2016.
2. Commission NH. China's health statistics yearbook 2018. Peking: Peking Union Medical College Press; 2018.

3. Mossialos E, Wenzl M, Osborn R, Sarnak D, editors. 2015 International profiles of health care systems. New York: Commonwealth Fund; 2016.
4. Fang H, Eggleston K, Hanson K, Wu M. Enhancing financial protection under China's social health insurance to achieve universal health coverage. BMJ. 2019;365:l2378.
5. Meng Q, Mills A, Wang L, Han Q. What can we learn from China's health system reform? BMJ. 2019;365:l2349.
6. Nofri EM. The Chinese healthcare system; how it works and future trends [online]. Available from: http://www.albertoforchielli.com/2015/11/13/the-chinese-healthcare-system-how-it-works-and-future-trends/. 2015.
7. Tan X, Liu X, Shao H. Healthy China 2030: a vision for health care. Value Health Reg Issues. 2017;12:112–4.
8. Xie F, Zhang D, Wu J, Zhang Y, Yang Q, Sun X, et al. Design and implementation of the first nationwide, web-based Chinese Renal Data System (CNRDS). BMC Med Inform Decis Mak. 2012;12:11.
9. Zhang L, Wang F, Wang L, Wang W, Liu B, Liu J, et al. Prevalence of chronic kidney disease in China: a cross-sectional survey. Lancet. 2012;379(9818):815–22.
10. Zhang L, Long J, Jiang W, Shi Y, He X, Zhou Z, et al. Trends in chronic kidney disease in China. N Engl J Med. 2016;375(9):905–6.
11. Yang L, Xing G, Wang L, Wu Y, Li S, Xu G, et al. Acute kidney injury in China: a cross-sectional survey. Lancet. 2015;386(10002):1465–71.
12. Lv J, Zhang H, Wong MG, Jardine MJ, Hladunewich M, Jha V, et al. Effect of oral methylprednisolone on clinical outcomes in patients with IgA nephropathy: the TESTING randomized clinical trial. JAMA. 2017;318(5):432–42.
13. Heerspink HJL, Parving HH, Andress DL, Bakris G, Correa-Rotter R, Hou FF, et al. Atrasentan and renal events in patients with type 2 diabetes and chronic kidney disease (SONAR): a double-blind, randomised, placebo-controlled trial. Lancet. 2019;393(10184):1937–47.
14. Perkovic V, Jardine MJ, Neal B, Bompoint S, Heerspink HJL, Charytan DM, et al. Canagliflozin and renal outcomes in type 2 diabetes and nephropathy. N Engl J Med. 2019;380(24):2295–306.
15. Chen N, Hao C, Liu BC, Lin H, Wang C, Xing C, et al. Roxadustat treatment for anemia in patients undergoing long-term dialysis. N Engl J Med. 2019;381(11):1011–22.
16. Chen N, Hao C, Peng X, Lin H, Yin A, Hao L, et al. Roxadustat for anemia in patients with kidney disease not receiving dialysis. N Engl J Med. 2019;381(11):1001–10.
17. Su Q, Hu F, Ge X, Lei J, Yu S, Wang T, et al. Structure of the human PKD1-PKD2 complex. Science. 2018;361(6406):eaat9819.
18. Yu XQ, Li M, Zhang H, Low HQ, Wei X, Wang JQ, et al. A genome-wide association study in Han Chinese identifies multiple susceptibility loci for IgA nephropathy. Nat Genet. 2011;44(2):178–82.
19. Coresh J, Selvin E, Stevens LA, Manzi J, Kusek JW, Eggers P, et al. Prevalence of chronic kidney disease in the United States. JAMA. 2007;298(17):2038–47.
20. Hallan SI, Coresh J, Astor BC, Asberg A, Powe NR, Romundstad S, et al. International comparison of the relationship of chronic kidney disease prevalence and ESRD risk. J Am Soc Nephrol. 2006;17(8):2275–84.
21. Wang F, He K, Wang J, Zhao MH, Li Y, Zhang L, et al. Prevalence and risk factors for CKD: a comparison between the adult populations in China and the United States. Kidney Int Rep. 2018;3(5):1135–43.
22. Wang F, Zhang L, Wang H. Awareness of CKD in China: a national cross-sectional survey. Am J Kidney Dis. 2014;63(6):1068–70.
23. Plantinga LC, Boulware LE, Coresh J, Stevens LA, Miller ER 3rd, Saran R, et al. Patient awareness of chronic kidney disease: trends and predictors. Arch Intern Med. 2008;168(20):2268–75.
24. Lysaght MJ. Maintenance dialysis population dynamics: current trends and long-term implications. J Am Soc Nephrol. 2002;13(Suppl 1):S37–40.
25. Wang F, Yang C, Long J, Zhao X, Tang W, Zhang D, et al. Executive summary for the 2015 Annual data report of the China kidney disease network (CK-NET). Kidney Int. 2019;95(3):501–5.
26. Zhang L, Zuo L. Current burden of end-stage kidney disease and its future trend in China. Clin Nephrol. 2016;86(2016)(13):27–8.
27. Center BHQCal. The annual data report of Beijing Hemodialysis Registry, 2012. Chin J Blood Purif. 2012;11(z1):42.
28. Zhang W, Qian J. Current status of dialysis therapy in Shanghai (results from Shanghai Renal Registry, 2011). Chin J Blood Purif. 2012;11(5):233–6.
29. Yamagata K, Yagisawa T, Nakai S, Nakayama M, Imai E, Hattori M, et al. Prevalence and incidence of chronic kidney disease stage G5 in Japan. Clin Exp Nephrol. 2015;19(1):54–64.
30. Liu ZH. Nephrology in China. Nat Rev Nephrol. 2013;9(9):523–8.
31. Commission NHaFP. National medical service and quality safety report, 2016. Beijing: People's Medical Publishing House; 2016. 510–28 p.
32. Xie Y, Chen X. Epidemiology, major outcomes, risk factors, prevention and management of chronic kidney disease in China. Am J Nephrol. 2008;28(1):1–7.
33. Saran R, Li Y, Robinson B, Ayanian J, Balkrishnan R, Bragg-Gresham J, et al. US renal data system 2014 annual data report: epidemiology of kidney disease in the United States. Am J Kidney Dis. 2015;66(1 Suppl 1):Svii, S1–305.
34. Wang J, Zhang L, Tang SC, Kashihara N, Kim YS, Togtokh A, et al. Disease burden and challenges of chronic kidney disease in North and East Asia. Kidney Int. 2018;94(1):22–5.
35. Hu F. The trends of obesity and type 2 diabetes in China and its policy implications (author's transl). Chin J Intern Med. 2014;53(1):5–8.
36. Group TNDPaCC. A mass survey of diabetes mellitus in a population of 300000 in 14 provinces and municipalities in China (author's transl). Zhonghua Nei Ke Za Zhi. 1981;20(11):678–83.
37. Wang L, Gao P, Zhang M, Huang Z, Zhang D, Deng Q, et al. Prevalence and ethnic pattern of diabetes and prediabetes in China in 2013. JAMA. 2017;317(24):2515–23.
38. Huang YM, Xu D, Long J, Shi Y, Zhang L, Wang H, et al. Spectrum of chronic kidney disease in China: a national study based on hospitalized patients from 2010 to 2015. Nephrology (Carlton). 2019;24(7):725–36.
39. Barsoum RS. Chronic kidney disease in the developing world. N Engl J Med. 2006;354(10):997–9.
40. Dialysis and Transplantation Registration Group, CSoN, CMA. The report about the registration of dialysis and transplantation in China 1999. Chin J Nephrol. 2001;17:77–9.
41. Li J, Cui Z, Long J, Huang W, Wang J, Zhang H, et al. Primary glomerular nephropathy among hospitalized patients in a national database in China. Nephrol Dial Transplant. 2018;33(12):2173–81.
42. Xu X, Wang G, Chen N, Lu T, Nie S, Xu G, et al. Long-term exposure to air pollution and increased risk of membranous nephropathy in China. J Am Soc Nephrol. 2016;27(12):3739–46.
43. Gharavi AG, Kiryluk K, Choi M, Li Y, Hou P, Xie J, et al. Genome-wide association study identifies susceptibility loci for IgA nephropathy. Nat Genet. 2011;43(4):321–7.
44. Kiryluk K, Li Y, Scolari F, Sanna-Cherchi S, Choi M, Verbitsky M, et al. Discovery of new risk loci for IgA nephropathy implicates genes involved in immunity against intestinal pathogens. Nat Genet. 2014;46(11):1187–96.
45. Zhu L, Zhai YL, Wang FM, Hou P, Lv JC, Xu DM, et al. Variants in complement factor H and complement factor H-related protein genes, CFHR3 and CFHR1, affect complement activation in IgA nephropathy. J Am Soc Nephrol. 2015;26(5):1195–204.
46. Xu R, Feng S, Li Z, Fu Y, Yin P, Ai Z, et al. Polymorphism of DEFA in Chinese Han population with IgA nephropathy. Hum Genet. 2014;133(10):1299–309.

47. Qi YY, Zhou XJ, Cheng FJ, Hou P, Zhu L, Shi SF, et al. DEFA gene variants associated with IgA nephropathy in a Chinese population. Genes Immun. 2015;16(3):231–7.
48. Novak J, Julian BA, Mestecky J, Renfrow MB. Glycosylation of IgA1 and pathogenesis of IgA nephropathy. Semin Immunopathol. 2012;34(3):365–82.
49. Xu LX, Zhao MH. Aberrantly glycosylated serum IgA1 are closely associated with pathologic phenotypes of IgA nephropathy. Kidney Int. 2005;68(1):167–72.
50. Li GS, Zhang H, Lv JC, Shen Y, Wang HY. Variants of C1GALT1 gene are associated with the genetic susceptibility to IgA nephropathy. Kidney Int. 2007;71(5):448–53.
51. Li GS, Zhu L, Zhang H, Lv JC, Ding JX, Zhao MH, et al. Variants of the ST6GALNAC2 promoter influence transcriptional activity and contribute to genetic susceptibility to IgA nephropathy. Hum Mutat. 2007;28(10):950–7.
52. Zhu L, Tang W, Li G, Lv J, Ding J, Yu L, et al. Interaction between variants of two glycosyltransferase genes in IgA nephropathy. Kidney Int. 2009;76(2):190–8.
53. Hou JH, Le WB, Chen N, Wang WM, Liu ZS, Liu D, et al. Mycophenolate Mofetil combined with prednisone versus full-dose prednisone in IgA nephropathy with active proliferative lesions: a randomized controlled trial. Am J Kidney Dis. 2017;69(6):788–95.
54. Li X, Liu Y, Lv J, Shi S, Liu L, Chen Y, et al. Progression of IgA nephropathy under current therapy regimen in a Chinese population. Clin J Am Soc Nephrol. 2014;9(3):484–9.
55. Lien YH. Patiromer: can less be better than more? Am J Med. 2018;131(5):459–60.
56. van Donkelaar A, Martin RV, Brauer M, Boys BL. Use of satellite observations for long-term exposure assessment of global concentrations of fine particulate matter. Environ Health Perspect. 2015;123(2):135–43.
57. Wang J, Cui Z, Lu J, Probst C, Zhang YM, Wang X, et al. Circulating antibodies against thrombospondin type-I domain-containing 7A in Chinese patients with idiopathic membranous nephropathy. Clin J Am Soc Nephrol. 2017;12(10):1642–51.
58. Stanescu HC, Arcos-Burgos M, Medlar A, Bockenhauer D, Kottgen A, Dragomirescu L, et al. Risk HLA-DQA1 and PLA(2) R1 alleles in idiopathic membranous nephropathy. N Engl J Med. 2011;364(7):616–26.
59. Lv J, Hou W, Zhou X, Liu G, Zhou F, Zhao N, et al. Interaction between PLA2R1 and HLA-DQA1 variants associates with anti-PLA2R antibodies and membranous nephropathy. J Am Soc Nephrol. 2013;24(8):1323–9.
60. Cui Z, Xie LJ, Chen FJ, Pei ZY, Zhang LJ, Qu Z, et al. MHC class II risk alleles and amino acid residues in idiopathic membranous nephropathy. J Am Soc Nephrol. 2017;28(5):1651–64.
61. Rafique Z, Weir MR, Onuigbo M, Pitt B, Lafayette R, Butler J, et al. Expert panel recommendations for the identification and management of hyperkalemia and role of patiromer in patients with chronic kidney disease and heart failure. J Manag Care Spec Pharm. 2017;23(4-a Suppl):S10–S9.
62. Wang HY, Cui Z, Xie LJ, Zhang LJ, Pei ZY, Chen FJ, et al. HLA class II alleles differing by a single amino acid associate with clinical phenotype and outcome in patients with primary membranous nephropathy. Kidney Int. 2018;94(5):974–82.
63. Zhang XD, Cui Z, Zhang MF, Wang J, Zhang YM, Qu Z, et al. Clinical implications of pathological features of primary membranous nephropathy. BMC Nephrol. 2018;19(1):215.
64. Wang X, Cui Z, Zhang YM, Qu Z, Wang F, Meng LQ, et al. Rituximab for non-responsive idiopathic membranous nephropathy in a Chinese cohort. Nephrol Dial Transplant. 2018;33(9):1558–63.
65. Nie S, He W, Huang T, Liu D, Wang G, Geng J, et al. The spectrum of biopsy-proven glomerular diseases among children in China: a national, cross-sectional survey. Clin J Am Soc Nephrol. 2018;13(7):1047–54.
66. Li X, Liu Z, Wang L, Wang R, Ding G, Shi W, et al. Tacrolimus monotherapy after intravenous methylprednisolone in adults with minimal change nephrotic syndrome. J Am Soc Nephrol. 2017;28(4):1286–95.
67. Xie J, Wu X, Ren H, Wang W, Wang Z, Pan X, et al. COL4A3 mutations cause focal segmental glomerulosclerosis. J Mol Cell Biol. 2014;6(6):498–505.
68. Xie J, Hao X, Azeloglu EU, Ren H, Wang Z, Ma J, et al. Novel mutations in the inverted formin 2 gene of Chinese families contribute to focal segmental glomerulosclerosis. Kidney Int. 2015;88(3):593–604.
69. Zhang Q, Ma J, Xie J, Wang Z, Zhu B, Hao X, et al. Screening of ACTN4 and TRPC6 mutations in a Chinese cohort of patients with adult-onset familial focal segmental glomerulosclerosis. Contrib Nephrol. 2013;181:91–100.
70. Zhuo L, Huang L, Yang Z, Li G, Wang L. A comprehensive analysis of NPHS1 gene mutations in patients with sporadic focal segmental glomerulosclerosis. BMC Med Genet. 2019;20(1):111.
71. Zhao F, Zhu JY, Richman A, Fu Y, Huang W, Chen N, et al. Mutations in NUP160 are implicated in steroid-resistant nephrotic syndrome. J Am Soc Nephrol. 2019;30(5):840–53.
72. Han R, Hu S, Qin W, Shi J, Hou Q, Wang X, et al. C3a and suPAR drive versican V1 expression in tubular cells of focal segmental glomerulosclerosis. JCI JCI Insight. 2019;4(13):e130986.
73. Li L, Zhang T, Diao W, Jin F, Shi L, Meng J, et al. Role of myeloid-derived suppressor cells in glucocorticoid-mediated amelioration of FSGS. J Am Soc Nephrol. 2015;26(9):2183–97.
74. Wu J, Zheng C, Fan Y, Zeng C, Chen Z, Qin W, et al. Downregulation of microRNA-30 facilitates podocyte injury and is prevented by glucocorticoids. J Am Soc Nephrol. 2014;25(1):92–104.
75. Guo JR, Chen QQ, Lam CW, Wang CY, Wong VK, Chang ZF, et al. Profiling ribonucleotide and deoxyribonucleotide pools perturbed by gemcitabine in human non-small cell lung cancer cells. Sci Rep. 2016;6:37250.
76. Jakes RW, Bae SC, Louthrenoo W, Mok CC, Navarra SV, Kwon N. Systematic review of the epidemiology of systemic lupus erythematosus in the Asia-Pacific region: prevalence, incidence, clinical features, and mortality. Arthritis Care Res (Hoboken). 2012;64(2):159–68.
77. Seligman VA, Lum RF, Olson JL, Li H, Criswell LA. Demographic differences in the development of lupus nephritis: a retrospective analysis. Am J Med. 2002;112(9):726–9.
78. Han JW, Zheng HF, Cui Y, Sun LD, Ye DQ, Hu Z, et al. Genome-wide association study in a Chinese Han population identifies nine new susceptibility loci for systemic lupus erythematosus. Nat Genet. 2009;41(11):1234–7.
79. Yang W, Shen N, Ye DQ, Liu Q, Zhang Y, Qian XX, et al. Genome-wide association study in Asian populations identifies variants in ETS1 and WDFY4 associated with systemic lupus erythematosus. PLoS Genet. 2010;6(2):e1000841.
80. Yang W, Tang H, Zhang Y, Tang X, Zhang J, Sun L, et al. Meta-analysis followed by replication identifies loci in or near CDKN1B, TET3, CD80, DRAM1, and ARID5B as associated with systemic lupus erythematosus in Asians. Am J Hum Genet. 2013;92(1):41–51.
81. Xu R, Li Q, Liu R, Shen J, Li M, Zhao M, et al. Association analysis of the MHC in lupus nephritis. J Am Soc Nephrol. 2017;28(11):3383–94.
82. Li LH, Yuan H, Pan HF, Li WX, Li XP, Ye DQ. Role of the Fcgamma receptor IIIA-V/F158 polymorphism in susceptibility to systemic lupus erythematosus and lupus nephritis: a meta-analysis. Scand J Rheumatol. 2010;39(2):148–54.
83. Yang W, Zhao M, Hirankarn N, Lau CS, Mok CC, Chan TM, et al. ITGAM is associated with disease susceptibility and renal nephritis of systemic lupus erythematosus in Hong Kong Chinese and Thai. Hum Mol Genet. 2009;18(11):2063–70.
84. Zhou XJ, Cheng FJ, Qi YY, Zhao MH, Zhang H. A replication study from Chinese supports association between lupus-

risk allele in TNFSF4 and renal disorder. Biomed Res Int. 2013;2013:597921.
85. Zhou XJ, Nath SK, Qi YY, Cheng FJ, Yang HZ, Zhang Y, et al. Brief report: identification of MTMR3 as a novel susceptibility gene for lupus nephritis in northern Han Chinese by shared-gene analysis with IgA nephropathy. Arthritis Rheumatol. 2014;66(10):2842–8.
86. Parsa A, Lovett DH, Peden EA, Zhu L, Seldin MF, Criswell LA. Renin-angiotensin system gene polymorphisms predict the progression to renal insufficiency among Asians with lupus nephritis. Genes Immun. 2005;6(3):217–24.
87. Chan TM, Li FK, Tang CS, Wong RW, Fang GX, Ji YL, et al. Efficacy of mycophenolate mofetil in patients with diffuse proliferative lupus nephritis. Hong Kong-Guangzhou Nephrology Study Group. N Engl J Med. 2000;343(16):1156–62.
88. Isenberg D, Appel GB, Contreras G, Dooley MA, Ginzler EM, Jayne D, et al. Influence of race/ethnicity on response to lupus nephritis treatment: the ALMS study. Rheumatology (Oxford). 2010;49(1):128–40.
89. Tam LS, Li EK, Leung CB, Wong KC, Lai FM, Wang A, et al. Long-term treatment of lupus nephritis with cyclosporin A. QJM. 1998;91(8):573–80.
90. Chen W, Tang X, Liu Q, Chen W, Fu P, Liu F, et al. Short-term outcomes of induction therapy with tacrolimus versus cyclophosphamide for active lupus nephritis: a multicenter randomized clinical trial. Am J Kidney Dis. 2011;57(2):235–44.
91. Li X, Ren H, Zhang Q, Zhang W, Wu X, Xu Y, et al. Mycophenolate mofetil or tacrolimus compared with intravenous cyclophosphamide in the induction treatment for active lupus nephritis. Nephrol Dial Transplant. 2012;27(4):1467–72.
92. Bao H, Liu ZH, Xie HL, Hu WX, Zhang HT, Li LS. Successful treatment of class V+IV lupus nephritis with multitarget therapy. J Am Soc Nephrol. 2008;19(10):2001–10.
93. Liu Z, Zhang H, Liu Z, Xing C, Fu P, Ni Z, et al. Multitarget therapy for induction treatment of lupus nephritis: a randomized trial. Ann Intern Med. 2015;162(1):18–26.
94. Zhang H, Liu Z, Zhou M, Liu Z, Chen J, Xing C, et al. Multitarget therapy for maintenance treatment of lupus nephritis. J Am Soc Nephrol. 2017;28(12):3671–8.
95. Wang HY, Cui TG, Hou FF, Ni ZH, Chen XM, Lu FM, et al. Induction treatment of proliferative lupus nephritis with leflunomide combined with prednisone: a prospective multi-centre observational study. Lupus. 2008;17(7):638–44.
96. Li J, Cui Z, Long JY, Huang W, Wang JW, Wang H, et al. The frequency of ANCA-associated vasculitis in a national database of hospitalized patients in China. Arthritis Res Ther. 2018;20(1):226.
97. Chen M, Yu F, Zhang Y, Zhao MH. Clinical [corrected] and pathological characteristics of Chinese patients with antineutrophil cytoplasmic autoantibody associated systemic vasculitides: a study of 426 patients from a single centre. Postgrad Med J. 2005;81(961):723–7.
98. Chen M, Yu F, Zhang Y, Zou WZ, Zhao MH, Wang HY. Characteristics of Chinese patients with Wegener's granulomatosis with anti-myeloperoxidase autoantibodies. Kidney Int. 2005;68(5):2225–9.
99. Wang HY, Cui Z, Pei ZY, Fang SB, Chen SF, Zhu L, et al. Risk HLA class II alleles and amino acid residues in myeloperoxidase-ANCA-associated vasculitis. Kidney Int. 2019;96(4):1010–9.
100. Wu Z, Wu Q, Xu J, Chen S, Sun F, Li P, et al. HLA-DPB1 variant rs3117242 is associated with anti-neutrophil cytoplasmic antibody-associated vasculitides in a Han Chinese population. Int J Rheum Dis. 2017;20(8):1009–15.
101. Zhao MH, Chen M, Gao Y, Wang HY. Propylthiouracil-induced anti-neutrophil cytoplasmic antibody-associated vasculitis. Kidney Int. 2006;69(8):1477–81.
102. Chen M, Gao Y, Guo XH, Zhao MH. Propylthiouracil-induced antineutrophil cytoplasmic antibody-associated vasculitis. Nat Rev Nephrol. 2012;8(8):476–83.
103. Chen M, Yu F, Wang SX, Zou WZ, Zhao MH, Wang HY. Antineutrophil cytoplasmic autoantibody-negative pauci-immune crescentic glomerulonephritis. J Am Soc Nephrol. 2007;18(2):599–605.
104. Xing GQ, Chen M, Liu G, Heeringa P, Zhang JJ, Zheng X, et al. Complement activation is involved in renal damage in human antineutrophil cytoplasmic autoantibody associated pauci-immune vasculitis. J Clin Immunol. 2009;29(3):282–91.
105. Gou SJ, Yuan J, Chen M, Yu F, Zhao MH. Circulating complement activation in patients with anti-neutrophil cytoplasmic antibody-associated vasculitis. Kidney Int. 2013;83(1):129–37.
106. Li ZY, Chang DY, Zhao MH, Chen M. Predictors of treatment resistance and relapse in antineutrophil cytoplasmic antibody-associated vasculitis: a study of 439 cases in a single Chinese center. Arthritis Rheumatol. 2014;66(7):1920–6.
107. Chen M, Yu F, Zhao MH. Relapses in patients with antineutrophil cytoplasmic autoantibody-associated vasculitis: likely to begin with the same organ as initial onset. J Rheumatol. 2008;35(3):448–50.
108. Lai QY, Ma TT, Li ZY, Chang DY, Zhao MH, Chen M. Predictors for mortality in patients with antineutrophil cytoplasmic autoantibody-associated vasculitis: a study of 398 Chinese patients. J Rheumatol. 2014;41(9):1849–55.
109. Cui F, Shen L, Li L, Wang H, Wang F, Bi S, et al. Prevention of chronic hepatitis B after 3 decades of escalating vaccination policy, China. Emerg Infect Dis. 2017;23(5):765–72.
110. Si J, Yu C, Guo Y, Bian Z, Qin C, Yang L, et al. Chronic hepatitis B virus infection and risk of chronic kidney disease: a population-based prospective cohort study of 0.5 million Chinese adults. BMC Med. 2018;16(1):93.
111. Zhang X, Liu S, Tang L, Wu J, Chen P, Yin Z, et al. Analysis of pathological data of renal biopsy at one single center in China from 1987 to 2012. Chin Med J. 2014;127(9):1715–20.
112. Whiting DR, Guariguata L, Weil C, Shaw J. IDF diabetes atlas: global estimates of the prevalence of diabetes for 2011 and 2030. Diabetes Res Clin Pract. 2011;94(3):311–21.
113. Hu C, Jia W. Diabetes in China: epidemiology and genetic risk factors and their clinical utility in personalized medication. Diabetes. 2018;67(1):3–11.
114. Ma RCW. Epidemiology of diabetes and diabetic complications in China. Diabetologia. 2018;61(6):1249–60.
115. Tian Y, Jiang C, Wang M, Cai R, Zhang Y, He Z, et al. BMI, leisure-time physical activity, and physical fitness in adults in China: results from a series of national surveys, 2000–14. Lancet Diabetes Endocrinol. 2016;4(6):487–97.
116. Zhou L, Zeng XX, Fu P. Community hemodialysis in China: opportunities and challenges. Chin Med J. 2017;130(18):2143–6.
117. The Microvascular Complications Group of Chinese Diabetes A. Chinese clinical practice guideline of diabetic kidney disease. Chin J Diabetes Mellit. 2019;11(1):15–28.
118. American Diabetes A. 11. Microvascular complications and foot care: standards of medical care in diabetes-2019. Diabetes Care. 2019;42(Suppl 1):S124–S38.
119. Hou JH, Zhu HX, Zhou ML, Le WB, Zeng CH, Liang SS, et al. Changes in the spectrum of kidney diseases: an analysis of 40,759 biopsy-proven cases from 2003 to 2014 in China. Kidney Dis. 2018;4(1):10–9.
120. Anders HJ, Huber TB, Isermann B, Schiffer M. CKD in diabetes: diabetic kidney disease versus nondiabetic kidney disease. Nat Rev Nephrol. 2018;14(6):361–77.
121. Tsao YC, Chen JY, Yeh WC, Li WC. Gender- and age-specific associations between visceral obesity and renal function impairment. Obes Facts. 2019;12(1):67–77.
122. Chen HM, Li SJ, Chen HP, Wang QW, Li LS, Liu ZH. Obesity-related glomerulopathy in China: a case series of 90 patients. Am J Kidney Dis. 2008;52(1):58–65.
123. Gao B, Wu S, Wang J, Yang C, Chen S, Hou J, et al. Clinical features and long-term outcomes of diabetic kidney disease – a

prospective cohort study from China. J Diabetes Complicat. 2019;33(1):39–45.
124. Li G, Zhang P, Wang J, An Y, Gong Q, Gregg EW, et al. Cardiovascular mortality, all-cause mortality, and diabetes incidence after lifestyle intervention for people with impaired glucose tolerance in the Da Qing Diabetes Prevention Study: a 23-year follow-up study. Lancet Diabetes Endocrinol. 2014;2(6):474–80.
125. Li H, Jiang L. Catastrophic medical insurance in China. Lancet. 2017;390(10104):1724–5.
126. Wang Z, Chen Z, Zhang L, Wang X, Hao G, Zhang Z, et al. Status of hypertension in China: results from the China hypertension survey, 2012–2015. Circulation. 2018;137(22):2344–56.
127. Zhang L, Zhao MH, Zuo L, Wang Y, Yu F, Zhang H, et al. China kidney disease network (CK-NET) 2015 annual data report. Kidney Int Suppl. 2019;9(1):e1–e81.
128. Xu X, Qin X, Li Y, Sun D, Wang J, Liang M, et al. Efficacy of folic acid therapy on the progression of chronic kidney disease: the renal substudy of the China stroke primary prevention trial. JAMA Intern Med. 2016;176(10):1443–50.
129. Zhang W, Shi W, Liu Z, Gu Y, Chen Q, Yuan W, et al. A nationwide cross-sectional survey on prevalence, management and pharmacoepidemiology patterns on hypertension in Chinese patients with chronic kidney disease. Sci Rep. 2016;6:38768.
130. Zhou QG, Jiang JP, Wu SJ, Tian JW, Chen JH, Yu XQ, et al. Current pattern of Chinese dialysis units: a cohort study in a representative sample of units. Chin Med J. 2012;125(19):3434–9.
131. Joint Committee for Guideline R. 2018 Chinese guidelines for prevention and treatment of hypertension-A report of the revision committee of Chinese guidelines for prevention and treatment of hypertension. J Geriatr Cardiol. 2019;16(3):182–241.
132. Robson R, Collins J, Johnson R, Kitching R, Searle M, Walker R, et al. Effects of simvastatin and enalapril on serum lipoprotein concentrations and left ventricular mass in patients on dialysis. The Perfect Study Collaborative Group. J Nephrol. 1997;10(1):33–40.
133. Yoon HE, Kwon YJ, Shin SJ, Lee SY, Lee S, Kim SH, et al. Bioimpedance spectroscopy-guided fluid management in peritoneal dialysis patients with residual kidney function: a randomized controlled trial. Nephrology (Carlton). 2019;24(12):1279–89.
134. Tonelli M, Riella MC. World Kidney Day 2014: CKD and the aging population. Am J Kidney Dis. 2014;63(3):349–53.
135. Nie S, Feng Z, Tang L, Wang X, He Y, Fang J, et al. Risk factor analysis for AKI including laboratory indicators: a nationwide multicenter study of hospitalized patients. Kidney Blood Press Res. 2017;42(5):761–73.
136. Zhang L, Zhang P, Wang F, Zuo L, Zhou Y, Shi Y, et al. Prevalence and factors associated with CKD: a population study from Beijing. Am J Kidney Dis. 2008;51(3):373–84.
137. Zhang L, Zhao MH, Zuo L, Wang Y, Yu F, Zhang H, et al. China kidney disease network (CK-NET) 2015 annual data report. Kidney Int Suppl (2011). 2019;9(1):e1–e81.
138. Fassett RG. Current and emerging treatment options for the elderly patient with chronic kidney disease. Clin Interv Aging. 2014;9:191–9.
139. Wang H, Fang C, Cai L, Dong B, Deng J. Chronic kidney disease and cognitive impairment among the very old in China. Aging Clin Exp Res. 2016;28(3):475–82.
140. Liang S, Wang WL, Zhu FL, Duan SW, Sun XF, Chen XM, et al. Chinese observational prospective study of ageing population with chronic kidney disease (C-OPTION): a study protocol. BMJ Open. 2018;8(2):e019457.
141. Wang WL, Liang S, Zhu FL, Liu JQ, Wang SY, Chen XM, et al. The prevalence of depression and the association between depression and kidney function and health-related quality of life in elderly patients with chronic kidney disease: a multicenter cross-sectional study. Clin Interv Aging. 2019;14:905–13.
142. Li PK, Chow KM, Van de Luijtgaarden MW, Johnson DW, Jager KJ, Mehrotra R, et al. Changes in the worldwide epidemiology of peritoneal dialysis. Nat Rev Nephrol. 2017;13(2):90–103.
143. Ministry of Health PRC. Chinese national renal data system. (online). http://www.cnrds.net. 2018.
144. Kidney Transplant Quality Control Center of National Health Commission PRC. Chinese Scientific Registry of Kidney Transplantation. (online). http://www.csrkt.org. 2018.
145. Dialysis_and_Transplantation_Registration_Group. The report about the registration of dialysis and transplantation in China 1999. Zhonghua Shen Zang Bing Za Zhi. 2001;(2):77.
146. Ho Y-W, Chau K-F, Choy B-Y, Fung K-S, Cheng Y-L, Kwan T-H, et al. Hong Kong renal registry report 2012. Hong Kong J Nephrol. 2013;15(1):28–43.
147. Yang WC, Hwang SJ. Incidence, prevalence and mortality trends of dialysis end-stage renal disease in Taiwan from 1990 to 2001: the impact of national health insurance. Nephrol Dial Transplant. 2008;23(12):3977–82.
148. Bieber B, Qian J, Anand S, Yan Y, Chen N, Wang M, et al. Two-times weekly hemodialysis in China: frequency, associated patient and treatment characteristics and quality of life in the China dialysis outcomes and practice patterns study. Nephrol Dial Transplant. 2014;29(9):1770–7.
149. Lin X, Yan Y, Ni Z, Gu L, Zhu M, Dai H, et al. Clinical outcome of twice-weekly hemodialysis patients in shanghai. Blood Purif. 2012;33(1–3):66–72.
150. Yan Y, Wang M, Zee J, Schaubel D, Tu C, Qian J, et al. Twice-weekly hemodialysis and clinical outcomes in the China dialysis outcomes and practice patterns study. Kidney Int Rep. 2018;3(4):889–96.
151. Zhang W, Mei C, Chen N, Ding X, Ni Z, Hao C, et al. Outcomes and practice patterns with hemodiafiltration in Shanghai: a longitudinal cohort study. BMC Nephrol. 2019;20(1):34.
152. Zhao X, Wang M, Zuo L. Early mortality risk in incident Chinese hemodialysis patients: a retrospective cohort study. Ren Fail. 2017;39(1):526–32.
153. Cheng X, Nayyar S, Wang M, Li X, Sun Y, Huang W, et al. Mortality rates among prevalent hemodialysis patients in Beijing: a comparison with USRDS data. Nephrol Dial Transplant. 2013;28(3):724–32.
154. Yao Q, Zhang W, Qian J. Dialysis status in China: a report from the Shanghai dialysis registry (2000–2005). Ethn Dis. 2009;19(1 Suppl 1):S1–23–6.
155. Zuo L, Wang M, Hou F, Yan Y, Chen N, Qian J, et al. Anemia management in the China dialysis outcomes and practice patterns study. Blood Purif. 2016;42(1):33–43.
156. Chinese Hospital quality safety management part 2–20: patient service-hemodialysis. Zhongguo Xue Ye Jing Hua Za Zhi. 2019;18:517–23.
157. Kwong VW, Li PK. Peritoneal dialysis in Asia. Kidney Dis. 2015;1(3):147–56.
158. Yu X, Yang X. Peritoneal dialysis in China: meeting the challenge of chronic kidney failure. Am J Kidney Dis. 2015;65(1):147–51.
159. Mehrotra R, Devuyst O, Davies SJ, Johnson DW. The current state of peritoneal dialysis. J Am Soc Nephrol. 2016;27(11):3238–52.
160. Peng F, Li Z, Yi C, Guo Q, Yang R, Long H, et al. Platelet index levels and cardiovascular mortality in incident peritoneal dialysis patients: a cohort study. Platelets. 2017;28(6):576–84.
161. Jiang Z, Yu X. Advancing the use and quality of peritoneal dialysis by developing a peritoneal dialysis satellite center program. Perit Dial Int. 2011;31(2):121–6.
162. Yu X. How to set up PD centres: the Chinese perspective. http://www.thelancet.com/campaigns/kidney/updates/how-to-set-up-pd-centres-the-chinese-perspective.
163. Peng Y, Ye H, Yi C, Wu M, Huang X, Xiao X, et al. Changes in outcomes over time among incident peritoneal dialysis patients in Southern China. Perit Dial Int. 2019;39(4):382–9.
164. Ye H, Yang X, Yi C, Guo Q, Li Y, Yang Q, et al. Urgent-start peritoneal dialysis for patients with end stage renal disease: a 10-year retrospective study. BMC Nephrol. 2019;20(1):238.

165. Xu Y, Dong J, Zuo L. Is frequency of patient-physician clinic contact important in peritoneal dialysis patients? Perit Dial Int. 2009;29(Suppl 2):S83–9.
166. Li Y, Wang H, Wang Y, Zhou Z, Liu B, Yang W, et al. Long-term survival analysis of the elderly peritoneal dialysis patients. Chin J Nephrol. 2017;33(1):1–7.
167. Fang W, Ni Z, Qian J. Key factors for a high-quality peritoneal dialysis program--the role of the PD team and continuous quality improvement. Perit Dial Int. 2014;34(Suppl 2):S35–42.
168. Zhang X, Shou Z, Chen Z, Xu Y, Han F, Yin X, et al. The role of an integrated care model for kidney disease in the development of peritoneal dialysis: a single-center experience in China. Perit Dial Int. 2014;34(Suppl 2):S55–8.
169. Yu Y, Zhou Y, Wang H, Zhou T, Li Q, Li T, et al. Impact of continuous quality improvement initiatives on clinical outcomes in peritoneal dialysis. Perit Dial Int. 2014;34(Suppl 2):S43–8.
170. Yang X, Mao HP, Guo QY, Yu XQ. Successfully managing a rapidly growing peritoneal dialysis program in Southern China. Chin Med J. 2011;124(17):2696–700.
171. Ye H, Zhou Q, Fan L, Guo Q, Mao H, Huang F, et al. The impact of peritoneal dialysis-related peritonitis on mortality in peritoneal dialysis patients. BMC Nephrol. 2017;18(1):186.
172. Fang W, Qian J, Lin A, Rowaie F, Ni Z, Yao Q, et al. Comparison of peritoneal dialysis practice patterns and outcomes between a Canadian and a Chinese centre. Nephrol Dial Transplant. 2008;23(12):4021–8.
173. Yao Q, Dong J, Feng T, Lindholm B. What PD research in China tells us. Perit Dia Int. 2018;38(Suppl 2):S19–24.
174. Huang J, Wang H, Fan ST, Zhao B, Zhang Z, Hao L, et al. The national program for deceased organ donation in China. Transplantation. 2013;96(1):5–9.
175. Weaning China off organs from executed prisoners. Lancet. 2015;385(9962):1.
176. Huang J, Millis JM, Mao Y, Millis MA, Sang X, Zhong S. A pilot programme of organ donation after cardiac death in China. Lancet. 2012;379(9818):862–5.
177. Chinese Society of Organ Transplantation CMA. National guidelines for donation after cardiac death in China. Hepatobiliary Pancreat Dis Int. 2013;12(3):234–8.
178. A definition of irreversible coma. Report of the Ad Hoc Committee of the Harvard Medical School to Examine the Definition of Brain Death. JAMA. 1968;205(6):337–40.
179. Sixty-Third World Health Assembly WHO. WHO guiding principles on human cell, tissue and organ transplantation. Cell Tissue Bank. 2010;11(4):413–9.
180. Sun Q, Gao X, Wang H, Ko DS, Li XC. A new era for organ transplantation in China. Lancet. 2014;383(9933):1971–2.
181. The China Organ Transplant Response System COTRS. http://www.cot.org.cn. Available from: COTRS, http://www.cot.org.cn.
182. Ma LZL, Yu L, et al. A questionnaire survey on cognition and intention towards organ donation in driving license holders of Mainland China (in Chinese). Chin J Urol. 2014;35:10–4.
183. Liu JOY, Wu C, et al. Cognition in human organ transplantation: comparative study between medical and non-medical college students in Beijing (in Chinese). Organ Transplant. 2014;5:103–6.
184. Regulation on Human Organ Procurement and Allocation (Interim). Updated 2016 Jul 08. Available from: http://www.nhfpc.gov.cn/yzygj/s3585u/201308/8f4ca93212984722b51c4684569e9917.shtml.
185. Shang X, Zhang M. Body and organ donation in Wuhan. China Lancet. 2010;376(9746):1033–4.
186. Waikar SS, Curhan GC, Wald R, McCarthy EP, Chertow GM. Declining mortality in patients with acute renal failure, 1988 to 2002. J Am Soc Nephrol. 2006;17(4):1143–50.
187. Lewington AJ, Cerda J, Mehta RL. Raising awareness of acute kidney injury: a global perspective of a silent killer. Kidney Int. 2013;84(3):457–67.
188. Schissler MM, Zaidi S, Kumar H, Deo D, Brier ME, McLeish KR. Characteristics and outcomes in community-acquired versus hospital-acquired acute kidney injury. Nephrology (Carlton). 2013;18(3):183–7.
189. Finlay S, Bray B, Lewington AJ, Hunter-Rowe CT, Banerjee A, Atkinson JM, et al. Identification of risk factors associated with acute kidney injury in patients admitted to acute medical units. Clin Med (Lond). 2013;13(3):233–8.
190. Xu X, Nie S, Liu Z, Chen C, Xu G, Zha Y, et al. Epidemiology and clinical correlates of AKI in Chinese hospitalized adults. Clin J Am Soc Nephrol. 2015;10(9):1510–8.
191. Wang Y, Wang J, Su T, Qu Z, Zhao M, Yang L, et al. Community-acquired acute kidney injury: a nationwide survey in China. Am J Kidney Dis. 2017;69(5):647–57.
192. Xu X, Nie S, Zhang A, Mao J, Liu HP, Xia H, et al. Acute kidney injury among hospitalized children in China. Clin J Am Soc Nephrol. 2018;13(12):1791–800.
193. Hui WF, Chan WK, Miu TY. Acute kidney injury in the paediatric intensive care unit: identification by modified RIFLE criteria. Hong Kong Med J. 2013;19(1):13–9.
194. Tang X, Chen D, Yu S, Yang L, Mei C, Consortium IAbC. Acute kidney injury burden in different clinical units: data from nationwide survey in China. PLoS One. 2017;12(2):e0171202.
195. Wen Y, Jiang L, Xu Y, Qian CY, Li SS, Qin TH, et al. Prevalence, risk factors, clinical course, and outcome of acute kidney injury in Chinese intensive care units: a prospective cohort study. Chin Med J. 2013;126(23):4409–16.
196. Zhang Y, Jiang L, Wang B, Xi X. Epidemiological characteristics of and risk factors for patients with postoperative acute kidney injury: a multicenter prospective study in 30 Chinese intensive care units. Int Urol Nephrol. 2018;50(7):1319–28.
197. Wang N, Jiang L, Zhu B, Wen Y, Xi XM. Fluid balance and mortality in critically ill patients with acute kidney injury: a multicenter prospective epidemiological study. Crit Care. 2015;19:371.
198. Wang X, Jiang L, Wen Y, Wang MP, Li W, Li ZQ, et al. Risk factors for mortality in patients with septic acute kidney injury in intensive care units in Beijing, China: a multicenter prospective observational study. Biomed Res Int. 2014;2014:172620.
199. Wang D, Guo Y, Zhang Y, Li Z, Li A, Luo Y. Epidemiology of acute kidney injury in patients with stroke: a retrospective analysis from the neurology ICU. Intern Emerg Med. 2018;13(1):17–25.
200. Qin JP, Yu XY, Qian CY, Li SS, Qin TH, Chen EZ, et al. Value of kidney disease improving global outcomes urine output criteria in critically ill patients: a secondary analysis of a multicenter prospective cohort study. Chin Med J. 2016;129(17):2050–7.
201. Li Y, Wang J, Bai Z, Chen J, Wang X, Pan J, et al. Early fluid overload is associated with acute kidney injury and PICU mortality in critically ill children. Eur J Pediatr. 2016;175(1):39–48.
202. Li JG, Qu D, Li Y, Wang F, Guo LY, Wang JJ, et al. Acute kidney injury in critically ill children infected with influenza A virus (H1N1) and enterovirus 71. Zhonghua Er Ke Za Zhi. 2011;49(11):839–42.
203. Wang F, Hong D, Wang Y, Feng Y, Wang L, Yang L, et al. Renal replacement therapy in acute kidney injury from a Chinese cross-sectional study: patient, clinical, socioeconomic and health service predictors of treatment. BMC Nephrol. 2017;18(1):152.
204. Zhou Y, Zhou F, Wang X, Chang P, Zhang L, Yao Q, et al. Practice of extracorporeal therapies for septic acute kidney injury patients in intensive care units in Mainland China. Blood Purif. 2019;47(Suppl 3):1–6.
205. Fan H, Zhao Y, Chen GD, Sun M, Zhu JH. Health insurance status and risk factors of mortality in patients with septic acute kidney injury in Ningbo, China. J Int Med Res. 2019;47(1):370–6.
206. Clark WR, Ding X, Qiu H, Ni Z, Chang P, Fu P, et al. Renal replacement therapy practices for patients with acute kidney injury in China. PLoS One. 2017;12(7):e0178509.

207. Ao X, Zhong Y, Yu XH, Marshall MR, Feng T, Ning JP, et al. Acute peritoneal dialysis system for neonates with acute kidney injury requiring renal replacement therapy: a case series. Perit Dial Int. 2018;38(Suppl 2):S45–52.
208. Wu Y, Chen Y, Li S, Dong W, Liang H, Deng M, et al. Value of electronic alerts for acute kidney injury in high-risk wards: a pilot randomized controlled trial. Int Urol Nephrol. 2018;50(8):1483–8.
209. China NHCotPsRo. Annals of heath statistics. 2018.
210. Osman MA, Alrukhaimi M, Ashuntantang GE, Bellorin-Font E, Benghanem Gharbi M, Braam B, et al. Global nephrology workforce: gaps and opportunities toward a sustainable kidney care system. Kidney Int Suppl (2011). 2018;8(2):52–63.
211. Science. IoMICAoM. Study of science and technology evaluation metrics of hospitals in China 2018. Nephrology.
212. Leung CB, Cheung WL, Li PK. Renal registry in Hong Kong-the first 20 years. Kidney Int Suppl (2011). 2015;5(1):33–8.
213. Hong Kong Hospital Authority Renal Registry. 2016.
214. Chau KF. Living-related renal transplantation in Hong Kong. Hong Kong Med J. 2018;24(1):4–5.

# Nephrology in India

# 21

Joyita Bharati and Vivekanand Jha

| | |
|---|---|
| Area[1] | 3.287 million Km$^2$ |
| Population[1,2] | 1.353 billion (2018) |
| Capital | New Delhi |
| Three most populated cities[1] | 1. Mumbai<br>2. Delhi<br>3. Bangalore |
| Official languages | Hindi, English |
| Gross domestic product (GDP)[2] | 2.719 trillion USD (2018) |
| GDP per capita[2] | 2009.979 USD (2018)<br>7762.882 Int$ (PPP, 2018) |
| Human development index (HDI)[2] | 0.647 (129th position, 2019) |
| Official currency | Indian Rupee (INR) |
| Total number of nephrologists[3] | 1639 (in 2016) |
| National society of nephrology | Indian Society of Nephrology<br>www.isn-india.org |
| Incidence of chronic kidney disease[3] | 2016 – 2545.5 pmp |
| Prevalence of chronic kidney disease[3] | 2016 – 33,509.6 pmp |
| Incidence of end-stage renal disease[4] | 2006 – 151 pmp (average crude incidence)<br>232 pmp (age-adjusted incidence) |
| Prevalence of end-stage renal disease (on dialysis) | 2017 – 130 pmp |
| Total number of patients on dialysis[3, 5] | 2016 – ~130,000<br>2017 – 174,478 |
| Number of patients on hemodialysis[3, 5] | 2016 – ~120,000<br>2017 – ~166,000 |
| Number of patients on peritoneal dialysis[3, 4] | 2016 – ~10,000<br>2017 – ~8500 |
| Number of renal transplantations per year[3] | 2017 – 6587 |

1. Censusindia.gov.in (2011)
2. The World Development Report (https://data.worldbank.org/products/wdi)
3. Jha V, Ur-Rashid H, Agarwal SK, et al. The state of nephrology in South Asia. Kidney Int. 2019;95:31–7
4. Modi GK, Jha V. The incidence of end-stage renal disease in India: a population-based study. Kidney Int. 2006; 70: 2131–3
5. Varughese S, Abraham G. Chronic kidney disease in India: a clarion for change. Clin J Am Soc Nephrol. 2018;13:802–4

## Introduction

India contributes to 17.75% of the world population with 1.35 billion people spread over 3.287 million square kilometers. Although the climatic conditions vary in the different zones of the country, on the whole India is considered a tropical country. Geographically, the tropical region is limited to an area on either side of the equator limited by the Tropic of Cancer and Capricorn, respectively. A tropical area is characterized by a direct overhead presence of the sun at least once a year. The level of rainfall varies from 750 mm in the peninsular India to 2000 mm per year in the tropical rainforests [1]. Although urban population has swiftly risen due to migration, about two-thirds of the population in India still live in rural areas.

## Economic and Health Indicators

India is classified by the World Bank as a lower middle-income country based on the gross national income per capita. In addition, there exists a huge socioeconomic stratification, with the richest 1% holding more than half of the country's total wealth. This increases the disparity in access to healthcare, with the poor being severely disadvantaged.

While the gross domestic product (GDP) has risen in the recent years, the overall health expenditure constitutes a miniscule proportion (3.9% of the GDP) [2]. Only 30% of the health expenditure is borne by the public sector.

J. Bharati
Postgraduate Institute of Medical Education and Research, Chandigarh, India

V. Jha (✉)
International Society of Nephrology, Brussels, Belgium

George Institute for Global Health, UNSW, New Delhi, India

Faculty of Medicine, Imperial College, London, UK

Manipal Academy of Higher Education, Manipal, India



J. A. Moura-Neto et al. (eds.), *Nephrology Worldwide*, https://doi.org/10.1007/978-3-030-56890-0_21

Out-of-pocket expenditure constitutes 70% of the current health expenditure in India. It has been estimated that about 7% of the population is pushed below poverty threshold every year due to medical expenses [3]. Despite substantial improvement in health indicators over the last 50 years, the maternal, infant, and under 5 mortality rates remain unacceptably high. The doctor-patient ratio is 0.8 per 1000, substantially lower than that recommended by the World Health Organization (1:1000). Only about 15% of the population is covered under various health insurance schemes. Most of insurance coverage is by government-sponsored schemes and some by private insurers. The union government launched the National Health Protection Mission in 2018 with an aim of covering poor families for expenses incurred during hospitalization at secondary and tertiary healthcare centers.

In recent decades, noncommunicable diseases have overtaken infections as the dominant cause of death and disability in India. The union government has announced a national policy for prevention and control of NCDs. However, kidney diseases have not been included in the noncommunicable disease program despite being a major public health problem (see below).

## Brief History of Nephrology in India

Nephrology, as a specialty of internal medicine, was nonexistent until 1960s in India. The first systematic study of renal diseases, which involved reporting of 50 successful renal biopsies, was done by Dr. Kirpal Singh Chugh, fondly called the Father of Nephrology in India in the 1950s [4]. The Indian Society of Nephrology was formed in 1970 to create a common forum for nephrologists across the nation. The society encourages collaboration between centers across the country and worldwide in terms of research and harmization of clinical practice. The first hemodialysis was done using Kolff twin coil dialysis machine, given as a gift to Christian Medical College, Vellore, for treating a patient with chronic uremia in 1961. Long-term dialysis using Kiil dialyzers started later in 1968 with arteriovenous shunts made of silastic tubing as vascular access. Less than 10 centers performed dialysis those days as compared to close to 5,000 dialysis centers currently. The existing infrastructure, however, is inadequate to meet the demands of >200,000 new patients developing kidney failure every year. Peritoneal dialysis (PD) was first performed in 1964 using polythene tubing as catheters and dialysate was prepared in-house. However, chronic PD was not popular until late 1990s. The first successful kidney transplant was done in 1971. Currently, over 250 centers perform kidney transplantation, mostly using kidneys from living donors. The deceased donor transplantation (DDT) rate in India is among the lowest in the world despite large numbers of potential organ donors. Inadequate sharing among hospitals, lack of trained transplant coordinators, and awareness among the general public are the main reasons for inadequacy of the DDT program. However, a few states and union territories (Tamil Nadu, Kerala, Pondicherry, Chandigarh) have shown improvement in organ retrieval rates over the last decade. Nephrology training started in India with a 2-year course at the Postgraduate Institute of Medical Education and Research, Chandigarh, in 1969. Currently, there are 72 centers enrolling approximately 180 students each year for a nephrology fellowship training [2].

## Measurement of Kidney Function

Serum creatinine is measured by either the Jaffe method or enzymatic method in Indian laboratories. There are limitations in the interpretation of serum creatinine. Firstly, different manufacturers use different assays for the same method, for example, two laboratories may be doing the Jaffe method for serum creatinine measurement but each with a different assay. Standardization to an IDMS reference measurement procedure, as recommended in the 2012 KDIGO Guidelines for chronic kidney disease definition and classification, is not routine in a large proportion of Indian laboratories. This limits the generalizability of serum creatinine with that of the world population, particularly for lower range of values [5]. The glomerular filtration rate (GFR) is estimated from serum creatinine-based equations which consider variability of serum creatinine due to age, gender, and ethnicity. Most commonly used eGFR equations are the Chronic Kidney Disease Epidemiology Collaboration (CKD-EPI equation) and Modification of Renal Diet (MDRD equation). These equations have not been validated in the Indian population. In a recently reported study on 130 healthy individuals and stable CKD patients from North India, CKD-EPI (creatinine) and MDRD were found to overestimate GFR measured by inulin clearance [6]. eGFR values derived using the CKD-EPI (cystatin) equation were closest to measured GFR (mGFR). Another interesting finding was the relatively low measured GFR in the healthy population ($79.44 \pm 20.19$ ml/min/1.73 $m^2$, range: 41.90–134.50 ml/min/1.73 $m^2$). Similar values of measured GFR have been previously reported from other centers in India [7, 8]. Low mGFR in apparently healthy Indians was postulated to be due to low protein intake and small and thin body habitus [6]. The measured creatinine excretion rates were lower than what has been reported for Japanese participants. The impact of having a low GFR on the future risks of renal failure or mortality in apparently healthy Indians is not studied. Decisions regarding kidney donation are made without really knowing the long-term implications of donation at such GFR levels. It is possible that perfectly healthy individuals are not accepted as donors because of the mGFR being below the cutoffs described in the western population, or donors with falsely elevated eGFR may be accepted for kidney donation in centers where GFR is not measured.

## Acute Kidney Injury in India

India, being a tropical country, is a host to many different flora and fauna with whom human inhabitants interact regularly. Kidneys are often involved in tropical infections, as a result of organisms directly affecting the kidneys, renal hypoperfusion (as a part of multiorgan dysfunction or diarrhea), and/or through postinfectious autoimmunity. Poor sanitation and hygiene predispose to contamination of food and water and breeding of vectors, even in urban areas. On top of that, there is a shift of wild animals and vectors from forests to urban areas as a result of deforestation. India is one of the top hotspots for zoonotic diseases with reemergence of the previously reported conditions like cutaneous leishmaniasis or highly infectious diseases including Nipah virus, leptospirosis, and scrub typhus [9].

The epidemiology of AKI in India is different from that seen in developed countries with temperate ecosystems. AKI is most often community-acquired (due to factors in the local environment) in otherwise healthy and young middle-age population. The common culprits are infection, toxins in traditional remedies or pesticides, snake or insect bite, and/or pregnancy-related. Patients usually have a single identifiable cause of AKI and present late to the hospital [10].

Snakebite is considered a neglected tropical disease and a public health problem in India. South Asia contributes to 70% of global snakebite annually [11]. Urban-rural divide and geographical biodiversity contribute to increased human exposure to venomous snake species. Agricultural occupation, delayed treatment with antidotes, and inadequate care at primary healthcare contribute to the rising snakebite-related complications. About 70–80% of deaths due to snakebite occur before patients reach the hospital, and nearly all snakebite deaths occur in rural areas [12]. Snakebites peak during monsoons and specifically in field workers [13]. AKI typically occurs in up to one-third of patients bitten by a venomous snake, commonly hemotoxic venom. Viper bites are the most common cause of snakebite-related AKIs in India. Hemolysis, hypotension, and thrombotic microangiopathy, either singly or in combination, result in acute tubular necrosis or in severe cases acute cortical necrosis [14].

The burden of pregnancy-related AKI is still substantial in India with a previously reported prevalence of 22% [15]. The incidence of pregnancy-related AKI has decreased from 15% in 1990s to 1.5% in the last decade [16, 17]. Decreased incidence of postabortal AKI following the legalization of abortion mandating hospital care has made a huge difference in the epidemiology of pregnancy-related AKI. However, puerperal sepsis-associated AKI was reported to be increased in the year 2003–2014 (~26%) as compared to 1982–1991 (~9%) [16]. Puerperal sepsis and obstetric hemorrhage now constitute most of the cases of pregnancy-related AKI [16]. About 60–70% of the patients with pregnancy-related AKI require dialysis, and a substantial proportion do not recover kidney function [16–19]. Renal cortical necrosis results from uncontrolled blood loss, sepsis, or preeclampsia, either in the antepartum or postpartum period. Underlying the complement pathway abnormality resulting in severe thrombotic microangiopathy, thereby renal cortical necrosis was suggested as a possibility [18]. While the overall incidence of renal cortical necrosis of obstetric etiology has decreased, the absolute numbers continue to be high [19]. Postpartum thrombotic microangiopathy is increasingly being recognized as an important cause of renal cortical necrosis [18–20]. In a large recent series, 43% of patients with postpartum renal cortical necrosis had postpartum hemorrhage preceding AKI, and the majority (95.2%) had laboratory features of thrombotic microangiopathy [13]. Pregnancy-related complications are important public health issues owing to its impact on maternal and fetal mortality rates. In addition, the burden of dialysis in these young patients is disturbing. Although the current maternal mortality rate (5.79%) has decreased significantly in India [16], it is still a nuisance among the vulnerable poor section of the society who do not get to avail high-quality obstetric care.

Renal replacement therapy (RRT) practices for AKI vary across different regions and between private and public hospitals in India. The need for RRT in patients with AKI is usually considered lower in India (up to 30%) as compared to developed countries. Most of the centers have use of intermittent hemodialysis (including slow low-efficiency hemodialysis) as the only RRT modality in AKI [21, 22]. Convective therapies such as continuous veno-venous hemofiltration (CVVH) are barely used due to high costs of equipment and inadequate man power. CVVH was found to be comparable to acute peritoneal dialysis (PD) in small groups of hemodynamically unstable patients with AKI [23, 24].

## Chronic Kidney Disease in India

With an increasing incidence worldwide, awareness about CKD and the associated burden on the nation have risen in India. CKD is recognized as a major noncommunicable disease across the globe that contributes to premature death [25]. With the increasing burden of hypertension and diabetes [26] across all socioeconomic strata in India, the prevalence of CKD is expected to rise further. The prevalence of CKD was reported to be between 13% and 17.2% based on detection of urine protein and MDRD or CKD-EPI eGFR (<60 ml/min/1.73 $m^2$) [27, 28]. The prevalence varies across different regions across the country. Nationwide data on the prevalence and etiology of CKD do not exist. The first effort was the creation of the Indian CKD registry by the Indian Society of Nephrology in 2005 with an aim of nationwide data collection. In its first report, 52,273 adult patients from 188 centers across all zones of the country were analyzed [29]. While diabetic nephropathy constituted majority (31.3%) of CKD in all geographical areas, CKD of unknown etiology (CKDu) was seen in 16% of the patients [29].

The southern state of Andhra Pradesh and some parts of Odisha have reported rising numbers of CKD of unknown origin, attributed to environmental triggers. In a recent study from Uddanam, part of Andhra Pradesh, out of 2210 subjects, CKD was diagnosed in 403 (18.23%), and 73% of them did not have any known risk factors for CKD [30]. Multiple factors, which include pesticides; heavy metals such as cadmium, arsenic, and fluoride; intake of over-the-counter painkillers; and dehydration coupled with hot working conditions, are suspected to contribute to the development of CKDu. Renal histology in these patients is a characteristic of chronic interstitial nephritis. The disease is typically paucisymptomatic until advanced stage, resulting in missed diagnosis. A substantial proportion of these individuals are young, in productive years of their lives. The development of kidney failure takes them out of the workforce, often plunging these families in economic distress.

Renal injury from herbal remedies and heavy metals is unique to the country's population which relies on traditional medicines to a large extent. Herbal medicines are usually not tested for content safety. Potentially toxic ingredients like heavy metals are used to increase their efficacy. Aristolochic acid-induced nephropathy is one such well-described example in the Chinese and Balkan belt (Romania, Croatia, Bosnia, Serbia, and Bulgaria) population. The contribution of herbal remedies and heavy metals to CKDu in India has been speculated [31]. Heavy metals, specifically mercury, in traditional remedies (Ayurveda and Siddha system of medicine) have been recently described to cause membranous nephropathy in Indians [32].

Over half of the patients with CKD in India come to medical attention only after they have developed advanced renal failure that requires dialysis. An urban population-based study revealed an age-adjusted ESRD incidence rate of 232 per million population, suggesting that over 200,000 new patients may be developing ESRD annually in India and 174,478 patients are on chronic dialysis [33, 34]. Similar to the western population, diabetic nephropathy was the commonest cause among new ESRD patients. However, Indian patients are younger at diagnosis of ESRD. Lack of awareness about kidney disease, screening for CKD, and access to healthcare are postulated to be the possible reasons. The burden of CKD in India, measured in terms of death rate and disability-adjusted life years, has increased over the last two decades. Estimated age-standardized annual death rate due to CKD in 2016 was 17.81 per 100,000 persons in India according to the Global Burden of Disease Study, [35] and CKD was ranked eighth among the causes of death [36]. This figure is unlikely to represent the true burden of CKD-related deaths due to the poor reporting system in the country. According to the Million Death Study, which determined the cause of death by verbal autopsy, chronic kidney disease was responsible for about 3% of all causes of death in the age-group of 15–69 years [37]. Majority (>50%) of deaths occur at home with a high likelihood of misclassification of the cause of death by questionnaire-based surveys [38]. CKD-related deaths were found to have regional differences, with age-standardized renal death rates being highest in the southern and eastern states [37]. Diabetes was the strongest predictor of renal failure deaths. The growing prevalence of CKDu in the several states may add to the CKD burden. The national programs for noncommunicable diseases do not include regular screening for CKD, even in a high-risk population. Little is known about the prevalent treatment patterns, especially about implementation of evidence-based guidelines for management of kidney disease in India [39].

## Renal Replacement Therapy in India

High costs, chronic nature of treatment, and lack of availability in large parts of the country make access to renal replacement therapy difficult for a large proportion of cases in India. Hemodialysis is the most common modality followed by renal transplantation. There are about 174,478 patients on HD, and <5% patients are undergoing peritoneal dialysis [2]. Dialysis is expensive for most families, with the median dialysis-related expenditure exceeding household nonsubsistence expenditure [40]. The mean cost of HD borne by the government health system in a public sector hospital was reported to be INR 4,148 (US$ 64) per HD session. Most of it is on human resource followed by building infrastructure. The mean out-of-pocket expenditure (OOPE) by the patient per HD session was INR 2,838 (US$ 44). Majority of the OOPE is on medicines followed by travel [41]. As a result, over 80% of families of patients requiring RRT incur catastrophic healthcare expenditure (>40% of nonfood expenditure) [42].

The existing number of hemodialysis (HD) facilities is insufficient to cater to the growing incidence of ESRD. Many young ESRD patients are forced to lose their jobs and social role. Only a minority of patients receive thrice a week HD, with twice a week frequency being the most prevalent practice comprising about 79–100% in reports from South India [43, 44]. A substantial proportion receive HD even less frequently, including a "as-needed" basis because of financial constraints. Home hemodialysis is rare, with the estimated number being less than 100 patients. The quality of care is further compromised by the inability to receive ancillary treatment, like that for anemia and mineral and bone disease. The Indian Society of Nephrology has issued guidelines for setting up dialysis units [45]. Dialyzer reuse is allowed and widely practiced. Dialyzers are reprocessed by chemical disinfectants and tested for performance using automated machines or manually. Based on the performance of dialyzer after reprocessing, they are discarded or reused. A dialyzer is typically reused up to ten times in some centers. A typical dialysis unit in India has one dialysis doctor (a nephrologist in most urban centers or an internist in peripheral centers), one dialysis technician or nurse, and a dialysis attendant/sanitation personnel. The patient to technician/nurse ratio of 3:1 is recommended by the guideline. A typical renal nurse in a public hospital gets about 60,000 INR per month as salary.

Both the central and state governments have started a variety of health insurance schemes for covering the costs of dialysis [41]. The National Dialysis Service was announced by the central government in 2016 with an aim to cover all 688 districts in India [46]. A few states like Andhra Pradesh (AP) and Tamil Nadu have been running such schemes for approximately 10 years. Since there are not enough facilities in public hospitals, most units are run by private entities under a public-private partnership model [47]. A recently published analysis of insurance claims in AP showed that even though the number of patients accessing HD increased on a year-by-year basis, the outcomes remained dismal. The median survival on dialysis was just about 6 months, and over 60% of patients "dropped out" of the program [48]. Out-of-pocket expenditure on associated medications, travel, and loss of income were speculated to be the reasons for these dropouts. In 2018, the AP government introduced a "pension scheme" to reduce out-of-pocket costs and improve the sustainability of dialysis programs. Research is also underway for development of technologies to reduce cost of HD [47].

Peritoneal dialysis (PD) is vastly underutilized in India despite its theoretical advantages in resource-constrained settings, with <10% of all dialysis patients being on this modality. Most patients who choose PD receive full reimbursement of costs from their employers (through Central Government Health Scheme) as the expenses involved are higher (approximately US $500/month) than that in maintenance hemodialysis (US $10–65/session, mostly twice a week) [49]. Reducing the current high price of PD bags by setting up indigenous manufacturing facilities and introducing quality improvement programs that improve technique survival would help in popularizing this treatment option [47]. A couple of PD manufacturers had started an innovative payment model for PD in 2003. In this "once-in-a-lifetime payment" scheme, a legal agreement between the patient and PD provider would enable the patient to avail lifelong supplies of PD bags for approximately US$15,500 [49]. The scheme was abandoned after a few years, however. The Government of India recently announced the inclusion of PD in the National Dialysis Program, which may improve penetration of PD in the country. Operational guidelines that describe the practical modalities of its implementation are yet to be released, however.

Of the 200,000 new ESRD patients, only about 8000 receive renal transplantation in India, mostly from living kidney donors [50]. On an average, about 8–8,000 patients get a kidney transplant every year [2]. Paradoxically, state coverage of the costs of treatment for kidney transplant is limited, with there being no national policy analogous to that for dialysis. Exceptions include the states of Tamil Nadu and Pondicherry, where patients are eligible to receive free care for surgery as well as postsurgical care including immunosuppressive therapy. Data on allograft survival on patients following renal transplant is fairly uniform across the country. While 1-year and 5-year death-censored allograft survival after live-related transplant in a referral center in North India were 94% and 79% [51], a report from South India showed 1-year and 5-year survival to be 92% and 75%, respectively [52]. Deceased donor transplant programs are poorly developed in most states. Notable has been the policy of providing free transplantation facility for the underprivileged and public-private partnership in organ sharing advocated by the state government of Tamil Nadu [53]. Modern monitoring practices, such as measurement of donor-specific antibodies using single antigen beads, are slowly receiving greater uptake as the costs come down. The practice of transplantation across the ABO blood group barrier has also become fairly widespread in recent years. Protocols followed for immunosuppression induction and maintenance after transplant are as per international recommendation. Majority of low-risk patients (first transplant, absence of sensitization, and/or living related donors) are not given induction therapy (with either depleting agents or basiliximab). In addition, owing to the expenses involved in these induction agents, many patients are given tailored dose to optimize cost. Maintenance immunosuppression comprises of combination of calcineurin inhibitors, mycophenolate mofetil, and steroids. All immunosuppressive drugs are manufactured as generic drugs by local pharmaceuticals and are available at a significantly reduced cost. The immunosuppressive drugs are largely self-funded by patients, except in the southern states where the government pays for medicines, investigations, and follow-up. On a long term, renal transplant is still a cheaper alternative to chronic dialysis in India [52].

## Comorbidities and Infections in Patients on RRT

Despite improvement in ESRD care, ~10% of patients on HD in India die within a year of starting treatment [54, 55]. Ischemic heart disease and infections together comprise 60% of overall mortality in patients on HD in India [55]. A significant number of patients choose nontunelled catheters owing to cost constraints and develop catheter-related bloodstream infections. Apart from bacterial catheter-related infections, 7–10% of patients on maintenance HD acquire tuberculosis, and 10–13% acquire chronic viral infections such as hepatitis B and hepatitis C [56]. Infections account for the most number of deaths with functioning graft in India, with 36% of deaths attributable to sepsis/infection as found in a study conducted in North India. Most of the deaths due to infections occurred within the first 5 years of transplant [57].

## Renal Diseases in Childhood

Nephrotic syndrome is the most common (about 40–50%) renal disease seen in a pediatric nephrology unit in India. About 5–10% of them are steroid-resistant nephrotic syndrome [58]. AKI following tropical fever is common in children as well. Hemolytic uremic syndrome (HUS) is a frequent cause of AKI, and a majority (50%) of them were found to be anti-factor H-related atypical HUS [59]. The prevalence of risk factors of CKD such as low birth weight is widespread. The exact burden of CKD in children is not known as nationwide registry is not yet available. Among various causes of CKD, obstructive uropathy due to posterior urethral valve is the commonest followed by chronic glomerulonephritis, reflux nephropathy, and others [60]. Most children present late with 25–50% already in end-stage renal failure at presentation [60, 61]. A dedicated hemodialysis unit for pediatric patients is largely restricted to a handful of centers in only metropolitan cities. Majority of children opt out either due to financial constraints or vascular access issues. PD is the most frequently utilized modality of RRT in children [58]. Few centers do pediatric renal transplant across the country, most being live-related, and graft survival at 1 year is up to 90% [62].

## Nephrology Practice in India

According to a recent report, there were 1,639 trained nephrologists (members of the Indian Society of Nephrology) in India in 2016, and approximately 170 are being enrolled every year for nephrology fellowship across 72 centers [2]. Most of the nephrologists are concentrated in large cities. Awareness of guideline-based care for early stage kidney disease that can be managed in the community is low among primary care physicians, resulting in poor quality of care. As a result, patients living in remote rural areas have to travel large distances to receive specialist care. Nephrologist shortage is compounded by low numbers of appropriately trained allied health professionals like nurses and dialysis technicians. The remuneration of the healthcare professional is quite variable. For example, the average monthly salary of a nurse in a public sector hospital is about 2500–3300 Int$, whereas the corresponding figure in a private hospital is 1300–1800 Int$. A large proportion of the dialysis units that have been set up under the public-private partnership (PPP) model are staffed primarily by paramedical personnel, under the supervision of a physician.

## Future Perspectives of Nephrology in India

Despite substantial challenges, the commitment by the Indian government to provide universal healthcare to its citizens presents opportunities to introduce several reforms to improve the care of patients with or at risk of kidney diseases [63]. These include improved focus on early prevention and health promotion, improving care for kidney diseases in advanced stages and the generation of evidence to inform policy interventions. Stakeholders must work together to ensure resources are used in a valuable and ethical way so that effective and sustainable models of care can be developed.

Of particular urgency is the need to generate evidence to support these initiatives. Areas where such evidence is needed include linking health promotion to improved health and economic outcomes regarding kidney diseases; measuring effectiveness, scalability, sustainability, and safety of all initiatives implemented to improve care of patients with kidney disease, whether in primary care (e.g., case-finding initiatives, task-shifting allowing community health workers to provide essential preventative care) or for advanced stage disease (e.g., better access to home-based peritoneal dialysis and supportive care where clinically appropriate); continuous monitoring of quality of care; and costs to assess the impact of different financing mechanisms so that financial protection of patients can be balanced with sustainability of health systems. Research is needed to identify novel risk factors that cause kidney disease including those related to upcoming challenges like climate change and COVID-19 pandemic. Barriers to access need to be removed in a socially participative model that responds to the needs of the most vulnerable and the worst off. A recent survey conducted among the Indian nephrologists identified the development of guidelines for prevention of kidney disease at primary care level, developing research capacity in kidney disease, improved support for deceased donation programs, adapting kidney disease treatment guidelines for local application, advocating development of sustainable dialysis programs, and setting up open access national dialysis registries as priority areas worthy of attention.

## Conclusions

Renal services in India are characterized by increasing disease burden and a rapidly growing demand for service and research in the face of inadequate financial and manpower capacity. Increasing number of trained nephrologists, improved evidence base that can inform policy, growing government support to improve care for kidney disease at all levels including renal replacement therapy, and development of locally appropriate models of service delivery offer hope for the future of nephrology in India.

## References

1. State of the Tropics 2014 Report. Townsville: James Cook University; 2014.
2. Jha V, Ur-Rashid H, Agarwal SK, et al. The state of nephrology in South Asia. Kidney Int. 2019;95:31–7.
3. Selvaraj S, Farooqui HH, Karan A. Quantifying the financial burden of households' out-of-pocket payments on medicines in India: a repeated cross-sectional analysis of National Sample Survey data, 1994–2014. BMJ open. 2018. https://doi.org/10.1136/bmjopen-2017-018020.
4. Chugh KS. Five decades of Indian nephrology: a personal journey. Am J Kidney Dis. 2009;54(4):753–63.
5. Delanaye P, Cavalier E, Pottel H. Serum creatinine: not so simple! Nephron. 2017;136:302–8.
6. Kumar V, Yadav AK, Yashuda Y, et al. Existing creatinine-based equations overestimate glomerular filtration rate in Indians. BMC Nephrol. 2018;19:22.
7. Mahajan S, Mukhiya GK, Singh R, et al. Assessing glomerular filtration rate in healthy Indian adults: a comparison of various prediction equations. J Nephrol. 2005;18(3):257–61.
8. Barai S, Gambhir S, Prasad N, et al. Levels of GFR and protein-induced hyperfiltration in kidney donors: a single-center experience in India. Am J Kidney Dis. 2008;51(3):407–14.
9. Dhiman RC, Tiwari A. Emergence of zoonotic diseases in India: a systematic review. Med Rep Case Stud. 2018;3(3):163.
10. Jha V, Parameswaran S. Community-acquired acute kidney injury in tropical countries. Nat Rev Nephrol. 2013;9(5):278–90.
11. Mohapatra B, Warrell DA, Suraweera W, Million Death Study Collaborators, et al. Snakebite mortality in India: a nationally representative mortality survey. PLoS Negl Trop Dis. 2011;5(4):e1018. https://doi.org/10.1371/journal.pntd.0001018. pmid:21532748.
12. Ralph R, Sharma SK, Faiz MA, et al. The timing is right to end snakebite deaths in South Asia. BMJ. 2019;364:k5317.
13. Chugh KS. Snake-bite-induced acute renal failure in India. Kidney Int. 1989;35:891–907.
14. Chugh KS, Pal Y, Chakravarty RN, et al. Acute renal failure following poisonous snakebite. Am J Kidney Dis. 1984;4:30–8.
15. Chugh KS, Singhal PC, Sharma BK, et al. Acute renal failure of obstetric origin. Obstet Gynecol. 1976;48(6):642–6.
16. Prakash J, Pant P, Prakash S, et al. Changing picture of acute kidney injury in pregnancy: study of 259 cases over a period of 33 years. Indian J Nephrol. 2016;26(4):262–7.
17. Mahesh E, Puri S, Varma V, et al. Pregnancy-related acute kidney injury: an analysis of 165 cases. Indian J Nephrol. 2017;27:113–7.
18. Ramachandran R, Nayak S, Anakutti HP, et al. Postpartum renal cortical necrosis is associated with atypical hemolytic uremic syndrome in developing countries. Kidney Int Rep. 2019;4(3):420–4.
19. Prakash J, Vohra R, Wani IA, et al. Decreasing incidence of renal cortical necrosis in patients with acute renal failure in developing countries: a single-centre experience of 22 years from Eastern India. Nephrol Dial Transplant. 2007;22:1213–7.
20. Bhaduaria D, Kaul A, Lal H, et al. Acute cortical necrosis in pregnancy still an important cause for end-stage renal disease in developing countries. Saudi J Kidney Dis Transpl. 2019;30(2):325–33.
21. Eswarappa M, Gireesh MS, Ravi V, Kumar D, Dev G. Spectrum of acute kidney injury in critically ill patients: a single center study from South India. Indian J Nephrol. 2014;24:280–5.
22. Korula S, Balakrishnan S, Sundar S, Paul V, Balagopal A. Acute kidney injury-incidence, prognostic factors, and outcome of patients in an Intensive Care Unit in a tertiary center: a prospective observational study. Indian J Crit Care Med. 2016;20:332–6.
23. Jaryal A, Vikrant S. A study of continuous renal replacement therapy and acute peritoneal dialysis in hemodynamic unstable patients. Indian J Crit Care Med. 2017;21(6):346–9.
24. George J, Varma S, Kumar S, Thomas J, Gopi S, Pisharody R. Comparing continuous venovenous hemodiafiltration and peritoneal dialysis in critically ill patients with acute kidney injury: a pilot study. Perit Dial Int. 2011;31:422–9.
25. Jha V, Garcia-Garcia G, Iseki K, et al. Chronic kidney disease: global dimension and perspectives. Lancet. 2013;382:260–72.
26. Anjana RM, Pradeepa R, Deepa M, et al. Prevalence of diabetes and prediabetes (impaired fasting glucose and/or impaired glucose tolerance) in urban and rural India: phase I results of the Indian Council of Medical Research-India Diabetes (ICMR-INDIAB) study. Diabetologia. 2011;54:3022–7.
27. Varma PP, Raman DK, Ramakrishnan TS, Singh P, Varma A. Prevalence of early stages of chronic kidney disease in apparently healthy central government employees in India. Nephrol Dial Transplant. 2010;25:3011–7.
28. Singh AK, Farag YM, Mittal BV, et al. Epidemiology and risk factors of chronic kidney disease in India – results from the SEEK (Screening and Early Evaluation of Kidney Disease) study. BMC Nephrol. 2013;14:114.
29. Rajapurkar MM, John GT, Kirpalani AL, et al. What do we know about chronic kidney disease in India: first report of the Indian CKD registry. BMC Nephrol. 2012;13:10.
30. Tatapudi RR, Rentala S, Gullipalli P, et al. High prevalence of CKD of unknown etiology in Uddanam, India. Kidney Int Rep. 2018;4(3):380–9.
31. Jha V. Herbal medicines and chronic kidney disease. Nephrology (Carlton). 2010;15(2):10–7.
32. Doshi M, Annigeri RA, Kowdle PC, Rao BS, Varman M. Membranous nephropathy due to chronic mercury poisoning from traditional Indian medicines: report of five cases. Clin Kidney J. 2019;12(2):239–44.
33. Modi GK, Jha V. The incidence of end-stage renal disease in India: a population-based study. Kidney Int. 2006;70(12):2131–3.
34. Kher V. End-stage renal disease in developing countries. Kidney Int. 2002;62(1):350–62. https://doi.org/10.1046/j.1523-1755.2002.00426.x.
35. Xie Y, Bowe B, Mokdad A, et al. The global, regional, and national state of chronic kidney disease epidemiology from 1990 to 2016: an analysis of the Global Burden of Disease Study. Kidney Int. 2018;94:567–81.

36. GBD 2015 Mortality and Causes of Death Collaborators. Global, regional, and national life expectancy, all-cause mortality, and cause-specific mortality for 249 causes of death, 1980–2015: a systematic analysis for the Global Burden of Disease Study 2015. Lancet. 2016;388:1459–544.
37. Dare AJ, Hang Fu S, Patra J, et al. Renal failure deaths and their risk factors in India 2001–13: nationally representative estimates from the Million Death Study. Lancet Glob Health. 2016;5:89–95.
38. Gajalakshmi V, Peto R. Verbal autopsy of 80,000 adult deaths in Tamil Nadu, South India. BMC Public Health. 2004;4:47. https://doi.org/10.1186/1471-2458-4-47.
39. Jha V, Arici M, Collins AJ, et al. Understanding kidney care needs and implementation strategies in low- and middle-income countries: conclusions from a "Kidney Disease: Improving Global Outcomes" (KDIGO) Controversies Conference. Kidney Int. 2016;90(6):1164–74.
40. Bradshaw C, Gracious N, Narayanan R, et al. Paying for hemodialysis in Kerala, India: a description of household financial hardship in the context of medical subsidy. Kidney Int Rep. 2019;4(3):390–8.
41. Kaur G, Prinja S, Ramachandran R, et al. Cost of hemodialysis in a public sector tertiary care hospital of India. Clin Kidney J. 2018;11(5):726–33.
42. Ramachandran R, Jha V. Kidney transplantation is associated with catastrophic out of pocket expenditure in India. PLoS One. 2013;8(7):e67812. https://doi.org/10.1371/journal.pone.0067812.
43. Lakshminarayana GR, Sheetal LG, Mathew A, et al. Hemodialysis outcomes and practice patterns in end-stage renal disease: experience from a Tertiary Care Hospital in Kerala. Indian J Nephrol. 2017;27:51–7.
44. Hemachandar R. Practice pattern of hemodialysis among end-stage renal disease patients in Rural South India: a single-center experience. Saudi J Kidney Dis Transpl. 2017;28:1150–6.
45. Indian Society of Nephrology guidelines for hemodialysis units. Indian J Nephrol Suppl. 2012;22:S1–45.
46. Ministry of Health and Family Welfare. National dialysis program under national health mission. New Delhi: Government of India; 2016.
47. Jha V. Setting up a national dialysis service in India – change, choice and principles. Nephrology (Carlton). 2016;21(11):913–5.
48. Shaikh M, Woodward M, John O, et al. Utilization, costs and outcomes for patients on publicly funded hemodialysis in India. Kidney Int. 2018;94:440–5.
49. Reddy YNV, Abraham G, Mathew M, Ravichandran R, Reddy YNV. An Indian model for cost-effective CAPD with minimal man power and economic resources. Nephrol Dial Transplant. 2011;26(10):3089–91.
50. Kapoor K, Sharma A, Kenwar DB, Singh S, Navdeep. Deceased donor renal transplantation: a single tertiary care center experience. Transplantation. 2018;102:496–7.
51. Mukhopadhyay P, Gupta KL, Kumar V, et al. Predictors of allograft survival and patient survival in living donor renal transplant recipients. Indian J Transplant. 2017;11:42–8.
52. Abraham G, John GT, Shroff S, et al. Evolution of renal transplantation in India over the last four decades. Clin Kidney J. 2010;3:203–7.
53. Abraham G, Vijayan M, Gopalakrishnan N, et al. State of deceased donor transplantation in India: a model for developing countries around the world. World J Transplant. 2016;6(2):331–5.
54. Rao M, Juneja R, Shirly RB, Jacob CK. Haemodialysis for end-stage renal disease in Southern India – a perspective from a tertiary referral care centre. Nephrol Dial Transplant. 1998;13:2494–500.
55. Chandrashekhar A, Ramakrishnan S, Rangarajan D. Survival analysis of patients on maintenance hemodialysis. Indian J Nephrol. 2014;24(4):206–13.
56. Jha V, Chugh S, Chugh KS. Infections in dialysis and transplant patients in tropical countries. Kidney Int. 2000;57(74):S-85–93.
57. Angell B, Jha V. Universal care for kidney diseases: sustainable development or path to financial ruin? Kidney Int Rep. 2019;4(3):361–4.
58. Kanitkar M. Chronic kidney disease in children: an Indian perspective. Med J Armed Forces India. 2009;65:45–9.
59. Sinha A, Gulati A, Saini S, Indian HUS Registry, et al. Prompt plasma exchanges and immunosuppressive treatment improves the outcomes of anti-factor H autoantibody-associated hemolytic uremic syndrome in children. Kidney Int. 2014;85:1151–60.
60. Hari P, Singla IK, Mantan M, Kanitkar M, Batra B, Bagga A. Chronic renal failure in children. Indian Pediatr. 2003;40:1035–42.
61. Gulati S, Mittal S, Sharma RK, Gupta A. Etiology and outcome of chronic renal failure in Indian children. Pediatr Nephrol. 1999;13:594–6.
62. Gulati S, Kumar A, Sharma RK, et al. Outcome of pediatric renal transplants in a developing country. Pediatr Nephrol. 2004;19:96–100.
63. Prakash J, Ghosh B, Singh S, Soni A, Rathore SS. Causes of death in renal transplant recipients with functioning allograft. Indian J Nephrol. 2012;22(4):264–8.

# Nephrology in Indonesia

# 22

Aida Lydia, I Gde Raka Widiana, Ria Bandiara, Afiatin, Zulkhair Ali, Pringgodigdo Nugroho, and Eka Laksmi Hidayati

| | |
|---|---|
| Area[1] | 1,913,578.68 km$^2$ |
| Population[2] | 267,663,435 (2018) |
| Capital | Jakarta |
| Three most populated cities[3] | DKI Jakarta<br>West Java<br>Banten |
| Official language | Bahasa Indonesia |
| Gross Domestic product[2] | 1.042 trillion USD (2018) |
| GDP per capita[2] | 3893.596 USD (2018) |
| Human Development Index (HDI)[4] | 0.694 (2017) |
| Official currency | Indonesian rupiah (Rp, IDR) |
| Total number of nephrologists | 144 |
| National Society of Nephrology | Indonesian Society of Nephrology (InaSN)/Perhimpunan Nefrologi Indonesia (Pernefri)<br>www.pernefri.org |
| Incidence of end-stage renal disease | 2018 – 251 pmp |
| Prevalence of end-stage renal disease (on dialysis) | 2018 – 499 pmp |
| Total number of patients on dialysis (all modalities) | 2017 – 79,629<br>2018 – 134,247 |
| Number of patients on hemodialysis | 2017 – 77,892<br>2018 – 132,142 |
| Number of patients on peritoneal dialysis | 2017 – 1737<br>2018 – 2105 |
| Number of renal transplantations per year | 2017 – 141<br>2018 – 142 |

Table References

[1]Badan Pusat Statistik. Luas Daerah dan Jumlah Menurut Provinsi, 2002–2016. [Internet]. Accessed in November 2019. Available from: https://www.bps.go.id/statictable/2014/09/05/1366/luas-daerah-dan-jumlah-pulau-menurut-provinsi-2002-2016.html

[2]World Bank. Indonesia. [Internet]. Accessed in November 2019. Available from: https://data.worldbank.org/country/indonesia

[3]Badan Pusat Statistik. Kepadatan Penduduk Berdasarkan Provinsi, 2000–2015. [Internet]. Accessed in November 2019. Available from: https://www.bps.go.id/linkTableDinamis/view/id/842

[4]United Nations Development Programme. Human Development Reports – Indonesia. Accessed in November 2019. Available from: http://hdr.undp.org/en/countries/profiles/IDN

## Introduction

Indonesia is the world's fourth most populous country with an estimated population of 270 million in 2019, 10 million higher than the 2016 estimate of 260 million [1]. Indonesia nowadays is a developing country facing a double burden of infectious and chronic noncommunicable diseases. In the two decades since 1990, chronic noncommunicable diseases have been topping the national chart of the causes of death and disease [2].

Chronic kidney disease (CKD) is currently one of the major health challenges faced by Indonesia. Impaired kidney function was the number ten risk factor contributing to dis-

A. Lydia (✉) · P. Nugroho
Division of Nephrology and Hypertension, Department of Internal Medicine, Faculty of Medicine Universitas Indonesia – Dr. Cipto Mangunkusumo General Hospital, Jakarta, Indonesia

I. G. R. Widiana
Division of Nephrology and Hypertension, Department of Internal Medicine, Faculty of Medicine Universitas Udayana – Sanglah General Hospital, Bali, Indonesia

R. Bandiara · Afiatin
Division of Nephrology and Hypertension, Department of Internal Medicine, Faculty of Medicine Universitas Padjadjaran – Dr. Hasan Sadikin General Hospital, Bandung, West Java, Indonesia

Z. Ali
Division of Nephrology and Hypertension, Department of Internal Medicine, Faculty of Medicine Universitas Sriwijaya – Dr. Mohammad Husein General Hospital, Palembang, Indonesia

E. L. Hidayati
Division of Nephrology and Hypertension – Department of Child Health, Faculty of Medicine Universitas Indonesia – Dr. Cipto Mangunkusumo General Hospital, Jakarta, Indonesia



J. A. Moura-Neto et al. (eds.), *Nephrology Worldwide*, https://doi.org/10.1007/978-3-030-56890-0_22

ease burden in 2016 [2]. Meanwhile, end-stage renal disease (ESRD) was the third largest healthcare expense, after heart disease and cancer, in nationwide health insurance scheme conducted by the Indonesian National Health Insurance System (INHIS) [3]. With the current dialysis coverage, more than 1.5 trillion IDR (1 USD = ~13,500 IDR) was spent in 2014.

A nationwide household survey in 2018 on basic health showed that 0.38% of the Indonesians are at risk of developing ESRD [4]. The data shows an increasing number since the 2013 survey, which showed that 0.2% of the population were at risk [5]. The survey is consistent with the ESRD findings from the Indonesian Renal Registry (IRR), an annual report that describes the CKD statistics in Indonesia. The 2018 report shows that the incidence rate of ESRD increased from 108 pmp in 2014 to 251 pmp in 2018. Meanwhile, the prevalence rate increased from 158 pmp in 2014 to 499 pmp in 2018 [6]. The increased prevalence and incidence of ESRD prompted the increased demand for renal replacement therapy (RRT), which consisted of three options commonly available: hemodialysis (HD), peritoneal dialysis (PD), and renal transplantation.

The growing burden of CKD and consequent increased need for RRT in Indonesia provides challenges for the nation's healthcare professionals in nephrology.

## A Short History of Indonesian Society of Nephrology (InaSN)

The development of the medical fields on nephrology and hypertension in Indonesia is inseparable from the historical development of internal medicine at the Faculty of Medicine of Universitas Indonesia. After the end of the Dutch colonization, the Department of Internal Medicine at the Dr. Cipto Mangunkusumo General Hospital, Faculty of Medicine Universitas, Indonesia, was led by Dr. Aulia, an internist who had received his education during the Dutch colonization at the School tot Opleiding van Inlandsche Artsen (STOVIA), which means "School for Native Physician," in 1949–1955.

In order to keep up with the ever-growing global development of internal medicine, some experts felt that it was necessary to pay greater concern on the medical fields of specific body organs. Therefore, branches of internal medicine subspecialties were developed, such as pulmonology, cardiology, nephrology, hepatology, etc.

For nephrology and hypertension, Dr. Aulia appointed Dr. Oei Eng Tie to give special attention for renal diseases and hypertension cases. The efforts were then continued by Dr. Busjra Zahir. Medical service and outpatient care for kidney diseases and hypertension were performed at the outpatient clinic of Dr. Cipto Mangunkusumo General Hospital twice a week. Later on, Dr. Zahir was elected to be the rector at the University of Andalas in Padang, West Sumatera; therefore, the clinic was then led by Dr. R. P. Sidabutar. Afterward, the Division of Nephrology and Hypertension was established and operated under the supervision of the Department of Internal Medicine in 1966.

The main concern in nephrology at the time was kidney failure. In order to manage the problem, the development of PD care was initiated in 1969. Only after the arrival of the first dialysis machine from abroad in 1970, the first HD was performed. Starting in 1971, the chronic HD program officially started.

The development of nephrology care in Jakarta was then followed by other big cities in Java and Sumatera. Experts in internal medicine from Jakarta branch moved out to other cities and became pioneers and founders of local universities and faculty of medicines such as in Yogyakarta, Surabaya (East Java), Semarang (Central Java), Bandung (West Java), and Medan (North Sumatera). A further increase in the number of internists led to the development of nephrology and hypertension care in Makassar (South Sulawesi), Manado (North Sulawesi), Malang (East Java), Solo (Central Java), Padang (West Sumatera), and Denpasar (Bali).

The Faculty of Medicine of Universitas Indonesia, located in the capital city of Jakarta, had become a role model in nephrology for other areas alongside Universitas Airlangga in Surabaya. Furthermore, the cities maintained good relationships with experts from the Netherlands and the United States of America (USA) to support the growing nephrology and hypertension care of both universities. This was followed by networking with Australia and other neighboring countries. The event of the First Asian Colloquium in Nephrology, which was held in Singapore in 1974, was attended by many Indonesian physicians who had their main interest in nephrology and hypertension.

After receiving an invitation from the First Asian Colloquium in Nephrology in Singapore 1974, Dr. R. P. Sidabutar, through the Indonesian Society of Internal Medicine (InaSIM), urged the local InaSIM branches throughout Indonesia to send their delegations to attend the event. Senior experts in internal medicine of some big cities in Java and Sumatera sent off their assistants to participate in the event. After witnessing that most participants were sent by a scientific organization in nephrology from their countries, Dr. R. P. Sidabutar encouraged experts and doctors with interests in nephrology to form a scientific organization, with the hope of shaping a better nephrology care in Indonesia.

October 5, 1976, was a historical day, and, though there were only ten doctors who had interest in nephrology and hypertension from Jakarta, Bandung, Semarang, Surabaya, and Medan, the Indonesian Society of Nephrology (InaSN) was founded at Sari Pan Pacific Hotel in Jakarta, which was then acknowledged by the Indonesian Medical Association (IMA) as a society of doctors with common interest on nephrology and hypertension.

Members of the society included members from Jakarta, who were Dr. R. P. Sidabutar, Dr. Pudji Rahardjo, Dr. H. M. S. Markum, Dr. Roemiati Oesman, Dr. Jose Roesma, and Dr. Enday Sukandar from Bandung, West Java; Dr. Imam Parsoedi from Semarang, Central Java; Dr. I Made Sukahatya and Dr. Soewanto from Surabaya, East Java; and Dr. Harun Rasyid Lubis from Medan, North Sumatra, the only member from outside of Java. On the first InaSN Congress, October 5, 1976, the Committee of InaSN was officially introduced as well as a plan of drafting bylaws.

The early development of InaSN cannot be separated from the role of InaSIM and Dr. R. P. Sidabutar, who was at that time the medical education chief in InaSIM. Dr. R. P. Sidabutar tried to establish interests on nephrology and hypertension, particularly with internists who lived outside Jakarta, by giving lectures in nephrology and hypertension. Every time they visited other areas, Dr. R. P. Sidabutar and his assistants, such as Dr. Pudji Rahardjo, Dr. H. M. S. Markum, and Dr. Jose Roesma, were always on the search for doctors who had interest in pursuing further education in nephrology and hypertension. They subsequently sent those doctors to the InaSN headquarters that were located in the 2nd Pavilion of Dr. Cipto Mangunkusumo General Hospital, Jakarta.

Thanks to the efforts made by Dr. R. P. Sidabutar, InaSN has progressed and soared to international level with his persistent efforts since 1965, by building correspondences with experts in nephrology worldwide, including from the Netherlands, England, Germany, and Japan, and establishing networking by sending his assistants to have further education abroad. His persistence and diplomatic skills in establishing networks with foreign countries had propelled InaSN into the international realm with ease. On the event of the Second Asian Colloquium in Nephrology in 1976 in Bangkok, InaSN participated as an organization of nephrology and hypertension representing Indonesia. It was then officially accepted as a member of International Society of Nephrology (ISN) in Montreal, Canada, in June 1978 as stipulated in the congress.

Meanwhile, InaSN had its homeward progress to other big cities such as in Bali, Sulawesi (Makassar and Manado) and Sumatera (Medan, Padang, and Palembang), and Java (Jogjakarta and Solo). The second InaSN Congress was held on September 27, 1981, and the Indonesian Kidney Foundation was proclaimed and a founding board established, consisting of five doctors from various expertise: Dr. R. P. Sidabutar, Dr. Hermanses (pediatrics), Dr. Djoko Rahardjo (urology), Dr. Soetisna Himawan (pathology anatomy), and Dr. Nico Lumenta (representing private hospital). On this second congress, Prof. Dr. Busjra Zahir signed and legalized 14 members of InaSN with a nephrologist title, and other 14 members were legalized as nephrology consultants.

InaSN also pioneered the development of the Asian Transplantation Society, with the first congress being carried out in Bali 1989, in which Dr. R. P. Sidabutar was the Executive Committee President, whereas the best achievement of InaSN was to successfully manage the event of the 13th Asian Colloquium in Nephrology (ACN) in Bali on November 23 to 25, 2000. The event was a collaborative work with Australian and New Zealand Society of Nephrology (ANZSN). The event, which was initiated by Dr. Wiguno Prodjosudjadi, successfully united 3000 experts in nephrology and hypertension across Asia Pacific region and provided the best speakers from various countries. During the ACN, a Manifest of Understanding was also signed to allow Indonesian nephrologists to have an opportunity for further studies in Australia or Japan for 3–6 months. After the ACN event in Bali, InaSN has become widely known overseas. InaSN also fully supported the implementation of the first kidney transplantation in Indonesia at Dr. Cipto Mangunkusumo General Hospital in Jakarta in 1977. Prof. Kazuo Ota from Japan who led the procedure was a special member of InaSN. The donors were brother and sister and the first transplantation was done successfully.

Dr. R. P. Sidabutar passed away in 1995. His leadership in InaSN was continued by Dr. Pudji Rahardjo, continuing all programs initiated by the former leader until 1998. Afterward, the InaSN leadership was continued by Dr. Wiguno Prodjosudjadi between 1999 and 2005. During that time, InaSN achieved a lot of progress in various fields. Various programs have been developed such as the Sister Renal Center Program, encouraging young nephrologists to participate in the ISN fellowship program, improving the education program for nephrologists and the InaSN organization system. The leadership of InaSN continued successively by Dr. Suhardjono and Dr. Dharmeizar Bahar, and now InaSN is led by Dr. Aida Lydia. Hopefully InaSN will further contribute to the improvement of kidney health in Indonesia.

## Renal Diseases in Indonesia

Indonesia is a tropical country with warm and humid atmosphere. Its tropical ecology provides a large plant and animal reservoir that ensures the development, persistence, and evolution of a dense microbiological environment. This causes widespread distribution of diseases transmitted from plants, animals, and microbial toxins, as well as common viruses and bacteria. This is further complicated by genetic variation and traditional beliefs and practices with regard to medical treatment. These tropical infections and administration of certain herbal or other traditional medicine, which may be nephrotoxic, can predispose to acute kidney injury (AKI) [7]. As reported by Sitprija in 1996, infections are the most common cause of AKI in the rural area where the majority of the population resides. Falciparum malaria, leptospirosis, typhoid fever, and diarrheal diseases are typical etiological factors [8].

The InaSN has established a registry compiling data of dialysis, renal transplantation, as well as epidemiological data of kidney disease and hypertension from all over Indonesia. This so-called Indonesian Renal Registry (IRR) has been published annually for the past 10 years and includes data from 651 among 797 renal units in Indonesia [6].

According to the IRR, HD patients in Indonesia come from three types of diseases, namely, AKI, chronic kidney disease (CKD) stage 5, and acute-on-chronic kidney disease. Incidence CKD stage 5 is the most common cause of HD (27,637 people, 90%), followed by AKI (2375 people, 8%) and acute-on-chronic kidney disease (593 people, 2%) in 2009 [9]. The 2018 annual report showed a CKD stage 5 incidence increase to 60,852 people (92%), followed by AKI (3822 people, 6%) and acute-on-chronic kidney disease (1273 people, 2%) [6].

According to the Basic Health Research (RISKESDAS) 2018, the prevalence of CKD in Indonesia was 3800 pmp. This is an increase when compared to RISKESDAS 2013, which reported a prevalence of 3000 pmp [4]. IRR reported that until 2017, there were 77,892 people with ESRD undergoing HD, while the number of new cases of ESRD was 30,831 in 2017. IRR reported that until 2018, there were 132,142 people with ESRD undergoing HD, while the number of new cases of ESRD was 60,852. According to Sitprija V, Indonesia had the largest number of people undergoing HD compared to other countries in Southeast Asia in 2003 [7].

The most common CKD etiology is hypertensive nephrosclerosis (36%), followed by diabetic nephropathy (29%) and primary glomerulopathy (12%), among many others [3]. A community screening of CKD in Indonesia that was conducted in four major cities in Indonesia (Jakarta, Yogyakarta, Surabaya, and Bali) reported a high prevalence of CKD among patients with hypertension and diabetes. Of 9412 subjects, CKD was found in 12.5% of the patients with hypertension, proteinuria, and/or diabetes [9].

AKI is most commonly reported to be found in people with malignancy (21%), followed by cardiovascular disease (15%), other urinary tract diseases (10%), gastrointestinal disease (8%), cerebrovascular disease (4%), tuberculosis (3%), hepatitis B (2%), hepatitis C (2%), and others [6].

Acute-on-chronic kidney disease is mostly found in hypertensive kidney disease (30%), followed by diabetic nephropathy (18%), obstructive nephropathy (16%), and primary glomerulopathy and others (11%). Regarding comorbidity, IRR reports that cardiovascular disease is the most prevalent (23%), followed by malignancy (19%), other urinary tract diseases (14%), cerebrovascular disease (8%), gastrointestinal disease (5%), tuberculosis (4%), and others. The most common cause of death was cardiovascular complications (37%), followed by sepsis (10%), cerebrovascular disease (9%), and gastrointestinal bleeding (2%). The most common reasons for cessation of HD were death (70%) and dropped out due to unknown causes. There is a possibility that these unknown dropouts are due to difficulties in finding and reaching HD units. Some medical centers are situated so far that it may take hours for patients to reach via multiple modes of transportation (ferry boat, chartered cars, etc.); besides, many factors such as weather or geographical challenges might hinder patients from getting proper treatment [6].

## Renal Replacement Therapy in Indonesia

All RRT modalities are available in Indonesia, namely, HD, CAPD, and kidney transplantation. In Indonesia, HD therapy was initiated in the late 1970s and PD program started at the late 1980s. Most of the patients with ESRD are on HD treatment (98%), while the rest are on PD or kidney transplantation [6].

Since 2014, Indonesian government has launched a comprehensive universal health coverage program called the Indonesian National Health Insurance System (INHIS). There are specific grouping codes for each modality of RRT in Indonesian Case-Based Grouping stated by the Ministry of Health [10].

## Resource for Nephrology Care

In Indonesia, there are only 154 nephrologists for the 268 million population, which translates to 0.57 nephrologist pmp [6]. Due to the lack of nephrologists, both by number and by distribution, Indonesian nephrologists need to delegate some of their competencies to other dialysis-trained medical professionals, such as general internists and general practitioners. For this reason, the InaSN has carried out a dialysis training program for internists and general practitioners to be certified for dialysis (HD and PD) treatment. Currently, there are 665 certified dialysis internists, 995 certified general practitioners, and 7249 certified dialysis nurses in 905 dialysis centers, treating 132,142 patients with HD and 2105 patients with PD. Certified dialysis internists are trained to have the competency as standing doctors responsible for the care of dialysis patients in both out- and inpatient setting. Certified general practitioners are general physicians who are trained for dialysis and have the competency as doctors on duty, capable of managing certain medical problems during their dialysis shift that need immediate attention. Likewise, there is an insufficient number of medical staff and dialysis centers to provide adequate treatment for all patients [6].

## Dialysis Unit

The Ministry of Health's (MoH) regulation on dialysis service in Indonesia was first launched in 1998. For a dialysis unit to be established, it must meet some requirements that include medical staff, building facilities, machines, and standard operational procedures, among others. The MoH has published a guideline book entitled *Pedoman Pelayanan Dialisis di Indonesia* which translates to *Indonesian Dialysis Service Guidelines* for the hospitals and other healthcare facilities that provide dialysis services. This book consists of national standards for medical staff, dialysis room, water treatment, water loop, storage, sink, infectious room, medical record, as well as the monitoring and evaluation of the dialysis service [11].

The minimum requirements of medical staff are nephrologist or certified dialysis internist as a standing physician, certified dialysis general practitioner, and certified dialysis nurse as staff who delivers the treatment. In case a dialysis unit has no nephrologists, the InaSN will assign a nephrologist from the nearby area to supervise the unit [11]. According to the 11th annual IRR report (2018), the dialysis service data showed as follows (Table 22.1) [6].

## Reimbursement Policy

As mentioned earlier, RRT is covered by the INHIS with specific grouping code for each modality of RRT: HD, PD (CAPD), and kidney transplantation. The reimbursement systems are as follows:

- Primary healthcare: paid by capitation.
- Secondary or tertiary healthcare (hospital): paid by Indonesian Case-Based Groups (Ina CBGs), Ina CBGs regulation is stated by the MoH. The scheme of Ina CBGs is based on:
  1. Hospital classes A, B, C, and D

**Table 22.1** The annual report of Indonesian Renal Registry (IRR) 2018: dialysis staff [6]

| Region | Province | Dialysis unit | Nephrologist | Dialysis-certified internist | Dialysis-certified GP | Dialysis-certified nurse |
|---|---|---|---|---|---|---|
| West | Aceh | 15 | 4 | 16 | 9 | 170 |
| West | North Sumatra | 52 | 7 | 33 | 41 | 513 |
| West | Riau | 20 | 1 | 19 | 15 | 136 |
| West | West Sumatra | 16 | 4 | 8 | 13 | 115 |
| West | Riau Islands | 14 | 1 | 15 | 12 | 123 |
| West | Jambi | 6 | 1 | 6 | 7 | 50 |
| West | Bengkulu | 7 | Supervised by West Sumatra | 8 | 10 | 77 |
| West | South Sumatra | 27 | 4 | 20 | 21 | 208 |
| West | Bangka Belitung Islands | 4 | 1 | 3 | 2 | 49 |
| West | Lampung | 25 | 2 | 15 | 29 | 218 |
| Central | Banten | 36 | 4 | 26 | 50 | 283 |
| Central | Jakarta | 135 | 39 | 58 | 138 | 997 |
| Central | West Java | 168 | 14 | 130 | 202 | 1096 |
| Central | Central Java | 116 | 14 | 101 | 128 | 1163 |
| Central | Yogyakarta | 46 | 9 | 34 | 42 | 346 |
| Central | East Java | 102 | 15 | 79 | 64 | 893 |
| East | Bali | 37 | 7 | 24 | 36 | 342 |
| East | West Nusa Tenggara | 6 | 1 | 6 | 6 | 45 |
| East | East Nusa Tenggara | 7 | 1 | 7 | 6 | 41 |
| East | West Kalimantan | 3 | Supervised by Jakarta | 3 | 3 | 21 |
| East | East Kalimantan | 17 | 1 | 17 | 13 | 133 |
| East | Central Kalimantan | 4 | Supervised by East Java | 4 | 6 | 33 |
| East | South Kalimantan | 10 | 1 | 9 | 11 | 106 |

2. Class of service: 1, 2, or 3 (class 1 can be upgraded to VIP with co-sharing by the patient)
3. Outpatient or inpatient service

## Hemodialysis

In Indonesia, a majority (98%) of ESRD patients are on HD, IRR 2018 (Fig. 22.1) [6].

Incidence and prevalence of HD patient have increased consistently in Indonesia, IRR 2018 (Fig. 22.2) [6].

Indonesian Statistic Bureau has reported that the Indonesian population was 258.7 million in 2016 and increased to 265 million in 2018 and predicted to be 296 million by 2030. This situation poses big challenges for nephrology health service [12]. RISKESDAS 2018 report found that the prevalence of CKD was 0.38%, and 19.33% of them were on dialysis treatment [13]. Survival rate at 60 months is 53.7% [13]; it is higher than the United States (37%) and almost the same as Malaysia (50%) and Europe (52%). IRR 2018 annual report showed an increase in new cases, from 15,128 in 2013 to 66,433 in 2018, and current active patients from 15,128 in 2013 to 134,247 in 2018 yielding a prevalence rate of 499 pmp and an incidence rate of 251 pmp by 2018. By the end of 2019, the current active number of HD patients in Indonesia was predicted to be about 147,340, with 90% of them being covered by INHIS [6].

In Indonesia, in addition to HD, there are other RRT techniques used for ESRD patients such as hemodiafiltration (HDF) and hemoperfusion reinfusion (HFR), although they are only a small number. The development of continuous renal replacement therapy (CRRT) may allow the hemodynamically unstable patients undergoing critical care to get RRT. Initiation of CRRT should be done by a team consisting of intensivist, nephrologist, nutritionist, critical care nurse, and pharmacist. Currently, the CRRT devices in Indonesia are scarce and are limited to the tertiary hospitals in Jakarta, thus inhibiting the nationwide intensivist or nephrologist to gain experience in utilizing CRRT devices. The limitation is related to tremendous cost of CRRT, which may further burden the insurance scheme.

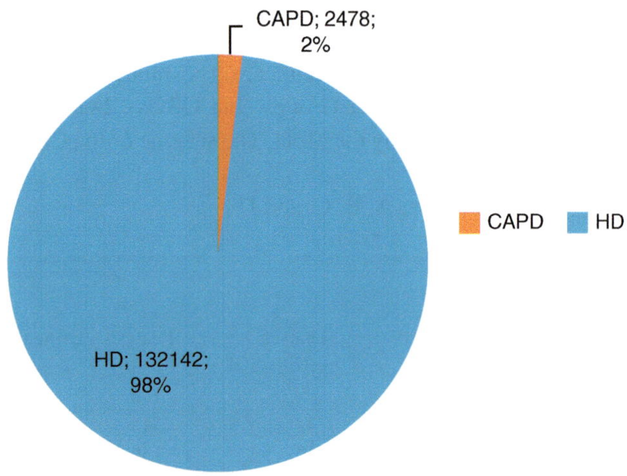


**Fig. 22.1** Renal replacement therapy in Indonesia [6]

## Peritoneal Dialysis

PD is not very popular as a treatment choice for ESRD patients in Indonesia; the prevalence was only 2% in 2018. CAPD is the only type of PD system available in Indonesia [6]. Some factors were identified that are related to the small uptake of PD patient in Indonesia: reimbursement value, Indonesian geography, number of available trained medical staff, and logistic issues. The current reimbursement of CAPD only covers for PD solution bags and minicaps for 1 month; laboratory examination, oral medication, and erythropoiesis-stimulating agents are not covered. The study conducted in 2016 showed that PD-first policy, in which

**Fig. 22.2** Incidence and prevalence of ESRD requiring dialysis [6]

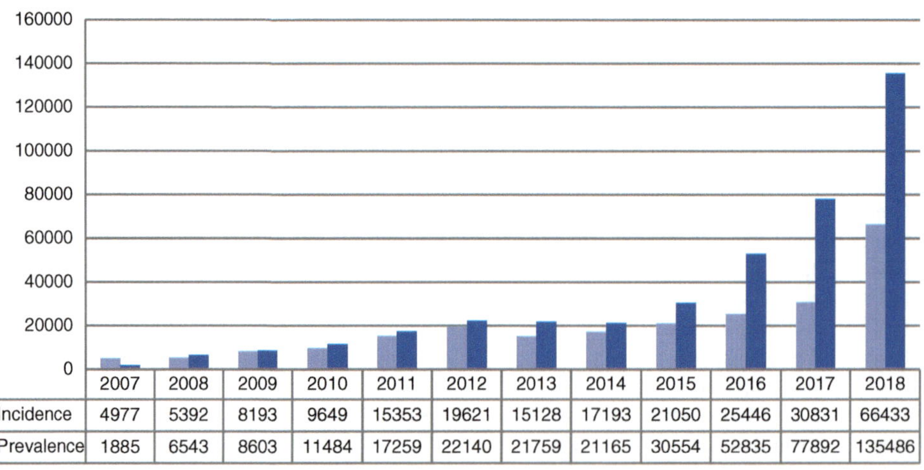


| | 2007 | 2008 | 2009 | 2010 | 2011 | 2012 | 2013 | 2014 | 2015 | 2016 | 2017 | 2018 |
|---|---|---|---|---|---|---|---|---|---|---|---|---|
| Incidence | 4977 | 5392 | 8193 | 9649 | 15353 | 19621 | 15128 | 17193 | 21050 | 25446 | 30831 | 66433 |
| Prevalence | 1885 | 6543 | 8603 | 11484 | 17259 | 22140 | 21759 | 21165 | 30554 | 52835 | 77892 | 135486 |

ESRD patients are offered PD as initial care followed by HD if complications occur, was found to be more cost-effective compared to the HD-first policy in INHIS setting [14]. IRR 2018 report showed the mapping of CAPD patients in Indonesia (Fig. 22.3) [6].

The MoH Research Department made a health economics study entitled "Economic Evaluation of Policy Options for Dialysis in End-Stage Renal Disease Patients Under the Universal Health Coverage in Indonesia." It was found that the budget impact analysis indicated that the required budget for the PD-first policy is 43 trillion IDR for 53% coverage and 75 trillion IDR for 100% coverage in 5 years, which is less than the HD-first policy, i.e., 88 trillion IDR and 166 trillion IDR. The PD-first policy was found to be more cost-effective compared to the HD-first policy [14]. Budget impact analysis provided evidence on the enormous financial burden for the country if the current practice, where HD dominates PD, continues for the next 5 years. Based on this study, MoH made a breakthrough program to increase uptake of CAPD patient; the first step is the Increasing Uptake of CAPD Pilot Project in West Java on May 2018. This pilot project ended on June 2019 and is still being evaluated [14]. The results have not yet been published as of December 2019; however, the MoH has already made a statement that they would prepare a budget for increasing the uptake for the CAPD program in 2020. West Java province has already this program with an advanced training of CAPD for internists and nurses (40 medical professionals from ten hospitals).

## Renal Transplantation in Indonesia

The first renal transplantation was performed on November 11, 1977, in Dr. Cipto Mangunkusumo General Hospital and was supervised by Professor Ota, a Japanese urologist from Tokyo Women's Medical College. During 1977–1985, the number of transplantation procedures was still less than five per year in two hospitals, Dr. Cipto Mangunkusumo General Hospital and PGI Cikini Hospital. There were less than ten surgeons who were able to perform the procedure. Back then, Indonesia was yet to have any judicial and religious consensus regarding renal transplantation. The experts continued to share their knowledge in renal transplantation procedure with other experts outside of Jakarta. After this point, Kariadi Hospital and Telogorejo Hospital in Semarang successfully handled some transplantations. However, the rate of renal transplantation was still less than 20 in a year [15, 16].

The first law regulating surgical procedure in deceased body and transplantations of human tissues was issued by the government, as in Government Regulation (Peraturan Pemerintah) No. 18/1981. It provided the first guideline for the use of organs from deceased and living-unrelated donors,

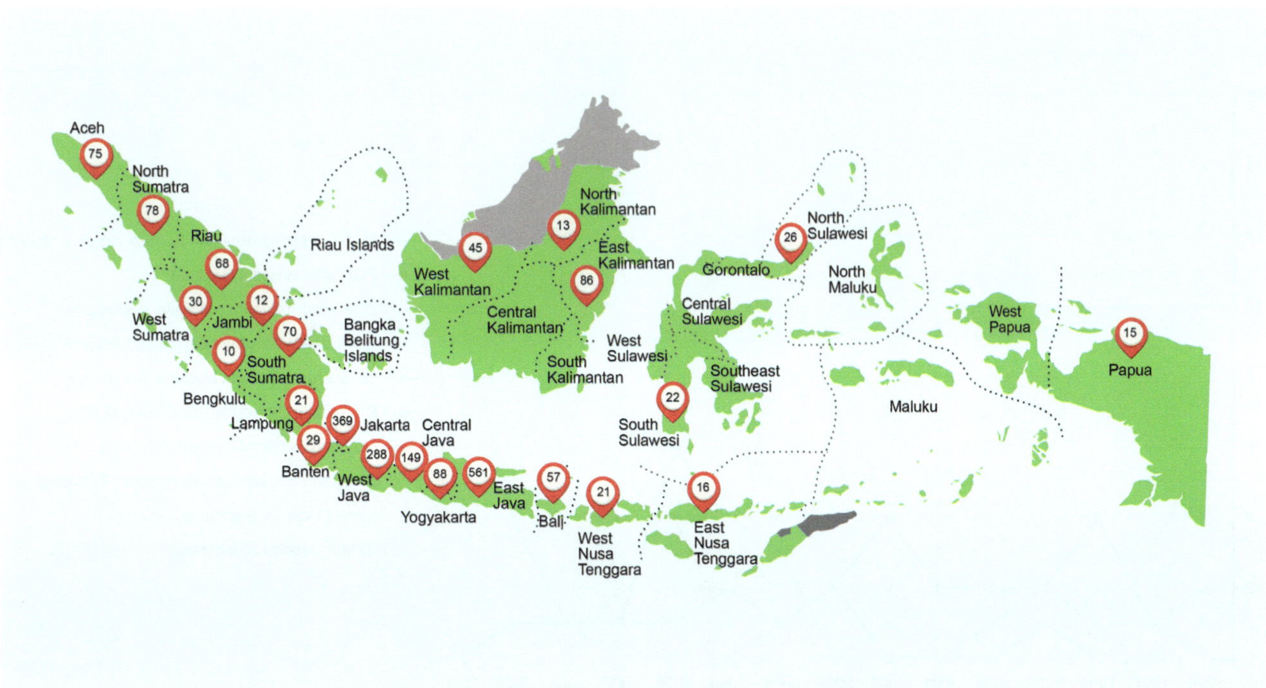


Fig. 22.3 Mapping of CAPD patients in 2018 [6]

supported by an international consensus from the Society of Transplantation.

In the early 1990s, centers for renal transplantation opened in numerous big cities, such as Bandung, Semarang, Yogyakarta, and Medan. Although the growth of renal transplantation in Indonesia was relatively slow, it had doubled compared to the previous decades. According to Markum [15], numerous factors that affected the rate of organ transplant donor in Indonesia were donor availability, availability of living donors, the hesitancy of using deceased organ donors, and the cost of transplantation. In this period, several regulations strengthened the economic and health programs, such as the earlier form of health insurance and well-distributed health services through primary healthcare centers. The law about organ transplantation was revived in Law (Undang-Undang) No. 23 in 1992, which explained about humanitarian purposes of organ transplantation and the prohibition of transplant organ commercialization. Later in 1995, religious leaders and medical experts made a consensus named *Kesepakatan Kemayoran* (Kemayoran Agreement), in which it was concluded that renal transplantation was one of the RRT options for ESRD, and the usage of deceased organ donor was permitted from the perspective of all official religious, medical, and cultural point of view. It was then formulated at the 2nd Indonesian Society of Nephrology (*Perhimpunan Nefrologi Indonesia* – Pernefri) and National Kidney Foundation (*Yayasan Ginjal Nasional* – YAGINA) symposium [15–17].

A new transplantation law was issued by the government to further prevent the commercial motivation of renal transplantation, as stated in Undang-Undang No. 36 in 2009. Improvement also came from the health insurance in 2005. Undang-Undang No. 40 in 2004 about National Social Security System (Sistem Jaminan Sosial Nasional) was created to ensure that vulnerable population, such as the impoverished, were guaranteed healthcare services. After that, renal transplantation started to increase especially in Dr. Cipto Mangunkusumo General Hospital, although the rate of transplantation was still relatively low compared with the present times. This happened because transplantation was still considered as a special procedure, requiring expensive resources, and there was no clear standard operating procedure (SOP). Fortunately, the distribution of transplantation skills and knowledge is still going strong, proven by the initiation of kidney transplantation in Malang, Solo, and Padang [16]. Figure 22.4 shows the trend of renal transplantation in Indonesia from 1996 to 2010.

The year of 2011 was a very important milestone for the development of renal transplantation in Indonesia. The rate of renal transplantation in Dr. Cipto Mangunkusumo General Hospital rose dramatically in this period. The first laparoscopic living donor nephrectomy (LLDN) was successfully performed at Dr. Cipto Mangunkusumo General Hospital in November 2011. LLDN was generally considered to cause less postoperative pain, post-operational morbidity, and better recovery and downtime [16].

Another breakthrough of Indonesia's renal transplantation in this period was the first pediatric renal transplantation in March 2013 [18]. Pediatric transplantation was known to be more complicated than adult organ transplantation. The factors that need to be considered before doing a transplanta-

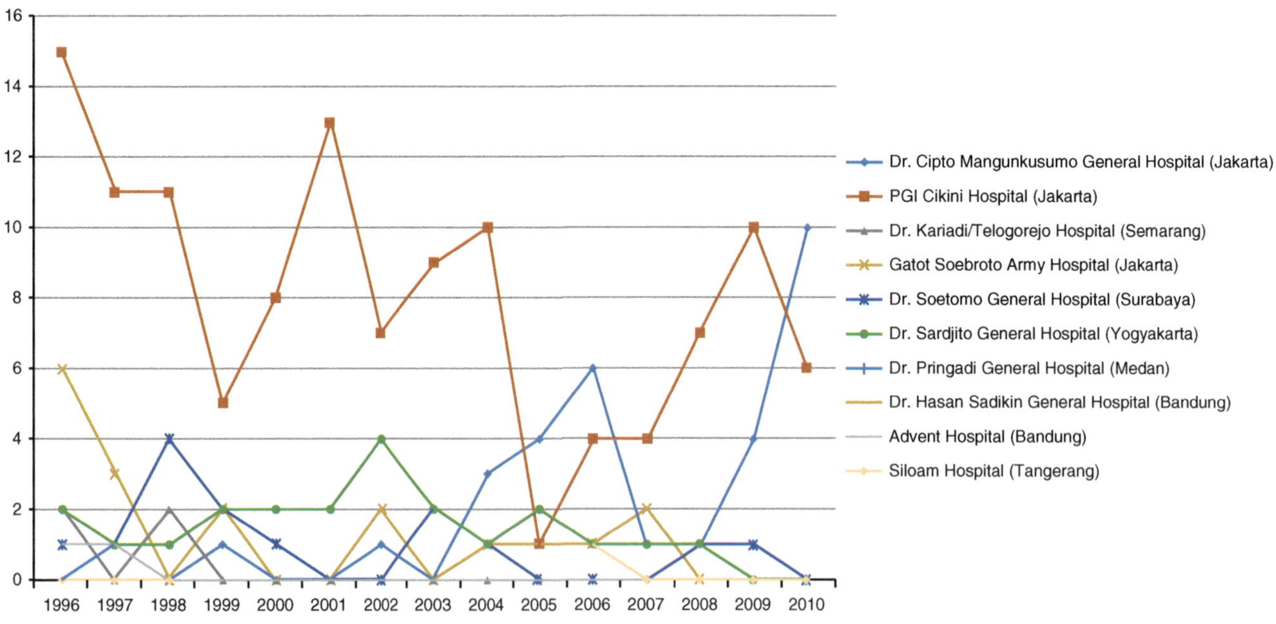


**Fig. 22.4** Trend of renal transplantation in Indonesia [16]

Table 22.2 General hospitals providing renal transplantation services

| No | Hospital | Year 2015 | 2016 | 2017 | 2018 | 2019 |
|---|---|---|---|---|---|---|
| 1 | Dr. Zainoel Abidin General Hospital, Aceh | 0 | 1 | 1 | 1 | 1 |
| 2 | Dr. M. Djamil General Hospital, Padang | 1 | 0 | 2 | 3 | 11 |
| 3 | H. Adam Malik General Hospital, Medan | 0 | 1 | 2 | 0 | 1 |
| 4 | Dr. Mohammad Hoesin General Hospital, Palembang | 0 | 1 | 2 | 1 | 0 |
| 5 | Dr. Cipto Mangunkusumo General Hospital, Jakarta | 125 | 115 | 114 | 108 | 63 |
| 6 | Dr. Hasan Sadikin General Hospital, Bandung | 1 | 0 | 0 | 0 | 0 |
| 7 | Dr. Moewardi General Hospital, Surakarta | 3 | 1 | 1 | 0 | 0 |
| 8 | Dr. Kariadi General Hospital, Semarang | 4 | 3 | 7 | 9 | 21 |
| 9 | Dr. Sardjito General Hospital, Yogyakarta | 0 | 0 | 2 | 12 | 14 |
| 10 | Dr. Soetomo General Hospital, Surabaya | 41 | | | | |
| 11 | Dr. Saiful Anwar General Hospital, Malang | 2 | 2 | 5 | 0 | 20 |
| 12 | Sanglah General Hospital, Denpasar | 0 | 1 | 5 | 8 | 2 |
| 13 | Prof. Dr. R. D. Kandou General Hospital, Manado | 0 | | | | |
| 14 | Prof. Dr. Wahidin Sudiro Husodo, Mojokerto | 0 | | | | |
| 15 | PGI Cikini Hospital, Jakarta | 342 | | | | |
| 16 | Gatot Soebroto Army Hospital, Jakarta | 51 | | | | |

tion to children are the prescription of chronic immunosuppression, immune response, dosage changes, risk of posttransplant viral infections, and lymphoproliferative disorders (LPD) [16].

In 2014, the Ministry of Health appointed 16 general hospitals to begin renal transplantation services (Table 22.2). Dr. Cipto Mangunkusumo General Hospital then established a multidisciplinary renal transplantation team to manage the high number of renal transplantation demand and provide comprehensive service to patients with ESRD. The team consisted of nephrologist, urologist, cardiologist, pulmonologist, anesthesiologist, clinical and anatomical pathologist, radiologist, pediatrician, forensics and medicolegal team, and nutritionists. Renal transplantation program in Aceh, Medan, Padang, Palembang, Solo, Malang, and dan Denpasar has been supervised by Dr. Cipto Mangunkusumo General Hospital until now. In the same year, the Indonesia Transplantation Society was established by multidisciplinary physicians involved in organ transplantation.

Based on the *Peraturan Menteri Kesehatan Republik Indonesia No. 38 Tahun* 2016, the Ministry of Health established the National Committee on Transplantation as a committee for hospitals that provide organ transplantation program in 2016. The revision of the reimbursement for renal transplantation in Indonesia was made by the INHIS, due to the high long-term cost of HD. Later on, the INHIS endorsed renal transplantation as the recommended ESRD treatment [16].

As of today, there is still no specific management or organization that helps facilitate for those people who want to be organ donors. The management of organ transplantation is mainly conducted by the related hospital [15–17].

Most of the kidney transplantations are performed at Dr. Cipto Mangunkusumo General Hospital. Overall, there have been 734 renal transplantation procedures performed at Dr. Cipto Mangunkusumo General Hospital from January 2010 to July 2019 (Fig. 22.5). Thirteen pediatric renal transplantations have been performed until August 2019. All recipients received transplantation from living donors and more than 70% were emotional-related donors [18].

A serial study from 2011 to 2017 by Marbun et al. [19] has shown that from 492 renal transplantation procedures with living-related donors, 335 recipients (70.7%) and 317 donors (66.9%) were male. The mean age of recipient was 47 (13.18) years and the median age of the donors was 30 years (17–66 years). Most of patients (93.9%) had undergone HD. Family relationship with recipients was found in 119 patients (25.1%), while the rest was emotionally related (Table 22.3).

As seen in Figs. 22.6 and 22.7, patients and graft survival trends are getting better every year. But according to a study by Marbun et al. [19], the survival rates in the first 3 years compared to the first year were 90.6% to 92% for graft survival and from 79.7% to 87% for patient survival. Some factors that were suspected to affect the patient survival rate were serum creatinine levels ($p = 0.0001$), comorbidity (diabetes mellitus $p < 0.01$), and surgical complications (RR = 5.64) [20–22].

The dominant factors from recipient that may affect survival include comorbidity, infectious disease, and unrelated donors. Other factors that should be considered are patients' compliance after transplantation such as the usage of immunosuppressant drugs and healthy lifestyle. In some cases, compliance may be affected by the problem of drug availability and distance between patients' residence and transplant hospital [19]. Table 22.4 shows graft failure rate after kidney transplantation from 2013 to 2018.

Although Indonesia renal transplantation program has much improved, it is still less well-developed than other ESRD modalities. Patients' preferences due to social and religious views, medical conditions, accessibility to treatment, and healthcare insurance definitely play a role. Support from the government is much needed, especially in order to make new laws and continuous national health insurance support. There's still a long way to increase the quantity and quality of the renal transplantation program. We have to develop more advance technology and research, to build

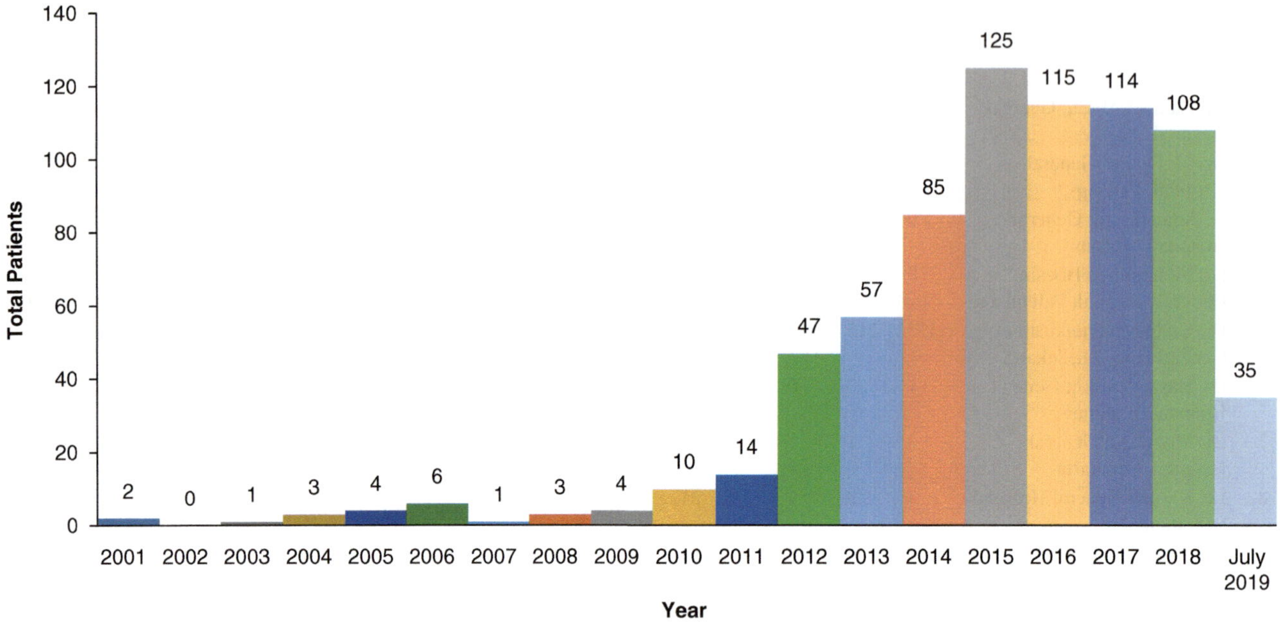


Fig. 22.5 Annual rate of adult renal transplantation in Dr. Cipto Mangunkusumo General Hospital, Jakarta [18]

Table 22.3 Characteristic of renal transplant patients from January 2011 to May 2017 [19]

| Characteristic (*n* = 474) | Value |
|---|---|
| Recipient age (years), mean (SD) | 47 (13.18) |
| Donor age (years), median (range) | 30 (17–66) |
| Recipient sex, *n* (%) | |
| Male | 335 (70.7) |
| Female | 139 (29.3) |
| Dialysis type, *n* (%) | |
| Hemodialysis | 445 (93.9) |
| CAPD | 16 (3.4) |
| Preemptive transplantation | 13 (2.7) |
| Cross-matching | |
| 0–10% | 4 (0.8) |
| 10–20% | 69 (14.6) |
| 20–30% | 247 (52.1) |
| >30–40% | 57 (12.0) |
| Data is not available | 97 (20.5) |
| Recipient-donor relationship, *n* (%) | |
| Related | 119 (25.1) |
| Unrelated | 355 (74.9) |

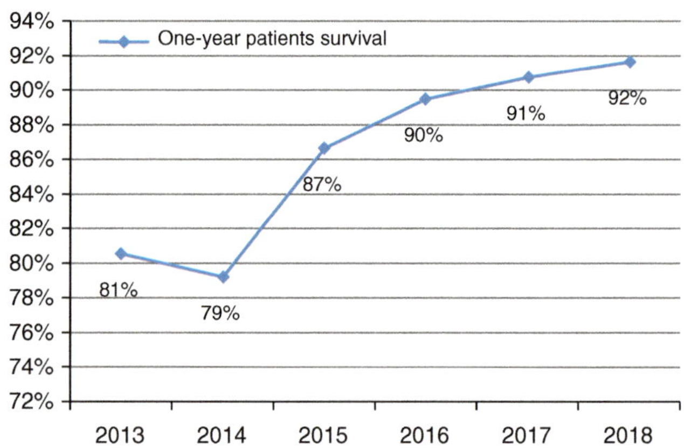


Fig. 22.6 Patient survival rate within 1 year after transplantation in Dr. Cipto Mangunkusumo General Hospital, Jakarta [18]

donor and organ procurement programs, and also to share the skills and knowledge among centers.

## Nephrology Practice in Indonesia

### Nephrologist and Medical Education of Nephrologist in Indonesia

There are currently 133 board-certified nephrologists in Indonesia. The number is scarce when compared to Indonesian huge population. The nephrologists are full members of Indonesian Society of Nephrology or InaSN (Perhimpunan Nefrologi Indonesia – Pernefri). InaSN is the national professional organization for nephrologist, established on October 5, 1976. IRR was an accomplishment of the InaSN, introduced first time in 2007.

The board-certified nephrologists in Indonesia spend years in medical school to become a nephrologist. The study period of the undergraduate program in medical school is at least 3.5 years of preclinical studies, followed by a 2-year clinical phase [23]. Then, the prospected nephrologist needs to take 5-year postgraduate medical education in internal medicine to be eligible to take the 3-year subspecialties training in nephrology and hypertension. The medical schools that are qualified to provide subspecialties training,

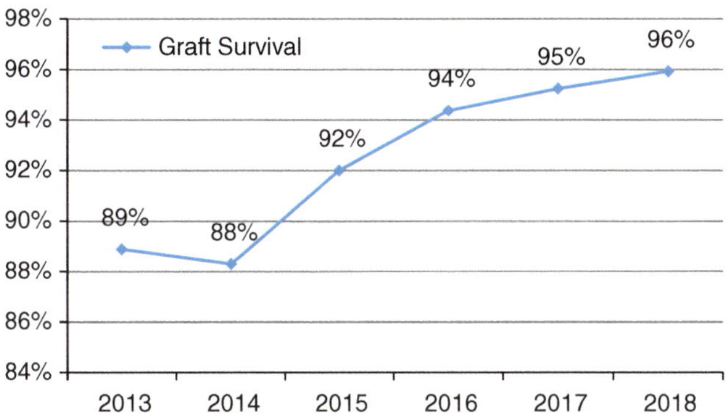


**Fig. 22.7** Graft survival rate within 1 year after transplantation in Dr. Cipto Mangunkusumo General Hospital, Jakarta [18]

**Table 22.4** Chronic rejection rate after renal transplantation [18]

| | 2013 | 2014 | 2015 | 2016 | 2017 | 2018 |
|---|---|---|---|---|---|---|
| Graft failure | 4 | 9 | 12 | 15 | 18 | 20 |
| Graft function | 32 | 68 | 138 | 252 | 361 | 472 |
| Total Patients | 36 | 77 | 150 | 267 | 379 | 492 |
| Failure Rate | *11%* | *12%* | *8%* | *6%* | *5%* | *4%* |

especially in nephrology, are limited in Indonesia because the institution must fulfill certain accreditation requirements to be deemed qualified.

## Health Professionals Associated with Nephrology Practices in Indonesia

As mentioned earlier, there are other physicians who contribute and are associated with nephrology practices in Indonesia. In 2019, there were 555 general internists who have taken a short dialysis therapy course in order to provide service in a HD unit under supervision of a nephrologist. There are also pediatric nephrologists and urologists who work in surgery for renal transplantation and vascular surgeons who work in surgery for dialysis access in patients undergoing HD. Currently, there are 45 pediatric nephrologists in Indonesia. An aspiring pediatrician who wants to be a pediatric nephrologist needs to take the 2-year subspecialties training in nephrology after completing 4-year residency in pediatrics.

IRR 2018 reported that there were 7660 dialysis nurses nationwide [6]. The report also explained that more than 2000 additional dialysis nurses are needed to overcome the scarcity of the dialysis nurse currently. The need is growing, expecting the increment of dialysis unit worldwide in the period of nationwide health insurance scheme conducted by the Indonesian National Health Insurance.

The undersupply of nephrologist and dialysis nurse in Indonesia nowadays creates a major challenge for nephrology practices in the country. The supply for these professionals requires careful calculation for the professional expected income, which is determined by some factors: the local regulation of healthcare facility (determined by initial employment contract and given in remuneration, fee for services, or revenue sharing), professional organization guidance, and the type of healthcare facility.

## Working in Indonesia as a Foreign Nephrologist

One of the biggest challenges in globalization was the chance for the importation of foreign nephrologist to work and give medical services in Indonesia. This opportunity shall lead to prospected transfer of medical knowledge, experience, and technology. Health services in international trade is one of the components of services trade, which is currently regulated in bilateral and ASEAN regional agreements. The influx of foreign health professional is regulated according to domestic regulation in Indonesia.

According to *Undang-Undang* 13/2003 about labor, which is explained in the Decree of Ministry of Labour and Transmigration No. 2/2008, MoH has a role as promotor to the application of working license for foreigner. According to the Decree of No. 67/2013, the MoH also has the role to permit foreigner health professionals for knowledge and technology transfer, education and training, research on health services, and/or social services.

Besides qualifying in nephrology, foreign nephrologists who want to work in Indonesia are demanded to satisfy the labor-normative and health technical requirement. The requirements consist of certificate of competence, temporary registration certificate of doctor, medical practice license, and certificate of Bahasa Indonesia language proficiency. Certificates of competence are obtained by foreign nephrologists after passing the competency evaluation by the Indonesian Medical Council. The certificate is the prerequisite requirement to obtain temporary registration certificate of doctor, which is 1-year valid and may be extended for another 1 year. Both certificates may be used to procure the medical practice license in the corresponding regional public health office.

## Future Perspective of Nephrology in Indonesia

In 2013, the president of the Republic of Indonesia issued a President Decree No. 12/2013, as amended by President Decree No. 111/2013, regarding healthcare insurance managed by the newly established Indonesian National Health Insurance System (INHIS). Both the Healthcare and Worker Social Security schemes are compulsory for all workers. The healthcare insurance program is handled by INHIS. Employees are required to participate and contribute to this healthcare scheme. Indonesian citizens and all residents of Indonesia, including long-term expatriate employees, are required to join. Registration with INHIS covers the whole family. Only one spouse is required to contribute to gain family coverage. By the end of 2019, all Indonesians would have universal healthcare coverage [24, 25]. This healthcare insurance covers dialysis treatment. During 2014, INHIS reported that kidney failure patients claims were placed at the second place in the list of catastrophic diseases, after heart diseases. It is shown that 2,165,507,578,258 IDR or around 161,606,000 USD were claimed by kidney failure patients during 2014. This claim tends to increase throughout the years [26]. Most of INHIS funding comes from the national budget or regional government budget targeting to support poor populations and from civil servants, public fund as subscription of individuals or private company workers. This fund will mostly go to secondary or tertiary centers where dialysis services are running [25, 26].

HD is a health service with characteristic of high cost, high volume, and high risk; therefore, it needs standardized service through evidence-based national clinical guideline and implemented as hospital standard procedure. It should be supported by well-organized dialysis unit and competent human resources. The basic of HD should be aimed at good outcomes and manifested reduced mortality with low cardiovascular complication, good nutritional status, and optimal quality of life. It may be achieved by targeted Kt/V, maintenance of vascular access, and adapted technology of dialysis machine and dialyzer. Implementation of health technology assessment and anti-fraud regulation on this technology application will lead to a cost-effective service in expensive dialysis treatment [27, 28]. The human resources involved in one dialysis unit in Indonesia, which are regulated by the Indonesian Society, are nephrologist, internist with 3 months of dialysis training, and general practitioner with 3 months of dialysis training [27, 29]. Most of the financial support for HD treatment comes from INHIS (the Indonesian National Health Insurance System). Nowadays, more than 80% of Indonesian population has been covered by this insurance agency. A minority of the population is supported by regional health insurance, other commercial insurance, and fee for service [30].

In order to choose more cost-effective treatment in dialysis service, MoH performed HTA (health technology assessment) in 2015 and evaluated cost-effectiveness between HD and CAPD. The result was that PD is more cost-effective when compared to HD. In order to improve an affordable treatment as well as improve access care for RRT, then PD-preferred policy is encouraged. The MoH has just started a pilot PD program in some region of West Java [30].

Studies in some countries have shown that kidney transplantation is more cost-effective than dialysis treatment [31–33]. Indonesian MoH in conjunction with 13 major hospitals in Indonesia has launched a development kidney transplantation program. A National Committee of Organ Transplantation was established in 2016 in order to regulate organ transplantation, including the kidney. Although deceased kidney transplantation national program is still in infancy, the government has committed to pursue this program by dispatching a team of doctors to Spain for deceased organ transplantation.

The treatment of kidney disease is a complex problem. In addition to great burden of kidney disease, high technology and human resources are involved in the management of the disease. Indonesian Society of Nephrology has developed short- and long-term programs in conjunction with MoH, including unleashing the PD-preferred program for the endorsement of CAPD, early detection and preventive program for CKD in the community and primary healthcare, and development of kidney transplantation in some tertiary hospitals. Indonesian Society of Nephrology is involved on collaborative studies with ANZSN (Australian and New Zealand Society of Nephrology) and ISN on randomized controlled trials with HD patients. In cooperation with the Taiwan Society of Nephrology, Indonesian Society of Nephrology is developing a preventive kidney disease program in Indonesia. An interventional nephrology society has been established recently, aiming to develop training for doctors who are interested in enrolling in education and training in nephrology. New developed educational curriculum to become nephrology consultant, targeting physicians, has been proposed to the Collegium of Internal Medicine.

## Pediatric Nephrology in Indonesia

Pediatric nephrology care in Indonesia varies, ranging from province with comprehensive care that provides all RRT to others offering no possibilities to provide dialysis or transplantation to children with ESRD. Most children are dialyzed in adult centers; there is only one center in the capital city Jakarta that has a pediatric dialysis unit separated from the adult unit. In 2017, there were 14 pediatric nephrology centers in major cities [34].

Nephrotic syndrome is the most common pediatric kidney disease in Indonesia, although the precise incidence is unknown. Steroid-resistant nephrotic syndrome is still a problem, since a small number of cases become end-stage renal disease within 10 years. AKI also remains an important problem, whose etiology includes post-streptococcal acute glomerulonephritis, severe hypovolemia from acute gastroenteritis, sepsis, and post-cardiac operation cases.

An impressive improvement has been made in the care of pediatric renal diseases during the past few decades. A total of 220 children underwent RRT in a pediatric nephrology center in 2017 [34]. Pediatric living donor kidney transplantation program was initiated in 2013 [35], and until 2019 there have been 17 children transplanted (unpublished data from Pediatric Nephrology Working Group of Indonesian Pediatric Society). The leading causes of ESRD in pediatric patients are glomerulonephritis (49.5%) and congenital anomalies of kidney and urinary tract (CAKUT) (26.4%) [35].

RRT in children remains inaccessible in most of our country especially in the area with no pediatric nephrology center. High cost of renal healthcare makes management of either acute or chronic RRT in children in Indonesia faced with diverse challenges, which contribute to the overall poor outcome of renal disease as well as the high general mortality and morbidity in the region. Future development is to formulate policies to improve pediatric nephrology services, including to alleviate the inaccessibility and unsustainability of RRT in children in such resource-limited setting.

**Conflicts of Interest** The authors declare that they have no conflict of interest.

## References


1. United Nations Department of Economic and Social Affairs. World population prospects. Available on https://population.un.org/wpp/Publications/Files/WPP2019_Highlights.pdf. Accessed on 12 Aug 2019.
2. Mboi N, Surbakti IM, Trihandini I, Elyazar I, Smith KH, Ali PB, Kosen S, Flemons K, Ray SE, Cao J, Glenn SD, Miller-Petrie MK, Mooney MD, Ried JL, Ningrum DNA, Idris F, Siregar KN, Harimuti P, Bernstein RS, Pangetsu T, Sidharta Y, Naghavi M, Murray CJL, Hay SI. On the road to universal health care in Indonesia, 1990–2016: a systematic analysis for the Global Burden of Disease Study 2016. Lancet. 2018; https://doi.org/10.1016/S0140-6736(18)30595-6.
3. National Healthcare Security Agency. Realization data of catastrophic service in year 2016. Article in Bahasa Indonesia. Pembiayaan pelayanan kesehatan penyakit kronis dan Katastropik Era JKN di Rumah Sakit. Presented at the National Forum of Indonesian Hospital Association and Palembang Hospital Expo; 2017.
4. National Institute of Health Research and Development. Basic Health Survey. Article in Bahasa Indonesia. Riset Kesehatan Dasar. 2018.
5. National Institute of Health Research and Development. Basic Health Survey. Article in Bahasa Indonesia. Riset Kesehatan Dasar. 2013.
6. Indonesian Society of Nephrology. 11th Report of Indonesian Renal Registry. Article in Bahasa Indonesia. 2018.
7. Sitprija V. Nephrology in South East Asia: fact and concept. Kidney Int. 2003;63(S83):S128–30.
8. Sitprija V. The future of tropical nephrology: a personal view. Nephrology. 1996;2:143–4.
9. Prodjosudjadi W, Suwitra K, Widiana IGR, Loekman JS, Nainggolan G, Prasanto H, et al. Detection and prevention of chronic kidney disease in Indonesia: initial community screening. Nephrology (Carlton). 2009;14:669–74.
10. Agustina R, Dartanto T, Sitompul R, Susiloretni KA, Suparmi, Achadi EL; On behalf of the Indonesian Health Systems Group, et al. Universal health coverage in Indonesia: concept, progress, and challenges. Published online 19 Dec 2018. https://doi.org/10.1016/S0140-6736(18)31647-7.
11. Departemen Kesehatan Republik Indonesia. Pedoman Pelayanan Dialisis di pelayanan kesehatan. 2008.
12. Biro Pusat Statistik. Proyeksi Penduduk menurut provinsi. Melalui https://www.bps.go.id/statictable/2014/02/18/1274/proyeksi-penduduk-menurut-provinsi-2010%2D%2D-2035.html.
13. Purnama D, Riono P, Farid MN. The impact of diabetes mellitus and hypertension as comorbid on survival rate chronic kidney disease on chronic hemodialysis patients (Indonesian Renal Registry Report Analysis 2007–2012). J Hypertens Suppl. 2015;33:e13–4.
14. Afiatin KLC, Kristin E, Masytoh LS, Herlinawaty E, Werayingyong P, et al. Economic evaluation of policy options for dialysis in end-stage renal disease patients under the universal health coverage in Indonesia. PLoS One. 2017;12(5):e0177436. https://doi.org/10.1371/journal.pone.0177436.
15. Markum HM. Renal transplantation problem in Indonesia. Acta Med Indones. 2004;36(3):184–6.
16. Mochtar CA, Alfarissi F, Soeroto AA, Hamid ARAH, Wahyudi I, Marbun MBH, et al. Milestones of kidney transplantation in Indonesia. Med J Indones. 2017;26(3):229–36.
17. Prodjosudjadi W, Suhardjono A. End stage renal disease in Indonesia: treatment development. Spring. 2009;19(Suppl 1):33–6.
18. Indonesian Society of Transplantation. The registry of renal transplantation.
19. Marbun MBH, Susalit E, Umami V. 7 Years experience of living donor kidney transplantation in Indonesia: a retrospective cohort study. Acta Med Indones. 2018;50(2):119–24.
20. Sayyadi H, Zayeri F, Baghestani AR, Baghfalaki T, Afshari AT, Mohammad Rahimi M, et al. Assessing risk indicators of allograft survival of renal transplant: an application of joint modeling of longitudinal and time-to-event analysis. Iran Red Crescent Med J. 2017;19(3):1–9.
21. de Oliveira MIG, Dos Santos AM, Salgado FN. Survival analysis and associated factors to mortality of renal transplant recipients in a University Hospital in Maranhão. J Bras Nefrol. 2012;34(3):216–25.
22. Fuggle SV, Allen JE, Johnson RJ, Collett D, Mason PD, Dudley C, et al. Factors affecting graft and patient survival after live donor kidney transplantation in the UK. Transplantation. 2010;89(6):694–701.
23. Mustika R, Nishigori H, Ronokusumo S, Scherpbier A. The odyssey of medical education in Indonesia. The Asia Pacific Scholar. 2 January 2019. https://doi.org/10.29060/TAPS.2019-4-1/GP1077.
24. BPJS Kesehatan: a new medicare system? IES Bulletin February 2014 1. IES Bulletin, February 2014 KPMG Advisory Indonesia.
25. BPJS: transaction of BOA 31 December 2014.
26. Dialysis treatment in Indonesia: focus on Bali. IOP Conference Series Materials Science and Engineering, 434:012334, December 2018. https://doi.org/10.1088/1757-899X/434/1/012334.
27. Guideline on hemodialysis services on health care facilities. Directorate of Bina Pelayanan Medik-Specialistik, Directorate General of Bina Pelayanan Medik Ministry of Health. 2008.
28. Prevention and law enforcement system of fraud in health services. Laksono Trisnantoro, Hanevi Jasri, Puti Aulia Rahman. Center of Health Policy and Management Faculty of Medicine University of Gadjah Mada Yogyakarta. Jakarta, 11 September 2014.
29. Regulation of Minister of Health Republic of Indonesia Number 812, 2010 about dialysis services on health care facilities (Ina).
30. Health technology assessment development in Indonesia: progress and challenges. Health Technology Assessment Commission, Ministry of Heath Republic of Indonesia, March 2016.

31. Sanchez-Escudo A, Alsina A, Diekmann F, Revuelta I, Esforzado N, Ricart MJ, Cofan JV, Torregrosa JV, Campistol JM, Oppenheimer F, dan Fernandez E. Economic analysis of the treatment of end-stage renal disease treatment: living-donor kidney transplantation versus hemodialysis. Transplant Proc. 2015;47:30–3.
32. Purnell TS, Auguste P, Crew DC, Lamprea-Montealegre J, Olufade T, Geer R, Ephraim P, Shey J, Kostecki D, Powe NR, Rabb H, Jaar B, dan Boulware LE. Comparison of life participation activity among adults treated by hemodialysis, peritoneal dialysis, and kidney transplantation: a systematic review. Am J Kidney Dis. 2013;62(5):953–73.
33. Dominguez J, Harrison R, dan Atal R. Cost-benefit estimation of cadaveric kidney transplantation: the case of developing country. Transplant Proc. 2011;43:2300–4.
34. International Pediatric Nephrology Association. IPNA Global RRT Registry Annual Report 2017. International Pediatric Nephrology Association. 2017. Available from: http://www.czech-in.org/ipna/Annual_Report_2017.pdf.
35. Pardede SO, Hidayati EL, Ambarsari CG, Puspitasari HA, Trihono PP, Tambunan T. Pengalaman transplantasi ginjal pada anak di Jakarta. Sari Pediatri. 2019;21:44–9.

# 23 Nephrology in Iran

Behrooz Broumand

## Abbreviations

| | |
|---|---|
| AIDS | Acquired immunodeficiency syndrome |
| AKI | Acute kidney injury |
| AMS | Academy of Medical Sciences |
| CAPD | Continuous ambulatory peritoneal dialysis |
| CKD | Chronic kidney disease |
| CRF | Chronic renal failure |
| CVD | Cardiovascular disease |
| DATPA | Dialysis and Transplant Patients Association |
| DDRT | Deceased donor renal transplantation |
| eGFR | Estimated glomerular filtration rate |
| ERA-EDTA | European Renal Association-European Dialysis and Transplant Association |
| ESRD | End-stage renal disease |
| FMF | Familial Mediterranean fever |
| GBD | Global Burden of Disease |
| GCS | Golestan Cohort Study |
| GDP | Gross domestic product |
| HCV | Hepatitis C virus |
| HD | Hemodialysis |
| HDI | Human development index |
| HIV | Human immunodeficiency virus |
| IDMP | Iranian Donor Maintenance Project |
| IF | Impact factor |
| IIEP | Iranian Interviewers Education Program |
| IJKD | Iranian Journal of Kidney Diseases |
| IPDDP | Iranian Possible Donor Detection Project |
| IrODaT | Iran's Office of Dialysis and Transplantation |
| IrSN | Iranian Society of Nephrology |
| ISI | International Scientific Indexing |
| ISN | International Society of Nephrology |
| ISOD | Iranian Society of Organ Donation |
| KDOQI | Kidney Dialysis Outcome Quality Initiative |
| km$^2$ | Square kilometer |
| LPP | Lifestyle Promotion Project |
| LRD | Living-related donor |
| LURD | Living-unrelated donor |
| MCTSD | Management Center for Transplantation and Special Diseases |
| MoH | Ministry of Health |
| NCD | Noncommunicable disease |
| OD | Organ donation |
| OPU | Organ procurement units |
| RRT | Renal replacement therapy |
| UNOS | United Network for Organ Sharing |
| WKD | World Kidney Day |

| | |
|---|---|
| Area | 1,648,195 km$^2$ |
| Population[1] | 81,672,342 (2016) |
| Capital[1] | Tehran |
| Three most populated cities: | 1. Tehran 8,154,051<br>2. Mashhad 2,749,374<br>3. Isfahan 1,756,126 |
| Official language | Farsi |
| Gross Domestic Product (GDP)[2] | 454.013 billion USD (2017) |
| GDP per capita[2] | 5627.749 USD (2017) |
| Human Development Index (HDI)[2] | 0.798 (2017) |
| Official currency | Rial (each Toman is 10 Rials) |
| Total number of nephrologists | 340 adult nephrologists<br>55 pediatric nephrologists |
| National society of nephrology | Iranian Society of Nephrology<br>www.isn-iran.ir |
| Incidence of end-stage renal Disease[3] | 2018 – 109.9 pmp |
| Prevalence of end-stage renal Disease[3] (including patients with a functioning kidney transplant) | 2018 – 892 pmp |
| Total number of patients on dialysis[3] (all modalities) | 2017 – 34,931<br>2018 – 35,744 |
| Number of patients on hemodialysis[3] | 2017 – 31,421<br>2018 – 34,059 |
| Number of patients on peritoneal dialysis[3] | 2017 – 1755<br>2018 – 1685 |

B. Broumand (✉)
Pars Hospital, Tehran, Iran

Iranian Society of Nephrology (IrSN), Tehran, Iran

Iran University of Medical Sciences, Tehran, Iran


J. A. Moura-Neto et al. (eds.), *Nephrology Worldwide*, https://doi.org/10.1007/978-3-030-56890-0_23

| | |
|---|---|
| Number of renal transplantations per year | 2017 – 931 live donors; 1351 deceased donors<br>2018 – 1018 live donors; 1263 deceased donors |

1. Roudi F et al. Iran's population dynamics and demographic window of opportunity Iranian studies Stanford.edu/Iran 2040 Project Paper No. 4 October 2017
2. World Bank Country Classifications, 2018 https://data.worldbank.org/indicator/NY.GDP.MKTP.CD?locations=IR
3. Aghighi M, et al. Dialysis in Iran, Int J Kidney Dis. 2008; 2:11–5

## Introduction

Iran is the second most populated country in the Middle East. Based on the 2016 census, the population of Iran is 81,672,342 [1]. Iran has an area of 1,648,195 km$^2$ (636,372 mi$^2$) with 31 provinces. According to the same census, 74% of Iran's population is distributed in urban areas and 25.9% in rural areas. Iran's elderly population has also been gradually increasing since 1986: the 30–64 age group population having increased from 25.1% to 44.8% in 2016 and the population over 65 years of age having grown from 3.1% to 6.1% (Statistical Center of Iran, accessed August 2017, https://www.amar.org.ir).

The system of government in Iran is that of an Islamic Republic where the government is composed of a supreme leader, president, parliament, cabinet of ministers, as well as several councils, such as the Expediency Council, all of whom share power. All health issues are administered by the Ministry of Health (MoH), the head of which holds a cabinet position. All patients with end-stage renal disease (ESRD) and on any form of renal replacement therapy (RRT) are provided full coverage by a national insurance at minimal to no cost. Health issues need to be looked at in the context that the Iranian currency (Rial) has sometimes experienced free-fall, making it hard for the Iranian citizen to purchase any imported medications or medical instruments other than those fully covered by the national healthcare system.

The World Bank has categorized Iran as a higher middle-income country with a gross domestic product (GDP) exceeding 454 billion USD in 2017 and a GDP per capita of approximately 5593 USD [2]. The total health expenditure estimate of the GDP was 5.8% in 2006 (Plan and Budget Organization Newsletter, March 2006) and increased to 9.9% in 2017 (Plan and Budget Organization Newsletter, May 2019). The World Bank, Washington DC, confirmed similar data in 2017.

## Brief History of Nephrology in Iran

Nephrology is a branch of medicine that concentrates on the well-being of the kidneys. In 1827, Richard Bright described features of kidney disease in his book *Reports of Medical Cases*. Thereafter, for 100 years kidney disease was named Bright's disease universally. The term "nephrology" was used first at a conference in September 1960, being accepted all over the world and replacing the term "Bright's disease."

The situation with kidney disease was the same in Iran. Prior to 1960, the term nephrology was not being used and only some internists were involved in the care of patients that were presenting with discoloration of the urine, oliguria, and edema. These physicians were called kidney doctors instead of nephrologists. Some university professors like the late Dr. Mehdi Azar (specialized in adults) and Professor Mohammad Gharib (pediatrics) were more involved in the management of patients with kidney disease until 1960. At the time, several beds in the Internal Medicine and Pediatric ward in Tehran University Hospital, then called Hezar Takhtekhab (1000 bed hospital), were devoted to kidney patients. After 1960, some of the medical graduates of Tehran University who had spent some time in Europe or the United States and had focused part of their training on the treatment of kidney disease returned to Iran and indeed composed the primary nucleus for the field of nephrology in Iran.

Modern nephrology began in Iran in the early 1960s after the return of a number of nephrology specialists from France, England, Germany, and the United States. Dr. Abdol-Hossein Samiee was the first American-trained nephrologist who provided a great deal of care for kidney and dialysis patients in the country. In 1961, Dr. Ahmad Farhad Motamed and Dr. Abdol-Mohammad Rafat founded an association with ten members, which was in fact the first Iranian Nephrology Society. The group held monthly meetings but until the mid-1970s was not very active due to the small number of members. In 1972, ten well-known physicians (Dr. Esfandiar Bodaghi, Dr. Mehdi Ghavamian, Dr. Noreldin Hadavi, Dr. Bijan Nikakhtar, Dr. Hooshang Saadat, Dr. Abdolsamad Raafat, Dr. Mansoor Hashemi Rad, Mehdi Khanmohammadi, and a few others) who were involved in the care of renal patients established a group, which later became known as the Iranian Society of Nephrology (IrSN), with main activities of monthly conferences in university hospitals, presenting and discussing difficult cases of patients with renal diseases and hypertension. Dr. Nour-Aldin Hadavi was elected and remained the president of the society until 1975.

Then, Dr. Behrooz Broumand returned from the United States as the first American board-certified internist-nephrologist and was elected as the president of the IrSN with 26 members. As the society became more active, it started having weekly case review meetings and renal pathology conferences to discuss and interpret renal biopsy with pathologists from the Medical College of the Tehran University. The first international congress on hypertension with around 500 participants was held in Iran by the IrSN in February 1977. The society continued its activities until 1980. When the Iran-Iraq War began, the IrSN slowly halted, similar to that of many other Iranian scientific societies in the country. In 1992, the IrSN was formally re-established with approved bylaws by the MoH. Dr. Ahad Jaafari Ghods, an American-trained nephrologist, as president and Dr. Ali Nobakht Haghighi as secretary-general were elected and served in these positions in the new IrSN for three consecutive 2-year terms. Dr. Ghods was the chairman of the 1st–6th International Congresses of Nephrology, Dialysis, and Transplantation in Iran, which were held from 1991 through 2000, roughly every 2 years.

In 2000, Dr. Behrooz Broumand was re-elected as president of the society and served for 6 years until 2006, with Dr. Ezatollah Abdi as the secretary-general of the society. Dr. Broumand hosted the 7th–10th International Congresses of Nephrology, Dialysis, and Transplantation in Iran, roughly every 18 months, as well as a joint conference between the IrSN and the European Renal Association-European Dialysis and Transplant Association (ERA-EDTA) in May 2001. The 10th Congress of Nephrology was held in Urumia (a midsize city in northwest Iran). During the period of 1992–2002, the board-certified internists who had served as associate members in the IrSN for 10 years were recognized as eligible for the board of nephrology certification, and after passing the board exam, ten Iranian board-certified nephrologists were introduced as members to the society. Nephrology training officially started at the Tehran University and the Iran University of Medical Sciences, each with a 2-year curriculum for Iranian board-certified internist to become nephrologists. Around 20 internists are annually accepted into the nephrology fellowship programs in ten medical schools in Iran. Between November 2006 and 2019, the IrSN has had several presidents including Dr. Ezzat Abdi, Dr. Mohammad Reza Ganji, and Dr. Mohsen Nafar.

By 2018, the IrSN was composed of 395 nephrologists (340 adult and 55 pediatric nephrologists) and 35 associated members. Every 2 years, the society holds national nephrology congresses in Tehran and the international congresses in other cities of Iran, with the presence of prominent Iranian and international speakers providing the news and updates in nephrology to the Iranian and international nephrologists. Since 2001, all the members of the IrSN have been registered in the International Society of Nephrology (ISN) in a collective membership program with a reduced rate for membership. Today, Iran has one of the largest member groups in the ISN. Since 1991, many of annual conferences of nephrology in Iran have been endorsed by the ISN. The ISN has supported the presence of three international speakers at a number of the IrSN international congresses through endorsement and CME credits. For instance, an ISN-CME conference was held in Tehran and Isfahan in 2014 with the collaboration of international and Iranian speakers. Each year, members of the IrSN actively hold the World Kidney Day (WKD) in various cities of Iran in collaboration with the ISN. As of April 2019, the IrSN has been recognized by the ISN to have enough clout, stature, and depth of expertise to host ISN-supported nephrology fellows from other countries. Today, there is one young physician from the Avicenna University of Dushanbe city in Tajikistan being trained in the Iran University of Medical Sciences at Hasheminejad kidney training center.

The major nephrology problem in Iran is the nonexistence of renal pathology. The biopsies are being interpreted by general pathologists and usually by light microscopy. Some university hospitals are equipped with immunofluorescence microscopy, but electron microscopy is only available in the Imam Khomeini Hospital in Tehran which was previously called the Hezar Takhtekhab Hospital. Much effort has been spent on creating a nephro-pathology fellowship training program in one of the university hospitals, but these efforts have been unsuccessful to date due to difficulty in recruiting fellows which in turn is due to the poor financial prospect for a pathologist devoting his/her efforts exclusively to renal pathology.

The *Iranian Journal of Kidney Diseases* (www.IJKD.org), the official publication of the IrSN and a peer-reviewed journal in English, is indexed in PubMed International Scientific Indexing (ISI), Scopus, and Google Scholar. The recent impact factor (IF) of the *IJKD* is 0.979, and it is available free of charge online globally. The aim of the *IJKD* is to provide the worldwide nephrology community the possibility to read and reflect on the experience and knowledge of the Iranian kidney scientists and clinicians. It has been published quarterly since 2007 and every 2 months since January 2011. The journal's objective is to serve as a focal point for debate and exchange among researchers at a global level. Original papers, case reports, and reviews on all aspects of kidney disease, hypertension, diabetes mellitus, dialysis, and transplantation are published in the *IJKD*. Contributions on basic science research, clinical practice, and renal health socioeconomics are also welcomed by the editors of the journal. Several handbooks have been published by the IrSN including the *Essentials of Chronic Renal Disease*, as well as dialysis and management guidelines in renal transplantation.

## The Progress of Dialysis in Iran

In 1970, Professor Mehdi Azar arranged for Dr. Mehdi Ghavamian, his former assistant in Hezar Takhtekhab Hospital in Tehran Medical School, to travel to the Cleveland Clinic in the United States to be trained in ESRD and hemodialysis (HD) with Professor Willem J. Kolff who was then one of the pioneers of HD. Meanwhile, the first dialysis ward was established by Dr. Azar in Hezar Takhtekhab Hospital (called Pahlavi Hospital at the time), and Dr. Ghavamian introduced the newly developed HD under the supervision of Dr. Azar. By 1972, there were small dialysis wards in Hezar Takhtekhab Hospital as well as two other university hospitals in Tehran: Dariush Kabir and Sina. At the time, due to the scarcity of nephrologists in Iran, it was not feasible to expand RRT to other major cities in Iran.

With the MoH cooperation in 1974, ten general physicians were assigned to be trained in the management of ESRD at the Behavar Hospital where Dr. Broumand supervised a 20-bed dialysis ward and a 24-bed nephrology ward. This training program led to the opening of dialysis wards in several other cities including Isfahan, Tabriz, Mashhad, Shahi, Urumia, Yazd, Kerman, and Kermanshah. The young physicians had 6 months of intense training to run dialysis units in those cities.

Another major problem was the lack of qualified nurses familiar with ESRD requiring RRT. Dr. Broumand started a program to teach nephrology courses focused on dialysis at the Azarmidokht nursing school of the MoH and first trained 12 registered nurses to work in Behavar Hospital, a hospital belonging to the MoH. The total number of patients under maintenance HD was 109 in 1976 [3], whereas data available as of 2019 shows that the number of patients under maintenance HD has increased to 34,059, with 7248 dialysis machines at 758 wards in Iran.

## Achievements of the Iranian Nephrologists in the ISN

Dr. Behrooz Broumand served as a member of the ISN Middle East board from 2011 to 2017. He was then replaced by Dr. Mohammad R. Ganji, followed by Dr. Shahrzad Ossareh from 2017 on. Prof. Behrooz Broumand was awarded the Pioneer of Nephrology in the Middle East at the ISN World Congress in Cape Town, South Africa, in 2015. Prof. Shahrzad Ossareh (the director of the Nephrology Fellowship Program at the Iran University of Medical Sciences/Hasheminejad Kidney Center and council member of the Iranian Society of Nephrology) was elected as an ISN counselor representing the Middle East region and serving as the co-chairwoman of the ISN Middle East Regional Board in March 2017 and in April 2019, finally becoming the chair of the ISN Middle East Regional Board.

On December 26, 2003, a magnitude 6.5 earthquake devastated the small city of Bam in southeast Iran. Incidentally, the IrSN annual meeting was being held in the city of Zahedan about 115 miles away. Bam's earthquake was felt in Zahedan, and within a few hours, many victims of the earthquake were transferred to the hospitals in Zahedan. Dr. Behrooz Broumand, the president of the IrSN at the time, and Dr. Ali Nobakht Haghighi, then secretary-general of the Iranian Academy of Medical Sciences, called for an emergency IrSN council meeting and established a Renal Disaster Relief Task Force composed of the members of the IrSN to prevent and treat acute kidney injury (AKI) in the victims of Bam's earthquake. The earthquake resulted in 26,271 deaths and around 200 victims with crush syndrome receiving dialysis treatment. Once the IrSN communicated with the ISN Renal Disaster Relief Task Force, several international nephrologists experienced in crush syndrome including Dr. Vanholder R, Dr. Van Biesen W, Professor Lameire N, and Dr. Sever MS arrived in Bam and cooperated with the IrSN to create a protocol for the management of earthquake victims and prevention of AKI following crush syndrome [4].

A few weeks later, an ISN handbook on the guidelines for prevention of AKI entitled *Recommendations for the Management of Crush Victims in Mass Disasters* was sent by the ISN to the IrSN and was translated into Farsi/Persian and published by the IrSN. Dr. Iraj Najafi from the IrSN was appointed as the director of the IrSN Renal Disaster Relief Task Force. Later, in January 2004, the IrSN president Dr. Broumand and Dr. Nobakht, both permanent members of the Iranian Academy of Medical Sciences, organized a 2-day meeting in Tehran on the management of earthquake victims.

## Renal Diseases in Iran

All types of kidney disease exist in Iran. Renal injury following hypertension and diabetes mellitus are the most common causes of renal disease [5], followed by different glomerular diseases, either primary or secondary such as systemic immunological diseases (lupus nephritis and vasculitis), obstructive and infectious renal diseases, different malignancies, analgesic nephropathy, and renal injury secondary to nephrotoxins including opium. In northwestern Iran, renal amyloidosis secondary to familial Mediterranean fever (FMF), a form of recessive hereditary nephritis such as Alport's syndrome with dominant autosomal recessive inheritance, is a common occurrence as in small remote villages, familial marriage between cousins and close relatives is common. There are reports about renal diseases following viral infections including AIDS [6] and following noncommunicable diseases [7]. Finally, trauma, especially in case of natural disaster such as earthquake, resulting in AKI and ESRD is reported [4]. The rate of CKD incidence in different provinces of Iran is different with the highest prevalence being in Khorasan and the lowest in the Alborz province. In a large population-based study, the overall prevalence of CKD reported was 18.9% [8], whereas in the Golestan Cohort Study (GCS), a prevalence of 23.7% (26.6% in women and 20.6% in men) was reported [5].

Iran could be considered a fast-emerging economy [2]. The fraction of GDP allocated to total health expenditure has risen from 5.8% in 2006 to 9.9% in 2019 (2019 Newsletter Plan and Budget Organization of Iran), as it would be expected in any other similar country in the world facing an increasing burden of CKD. To describe the burden of CKD in any country, a good renal registry is required, which at present is not available in Iran. A few national and provincial (state-level) studies that may elucidate the status of CKD and its risk factors in Iran have been reported [8–11]. Well-known risk factors of noncommunicable diseases such as diabetes mellitus and arterial hypertension have been shown to be increasing as there is an increase in the age of the population living in urban areas. GCS is the largest prospective cohort observational study in Iran having enrolled 11,409 participants aged 45–70 [5]. In the second phase of this study, gender, age, literacy, residence, anthropometric measurements, smoking, opium use, self-reported history of cardiovascular disease (heart disease and/or stroke), hypertension, diabetes, and lipid profile were the predictors of interest. The outcomes of interest were eGFR and CKD defined as eGFR < 60 ml/min/1.73 m$^2$. The prevalence of CKD was 23.7% (26.6% in women, 20.6% in men). The prevalence of CKD stages 3a, 3b, 4, and 5 were 20.0%, 3.3%, 0.4%, and 0.1%, respectively. Female gender, older age (greater than 65), urban residence, CVD history, hypertension or diabetes, larger body mass and surrogates of body fat, and opium abuse were all associated with CKD.

Opium had a significant positive association with CKD in an adjusted model. The clinical manifestation of kidney disease in opium-addicted patients is similar to that of other patients except that there are several reports of high incidence of renal and urological malignancies in patients with opium addiction. There are no studies on the prevalence of opium addiction in the general Iranian population, although the statistics reveal that opium addiction is the main modality of illicit substance use in all provinces of Iran. Well-designed studies on this latter topic are currently lacking in Iran.

All anthropometric measurements had positive linear association with CKD. Being literate had inverse association. Gender had a significant interaction with anthropometric indices, with higher odds ratios among men compared to women. A significantly high association was observed between the rate of change in waist circumference and systolic blood pressure with the risk of CKD. One in four people in this cohort had low eGFR. Overweight, obesity, diabetes, hypertension, and dyslipidemia are major risk factors for CKD [5]. Gender had a significant association with CKD in both crude and adjusted models, with men being less likely to have CKD.

Higher incidence of CKD in GCS compared to a few other reports can be due to high prevalence of untreated hypertension and diabetes in this cohort of approximately 54,000 patients, which incidentally was originally designed to study factors relevant to the cancer of esophagus, as well as high opium use and high prevalence of overweight and obesity.

The Global Burden of Disease (GBD) study reveals that mortality due to CKD in Iran increased from less than 1% in 1990 to over 2% in 2013, and low glomerular filtration rate (GFR) is the main risk factor of mortality and morbidity in Iran [12]. Considering Iran's aging population and the increasing prevalence of other risk factors of CKD such as obesity, hypertension, diabetes, and cardiovascular disease, Iran is likely to face a higher burden of CKD in the near future.

GCS has shown that diabetes mellitus and hypertension are the most common causes of CKD. Importance of DM and high BP beyond CKD is likely secondary to increasing incidence of CVD in the older population and secondary to advancing age. High systolic blood pressure has been the leading cause of death accounting for 80,000 deaths in Iran in 2011 [11]. One report indicates that CVD occurs in a relatively younger population in Iran than in high-income countries [13]. Recently, like other countries in the globe, CKD following viral diseases such as HIV and HCV is becoming more of a problem. A report from biobehavioral studies in Iran revealed the prevalence of HIV in about 4.5% of female workers [6].

It is known that hypertension is the strongest modifiable risk factor of CVD and CKD. More than 50% of Iranians older than 55 years have been found to be hypertensive according to the GCS study [5]. Early CKD detection can help prevent the progress of CKD significantly. A major difficulty in detection and management of hypertension in many remote small villages in Iran is that they have no physician or medical facilities. Since more than 50% of Iranians older than 55 years of age were found to be hypertensive in the GCS study, and that hypertension is the strongest modifiable risk factor for both CVD and CRF [14], the Iranian healthcare system has created a unique category of caregivers who are at somewhat similar to the category of Nurse's Aids in the United States system, named Behvarz (literally translated as health promoter) [15, 16]. By making the diagnosis, proper management, and control of hypertension and diabetes mellitus [15], this program decreased the incidence of CKD in the remote areas between 1996 and 2002 [16]. This program still continues in many remote areas in Iran.

Considering that a major problem in early detection of CKD is the lack of ESRD data, efforts to solve this problem were initiated by conducting larger national population-based studies on determinants of CKD and establishing a renal registry in Iran. It is well known that the general public needs education about the hazards of hypertension. Therefore, a national mobilization project to measure the blood pressure of 20 million Iranians between ages 30 and 75 was organized by the MoH. This study was done from June 8, 2019, until July 6, 2019, in public outlets and by various official institutions, and the IrSN played a very active role in guiding it. This project is being named the "National

Screening Days for the Detection of and Education about Hypertension," which also educated the public about the influence of physical activity and diet to prevent obesity, hypertension, and as a result ESRD in Iran (May 2019 by the MoH).

In addition, efforts to encourage a healthier lifestyle are being carried out in different parts of Iran including Tabriz in the East Azerbaijan province. As reported by the Tabriz Health Services Management Research Center (the Faculty of Management and Medical Informatics), the Lifestyle Promotion Project (LPP) was designed as a prospective study aimed at implementing healthy lifestyle interventions and the monitoring of noncommunicable disease (NCD) risk factors. The interventional phase of the study is aimed at lifestyle modification of the general population. The experience with the LPP in Iran may support the idea that a well-organized, fully evidence-based, and well-developed community-based program could be affordable and able to reduce noncommunicable disorders and its consequences in developing countries [7–14].

## Renal Replacement Therapy in Iran

### Hemodialysis

The program of chronic maintenance HD began and gradually developed between 1967 and 1976 in several governmental and private hospitals. Starting with the establishment of the Behavar Dialysis Center in 1975, now called the "Center for the Management of Special Diseases," dialysis facilities were developed throughout the country. The statistics of October 2018 revealed that there are currently 34,059 patients in 758 wards in the country undergoing maintenance HD. According to the general manager of the Organ Transplant Administration and Disease Treatment Center, Dr. Shadnoosh, in an interview with Shafaonline (Shafaonline.Ir) on May 31, 2019, 16,000 dialysis treatments are being delivered in Iran every day and 10 patients expire daily. The cost of each dialysis is 500,000 Tomans (almost equivalent to 45 USD based on the conversion rate of Rial to USD as of December 2019), and 3000 new patients are being added to the HD patient population each year.

All patients undergoing maintenance HD have access to erythropoietin and similar drugs, and patients receive such medications if they are anemic. These medications are provided based on a prescription by the nephrologist at the time of dialysis, and their costs are fully covered by the special national insurance for ESRD patients, which also fully covers the costs of dialysis. If a CKD patient is not under maintenance dialysis and is anemic, erythropoietin could be purchased at a highly reduced price of 19,000 Tomans (1.5 USD in 2019) for every 4000 units. Iron panel, including serum ferritin, is measured in all patients, and intravenous iron (Venofer) is administered when necessary, restoring values to normal levels and anemia being resolved. For patients with hyperparathyroidism (PTH > 300), active vitamin D or oral and IV calcitriol will be administered according to the guidelines of the Kidney Dialysis Outcome Quality Initiative (KDOQI guidelines).

No reuse of dialyzers is allowed in Iran today. It was only allowed during the difficult period of the 1980–1988 Iran-Iraq War, due to the economic problem and shortage of dialysis supplies. At the time, all dialyzers were imported from abroad. Today, all dialyzers are manufactured domestically, and therefore no reuse of them is necessary.

The dialysis team is composed of a nephrologist for every 15 beds/patients, one registered nurse for every 3–4 patients, one dialysis technician for every six patients, and one renal dietitian for every dialysis unit composed of 15–20 beds. Psychiatrists and psychologists are consulted only when needed. We prefer the ratio of one registered nurse for 3–4 patients in order to maintain high quality of care. This has been the norm particularly at the dialysis centers at university hospitals in medium-to-large metropolitan areas. In underserved areas in remote small town in Iran, a dialysis center may only be staffed with dialysis technician and no registered nurses or even a nephrologist.

The quality of dialysis treatment is under the auspices and supervision of the MoH. The MoH Dialysis Center was established in 1974 and gradually has had its structure and responsibilities changed. By changing the tasks, the name of the center was first changed to the Dialysis and Organ Transplantation Center in 2000, and then to the Management Center for Transplantation and Special Diseases (MCTSD) with tasks and responsibilities much more extensive than just the management of kidney diseases. Now, the main responsibilities of the MCTSD are RRT policy making, programming, and supervising. HD condition is evaluated using two sets of statistics: (1) quantitative indices (these include the number of dialysis sessions/week and the type of HD machines and patient/machine ratio) and (2) qualitative indices (these include the kind of buffer used, dialyzer type, dialysis adequacy, and water purification).

Surveillance and assessment of dialysis adequacy is one of the objectives at the MCTSD, which was started in 2007. The main objective is to implement assessment of dialysis adequacy (Kt/V) in HD centers as a routine activity [3]. In the Tehran (the capital) province, it has been shown that the duration of each dialysis treatment is 234. ± 17.4 min. The mean Kt/V, as a measure of adequacy of dialysis, is 0.97 ± 0.25. Bicarbonate-based HD was started in 2000 as a pilot study in nine dialysis centers, and the number of centers using bicarbonate-containing dialysate gradually increased to a point that, at present, all centers in Iran use bicarbonate-containing dialysate. High-flux dialyzers are being used at present to improve the quality of dialysis in most dialysis centers. Almost all dialysis centers are equipped with advance water treatment and reverse osmosis [17]. The results of these quality control studies were reported in several papers. Data of 560 hemodialysis patients in the Hasheminejad Hospital were used to evaluate 9-year survival rates and predictors of mortality. Survival rates were 91.9%, 66.0%, 46.3%, and 28.5% at 1, 3, 5, and 9 years, respectively, in all patients and 90.8%, 61.6%, 42.1%, and 28.0% in 395 incident patients starting HD after 2004 [17]. According to data published by the MCTSD, the mortality in patients undergoing maintenance HD in Iran is 14.2%, well within the range of the worldwide mortality in the dialysis patients of 10–15%.

An overall anti-HCV antibody prevalence of less than 1% was reported in the general population of Iran. The most dominant genotype of HCV in Iran was subtype 1a (44.9%) followed by 3a (39.6%) and 1b (11.3%) among the general population. The overall prevalence of HCV infection among HD patients in Iran according to the last decade's publications was estimated as 12% (95% CI: 9–15%) [18].

## Peritoneal Dialysis

Peritoneal dialysis (PD) started as acute intermittent peritoneal dialysis (IPD) with Baxter catheter in 1975 in Tehran Behavar Hospital, which was later renamed as Hasheminejad Hospital. In 1978, continuous ambulatory peritoneal dialysis (CAPD) was first started in Mashhad, Iran's second largest metropolitan area, and later in Tehran (the largest) and Isfahan (the third largest metropolitan area). In collaboration with other Iranian nephrologists, Dr. Iraj Najafi used the PD registry established in Tehran to conduct and publish several studies on various PD aspects [9]. In 2009, while the prevalence of ESRD was 507 per million of population (pmp), the reported CAPD prevalence was 4.1% of the RRT. At the end of 2018, the prevalence of ESRD in Iran was 892 pmp, and the CAPD was 20 pmp (2.2%). Currently, 1721 CAPD patients are being treated in 75 PD centers with the most active being the Alzahra Hospital in Esfahan with 130 patients, Imam Reza Hospital in Tabriz with 130 patients, Shahid Sadoughi Hospital in Yazd with 110 patients, Shafa Hospital in Kerman with 100 patients, and Imam Reza Hospital in Mashhad with 63 patients. The most common causes of ESRD in patients under CAPD are diabetes mellitus (33.5%), hypertension (24.4%), and glomerulonephritis (8.2%). The mean age of CAPD patients is 46 years [9].

The most common cause of change in modality of dialysis has been peritonitis (17.6%) with *Staphylococcus* (coagulase-negative and *S. aureus*) being the most prevalent causative organism in peritonitis episodes.

In a comprehensive review of the PD outcomes in Iran reported in 2013, patient survival was calculated using the Kaplan-Meier technique. Patients were included if they had been on PD for at least 90 days. As a result of the study, the overall patient mortality was 25%, with more than 93% of deaths not being directly related to PD complications such as peritonitis and sepsis. The main causes of death were cardiac events (46%), cerebral stroke (10%), and infection (8%). Overall, the mean patient survival at 1, 3, and 5 years was 89%, 64%, and 49%, respectively [9]. Diabetic patients and those more than 40 years of age had a lower survival at all-time points. In univariate analysis, age, ESRD etiology, education, marital status, appetite, edema, and type of selection (positive or negative) were the factors that significantly affected patient survival. In Iran, patients are initially educated about PD by a registered nurse specially trained in CAPD as well as additional assistance through nursing aids.

The ESRD prevalence and incidence rates have been increasing in Iran from 238 pmp and 49.9 pmp in 2000 to 357 pmp and 63.8 pmp in 2006, respectively. In 2012, the prevalence of kidney transplant patients was 463 pmp, HD 411 pmp, and CAPD 19 pmp (with incidence being 9 pmp) [9]. In 2018, while the prevalence of ESRD was reported to be 892 pmp, the most common RRT was kidney transplantation (50.1%), followed by maintenance HD (45.8%) and CAPD (4.1%). Currently, all patients with ESRD, renal transplant recipients, and patients undergoing dialysis belong to a group of patients called patients with special disease and are eligible for government-provided medical insurance.

## Renal Transplantation

The ideas for transplantation have prevailed since ancient times, reflected in some notable Iranian artworks resembling chimeras such as the griffin (an imaginary figure with the head of a human and the body of an animal, or vice versa). Indeed, the evidence for the idea of xenotransplantation dates back to early days of Iranian dynasties as far back as the days of Achaemenidae (from the Achaemenian dynasty) recorded by the engravings of many mythologic chimeras still present in Persepolis (the Persian palace dating back to 2500 years ago). In support of this claim, a report of medical practice from the medieval times as reported by Seyyed Esmail Jorjani (1042–1136 AD) in his book *Zakhireye Khwarazmshahi* appears to be one of the earliest documentations of xenotransplantation specifically noting that dog bones could be used to cure human bone fractures [19].

Kidney transplantation in Iran started almost 10–20 years following the rest of the world. The first living-related kidney transplant was performed at Shiraz University Hospital in 1967, followed by 112 renal transplantations from living-related donors in Tehran within 2 years. Two cadaver kidneys were transplanted in Shiraz and Tehran in 1968 [20], 14 cadaver kidneys were imported via the Euro Transplantation

Network and were transplanted from 1968 to 1979. Interestingly, two of these kidneys were harvested in Hennepin County in Minneapolis, United States, and were considered unsuitable for any candidates in the United States (those days the donors and recipients had to have compatible blood groups). As kidneys were shipped after 24 h in preservative solution in Europe, the transplant teams did not accept those kidneys. At that time, the Behavar Hospital was in contact with the Euro Transplantation Network and the information on its patients' blood group available to the Euro Network. As there were two recipients with the same blood group waiting in Iran for transplantation, those kidneys were flown to Tehran via Germany in 1977 and transplanted successfully after 74 h of cold ischemia time. One of those kidneys was transplanted to a 16-year-old girl on maintenance dialysis in Behavar Hospital in Tehran. This kidney functioned well for 20 years until the recipient developed myocardial infarction. The report is available in Eugene Register-Guard of April 18, 1977 (Fig. 23.1) [21]. In the 1980s, the process of kidney transplantation was slow in Iran as a result of the 1979 revolution and the ensuing Iran-Iraq War. Between 1980 and 1985, around 429 Iranian patients traveled abroad, mostly to the United Kingdom and occasionally to India, to be transplanted from either a living-related donor traveling with the recipient or to purchase a kidney from the destitute indigent donors in India. These transplants often had a poor outcome.

In late 1985, Professor Iraj Fazel, an American-trained vascular surgeon, initiated an organized kidney transplantation program in a major university hospital. Dr. Fazel's team succeeded to carry out two to four transplantations per week [22]. Within 8 months, several general surgeons and urologists had been trained for kidney transplantation. These recently trained transplant surgeons started performing transplantation in another university hospital. From late 1985 to 1987, 274 renal transplants were carried out from living-related donors (LRDs) in just two transplant centers. In 1994, the Scientific Society of Iran's Organ Transplantation was established with Professor Iraj Fazel at its helm, with the goal of expanding the science of transplantation. In October 1994, the second Middle East Society of Organ Transplantation Conference was held in the city of Isfahan, which helped increase awareness about the field of transplantation in Iran. Meanwhile, chronic HD facilities were expanding significantly, and as a result, the number of patients on the waiting list for kidney transplantation was also increasing.

Since there was a shortage of LRDs, a government-regulated and government-funded living-unrelated donor (LURD) program with compensation for the donors began in 1997 to end the expensive transplant tourism that included trips by the donors from Iran to the United Kingdom or to India with mostly poor outcomes [22]. When renal transplantation was needed and the recipient had no living-related donors, the recipient would be referred to the Dialysis and Transplant Patients Association (DATPA). DATPA is a charitable organization composed of ESRD patients and some nephrologists that was founded in 1997 to help search for suitable unrelated donors. The workup would be carried out by a nephrologist at DATPA to make sure that the vendor is compatible and suitable and has no contraindication for donation. When the vendor was found to be suitable, both the vendor and the recipient would be referred to one of the transplant centers. Following transplantation, donors would receive a government allowance of 1,000,000 Tomans (equivalent to 1200 USD in 1997) plus medical insurance coverage for 1 year for the donor. In addition, DATPA always arranged a meeting between the recipient and the selected donor for more money, usually four times higher than the government allowance. Today, in 2019, this extra requested money by the vendors could be as much as 180 million Tomans or approximately 15,000 USD (please note there has been 1600% inflation in the value of USD in Iran). So, in 2019, a vendor could ask for up to 100 times more in terms of the Iranian currency than he did in 1997. According to the Iranian law, this process could just be carried out between two Iranian citizens.

As Dr. Francis L. Delmonico clearly stated in his article in *Kidney International*, "the experience of Iran and the rest of the world has clearly shown that vendors are poor, hapless, jobless, indebted, and largely destitute. It is this social condition that compels the vendor to sell a kidney" [23]. However, the cadaver kidney was not adequately available and public acceptance for retrieving organs from deceased donors required long periods of preparation and education. In addition, the brain death concept needed religious and legal approval. In 1989, a fatwa (religious approval) was issued by late Imam Khomeini at the request of Dr. Iraj Fazel, the

**American's kidney flow to Tehran for transplants**

MINNEAPOLIS (UPI) - Kidneys removed from a suicide victim t the Hennepin County Medical Center were flown-to Tehran. Iran, and transplanted into two person, all within 48 hours the center said today.

"Euro Transplant in Leyden, Holand, which coordinated the arrange -ments, called us and saidthe kidneys were transplanted and were working beautifully," a spokesman at the medical center said.

The sucide victim was brought into the center last Tuesday and died at 6:50 p.m He left Instructions that his kidneys be donated for a transplant.

"Its's difficult to find recipients for a donor with his A-B blood type," a spokesman for the center said, "We have a computer system for finding recipients but none was waiting for this type in the Unites States.

" So we called Euro Transplant and made arrangements to ship them to Germany. Dr. Robert Christian Andersen removed the kidneys from the donor about 1 a.m. Wednesday and they were flown out of Chicago about 5 p.m. that day to Frankfurt, Germany.

"The doctor there did not want to use them because we had shipped them on ice in a preservatives solution. Some surgeons don't like to transplant kidneys that have been on ice very long."

"So Euro Transplant called Tehran and arranged to send the kidneys there. They reported that a Dr. Nibkin and team of surgeons transplanted the kidneys into two recipients in operations that took several hours on Thursday.

Euro-Transplant reported the kidneys began functioning immediately.

A doctor on the National Dialysis Committee in Iran said 120 persons in Iran were on the waiting list to undergo kidney transplant operations.

**Fig. 23.1** Media coverage of one of the earliest deceased kidney transplantations in Iran founder of renal transplantation in Iran. This fatwa, the first one regarding this matter in the Shia Islam tradition, confirmed the validity of brain death from the religious standpoint. This was a giant step forward because the legal courts needed religious validation before legislation.

After two rejections by the house of representatives of the Islamic Republic of Iran, the Brain Death Act for organ transplantation was finally approved by the parliament of Iran in June 2000. Following this approval, cadaver organ harvest and transplantation from deceased donors became a safe practice for medical professionals. A ratification was also issued by the cabinet on May 22, 2002, was issued as follows: "Brain death should be confirmed by four specialists" including: one neurosurgeon, one neurologist, one internist and one anesthesiologist, independently. After confirmation of brain death by these specialists, one forensic specialist should also confirm the legal process. All the possible donors should be reported to organ procurement units (OPU) by the hospitals. The management, allocation of organ donation, and transplantation program should be done according to the regulations of the Ministry of Health's Transplant Management Center. Deceased donation and transplantation expenses should be covered by the MoH.

Following this cabinet act, a parliamentary act issued to facilitate and legalize organ harvesting from brain death individuals clarified that only well-equipped governmental hospitals approved by the MoH have the permission to harvest organs after family consent was obtained. Furthermore, brain death confirmation should be done by specialists who have been appointed by the MoH for 4 years, and the members of this team could not be involved in the transplantation program.

Following these two acts, the Iranian Network for Transplantation and Organ Procurement was established. These acts helped expand heart, lung, and liver transplantation programs in Iran as well [24]. By 2003, 82% of kidney transplantations performed in Iran were from living-unrelated donors, 8% from living-related donors, and 10% from cadaver donors. Reported experience about transplantation in Iran showed that until 2006 the highest global number of living-unrelated donors for renal transplantation was in Iran [25].

Although cadaver organ donation had started following the cabinet ratification in 2002, the rate of organ donation was still too low. Hence, the MoH assigned several experts in organ procurement to establish the Iranian OPU for transplantation. In 2015, the Iranian Society of Organ Donation (ISOD) was established (http://www.ehda.center). As a result of their activities, the rate of organ procurement from brain death donors increased from 0.2 pmp in 2000 to 11.57 pmp in 2017 – data provided by Iran's Office of Dialysis and Transplantation (IrODaT) (Fig. 23.2).

According to the ISOD, this great achievement became possible by starting the following programs: (1) the Iranian

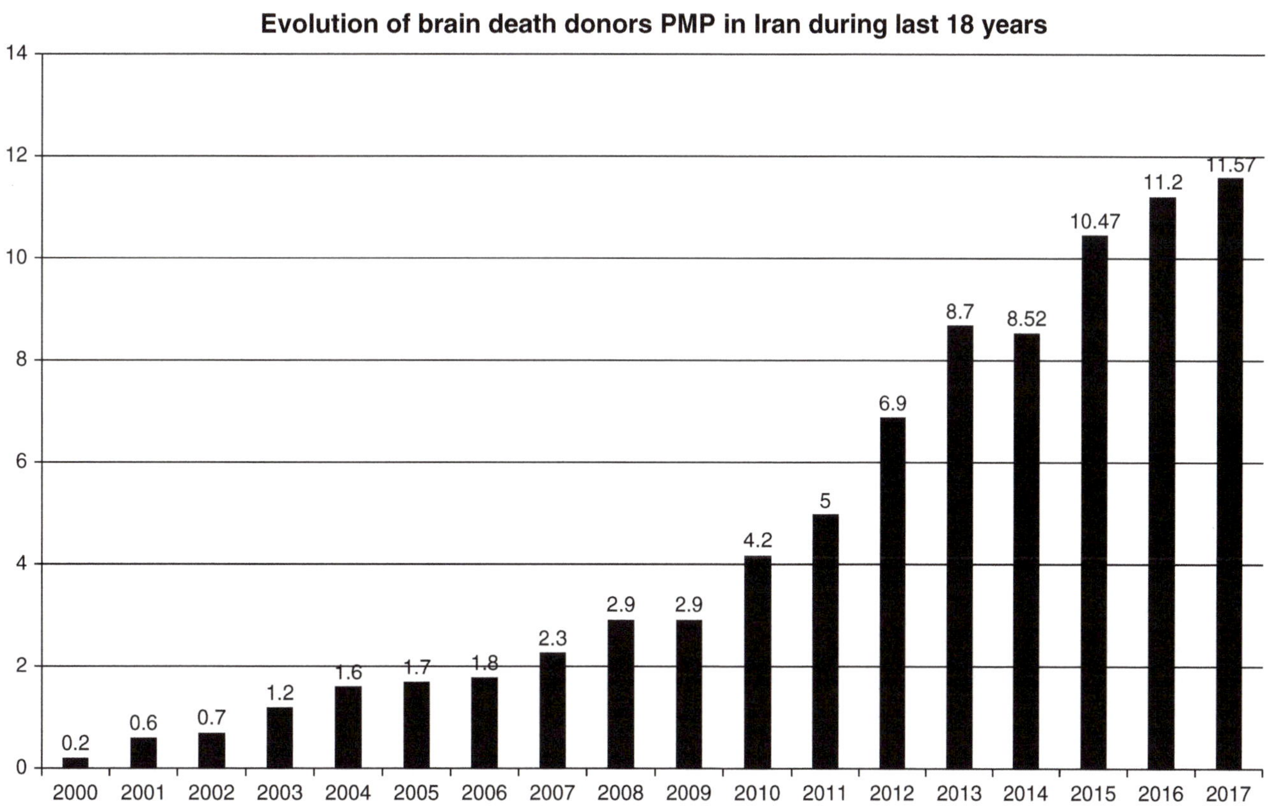


**Fig. 23.2** Inverse correlation between the increase in the deceased donor kidneys and the living donors in renal transplant in Iran

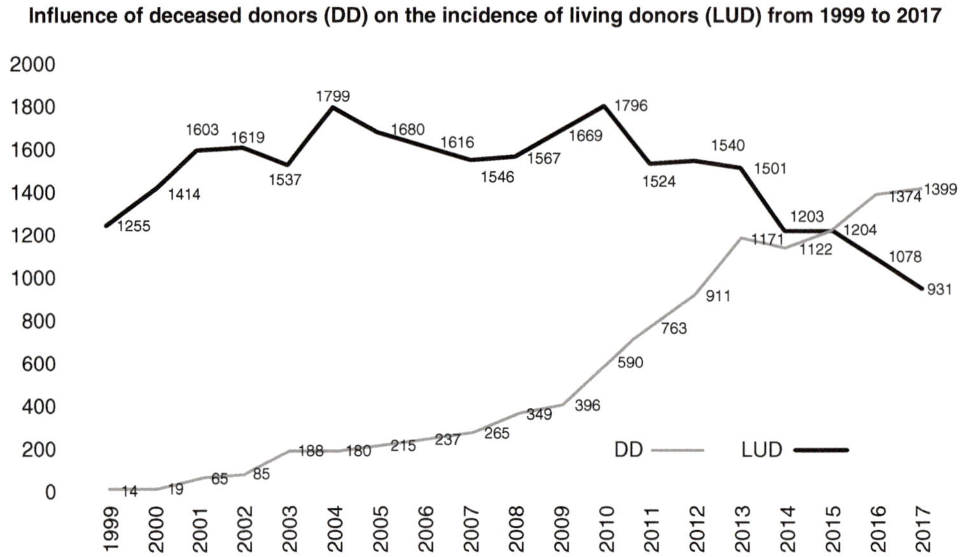


**Fig. 23.3** Influence of deceased donors on the incidence of living kidney donors. (Data distributed by Iran's Office of Dialysis and Transplantation – IrODaT)

Possible Donor Detection Project (IPDDP) established in 2009, (2) the Iranian Interviewers Education Program (IIEP) established in 2009, and (3) the Iranian Donor Maintenance Project (IDMP) established in 2010. This level of intense attention and organization has been allocated to the brain-dead cases because such donors often suffer from many imbalances including hemodynamic, electrolyte, hormonal, and many other issues. Close management of these cases is crucial. For instance, in the IDMP program, all the Glasgow Coma Scale-3 (GCS-3) cases that had two or less reflexes were closely observed, and one trained coordinator stayed at beside until organ donation took place. With appropriate skills and proper necessary management of potential donors, organ donation rate has increased to up to 25% in some hospitals.

According to the reports by the ISOD, there are 3000 cases of brain death in Iran each year from which 1000 kidneys are retrieved for transplantation [26]. The ISOD became more successful and efficient by providing donation cards to general public with this sentence printed on the donation card: "When my time comes, I would like to give life to others." The achievement of the ISOD was very impressive after distributing the donor cards [27]. Another efficient recruitment technique was creating a system where anyone could register for organ donation simply by inserting a four-digit unique verified code in their mobile phone.

At the beginning, the absence of infrastructure for the deceased donor (DDRT) program made its progress slow. The need for transplant and the pressure from recipients made the so-called Iranian model of renal transplantation with payments to the LURT donors the main modality of transplantation. This situation resulted in transplant commercialism and transplant tourism in Iran. With the establishment of the deceased donor renal transplantation (DDRT) program in 1988 and the successful efforts of the Iranian Society of Organ Donation (ISOD), the pattern of transplantation has reversed in favor of DDRT since 2015 (Fig. 23.3) [27].

To prevent transplant tourism, in 1992, the high council of organ transplantation in the MoH and Medical Education ruled to forbid foreign nationals to be transplanted in Iran unless they present living-related donor of their own nationality and approved by the MoH. Since April 2010, following the Istanbul Declaration, and to respect its contents, kidney transplantation of foreign individuals was completely removed from transplantation activities in Iran. Despite the tireless efforts to encourage and promote cadaver organ donation, the large gap between available organs and the demand makes the unrelated donation an alternative unpleasant choice.

To support the LRD and their recipients, a state insurance system was initiated and a reward was offered to the volunteer donors following the transplant procedure. Although the monetary compensation by the government was acceptable by the living-unrelated donors at the beginning, it gradually lost its real value due to the annual inflation so that in the present day the sum being asked by the vendor to sell their kidney is unaffordable by most recipients.

In order to regulate this new situation and to prevent transplant tourism and commercialism, and to respect the ethical and social importance of this issue, the Iranian Society of Organ Transplantation presented this matter to the Bioethics section of the Academy of Medical Siences (AMS) of Iran. The AMC established a committee that started a series of meetings. The committee was composed of medical specialists, legal experts, philosophers, sociologists, psychiatrics, and clergies. Following detailed discussions in several sessions, the committee released the following statement on February 4, 2008: Since the protection of lives of human beings should be considered the most fundamental moral principle, which is, by the way, subject to different cultural and social interpretations, and to offer the best and advanced medical services to the patients, the Bioethics Committee of the Academy of Medical Sciences of Iran declared that the act of kidney donation from living-related and living-unrelated volunteers is generally acceptable, and offering a reward as a gratitude or gift or compensation is not considered unethical and should not discourage this noble act of giving as long as the following conditions are met:

1. The donor is truly willing to donate a kidney in the right mind and free from coercion by the living-unrelated donor.
2. The donor undergoes complete medical and psychological evaluation and is found to be fit for the procedure.
3. There is no contraindication for the operation.
4. The donor is able to get long-term medical attention.
5. The medical team has no part (personal stake) in the process of donation.
6. The donor and recipient should be from the same nationality (tourist transplantation is forbidden).
7. No one under age of 18 and over 45 years should be accepted for donation.
8. A national committee assigned by the Ministry of Health and Medical Education with the cooperation of the Iranian Transplantation Society will regulate and supervise the renal transplantation centers nationwide [28].

Indeed, the ISOD by collecting data, allocating retrieved organs, education, and research functioned like the United Network for Organ Sharing (UNOS) equivalent in Iran and worked toward having a registry of renal transplantation in the near future. In September 2017, a mutual agreement protocol was signed between the undersecretary of the MoH and the chief of ISOD council to coordinate the education of public on organ donation and teach social workers how to obtain consent from relatives of donors with brain death.

To achieve this goal, the ISOD established three committees: (1) the scientific committee to regulate education of medical personnel and research for increasing organ donations, with special attention to the cultural aspects of organ extraction from cadavers for transplantation; (2) the social workers' committee, especially for training of new transplant social workers concentrating on the living-unrelated donors; and (3) cultural and art committee to increase the knowledge of the public about organ donation, creating educational films, videos, and shows and infomercials by artists and celebrities. This cultural effort helped the social workers obtain more consent for use of cadaver donors. In an 18-month period of organ donation drive, 353 potential brain-dead organ donors were referred to organ procurement units. The mean age of the cases was 42.6, and 62% were male. The main causes of brain death were cerebrovascular accidents and trauma (41.2% and 32.6%, respectively). The family consent rate was 84.4%, and 55 families rejected the request for organ donation. The leading cause for family refusal was religious beliefs, mainly from Sunni families (43.6% denials by Sunnis vs. 8.6% denials by Shiites in 2009). Brain death denial reduced significantly from 44.4% in 2009 to 12.7% in 2015 and 2016 ($P < 0.001$) [29].

Indeed, the transplantation in Iran has been organized and progressed according to the need and the available facilities of the time. The Iranian transplant surgeons first started with the living-related transplantations. Then, due to the shortage of enough related donors and with the demand to decrease the mortality of the candidate recipients, the process of living-unrelated transplantation was also added to the transplant program.

While the number of LURDs increased, LRD's decreased simultaneously. In reality after 1 year of using living-unrelated donors, no real significant rise was seen in the total number of transplantations because living-related donors decreased just as much as LURDs increased, so for several years total transplantation remained the same [20].

Finally, as a result of successful expansion of the deceased donor program, living-unrelated use trended downward starting in 2015 as shown in Fig. 23.3. As the Iranian Society of Organ Transplantation has declared, occasionally, there were misuses of the facilities in Iran for transplantation and tourism; thus, the Transplant Office of the MoH managed to prevent transplantation of non-Iranians to Iranians in accordance to the Istanbul Declaration to fight transplantation tourism and commercialism. As a matter of fact, by the time Iran implemented these changes, other countries had also concluded that the promise of eliminating a waiting list for transplantation through mostly an LURD program was not possible.

In a *New York Times* article on the topic of elimination of the transplant waiting list, a commentator debated: "Such claims about the Iranian waiting list, which are commonly invoked in support of kidney markets in the United States and elsewhere, are simply false. People with ESRD living in the United States are more likely to receive a transplant than those living in Iran." As a document of their statement in Table 2 of this *New York Times* article, they reported 17,910 patients on the wait list for transplantation in 2011, while in that same year just 2273 kidney transplantations were carried out in Iran [30].

Although many patients with ESRD have received transplants through the paid living donors, the Iranian model has now been shown to have serious flaws and potentially inhibiting factors and is being replaced by a substantial growth in the deceased donor program in Iran [31]. It was shown by several researchers that elimination of the waiting list for transplantation was not real [30]. If, indeed, the number of patients who need transplantation under maintenance dialysis is considered, the waiting list had not even changed, and if one looked more carefully, indeed, the number had increased [30]. Direct monetary relation between the donor and the recipient with resultant commercialization and exploitation of the poor and the suppression of the living-related and altruistic donations all argued that the Iranian model should be abandoned.

Indeed, the experience of the Shiraz team (sixth largest metropolitan area in Iran) proved that the best way to stop monetary transplant is expanding transplant organ from deceased donors together with refusing to transplant kidney from LURD. The admirable policy of transplantation in Shiraz was a big push for success of the DD transplantation in Iran and resulting in a significant decline in transplant commercialism. The Shiraz experience provides an opportunity for an evidence-based analysis of the potential contributors to the growth of the DD program in this city compared with other areas in the country. In the year 2011, the national kidney transplant rate was 30 pmp. In the same year, 255 kidney transplants were performed in Shiraz, yielding a rate of 37 pmp from DDs in the Shirazi transplant population. The latest data provided by Abu Ali Sina Hospital which is a 700-bed transplant hospital specialized in a variety of transplantations (Fig. 23.4) shows that from 1993 until June 15, 2019, a total of 4617 kidney transplantations were performed. In fact, since 2008, no LURD transplants were carried out in Shiraz (Fig. 23.5).

Another valuable achievement of the Shiraz Transplant Society is its publication of the *International Journal of Organ Transplantation Medicine* (*IJOTM*), which is the offi-

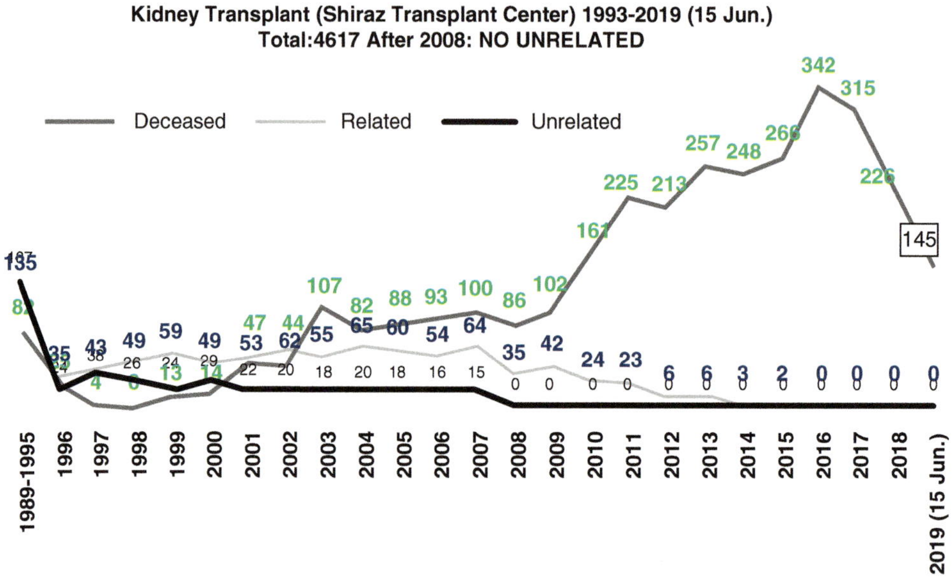


**Fig. 23.4** Statistics on kidney transplant numbers in Shiraz, Iran

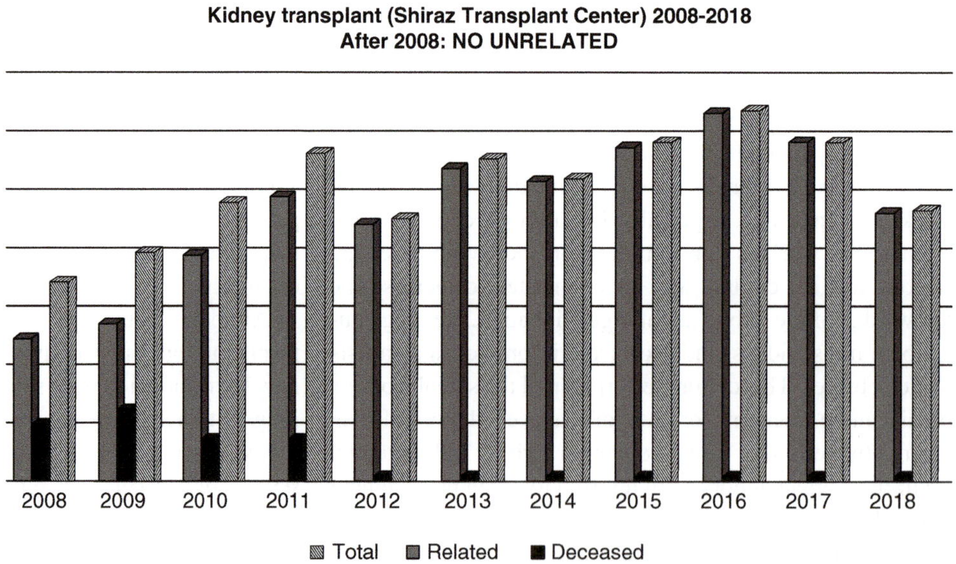


**Fig. 23.5** Sources of kidney for transplantations in Shiraz-Iran by year

cial journal of the Iranian Society of Organ Transplantation and the Avicenna Organ Transplant Institute. Electronic *IJOTM* is available online at www.ijotm.com, free of charge. Avicenna Organ Transplant Institute is planning to establish a college for educating fellows from Iran and the neighboring countries, and as a step in that direction to date, Avicenna has already trained several young applicants from Tajikistan, Uzbekistan, and Afghanistan, and some have already started performing kidney and liver transplantations in their countries. Indeed, Avicenna hospital is devoted to all kinds of transplantation and achieved the highest number of liver transplantations in the world for 2018.

## Practice of Nephrology in Iran

Within developing countries, each country has a different training system for nephrologists. In Iran, for example, there was no such thing as a nephrology training program in the past. Training in the field of nephrology was only started in Iran in 1980. The initial nephrologists' training was informal, as they were only physicians able to treat kidney diseases and acted as nephrologists, until the American- and European-trained nephrologists returned to Iran and official formal training programs began. In recent years, candidates first have become board eligible in internal medicine and then complete a 2-year nephrology fellowship. Today, even major cities other than the capital (Tehran), Shiraz, Tabriz, Mashhad, Isfahan, Kermanshah, Sari, and Rasht contain many physicians who practice nephrology but are not board certified.

Iran currently has about 350 formally trained adult nephrologists, and the majority of them work in the major metropolitan areas such as Tehran, Isfahan, Tabriz, Shiraz, and Mashhad. The current training is composed of 3 years of postgraduate training in internal medicine and 2 years in nephrology. However, since the compensation for the practice of nephrology is little, these training programs do not have enough applicants. Therefore, the MoH is planning to reduce the training to a total of 4 years of combined internal medicine/nephrology postgraduate training. However, some of the most rigorous medical students still do not apply to nephrology due to low pay for nephrologists. Low to unsatisfactory reimbursements for the nephrologists is the biggest danger to the field of nephrology in Iran. The latest development to accomplish the required manpower in December 2019, in case of remote places that do not have access to nephrologists, a 96 h training period in both the theory and practice of dialysis has been designed through which the general practitioners may obtain a 1-year permit to visit and treat dialysis patients. In situations where this continued need is demonstrated and proven, the permit may be renewed for one additional year.

The number of adult nephrologists in Iran in 2019 was 350 for a population of 81 million or 4.19 pmp. In order to comply with its needs, Iran still needs to train more nephrologists. According to the IrSN, the number of nephrology fellows (trainees) in Iran is now 40, which corresponds to 0.49 pmp. More nephrology training programs are needed in order to increase this ratio to 1 pmp. This goal is hard to achieve as the number of applicants to nephrology fellowships is decreasing because of the low salaries offered to nephrologists in Iran. The average income of a nephrologist in Iran is 10 million Tomans per month (or 800–900 US dollars per month), which is even less than those of the other subspecialties such as GI or cardiology. The Scientific Society of Nephrology is trying to find a solution to this problem and is currently working hard to collaborate with the rest of the world's scientific community and to help train fellows from other Persian (Farsi)-speaking countries in the art and science of nephrology.

For pediatric nephrologists, the training is 3 years of training in pediatrics and 2 years of nephrology. At present, the majority of the seats on the board of directors of the IrSN, five out of seven, are being held by women. The nephrology registered nurses did not have a formal training until approximately 10 years ago. Back then, the nurses only did a brief training period. Today, nurses are trained in dialysis and RRT skills. Currently, there is a shortage of nephrology nurses in Iran. As described earlier in the text, renal pathology fellowship does not exist in Iran yet, but plans are in place to create one.

## Highlights of Nephrology in Iran

### Renal Transplant Surgery in Iran

In the subspecialty of transplantation surgery, except for transplantation specialists such as Dr. Malek-Husseini, who trained in liver and kidney transplantation in Pittsburgh, United States, and is known for having performed the largest number of liver transplantations in the world in 2018, there are only general surgeons or urologists who work side by side with the transplant surgeons and learned their skills by performing transplantations.

### World Kidney Day in Iran

Another significant achievement of the IrSN is raising public education and awareness. Since 2008, the World Kidney Day (WKD) has been held in Iran every year [3]. The third WKD was celebrated on the second Thursday of March in 2008 (13/03/2008) and delivered lectures about the "Amazing Kidney" in several hospitals, city halls, and official ministries. With the support of famous athletes and celebrities, the WKD was celebrated on the streets of major cities and attracted the attention of the general population and educated them about the importance of the kidney. The fourth WKD was celebrated in Iran in 2009 with a focus on hypertension, a focus on kidney disease and diabetes mellitus in 2010, and interaction between kidney and heart in 2011, each year following the agenda suggested by the WKD organizing committee [3]. The last WKD was held in 2019 with the theme "Kidney Health for Everyone Everywhere." In its February issue, the *IJKD* published the content suggested by the WKD organization in its editorial section.

## Conclusion

The science of renal disease is relatively new globally, especially in Iran, where unusual events took place such as a cultural revolution in 1979 (which closed all universities and halted education in all medical schools as a result) and 8 years of war between Iran and Iraq (1980–1988) that led many physicians, including nephrologists and a few transplant surgeons, to leave the country. These events influenced all aspects of health, medical education, and management in Iran. All varieties of RRT slowed down. Other negative influencers included health policies and the less-than-satisfactory reimbursement of physicians. In Iran, the average compensation for a transplant physician in 2019, regardless of their subspecialty, was between 6000 and 30,000 US dollars. Finally, in spite of all of these difficulties, the future perspective of nephrology and RRT in Iran is bright, as dedicated young nephrologists are trying very hard to keep up with the scientific and clinical advances in the rest of the world and especially Persian-speaking countries in medical education and also in the art of nephrology.

**Acknowledgment** The author thanks Parmees P. Fazeli in Fayetteville, NY, and Vesta Broumand in San Antonio, Texas, for editorial contributions.

**Conflicts of Interest** The author declare that he has no conflict of interest.

## References

1. Roudi F, et al. Iran's population dynamics and demographic window of opportunity Iranian studies Stanford.edu/Iran 2040 Project Paper No. 4 October 2017.
2. World Bank Country Classifications, 2018. https://datahelpdesk.worldbank.org/knowledgebase/articles/906519.
3. Aghighi M, et al. Dialysis in Iran. Iran J Kidney Dis. 2008;2(1):11–5. ISSN:1735-8604. www.ijkd.org.
4. Hatamizadeh P, et al. Epidemiologic aspects of the Bam earthquake in Iran: the nephrologic perspective. Am J Kidney Dis. 2006;47(3):428–38. https://doi.org/10.1053/j.ajkd.2005.11.019.
5. Sepanlou SG, et al. Prevalence and determinants of chronic kidney disease in northeast of Iran: results of the Golestan cohort study. PLoS ONE. 2017. https://doi.org/10.1371/journal.pone.0176540.
6. Haghdoost AA, et al. Modeling of HIV/AIDS in Iran up to 2014. JAIDS. 2011;3:231–3910. https://doi.org/10.5897/jahr11.030.
7. Tabrizi JS, et al. Prevention and control of non-communicable diseases in Iranian population: life style promotion project phase II: study protocol. Iran J Public Health. 2018;47(9):1397–405.
8. Hosseinpanah F, et al. High prevalence of chronic kidney disease in Iran: a large population-based study. BMC Public Health. 2009;9:44. https://doi.org/10.1186/1471-2458-9-44.
9. Najafi I, et al. Seventeen years' experience of peritoneal dialysis in Iran first official report of the Iranian peritoneal dialysis registry. Perit Dial Int. 2014;34(6):636–42. https://doi.org/10.3747/pdi.2012.00054.
10. Hassannia T, et al. National and sub-national prevalence, trend, and burden of end stage renal diseases (ESRD) in Iran 1990–2013; the study protocol. Arch Iran Med. 2014;17(12):800–3.
11. Farzadfar, et al. National and subnational mortality effects of metabolic risk factors and smoking in Iran: a comparative risk assessment. Popul Health Metrics. 2011;9(1):55. https://doi.org/10.1186/1478-7954-9-55.
12. Broumand B. Diabetes: changing the fate of diabetics in the dialysis unit. Blood Purif. 2007;25(1):39–47. https://doi.org/10.1159/000096396.
13. Sarafzadegan N, et al. Cardiovascular disease in Iran in the last 40 years: prevalence, mortality, morbidity, challenges and strategies for cardiovascular prevention. Arch Iran Med. 2019;22(4):204–10. PMID: 31126179.
14. Global, regional, and national incidence, prevalence, and years lived with disability for 301 acute and chronic diseases and injuries in 188 countries, 1990–2013: a systematic analysis for the Global Burden of Disease Study 2013. Lancet. 2015;386(9995):743–800. https://doi.org/10.1016/S0140-6736(15)60692-4
15. Farzadfar F, et al. Effectiveness of diabetes and hypertension management by rural primary health-care workers (Behvars worker) in Iran: a nationally representative observational study. Lancet. 2012;379(9810):47–54. https://doi.org/10.1016/S0140-6736(11)61349-4.
16. Javanparast S, et al. The experience of community health workers training in Iran: a qualitative study. BMC Health Serv Res. 2012;12:291. https://doi.org/10.1186/1472-6963-12-291.
17. Ossareh SH, Farrokhi F, Zebarjadi M. Survival of patients on hemodialysis and predictors of mortality a single-centre analysis of time-dependent factors. Iran J Kidney Dis. 2016;10(6):369–80.
18. Ashkani-Esfahani S, et al. Prevalence of hepatitis C virus infection among hemodialysis patients in the Middle-East: a systematic review and meta-analysis. World J Gastroenterol. 2017;23(1):151–66. https://doi.org/10.3748/wjg.v23.i1.151.
19. Broumand B. Progress of nephrology in Iran. In: Proceedings of COMGAN meeting in world nephrology. Berlin, June 7, 2002.
20. Broumand B. Living donors: the Iran experience. Nephrol Dial Transplant. 1997;12(9):1830–1. https://doi.org/10.1093/ndt/12.9.1830.
21. Broumand B. The global registry: hope for the future: experimental and clinical transplantation. Exp Clin Transplant. 2015;(Suppl 1):4–8. PMID: 25894119.
22. Fazel I. Renal transplantation from living related and unrelated donors. Transplant Proc. 1995;27(5):2586–7. PMID: 7482839.
23. Delmonico FL. The alternative Iranian model of living renal transplantation. Kidney Int. 2012;82(6):625–6. https://doi.org/10.1083/ki.212.247.

24. Broumand B. Transplantation in Iran. Exp Clin Transplant. 2005;1:333–7. PMID: 15989679.
25. Ghods, et al. Iranian model of paid and regulated living unrelated kidney donation. Clin J Am Soc Nephrol. 2006;1(6):1136–45. https://doi.org/10.2215/CJN.00700206.
26. Broumand B, et al. Commendable developments in deceased organ donation and transplantation in Iran. Transplantation. 2013;96:765–6. PMID: 24162245. https://doi.org/10.1097/01.tp.0000436099.27866.30.
27. Saidi RF, et al. Current challenges of kidney transplantation in Iran moving beyond the "Iranian model". Transplantation. 2018;102(8):1195–7. PMID: 30044359. https://doi.org/10.1097/TP.0000000000002212.
28. Nobakht A, et al. Organ transplantation in Iran before and after Istanbul declaration, 2008. Int J Organ Transplant Med. 2011;2(1):1–2. PMID: 25013587 PMCID: 4089250.
29. Mojtabaee M, et al. Update on causes of family refusal for organ donation and the related factors: reporting the changes over 6 years. Transplant Proc. 2018;50(1):10–3. PMID: 29407290. https://doi.org/10.1016/j.transproceed.2017.11.021.
30. The Declaration of Istanbul. Incentives, kidney donation, and the myth of the Iranian waiting list. 2014. Available at: https://www.declarationofistanbul.org/resources/recommended-reading/reports-and-reviews-of-national-and-regional-experience/629-incentives,-kidney-donation,-and-the-myth-of-the-iranian-waiting-list.
31. Ghahramani N. Paid living donation and growth of deceased donor programs. Transplantation. 2016;100(6):1165–9. https://doi.org/10.1097/TP.0000000000001164. PMID: 27203584.

# Nephrology in Israel

# 24

Suheir Assady, Geoffrey Boner, Miriam Davidovits, Victor Frajewicki, Ruth Rachamimov, Daniel Landau, Eliezer Golan, and Talia Weinstein

| | |
|---|---|
| Area[a] | 22,072 km$^2$ |
| Population[b] | 8,899,796 (2018) |
| Capital | Jerusalem |
| Three most populated cities[b] | 1. Jerusalem<br>2. Tel Aviv<br>3. Haifa |
| Official languages | Hebrew, Arabic |
| Gross Domestic Product (GDP)[c] | 369.69 billion USD (2018) |
| GDP per capita[c] | 41,614 USD (2018) |
| Human Development Index (HDI)[d] | 0.906 (22nd, 2019) |
| Official currency | New Israeli Shekel (NIS) |
| Total number of nephrologists[e] | 294 – registered<br>150 – estimated active |
| National society of nephrology | The Israeli Society of Nephrology and Hypertension (ISNH)<br>www.isnh.org.il |
| Incidence of end-stage renal disease[f] | 2018 – 226 pmp |
| Prevalence of end-stage renal disease[f] (including patients with a functioning kidney transplant) | 2018 – 1229 pmp |
| Total number of patients on dialysis (all modalities)[f] | 2017 – 6700<br>2018 – 6687 |
| Number of patients on hemodialysis[f] | 2017 – 6238<br>2018 – 6211 |
| Number of patients on peritoneal dialysis[f] | 2017 – 462<br>2018 – 476 |
| Number of renal transplantations per year[g] | 2017 – 369<br>2018 – 399 |

a. Israel in figures, selected data from the statistical abstract of Israel 2018. Central Bureau of Statistics. Available at: https://www.cbs.gov.il/he/publications/DocLib/isr_in_n/isr_in_n18e.pdf. Accessed September 16, 2019
b. Central Bureau of Statistics. Available at: https://www.cbs.gov.il/he/Documents/2018_קובץ_ישובים.xlsx. Accessed September 16, 2019
c. World Bank: countries and economies. Available at: https://data.worldbank.org/country/israel. Accessed September 16, 2019
d. United Nations Development Programme, Human Development reports. Available at: hdr.undp.org/en/countries/profiles/ISR. Accessed February 15, 2020
e. Israel Medical Association (personal communication)
f. Annual Reports of the Israeli Center for Disease Control, Ministry of Health (personal communication)
g. ADI – National Transplant Center, Ministry of Health. Available at: https://www.health.gov.il/Subjects/Organ_transplant/transplant/Pages/default.aspx. Accessed September 16, 2019

S. Assady (✉)
Rambam Health Care Campus, Haifa, Israel

Technion – Israel Institute of Technology, Haifa, Israel

The Israeli Society of Nephrology and Hypertension, Ramat Gan, Israel
e-mail: s_assady@rambam.health.gov.il

G. Boner
Rabin Medical Center, Petah Tikva, Israel

Tel Aviv University, Tel Aviv, Israel
e-mail: gboner1@013.net

M. Davidovits · D. Landau
Schneider Children's Medical Center, Petah Tikva, Israel

Tel Aviv University, Tel Aviv, Israel
e-mail: Mdavidovits@clalit.org.il; Danny_L@clalit.org.il

V. Frajewicki
The Israeli Society of Nephrology and Hypertension, Ramat Gan, Israel

Carmel Medical Center, Haifa, Israel
e-mail: vfraje@clalit.org.il

R. Rachamimov
The Israeli Society of Nephrology and Hypertension, Ramat Gan, Israel

Tel Aviv University, Tel Aviv, Israel

The Israeli Transplantation Society, Ramat Gan, Israel

Rabin Medical Center, Petah Tikva, Israel
e-mail: rutir@clalit.org.il

E. Golan
The Israeli Society of Nephrology and Hypertension, Hafia, Israel

Tel Aviv University, Tel Aviv, Israel
e-mail: golane@tauex.tau.ac.il

T. Weinstein
The Israeli Society of Nephrology and Hypertension, Ramat Gan, Israel

Tel Aviv University, Tel Aviv, Israel

Sourasky Medical Center, Tel Aviv, Israel
e-mail: taliaw@tlvmc.gov.il; tweinste@tauex.tau.ac.il


J. A. Moura-Neto et al. (eds.), *Nephrology Worldwide*, https://doi.org/10.1007/978-3-030-56890-0_24

## Introduction

The State of Israel is situated in the Levant, the Eastern Mediterranean region of Western Asia. Israel is a parliamentary democracy with universal suffrage. It is governed by a 120-member parliament, known as the Knesset. The Prime Minister is the head of the government and the President of Israel is the head of state, with limited and largely ceremonial duties [1]. There are 255 local authorities distributed in six districts (Jerusalem, Tel Aviv, Haifa, Northern, Southern, and Central) [2]. They are divided according to their municipal status into municipalities, local councils, and regional councils. The local authorities are responsible for municipal services, as prescribed by the law, such as education and sanitation.

According to the classification system of the World Bank [3, 4], Israel is considered as a high-income country with a 2018 gross national income per capita of 40,850 current USD. Prominently, Israel is spiritually significant for the world's three major monotheistic religions: Judaism, Christianity, and Islam. The Bahá'í World Centre is also situated in Israel, in two cities, Acre and Haifa. Israel has a rich history for the past millennia. Because of massive immigration, the population is multicultural and multilinguistic. About 21% of the population is of Arab ethnicity and 79% is of Jewish ethnicity [1]. The above table summarizes the main general information about Israel [1, 4–7].

According to the State Health Insurance Law, the state is responsible for insuring the health of all residents according to a defined basket of health services. Overall, the general health status in Israel is favorable [8]. Life expectancy is 80.7 years for men and 84.6 years for women, which is substantially higher than that in neighboring countries, and ranking 8th among Organisation for Economic Co-operation and Development (OECD) countries [8–10]. Several unique characteristics have affected Israel's age pattern, the most notable of which is immigration [10]. Infant mortality rate, an important health indicator, is 3 per 1000 live births, among the best in the world [1, 11]. However, despite population growth and increased demand, the relative expenditure on healthcare has stayed largely static over the past decade [8]. In 2018, the national expenditure on health was NIS 95.3 billion (7.5% of gross domestic product). Notably, 82.8% of all households purchased supplementary health insurance [1]. Compared with OECD countries, there are fewer acute hospital beds and lower relative numbers of employed physicians and nurses in health services (in 2018, rates per 1000 residents were 1.8, 3.1, and 4.6, respectively).

Unfortunately, inequalities in noncommunicable diseases do exist between the subpopulations of Israel, across different socioeconomic levels, and between urban and peripheral regions [12]. Age-adjusted mortality rates from heart disease, stroke, or diabetes remain higher in Arabs, whereas the age-adjusted incidence and mortality of cancer are higher among Jews. The Ministry of Health (MoH) acknowledges the wide gaps between certain sectors of the population. Since 2010, the MoH has launched several comprehensive programs to overcome hurdles leading to health disparities [10, 12].

## Brief History of Nephrology in Israel

Nephrology was recognized worldwide as a new specialty in the 1960s and 1970s, following the recognition that hemodialysis (HD) could be used to treat end-stage renal disease (ESRD) [13]. In the initial practices using HD, it was performed to treat acute kidney injury (AKI) [14]. Following the successful treatment of ESRD, new clinical units were established. Nephrologists started treating chronic kidney disease (CKD) and hypertensive patients and to carry out research in these fields.

Israel gained its independence in 1948, but medical facilities had been established several years before. They expanded after 1948 to provide medical care for the entire population [8].

HD was first utilized for treating AKI in Israel in 1947 by Kurt Steinitz (1907–1966). Kurt Steinitz was born in Breslau and worked for a period in Turkey, publishing his research related to kidney physiology [15, 16]. He immigrated to Palestine in 1943, and following the description of dialytic treatment of patients by WJ Kolff and N. Alwall, he decided to build a device similar to that of Alwall (a vertical drum dialyzer). With the help of collaborators at the Technion in Haifa, he built an Alwall type dialyzer and treated three patients at the Rothschild hospital (now Bnei Zion) in Haifa [17]. The treatment with HD resulted in a substantial decline in the blood urea; however, the first two trauma patients died. The third patient was a young woman, who had an extrauterine pregnancy and had developed AKI following a mismatched blood transfusion. She was dialyzed three times at the end of September 1948 before gaining consciousness. She recovered, lived a long life, and gave birth to two children. Unfortunately, due to financial constrictions and lack of support, K. Steinitz was unable to continue with his work in dialysis.

David Ullmann (1908–1975) was the true pioneer of nephrology in Israel. He was born in Würzburg, studied in Würzburg and Dusseldorf, and immigrated to Palestine in 1934, initially working as a chemist in a paint factory. In 1940, he joined the Department of Internal Medicine at Hadassah University Hospital in Jerusalem, where he spent most of his career. Early on, he was active in the investigation of renal disease and in 1948 published an article on parathyroid activity in renal failure due to a congenital anomaly [18]. During the period 1949–1951, he completed a fellowship at the Montefiore hospital in New York, one of the first centers to investigate water and electrolyte balance in man.

Among his publications, he described the effects of mercurial diuretics on renal function [19]. On his return to Jerusalem, he was able to establish a "kidney unit" within the framework of the Department of Medicine in Hadassah hospital. The research in this unit focused on the excretion of nonionic substances, the effects of antihypertensive substances on renal function, renal excretion of salt and water by hypertensive patients, the effects of volume expansion on electrolyte excretion, and the pathophysiology of toxemia of pregnancy. In 1957, following a trip overseas, he obtained an artificial kidney apparatus (Travenol 100-liter tank for use with the Kolff twin-coil disposable dialyzer), as a gift from Dr. EA Friedman of Brooklyn, and established the first and only HD unit in Israel at that time [20]. Over the next few years, similar units for the treatment of acute renal failure were established by JB Rosenfeld at the Beilinson hospital (now part of the Rabin Medical Center) and by HE Eliahou at the Tel Hashomer hospital (now Sheba Medical Center).

In 1960, the Seattle group of Scribner reported on the use of HD to treat patients with ESRD [13]. The directors of the three HD units in Israel carried out the necessary adaption of equipment and staff and the first ESRD patients were treated with HD at Beilinson in 1963, Hadassah in 1964, and Tel Hashomer in 1965. In 1965, D. Erlik of the Rambam hospital in Haifa obtained a donation, which enabled O. Better to set up the first HD unit in the north of the country (Fig. 24.1). As HD became an accepted method for the treatment of ESRD and as more patients were accepted for treatment, dialysis units were opened at other hospitals, until there was a unit at every general hospital in Israel.

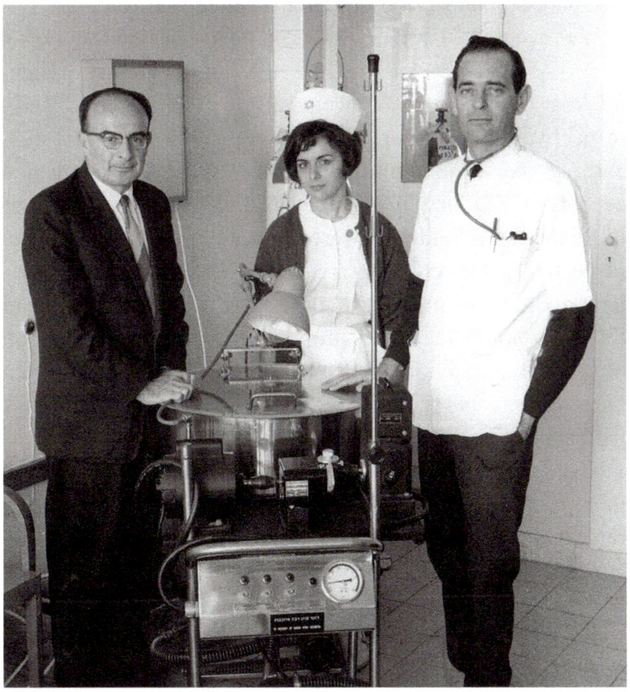

Fig. 24.1 First dialysis machine at Rambam Medical Center, Haifa, Israel, 1965. Left to right: David Erlik, MD, the first surgeon to transplant a kidney from a deceased donor in Israel; Ilana Ungerman, RN; Ori Better, MD, Director of Nephrology at Rambam, 1965–1993, the first recipient of the ISN Bywaters Award

One of the important developments, which was responsible for the general acceptance of HD as a feasible treatment for ESRD, was the description of the use of a surgically created arteriovenous fistula (AVF) as an access to the vasculature [21]. B. Hurwich, who was one of the authors of the seminal paper, immigrated to Israel and became director of nephrology at the Shaare Zedek Medical Center.

The acceptance of new patients requiring HD treatment was limited by the lack of equipment and disposables in the various hospitals. An attempt was made in 1974 to engage the MoH Director-General, B. Padeh, who was unable to provide the necessary funding and, within days of the meeting, resigned from this position. B. Modan, who became MoH Director-General in 1979, decided that dialytic treatment would be provided to every ESRD patient. Following this decision, there was a rapid increase in the number of treated patients. New units opened within hospitals and in the community, in parallel with the expansion of specialist clinics for the investigation and treatment of renal disease and hypertension, and the development of both basic and clinical research.

There were sporadic attempts to introduce peritoneal dialysis (PD) as a chronic treatment for ESRD. L. Gotloib at the Afula hospital was one of the first proponents of this treatment. However, it was only after the description of continuous ambulatory peritoneal dialysis (CAPD) and the introduction of CAPD at Beilinson and Tel Hashomer, and later at Be'er Sheva', that this method of treatment became routine in Israel [22].

The 1960s saw the launch of research and collaboration between the units. The Israeli Society of Nephrology and Hypertension (ISNH) was established in 1964. The Society subsequently held annual meetings with the presentation of scientific papers. There was also an active "Salt and Water Club," which met regularly to discuss various subjects. Pediatric nephrology became an independent specialty inspired by C. Boichis, H. Stark, and A. Drukker.

The 1950s also saw the introduction of renal transplantation as a means of ESRD treatment, initially by means of living donors and at a later stage utilizing deceased donors [23]. In 1964, M. Levi, a cardiac surgeon, performed a living donor kidney transplant (mother to son) at the Beilinson hospital. The recipient survived more than 30 years after the transplant. In 1966, D. Erlik, a general surgeon at the Rambam hospital, performed the first deceased kidney transplant [24]. These early attempts led eventually to the founding of transplant units at Beilinson, Hadassah, Tel Hashomer, Rambam, Soroka, and Sourasky hospitals, as well as tissue-typing laboratories and an administrative center for organ sharing (Israel Transplant). In 1994, the National Transplant Center was established by the MoH in order to establish a neutral, national body to manage and coordinate the organ donation system in Israel.

B. Modan, an epidemiologist at Tel Hashomer, received in the 1960s a NIH grant to investigate dialysis requirements in Israel in order to provide estimates on dialysis requirements throughout the world. Modan and colleagues examined the files of all patients hospitalized during 1965–1966, who had a blood urea nitrogen level above 60 mg/dl. They reported that the annual incidence of ESRD requiring maintenance dialysis was 70 new patients per million population (pmp), in ages 15–59 years [25].

In 1973–1974, the Israel Transplantation and Dialysis Association was established, creating a central registry of patients being treated for ESRD. Previously, the units had reported to the European Dialysis and Transplant Association (EDTA). At the end of September 1975, there were 350 patients being treated in 20 dialysis units, with a mean of 17 patients per unit, of whom 14 were on home HD and 4 on PD. During a 1-year period, 161 new patients were introduced, 28 were transplanted, and the net increase in the number of patients was 100 [26].

Today, the Israeli nephrology community participates in the activities of nephrology throughout the world. In 1974, the annual conference of the EDTA (now the European Renal Association-European Dialysis and Transplant Association, or ERA-EDTA) was held in Israel. This was followed by the conference of the International Pediatric Nephrology Association (IPNA) in 1975 and the World Congress of the International Society of Nephrology (ISN) in 1993.

The pioneer work by the physicians mentioned in this short description and many others resulted in the Israeli nephrology community being at the world forefront in providing dialysis treatment for ESRD patients, caring for patients with renal disease and hypertension, and for conducting both clinical and basic research.

## Renal Diseases in Israel

In 2013, CKD was the seventh leading cause of death in Israel, accounting for 3.7% of all deaths, after cancer (25%), heart disease (15.9%), diabetes and stroke (5.6% each), sepsis (5.2%), and accidents (4.2%) [27].

*Epidemiology* In Israel, as in many other countries, population-based cohort studies on the incidence and prevalence of AKI are scarce and imprecise, because of inconsistent definitions, underreporting, and lack of national surveys. In a 1-year retrospective cohort study from a single center in northern Israel, Shema and associates reported that the annual incidence rate of AKI among hospitalized adult patients was 1–5.1%, depending on the AKI definition that was used [28].

The actual number of prevalent patients with CKD at each eGFR stage of the Kidney Disease: Improving Global Outcomes (KDIGO) classification in Israel is uncertain. It is likely to be in line with global estimates [29]. However, no Israeli CKD registry for CKD G1–G4 exists. Recently, a large cohort from Maccabi Healthcare Services (1,011,789 adult Israeli individuals without CKD, of whom 72,480 were diabetics) participated in a multinational longitudinal study (the CKD Prognosis Consortium), aiming to develop equations that predict the 5-year risk of developing CKD (defined as eGFR $\leq$ 60 ml/min/1.73 m$^2$) [30]. Of note, baseline characteristics differed between the two subgroups of the Israeli cohort. Baseline features of the nondiabetic participants show the following: the cohort mean age was 43 ± 15 years, 58% of whom were females, mean eGFR at the start of the study 104 ± 17 ml/min/1.73 m$^2$, 6% with a history of cardiovascular disease (CVD), 23% had hypertension, 25% were ever smokers, and mean body mass index (BMI) was 27 ± 5 kg/m$^2$. In comparison, baseline characteristics of the diabetic participants indicate older age (60 ± 13 years), male preponderance (55%), lower eGFR at the start (92 ± 15 ml/min/1.73 m$^2$), and increased associated comorbidities: a history of CVD in 25%, hypertension in 75%, 30% were ever smokers, and mean BMI was 31 ± 6 kg/m$^2$. Accordingly, in nondiabetic cohort, the cumulative incidence rates of confirmed events of CKD at different stages (defined as eGFR $\leq$60, $\leq$45, and $\leq$30 ml/min/1.73 m$^2$), during a 5.3-, 5.4-, and 5.5-year follow-up period, were 1.29%, 0.696%, and 0.172%, respectively. In comparison, during a follow-up of 5.7, 6.3, and 6.7 years, the cumulative incidence rates of confirmed events of CKD for eGFR $\leq$60, $\leq$45, and $\leq$30 ml/min/1.73 m$^2$ in diabetic individuals were 19.73%, 7.8%, and 2.5%, respectively. These figures are striking and need further evaluation. Based on this study of the CKD Prognosis Consortium [30], we anticipate that the proposed risk equations will soon be used as an individual risk assessment tool for CKD to help clinicians adapt primary preventive measures for at-risk patients and health policy planning.

Estimates of the prevalence and incidence of ESRD are more reliable because each patient who has receiving renal replacement therapy (RRT) is listed in a national database, which will be discussed later.

*Causes of Chronic Kidney Diseases* Diabetes mellitus is the main cause of CKD in adults. However, genetic disorders have received much attention in pediatric and adult nephrology in Israel, because of the demographic strata of the country. The genetic preponderance of the different ethnic groups in Israel has been shaped by their history and cultural practices [31, 32]. In one study of Palestinian Arabs, more than

40% of the marriages were between relatives, and of these, 50% between first cousins [33]. In the Bedouin society, 40% of women of childbearing age are married to first cousins [34]. Nevertheless, a comprehensive recent study, conducted in a single Muslim village in Israel, demonstrated significant sociodemographic changes during a 50-year time period [35]. A shift from the practice of marrying a first cousin to marrying a remote relative was noted. There was a significant reduction in the mean number of children born per woman and in parallel, the mean age of first-time mothers increased progressively. The impact of these changes on future incidence of recessively inherited diseases among this population is of much interest.

In contrast, the consanguinity rate among Israeli Jews is reported to be 2.3%, and of these, first-cousin marriages account for 0.8%. The highest consanguinity rate among Israeli Jews (7.1%) is found among Eastern Jews [36]. A comprehensive list of genetic kidney diseases of Israeli and Middle Eastern subpopulations was reviewed by Assady and colleagues [32] and partly detailed below in the pediatric nephrology section.

In northern Israel, the main indication to perform kidney biopsy was nephrotic range proteinuria, and membranous nephropathy was the main diagnosis (personal communication). Of note, initiatives have recently been launched under the auspices of the ISNH, to detect the genetic basis for ESRD in Israel and to establish a kidney biopsy registry.

## Renal Replacement Therapy in Israel

All modalities of RRT are accessible to every patient with ESRD in Israel. Since 1995, the National Health Insurance law regulates the rights of residents in Israel, the basket of health services, and supplemental insurance. According to the law, RRT is included in the list of "Severe Diseases" and is funded differentially [37, 38]. Therefore, each Israeli resident who requires RRT is entitled to receive the treatment, free of charge, regardless of their socioeconomic status. Dialysis health basket is comprehensive, including dialysis treatments, hospitalizations, surgical interventions such as creation and maintenance of vascular access, and partial coverage of transportation to and from the dialysis center. Dialysis patients are not required to pay for medications, such as erythropoietin-stimulating agents (ESA), heparin, vitamin D derivatives and analogues, calcimimetics, and all other medications administered during dialysis. There is a payment "ceiling" for nutritional preparations included in the health basket. Cyclers used in PD are also fully covered. At this time, there is an initiative to develop and expand home HD, which will also be provided at no cost.

When traveling abroad, dialysis patients are eligible for reimbursement for dialysis treatments done on-site in accordance with the cost of treatment in Israel. In addition, dialysis patients are exempt from paying income tax and receive a special status in the National Insurance program.

*Epidemiology* As described previously, RRT was initiated in Israel during the 1960s. In parallel, a registry of patients being treated for ESRD was founded [26]. Unfortunately, the data regarding the years up to 1990 were partially lost.

The Israel Renal Registry (IRR) was established by the ISNH during the 1990s. The IRR cooperates with the Israel Center for Disease Control (ICDC) of the MoH. Each patient initiating RRT is reported to the ICDC by the treating unit, on a special form with the following data: demographics; primary renal disease using the coding system of the ERA-EDTA Registry; type of RRT (in-center HD, online hemodiafiltration (HDF), home HD, or PD); type of vascular access used to initiate HD/HDF; and viral positivity for hepatitis B (HBV), hepatitis C (HCV), and human immunodeficiency virus (HIV).

The information is analyzed by the ICDC staff. Each year, the data is summarized and reported to the various dialysis units, as well as to the MoH Director-General. The national data is also presented to members of the ISNH during the annual conference. The results were published in Hebrew for the years 1990–2007 [39] and then updated up to 2010 [40] and 2015 [41]. The next update will cover up to 2020 and is expected to be published in 2021–2022.

The IRR/ICDC also cooperates with international registries, such as the ERA-EDTA Registry and the United States Renal Data System (USRDS). Due to the regulatory limitations, we provide aggregated data instead of individual patient data, which was transferred to the ERA-EDTA Registry during the 1970s.

As shown in Table 24.1, the number of new patients increased from 1990 to 2000 and then plateaued. The rate pmp reflects the increase in the Israeli population (from 4,821,700 at the end of 1990 to 8,899,796 inhabitants at the end of 2018) and the aging of the Israeli population [10]. In 1990, the mean and median age of incident ESRD patients were 55.4 and 60 years, respectively, while in 2018 this rose to 66.55 and 68.54 years, respectively.

In contrast to the incidence of RRT, the prevalence of patients receiving dialysis did not plateau, probably reflecting aging of the population, improvement of treatment over the years, and the low number of kidney transplants (Table 24.1). The mean age of prevalent patients in 1990 was 55.82 and the median 59.01 years, while in 2018 they were 66.6 ± 14.72 and 68.55 years, respectively.

Remarkably, there is a male majority among ESRD patients (61%) and a growing number of patients older than

**Table 24.1** The incidence and prevalence of dialysis in Israel

| Year | New patients | Incidence rate (pmp) | Number of patients | Prevalence rate (pmp) |
|---|---|---|---|---|
| 1990 | 527 | 113 | 1558 | 334 |
| 1991 | 577 | 117 | 1677 | 339 |
| 1992 | 585 | 114 | 1793 | 350 |
| 1993 | 633 | 120 | 1939 | 368 |
| 1994 | 680 | 126 | 2113 | 391 |
| 1995 | 749 | 135 | 2284 | 412 |
| 1996 | 796 | 140 | 2468 | 434 |
| 1997 | 912 | 156 | 2688 | 461 |
| 1998 | 934 | 156 | 2854 | 478 |
| 1999 | 1100 | 180 | 3145 | 513 |
| 2000 | 1092 | 174 | 3398 | 540 |
| 2001 | 1152 | 179 | 3605 | 560 |
| 2002 | 1178 | 179 | 3769 | 570 |
| 2003 | 1257 | 188 | 4009 | 599 |
| 2004 | 1284 | 189 | 4235 | 622 |
| 2005 | 1290 | 186 | 4413 | 637 |
| 2006 | 1357 | 192 | 4603 | 653 |
| 2007 | 1388 | 193 | 4800 | 669 |
| 2008 | 1387 | 188 | 5052 | 685 |
| 2009 | 1429 | 198 | 5273 | 729 |
| 2010 | 1375 | 182 | 5479 | 726 |
| 2011 | 1407 | 190 | 5692 | 723 |
| 2012 | 1418 | 181 | 5795 | 729 |
| 2013 | 1509 | 186 | 5896 | 725 |
| 2014 | 1727 | 201 | 6287 | 758 |
| 2015 | 1558 | 186 | 6434 | 768 |
| 2016 | 1582 | 185 | 6566 | 768 |
| 2017 | 1637 | 186 | 6700 | 762 |
| 2018 | 1628 | 181 | 6687 | 752 |

85 years (321 males and 210 females), accounting for 7.9% of dialysis patients in 2018.

*Etiology* The primary causes of ESRD are detailed in Fig. 24.2. As in many countries, diabetic kidney disease (DKD) is the leading cause of ESRD in Israel. However, the interpretation of this data could be misleading. It is well known that a proportion of diabetic patients with CKD may have various etiologies for their kidney failure [42] and most of them do not perform a kidney biopsy. Therefore, the reported DKD is mostly a presumed rather than a biopsy-proven diagnosis.

*Dialysis Practice* HD is by far the preferred treatment modality of the Israeli ESRD patients. In 2018, 87.83% of patients were on HD, of whom only two patients were on home HD, and 5.05% on post-dilution online HDF. PD comprised the RRT modality in 7.12% of patients, consisting of CAPD in 56.51% and automated PD (APD) in 43.29%. Of note, in 1994, PD accounted for 33.8% of dialysis therapy in incident patients and 25% in prevalent patients [41]. This decline in the proportion of patients treated by PD in Israel over the past two decades parallels the trend observed in many developed countries worldwide, as described by Li et al. [43] and Jain et al. [44].

At the end of 2018, 50.4% of the 6211 HD patients were treated in 45 community-based HD facilities, dispersed throughout the country, which had been previously operated

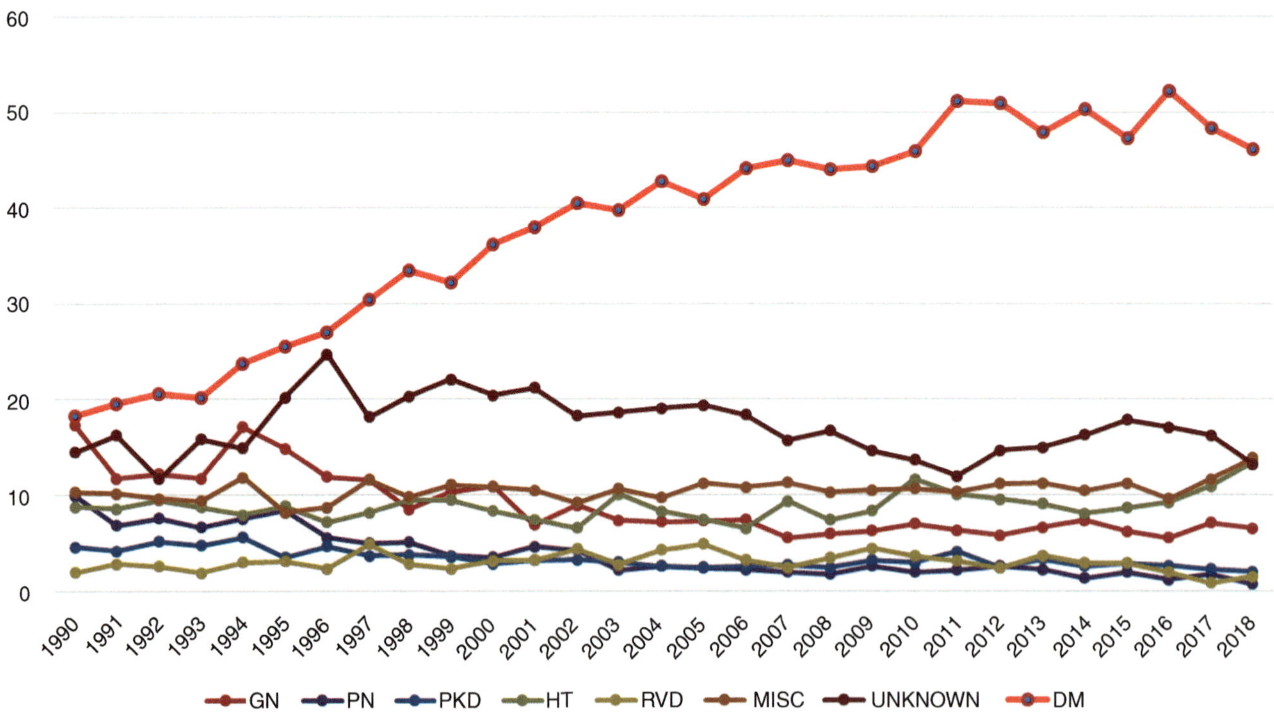


**Fig. 24.2** Primary cause of end-stage renal disease in Israel. GN glomerulonephritis, PN pyelonephritis, PKD polycystic kidney disease, HT hypertension, RVD renovascular disease, DM diabetes mellitus, MISC miscellaneous

by local dialysis owners. However, since 2016, an international dialysis provider, Fresenius Medical Care, has become the owner of 30 of them. The remaining patients, usually with comorbidities and less stable, were treated in 35 in-hospital facilities. The vascular access encompassed native AVF in 59.6%, AV grafts in 8.04%, permcaths in 32.13%, and temporary HD catheters in 0.23% of HD patients. The standard HD prescription is mostly 4 h, thrice weekly, and a blood flow of 300–400 ml/min. However, very elderly patients are often prescribed fewer weekly hours and reduced blood flow if comorbidities exist. There is also one unit that performs thrice weekly nocturnal dialysis. HDF is conducted in a few centers, and prescription targets convection volumes of more than 21–22 liters per session. However, the achievability of the recommended convection volume was neither investigated nor reported to the IRR.

PD treatment is offered by 20 nephrology institutes in general hospitals. They usually utilize conventional dextrose-based PD solutions. Sixteen units report using icodextrin and five use amino acid-based PD solution (Nutrineal®).

The ISNH publishes position papers and national guidelines, which are updated periodically, in line with KDIGO guidelines, and are implemented in all dialysis facilities. They address standards of therapy of anemia, CKD-associated mineral bone disorders (CKD-MBD), viral infection control and vaccination, hypertension, and quality of care. The MoH has strict regulations regarding the infrastructure and quality of dialysis water and dialysates. The Quality and Service Administration of the MoH leads the national quality indicators program, which includes Kt/V among others, and performs audits for all hospitals and dialysis facilities, ensuring safety and quality of care. It also conducts investigation and analysis of information on mortalities, adverse events, and cases of medical negligence [45].

In 2017, a steering committee composed of the ISNH leading nephrologists, nurses, dietitians, social workers, representatives of the public, patients, and the MoH-Quality and Service Administration recommended standards of quality in the field of dialysis. It includes both PD and HD. Based on these recommendations, a national peer-review audit was conducted between September and December 2017 and a full report was published in 2019. Analysis of the information—gathered from various sources: interviews with multidisciplinary teams in 44 dialysis units, 1238 patient medical record reviews, 165 inspections, and 764 patient interviews—revealed a 92% compliance rate. Adherence to HD water and PD quality standards were the highest (98%).

Apparently, implementation of routine viral testing, strict isolation measures, HBV vaccination, no reuse of dialyzers, and ESA administration with few blood product transfusion requirements have resulted in a low prevalence of both HBV (1.7–2%) and HCV (3.7–5.7%) infection among Israeli patients receiving dialysis between 2005 and 2010, according to the 2012 ICDC report [40]. At the end of 2018, 87 patients were reported to be positive for HBV, 47 for HCV, and 10 for HIV. It is expected that within a few years, HCV infection will be eliminated from ESRD patients as many of them are offered direct-acting antiviral oral therapies. Seventeen patients were treated during 2018 and reported as sustained viral response.

The unadjusted 1-year, 2-year, 3-year, and 10-year survival rates among Israeli dialysis patients were 86.6%, 73%, 61.3%, and 15%, respectively, from 1990 to 2015 [41]. Interestingly, there appears to be a survival advantage for Arab over Jewish patients on maintenance dialysis in Israel, in contrast to the life expectancy of Arabs in the general population which is 3–4 years lower than that of the Jewish population [10, 12, 46].

In the setting of AKI, HD but not PD is utilized. Nephrologists' involvement varies and can have an impact if the intensive/intermediate care unit (ICU) is not completely independent. Generally, ICU physicians and nurses are qualified to perform continuous veno-venous hemofiltration (CVVH), hemodialysis (CVVHD), and hemodiafiltration (CVVHDF). Depending on the policies of each hospital, either nephrology or ICU personnel evaluate patients and perform these continuous therapies. However, intermittent RRT, HD and sustained low-efficiency daily dialysis (SLEDD), are under the responsibilities of nephrologists.

## Kidney Transplantation in Israel

Currently, six adult transplant centers are active in Israel. They include Soroka Medical Center in the south, Rambam Health Care Campus in the north, Hadassah University Hospital in Jerusalem, and three in the center of Israel, Rabin, Sheba, and Sourasky Medical Centers. In addition, two centers perform pediatric kidney transplantation (see below). A supporting central tissue-typing laboratory was established at the Sheba Medical Center. In 1994, the MoH set up a National Transplant Center [47]. In 2008, the Israeli Knesset passed two laws, one regulating organ transplantation and the other defining brain death.

*Israel Transplant Law 2008* This Israel Transplant Law was introduced in order to regulate the transplantation of organs both from live and deceased donors [48, 49]. The law defined the legality of the transplants and stated that any commercialization of transplantation was illegal and subject to legal procedures. However, the law does allow remuneration for loss of income and other costs to living donors. The performance of a transplant in a foreign country is sanctioned only if the country has similar strict regulations. In the same year, the Istanbul Declaration was passed with similar restrictions on organ trafficking [50, 51]. Based on the legal aspects, the MoH published the requirements for the use of kidneys from living altruistic donors. These regulations require physical and psychological testing, followed by a decision of a national statutory committee. Of note, living organ donors in Israel are exempted from paying health insurance for a 36-month period, if the following conditions are met: the organ recipient is an Israeli resident and the donation took place in Israel as of 2010 onwards [52].

*Brain-Respiratory Death Act 2008* This law defines brain death and regulates the requirements for transplanting organs from deceased donors [53]. The directives based on this law require that there is a complete cessation of spontaneous respiration. The diagnosis requires the use of an apnea test and mandatory performance of ancillary testing or brainstem auditory evoked potentials [54].

*National Transplant Center* The center was assigned important tasks in the regulation of transplants in Israel. These include (1) the enrollment of all potential recipients for organ transplantation, (2) coordinating the acquisition of organs from deceased donors from the various hospitals in Israel, (3) promoting living organ donations, (4) allocating organs to specific recipients, (5) publicizing the need for organ donors, and (6) the establishment of a donor card and maintaining the list of potential donors. All personnel in the Transplant Center are MoH employees. There is a steering committee, with representatives of the organizations promoting transplants (the transplant center, the central laboratory, transplant surgeons and physicians from various specialties). There are subcommittees for the various transplant organs, and each chairperson serves on the steering committee. These are responsible for establishing the guidelines regarding the organ allocation and for quality control in the transplant centers, as well as providing the information required for informed consent by recipients and living donors.

*Allocation of Organs for Transplantation* As Israel is a small country, it was decided initially that transplants would be offered primarily to patients on dialysis treatment. All patients on dialysis are entitled to be included on the list of potential transplant recipients. According to international and Israeli guidelines, the patient must undergo a series of examinations in order to ascertain his or her suitability to be listed. Each dialysis unit is responsible to oversee the performance of these examinations and then to refer the patient to a transplant center at the patient's choice, before being registered at the National Transplant Center. All potential recipients are listed according to a graded point system. The points are granted according to the following criteria: (1) age (most points are given to the youngest patients and no points to the elderly ones), (2) time on dialysis (most points are given to patients on dialysis for the longest period and none to those initiating dialysis), (3) preformed antibodies (points are given to the patients with high levels), and (4) tissue-typing matching (points are given for a DR locus match). Following the implementation of the Transplant Law in 2008, additional points are given to dialysis patients who donated an organ or had a first-degree relative who donated an organ. Points are also given to patients who have signed a donor card or have a relative who has signed the donor card. When a kidney becomes available for transplantation, the recipients with a matching blood group are listed according to the total number of points and the organ is offered to the patient with the most points. There is also a program for allocating kidneys from deceased donors over the age of 60 to suitable recipients over the age of 60.

*Acquiring Organs for Transplantation* The National Transplant Center communicates with transplant nurse coordinators at all general hospitals in Israel. These coordinators are informed of all potential donors within their respective hospitals. They follow the status of the potential donors and discuss the possibility of organ donation with the family. If the patient is pronounced brain-dead and the family has consented to a donation, the Israel Transplant Center is informed. Blood and/or a lymph node are sent to the Central Tissue-typing laboratory. Upon receiving the tissue typing, an allocation decision is made based on suitable recipients listed according to the number of points. The dialysis unit where the patient is treated is informed of a possible transplantation. When a final decision is made, the patient travels to the hospital where he is registered as a transplant recipient. Preemptive transplantation is performed only if a living donor is available. Therefore, there are no preemptive deceased donor transplants and time on dialysis is equal to time on the waiting list, except if the patient suffers from type 1 diabetes mellitus and needs combined pancreas and kidney transplants.

*Kidney Transplantation***:** *The Role of Nephrologists* The assessment of the suitability of patients for transplantation is carried out by the nephrologists and nurses dedicated to this task. Living-related donors are examined by the nephrologists in the transplant center. They undergo psychosocial examination by a social worker and psychologist/psychiatrist evaluation. Donors who are not related to the recipient undergo a psychological examination at an independent institution and are then referred to a national statutory committee for the final decision.

Nephrologists and transplant coordinators at the various transplant centers are responsible for the follow-up of all transplanted patients during hospitalization and at the outpatient clinics.

**Table 24.2** Total number of wait-listed transplant candidates and kidney transplants in Israel

| Numbers at end of year | 2009 | 2010 | 2011 | 2012 | 2013 | 2014 | 2015 | 2016 | 2017 | 2018 |
|---|---|---|---|---|---|---|---|---|---|---|
| Wait-listed | 690 | 733 | 729 | 755 | 762 | 849 | 843 | 847 | 840 | 813 |
| Deceased donors | 83 | 56 | 97 | 57 | 112 | 71 | 105 | 109 | 128 | 148 |
| Living donors | 69 | 78 | 119 | 108 | 134 | 135 | 174 | 222 | 222 | 231 |
| Kidney + liver | 3 | 4 | 8 | 3 | 1 | – | 4 | 5 | 8 | 8 |
| Kidney + pancreas | 7 | 3 | 12 | 7 | 10 | 5 | 6 | 10 | 9 | 7 |
| Two kidneys | – | 2 | 5 | 3 | 5 | 5 | 5 | 6 | 2 | 5 |
| Total | **162** | **143** | **241** | **178** | **262** | **216** | **294** | **352** | **369** | **399** |
| Total/million inhabitants | **21.64** | **18.76** | **31.03** | **22.5** | **32.51** | **26.29** | **35.08** | **41.19** | **42.35** | **44.91** |

*The Israeli Transplantation Society* The Israeli Transplantation Society (IST) represents all the professions who participate in transplantation. The IST organizes scientific meetings and has an annual conference. It publishes the Society Position on important subjects. Numerous nephrologists are active members of the IST. The present chairwoman of the Society is a nephrologist.

*The Number of Kidney Transplants in Israel* Until 2010, the number of both deceased donor and living donor kidney transplants was relatively low, with a total of about 150–160 per year or about 20 pmp (Table 24.2). During the last decade, there has been a steady increase in the number of transplants, especially from living donors, so that in 2018 the number of kidney transplants was 399, almost 45 pmp. Sixty-one percent of single-kidney transplants were from living donors. There are several reasons for this twofold increase in the number of kidneys. Public awareness of the importance of kidney transplant, following use of the media by the National Transplant Center, has resulted in more people signing donor cards and more families allowing the use of organs from their deceased loved ones. In fact, there is a 60% acquiescence rate on approaching the families of potential donors. Public awareness has also resulted in a sharp increase in the number of living donors. An additional important factor was the establishment in 2009, by a Rabbi, himself a kidney recipient, of a community-based organization for facilitating living donors from the religious sector of the population [55]. The number of potential recipients for a transplant increased annually until 2014, when there were 849 patients on the waiting list. Since then, the number has stabilized and even decreased to 813 by the end of 2018.

*Outcome* The outcome of kidney transplant in adults is favorable after the introduction of modern immunosuppressive drugs, which are available and provided free of charge. All centers use high-dose steroids with either IL-2 receptor antagonist or anti-thymocyte globulin for induction. Highly sensitized patients may receive plasmapheresis, immunoglobulins, or rituximab before transplantation. Maintenance therapy usually consists of a combination of calcineurin inhibitors (mostly tacrolimus) or mammalian target of rapamycin inhibitors with steroids and mycophenolate. The minority of patients are on steroid-free regimens.

According to the 1990–2017 kidney transplant data, death-censored renal allograft half-lives (t ½) from deceased donors, one haplotype living donor, and HLA-identical sibling were 15.7 years, 18.3 years, and 35.2 years, respectively (personal communication).

## Pediatric Nephrology in Israel

Israel's child population is over 2.85 million according to the last 2016 census. Since 1995, when a National Health Insurance law was ratified by the Israeli Parliament, all Israeli children have free access to preventive care—including immunizations and prenatal care—as well as curative medical care. General and comparative national health indicators in Israel are very good. Between 1955 and 2000, the overall infant mortality rate declined sevenfold in all Israeli communities, exceeding the goal set by the World Summit for Children in 1990 [56]. These major achievements have been ascribed to an extensive primary care infrastructure, where doctor visits are free. Secondary healthcare (including subspecialty consultations) is also relatively affordable, around 10 USD per visit. Tertiary care is mainly offered in regional hospitals, which are owned by the state or by nonprofit organizations. Pediatric nephrology services are provided by experts who practice in these hospitals.

The pediatric nephrology subspecialty was recognized by the Israel Medical Association (IMA) Scientific Council, which supervises all postgraduate medical training for the MoH, in 1994. In the 1970s, most of the specialists were trained abroad. There are currently more than 30 certified pediatric nephrologists in Israel, who are organized in the Israeli Society of Pediatric Nephrology. This provides a rate of 1.05 pediatric nephrologists per 100,000 children, higher than the 0.5 rate for the United States [57]. This service is accompanied by a broad supportive infrastructure, including imaging and laboratory systems, trained nurses, and supporting medical personnel. All this has enabled the provision of good and accessible medical care, including dialysis and transplantation for pediatric ESRD patients.

## Pediatric Chronic Kidney Disease

Estimates of pediatric CKD prevalence are substantially below those noted for adults. For example, the prevalence of pediatric CKD (stage >2) in two European countries (Italy and Spain) has been estimated to be no more than 75 cases pmp. However, such estimates were based on CKD detected by tertiary care centers, probably in higher stages. Current literature evidence hints for under-detection of childhood CKD in a sizeable enough fraction that would contribute to the rise in the young adult CKD prevalence. A recent true population frequency study in Turkey demonstrates that the prevalence of childhood CKD approaches 1% [58]. Data from Israel supports this finding. Landau et al. [59] reviewed all detected cases of pediatric CKD (stages 1–5) in southern Israel during a 15-year period and then prospectively summarized the incidence and prevalence of CKD during the subsequent 2 years. In December 2008, the prevalence was 795 cases pmp for all CKD and 331 pmp for CKD stage 2 and above. Calculated annual CKD incidence was 46 pmp. Pediatric CKD resulted mainly from renal hypodysplasia (35%), genetic renal diseases (28%), glomerulonephritis (15%), and obstructive uropathy (13%). CKD stage 1 comprised 50% of the cohort; stages 2–4 and stage 5 were 30% and 20%, respectively. Thus, pediatric CKD prevalence may be underestimated [59]. In population-based, retrospective cohort studies, overweight, obesity, normal renal function with a history of any childhood kidney disease, and persistent asymptomatic isolated hematuria detected in 17-year-old young conscripts to the Israeli army were strongly associated with an increased cumulative incidence of treated ESRD, with crude hazard ratios of 3, 6.89, 4.19, and 18.5, respectively [60–62]. Thus, early detection and treatment of pediatric CKD and its complications may have a significant impact beyond the pediatric age.

## Genetic Kidney Diseases

Genetic kidney diseases (GKDs) are pathological renal conditions caused by an absent or defective gene or by a chromosomal aberration. They may manifest as steroid-resistant nephrotic syndrome, as a specific tubular transport defect (e.g., Bartter syndrome), or as a major disarrangement in kidney structure (e.g., polycystic kidney disease). Some GKDs may lead to secondary renal inflammation and fibrosis (e.g., nephronophthisis, atypical HUS). Most of the GKDs are inherited in a recessive mechanism, present in early childhood, and are therefore a well-known entity to the pediatric nephrology community. Given the high rate of consanguinity in several communities in Israel (both Jews and Arabs) and because of the availability of high-quality and easily accessible medical care, many GKDs have been described in Israel, including novel mutations [32, 63]. Since the prevalence of rare GKD is difficult to assess, Landau et al. calculated that in southern Israel, where consanguinity is particularly prevalent, the GKD/ESRD prevalence ratio was close to 4:1.

## Pediatric Dialysis Services

While the Arab minority comprises approximately 21% of the population, the prevalence of ESRD for the decade from 2004 to 2013 was 43.1 pmp for non-Jewish children (overwhelmingly of Arab ethnicity) compared to only 13.3 pmp for the population as a whole. Chronic dialysis services for children are provided in five hospital-based pediatric units dispersed in the country: four of them provide both HD and PD and one provides PD only. At the end of 2018, 44 children (roughly 15 per million children, like other Western countries) were treated with chronic dialysis, of whom 33 patients received HD and the remaining utilized PD [64, 65].

## Pediatric Transplantation

The Pediatric Renal Transplant Program in Israel was initiated at Beilinson Medical Center (later Schneider Children's Medical Center) in 1981. Until 2013, this was the only government-approved pediatric renal transplant program in Israel. Since the beginning of the program through the end of 2013, 420 children received a total of 469 grafts including 42 with two grafts and 7 with three grafts; 296 transplantations were in children of Jewish origin and 173 in Arab children. The proportion of children younger than 6 years was 21.6%. The proportion of deceased donor (DD) transplantations was higher in the Arab subpopulation: 76.3% vs 53% ($p < 0.002$). In 88 cases (18.8% of the total number of transplants), preemptive transplantation of living donor (LD) kidneys was performed; the remaining 381 transplantations were performed in children after they started dialysis. The mean waiting time on dialysis did not differ significantly between Arab and Jewish children: 20.2 ± 18.1 and 16.4 ± 21.0 months, respectively ($p = 0.52$).

Twenty-year patient survival was 91.6% for living donor and 86.8% for DD recipients. These results compare favorably to those reported in the United States by the North American Pediatric Renal Trials and Collaborative Studies

(NAPRTCS) [66] and those reported by other centers around the world. Respective 20-year death-censored graft survival was 52% and 44%, and expected half-life 28.7 and 17.8 years. These outcomes of graft survival compare with the recently reported data from a single-center experience in France [67], the NAPRTCS registry and from the Scientific Registry of Transplant Recipients (SRTR) [68]. Long-term graft survival improved significantly with each decade of transplantation for recipients of both LD and DD allografts. The improvement in outcome is most likely attributable to more potent immunosuppressive protocols along with infection surveillance and management, similar to reports in the literature [69, 70]. As in other published reports of long-term renal allograft survival [71, 72], chronic allograft nephropathy remains the major cause of graft loss in these patients.

There is no impact of recipients' age at transplantation on graft survival. This differs from the NAPRTCS and SRTR data [73], which show poorer long-term graft survival among adolescents than among younger recipients. The discrepancy in results may be due to the greater incidence of nonadherence reported among adolescents in those studies. Here there were no such differences in adherence, nor was this reported in studies from centers in Europe [71] or Japan [72]. Differences in outcome may be related to cultural differences. Increased parental supervision extending into adult life in a more traditional culture may explain the more favorable outcome in the Israeli teenage group compared to other studies. Moreover, the Israeli social health system, which covers all healthcare expenses, including medications and clinical visits, regardless of socioeconomic status may also play a role. The percentage of LD transplants in our cohort was 38.4%. This is low compared to the United States, where LD transplants provide more than 50% of the kidneys transplanted in children, and in some countries in Europe, where as many as 80% of grafts of the pediatric kidney transplants are from LD [73]. The scarcity of living donors in Israel results in a rather long waiting time of 22 months among Israeli pediatric ESRD population. More recently, we noted an increasing proportion of living donation, reaching 49%, which should reduce waiting time and further improve results. The increase in living donation is presumably related to the changes in the law regulating organ donation in 2008. Increased living donation should reduce waiting time and further improve results for transplant recipients.

Graft survival does not differ between the Arab and Jewish children, in contrast to ethnic disparities reported in the United States, Europe, and New Zealand [74–77]. This could be attributed to equality of access to pre- and post-transplant healthcare. The genetic similarities of the two populations, Arabs and Jews, which lead to similarities in immunologic responses, may also explain comparable results. The long-term data demonstrate positive and improving results over time in a national center of pediatric kidney transplantation.

## Nephrology Practice in Israel

The ISNH is a branch of the IMA. It was founded in 1964 to bring together physicians and allied scientists interested in nephrology and arterial hypertension and represent them at the IMA, official institutions, and national and international forums. Its goals include, among others:

- Professional evolvement of medical disciplines related to nephrology and hypertension
- Education and empowerment of the future generation of physicians engaged in the practice of nephrology and hypertension
- Establishment and monitoring of procedures and standards of care
- Promotion of collaborative clinical and basic research

Currently, the Society has several sections including HD, PD, transplantation, hypertension, research, and a regional Israeli-Palestinian nephrology forum. During 2019, the ISNH had 318 members; of them, 294 are physicians and 24 nonphysicians, mainly basic scientists. Interestingly, 92 members of the Society are retired and 10 are pediatric nephrologists.

The body authorized by law to grant licenses to practice medicine in Israel is the MoH. Nephrology training programs are offered as a subspecialty (after residency in medicine or pediatrics) in accredited nephrology institutes in general hospitals and continue for 2.5 years. At the end of the fellowship, it is mandatory to pass a two-part board examination to acquire approved certification in nephrology from the Scientific Council of the IMA. Since nephrology is contemplated as a complex profession, with a hard fellowship and less attractive remuneration, the new generation of young physicians hesitates to pursue this track. In 2019, there were 26 trainees at different stages of their fellowship being conducted in 19 general hospitals.

Physicians who graduated and are certified as specialists abroad, and practiced clinical medicine for 14 years or more, apply to the MoH and to the IMA's Scientific Council for recognition of their specialty. They are usually required to successfully complete an observation period at a department in an accredited institution. Otherwise, foreign nephrologists might be asked to complete one- or two-part board examination.

It is estimated that 150 active ISNH members, i.e., 17 pmp, are practicing nephrologists, mainly in general hospitals. Indeed, most nephrologists develop their entire professional career in hospitals. Working in such a setup, they are exposed to the multifaceted fields of nephrology, such as intensive care nephrology, out- and inpatient HD, PD, transplantation, clinical nephrology, hypertension, pregnancy-related kidney diseases, and more. A nephrologist in Israel may engage in one or more professional activities, such as renal consultant, senior staff physician in in-hospital or ambulatory dialysis unit, transplantation unit, outpatient clinics, and ICUs, which can be combined with clinical or translational research. Five Israeli medical centers have active kidney transplantation programs. Interventional procedures such as kidney biopsies are mainly performed by nephrologists and less by interventional radiologists. In a few centers, nephrologists are also responsible for insertion of long-term HD tunneled catheters (permcaths) and PD catheters.

Prior to 1995, Israel had a voluntary health insurance system. A law sanctioned in 1994, the National Health Insurance, made health insurance both compulsory and universal, with four general health providers (health funds) [78].

In addition to hospital-based services, ambulatory nephrology care is managed by each of these providers. Not surprisingly, there is a shortage of nephrologists, taking into account (1) the growing number of patients with CKD, including dialysis patients; (2) aging of the population; (3) increasing tasks not only in hospitals but also in community clinics; and (4) few new posts for nephrologists which have been created over the past 5 years. Financially, salaries in the field may vary, but the basic pay is relatively low and is supplemented by "extra" work, mainly "on duty" jobs in hospitals. A significant number of nephrologists have complementary occupations in health funds, private dialysis clinics, or other positions.

A shortage of dialysis nurses is also noted, especially in areas in the south and east of the country. Today, nursing studies take 4 years in most universities. Nurses need to undertake postgraduate studies to accomplish a nephrology specialization before they engage in dialysis activities. Israeli regulation determines a ratio of 1 nurse to 4 HD patients. Nurses working in the private dialysis sector may travel long distances to provide the adequate number of nurses in peripheral dialysis units.

There is an unmet need for allied healthcare professionals in nephrology. Israeli regulation clearly states criteria for dietitian consultations and frequency of visits in ESRD. There is scarcity of nephrology dietitians. Historically, they were hired part-time, both in the hospital setup and in community-based dialysis units. Therefore, necessity for dietitians is high because of an enormous workload. Likewise, nephrology social workers were historically hired in part-time jobs and still are the most unpaid sector in nephrology care. Alongside a shortage of professionals, the growing complexity of ESRD in the elderly has become a real challenge for health policy leaders.

## Highlights of Nephrology in Israel

### Management of Crush Injury

Due to military conflicts, nephrologists in Israel gained expertise in the management of casualties with crush injuries and subsequent devastating AKI, hemodynamic instability, and electrolyte disturbances. Ori S. Better, together with international colleagues, has coined protocols for prevention of developing AKI in traumatic rhabdomyolysis [79–81]. He received the 1991 ISN Bywaters Award for his major contributions to AKI research.

### CKD-MBD Research

The Minerva Center for Calcium and Bone Metabolism at Hadassah University Hospital directed by Justin Silver and Tally Naveh-Many has published cutting-edge research, illuminating the role of phosphate, parathyroid hormone (PTH), fibroblast growth factor 23, and vitamin D in the pathogenesis of mineral and bone disorders in CKD. For decades, they have provided novel insights into the regulation of PTH in health and disease, which helped devise rational therapy for secondary hyperparathyroidism and transformed clinical approach worldwide [82].

## Future Perspectives of Nephrology in Israel

The nephrology community in Israel, led by the ISNH, set major goals to establish screening programs for early identification and treatment of CKD, to implement national quality measures for the treatment of ESRD, and to increase the consent of deceased kidney donors as well as living-related donors and paired-exchange kidney transplantation programs.

In Israel, about half of ESRD patients are treated in hospital centers, and a half in community centers. In principle, the healthier and more independent patients are treated in the community centers. The ISNH has initiated a program to implement national quality measures, with the purpose of unifying the standard of care. These measures include parameters such as Kt/V, hemoglobin, calcium, infection rate, and number of transplant candidates in each unit.

CKD is often clinically silent and traditional clinical data alone cannot differentiate disease subtypes. There is an urgent need to expand medical examination for all young adults including those who are not recruited for army service to detect silent kidney diseases and risk factors. The ISNH is also in the process of establishing a national registry to identify subjects with genetic diseases within the population of young patients with CKD.

An additional quest of the ISNH is to increase the number of ESRD patients treated at home. Currently, less than 10% are using home modalities, mainly PD. We are planning to integrate home HD into the ESRD program and are striving to increase the number of peritoneal dialysis patients by utilizing assisted PD.

Finally, the aging of the population and the exceptional growth in the absolute number of older people with CKD and RRT provide an impetus to develop home and community services, which are viewed as the best economically and humane solutions.

## Conclusion

Israel is a relatively small country, which has kept a high standard of medical care since its establishment. The burden of kidney diseases is high in Israel. Practicing nephrologists are familiar with the genetic background, social habits, and diverse culture of their patients. The emerging epidemic of diabetes mellitus is significant, being the major cause of CKD in Israel. The prevailing genetic kidney diseases in the various population subgroups are also of much importance. All patients reaching ESRD are entitled to receive RRT, which is fully reimbursed. Today, approximately 50% of patients are dialyzed within their community. Early sporadic attempts were made to introduce kidney transplantation, but it was only in the 1990s, with the establishment of the National Transplant Center, that kidney transplantation was conducted on a national level. The enactment of the Transplant and Brain Death laws in 2008 was pivotal in encouraging the acceptance of deceased donor and living donor transplantation, which has led to a continuous growth in both types, and since 2014, the number of candidate transplant recipients has plateaued. Many nephrologists developed an interest in basic and clinical research, conducted within the hospital institutes or in cooperation with researchers from local and international universities.

Despite this success story in clinical care and research, and involvement in the global nephrology community over the past 60 years, there is still much to achieve. First and foremost is to attract young physicians to specialize in nephrology, to provide them with positions, and to encourage them to devote time to high-quality research. Additional needs include (1) addressing issues related to geriatric nephrology and onco-nephrology; (2) expanding both in-center convective dialysis and home dialysis modalities; (3) encouraging organ donation through deceased donors, living-related donors, and paired-exchange kidney transplantation programs; (4) establishing nationwide screening of subpopulations at risk for CKD and genetic screening as well as increasing awareness of the public to endorse a healthy lifestyle and periodic physical examination, among others; and (5) educating our medical colleagues for early referral of kidney patients to dedicated nephrology clinics.

**Acknowledgment** The authors are deeply grateful to Prof. Lital Keinan-Boker and Rita Dichtiar, ICDC, MoH, who provided the ESRD data.

**Conflicts of Interest** The authors declare that they have no conflict of interest.

## References

1. Israel in figures, selected data from the statistical abstract of Israel 2018. Central Bureau of Statistics. Available at: https://www.cbs.gov.il/he/publications/DocLib/isr_in_n/isr_in_n18e.pdf. Accessed 16 Sept 2019.
2. State of Israel, districts, sub-districts and natural regions, The Central Bureau of Statistics Jerusalem, 2005. Available at: https://www.science.co.il/israel/maps/Israel-districts.pdf. Accessed 16 Sept 2019.
3. World Bank: how we classify countries. Available at: http://data.worldbank.org/about/country-classifications. Accessed 16 Sept 2019.
4. World Bank: countries and economies. Available at: https://data.worldbank.org/country/israel. Accessed 16 Sept 2019.
5. Central Bureau of Statistics. Available at: https://www.cbs.gov.il/he/Documents/2018_קובץ_ישובים.xlsx. Accessed 16 Sept 2019.
6. United Nations Development Programme, Human Development reports. Available at: hdr.undp.org/en/countries/profiles/ISR. Accessed 16 Sept 2019.
7. ADI – National Transplant Center, Ministry of Health. Available at: https://www.health.gov.il/Subjects/Organ_transplant/transplant/Pages/default.aspx. Accessed 16 Sept 2019.
8. Clarfield AM, Manor O, Nun GB, Shvarts S, Azzam ZS, Afek A, et al. Health and health care in Israel: an introduction. Lancet. 2017;389(10088):2503–13.
9. Organisation for Economic Co-operation and Development: Health Data. Available at: https://data.oecd.org/healthstat/life-expectancy-at-birth.htm#indicator-chart. Accessed 2 Oct 2019.
10. Dwolatzky T, Brodsky J, Azaiza F, Clarfield AM, Jacobs JM, Litwin H. Coming of age: health-care challenges of an ageing population in Israel. Lancet. 2017;389(10088):2542–50.
11. Rubin L, Belmaker I, Somekh E, Urkin J, Rudolf M, Honovich M, et al. Maternal and child health in Israel: building lives. Lancet. 2017;389(10088):2514–30.
12. Muhsen K, Green MS, Soskolne V, Neumark Y. Inequalities in non-communicable diseases between the major population groups in Israel: achievements and challenges. Lancet. 2017;389(10088):2531–41.
13. Scribner BH, Buri R, Caner JE, Hegstrom R, Burnell JM. The treatment of chronic uremia by means of intermittent hemodialysis: a preliminary report. Trans Am Soc Artif Intern Organs. 1960;6:114–22.

14. Kolff WJ, Berk HT, ter Welle M, van der LA, van Dijk EC, van Noordwijk J. The artificial kidney: a dialyser with a great area. Acta Med Scand. 1944;CXVII:121–34.
15. Steinitz K. A colorimetric method for the determination of inulin in blood, plasma and urine. J Biol Chem. 1938;126:589.
16. Steinitz K, Turkand H. The determination of the glomerular filtration by the endogenous creatinine clearance. J Clin Invest. 1940;19(2):285–98.
17. Levy N. Dr. Kurt Steinitz (1907–1966) and the 60th anniversary of the first hemodialysis in the Middle East. Harefuah. 2010;149(2):108–10, 23.
18. Ullmann TD, Schorr S. Renal dwarfism with hyperparathyroidism in a case of congenital familial malformation of the kidneys. Ann Intern Med. 1948;29(4):715–30.
19. Weston RE, Grossman J, Lehman RA, Ullmann TD, Halperin JP, Leiter L. Renal extraction and excretion of mercury in man following intravenously administered mercurial diuretics. J Clin Invest. 1951;30(11):1221–7.
20. Ullmann TD, Czaczkes WJ, Ben-Ishay D. The use of the artificial kidney in the treatment of acute renal failure. Harefuah. 1962;62:363–8.
21. Brescia MJ, Cimino JE, Appel K, Hurwich BJ. Chronic hemodialysis using venipuncture and a surgically created arteriovenous fistula. N Engl J Med. 1966;275(20):1089–92.
22. Shohat J, Boner G, Rosenfeld J, Waller A, Iaina A, Eliahou HE. Continuous ambulatory peritoneal dialysis- a new dimension in the treatment of end-stage renal disease. Isr J Med Sci. 1982;18(10):1014–8.
23. Hume DM, Merrill JP, Miller BF, Thorn GW. Experiences with renal homotransplantation in the human: report of nine cases. J Clin Invest. 1955;34(2):327–82.
24. Erlik D, Better OS, Shramek A, Richter-Levin D, Hemli JA, Barzilai A. Cadaveric renal transplantation in man: first report from Israel. Isr J Med Sci. 1967;3(1):88–92.
25. Modan B, Boichis H, Bott-Kanner G, Barell V, Bar-Noach N, Eliahou HE. An epidemiologic study of renal failure. I. The need for maintenance hemodialysis. Am J Epidemiol. 1975;101(4):276–80.
26. Boner G, Elster Z. Renal transplantation and dialysis in Israel, 1974–75. Report of the Israel transplantation and dialysis association. Isr J Med Sci. 1977;13(1):65–75.
27. Israeli Center for Disease Control, Ministry of Health – Chronic diseases. Available at: https://www.health.gov.il/English/MinistryUnits/ICDC/Chronic_Diseases/Pages/default.aspx. Accessed 16 Sept 2019.
28. Shema L, Ore L, Geron R, Kristal B. Hospital-acquired acute kidney injury in Israel. Isr Med Assoc J. 2009;11(5):269–74.
29. Levin A, Tonelli M, Bonventre J, Coresh J, Donner J-A, Fogo AB, et al. Global kidney health 2017 and beyond: a roadmap for closing gaps in care, research, and policy. Lancet. 2017;390(10105):1888–917.
30. Nelson RG, Grams ME, Ballew SH, Sang Y, Azizi F, Chadban SJ, et al. Development of risk prediction equations for incident chronic kidney disease. JAMA. 2019;322:2104–14.
31. Shalev SA, Zlotogora J, Shalata A, Levy-Lahad E. Medical genetics in Israel's diverse population. Lancet. 2017;389(10088):2453–5.
32. Assady S, Ramadan R, Frishberg Y. Global considerations in kidney disease: near and Middle East. Brenner and Rector's, the kidney. 11th ed. Philadelphia: Elsevier Inc.; 2019.
33. Zlotogora J. Molecular basis of autosomal recessive diseases among the Palestinian Arabs. Am J Med Genet. 2002;109(3):176–82.
34. Raz AE, Atar M, Rodnay M, Shoham-Vardi I, Carmi R. Between acculturation and ambivalence: knowledge of genetics and attitudes towards genetic testing in a consanguineous bedouin community. Community Genet. 2003;6(2):88–95.
35. Zlotogora J, Shalev SA. Marriage patterns and reproductive decision-making in the inhabitants of a single Muslim village during a 50-year period. Hum Hered. 2014;77(1–4):10–5.
36. Cohen T, Vardi-Saliternik R, Friedlander Y. Consanguinity, intracommunity and intercommunity marriages in a population sample of Israeli Jews. Ann Hum Biol. 2004;31(1):38–48.
37. Israeli Center for Disease Control, Ministry of Health – Registry of severe diseases. Available at: https://www.health.gov.il/English/MinistryUnits/ICDC/disease_Registries/Pages/Registration_Control_diseases.aspx. Accessed 16 Sept 2019.
38. Rosen B, Waitzberg R, Merkur S. Israel: health system review. Health Syst Transit. 2015;17(6):1–212.
39. Renal replacement therapy in Israel, 1990–2007. Israel Ministry of Health and the Israel Society for Nephrology and Hypertension, ICDC Publication No. 324. Jerusalem, Israel, November 2009.
40. Renal replacement therapy in Israel, 1990–2010. Israel Ministry of Health and the Israel Society for Nephrology and Hypertension [ICDC Publication No. 350, December 2012, in Hebrew]. Available at: http://www.isnh.org.il/RRTI1990_2010.pdf. Accessed 21 Feb 2017.
41. Renal replacement therapy in Israel, 1990–2015. Israel Ministry of Health and the Israel Society for Nephrology and Hypertension [ICDC Publication No. 367, January 2018, in Hebrew]. Available at: https://www.health.gov.il/PublicationsFiles/RRT1990_2015.pdf. Accessed 27 May 2018.
42. Sharma SG, Bomback AS, Radhakrishnan J, Herlitz LC, Stokes MB, Markowitz GS, et al. The modern spectrum of renal biopsy findings in patients with diabetes. Clin J Am Soc Nephrol. 2013;8(10):1718–24.
43. Li PK, Chow KM, Van de Luijtgaarden MW, Johnson DW, Jager KJ, Mehrotra R, et al. Changes in the worldwide epidemiology of peritoneal dialysis. Nat Rev Nephrol. 2017;13(2):90–103.
44. Jain AK, Blake P, Cordy P, Garg AX. Global trends in rates of peritoneal dialysis. J Am Soc Nephrol. 2012;23(3):533–44.
45. Quality assurance and service. Ministry of Health. Available at: https://www.health.gov.il/English/Topics/Quality_Assurance/Pages/default.aspx. Accessed 11 Nov 2019.
46. Kamyar KZ, Eliezer G, Tamy S, Elani S, Norris KC, Kopple JD. Survival disparities within American and Israeli dialysis populations: learning from similarities and distinctions across race and ethnicity. Semin Dial. 2010;23(6):586–94.
47. National Transplant Center, Ministry of Health. Available at: https://www.health.gov.il/English/MinistryUnits/HealthDivision/MedicalAdministration/Transplant/Pages/default.aspx. Accessed 2 Oct 2019.
48. Jotkowitz A. Notes on the new Israeli organ donation law-2008. Transplant Proc. 2008;40(10):3297–8.
49. Israel Transplant Law-Organ Transplant Act 2008 (in Hebrew).
50. The Declaration of Istanbul on organ trafficking and transplant tourism. International summit on transplant tourism and organ trafficking. Kidney Int. 2008;74(7):854–9.
51. The declaration of Istanbul on organ trafficking and transplant tourism. Clin J Am Soc Nephrol. 2008;3(5):1227–31.
52. National Insurance Institute of Israel. Available at: https://www.btl.gov.il/English%20Homepage/Insurance/Health%20Insurance/Pages/exempt.aspx. Accessed 2 Oct 2019.
53. Brain-Respiratory Death Act 2008 (Israel). Book of statutes 327 (in Hebrew).
54. Cohen J, Ashkenazi T, Katvan E, Singer P. Brain death determination in Israel: the first two years experience following changes to the brain death law-opportunities and challenges. Am J Transplant. 2012;12(9):2514–8.
55. Wasser WG, Boner G, Koslowsky M, Lazar A. Emergence of an Israel faith-based community organization facilitating live donor kidney transplantation. BMC Nephrol. 2018;19(1):128.

56. Amitai Y, Haklai Z, Tarabeia J, Green MS, Rotem N, Fleisher E, et al. Infant mortality in Israel during 1950–2000: rates, causes, demographic characteristics and trends. Paediatr Perinat Epidemiol. 2005;19(2):145–51.
57. Ku E, Johansen KL, Portale AA, Grimes B, Hsu CY. State level variations in nephrology workforce and timing and incidence of dialysis in the United States among children and adults: a retrospective cohort study. BMC Nephrol. 2015;16:2.
58. Soylemezoglu O, Duzova A, Yalcinkaya F, Arinsoy T, Suleymanlar G. Chronic renal disease in children aged 5–18 years: a population-based survey in Turkey, the CREDIT-C study. Nephrol Dial Transplant. 2012;27(Suppl 3):iii146–51.
59. Landau D, Schreiber R, Kleinman A, Vodonos A, Shalev H. Pediatric chronic kidney disease rates in southern Israel are higher than reported. F1000Res. 2013;2:186.
60. Vivante A, Golan E, Tzur D, Leiba A, Tirosh A, Skorecki K, et al. Body mass index in 1.2 million adolescents and risk for end-stage renal disease. Arch Intern Med. 2012;172(21):1644–50.
61. Vivante A, Afek A, Frenkel-Nir Y, Tzur D, Farfel A, Golan E, et al. Persistent asymptomatic isolated microscopic hematuria in Israeli adolescents and young adults and risk for end-stage renal disease. JAMA. 2011;306(7):729–36.
62. Calderon-Margalit R, Golan E, Twig G, Leiba A, Tzur D, Afek A, et al. History of childhood kidney disease and risk of adult end-stage renal disease. N Engl J Med. 2018;378(5):428–38.
63. Finer G, Shalev H, Landau D. Genetic kidney diseases in the pediatric population of southern Israel. Pediatr Nephrol. 2006;21(7):910–6.
64. Walker RG. Paediatric report. In: Disney APS, editor. The twenty-second report: Australia and New Zealand dialysis and transplant registry. Adelaide: ANZDATA Registry; 1999. p. 90–7.
65. US Renal Data System 2018 Annual Data Report: Epidemiology of Kidney Disease in the United States. Available at: https://www.usrds.org/2018/view/v2_07.aspx?zoom_highlight=pediatric. Accessed 4 Dec 2019.
66. Hart A, Smith JM, Skeans MA, Gustafson SK, Stewart DE, Cherikh WS, et al. OPTN/SRTR 2014 annual data report: kidney. Am J Transplant. 2016;16(Suppl 2):11–46.
67. Harambat J, Ranchin B, Bertholet-Thomas A, Mestrallet G, Bacchetta J, Badet L, et al. Long-term critical issues in pediatric renal transplant recipients: a single-center experience. Transpl Int. 2013;26(2):154–61.
68. Van Arendonk KJ, Boyarsky BJ, Orandi BJ, James NT, Smith JM, Colombani PM, et al. National trends over 25 years in pediatric kidney transplant outcomes. Pediatrics. 2014;133(4):594–601.
69. Holmberg C, Jalanko H. Long-term effects of paediatric kidney transplantation. Nat Rev Nephrol. 2016;12(5):301–11.
70. LaRosa C, Baluarte HJ, Meyers KE. Outcomes in pediatric solid-organ transplantation. Pediatr Transplant. 2011;15(2):128–41.
71. Tangeraas T, Bjerre A, Lien B, Kyte A, Monn E, Cvancarova M, et al. Long-term outcome of pediatric renal transplantation: the Norwegian experience in three eras 1970–2006. Pediatr Transplant. 2008;12(7):762–8.
72. Yamada A, Tashiro A, Hiraiwa T, Komatsu T, Kinukawa T, Ueda N. Long-term outcome of pediatric renal transplantation: a single center study in Japan. Pediatr Transplant. 2014;18(5):453–62.
73. Andreoni KA, Forbes R, Andreoni RM, Phillips G, Stewart H, Ferris M. Age-related kidney transplant outcomes: health disparities amplified in adolescence. JAMA Intern Med. 2013;173(16):1524–32.
74. Patzer RE, Mohan S, Kutner N, McClellan WM, Amaral S. Racial and ethnic disparities in pediatric renal allograft survival in the United States. Kidney Int. 2015;87(3):584–92.
75. Patzer RE, Sayed BA, Kutner N, McClellan WM, Amaral S. Racial and ethnic differences in pediatric access to preemptive kidney transplantation in the United States. Am J Transplant. 2013;13(7):1769–81.
76. Tjaden LA, Noordzij M, van Stralen KJ, Kuehni CE, Raes A, Cornelissen EA, et al. Racial disparities in access to and outcomes of kidney transplantation in children, adolescents, and young adults: results from the ESPN/ERA-EDTA (European Society of Pediatric Nephrology/European Renal Association-European Dialysis and Transplant Association) registry. Am J Kidney Dis. 2016;67(2):293–301.
77. Grace BS, Kara T, Kennedy SE, McDonald SP. Racial disparities in pediatric kidney transplantation in New Zealand. Pediatr Transplant. 2014;18(7):689–97.
78. Rights of the insured under the National Health Insurance Law. Ministry of Health. Available at: https://www.health.gov.il/English/Topics/RightsInsured/RightsUnderLaw/Pages/default.aspx. Accessed 11 Nov 2019.
79. Better OS, Stein JH. Early management of shock and prophylaxis of acute renal failure in traumatic rhabdomyolysis. N Engl J Med. 1990;322(12):825–9.
80. Better OS, Rubinstein I, Reis DN. Muscle crush compartment syndrome: fulminant local edema with threatening systemic effects. Kidney Int. 2003;63(3):1155–7.
81. Sever MS, Vanholder R. Recommendation for the management of crush victims in mass disasters. Nephrol Dial Transplant. 2012;27(Suppl 1):i1–67.
82. Silver J, Naveh-Many T. Phosphate and the parathyroid. Kidney Int. 2009;75(9):898–905.

# Nephrology in Japan

# 25

Ikuto Masakane, Norio Hanafusa, Mariko Miyazaki, Junichi Hoshino, and Hayato Nishida

| | |
|---|---|
| Area | 378,000 Km$^2$ |
| Population[1] | 126,453,000 (2018) |
| Capital | Tokyo |
| Three most populated cities | 1. Tokyo (9,272,740)<br>2. Yokohama (3,724,844)<br>3. Osaka (2,691,185) |
| Official language | Japanese |
| Gross Domestic Product (GDP)[1] | 4.971 trillion USD (2018) |
| GDP per capital[1] | 39,306 USD, 2018 IMF |
| Human Development Index (HDI) | 0.909 (2018) |
| Official currency | Yen |
| Total number of nephrologists | 5317 (JSN board-certified nephrologists, as of 2019)<br>5898 (JSDT board-certified fellows, as of 2019)<br>441 (JSCRT board-certified fellows, as of 2019) |
| National Society of Nephrology | Japanese Society of Nephrology (JSN), Japanese Society for Dialysis Therapy (JSDT), Japanese Society for Clinical Renal Transplantation (JSCRT)<br>www.jsn.or.jp; www.jsdt.or.jp |
| Incidence of End-Stage Renal disease[2] (on dialysis) | 2017 – 323 pmp<br>2018 – 320 pmp |
| Prevalence of End-Stage Renal disease[2] (on dialysis) | 2017 – 2640 pmp<br>2018 – 2687 pmp |
| Total number of patients on dialysis[2] (all modalities) | 2017 – 334,505<br>2018 – 339,841 |
| Number of patients on hemodialysis[2] | 2017 – 325,415<br>2018 – 330,396 |
| Number of patients on peritoneal dialysis[2] | 2017 – 9090<br>2018 – 9445 |
| Number of renal transplantations per year[3,4] | 2017 – 1742<br>2018 – 1865 |

*Table References*

[1]Statistical Bureau, Ministry of Internal Affairs and Communications. https://www.stat.go.jp/english/data/jinsui/tsuki/index.html (04 May 2019 last access)

[2]Annual Dialysis Data Report 2017, JSDT Renal Data Registry [1]

[3]Annual Dialysis Data Report 2017, JSDT Renal Data Registry [2]

[4]Fact book 2018 of organ transplantation in Japan http://www.asas.or.jp/jst/pdf/factbook/factbook2018.pdf (04 May 2019 last access)

I. Masakane (✉)
Department of Nephrology, Yabuki Hospital, Yamagata, Japan
e-mail: imasakan.aipod@seieig.or.jp

N. Hanafusa
Department of Blood Purification, Tokyo Women's Medical University, Tokyo, Japan

M. Miyazaki
Department of Nephrology, Endocrinology, and Vascular Medicine, Tohoku University Graduate School of Medicine, Sendai, Japan

J. Hoshino
Nephrology Center, Toranomon Hospital, Tokyo, Japan

H. Nishida
Department of Urology, Yamagata University Faculty of Medicine, Yamagata, Japan

## Introduction

Japan is located in the east edge of Asia and Japan is totally surrounded by the sea; its western coastline faces the Sea of Japan and its east coastline faces the Atlantic Ocean. Japan is composed of four main islands, Hokkaido, Honshu, Shikoku, and Kyushu, and other numerous islands, which are finally counted down to 6852. Therefore, Japan is completely isolated from the neighboring countries by the sea. The Japanese population has been decreasing with an annual reduction rate of −0.1 ~ 0.2% since 2010; the fixed population was 128,057,352 in 2010 and 126,443,180 in 2018.

The official currency is the yen, introduced in 1871 and symbolized as JPY, In February 2020, JPY 1.00 was worth 0.0091 US dollar and 0.0082 euro. The Japanese gross domestic product (GDP) was 4.972 trillion in 2018, which makes Japan the third largest economy in the world. Japan is one of the matured countries with a population decline and economical shrinkage in the future. Being isolated from the neighboring countries by sea, 98% of Japanese population speaks Japanese, as the official language.


J. A. Moura-Neto et al. (eds.), *Nephrology Worldwide*, https://doi.org/10.1007/978-3-030-56890-0_25

The Japanese political regime is a parliamentary democratic one, ruled by the prime minister with the emperor as a symbol of the state. Japan has 47 prefectures as a local political matrix, but the independency of each prefecture from the nation government is not so strong when compared with the state system or federal system. There are 1741 municipalities, and the 3 most populated are Tokyo, Yokohama, and Osaka. The country is also divided into nine major regions: Hokkaido, Tohoku, Kanto, Chubu, Kansai, Chugoku, Shikoku, and Kyusyu/Okinawa. Although the regions have no political or legislative autonomy, there are some cultural, geographical (climate, vegetation), and economic similarities among the states within each region. The differences in culture and accent actually exist among the regions; however, the diversity is not so accentuated as compared with other mixed-race nations.

Historically, the Yamato race, which was the major ancestor of the Japanese, and other some indigenous races lived in the ancient Japan. In the early history of Japan, there were many local kings or strong men, and they repeatedly fought each other. They were united into one country as the primer of Japan by Toyotomi in 1590, and it was followed by the long and stable Edo era. The current parliamentary democratic political system with one era per emperor started at 1889, when "the Constitution of the Japanese Empire (Meiji Constitution)" was built. Japan is a unique country that has not experienced a major invasion by the neighboring countries because of its unique geographic situation.

The first public medical insurance system was introduced in 1922, but this system only covered company workers. Since 1935, several local systems, which were intended to cover the general population, were introduced and modified. Finally, in 1961 the current national health insurance system in which each Japanese residence must be included into one public health insurance system was established. In the current system, the patient's self-pay rates are 20% for less than 6 years old, 30% for 6 to less than 70 years old, 20% for 70 to less than 75 years old, and 10% for greater than 75 years old. All Japanese people can freely visit any types of medical facilities; however, if they want to visit a university or regional general hospital, they have to contribute a minor additional payment.

## Brief History of Nephrology in Japan

### History of Chronic Kidney Diseases

Richard Bright (1789–1858) is widely regarded as the founder of the nephrology specialty. His name was given to Bright's disease, which was classified as follows: nephrotic syndrome, glomerulonephritis, and sclerosing glomerulonephritis or atrophic kidney [3]. In Japan, the first kidney biopsy was performed by Kinoshita in 1954, and it was the beginning of clinical nephrology based on kidney pathology findings [4]. The Japanese Society of Nephrology (JSN) was established in 1959, earlier than International Society of Nephrology (1960) and American Society of Nephrology (1967), and the official journal entitled *Japanese Journal of Nephrology* was also launched in 1959. In the 1960s, acute nephritis was the most serious problem leading to students' long absence from school, and it evoked the feasibility of an early and routine test for pediatric kidney diseases. In 1974, the mandatory urine test system was established, as first in the world, and thereafter many kidney diseases could be detected in their early stages. The patients who are checked in these opportunities can smoothly receive further examinations including kidney biopsy because of the public health insurance system. Thereby, the mainstreams of the nephrology based on the kidney pathology were established in Japan.

Under these conditions, several kidney diseases classifications were introduced. Ueda et al. [5] proposed a classification of nephrotic syndrome in 1962. Kinoshita et al. [6] also classified kidney disease into nonprogressive sub-chronic glomerulonephritis (GN) and progressive chronic GN according to the clinical course and pathology. Furthermore, they divided glomerular diseases into nephrotic syndrome and GN, and they recommended to use corticosteroids for nephrotic syndrome. In 1968, Oshima et al. [7] revised the classification, and they classified the nephritis with heavy proteinuria and hypoproteinemia into chronic GN. JSN expressed their appreciation to Dr. Ueda and Dr. Oshima for the distinguished contributions to the development of nephrology in Japan, and they created the "Ueda Award" and the "Oshima Award" for encouraging excellent young nephrologists.

Other several unique findings have also been introduced from Japan. Suwa et al. [8] proposed the glomerular sclerosis index for the quantitative evaluation of kidney biopsy in 1968, and the index has been used until now. Renal tubular acidosis secondary to Sjogren's syndrome was reported from Japanese nephrologists in 1970 [9]. Lipoprotein glomerulopathy which is one of the hereditary glomerulopathies with unique features of glomerular lipoprotein thrombi was reported in 1989 [10]. IgG4-related tubulointerstitial nephritis was first reported by Saeki et al. [11] in 2010, and the diagnostic criteria for IgG4-related kidney disease were published in 2011. One more recent contribution from Japan was the creation of an accurate glomerular filtration rate (GFR) estimation formula for the Asian population [12]. Three hundred and fifty participants from 80 medical centers in Japan participated in the trial to validate the estimated GFR based on creatinine and inulin in 2009; the elements composing the formula were serum creatinine, age, and gender [12].

The prevalence of ESRD on dialysis and KT have been surveyed by the JSDT Registry and the Japanese Society for Clinical Renal Transplantation (JSCRT); however, a nationwide CKD registry has not yet been established. The prevalence of overall CKD in the adult Japanese population has been estimated as 11%, out of 574,000 people participating in the annual health checkup program [13]. In order to outline CKD population in Japan, several registries have been started, such as the Japan Renal Biopsy Registry (J-RBR) in 2007 and the Japan Kidney Disease Registry (J-KDR) in 2009, both established by JSN [14]. However, these registries were not enough to grasp the overall features of CKD in Japan, so it is necessary to conduct a nationwide CKD epidemiological surveillance.

In 2018, the government released the next 10-year plan to prevent and manage CKD. The first topic of it was education about CKD for the general population, CKD prevention, early CKD diagnosis, appropriate intervention, and renal replacement therapy (RRT). To achieve these goals, JSN released the CKD guidelines for general practitioners (GPs) and general population [15]. The second topic was the cooperation between GPs and nephrologists. The third topic was promoting research activities in the genetic field, regenerative medicine, developing new drugs, and megadata-based medicine. These nationwide approaches are expected to clarify the outline of CKD in Japan and improve its outcome in the future.

## Dialysis History

The history of dialysis therapy was reviewed at the time of the JSDT 50th anniversary in 2018 and the memorial book published in 2019 [16]. The following brief history of dialysis therapy in Japan is an excerpt of the book.

The first dialysis therapy performed in Japan dates back to the Korean War. The soldiers who suffered from crush syndrome were transferred to the Army base in Kyushu or the Army hospital in Tokyo, where they could receive hemodialysis (HD) with use of Kolff-Brigham dialyzer. The Kolff-Brigham dialyzer was then introduced to Kyushu University. However, the dialyzers imported were expensive, and studies researching the production of original types of dialyzers began in this era. These studies were publicized in 1954–1957 by the investigators at the Departments of Surgery at the University of Tokyo and Gunma University. Thereafter, the economic development of Japan enabled the import of dialyzers, which were mass-produced and commercially available in oversea countries. Such a trend promoted the wider use of HD treatment for CKD stage 5.

The first chronic HD treatment program was initiated in 1963. First home HD was performed in 1964, and overnight HD performed in 1965. At the beginning of HD history, imported dialyzers were used. However, the first dialyzer was produced domestically in 1965. In 1967, CKD stage 5 therapy began to be reimbursed by the public health insurance system, and then the number of CKD patients started expanding. HD machines production manufacturing domestically was initiated in 1969. Although HD became widely available, the prognosis was poor, and the average survival only 2.5 years in 1968. The HD cost, which the patients payed from their pocket, started being covered by the government as a form of the Services and Supports for Persons with Disabilities in 1972. Since then, the medical cost for dialysis treatment has been covered by the government.

The first hollow-fiber dialyzer was produced in 1971, and they started being produced domestically in 1972. Together with that, the cellulose membrane was gradually replaced by the synthetic membrane materials. The ultrafiltration (UF) mechanism was further improved, and automated UF controller developed in 1983, and the safety management levels have been improved much.

The first dialysis fluid, bicarbonate-containing dialysate, was on the market in 1967, whereas the acetate-containing dialysis fluid was introduced in 1969 and widely used until the 1980s when acetate intolerance was recognized, and the bicarbonate dialysis fluid resumed to be used. At the same time, the dialysis fluid production system was also improved with reverse osmosis water purification, and centralized dialysis fluid delivery system (CDDS) [17] implemented. The standard for dialysis fluid quality was established by JSDT in 1995 [18]. The current biological and chemical contamination of dialysis fluid guideline was published by JSDT in 2016 [19]; the efforts to improve the quality of dialysis fluid have been a continuous undertaking.

Hemodiafiltration (HDF) treatment was proven to enhance the removal of middle molecular uremic toxins. Online HDF in Japan was started around 1995 when the treatment was not approved officially by the government. However, the machines which can perform online HDF were approved in 2010 and the online HDF itself also approved, started being reimbursed in 2012. After that, the numbers of the patients receiving this therapy have dramatically increased. Moreover, intermittent infusion HDF (IHDF) was firstly reported in 2007 [20, 21], and the JSDT guideline determined the IHDF requirements in 2013 [22]. Since then, this modality has also become popular. As of 2017, a total of 70,604 and 17,105 patients are receiving online HDF and IHDF, respectively, among a total of 334,505 HD patients [2].

The surgeons at Nagasaki University started continuous PD (CPD) for acute kidney injury (AKI) in 1959, and PD started being performed for CKD patients in 1963 because the modality did not require expensive dialyzers or machines.

However, the modality presented several problems such as the difficulty during procedures, low uremic toxins removal rates, and catheter-related complications. After that, PD began to be reimbursed in 1982. The PD patients increased at first, but the number of 9858 PD patients in 2009 turned into decline just after the report of a serious PD complication, namely, encapsulating peritoneal sclerosis (EPS) [23]. In the last couple of years, the number of PD patients started augmenting again, as biocompatible PD solutions and icodextrin were launched in Japan in the early 2000s and the incentives for PD established in 2018.

The Society of Internal Organs was established in 1957, and it has developed into JSAIO. The first meeting regarding dialysis therapy was held in 1968 named as Society for Artificial Kidney; the society evolved into JSDT. *Therapeutic Apheresis and Dialysis* (TAD) has become the official journal of JSDT in 2003, and another English official journal of RRT was also commenced in 2015. JSDT has published as many as 22 guidelines regarding the clinical practice of dialysis therapy since 2004, when the first version of anemia guideline was published. Most of them were translated into English and published either in TAD or RRT [24]. Notably, JSDT implemented the renal data registry for dialysis patient in 1968; at first, the registry system only covered a facility survey. Individualized patient data collection was initiated in 1983; and since then, the same structure of the registry has been maintained. The individual data had been interlinked to each year from 2001 to the present, and over 950,000 individual data were stored in the JRDR data at the end of 2018.

Clinical engineer, as the professional in charge of dialysis therapy from the perspective of technology, was approved by the Japanese government in 1987. These professionals have played a tremendous role in the development and improvement of dialysis therapy. Several academic societies are run by them and the scope has been widened outside of dialysis therapy.

## Kidney Transplantation History

The first KT in Japan, autotransplantation of dogs, was reported by Yamauchi [25] at the congress of the Japan Surgery Society in 1910. The first human KT was performed in 1956 by Kusunoki et al. [26, 27]. The recipient was a 30-year-old man who attempted to commit suicide by bichloride mercury intoxication and developed AKI. A graft kidney was removed from a 56-year-old man due to severe idiopathic renal bleeding and was transplanted into the left femoral space of the patient. About 50–200 mL urine output per day from the transplanted kidney was observed; however, the grafted kidney was removed 4 days after transplantation because bleeding from the wound was getting worse and urine output from the native kidneys increasing, which indicated recovery from AKI. First cases of cadaveric KT in Japan were reported by Shikata et al. in 1964 [28].

The first KT for an ESRD patient in Japan was performed by Takahashi et al. [27] in 1964, and it was also the first KT in Japan, in which azathioprine (AZP) was administered as immunosuppressive medicine. The transplant surgery was successfully finished; however, transplanted kidney did not function due to renal artery occlusion so the recipient died 9 days after surgery. Even though this first living KT in Japan failed, the number of institutions starting KT as well as clinical KT cases was gradually increasing, and a few cases of long-term survival were reported after AZP appearance in the late 1960s. The Japanese Society for Transplantation was established in 1965, and the predecessor of the Japanese Society for Clinical Renal Transplantation in 1969 with the aim of discussing limited KT cases to improve KT outcomes. As in the rest of the world, the appearance of ciclosporin dramatically improved the short-term graft survival in Japan as well [29]. At the same time, mizoribine, which is an antiproliferative agent with less hepatotoxicity and bone marrow suppression compared to AZP, was developed in Japan and was approved for clinical use in 1984 [30, 31]. Tacrolimus, which has been used worldwide as one of the most important immunosuppressants in KT, was discovered as a substance produced from one of actinomycetes identified from the soil at the foot of Mt. Tsukuba at Ibaraki Prefecture in Japan in 1987. Ochiai et al. [32] demonstrated that tacrolimus had powerful immunosuppressive effect, and it was approved as an immunosuppressant in KT in 1996, after clinical evaluation of its immunosuppressive effect on KT [33].

Even though the Japanese first law of cadaveric kidney and cornea donation was enacted, cadaveric organ donation did not increase. To compensate for the lack of organ donation, two methods were taken into practice in Japan. One was ABO-incompatible living transplantation to expand the indication for living kidney donor transplantation. The first ABO-incompatible living kidney transplantation was successfully performed with the use of double filtration plasmapheresis (DFPP) combined with immunoadsorption for pretransplant removal of anti-ABO blood type antibodies and splenectomy at the time of transplantation [34]. ABO-incompatible KT has been performed continuously, and it accounts for about 30% of living kidney transplantation nowadays [35]. The other taken practice was shipped kidney for transplantation from the USA to Japan [36]. In May 1981, Terasaki initiated the sending of kidneys from the USA to Japan for the purpose of trying to change the negative attitude of Japanese citizens toward the postmortem donation of their organs. About 160 kidneys were sent to 10 centers throughout Japan during the following 2 years.

The number of KT in Japan has gradually increased with the progress that has evolved in the clinical aspects; conversely, organ donation from cadaveric donor has not increased [35]. The organ transplant law was enacted in 1997, which paved the way for heart, lung, liver, kidney, pancreas, and small intestine transplants from heart-beating donors; however, the number of organ donations from heart-beating donor did not increase because heart-beating organ donation was only possible if the patients had expressed in writing in advance their willingness to donate their organs and their family members approved the organ donations [37]. The organ transplant law was revised in 2010, which has made it possible to procure organs from heart-beating donors who had not expressed their readiness to donate. Cadaveric KT from heart-beating donors has gradually increased; however, the total number of cadaveric kidney transplantations still remains low due to decline in organ donation from non-heart-beating donors [35].

## Kidney Diseases in Japan

### Outline of CKD in Japan

The definition of CKD was proposed in 2002 when the rapid increase of dialysis patients became a serious problem worldwide [38]. CKD patients have a higher risk of developing cardiovascular diseases (CVD), and it accelerates the mortality risk for ESRD patients. The diagnosis and evaluation can be simply defined by proteinuria and eGFR, which is calculated based on serum creatinine, gender, and age [12]. The JSN scientific committee published and updated the CKD guidelines, targeting both nephrologists and GPs [15]. The prevalence of CKD patients in Japan was estimated by Imai et al. [13], and the results shown in this study had a great impact for the promotion of CKD prevention. The prevalence of CKD stages 3–5, defined as an eGFR of less than 60 ml/min per 1.73 $m^2$, was 13% of the Japanese adult population – approximately 13.3 million people were predicted to have CKD. The prevalence of CKD stage 3 was 10.5%, much higher than that of the USA at 4.5% [39].

In Japan, lifelong health checkup systems and the public health insurance system have been well established, so many CKD patients, who are usually asymptomatic, are found and sent to further examinations. The frequency of CKD in Japanese general population was evaluated in a famous Japanese cohort study named as the "Hisayama study" [40]. They reported that the prevalence of CKD increased significantly in men, but not in women over the last three decades in a general Japanese population as follows: 13.8% (1974), 15.9% (1988), and 22.1% (2002) in men and 14.3% (1974), 12.6% (1988), and 15.3% (2002) in women. CKD stages 3–5 increased over the three decades in both genders.

The risk of CVD in Japanese CKD patients was evaluated by the Gonryo study [41] and the CKD Japan Cohort Study (CKD-JAC) [42]. The risk of CVD depends on the underlying disease: diabetic nephropathy and hypertensive nephrosclerosis showed more unfavorable outcome than primary glomerular disease [41]. On the contrary, the risk of cardiovascular events increased as the eGFR decreased, with a significant difference only between CKD stage 5 and CKD stage 3a with the hazard ratio of 3.16 and 95% confidence interval of 1.28–7.76 [42].

### Primary Glomerular Diseases

The Japan Renal Biopsy Registry (J-RBR) was established to evaluate the CKD primary diseases, collecting data of clinical and pathological findings since 2007. The first report from J-RBR showed that the indications for a kidney biopsy were different among countries; it was performed based on wider indications in Japan than those in the USA or other countries. In this paper, the primary diseases of 2427 CKD patients were clarified by a kidney biopsy. The most frequent primary disease was IgA GN as 29.1%, the second vasculitis syndrome 9.9%, and the third membranous nephropathy 7.6% [14, 43] (Fig. 25.1). The proportion of diabetic nephropathy was just 4.8% because the patients with a typical clinical course of diabetic nephropathy were not usually indicated for a kidney biopsy in Japan.

### Diabetic Kidney Disease

As previously addressed, diabetic nephropathy has been the leading cause of the incident dialysis patients since 1998 and of the prevalent dialysis patients since 2011. Recently, the concept of diabetic kidney disease (DKD) has been proposed to clarify the diversity of the progression of CKD in patients with diabetes. "Diabetic nephropathy" has been usually used for CKD with a classic clinical course of massive proteinuria, retinopathy, and hypertension. However, we occasionally encountered many types of diabetic CKD patients without the above classic manifestations. In Japan, the relationship between the pathological findings of the kidney, clinical manifestations, and outcome are evaluated. Non-proteinuric DKD patients had better control of blood pressure and didn't have the typical morphological changes. The risk of CKD progression and all-cause mortality were lower in non-proteinuric DKD [44]. Histological differences of the vascular damages and the risk of CVD between DKD and nephrosclerosis analysis have been well evaluated in Japan [45, 46].

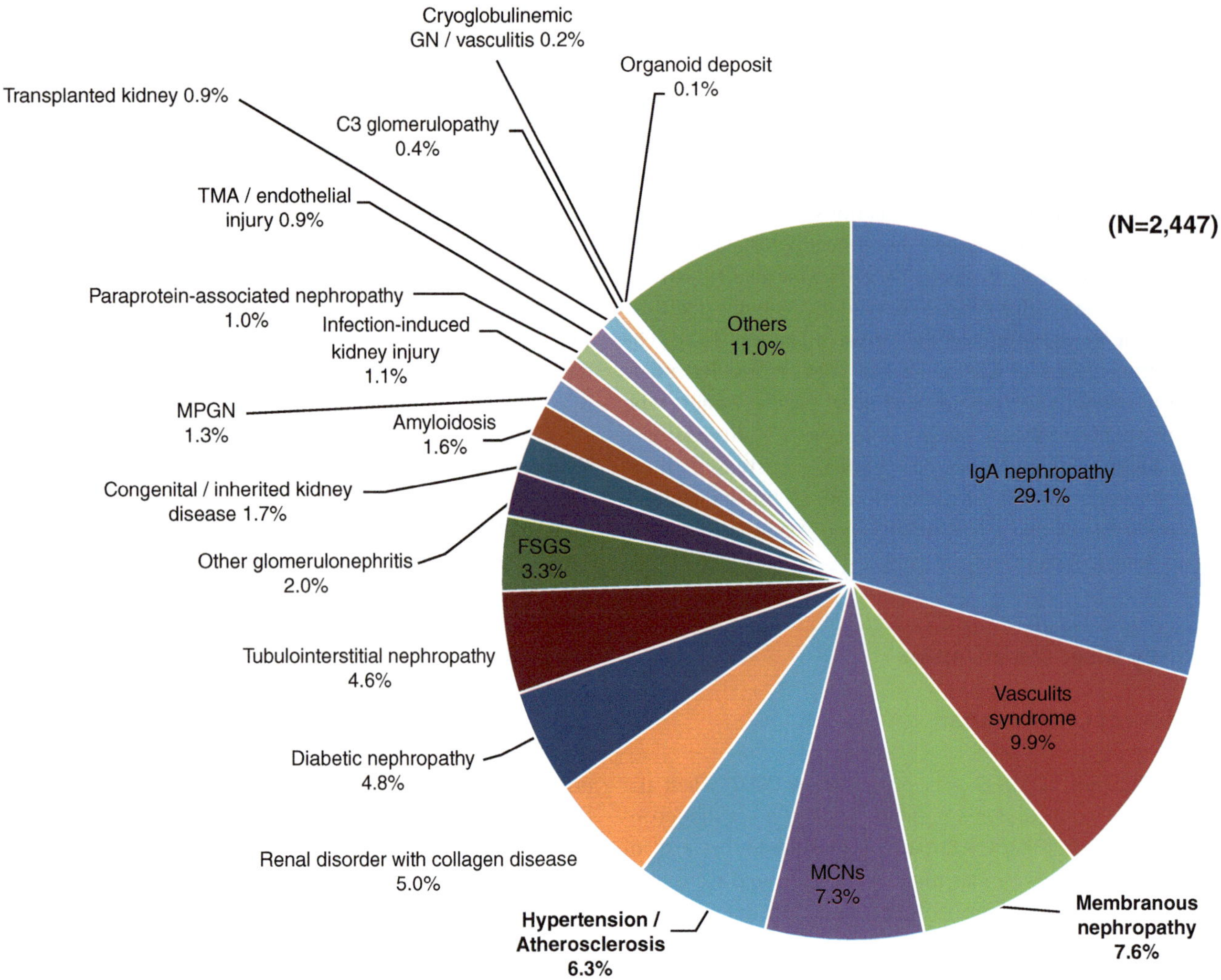


**Fig. 25.1** Final diagnosis by a kidney biopsy. Committee for Standardization of Renal Pathological Diagnosis and Committee for Kidney Disease Registry, Japanese Society of Nephrology, Japan renal biopsy registry and Japan kidney disease registry: committee report for 2018 [43]. https://cdn.jsn.or.jp/news/190625_kp.pdf

Various medicines have been used for DKD and comorbidities to prevent the progression of CKD. RAS inhibitors are now essential for CKD management as Taguma et al. [47] reported that captopril was effective to reduce proteinuria in advanced DKD patients. SGL2 inhibitors have been also used for DKD not only to control the blood glucose but also to preserve the residual kidney function (RRF) and protect CKD events. Statins and non-purine-type xanthine oxidase inhibitors, which were originally discovered in Japan [48, 49], were widely used to treat the comorbidities in DKD as well as CKD. These drugs have been expected to reduce proteinuria and preserve RRF.

## Other Kidney Diseases

Polycystic kidney disease (PCKD) is the fourth most frequent cause of ESRD with a prevalence of 3.6% and an incidence of 2.5% PCKD patients newly started dialysis during 2016 according to the 2018 JSDT registry report [2, 50]. Vasopressin 2 antagonist, tolvaptan, was officially approved by the government to prevent the enlargement of the kidneys and the decline of kidney function for PCKD patients in 2014. The payments are almost fully covered by the public health insurance system for the patients with intractable diseases.

Fabry disease is one of the hereditary enzyme deficiency diseases, "lysosome disease" in which multi-organs such as the kidney, heart, and neural system are affected. Enzyme (recombinant human alpha-galactosidase A, r-alphaGalA) replacement therapy was approved by the government in 2004. Now two types of r-alphaGalA are available, agalsidase alfa and agalsidase beta. The payments are also covered by the same insurance system as PCKD.

Drug-induced kidney disease or polypharmacy is another difficult issue, especially in elderly people with normal kidney function as well as with CKD. As previously addressed, people in Japan can freely have access to any type of medical facilities and are fully covered by the public insurance system. The self-payments are cheaper for elderly patients than young patients as previously addressed in the "Introduction," so the risks of polypharmacy and drug-induced kidney disease are higher in elderly. There have been many attempts, in collaboration among doctors, pharmacists, visiting nurses, and social workers, to prevent CKD patients from drug adverse effects and polypharmacy.

## Action Plan Against CKD

In 2008, the Japanese government took actions against CKD in order to inhibit an increase of ESRD patients. These actions partially succeeded after 10 years as the age-specific incidence of ESRD decreased in the 74-year-old or younger population [51]. However, the total number of incident dialysis patients is still increasing, and new actions are being taken against lifestyle-related diseases since 2018. The main purpose of these actions is to inhibit the progression of DKD, by organizing the local collaboration among nephrologists, diabetologists, GPs, and other healthcare providers. The goal of our efforts for the next 10 years is to reduce the incidence of ESRD by 15%, from 40,000 to 35,000 by 2028.

## Renal Replacement Therapy in Japan

### Overview of Chronic Dialysis

The annual dialysis JSDT data report is the most accurate information overviewing the present status of chronic dialysis therapy in Japan. The annual JSDT data collection has been performed since 1968, and the JSDT Renal Data Registry (JRDR) has more than 900,000 dialysis patients' cohort data. However, JSDT has been collecting only data of chronic dialysis patients, but not of patients treated with KT. RRT medical costs for HD or HDF, PD, and KT have been reimbursed by the governments. The average costs are around 40,000–50,000 US dollars for in-center HD, 50,000–55,000 HDF, 45,000–50,000 PD, and 45,000–50,000 HHD per year. For KT it is 65,000–85,000 in the first year and 13,000–17,000 in the following years. The patient has to pay 0/2500/5000/10,000/20,000 JPY (0/23/46/92/184 USD) per month, according to their incomes. Dialyzer or bloodlines reuse is not permitted neither in in-center HD nor HHD in Japan. There are no RRT first-treatment policies in Japan, so patients and doctors can freely choose any type of RRT, if no contraindications.

At the end of 2018, there were 339,841 chronic dialysis patients in 4402 dialysis facilities in Japan [2]. The majority of the dialysis facilities (78%) are private hospitals and dialysis clinics, and 85% of all dialysis patients are treated in private dialysis facilities. Nephrologist, nurse, clinical engineer who has a national license for the specialist of medical devices, dietitian, and social worker are generally involved in dialysis care in the Japanese dialysis facilities. There are few rules to regulate the allocation of medical staffs including doctors, but the director of a dialysis facility must be one. Moreover, at least one doctor must be present at the dialysis facility when the dialysis treatment is being performed. The average number of dialysis staffs are two nurses or clinical engineers for each ten dialysis patients. Even if a doctor were not nephrologist, the doctor could open a dialysis clinic. A clinical engineer, a unique-to-Japan dialysis career within the national license system, is a specialist for medical devices and dialysis care. In Japan most of dialysis facilities used centralized dialysis fluid delivery system (CDDS), in which dialysis fluid is prepared at the central dialysis fluid delivering machine and delivered to bedside dialysis consoles. One CDDS can use only one type of dialysis fluid so the patients who are treated under one CDDS are treated by the same dialysis fluid composition.

The dialysis population in Japan has been getting older, as the average age of the incident dialysis patients in 2018 was 69.3 years for male, 71.6 years for female, and 70.0 in total. On the other hand, the average age of the prevalent dialysis patients in 2018 was 68.0 years for male, 70.3 years for female, and 68.8 in total. 65.4% of the prevalent dialysis patients were males. The average dialysis vintage was 6.8 years for males and 8.3 years for females, and the longest dialysis vintage was 50 years and 4 months. The annual crude death rate was 10.0% in 2018, and it has hovered between 9% and 10% since 1983 [2].

The incident dialysis patients CKD primary diseases distribution are as follows: diabetes at 42.5%, chronic GN 16.3%, nephrosclerosis 14.7%, and unknown cause 13.2%. Diabetes has been the most common primary disease in the incident dialysis patient group since 1998 [2]. The prevalent dialysis patients CKD primary diseases distribution are as follows: diabetes 39.0%, chronic GN 27.8%, nephrosclerosis 10.8%, and unknown cause 10.2%. Diabetes has been the most common primary disease in the prevalent dialysis patient group since 2011 [2].

Of all dialysis patients, 324,731 (97.1%) are treated by in-center HD/HDF, 684 (0.2%) patients on home hemodialysis (HHD), and 9090 (2.7%) patients on PD. Japan has one of the lowest home dialysis (HHD and PD) prevalence among all countries with home dialysis [52].

### In-Center Hemodialysis/Hemodiafiltration (HD/HDF)

As previously addressed, 97.1% of all dialysis patients are treated by in-center HD or HDF. HDF, especially of online HDF, has been prescribed in 37% of all in-center dialysis patients [2]. The standard in-center HD/HDF program is three times per week and 4–5 hours each session. More than 85% of all dialysis patients were treated under this program in 2017. The average dialysis time was 239 minutes in HD and 243 minutes in HDF. The average blood flow rate was

206 ml/min in HD and 224 ml/min in HDF. The average blood flow rate in Japan has been rather lower than in other parts of the world. The dialysis fluid flow rate is usually 500 ml/min.

Online HDF is a rapid emerging modality, which is aimed to remove low molecular weight proteins (LMWPs) efficiently, ameliorate the dialysis-related symptoms, and improve the survival of dialysis patients [53]. Online HDF got reimbursed by the government in 2010; and an additional payment of 500 JPY (4.5 US dollars) for each online HDF and IHDF session was introduced in 2012. After that, the number of dialysis patients treated with all types of HDF has rapidly increased up to 37% of all in-center HD/HDF patients by the end of 2018 [2]. The patients treated with online HDF in 2018 were 70.9% of all HDF patients, 26.0% of the patients treated with IHDF, and 3.1% of the patients treated with the conventional HDF [2]. Online HDF is generally performed by postdilution throughout the world, but in Japan it has been performed mostly by predilution in greater than 90% of all patients treated with online HDF [2]. The reason for that is closely related to the Japanese dialysis concept, which will be described later here, entitled as "Japanese Dialysis Concept."

There have been developed various membrane materials for dialysis, polysulfone (PS) being the most frequently used in the world. There are several unique membrane materials made in Japan, which have been available, such as polymethylmethacrylate (PMMA), polyether polymer alloy (PEPA), and polyether sulfone (PES). These membranes have unique properties as protein adsorption, high protein permeability, and better biocompatibility compared with previous membrane materials. In the 2017 JSDT registry, the distributions of dialysis membrane materials in HD were 56.5% PS, 16.4% PES, 15.6% cellulose triacetate (CTA), 4.1% PMMA, and 3.1% PEPA [2]. Abe et al. [54] reported that PMMA and PES had beneficial effects on patient survival using JRDR data.

### Home Hemodialysis (HHD)

HHD in Japan started in 1968 and it got reimbursed by the government in 1998. The number of the patients treated with HHD has been slowly increasing up to 720 patients at the end of 2018 [2]. The average age of the HHD patients was 55.2 years old, and they were 13 years younger than those in-center dialysis patients in the 2016 JSDT data [50]. Globally speaking, there are two major HHD programs: nocturnal HHD (NHD) and short daily HHD (SDHD). However, the frequently performed HHD program in Japan differs from them as they are performed 4–6 times per week and during 3–5 hours. The special dialysis machines for HHD have not been approved by the government, so the same individual dialysis machines as used in in-center dialysis have been generally used.

### Peritoneal Dialysis (PD)

PD in Japan started in 1963 and got reimbursed in 1982. The number of PD patients steeply increased until 1996, when the serious PD complication, encapsulating peritoneal sclerosis (EPS), became well known [23]. After the number of PD patients reaching a peak at 9858 in 2009, the number gradually decreased to 9090 patients in 2017 at the lowest. In 2018, with the additional reimbursement for proper introduction of PD and KT to the patient, the number of PD patients increased to 9445. The average age of PD patients is 63.8 years, 5 years younger than that of all dialysis patients. The average time on PD therapy is 3.1 years, and the patient distribution with long PD period greater than 8 years was only 7.1% [2].

The most unique point of the Japanese PD program is the combination therapy or hybrid therapy with in-center HD. Out of 9445 PD patients, a total of 1863 (19.7%) patients were under the combination therapy in 2018 with 1505 (16.6%) of them being treated with 1 HD session weekly [2]. Icodextrin solution was used in 54.4% of all PD patients, and the APD machine was used in 41.7% of the patients. 72.5% of the PD patients used aseptic PD bag connecting system by UV irradiation or heat sterilization.

## Acute Kidney Injury

There are no national registries of acute kidney injury (AKI) in Japan. Japanese Society for Blood Purification in Critical Care started collecting AKI data in 2019, but the results of the survey have not yet been published. Generally, AKI develops as a part of multi-organ failure after surgeries, sepsis, or other systemic diseases. Continuous renal replacement therapy (CRRT) such as continuous hemodiafiltration (CHDF) is usually performed for AKI mainly in an intensive care unit. The substitution fluid is conventional bottle type one, and online HDF is not usually performed for AKI. In cases of septic AKI by Gram-negative rods, endotoxin adsorbent column is occasionally used. In the case of acute hepatic failure, plasma exchange is generally performed as aimed for supplementing coagulation factors, and CHDF aimed for improving the conscious level. In several institutions, online HDF with large substitution volumes is prescribed in order to try improving the conscious level.

## Kidney Transplantation

The number of total kidney transplantations has gradually increased annually [35]. The total of 1742 in 2017 was the largest number of kidney transplantations performed in Japan; however, the number was much smaller than that of patients introduced to dialysis therapy. While cadaveric donation kidney transplantation is the mainstream in the world, in Japan it has not increased, and living donation kidney transplantation accounts for the majority. Organ donation from heart-beating donor is increasing little by little after revision of the Japanese law related to organ donation in 2010; on the other hand, donation from non-heart-beating donor, which had been majority until 2012, has gradually decreased. As a result, the total number of cadaveric kidney transplantations was limited to 198 cases in 2017. The duration of the waiting list period for about 12,000 candidates who have registered with Japan Organ Transplant Network has reached an average of 15 years. The main obstacle of organ donation in Japan is not the unique way of thinking, such as cannibalizing of one's own body or the body of a loved one. The option to donate organs from brain-dead patient is not regulated by the law in Japan and depends on the decision of the physicians in charge. Organ procurement organization, which plays an important role in organ donation, has not been established yet, and lots of institutions which were designated by the MoH to be qualified to participate in the organ donation program have not been prepared for organ donation. To increase organ donation in Japan, it is necessary to resolve these structural obstacles by both medical and political aspects.

In order to compensate such lack of cadaveric organ donation, ABO blood type-incompatible living-donated kidney transplantation has been established as a conventional treatment in Japan [37]. The number of kidney transplantations for this category has increased and reached 300 in 2010, which was about 20% of all cases of kidney transplantations in Japan, continuing to increase to more than 300 cases since then. Splenectomy was once considered essential to avoid antibody-mediated rejection in ABO-incompatible kidney transplantation. The efficacy and safety of desensitization protocol which includes induction therapy of low-dose rituximab has been well established, and patients and graft outcomes of ABO-incompatible KT are now comparable those of ABO-compatible kidney transplantations [55, 56].

Even though the rate of diabetes and elderly candidates have increased, patient and graft survival have gradually improved. Five-year patient survival from 2010 to 2016 was 97.1% in living donor transplantation and 93.1% in cadaveric donor transplantation, whereas the earlier results for the period 1983 to 2000 were 93.5% in living donor transplantation and 85.5% in cadaveric donor transplantation. Five-year graft survival from 2010 to 2016 was 94.3% in living donor transplantation and 88% in cadaveric donor transplantation, whereas the earlier results for the period 1983–2000 were 82.0% in living donor kidney transplantation and 64.8% in cadaveric donor kidney transplantation. Not only improvements of diagnosis and treatment for rejection, infectious diseases, and cardiovascular diseases but also increase of the number of preemptive living kidney transplantations (PEKT) have contributed to the improvement of kidney transplantation outcomes in Japan. A Japanese single-center cohort study showed that the rate of clinical events consisting of death with functioning graft, graft loss, and cardiovascular events was lower in PEKT patients than that in non-PEKT patients, even though long-term outcomes of HD patients in Japan are thought to be excellent [57, 58].

The number of living donor kidney transplantations has increased yearly in Japan. Both PEKT and the increasing number and improvement of outcomes of ABO-incompatible kidney transplantation have contributed to that. However, the number of cadaveric donor kidney transplantations is still very small, leading to the persistent need for further efforts to increase deceased donation in Japan.

## Nephrology Practice in Japan

### Medical Systems in Japan

The three most important features of the Japanese medical service are the health insurance system, easy access to facilities, and enhanced medical access to medical devices. In accordance with the Japanese government policy, all Japanese citizens are covered by the public health insurance system. Therefore, most clinical practices in nephrology, including dialysis care and kidney transplantation, are insured by government regulation. Patients with ESRD (Ccr $<$ 10 mL/min or serum creatinine $\geq$8.0 mg/dL) are categorized as "first class of physical disability," whose medical expenses related to kidney diseases are paid by the government. Dialysis patients in Japan are entitled to receive dialysis therapy forever, regardless of their income. In addition, CKD patients with some "intractable diseases" as defined by the Japanese government have all medical expenses fully paid by the government. Although the criteria for "intractable diseases" are complex, this system may ensure better survival for these patients, as effective drugs for these diseases are often expensive, such as tolvaptan for PCKD, immunosuppressants for SLE, and immunosuppressants for vasculitis. Moreover, there is a High-Cost Medical Expense Benefit system in Japan that sets a ceiling of payment according to patients' income. In this system if the patient has paid more than the limit of monthly payment, the patient could be refunded the additional payment over the limit [59].

The second important feature is the "free-access policy." Patients can choose any type of hospital or clinic with almost the same co-payment. University hospitals and general hospitals are always crowded because most of the CKD patients are elderly, with systemic complications, and desiring to be seen by different specialists in one institution. This free-access policy is the same in emergency medicine.

The third important feature in Japanese clinical practice is enhanced access to medical devices including computed tomography (CT) and/or magnetic resonance imaging (MRI), not only in large hospitals but also in some small clinics. This contributes to quick and accurate diagnosis of kidney diseases.

Although medical systems are universally available in Japan, these services are less accessible in some rural areas. These regional gaps can be observed not only in medical services but also in many other social services in Japan. With the increase in the elderly population in Japan, the amount of overall medical costs for kidney diseases has also been increasing every year, reaching about 1.5 trillion yens (14 billion US dollars) in 2014, corresponding to 3.75% of the total national healthcare costs. More than 80% of medical expenses are used for patients aged 65 or more, who are likely to have more critical and multiple complications.

## CKD Clinical Practice by Doctors and Medical Specialists

Many facilities provide CKD educational programs for renal patients, by multidisciplinary clinical teams of doctors, nurses, and dietitians; many of them also have additional educational programs for advanced CKD patients, mainly focusing on the choice of RRT as well as preservation of the remaining kidney function. These programs can be done in both outpatient services and during hospitalization. For medical specialists, the Japanese Society of Nephrology recently started a certified CKD educator program to encourage multidisciplinary CKD care and improve the quality of care [60].

## Nephrologists in Japan

If patients are hospitalized, it is usual to be treated by the same attending physician at the outpatient service. The main nephrology tasks for hospitalized patients are diverse, including internal medical care, kidney biopsy, vascular access (VA) surgery, VA angioplasty, VA catheter insertion, PD catheter insertion, and treatment of dialysis-related complications. Specialist consultation to other departments is also among the primary nephrology tasks in the hospitals. Kidney transplantation is usually performed by transplant surgeons and/or urology specialists. Nephrologists may sometimes care for patients after kidney transplantation, depending on the hospital. There are several certifications in nephrology, dialysis, and transplantation from each of the different academic societies. The pre-requirements for the nephrology board-certified examination in Japan are as follows: (a) those having Japanese medical license and those having board certified from the Japanese Society of Internal Medicine, the Japan Pediatric Society, the Japanese Surgical Society, or the Japanese Urological Association for certain years, (b) those working under the nephrologist training program more than 3 years at certified facilities, and (c) those being a member of the Japanese Society of Nephrology for more than 3 years. Usually, doctors need to work for long hours. They may receive a call from hospitals during the night and holidays when a patient's condition changed. The salary of nephrologists and other medical specialists are widely distributed, which totally depends on the institution's policy. The expected annual salary of doctors is approximately 15 million yen (136,000 US dollars); that of nurses is approximately 5 million yen (45,000 US dollars) in general. However, a rural doctor's salary is higher than for those working in large cosmopolitan hospitals, as the demand for doctors and medical staffs in rural areas is higher due to scarcity. However, both are considered as an above-average salary profession as well.

# Highlights of Nephrology in Japan

## Intensive Therapy of IgA Nephropathy

IgA nephropathy (IgAN) is one of the most common primary GN worldwide, especially in Asian countries. In the early stage of IgAN, recurrent benign hematuria is a major manifestation; however, the prognosis of IgAN is not benign. In the next stage of the disease, persistent proteinuria and hypertension worsen renal function, and finally 30–40% of the patients with IgAN end up with ESRD after 20 years [61]. Many of the IgAN patients in Japan have been initially identified during the annual health checkup programs performed in schools and offices and then diagnosed by a kidney biopsy.

Gross macrohematuria could occur during or after upper respiratory infection or tonsillitis, and tonsillectomy was occasionally performed as IgAN supportive treatment since the early 1970s. However, the efficacy of tonsillectomy alone was still controversial because well-designed studies with larger subjects and long observation period have not yet been conducted [62]. Recently, a multicenter retrospective cohort study in Japan found that tonsillectomy is associated with improved renal survival rates in patients with IgAN [63].

Corticosteroids are anti-inflammatory and immunosuppressive agents and have been administered to IgAN patients for 40 years. Kobayashi et al. [64] reported that the conventional oral administration of prednisolone to IgAN patients with proteinuria of 1 g/day or more could stabilize renal function and reduce proteinuria for 10 years. However, after corticosteroids withdrawal, the renal function worsened again. Katafuchi et al. [65] reported the results of a randomized controlled trial where the conventional low-dose prednisolone of 20 mg daily was effective for reducing proteinuria, but not effective to prevent the progression of IgAN.

In 1988, Hotta et al. [62] first successfully treated a young male IgAN patient with active necrotizing glomerular lesions and moderate proteinuria with a combination therapy of tonsillectomy and steroid pulse therapy. They reported the results of their new intensive treatment, which were better than previously reported [66]. IgAN patients ($n = 329$) in various disease stages were treated by the combination therapy between 1977 and 1995. The urinary pathological findings completely disappeared on 48% of the subjects, and none of them developed ESRD. They also reported the efficacy of the combination therapy; hematuria disappeared in more than 80% of the patients regardless of the histological lesions, but proteinuria remained according to the histological damages. They proposed the paradigm shift in the treatment of IgAN, from "slowing the progression of nephropathy" to "remission of nephropathy" [62]. Many Japanese nephrologists tried the combination therapy and realized its efficacy, and the new strategy for IgAN was rapidly spread to the entire Japan by the end of the 2000s [67]. Kawamura et al. [68] conducted a multicenter randomized controlled trial between tonsillectomy with steroid pulse therapy ($n = 33$) and steroid pulse therapy alone ($n = 39$). After 12-month observation, proteinuria was significantly reduced in the combined therapy. They proposed whether this antiproteinuric effect might improve kidney survival. There have been many basic studies which were intended to clarify the interaction between the tonsil, immune system, and kidney. Recently, the identification of Toll-like receptor 9 [69] and the overexpression of a proliferating inducing ligand has been demonstrated in the tonsils of IgAN patients [70]. These studies could explain the basic mechanism of the efficacy of the combination therapy with tonsillectomy and steroid pulse therapy in the future.

## Japanese Dialysis Concept

The survival rate of dialysis patients in Japan has been excellent when compared with European countries and the USA [57]; however, the reasons have not been fully clarified. We believe that some of them could be related to the unique dialysis system and to the concept of chronic dialysis in Japan. They are the centralized dialysis fluid delivery system (CDDS), excellent dialysis fluid quality, protein-permeable dialysis, and patient-centered dialysis care.

### CDDS and Dialysis Fluid Quality

In generally used dialysis fluid delivery systems, reverse osmosis (RO) water is provided from the RO machine placed in the central area to each patient's dialysis machine, and then the final dialysis fluid is made by mixing RO water with electrolyte concentrate and the buffer concentrate in the dialysis machine. The CDDS is a unique dialysis fluid delivery system, which has been developed in Japan and widely used in most of the Japanese dialysis facilities [17], where the final dialysis fluid is composed in the central area where the CDDS is placed and is directly provided to the individual dialysis console. The advantages of the CDDS are good cost performance, easy and efficient rinsing of the entire dialysis fluid delivery system, and, finally, enabling most of the dialysis facilities the possibility to use highly purified dialysis fluid. Even though JSDT has the strictest standard requirement for dialysis fluid bacteriological contamination in the world [19], the adherence rate for the standard dialysis fluid was 97.0% and 74.6% for the ultrapure dialysis fluid [2]. Based on the JRDR analysis report, there is a dialysis patient survival advantage when using ultrapure dialysis fluid when compared with the standard dialysis fluid [71]. In Japan there is a national license profession named "clinical engineer" who manages medical devices such as dialysis machines [72]. The clinical engineer has various important roles in maintenance dialysis therapy, especially in maintaining a high-quality level of the dialysis fluid delivery.

### Protein-Permeable Dialysis and HDF

Protein-permeable dialysis is a concept of chronic dialysis, enhancing the removal of larger low molecular weight protein (LMWP) as well as permitting some albumin leakage during a dialysis session [53]. Saito et al. [73] reported that renal anemia and joint pain associated with dialysis-related amyloidosis were ameliorated by HDF, with massive albumin leakage during a dialysis session. They hypothesized that protein-permeable dialysis might have some beneficial effects for the dialysis patients. After these experiences, various types of protein-permeable or protein adsorptive dialysis membranes have been developed to remove larger LMWPs. In Japan the dialysis membranes were classified into five categories in 2004 and reclassified into four categories in 2012; both classifications were based on the clearance of beta-2 microglobulin (2004, 2012) and sieving coefficient of albumin (2012) [53]. The dialysis membrane with higher protein permeability is better reimbursed by the government.

Online HDF is one of the options to remove larger LMWPs by convection. As previously addressed, predilution online HDF has been generally performed in Japan as greater than 90% of all online HDF treatments, even though postdilution is the major method prescribed elsewhere in the world [50]. In Japan, various types of protein-permeable dialyzers are available for online HDF; and the predilution mode is more suitable and safer to remove larger LMWPs, including some albumin with these membranes.

Several randomized controlled trials and systematic reviews have shown clinical advantages of postdilution online HDF; however, the hard evidence for the survival advantage of dialysis patients had not been established. Recently, Kikuchi et al. [74] reported that online predilution with large volume of substitution fluid has a survival advantage when compared with high-flux HD and low substitution volume online predilution HDF.

### Patient-Centered Dialysis Care

The principle of medicine in the twenty-first century is "patient-centeredness." However, what kind of actions should we take for patient-centeredness in the dialysis field? Recently, several approaches have been introduced to identify the outcomes of dialysis therapy, which would be beneficial for the patients or compatible to their life values [75]. These outcomes are either closely related to quality of life (QoL) or their feelings. Dialysis-induced fatigue or delayed recovery from fatigue has been reported as an independent prognostic factor [76], which deteriorates both the QoL and ADL of the patients. We established a dialysis practice pattern based on the patient's symptoms, which is called "patient-oriented dialysis" system (POD system) [53, 77]. In the POD system, 20 dialysis-related symptoms are systematically evaluated, and the dialysis prescriptions may be changed in order to improve the identified symptoms. Some of these symptoms, such as fatigue, skin itchiness, depressive sense, and dialysis-related hypotension, have been reported as a mortality risk factor. Saito et al. have reported improvement in the severe renal anemia and joint pain when utilizing postdilution HDF with massive albumin leakage during dialysis session in the early 1980s [73]. Thereafter, many Japanese nephrologists became interested in the relationship between the patients' symptoms and larger LMWPs removal. Online HDF provided improvement in dialysis-related hypotension, skin itchiness, and bone/joint pain. Sakurai reported that aggressive removal of larger LMWPs, with greater than 35% of alpha-1 microglobulin removal rate, could eliminate restless legs syndrome [78].

### Patients with Long Dialysis Vintage

Dialysis patients in Japan have a uniquely longer dialysis vintage. The Dialysis Outcomes and Practice Pattern Study (DOPPS) reported that the mean Japanese dialysis vintage was 8.9 years in 2011, which was the longest vintage compared to ten other DOPPS countries (www.dopps.org). In addition, the number of patients with long dialysis vintage is continuously increasing in Japan, although the mean age of all incident patients is also increasing annually (69.4 years at the end of 2016). It has been reported that the proportion of patients with vintages of 20 years or longer in Japan reached 8.3% of all dialysis patients at the end of 2016, whereas it was <1% at the end of 1992 [50].

In Japan, biocompatible membranes became standard in the 1980s, use of high-flux membranes became widespread in the 1990s, and reverse osmosis and endotoxin-retentive filters came into use in the late 1990s [79]. Based on the JSDT surveys, the proportion of dialysis clinics that attained an endotoxin concentration below 0.001 EU/mL (which is the requirement for ultrapure dialysis fluid according to the JSDT standard) stood at only 13.4% in 1999 [80], whereas it dramatically increased to 62.1% in 2010 [81]. With further development of these dialysis technologies, mortality has greatly improved since the 1980s. In 1985, it was reported that more than 10% of patients had a dialysis vintage of 10 years or longer [79]. On the other hand, the survival improvement yielded a new concept of dialysis-related complications: dialysis-related amyloidosis (DRA). In the 1980s, it was reported that more than 60% of patients with dialysis vintage of 16 years or longer had symptoms of dialysis-related amyloidosis [79]. Thereafter, it was recognized as one of the inevitable complications of long-term dialysis, especially for vintages >20 years [82]. Thanks to advances of dialysis technology, the risk of first-time carpal-tunnel surgery has almost halved in the last two decades, according to JRDR reports (1998–2010) [83]. However, it remains one of the important complications for longer vintage dialysis patients.

The main causes of death among deceased dialysis patients were heart failure (25.7%), followed by infectious disease (21.9%), malignant tumor (9.7%), and cerebrovascular disease (6.5%) in 2016 [50]. Among them, only infectious and tumor deaths had been consistently increasing since around 1993. Although these proportions were not specified for long-term dialysis patients, this data suggests that infectious disease and malignancy are important problems faced by long-term dialysis patients. In addition, with the increase in the mean age of prevalent dialysis patients, frailty also became an important problem. Accordingly, the concept of renal rehabilitation – including exercise therapy, diet therapy, education, and mental support – has become widespread among dialysis specialists to improve survival and quality of life.

## Future Problems and Perspectives of Nephrology in Japan

### Frail in Dialysis Patients

Age distribution of dialysis patients shows a rapid aging of this population in Japan [50]. The age increase of dialysis patients is due to an increase in new patients with 70 years of age or more [84]. The older dialysis patients often manifest nutritional derangement or wasting-related syndrome [85]. These malnutrition-wasting conditions are associated with worse activities in daily living, QoL, cardiovascular mortality, or even all-cause survival. There are similar, but distinctive, related-conditions: sarcopenia, dynapenia, protein-energy wasting (PEW), and frailty. Sarcopenia is translated as a decline in muscle mass, strength, and physical function. Dynapenia is mainly focused on muscle strength, which is a more powerful predictor of clinical outcomes than muscle mass. Comparative associations of muscle mass and muscle strength with mortality in dialysis patients have been shown by a Japanese investigator [86]. PEW, a condition in which the protein and/or energy reserve in the body decreases, has been described by the International Society of Renal Nutrition and Metabolism [87]. Many conditions related to kidney failure may cause PEW, which in its turn can lead to worse clinical outcomes.

Frailty encompasses a wide variety of conditions, which eventually result in a decline in both physical and mental functions. Physical frailty is most commonly recognized; cognitive, psychological, social, or even oral frailty can be associated with worse clinical conditions. Moreover, frailty implies reversibility, and appropriate intervention may technically reverse this condition. These four conditions share the phenotypes of malnutrition and wasting manifestation. Thus, these conditions should be managed.

Strategies against malnutrition and wasting conditions have been discussed extensively in the community of Japanese professionals in charge of dialysis clinical practice. A broad number of strategies have been investigated; the two main strategies which include dietary therapy and exercise training are now priority #1. More precisely, dietary therapy includes adequate protein intake and energy intake. The criteria for PEW include protein intake <0.8 g/kg/day and energy intake <25 kcal/kg/day, which reinforce the significance of maintaining dietary intake of protein and energy. Historically, the Japanese health insurance used to cover the meals during dialysis treatment offered by the facility until the year 2002. Thus, some facilities offer meals during the dialysis therapy or allow the patients to have the meals brought by the patients themselves even now. Such culture might be associated with the better survival of the dialysis patients. Two nephrology societies concerning kidney diseases, JSN [88] and JSDT [89], have published guidelines regarding nutritional management for CKD patients and patients on dialysis. The guidelines recommend detailed nutritional intake targets, including protein, energy, sodium, potassium, phosphorus, and fluid. Besides that, nephrologists should monitor the presence of malnutrition or wasting in prescribing dietary therapy. Even for predialysis patients who are supposed to receive a low-protein diet, the amount of protein can be increased when the patient manifests malnutrition and/or wasting. The point is to ensure adequate dietary energy intake when prescribing a low-protein diet.

On the other hand, exercise training has been prohibited for patients with an increase in proteinuria or reduced renal function in Japan, based on the fear of renal function deterioration or increased proteinuria. However, the evidence is accumulating that exercise training might preserve kidney function rather than deteriorating it. Moreover, many exercise training clinical trials of patients on dialysis revealed that the intervention improved exercise tolerance or physical function of the dialysis patients [90]. Therefore, the Japanese Society of Renal Rehabilitation decided to compile evidence regarding exercise training on patients with kidney disease as a form of a meta-analysis. The society issued a guideline regarding renal rehabilitation, especially focusing on exercise training in 2018 [91, 92]. This is the world-first evidence-based guideline concerning exercise training. A study was published demonstrating that more than 4000 steps on non-dialysis days were associated with a better survival [93]; exercise training both during dialysis and on non-dialysis days are now encouraged.

Another intervention against malnutrition and wasting conditions has been investigated, which includes modest ultrafiltration and removal of uremic solutes, ensuring dialysis length and biocompatible membrane materials. Future clinical trials are required to ensure adequate nutritional intake and to avoid wasting conditions in CKD patients.

## Conclusion

Many patients with kidney diseases, especially GN, have been detected in early stages by means of the mandatory annual health checkup. However, the number of patients who require dialysis treatment is still increasing. Academic societies and the Japanese government have started collaborative efforts to decrease the incidence of ESRD by managing the current status of expansion of kidney disease patients. On the other hand, the demographics or characteristics of the patients with kidney disease are dramatically changing during the past several decades in Japan, which is the reflection of low birth and death rates and the improvement of the noncommunicable diseases management. Thus, we, the Japanese nephrology community members, are facing changes in the framework of kidney diseases management. Knowledge obtained through such experience may be utilized by healthcare professionals in other nations as well as in the fields of other diseases.

## References

1. Nitta K, Masakane I, Hanafusa N, Taniguchi M, Hasegawa T, Nakai S, et al. 2017 Annual dialysis report, JSDT renal data registry. Ren Replace Ther. 2019;5:53.
2. Nitta K, Masakane I, Hanafusa N, Goto S, Abe M, Nakai S, et al. 2018 Annual dialysis report, JSDT renal data registry [in Japanese]. J Jpn Soc Dial Ther. 2019;52:679–754.

3. Bright R. Reports of medical cases. 1827. https://archive.org/details/34725085.5943.emory.edu/page/n21.
4. Kinoshita Y, Osawa G, Mikami A, T. M. About new anti-hypertensive drug, additionally about punched renal biopsy. Rinsho Shonika. 1954;9:735.
5. Ueda Y, Miyahara T, Sakai O, Fujinoki T, Kagawa K. Nephrosis-type nephritis--morphological considerations. Nihon Rinsho. 1966;24(4):635–42.
6. Kinoshita Y. Aspects of smoldering glomerulonephritis. In: Rea K, editor. Glomerulonephritis. Stuttgart: Georg Thieme; 1976. p. 79.
7. Oshima K. The classification and clinical feature. Jpn J Int Med. 1968;59:1043–57.
8. Suwa N, Takahashi T. Morphological and morphometrical analysis of circulation in hypertension and ischemic kidney. Fortschritte der morphologischen Pathologie. München, Germany: Urban & Schwarzenberg; 1971, p. 108–16.
9. Shioji R, Furuyama T, Onodera S, Saito H, Ito H, Sasaki Y. Sjogren's syndrome and renal tubular acidosis. Am J Med. 1970;48(4):456–63.
10. Saito T, Sato H, Kudo K, Oikawa S, Shibata T, Hara Y, et al. Lipoprotein glomerulopathy: glomerular lipoprotein thrombi in a patient with hyperlipoproteinemia. Am J Kidney Dis. 1989;13(2):148–53.
11. Saeki T, Nishi S, Imai N, Ito T, Yamazaki H, Kawano M, et al. Clinicopathological characteristics of patients with IgG4-related tubulointerstitial nephritis. Kidney Int. 2010;78(10):1016–23.
12. Matsuo S, Imai E, Horio M, Yasuda Y, Tomita K, Nitta K, et al. Revised equations for estimated GFR from serum creatinine in Japan. Am J Kidney Dis. 2009;53(6):982–92.
13. Imai E, Horio M, Watanabe T, Iseki K, Yamagata K, Hara S, et al. Prevalence of chronic kidney disease in the Japanese general population. Clin Exp Nephrol. 2009;13(6):621–30.
14. Sugiyama H, Yokoyama H, Sato H, Saito T, Kohda Y, Nishi S, et al. Japan renal biopsy registry and Japan kidney disease registry: committee report for 2009 and 2010. Clin Exp Nephrol. 2013;17(2):155–73.
15. Committee CGfCKDA. Evidence-based clinical practice guidelines for CKD 2018. Jpn J Nephrol. 2018;60(8):1037–193.
16. Therapy TJSfD. The Japanese Society for Dialysis Therapy, 50th Anniversary. The Japanese Society for Dialysis Therapy; 2019.
17. Kawanishi H, Moriishi M, Sato T, Taoka M. Fully automated dialysis system based on the central dialysis fluid delivery system. Blood Purif. 2009;27(Suppl 1):56–63.
18. Yamagami S. The report of technical committee for standard for safety of dialysis fluid. J Jpn Soc Dial Ther. 1995;28(11):1487–93.
19. Mineshima M, Kawanishi H, Ase T, Kawasaki T, Tomo T, Nakamoto H, et al. 2016 update Japanese Society for Dialysis Therapy Standard of fluids for hemodialysis and related therapies. Ren Replace Ther. 2018;4(1):15.
20. Eguchi K, Ikebe N, Konno Y, Yamada Y, Kaneko I, Mineshima M, et al. Development and clinical effectiveness of intermittent infusion hemodiafiltration (I-HDF) as a new HDF therapy. J Jpn Soc Dial Ther. 2007;40:769–74.
21. Mineshima M, Eguchi K. Development of intermittent infusion hemodiafiltration using ultrapure dialysis fluid with an automated dialysis machine. Blood Purif. 2013;35(Suppl 1):55–8.
22. Kawanishi H, Mineshima M, Tomo T, Minakuchi J. Functional classification of dialyzers (Hollow-fiber Type) in 2013 [in Japanese]. J Jpn Soc Dial Ther. 2013;46:501–6.
23. Kawaguchi Y, Kawanishi H, Mujais S, Topley N, Oreopoulos DG. Encapsulating peritoneal sclerosis: definition, etiology, diagnosis, and treatment. International Society for Peritoneal Dialysis Ad Hoc Committee on Ultrafiltration Management in Peritoneal Dialysis. Perit Dial Int. 2000;20 Suppl 4:S43–55.
24. Nitta K, Masakane I, Tomo T, Tsuchida K, Ikeda K, Ogawa T, et al. Policy for developing clinical practice guidelines of Japanese Society for Dialysis Therapy. Ren Replace Ther. 2017;3(1):34.
25. Yamauchi H. Organ transplantation. Jpn J Surg. 1910;11:45–8.
26. Inoue H, Suzuki A, Sato S, Hirokawa I, Kawaji K, Kusunoki T. Renal transplantation: experimental study and clinical experience. Urol Int. 1957;5(5):253–73.
27. Takahashi K. History of kidney transplantation and future perspectives [in Japanese]. Jin Touseki. 2013;75:13–29.
28. Shikata T, Inoue H. Clinical aspect of allo-transplantation of kidney [in Japanese]. Ishoku. 1967;2:34–41.
29. Ochiai T, Toma H, Takagi H, Oka T. The report of multicenter analysis of ciclosporin in kidney transplantation. [in Japanese]. Ishoku. 1986;21:255–78.
30. Uchida H, Yokota K, Akiyama N, Masaki Y, Aso K, Okubo M, et al. Effectiveness of a new drug, bredinin, on canine kidney allotransplant survival. Transplant Proc. 1979;11(1):865–70.
31. Sagawa S, Ishibashi M, Arima M, Usami M, Ngafune M, Sonoda T, et al. Research for development of a new immunosuppressant. [in Japanese]. Ishoku. 1978;13:271–6.
32. Ochiai T, Nagata M, Nakajima K, Suzuki T, Sakamoto K, Enomoto K, et al. Studies of the effects of FK506 on renal allografting in the beagle dog. Transplantation. 1987;44(6):729–33.
33. Group JFs. Japanese study of FK506 on kidney transplantation: results of late phase II study. Transplant Proc. 1993;25:649–54.
34. Takahashi K, Tanabe K, Ooba S, Yagisawa T, Nakazawa H, Teraoka S, et al. Prophylactic use of a new immunosuppressive agent, deoxyspergualin, in patients with kidney transplantation from ABO-incompatible or preformed antibody-positive donors. Transplant Proc. 1991;23(1 Pt 2):1078–82.
35. Yagisawa T, Mieno M, Ichimaru N, Morita K, Nakamura M, Hotta K, et al. Trend of kidney transplantation in Japan in 2018: data from the kidney transplant registry. Ren Replace Ther. 2019;5(1):14.
36. Ota K, Fuchinoue S, Nakamura M, Tokumoto T, Tanabe K, Toma H. Transplantation of kidneys donated from the USA: long-term results and viability testing using 31P-MRS. Transpl Int. 1997;10(1):7–12.
37. Yoshimura N, Okajima H, Ushigome H, Sakamoto S, Fujiki M, Okamoto M. Current status of organ transplantation in Japan and worldwide. Surg Today. 2010;40(6):514–25.
38. National Kidney F. K/DOQI clinical practice guidelines for chronic kidney disease: evaluation, classification, and stratification. Am J Kidney Dis. 2002;39(2 Suppl 1):S1–266.
39. Coresh J, Selvin E, Stevens LA, Manzi J, Kusek JW, Eggers P, et al. Prevalence of chronic kidney disease in the United States. JAMA. 2007;298(17):2038–47.
40. Nagata M, Ninomiya T, Doi Y, Yonemoto K, Kubo M, Hata J, et al. Trends in the prevalence of chronic kidney disease and its risk factors in a general Japanese population: the Hisayama study. Nephrol Dial Transplant. 2010;25(8):2557–64.
41. Nakayama M, Sato T, Sato H, Yamaguchi Y, Obara K, Kurihara I, et al. Different clinical outcomes for cardiovascular events and mortality in chronic kidney disease according to underlying renal disease: the Gonryo study. Clin Exp Nephrol. 2010;14(4):333–9.
42. Tanaka K, Watanabe T, Takeuchi A, Ohashi Y, Nitta K, Akizawa T, et al. Cardiovascular events and death in Japanese patients with chronic kidney disease. Kidney Int. 2017;91(1):227–34.
43. Committee for Standardization of Renal Pathological Diagnosis and Committee for Kidney Disease Registry JSoN. Japan renal biopsy registry and Japan kidney disease registry: committee report for 2018. 2018. https://cdn.jsn.or.jp/news/190625_kp.pdf.
44. Yamanouchi M, Furuichi K, Hoshino J, Toyama T, Hara A, Shimizu M, et al. Nonproteinuric versus proteinuric phenotypes in diabetic kidney disease: a propensity score-matched analysis of a nationwide, biopsy-based cohort study. Diabetes Care. 2019;42(5):891–902.
45. Uesugi N, Shimazu Y, Kikuchi K, Nagata M. Age-related renal microvascular changes: evaluation by three-dimensional digital imaging of the human renal microcirculation using virtual microscopy. Int J Mol Sci. 2016;17(11):1831.

46. Shimizu M, Furuichi K, Toyama T, Funamoto T, Kitajima S, Hara A, et al. Association of renal arteriosclerosis and hypertension with renal and cardiovascular outcomes in Japanese type 2 diabetes patients with diabetic nephropathy. J Diabetes Investig. 2019;10(4):1041–9.
47. Taguma Y, Kitamoto Y, Futaki G, Ueda H, Monma H, Ishizaki M, et al. Effect of captopril on heavy proteinuria in azotemic diabetics. N Engl J Med. 1985;313(26):1617–20.
48. Endo A. The discovery and development of HMG-CoA reductase inhibitors. J Lipid Res. 1992;33(11):1569–82.
49. Takano Y, Hase-Aoki K, Horiuchi H, Zhao L, Kasahara Y, Kondo S, et al. Selectivity of febuxostat, a novel non-purine inhibitor of xanthine oxidase/xanthine dehydrogenase. Life Sci. 2005;76(16):1835–47.
50. Masakane I, Taniguchi M, Nakai S, Tsuchida K, Wada A, Ogata S, et al. Annual dialysis data report 2016, JSDT renal data registry. Ren Replace Ther. 2018;4(1):45.
51. Wakasugi M, Kazama JJ, Narita I. Secular trends in end-stage kidney disease requiring renal replacement therapy in Japan: Japanese Society of Dialysis Therapy Registry data from 1983 to 2016. Nephrology (Carlton). 2019.
52. System USRD. Chapter II: International Comparisons; 2018.
53. Masakane I, Sakurai K. Current approaches to middle molecule removal: room for innovation. Nephrol Dial Transplant. 2018;33(Suppl 3):iii12–21.
54. Abe M, Hamano T, Wada A, Nakai S, Masakane I. High-performance membrane dialyzers and mortality in hemodialysis patients: a 2-year cohort study from the annual survey of the Japanese renal data registry. Am J Nephrol. 2017;46(1):82–92.
55. Takahashi K, Saito K, Takahara S, Fuchinoue S, Yagisawa T, Aikawa A, et al. Results of a multicenter prospective clinical study in Japan for evaluating efficacy and safety of desensitization protocol based on rituximab in ABO-incompatible kidney transplantation. Clin Exp Nephrol. 2017;21(4):705–13.
56. Okumi M, Toki D, Nozaki T, Shimizu T, Shirakawa H, Omoto K, et al. ABO-incompatible living kidney transplants: evolution of outcomes and immunosuppressive management. Am J Transplant. 2016;16(3):886–96.
57. Goodkin DA, Bragg-Gresham JL, Koenig KG, Wolfe RA, Akiba T, Andreucci VE, et al. Association of comorbid conditions and mortality in hemodialysis patients in Europe, Japan, and the United States: the Dialysis Outcomes and Practice Patterns Study (DOPPS). J Am Soc Nephrol. 2003;14(12):3270–7.
58. Goto N, Okada M, Yamamoto T, Tsujita M, Hiramitsu T, Narumi S, et al. Association of dialysis duration with outcomes after transplantation in a Japanese cohort. Clin J Am Soc Nephrol. 2016;11(3):497–504.
59. Ministry of Health LaW. High-cost medical expense benefit (Eligibility Certificate for Ceiling-Amount Application). 2019. https://www.mhlw.go.jp/seisakunitsuite/bunya/kenkou_iryou/iryou/kokusai/setsumeisiryo/dl/en09.pdf.
60. Nephrology JSo. Certified CKD educator program. 2019. https://j-ka.or.jp/educator/.
61. Koyama A, Igarashi M, Kobayashi M. Natural history and risk factors for immunoglobulin A nephropathy in Japan. Research Group on Progressive Renal Diseases. Am J Kidney Dis. 1997;29(4):526–32.
62. Hotta O. Use of corticosteroids, other immunosuppressive therapies, and tonsillectomy in the treatment of IgA nephropathy. Semin Nephrol. 2004;24(3):244–55.
63. Hirano K, Matsuzaki K, Yasuda T, Nishikawa M, Yasuda Y, Koike K, et al. Association between tonsillectomy and outcomes in patients with immunoglobulin A nephropathy. JAMA Netw Open. 2019;2(5):e194772.
64. Kobayashi Y, Hiki Y, Kokubo T, Horii A, Tateno S. Steroid therapy during the early stage of progressive IgA nephropathy. A 10-year follow-up study. Nephron. 1996;72(2):237–42.
65. Katafuchi R, Ikeda K, Mizumasa T, Tanaka H, Ando T, Yanase T, et al. Controlled, prospective trial of steroid treatment in IgA nephropathy: a limitation of low-dose prednisolone therapy. Am J Kidney Dis. 2003;41(5):972–83.
66. Hotta O, Miyazaki M, Furuta T, Tomioka S, Chiba S, Horigome I, et al. Tonsillectomy and steroid pulse therapy significantly impact on clinical remission in patients with IgA nephropathy. Am J Kidney Dis. 2001;38(4):736–43.
67. Matsuzaki K, Suzuki Y, Nakata J, Sakamoto N, Horikoshi S, Kawamura T, et al. Nationwide survey on current treatments for IgA nephropathy in Japan. Clin Exp Nephrol. 2013;17(6):827–33.
68. Kawamura T, Yoshimura M, Miyazaki Y, Okamoto H, Kimura K, Hirano K, et al. A multicenter randomized controlled trial of tonsillectomy combined with steroid pulse therapy in patients with immunoglobulin A nephropathy. Nephrol Dial Transplant. 2014;29(8):1546–53.
69. Sato D, Suzuki Y, Kano T, Suzuki H, Matsuoka J, Yokoi H, et al. Tonsillar TLR9 expression and efficacy of tonsillectomy with steroid pulse therapy in IgA nephropathy patients. Nephrol Dial Transplant. 2012;27(3):1090–7.
70. Muto M, Manfroi B, Suzuki H, Joh K, Nagai M, Wakai S, et al. Toll-like receptor 9 stimulation induces aberrant expression of a proliferation-inducing ligand by tonsillar germinal center B cells in IgA nephropathy. J Am Soc Nephrol. 2017;28(4):1227–38.
71. Hasegawa T, Nakai S, Masakane I, Watanabe Y, Iseki K, Tsubakihara Y, et al. Dialysis fluid endotoxin level and mortality in maintenance hemodialysis: a nationwide cohort study. Am J Kidney Dis. 2015;65(6):899–904.
72. Engineers JAfC. What is Japan Association for clinical engineers? 2019. https://www.ja-ces.or.jp/english/.
73. Saito A, Suzuki I, Chung TG, Okamoto T, Hotta T. Separation of an inhibitor of erythropoiesis in "middle molecules" from hemodialysate from patients with chronic renal failure. Clin Chem. 1986;32(10):1938–41.
74. Kikuchi K, Hamano T, Wada A, Nakai S, Masakane I. Predilution online hemodiafiltration is associated with improved survival compared with hemodialysis. Kidney Int. 2019;95(4):929–38.
75. Tong A, Manns B, Wang AYM, Hemmelgarn B, Wheeler DC, Gill J, et al. Implementing core outcomes in kidney disease: report of the Standardized Outcomes in Nephrology (SONG) implementation workshop. Kidney Int. 2018;94(6):1053–68.
76. Rayner HC, Zepel L, Fuller DS, Morgenstern H, Karaboyas A, Culleton BF, et al. Recovery time, quality of life, and mortality in hemodialysis patients: the Dialysis Outcomes and Practice Patterns Study (DOPPS). Am J Kidney Dis. 2014;64(1):86–94.
77. Masakane I. High-quality dialysis: a lesson from the Japanese experience: effects of membrane material on nutritional status and dialysis-related symptoms. NDT Plus. 2010;3(Suppl 1):i28–35.
78. Sakurai K. Biomarkers for evaluation of clinical outcomes of hemodiafiltration. Blood Purif. 2013;35(Suppl 1):64–8.
79. Hoshino J, Yamagata K, Nishi S, Nakai S, Masakane I, Iseki K, et al. Carpal tunnel surgery as proxy for dialysis-related amyloidosis: results from the Japanese society for dialysis therapy. Am J Nephrol. 2014;39(5):449–58.
80. Nakai S, Shinzato T, Sanaka T, Kikuchi K, Kitaoka T, Shinoda T, et al. An overview of dialysis treatment in Japan (as of Dec. 31, 1999). J Jpn Soc Dial Ther. 2001;34(7):1121–47.
81. Nakai S, Iseki K, Itami N, Ogata S, Kazama JJ, Kimata N, et al. An overview of regular dialysis treatment in Japan (as of 31 December 2010). Ther Apher Dial. 2012;16(6):483–521.
82. Koch KM. Dialysis-related amyloidosis. Kidney Int. 1992;41(5):1416–29.
83. Hoshino J, Yamagata K, Nishi S, Nakai S, Masakane I, Iseki K, et al. Significance of the decreased risk of dialysis-related amyloidosis now proven by results from Japanese nationwide surveys in 1998 and 2010. Nephrol Dial Transplant. 2016;31(4):595–602.

84. Hanafusa N, Nitta K, Tsuchiya K. The characteristics of the older dialysis population—heterogeneity and another type of altered risk factor patterns. Ren Replace Ther. 2017;3(1):29.
85. Hanafusa N, Tsuchiya K, Nitta K. Malnutrition-wasting conditions in older dialysis patients: an individualized approach. Contrib Nephrol. 2019;198:12–20.
86. Isoyama N, Qureshi AR, Avesani CM, Lindholm B, Barany P, Heimburger O, et al. Comparative associations of muscle mass and muscle strength with mortality in dialysis patients. Clin J Am Soc Nephrol. 2014;9(10):1720–8.
87. Fouque D, Kalantar-Zadeh K, Kopple J, Cano N, Chauveau P, Cuppari L, et al. A proposed nomenclature and diagnostic criteria for protein-energy wasting in acute and chronic kidney disease. Kidney Int. 2008;73(4):391–8.
88. Suzuki Y, Kimura K, Koya D, Yuzawa Y, Tsuruya K, Kanno Y, et al. Dietary recommendations for chronic kidney disease, 2014 [in Japanese]. Jpn J Nephrol. 2014;47:287–91.
89. Nakao T, Kanno Y, Nagasawa Y, Kanazawa Y, Akiba T, Sanaka T, et al. Standard for dietary therapy in chronic dialysis patients [in Japanese]. J Jpn Soc Dial Ther. 2014;40:478–90.
90. Sheng K, Zhang P, Chen L, Cheng J, Wu C, Chen J. Intradialytic exercise in hemodialysis patients: a systematic review and meta-analysis. Am J Nephrol. 2014;40(5):478–90.
91. Rehabilitation JSoR. Guideline for renal rehabilitation [in Japanese]. Tokyo: Nankodo; 2018.
92. Yamagata K, Hoshino J, Sugiyama H, Hanafusa N, Shibagaki Y, Komatsu Y, et al. Clinical practice guideline for renal rehabilitation: systematic reviews and recommendations of exercise therapies in patients with kidney diseases. Ren Replace Ther. 2019;5(1):28.
93. Matsuzawa R, Roshanravan B, Shimoda T, Mamorita N, Yoneki K, Harada M, et al. Physical activity dose for hemodialysis patients: where to begin? Results from a prospective cohort study. J Ren Nutr. 2018;28(1):45–53.

# Nephrology in Malaysia

# 26

L. S. Hooi, S. Bavanandan, G. Ahmad, Y. N. Lim, B. C. Bee, and Z. Morad

| | |
|---|---|
| Area[1] | 330,803 km$^2$ |
| Population[2] | 32.6 million (2018) |
| Capital | Kuala Lumpur (KL) |
| Three most populated cities[3] | 1. Kuala Lumpur<br>2. Penang<br>3. Johor Bahru |
| Official language | Malay |
| Gross Domestic Product (GDP)[4,5] | 314.5 billion USD (2017)<br>345.4 billion USD (2018) |
| GDP per capita[6] | 10,557 USD (2018) |
| Human Development Index (HDI)[7] | 0.802 (2018) |
| Official currency | Malaysian Ringgit (RM) |
| Total number of nephrologists[8] | 179 (adult)<br>17 (pediatric) |
| National society of nephrology | Malaysian Society of Nephrology<br>www.msn.org.my |
| Incidence of End-Stage Renal disease[9,10] | 2016 – 251 pmp<br>2017 – 252 pmp<br>2018 – 254 pmp (estimate) |
| Prevalence of End-Stage Renal Disease[9,10] | 2016 – 1345 pmp<br>2017 – 1356 pmp<br>2018 – 1375 pmp (estimate) |
| Total number of patients on dialysis (all modalities)[9, 10] | 2016 – 39,711<br>2017 – 41,607<br>2018 – 42,717 |
| Number of patients on hemodialysis[9, 10] | 2016 – 35,781<br>2017 – 37,324<br>2018 – 38,297 |
| Number of patients on peritoneal dialysis[9, 10] | 2016 – 3930<br>2017 – 4283<br>2018 – 4420 |
| Number of renal transplantations per year[9, 10] | 2016 – 82<br>2017 – 108<br>2018 – 85 |

[1]https://en.wikipedia.org/wiki/Malaysia. Accessed 17 Mar 2019.

[2]Department of Statistics Malaysia. https://www.dosm.gov.my/v1/index.php?r=column/ctwoByCat&parent_id=115&menu_id=L0pheU43NWJwRWVSZklWdzQ4TlhUUT09. Accessed on 17 Mar 2019.

[3]https://en.wikipedia.org/wiki/List_of_cities_in_Malaysia. Accessed on 25 May 2019.

[4]Department of Statistics Malaysia, https://dosm.gov.my/v1/index.php?r=column/cthemeByCat&cat=266&bul_id=SW5lOVJadmV1ckdQa09RVUlHbDFjQT09&menu_id=TE5CRUZCblh4ZTZMODZIbmk2aWRRQT09. Accessed on 10 June 2019 (average USD 1 = RM 4.3).

[5]Department of Statistics Malaysia, pocket statistics Q4 2018. Accessed 17 Mar 2019 (USD 1 = RM 4.14).

[6]Department of Statistics Malaysia, assessed 17 March 2019 (average USD 1 = RM 4.00).

[7]United Nations Development Programme, Human Development Reports 2018, http://hdr.undp.org/en/countries/profiles/MYS. Accessed 17 Mar 2019.

[8]National Specialist Register, Malaysia, https://www.nsr.org.my/list-1pview.asp?page=1. Accessed 17 Mar 2019.

[9]Personal communication – Registry manager, email: nrr@msn.org.my, 17 June 2019.

[10]Wong HS, Goh BL (eds). 24th Report of the Malaysian Dialysis and Transplant Registry 2016, Kuala Lumpur 2018, https://www.msn.org.my/nrr/mdtr2016.jsp.

## Introduction

Malaysia is a country in Southeast Asia, a constitutional federal monarchy with a democratically elected government run by a prime minister. The head of state is the king who is elected by and from nine hereditary rulers. The monarch changes every 5 years and the duties are largely ceremonial.

L. S. Hooi (✉)
Johor Bahru, Malaysia

S. Bavanandan
Department of Nephrology, Kuala Lumpur Hospital, Kuala Lumpur, Malaysia

G. Ahmad
Department of Cardiology, National Heart Institute, Kuala Lumpur, Malaysia

Y. N. Lim
Prince Court Medical Centre, Kuala Lumpur, Malaysia

B. C. Bee
Department of Nephrology, Selayang Hospital, Kepong, Selangor, Malaysia

Z. Morad
Ampang Puteri Hospital, Kuala Lumpur, Malaysia


J. A. Moura-Neto et al. (eds.), *Nephrology Worldwide*, https://doi.org/10.1007/978-3-030-56890-0_26

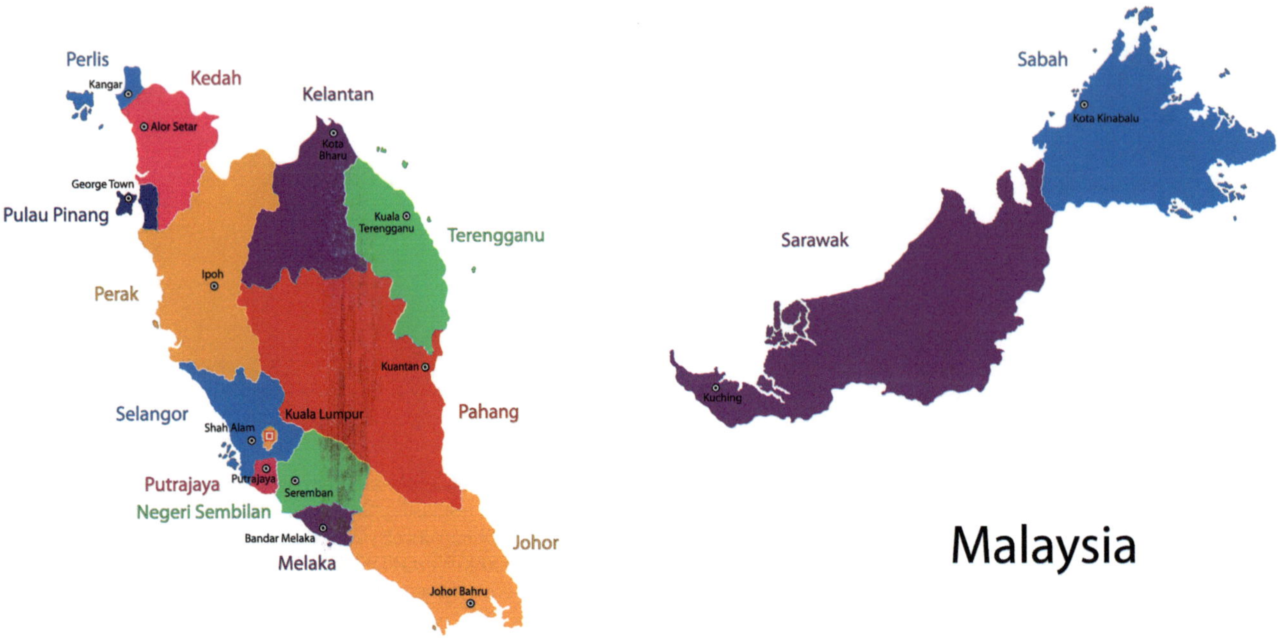


**Fig. 26.1** Map of Malaysia with states

Malaysia has 13 states and three federal territories. The capital city is Kuala Lumpur. Each state is run by an elected chief minister and state legislative assembly [1].

Geographically, it is made up of two parts: a peninsula which includes the southernmost point of continental Asia which is 138 km north of the equator and a part of the island of Borneo which it shares with Indonesia and Brunei. The peninsula is known as West Malaysia while the Malaysian part of Borneo is East Malaysia. Peninsular Malaysia has a land border with Thailand in the north and is connected to the island of Singapore by a causeway across a narrow strait in the south. The two parts of Malaysia are separated by the South China Sea [2] (Fig. 26.1).

Historically, Malaya was colonized by the Portuguese in 1511, the Dutch in 1641, and the British in 1824. During the nineteenth century, Chinese and Indians had migrated to the country to work in tin mines and rubber plantations. Japan occupied Malaya during the Second World War (1942–1945). The country gained independence from colonial British rule on 31 August 1957 [1]. This period is depicted in the literature of Somerset Maugham, Anthony Burgess, and Han Su-Yin.

The population of Malaysia has grown steadily since independence from 7.5 million in 1957 to 32.6 million in 2018. The country is multicultural, multiethnic, and multilingual consisting of 67% Malays, 25% Chinese, 7% Indians, and 1% others. The main religion is Islam, with freedom to practice others, e.g., Buddhism, Hinduism, and Christianity. The national language is Malay with English being the second language.

The climate is equatorial, hot, and humid throughout the year with an average temperature of 27 °C. The rainy seasons comprise the northeast monsoon (October to March) and southwest monsoon (May to September). There is 250 cm of rain a year. The country is not in the path of typhoons, hurricanes, or earthquakes, and the only natural disaster is occasional flooding usually during the northeast monsoon.

The official currency of Malaysia is the ringgit (RM). In November 2019, RM 1.00 was worth 0.24 US dollar, 0.22 Euro, 26.23 Japanese Yen, and 1.69 Chinese Yuan Renminbi. The gross domestic product (GDP) was RM 1429.8 billion in 2018 [3], and it is the 35th largest economy in the world [4].

It is an upper middle-income country, a growing, newly industrialized market economy. The average growth rate of GDP is 6.5% per annum since independence. The main earnings used to be from natural resources, e.g., tin and agriculture from rubber and palm oil. This has been superseded by the export of petroleum, manufacturing, and by tourism. The people enjoy a high standard of living with low income tax, low cost of local food, transport fuel and household essentials. There is fully subsidized public healthcare, and comprehensive social welfare benefit.

Healthcare in government clinics and hospitals is almost free, funded by the government, while there is a parallel system of private healthcare, which is funded by private insurance and out-of-pocket payments. The overall expenditure on health is 4.24% of GDP [5], which is rather low. Dialysis provision is a priority. Most politicians are supportive of increasing funding for dialysis as it is expensive and not affordable by the man in the street. Nephrology as a specialty is allocated an oversized portion of the healthcare budget, out of proportion to the number of patients treated. There is usually extra development allocation for building and equipment in the yearly federal budget. The rate of renal transplantation on the other hand is not limited by lack of funds but rather by cultural and religious norms that are hard to shift despite concerted efforts in the last few decades.

This chapter aims to give the reader an idea of nephrology as practiced in Malaysia from the 1960s until the present day (2019).

## Brief History of Nephrology in Malaysia

The first hemodialysis (HD) was done in Kuala Lumpur Hospital (HKL) in 1964 using a Kolff dialysis machine. This was for acute kidney injury (AKI) to stabilize patients before surgery for bilateral obstruction due to kidney stones. Peritoneal dialysis (PD) for AKI started in 1966 using a stiff catheter on an intermittent basis [6].

Long-term HD for end-stage renal disease (ESRD) in Malaysia started in 1967 on a single patient. In 1969, a small chronic HD program was started in HKL and it exists, today, as a large hemodialysis unit with 183 patients.

The first renal biopsy was done at the KL University Hospital in 1968 [7]. The renal histopathology service had grown first in the universities and then in Ministry of Health (MOH) hospitals. Lupus nephritis is common in Malaysia and early reports came from the KL University Hospital in the 1970s [8].

Nephrology as a discipline probably started with dialysis services at the Institute of Urology and Nephrology (IUN) at HKL in 1974. The Human Tissues Act legislation was introduced in the same year to enable organ retrieval from deceased donors for transplantation. This law serves the basis for the "opting-in" system of deceased organ donation, which remains to this day. The first living-related (sibling) donor kidney transplant was done in 1975 and the first deceased donor kidney transplant was performed in 1976, both at the IUN HKL [6].

Pediatric nephrology had its beginnings in the KL University Hospital in the 1960s [9]. The first pediatric kidney transplant was done in 1986 in HKL and, in 2000, a pediatric HD unit was started there.

As there was initially a lack of provision for dialysis for ESRD, a home HD program was started in 1979. Some patients were also dialyzing at their office, i.e., at their place of work. At its height there were more than 350 patients dialyzing at home or at work as no HD units existed outside Kuala Lumpur.

Continuous ambulatory peritoneal dialysis (CAPD) started at the KL University Hospital in 1980, followed by HKL in 1985. Automated PD (APD) for children started in 1991. CAPD extended out of Kuala Lumpur to several large state hospitals in 1992 and then decentralized to all government hospitals with nephrologists. Very few private centers offered CAPD. A nucleus of nephrologists and nurses were instrumental in this initial endeavor to expand the PD program, providing training and support in establishing PD units in other states of the country in the 1990s.

The first CAPD connectology was a single bag-spike system in the early 1980s (Travenol system with a connection shield), and then the UVXD (ultraviolet exchange device to sterilize the bag-spike junction) was used from 1987. The bags were still connected to the patient who had to roll up the bag and tie it to the waist. In 1993, the disconnect (UltraSet) system was introduced, and then, in 2001, a twin bag with pre-connected Y set (UltraBag, Baxter). These innovations reduced the rate of peritonitis as spiking of bags was no longer necessary.

The country used the Carex system by B. Braun for a short time. There was also the Fresenius ANDY-Disc followed by the Stay-Safe twin-bag system. The development of PD was further facilitated by the availability of automated cyclers. From the large and heavy Pax-X cyclers, we now have Baxter Homechoice, Homechoice Claria, Fresenius Sleep-Safe, and Sleep-Safe Harmony.

During the early years of the PD program, PD access procedures were performed by urologists. General surgeons were subsequently involved. In 2003, some nephrologists started placement of Tenckhoff catheters using the peritoneoscopic method. Over the years, increasing numbers of nephrologists have been trained to insert the PD catheter on their own. This has resulted in significant growth of the PD program. Serdang Hospital has been organizing an annual seminar and workshop on peritoneoscopic insertion of PD catheter, with participation of delegates from neighboring countries.

At present, the methods used for Tenckhoff catheter insertion at various PD centers are minilaparotomy, percutaneous Seldinger, peritoneoscopy, and laparoscopy [10]. In most state hospitals, the PD catheters are inserted by nephrologists using the peritoneoscopic and percutaneous techniques. Most surgeons still adopt the open minilaparotomy method for catheter placement. Selayang Hospital has become a tertiary referral center for laparoscopic PD access and salvage by surgeon for challenging abdomens. There has been a steady growth of PD utilization, from only 3 PD patients in 1981 to 4420 patients in 2018 ([6], Registry manager, email: nrr@msn.org.my, 25 November 2019, "personal communication").

The idea of setting up the Malaysian Society of Nephrology (MSN) was discussed at a meeting in 1983, and the inaugural general meeting was held the following year.

**Table 26.1** International and regional conferences hosted by MSN since its creation

| Year | Conference | Place |
|---|---|---|
| 1985 | 6th Asian Colloquium in Nephrology | Kuala Lumpur |
| 1998 | 12th Asian Colloquium in Nephrology | Kuala Lumpur |
| 2005 | Satellite Symposium on Acute Renal Failure post-World Congress of Nephrology | Penang |
| 2008 | 11th Asian Pacific Congress of Nephrology | Kuala Lumpur |
| 2012 | 14th Congress of the International Society of Peritoneal Dialysis | Kuala Lumpur |
| 2015 | 9th Congress of the International Society for Hemodialysis | Kuala Lumpur |
| 2017 | 1st Asia Pacific AKI CRRT Congress | Kuala Lumpur |
| 2019 | 4th Congress of Asian Pacific Society of Dialysis Access | Kuala Lumpur |
| 2019 | 3rd Asia Pacific AKI CRRT Congress | Kuala Lumpur |

MSN has hosted many international and regional conferences (Table 26.1) and will host the World Congress of Nephrology in 2022.

MSN has links with the International Society of Nephrology (ISN) and regional nephrology societies. It is a provider of continuing medical education (CME) through congresses every year, short courses, and workshops. It is the adviser for HD and PD standards, nephrology training, credentialing to the Ministry of Health and produces local clinical practice guidelines e.g. on chronic kidney disease.

The National Kidney Foundation of Malaysia (NKF) was started in 1969. It is a dialysis provider and a charitable organization promoting prevention and screening for kidney diseases. World Kidney Day, which takes place on the second Thursday of March, started in 2006 as an initiative of the ISN and International Federation of Kidney Foundations has been celebrated every year by NKF and MSN.

The Malaysian Society of Transplantation was inaugurated in 1994. It hosted the 8th Congress of the Asian Society of Transplantation (CAST) in 2003 and will host the 17th CAST in 2021.

The Dialysis and Transplant Register was started in 1992 in HKL; the first report of the Malaysian Dialysis and Transplant Registry (MDTR) was published in 1993, and it is still reporting today, more than 25 years later [11]. The Malaysian Registry of Renal Biopsy (MRRB) started reporting in 2005 [12], and the deceased donor kidney transplant waiting list linked to MDTR (Malaysian Organ Sharing System) started in 1999 [13]. Data on renal replacement therapy (RRT) in Malaysia are shared with the United States Renal Data System (USRDS) and with the Global Observatory on Donation and Transplantation.

In the 1980s, there was a pressing need for HD units. The first few were started outside KL in 1984 and all MOH hospitals had HD units by 2008. At the same time, nongovernmental organizations (NGOs) like NKF started HD units in the 1990s. Private HD units, which were few (first one started in 1985 at Pantai Hospital in KL), mushroomed in the 2000s. These developments paralleled the improving finances of the country and the willingness of the government to pay for dialysis. Financial subsidies were given to NGO centers from 1991 and payment to private centers for HD of government servants, their dependents, or those with social security followed.

For dialysis provision, the incidence rate increased from 13 pmp in 1990 to 101 pmp in 2005 and 251 pmp in 2018; the prevalence rate increased from 46 pmp in 1990 to 497 pmp in 2005 and 1319 pmp in 2018 ([6], Registry manager, email: nrr@msn.org.my, 25 November 2019, "personal communication"). The percentage of HD performed in government, NGO, and private centers gradually changed over the years. Initially, HD was provided predominantly by MOH centers. The percentage decreased when NGO and private centers started providing services from the early 1990s. Since 2007, the percentage of HD provided by private centers predominated (58% in 2018) (Registry manager, email: nrr@msn.org.my, 25 November 2019, "personal communication"). Despite the increase of HD centers nationwide, there remains inequitable distribution in favor of urban areas especially the West Coast of Peninsular Malaysia. This is being addressed by MOH with the setting up of 17 HD units in public health clinics in smaller towns and rural areas between 2006 and 2019.

In 2006, the government implemented the Private Healthcare Facilities and Services Act of 1998. A license is required to provide HD services in private premises.

Continuous renal replacement therapy (CRRT) for AKI started in HKL in 1984. The veno-venous approach was used, initially with a Nipro single pump system followed by the Gambro AK10. In 1993, the Hospal BSM machine was used and the first prototype of the Prisma machine was acquired in 1996. Commercially prepared bicarbonate solutions became available in 2000. Sustained low-efficiency daily dialysis (SLEDD) started in 2006. CRRT, SLEDD, and HD have superseded PD in intensive care units (ICUs) in major hospitals as modalities to treat AKI.

With the increase of services, there was a need for more nephrologists and nurses/medical assistants. The number of nephrologists has increased from a handful in 1985 to nearly 200 in 2019. Similarly, the number of renal-trained nurses/medical assistants has gone up from a handful in the mid-1980s to nearly 4000 in 2016.

Unlike the earlier years, when kidney transplantation from a living-related donor was the only treatment option to stay alive, the widespread availability of dialysis unfortunately led to a decrease in kidney transplants performed locally. KL University Hospital did its first kidney transplant in 1991 and Selayang Hospital in 1999. Deceased donor kidney transplants were not common due to lack of donors. Some living-donor transplants were done in private hospitals, including Prince Court Medical Centre in Kuala Lumpur, for patients with access to personal funding. The first laparoscopic living-related donor nephrectomy and the first robotic living-related donor nephrectomy were done in 2000 and 2006, respectively, in HKL. Primary immunosuppression was steroids and azathioprine in the 1980s. Cyclosporine was introduced in 1987, anti-thymocyte globulin (ATG) and OKT3 in 1989, tacrolimus and basiliximab in 1999, mycophenolate mofetil in 2000, sirolimus in 2006, and thymoglobulin in 2008. The first report of the National Transplant Registry [14], reporting on the annual incidence, prevalence, and clinical outcomes of organ transplants in the country, was published in 2003.

In the 1990s, many Malaysians travelled to India for living-unrelated donor kidney transplants. In the last few years, an increasing number of transplants from unrelated living donors were performed in Cambodia, Sri Lanka, and China. China was the source of many overseas transplants from deceased donors since the late 1990s, but this has almost stopped after a clampdown by the Chinese authorities. The international transplant community has outlawed these hazardous and unethical commercial kidney transplants. Current MOH policy requires such patients to pay for their own immunosuppressive medications.

There is an alarming increase in patients on dialysis with diabetes mellitus. The percentage of incident ESRD patients with diabetes, which has been more than 50% since 2002, has increased to 65% in 2016 [11]. Measures to curb the rising prevalence of diabetes are ongoing.

Several papers on nephrology topics from Malaysia have been published since 1960. In an era of large multicenter research trials, Malaysian nephrologists have embarked on three CAPD trials [15–17] and a lupus nephritis trial [18] within the country. They have also taken part in many well-known international trials [19–29].

The three randomized multicenter CAPD trials were done to compare new CAPD systems against the ones currently used. Their outcomes have been instrumental in changing the type of CAPD system being used in the country. From the earlier days when a handful of Malaysian centers took part in the RENAAL [19] and IDNT [20] trials on diabetic nephropathy, many centers became active especially in the SHARP trial [21] – the Study of Heart and Renal Protection. Subsequently, they continued to take part in large multinational or regional trials, e.g., FAVOURED [23], CANVAS [24], CREDENCE [25], SONAR [26], TRANSFORM [27], EMPA-KIDNEY [28], and IMPROVE [29].

MOH nephrologists published a practical pocket-sized book on RRT in 1999, which is used widely by nurses and doctors alike. This book had its fourth edition in 2017 [30]. Malaysia also participated in the Global Kidney Health Atlas on ESRD published by the ISN in 2019 [31].

## Renal Diseases in Malaysia

The MRRB has collected data since 2005 [12]. About half of native renal biopsies (43%) were for secondary glomerulonephritis (GN) – most commonly lupus nephritis (80%), diabetic nephropathy (11%), and post-infectious GN (4%). For primary GNs, the most common is minimal change disease (33%), followed by focal segmental glomerulosclerosis (31%), IgA nephropathy (21%), membranous GN (8%), non-IgA mesangial proliferative GN (3%), membranoproliferative GN (2%), idiopathic crescentic GN (1%), and ANCA-positive crescentic GN (1%).

## Lupus Nephritis

The most common serious GN seen in Malaysia is lupus nephritis. Observational series on this disease had been quite common from various centers in Malaysia [32–35]. The MRRB reported 2652 biopsies for lupus nephritis between 2005 and 2012 (8 years) in patients >15 years old. The mean age of adult patients with lupus nephritis at the time of biopsy was 30 years. The most predominant age group was between 15 and 25 years old, which accounted for 39% of cases. The onset of lupus above the age of 45 was uncommon and constituted 12% of cases [12].

Based on the MRRB report, lupus nephritis predominantly affected females; the female to male ratio was 6.6:1. In adult patients with lupus nephritis, 35% presented with urine abnormalities, 28% with nephrotic syndrome, 14% with a combination of nephritic and nephrotic features, and 9% with nephritic syndrome. Thirty-three percent had hypertension on presentation. Thirty-four percent had impaired kidney function (defined as eGFR <60 ml/min/1.73 m$^2$) at the time of presentation and 6.6% had eGFR <15 ml/min [12].

Seventy-nine percent of biopsy-proven lupus nephritis was proliferative (i.e., class III&III+V or IV&IV+V). Class IV and class IV in combination with class V lupus nephritis was the predominant histopathological diagnosis accounting for 57% of patients. Classification is a mix of WHO and ISN/RPS as different centers transitioned their reporting from one to the other in different years [36, 37].

Of the non-proliferative groups, class V and II+V contributed 11% of all cases. Mild forms of lupus nephritis, namely, class I and class II, made up 8%. A small number (1%) had advanced sclerosing lupus nephritis (class VI).

There was no correlation between histopathological findings and clinical presentation. However, incidence of impaired kidney function correlated with histology. The proportion of patients with eGFR <60ml/min/1.73 m2 was 65%, 43%, 22%, 18% and 10% for class VI, IV or IV+V, class III or III+V, class V or class V+II, and class II, respectively.

Presentation of lupus nephritis in Malaysia is usually with a severe proliferative form, sometimes with hypertension and impaired kidney function. It is now treatable with newer immunosuppressive drugs and steroids.

One of the earliest trials on proliferative lupus nephritis with mycophenolate mofetil (MMF) was a multicenter investigator-initiated randomized trial of 6 months of induction therapy using steroids and either MMF or intravenous cyclophosphamide in eight centers in Malaysia [18]. This trial started in 2001 and the 3-year follow-up ended in 2004. It showed no difference in remission rate for both therapies and resulted in MMF being registered by the Malaysian Drug Control Authority for the treatment of lupus nephritis in 2006, the first in the world. Some Malaysian centers took part in the Aspreva Lupus Management Study (ALMS), a large multinational trial of MMF versus intravenous cyclophosphamide for induction, and this reported the same outcome in 2009 [22]. Other multinational trials on lupus nephritis are underway.

## IgA Nephropathy

Of the primary GNs, IgA nephropathy (IgAN) is somewhat atypical in Malaysia. It is also uncommon. Over the 8-year period (2005–2012), there were 303 reported cases of IgAN. The mean age at biopsy was 33 years, and 81% were between ages 15 and 45 years. There is a female preponderance (57%). This is contrary to what has been reported in the literature but may reflect local nephrology practice where the threshold to biopsy females is lower due to the high incidence of lupus nephritis [12].

Asymptomatic urine abnormalities remain the most common presentation of IgAN (49%) but 24% had nephrotic syndrome. This is much higher than the 5% usually quoted in the literature [12] and may reflect relatively conservative local practices with regard to investigation of asymptomatic urine abnormalities. At presentation, hypertension was present in 44%, and 47% had eGFR <60 ml/min/1.73 $m^2$. Five-year renal and patient survival were 78% and 93% respectively [12].

The rate of progression to ESRD in 20–25 years is generally reported to be 25–30%, and the local rate measured over a shorter period seems higher. IgAN in Malaysia seem to have a different natural history and progression, and nearly a quarter are presenting with nephrotic range proteinuria.

## Chronic Kidney Disease

Chronic kidney disease (CKD) represents a major public health problem as it is common and has significant socioeconomic and health consequences. In 2011, the National Health and Morbidity Survey (NHMS) found that the prevalence of CKD among adults in West Malaysia was 9.07% [38]. Diabetes, hypertension, and older age were identified as risk factors. A second CKD prevalence study was conducted in 2018 to identify national trends and to extend the survey to include East Malaysia. This has shown a rise in CKD prevalence to 15.48% with majority of cases (6.48%) in CKD stage 3.

The rising trend in CKD prevalence is likely due to an aging population and increasing prevalence of noncommunicable diseases. In addition to the previous risk factors, increasing body mass index (BMI) was found to be associated with the development of CKD [39]. The NHMS has shown an alarming increase in the prevalence of diabetes in the population from 11.6% in 2006 to 17.5% in 2015. Hypertension prevalence has remained stable at 30.3% in 2015. However, the prevalence of overweight and obesity among adults has increased from 14.0% in 2006 to 17.7% in 2015 [40, 41].

Awareness of CKD among the Malaysian population is low and barely improved over the last 7 years (5% in 2018 versus 4% in 2011) [38, 39]. Efforts to control and monitor CKD have included the following measures:

1. Education of public and healthcare providers – a Renal Retardation Program that emphasized early detection and prevention of CKD for healthcare providers and a Kidney Care Program for public education was run in the form of roadshows in every state (2003–2008).
2. Development of local clinical practice guidelines on Management of Diabetic Nephropathy (2004) and Management of Adults with CKD (first and second editions, 2011 and 2018) [42].
3. Development of a National Strategic Action Plan for CKD in 2018 [43]. This has been adopted into the National Strategic Plan for Non-Communicable Disease in the country [44]. This action plan includes stakeholders in primary care, public health, nephrology, professional societies, and nongovernmental organizations. It aims to improve all levels of CKD care from prevention and early detection to the other end of the spectrum, i.e., renal replacement options.

The problem cannot be addressed by nephrologists alone but involves government policy and general practitioners. There have been declared a ban on smoking in all eateries in Malaysia and a "sugar tax" imposed on fizzy drinks or soda with a high sugar content in 2019 [45].

## Acute Kidney Injury (AKI) and Critical Care Nephrology

The causes of AKI are the same as in developed countries.

A prospective, multicenter, observational study of patients fulfilling the KDIGO (Kidney Disease Improving Global Outcomes) criteria for AKI has been conducted in five Malaysian tertiary hospitals for 3 months. Of 21,621 patients screened, 1527 developed AKI (incidence 7%); 209 (14%) developed in ICUs (incidence in ICU 26%). Sixty-one percent were males and the mean age on admission was 60 years. The most common comorbidities were hypertension (58%), diabetes mellitus (49%), ischemic heart disease (16%), and CKD (13%). The commonest causes of AKI were extrarenal infections (27%), pneumonia the most frequent, hypovolemia (14%), pyelonephritis or urinary tract infection (5%), and hemorrhage (5%). A total of 126 (8%) patients required dialysis, and of these, 62 (49%) were admitted into ICU. Acidosis (41%), uremia (27%), and electrolyte disturbances (13%) were the most common indications for initiation of dialysis. On discharge (1212, 79%) or transfer (20, 1%), 897 (73%) achieved full renal recovery, 206 (17%) had partial renal recovery, and 100 (8%) failed to recover. The mortality rate was 16%. Mortality was higher among those who required dialysis (44%) versus those who did not (13%). The median length of stay in hospital was 6 days [46].

In another observational study, on a large cohort in four ICUs in Malaysia, 24% of 26,663 adult patients had AKI (AKI being defined as twice the baseline creatinine or urine output of <0.5 ml/kg/h for 12 h). Of those with AKI, 48% died and 32% of the total cohort had sepsis. Those with AKI and sepsis had a more than threefold risk of mortality [47].

A single center report of AKI episodes requiring RRT in ICU showed that 56% were treated with CRRT, 27% SLEDD, and 17% HD [48].

In a recent survey of RRT practices for AKI in 19 ICUs, 58% used continuous veno-venous hemofiltration as the treatment of choice for AKI in critically ill patients. The mean blood flow rate and effluent flow rate used for CRRT were 189 ml/min and 31 ml/kg/h, respectively. Replacement fluid solutions containing both lactate and bicarbonate were commonly used during CRRT, applied both pre- and post-dilution [49]. Several machines are used for CRRT, including Prismaflex (Baxter), Multifiltrate (Fresenius), and Plasauto (Asahi).

Dialysis was first started in the country for the treatment of AKI, as it is considered eminently treatable and may return the patient to normal health. Resources for dialysis for patients with AKI are therefore provided as a priority and not denied when indicated.

## Pediatric Nephrology

Currently, Malaysia has 17 credentialed pediatric nephrologists for a child population of about ten million. To be credentialed, a pediatrician should have received at least 3 years of training in accredited centers, demonstrating satisfactory performance of patient management and procedures.

Pediatric nephrology centers are located mainly in the more developed parts of the country. Attempts are being made to have these centers located in the various regions of the country. In the interim, pediatric nephrology services are provided by visiting pediatric nephrologists as well as pediatricians with an interest in nephrology. Adult nephrologists who are more in numbers and distribution assist in provision of services to children particularly in the area of dialysis therapy.

The main kidney disease affecting children is idiopathic nephrotic syndrome – the majority of which are steroid sensitive, and other glomerulonephritides. With the country becoming more developed, acute psot-infectious GN due to streptococcal infection is uncommon, but that due to Henoch-Schönlein purpura is increasing in frequency [12]. Urinary tract infections and congenital hydronephroses are common conditions in children that are managed by pediatric nephrologists.

The incidence of RRT in children and young people (<20 years of age) varies from 10 to 12 per million age-related population (pmarp) with a prevalence of about 100 pmarp. However, in children <5 years of age, the incidence is only about 1–2 pmarp, those who are 5–10 years old 5 pmarp, 10–15 years old about 10 pmarp, and 15–20 years 20–25 pmarp [11]. This is partly due to the time needed for CKD to progress to ESRD. In addition, due to constraints of service, including insufficient pediatric nephrologists and that children can only be transplanted when they have achieved a body weight of 15 kg, children <5 years of age, particularly those <2 years of age, are not universally accepted for RRT.

For children and young people with ESRD, 42% are due to GN and 15% due to renal dysplasia with or without vesicoureteric reflux or urinary tract obstruction. Twenty-seven percent were reported to have unknown cause of CKD. These patients present late and investigations to find the cause are limited or not done [11].

The majority (80%) of children and young people on RRT are on dialysis. About 40% of new dialysis patients are accepted for HD. There are very few pediatric HD units. A significant number of bigger children and young people are dialyzed in adult units. Sixty percent of children and young people with ESRD are started on PD, with over 90% of them on CAPD [11].

Only about 1–2% of those on dialysis receive kidney transplants each year. About 60% of kidney transplants are deceased donor and 40% living-related donor transplantation. Patient survival at 5 years was 94% for transplant recipients and about 80% for those on dialysis. Graft survival was 90% at 1 year and 80% at 5 years [11].

## Renal Replacement Therapy

At the end of 2016, there were 41,525 people on RRT in Malaysia. The dialysis incidence rate was 248 pmp (HD 216 pmp, PD 32 pmp) and the kidney transplant incidence rate was 3 pmp. Prevalence rates were 1159 pmp for HD, 127 pmp for PD, and 59 pmp for kidney transplantation [11].

The highest treatment rates for dialysis are in the 55–64 and >65 years age groups. Eighty-seven percent of incident patients started center HD. Center HD accounts for 89% of prevalent patients, etc. It accounts for 89% of prevalent patients, with 10% on PD and 1% on home or "at work" HD.

The private sector provided 48%, government 31% and NGOs 21% of the dialysis. In 2016, about two-thirds of new patients had diabetes mellitus as the primary renal disease. Hypertension was the primary disease in 19% of new patients, GN and systemic lupus erythematosus (SLE) 3% and unknown primary renal disease 11% [11].

The number of HD and PD centers is 814 (26 pmp). Of these, 51 were PD centers and the rest HD. Of the PD centers, 41 were in the public sector and 10 in the private sector.

In contrast to the economically advantaged and urban West Coast states, where most patients are dialyzed in the private sector, the public sector provides dialysis to most patients in the economically disadvantaged (rural) East Coast states and East Malaysia.

The number of registered dialysis nurses/medical assistants in Malaysia increased from 1808 (62 pmp) in 2011 to 3920 in 2016 (127 pmp).

The annual mortality rate on dialysis in 2018 was 14.3%. The annual mortality rate among HD patients was 13.8%, while PD patients had a mortality rate of 18.5% in 2018 (Registry manager, email: nrr@msn.org.my, 25 November 2019, "personal communication"). From the MDTR report of 2016, cardiovascular disease remained the main cause, accounting for 33% of all deaths. Sepsis was the second most common cause of death, accounting for 28%. Death at home accounted for another 16% and many of these were probably due to cardiovascular events [11].

In 2018, 20.3% of the dialysis population was working either full time or part time, of which 59.8% was full time. Twenty-seven percent of males worked, while for females it was 12%. For patients on HD, 19.9% worked, 58% full time. Twenty-one percent of males worked compared to 11% females. For the much smaller cohort of PD patients 24% worked, 74.5% full time. Twenty-nine percent of males worked compared to 19% females (Registry manager, email: nrr@msn.org.my, 25 November 2019, "personal communication"). Calcium carbonate was the main phosphate binder for both HD patients (93%) and PD patients (84%). Lanthanum carbonate and sevelamer were rarely used due to cost constraints. Calcitriol was the main vitamin D analogue, used in 55% of HD patients and 38% of PD patients. About 1% of dialysis patients had a parathyroidectomy in 2016 [11].

## Peritoneal Dialysis

In 2018, there were 4420 patients on PD (49% male) (Registry manager, email: nrr@msn.org.my, 25 November 2019, "personal communication"). From the MDTR report of 2016, most patients (84%) were on CAPD, 13% were on APD, and 3% were on DAPD (daytime ambulatory peritoneal dialysis). Fifty-nine percent of patients were on Baxter and 41% on Fresenius PD fluids. APD patients were mainly (87%) being prescribed 10 l as total infusion volume daily. Most CAPD patients (90%) performed four exchanges per day and used 8 l (87%) total infusion volume daily. Assisted care contributed to 21% in CAPD patients compared to 41% in APD [11].

The median peritonitis rate was one in 42.3 patient-months with wide inter-center variation. Gram-positive organisms accounted for 32% of peritonitis with coagulase-negative *Staphylococcus* (CoNS) as the predominant gram-positive pathogen. Gram-negative peritonitis made up 31% with *E. coli* being the commonest organism. Peritonitis was caused by fungi in 3.8% and mycobacteria in 0.8%. The culture-negative rate was 24.5% [11].

The incidence of PD-related peritonitis has improved with better connectology and twin-bag system, patient care, and selection. CME from regular workshops and conferences have led to a better quality of trained nurses. Home visits should play an important role in the expansion and improvement of PD program. However, due to inadequate resources and increasing demand, home visits have been carried out on an ad hoc basis. These are arranged to counsel patients and family members and to check the home environment. Retraining of PD technique would be carried out as well for patients with episodes of peritonitis.

Technique survival was 80% at 1 year and 24% at 5 years. For PD technique survival in the first 5 years, the younger age group (age <14 years) fared better than older age groups after censoring for death and transplant. However, after 5 years, the older age groups had better technique survival. There was no difference in technique survival between diabetic and nondiabetic, and female patients performed better than their male counterparts. The top three reasons for PD dropout were death, peritonitis, and membrane failure [11].

For the prevalent patients of 2018, 11.6% have been on PD for 5 or more years (Registry manager, email: nrr@msn.org.my, 25 November 2019, "personal communication"). Thirty-five patients who were HIV positive were on PD in 2018 (Registry manager, email: nrr@msn.org.my, 25 November 2019, "personal communication").

The annual mortality rate of PD patients has been around 15–19% over the last 20 years. It is 4–5% higher compared to HD patients. The difference observed could be partly contributed by the negative selection of patients, e.g., using PD on patients with intolerance to HD or severe cardiovascular disease [11].

Eighty-three percent of patients were on erythropoietin (a median dose of 4500 U per week), with a median serum hemoglobin level of 10.2 g/dl. Fifteen percent were on intravenous iron. Patients on CAPD have a better quality of life than those on HD [50, 51].

In PD units, the current nurse ratio is of 1 to 30–40 patients (Dr Lily Mushahar, "personal communication").

Increasing the proportion of patients on PD could lead to a substantial saving in dialysis-related expenditure [52]. To achieve this objective, a PD-preferred or PD-first policy should be implemented. This idea has been proposed for the past 10 years, but only public hospitals have adhered to it. No financial incentives for PD are provided to the private sector. The uptake of PD may improve if doctors in the private sector are paid in a "bundle" for their patients on PD equivalent to what they receive for patients on HD [53].

## Maintenance HD, Including Convective Therapies

In 2018, there were 38,297 patients on HD. Males made up 54.6% (Registry manager, email: nrr@msn.org.my, 25 November 2019, "personal communication"). From the MDTR report of 2016, 85% had an arteriovenous (AV) fistula, 1.4% used AV grafts, 6.7% cuffed catheters, and 6.9% non-cuffed catheters. Ninety-one percent were on erythropoietin (a median dose of 5000 U per week) and 36% were on intravenous iron, with a median serum hemoglobin level of 10.3 g/dl [11].

Ninety-eight percent were on HD three times a week and 99% of all patients had a duration of four hours per session. Ninety-eight percent were on HD three times a week and 99% 4 hours duration per HD. Eighty-seven percent used synthetic dialyzer membranes and 13% modified cellulose. Mean and median delivered Kt/v was 1.4 and median urea reduction ratio (URR) was 72%.

Bicarbonate dialysate and reverse osmosis water treatment are universal. HD machines are supplied by multinational companies like Fresenius, B. Braun, Baxter, Nipro, and Toray. Reuse of dialyzers was reported in 15,794 patients and 65% reused >10 times. No one reused more than 13 times. Standards for delivering HD in Malaysia are in a document "The National Haemodialysis Quality Standards 2018" [54]. The two previous editions were in 1994 and 2012.

In the latest analysis done in 2017, the cost of a year on HD was RM 39,790, of which 37.6% was the cost of staff, 29.3% dialysis consumables, and 2.4% laboratory tests [55]. The other components included medications 9.1%, equipment 8.3%, overheads 4.4%, access surgeries 3%, hospitalization 2.2%, building and land 2%, clinic visits and referrals 1.1%, and radiology 0.6%. A reverse osmosis water system costs about RM 100,000 and a HD machine RM 45,000.

There are specific regulations on facility layout, staffing, and patient care. For every six dialysis patients, there is at least one renal-trained nurse/medical assistant in each shift. Each HD unit has a "person-in-charge" (PIC) who is a nephrologist. In areas where there is a critical need for HD services, the PIC may include a physician/pediatrician. If this is not possible, any doctor who has completed 200 hours of recognized training in hemodialysis treatment and maintains an affiliation with a nephrologist is the PIC. One of the many responsibilities of the PIC is ensuring that there are arrangements to provide immediate medical care when needed. There is no nephrologist-to-patient ratio at present, and he or she does not need to be in the unit at every shift.

Current regulations in Malaysia require all patients with hepatitis B or C to be segregated in separate rooms. Seroconversion to HCV is rare in HD units, and the overall HCV prevalence has dropped from 11% in 2007 to 2% in 2016. The HBV rate remains static at 3% [11]. Fifty patients who are HIV positive were on HD in 2018 (Registry manager, email: nrr@msn.org.my, 25 November 2019, "personal communication").

For the prevalent patients of 2018, 32.2% have been on HD for 5 or more years (Registry manager, email: nrr@msn.org.my, 25 November 2019, "personal communication").

There is no danger of foreign monopolies developing into the HD provision as MOH regulators demand that ownership of each center must be more than 50% local. The license holder must be a local doctor with training in HD or a nephrologist.

There were very few patients on hemodiafiltration (HDF): 124 were started, with a total of 439 prevalent in 2018 (Registry manager, email: nrr@msn.org.my, 25 November 2019, "personal communication").

## Dialysis Reimbursement

Malaysia, an upper middle-income country with a GDP per capita of USD 10,557 and a population of 32.6 million in 2018, has an active and growing RRT program. Funding for RRT has not been well structured; nonetheless, most patients with ESRD who are medically suitable receive treatment.

The government is the major player in funding RRT [56], and it does so through several agencies rather than a single dedicated bureau. These agencies include MOH, which runs the largest network of government dialysis centers, Ministry of Education (University Hospitals), Ministry of Defense, the Pension Division of the Public Services Department which pays for dialysis of government pensioners, and SOCSO which is a government body responsible for social security of workers. Together, these agencies fund 67% of all patients on maintenance dialysis. The remaining patients are funded by charitable bodies (13%), out-of-pocket expenses (15%), and others (5%).

The role of charitable bodies in funding HD in Malaysia is quite unique. The major charity bodies include the National Kidney Foundation of Malaysia, faith-based organizations, service clubs such the Rotary or Lions, and other groups. Many of these bodies do not just fund treatment but also set up HD centers to cater for the underprivileged who are not fortunate enough to get into government-funded centers. These organizations raise funds from the public and corporate bodies. In predominantly Muslim Malaysia, a major source of contribution for charity bodies is the *Zakat*, a tithe mandatory on all Muslims who have excess income. Contributions sometimes come in the form of HD machines or consumables. Most of these organizations also receive subsidy from the government to help pay for the cost of treatment. The governmental subsidy, which initially covered about 30% of the cost of treatment, had been increased in 2017 to cover 60%. Insurance payments play a minimal role in funding HD (0.5%). The government funds most patients on PD and patients who had kidney transplantation done in the country.

Two economic evaluations showed that the HD:PD cost ratio was almost equal. The cost per life year saved was RM 33,642 for HD and RM 31,635 for CAPD in 2011 (HD:PD 1.06) [57]. The cost per patient per year was RM 39,790 for HD and RM 37,576 for CAPD in 2017 (HD:PD 1.06) [49]. The cost per quality-adjusted life year gained was RM 46,594 for HD and RM 41,527 for CAPD in 2017 (HD:PD 1.12) [58]. The quality of life for PD was slightly better than HD but survival was better on HD.

The total number of patients on dialysis had gone up quickly and so had the ability to pay with a rising GDP. This was helped by the relative drop in prices of machines and disposables due to economies of scale and in some cases ability to assemble or produce the items within the country. Erythropoietin, which was very expensive, is now off-patent with the advent of biosimilar, which is cheaper.

## Renal Transplantation: Organ Procurement and Transplantation Policies

More than 40 years after the start of the local transplant program, the country is still struggling with low transplantation rates from both living and deceased donors. The rate of kidney transplantation from local donors had never exceeded 3 pmp, while the rate of deceased kidney donation had never exceeded 1 pmp. In contrast, the number of patients with ESRD treated with dialysis continues to rise annually, making Malaysia one of the countries in the top ten highest rates of incident and prevalent dialysis patients globally. Malaysia is ranked lowest in the international comparison for kidney transplantation rate per 1,000 dialysis patients, as reported by the United States Renal Data System [59].

In response, several initiatives have been implemented by the MOH. These include establishment of the National Transplant Council and National Transplant Technical Committee (NTTC), National Transplant Resource Center (NTRC) in 1997, and a National Policy on Cell, Tissue and Organ Transplantation in 2007 [60]. Tissue and Organ Procurement (TOP) teams were set up at major public hospitals. These were manned by nurses and doctors to identify patients in ICU as potential brain-dead organ donors, counsel family members on organ donation, and coordinate the organ retrieval process with the retrieval team.

Nurses, transplant coordinators, laboratory technologists, nephrologists, and surgeons were sent overseas for training in well-known organ procurement centers in Spain, Australia, and Turkey. A Renal Sistership Program exists between the Department of Nephrology HKL and Royal Prince Alfred Hospital in Sydney, Australia, aiming to assist the former to develop and improve kidney transplantation services. The program is sponsored and facilitated by the ISN and The Transplantation Society since 2015. Short training programs were arranged which enable experts to visit Kuala Lumpur and doctors to receive training in Sydney.

There was collaboration with official religious bodies at state and federal levels to increase public awareness regarding their view on organ donation and transplantation, especially from deceased donors. Religious edicts and opinions of authoritative scholars of Islam were published and disseminated for public information.

Malaysia is a signatory to the WHO Guiding Principles on Human Cell, Tissue and Organ Transplantation (2010), and a representative of the Malaysian Society of Transplantation participated in the Declaration of Istanbul on Organ Trafficking and Transplant Tourism in 2008.

A health economic research to assess the cost and utility of kidney transplantation in Malaysia was published in 2015.

The study which used micro-costing method showed that the cost per quality-adjusted life year in adults was USD 8826 (RM 30,224) for living-donor kidney transplant and USD 13,592 (RM 46,546) for deceased donor kidney transplant in adult patients [61].

When it comes to living-donor transplantation, many do not believe in it. In a recent study, a sample of Malaysians were surveyed asking their decision on becoming unrelated living kidney donors if the reward was financial incentives. From the 1310 respondents, 72% said "no" on becoming a living donor. The reason "I don't think humans can live with only one kidney" scored the highest (36%) [62].

## Clinical Transplant Practices and Outcomes

Most of the living-related kidney transplants performed were from genetically related pairs. Emotional donors were confined to spousal donation. The national transplant policy disallowed unrelated living donors until 2011 when an independent committee under MOH, Unrelated Transplant Approval Committee, was established to assess potential unrelated pairs for transplant approval [63]. However, the evaluation process was very thorough and strict conditions were applied making unrelated live kidney donation approval difficult to achieve. No altruistic live donor transplant, either directed or undirected, has taken place so far.

Kidney transplantation involving ABO-incompatible donors started in Prince Court Medical Centre in 2011. In subsequent years, HKL and University Hospital followed suit, using therapeutic plasma exchange and anti-CD20 agent rituximab pretransplant to reduce circulating anti-A or anti-B titers to levels below 1:8. Maintenance agents are like the ones for ABO-compatible transplants: tacrolimus, mycophenolate mofetil, and corticosteroids.

Transplantation for highly sensitized patients is not frequently performed due to limited resources, sub-optimal transplant immunology services, and inadequate clinical experience.

In the deceased donor transplant program, a national waiting list of patients is maintained by the MSN. The Malaysian Organ Sharing System (MOSS) was established in 1999 and changed to the electronic online version, eMOSS, in 2006. Suitable patients on dialysis up to 60 years of age and agreeable to be listed in the database were screened for exclusion criteria. At its peak, more than 20,000 patients were listed. A major revamp of the organ allocation system has been undertaken in 2019, given the low deceased organ donation rate and the number of available kidneys never exceeding 60 per year. This uses modified UNOS (United Network for Organ Sharing) criteria, incorporating Kidney Donor Profile Index (KDPI) and Estimated Post Transplant Survival (EPTS), in order to optimize the utility of the scarce kidneys and produce better allograft and recipient outcomes. The new allocation system is referred to as MyKAS (Malaysian Kidney Allocation System).

The total number of renal transplants done in Malaysia between 1975 and 2018 was 2001, of which 1447 were from living donors and 554 from deceased donors. Another 2160 had been done overseas (Registry manager, email: nrr@msn.org.my, 25 November 2019, "personal communication").

The number of functioning kidney transplants in 2018 was 1802 (Registry manager, email: nrr@msn.org.my, 25 November 2019, "personal communication"). From the MDTR report of 2016, the mean age for new transplant recipients was 44 years, 66% were male, 24% had diabetes, 6% were HBV positive, and 2% were HCV positive at the time of transplantation. Ninety-five percent of prevalent kidney transplant recipients were on prednisolone, 61% mycophenolic acid, 50% tacrolimus, 36% cyclosporine, and 12% azathioprine. Even though the use of proliferation signal inhibitors had gradually increased over the years, only 9% of prevalent patients were on everolimus or sirolimus in 2016 [11].

Annual transplant death rate between 2007 and 2016 remained stable in the region of 3%, while annual graft loss varied between 2 and 3% in the same interval. Graft survival rates (uncensored for death) were 92% at 1 year, 82% at 5 years, and 57% at 10 years posttransplantation. Patient survival of local living-donor kidney transplants was 98%, 96%, and 92% at 1 year, 5 years, and 10 years, respectively. For local deceased donor transplants, patient survival at 1 year and 5 years was lower at 92% and 85%, respectively. The most important causes of death at 30% were combined cardiovascular death and sudden death at home, followed by infection in 27% of patients [11].

Sixty-three percent of patients with renal transplants were working either full time or part time, 90% of which were full time. Seventy-five percent of males were working, while for females it was 45% (Registry manager, email: nrr@msn.org.my, 25 November 2019, "personal communication").

## Nephrology Practice in Malaysia

There is a shortage of nephrologists in Malaysia. Currently, there are 179 adult and 17 pediatric nephrologists, equivalent to six nephrologists per million population. They are distributed mainly in large centers with fewer numbers in remote and smaller towns. As there are 814 centers delivering RRT with only about 4000 trained medical assistants and nurses, there is also a shortage of staff with the same inequity of distribution.

To become a nephrologist, a fully registered medical practitioner must undergo a structured training in internal medicine for 3 years and obtain a recognized postgraduate qualification, e.g., MRCP (UK) or Master of Medicine (Internal Medicine). Nephrology training is on a modular system of 4 months each in large hospitals: two modules each for general nephrology, HD and kidney transplantation, one module each for PD, critical care nephrology, and an elective posting, the options of which include research methodology, renal histopathology, transplant immunology, pediatric nephrology, interventional nephrology, and advanced PD. To fulfill the criteria to train for such modules, the centers must have enough procedures and trainers. A trainee usually gets at least two trainers within the 3 years of training. Further training overseas is optional, dependent on funding and ability to obtain study leave. Various places where trainees had gone for their fellowship include the United Kingdom, Australia, Italy, Canada, Hong Kong, Singapore, and Japan.

Nephrology training is either within the local accredited universities or MOH hospitals with an exit examination at the end of it. The exit examination was started in 2003 in the MOH training program. This became a common exam with the universities in 2007, organized by the Malaysian Society of Nephrology.

In 2005, a subspecialty board for nephrology was set up by the Academy of Medicine. From 2017, the board is directly under the Malaysian Medical Council which also upkeeps the National Specialist Register (NSR). The training logbook, report, and exam results of each trainee are evaluated by the subspecialty board, and he/she is granted registration on NSR as a nephrologist hereafter.

Foreigners or foreign-trained Malaysians wishing to work in the country should be fully registered by MMC first. Their credentials in nephrology are reviewed on a case-by-case basis. There may be a need to do some modules that had not been done before. The applicant may be asked to go through the exit examination. There is also a need to be attached to a major center for 6 months for assessment as it is thought that familiarity with local conditions is necessary.

Nephrologists in Malaysia may hold licenses to run freestanding HD centers and have responsibilities rather like the Medical Director in a HD unit in the United States. They not only take care of patients but are also responsible for the smooth running of the HD center.

A post-basic renal nursing course started in HKL in 1984 as HD units are dependent on nurses and medical assistants to carry out the treatment. Other entities including private nursing schools and NKF have started these courses now. Medical assistants and nurses attend a 6-month renal nursing course after their basic certificate/diploma. They are in short supply. For the provision of HD services, there must be at least one renal-trained nurse/medical assistant in every shift with at least one staff who has a certificate in basic life support. The average pay of a renal-trained nurse/medical assistant is RM 48,000 per annum.

Almost all CAPD is done in MOH as there are no financial incentives for it to be provided in the private sector. Perhaps a different reimbursement system needs to be proposed to get CAPD off the ground in private practice. Increased uptake of PD may produce economic benefits and improve patients' access to dialysis [64].

In the case of critical care nephrology and dialysis in ICUs, there are centers where CRRT is done solely by nephrologists, centers where CRRT is run by intensivists or anesthetists, and centers where CRRT is done by both nephrologists and intensivists. This depends on the availability of one or the other. Nephrologists deliver almost all the HD, PD, and SLEDD in ICUs throughout Malaysia. Nephrology being an older specialty than intensive care in Malaysia, the balance is still on the side of more nephrologists doing CRRT. The transitioning to HD and SLEDD involves nephrologists. Management of AKI in the wards is the purview of nephrologists including management of severe diffuse proliferative or crescentic GN due to SLE, acute infections, heart failure, urological conditions due to kidney stones and cancers, and postoperative surgical acute tubular necrosis. Obstetric causes include HELLP (hemolysis, elevated liver enzymes, low platelet count) syndrome, preeclampsia, and abruptio placentae. If the hospital has a cardiothoracic unit, AKI due to post-CABG (coronary artery bypass grafting) cardiogenic shock is also commonly seen. Tumor lysis syndrome is managed in hospitals with large hematology/oncology units and liver failure in large tertiary hospitals and in those with liver units.

The pay for work in MOH for a nephrologist is low, but the range of conditions and experience is very broad. Remuneration in the private sector is higher for less work done with fewer inpatients and procedures. It is estimated that a moderately successful nephrologist in the private sector earns about RM 800,000 a year while those in the public sector earn about half of this. In Malaysia, 72% of all admissions and 85% of outpatient consults are in government hospitals [65]. A search of the National Specialist Register showed that 46% of all adult nephrologists and 65% of pediatric nephrologists work in the public sector (www.nsr.org.my assessed on 8 April 2019). The number of specialists in medicine in the private sector was estimated to be 46% in 2011 [66]. Some nephrologists in the public sector supplement their income by working sessions in the private sector. In the future, if a healthcare financing scheme gets underway, remuneration would be the same across both sectors. At present, there is a public-private partnership with unequal remuneration between sectors.

## Highlights of Nephrology in Malaysia

The rate of diabetes mellitus had gone up drastically over the years along with a rise in obesity and a stable high rate of hypertension of about 30% [40, 41]. It has been documented that diabetes is not well controlled in the country [67]. The challenge is to arrest the increase in these conditions along with promoting a healthy lifestyle in a hope of stopping the increasing incidence of diabetes and later ESRD.

## Future Perspectives of Nephrology in Malaysia

Initially, there was a rush to save lives and to provide dialysis. It is time to refine what is available and to look closely at quality of care. Nephrologists need to know about the management of chronic disease, diabetes, cardiovascular disease, and vascular access. There is a need for implementation of nutritional advice, management of CKD mineral bone disease, and palliative care by training more dietitians and doctors with such expertise.

## Conclusion

In summary, the challenges facing nephrology in Malaysia include the capacity to train enough nephrologists, physicians and dialysis personnel to care for patients, providing for an aging dialysis population with complex medical problems and reducing inequity in dialysis provision. This encompasses recording, auditing, and improving quality and outcome of dialysis, containing costs, encouraging kidney transplantation as the preferred option, and decreasing the incidence of diabetic ESRD.

## References

1. Malaysia. https://en.wikipedia.org/wiki/Malaysia. Accessed on 20 Nov 2019.
2. Map of Malaysia with states. https://id.maps-malaysia-my.com/malaysia-negara-peta. Accessed on 19 Nov 2019.
3. Department of Statistics Malaysia, pocket statistics Q4 2018. https://dosm.gov.my/v1/uploads/files/7_Publication/Infographic/PocketStats/Pocket_Stats_Q4-2018.pdf. Accessed 18 Nov 2019.
4. Economy of Malaysia. https://en.wikipedia.org/wiki/Economy_of_Malaysia. Accessed on 18 Nov 2019.
5. National Health Expenditure 1997–2017. http://www.moh.gov.my/moh/resources/Penerbitan/Penerbitan%20Utama/MNHA/Pembentangan_Mesyuarat_Jawatankuasa_Pemandu_MNHA_2018_-_National_Health_Expenditure_1997-2017_07122018.pdf. Accessed on 20 Nov 2019.
6. Lim YN, Bavanandan S, Tan CC, Zaki M, editors. Nephrology in Malaysia- celebrating 50 years of progress. Kuala Lumpur: Malaysian Society of Nephrology; 2009. ISSN 978-983-44909-0-4.
7. Prathap K, Looi LM. Morphological patterns of glomerular disease in renal biopsies from 1000 Malaysian patients. Ann Acad Med Singap. 1982;11(1):52–6.
8. Wang F, Wang CL, Tan CT, Manivasagar M. Systemic lupus erythematosus in Malaysia: a study of 539 patients and comparison of prevalence and disease expression in different racial and gender groups. Lupus. 1997;6(3):248–53.
9. Lam KL, Tan KK. Percutaneous renal biopsy as a diagnostic aid. J Singapore Paediatr Soc. 1968;10(2):118–22.
10. Goh BL. Nephrologist-initiated peritoneal dialysis catheter insertion programme: a new paradigm shift. Contrib Nephrol. 2017;189:79–8. Epub 2016 Dec 12. Review.
11. Wong HS, Goh BL, editors. 24th Report of the Malaysian Dialysis and Transplant 2016. 2018. https://www.msn.org.my/nrr/mdtr2016.jsp.
12. Rosnawati Y, Wan Jazilah WI, editors. 5th Report of the Malaysian Registry of Renal Biopsy 2012. 2014. https://www.msn.org.my/nrr/mrrb_2012.jsp.
13. Wong HS. Malaysian organ sharing system (MOSS). Med J Malaysia. 1999;54(4):537–8.
14. Hooi LS, Chandramalar R, editors. 12th Report of the National Transplant Registry Malaysia 2015. 2018. http://www.mst.org.my/ntrsite/donwload/report2015/2015_NTR_Full_Report.pdf.
15. Ong LM, Lim TO, Hooi LS, Morad Z, Tan PC, Wong HS, et al. A randomized, multicenter, open-label trial to establish therapeutic equivalence between the Carex and Ultra disconnect systems in patients on continuous ambulatory peritoneal dialysis. Perit Dial Int. 2003;23(Suppl 2):S139–43.
16. Wong HS, Ong LM, Lim TO, Hooi LS, Morad Z, Ghazalli R, et al. A randomized, multicenter, open-label trial to determine peritonitis rate, product defect, and technique survival between ANDY-Disc and UltraBag in patients on CAPD. Am J Kidney Dis. 2006;48(3):464–72.
17. Mak WY, Ong LM, Goh BL, Bavanandan S, Mushahar L, Chin TL, et al. Protocol for a randomised, open-label, parallel group, multicentre controlled study to evaluate the clinical performance and safety of Stay Safe Link compared with Stay Safe in patients with end-stage kidney disease on continuous ambulatory peritoneal dialysis. BMJ Open. 2019;9:e024589. https://doi.org/10.1136/bmjopen-2018-024589.
18. Ong LM, Hooi LS, Lim TO, Goh BL, Ahmad G, Ghazalli R, et al. Randomized controlled trial of pulse intravenous cyclophosphamide versus mycophenolate mofetil in the induction therapy of proliferative lupus nephritis. Nephrology (Carlton). 2005;10(5):504–10.
19. Brenner BM, Cooper ME, de Zeeuw D, Keane WF, Mitch WE, Parving HH, RENAAL Study Investigators, et al. Effects of losartan on renal and cardiovascular outcomes in patients with type 2 diabetes and nephropathy. N Engl J Med. 2001;345(12):861–9.
20. Lewis EJ, Hunsicker LG, Clarke WR, Berl T, Pohl MA, Lewis JB, Collaborative Study Group, et al. Renoprotective effect of the angiotensin-receptor antagonist irbesartan in patients with nephropathy due to type 2 diabetes. N Engl J Med. 2001;345(12):851–60.
21. Baigent C, Landray MJ, Reith C, Emberson J, Wheeler DC, Tomson C, SHARP Investigators, et al. The effects of lowering LDL cholesterol with simvastatin plus ezetimibe in patients with chronic kidney disease (Study of Heart and Renal Protection): a randomised placebo-controlled trial. Lancet. 2011;377(9784):2181–92.
22. Appel GB, Contreras G, Dooley MA, Ginzler EM, Isenberg D, Jayne D, Aspreva Lupus Management Study Group, et al. Mycophenolate

mofetil versus cyclophosphamide for induction treatment of lupus nephritis. J Am Soc Nephrol. 2009;20(5):1103–12.

23. Irish AB, Viecelli AK, Hawley CM, Hooi LS, Pascoe EM, Paul-Brent PA, Omega-3 Fatty Acids (Fish Oils) and Aspirin in Vascular Access Outcomes in Renal Disease (FAVOURED) Study Collaborative Group, et al. Effect of fish oil supplementation and aspirin use on arteriovenous fistula failure in patients requiring hemodialysis: a randomized clinical trial. JAMA Intern Med. 2017;177(2):184–93.
24. Neal B, Perkovic V, Mahaffey KW, de Zeeuw D, Fulcher G, Erondu N, CANVAS Program Collaborative Group, et al. Canagliflozin and cardiovascular and renal events in type 2 diabetes. N Engl J Med. 2017;377(7):644–57.
25. Perkovic V, Jardine M, Neal B, Bompoint S, Heerspink H, Charytan D, for the CREDENCE Trial Investigators, et al. Canagliflozin and renal outcomes in type 2 diabetes and nephropathy. N Engl J Med. 2019; https://doi.org/10.1056/NEJMoa1811744.
26. Heerspink HJL, Andress DL, Bakris G, Brennan JJ, Correa-Rotter R, Dey J, et al. Rationale and protocol of the Study Of diabetic Nephropathy with AtRasentan (SONAR) trial: a clinical trial design novel to diabetic nephropathy. Diabetes Obes Metab. 2018;20(6):1369–76.
27. Pascual J, Berger SP, Witzke O, Tedesco H, Mulgaonkar S, Qazi Y, TRANSFORM Investigators, et al. Everolimus with reduced calcineurin inhibitor exposure in renal transplantation. J Am Soc Nephrol. 2018;29(7):1979–91.
28. Herrington WG, Preiss D, Haynes R, von Eynatten M, Staplin N, Hauske SJ, et al. The potential for improving cardio-renal outcomes by sodium-glucose co-transporter-2 inhibition in people with chronic kidney disease: a rationale for the EMPA-KIDNEY study. Clin Kidney J. 2018;11(6):749–61.
29. Lioufas N, Toussaint ND, Pedagogos E, Elder G, Badve SV, Pascoe E, IMPROVE-CKD Writing Committee, et al. Can we IMPROVE cardiovascular outcomes through phosphate lowering in CKD? Rationale and protocol for the IMpact of Phosphate Reduction On Vascular End-points in Chronic Kidney Disease (IMPROVE-CKD) study. BMJ Open. 2019;9(2):e024382. https://doi.org/10.1136/bmjopen-2018-024382.
30. Hooi LS, Lily M, Ong LM, Visvanathan R, Wong HS, editors. Renal replacement therapy. 4th ed. Kuala Lumpur: Postgraduate Renal Society of Malaysia; 2017. ISBN: 978-983-44908-0-5.
31. Bello AK, Levin A, Lunney M, Osman MA, Ye F, Ashuntantang G, et al. Global kidney health atlas: a report by the International Society of Nephrology on the global burden of end-stage kidney disease and capacity for kidney replacement therapy and conservative care across world countries and regions. Brussels: International Society of Nephrology; 2019.
32. Wang F, Looi LM. Systemic lupus erythematosus with membranous lupus nephropathy in Malaysian patients. Q J Med. 1984;53(210):209–26.
33. Kong N, Cheong IK, Chong SM, Suleiman AB, Morad Z, Lajin I, et al. Pattern of lupus nephritis in Malaysia. Med J Malaysia. 1988;43(3):200–5.
34. Chan AY, Hooi LS. Outcome of 85 lupus nephritis patients treated with intravenous cyclophosphamide: a single centre 10-year experience. Med J Malaysia. 2000;55(1):14–20.
35. Yeap SS, Chow SK, Manivasagar M, Veerapen K, Wang F. Mortality patterns in Malaysian systemic lupus erythematosus patients. Med J Malaysia. 2001;56(3):308–12.
36. Churg J, Sobin LH. Renal disease: classification and atlas of glomerular disease. Tokyo, New York: Igaku-Shoin; 1982.
37. Weening JJ, D'Agati VD, Schwartz MM, Seshan SV, Alpers CE, Appel GB, International Society of Nephrology Working Group on the Classification of Lupus Nephritis, Renal Pathology Society Working Group on the Classification of Lupus Nephritis, et al. The classification of glomerulonephritis in systemic lupus erythematosus revisited. J Am Soc Nephrol. 2004;15(2):241–50.
38. Hooi LS, Ong LM, Ghazali A, Bavanandan S, Noor Aini A, Balkish N, et al. A population-based study measuring the prevalence of chronic kidney disease among adults in West Malaysia. Kidney Int. 2013;84(5):1034–40.
39. Bavanandan S, Saminathan T, Hooi LS, Yusoff MF, Ong LM, Shakira W, et al. Is chronic kidney disease on the rise in Malaysia? Findings from a nationwide study. SAT-212, poster session, 13 April 2019 12.27 pm, at World Congress in Nephrology, Melbourne 2019, Melbourne 12–15 April 2019.
40. Institute for Public Health (IPH). The Third National Health and Morbidity Survey (NHMSIII) 2006, Diabetes mellitus. Malaysia: Ministry of Health; 2008. ISBN: 978-983-3887-17-0.
41. Institute for Public Health (IPH). National Health and Morbidity Survey 2015 (NHMS 2015). Vol. II: Non-communicable diseases, risk factors & other health problems; Ministry of Health, Malaysia, MOH/S/IKU/52.15 (RR); 2015. ISBN: 978-983-2387-23-7.
42. Ministry of Health Malaysia. Management of chronic kidney disease in adults. In: Clinical practice guidelines 2018. 2nd ed. MOH/P/PAK/394.18(GU). ISBN: 978-967-2173-39-7. http://www.moh.gov.my/moh/penerbitan/CPG/CPG%20Management%20of%20Chronic%20Kidney%20%20Disease%20(Second%20Edition).pdf. Accessed on 14 May 2019.
43. Feisul IM, Bavanandan S, editors. Ministry of Health 2018. National Healthy Kidneys Action Plan (ACT-KID) 2018–2025. National Action Plan for Healthy Kidneys. 1st ed. 2018. ISBN 978-967-2173-58-8. http://www.moh.gov.my/moh/resources/Penerbitan/Rujukan/NCD/National%20Strategic%20Plan/act_kid-1-min.pdf. Accessed on 8 Apr 2019.
44. Ministry of Health, Malaysia 2016. National Strategic Plan for Non-Communicable Disease (NSPNCD) 2016–2025. 1st ed. 2016. ISBN 978-967-0769-82-0.
45. Ministry of Finance Malaysia. Budget 2019. http://www.treasury.gov.my/pdf/budget/speech/bs19.pdf. Accessed on 14 May 2019.
46. Goh CY, Visvanathan R, Ong LM, Manocha AB, Mushahar L, Goh BL, et al. A prospective multicenter, observational study to determine the incidence and outcome of acute kidney injury among hospitalized patients in Malaysia. KI Rep. 2017;2:S14.
47. Ralib AM, Nanyan S, Ramly NF, Lim CH, Tan CC, Mat Nor MB. Acute kidney injury in Malaysian intensive care setting: incidences, risk factors, and outcome. Indian J Crit Care Med. 2018;22(12):831–5.
48. Malini S, Rodiana I, Asmahani H, Jane S, Sara Y, Mulok H, et al. Acute renal replacement therapy in intensive care setting: a single tertiary centre experience. KI Rep. 2017;2:S39.
49. Jamal JA, Mat-Nor MB, Mohamad-Nor FS, Udy AA, Lipman J, Roberts JA. A national survey of renal replacement therapy prescribing practice for acute kidney injury in Malaysian intensive care units. Nephrology (Carlton). 2014;19(8):507–12.
50. Liu WJ, Musa R, Chew TF, Lim CT, Morad Z, Bujang A. Quality of life in dialysis: a Malaysian perspective. Hemodial Int. 2014;18(2):495–506.
51. Surendra NK, Abdul Manaf MR, Hooi LS, Bavanandan S, Mohamad Nor FS, Firdaus Khan SS, et al. Health related quality of life of dialysis patients in Malaysia: haemodialysis versus continuous ambulatory peritoneal dialysis. BMC Nephrol. 2019a;20:151. https://doi.org/10.1186/s12882-019-1326-x.
52. Bavanandan S, Ahmad G, Teo AH, Chen L, Liu FX. Budget impact analysis of peritoneal dialysis versus conventional in-center hemodialysis in Malaysia. Value Health Reg Issues. 2016;9:8–14.

53. Sloan C, Coffman C, Sanders L, Maciejewski M, Lee S-Y et al. Trends in peritoneal dialysis use in the United States after Medicare payment reform. Clin J Am Soc Nephrol. 2019;CJN.05910519. https://doi.org/10.2215/CJN.05910519.
54. Ong LM, Hooi LS, editors. The national haemodialysis quality standards 2018. MOH/P/PAK/395.18(QAP). ISBN 978-967-217322-9. Accessed at https://www.msn.org.my/msn/Doc/PublicDoc_PB/National_Haemodialysis_Quality_Standards_2018.pdf on 16 Nov 2019.
55. Surendra NK, Abdul Manap MR, Hooi LS, Bavanandan S, Mohamad Nor FS, Firdaus Khan SS, et al. The cost of dialysis in Malaysia: haemodialysis and continuous ambulatory peritoneal dialysis. Malaysian J Public Health Med. 2018;18(2):70–81.
56. Morad Z, Choong HL, Tungsanga K, Suhardjono. Funding renal replacement therapy in Southeast Asia: building public-private partnerships in Singapore, Malaysia, Thailand, and Indonesia. Am J Kidney Dis. 2015;65(5):799–805.
57. Hooi LS, Lim TO, Goh A, Wong HS, Tan CC, Ghazali A, et al. Economic evaluation of centre haemodialysis and continuous ambulatory peritoneal dialysis in Ministry of Health hospitals Malaysia. Nephrology (Carlton). 2005;10(1):25–32.
58. Surendra NK, Abdul Manaf MR, Hooi LS, Bavanandan S, Mohamad Nor FS, Firdaus Khan SS, et al. Cost utility analysis of end stage renal disease treatment in Ministry of Health dialysis centres, Malaysia: hemodialysis versus continuous ambulatory peritoneal dialysis. PLoS One. 2019b;14(10):e0218422. https://doi.org/10.1371/journal.pone.0218422. eCollection 2019.
59. United States Renal Data System 2018 annual data report. Vol. 2, Chapter 11 International comparisons. https://www.usrds.org/20px18/view/v2_11.as. Accessed on 2 May 2019.
60. National Organ, Tissue and Cell Transplantation Policy. Medical Development Division, Ministry of Health Malaysia. 2007. MOH/P/PAK/131.07 (BP).
61. Bavanandan S, Yap YC, Ahmad G, Wong HS, Azmi S, Goh A. The cost and utility of renal transplantation in Malaysia. Transplant Direct. 2015;1(10):e45. https://doi.org/10.1097/TXD.0000000000000553.
62. Tumin M, Rasiah R, Noh A, Satar NM, Chong CS, Lim SK, et al. Living kidney donation: the importance of public education. Clin Transpl. 2014;28(4):423–7.
63. Unrelated living organ donation, policy and procedures. Medical Development Division, Ministry of Health Malaysia. 2011. ISBN 978-983-3433-99-5.
64. Abdul Manaf MR, Surendra NK, Abdul Gafor AH, Hooi LS, Bavanandan S. Dialysis provision and implications of health economics on peritoneal dialysis utilization: a review from a Malaysian perspective. Int J Nephrol. 2017;5819629 https://doi.org/10.1155/2017/5819629. Epub 2017 Oct 31.
65. Health Facts 2017, Ministry of Health. http://vlib.moh.gov.my/cms/documentstorage/com.tms.cms.document.Document_77d75374-a0188549-16992bd0-76fb713b/HEALTH%20FACTS%202017.pdf. Accessed on 8 Apr 2019.
66. Faizah A, Kamilah D, Sivasampu S, Tahrani PK, Kasturi M. National Clinical Research Centre, Kuala Lumpur. Distribution of clinical specialists in Malaysian hospitals. http://www.crc.gov.my/nhsi/wp-content/uploads/document/Distribuation_of_Clinical_Specialist_in_Malaysia.pdf. Accessed on 15 May 2019.
67. Feisul MI, Azmi S, editors. National diabetes registry report, Vol. 1, 2009–2012. Kuala Lumpur: Ministry of Health Malaysia; 2013. www.moh.gov.my/index.php/pages/view/115?mid=53. Accessed on 15 May 2019.

# Nephrology in Pakistan

# 27

Rubina Naqvi and Seema Hashmi

| | |
|---|---|
| Area[1] | 770,875 Km$^2$ |
| Population[1] | 220.892 million (2020) |
| Capital | Islamabad |
| Three most populated cities | 1. Karachi<br>2. Lahore<br>3. Faisalabad |
| Official languages | English, Urdu |
| Gross domestic product (GDP)[2] | 312.57 billion USD (2018) |
| GDP per capita[2] | 1196.60 USD (2018) |
| Human development index (HDI) | 0.562 (2017) |
| Official currency | Pakistani rupee (PKR) |
| Total number of nephrologists | 150 |
| National society of nephrology | Pakistan Society of Nephrology<br>www.psn.com.pk |
| Incidence of end-stage renal disease | 2018 – 15 ppm |
| Prevalence of end-stage renal disease | 2018 – 49 ppm |
| Total number of patients on dialysis (all modalities) | 2017 – ~9000 – 10,000<br>2018 – ~10,000 – 10,500 |
| Number of patients on hemodialysis | 2017 – ~8800 – 9800<br>2018 – ~9800 – 10,300 |
| Number of patients on peritoneal dialysis | 2017 – ~150 – 200<br>2018 – ~150 – 200 |
| Number of renal transplantations per year | 2017 – ~350 – 500<br>2018 – ~350 – 500 |

1. https://www.worldometers.info/world-population/pakistan-population/
2. https://tradingeconomics.com/pakistan/gdp-per-capita

R. Naqvi (✉)
Department of Nephrology,
Sindh Institute of Urology and Transplantation (SIUT),
Karachi, Pakistan

S. Hashmi
Department of Pediatric Nephrology,
Sindh Institute of Urology and Transplantation (SIUT),
Karachi, Pakistan

## Introduction

Located on the continent of Asia, Pakistan covers 770,875 km$^2$ of land and 25,220 km$^2$ of water, making it the 36th largest nation in the world with a total area of 796,095 km$^2$ [1]. Pakistan shares an eastern border with India and a northeastern border with China. Iran makes up the country's southwest border, and Afghanistan runs along its western and northern edge. The Arabian Sea is Pakistan's southern boundary with 1064 km of coastline. Pakistan geologically overlaps with both Indian and Eurasian tectonic plates. The Northern areas have 5 of the world's 17 highest peaks, along with the highest range of mountains, the Himalayas and Karakoram, as well as extensive glaciers [2].

The country of Pakistan has a history that dates back to almost 2500 years B.C. In ancient times of the Indus valley civilization, it was considered to be one of the most advanced and highly developed civilizations. Finally, Pakistan became an independent state on August 14, 1947. It has four different provinces: Punjab, Khyber Pakhtunkhwa, Sindh, and Baluchistan.

According to the 2017 census, the country's population is 213.619 million [2]. As seen in Table 27.1, Pakistan has a growing population, with over 50% living in rural areas [3].

According to the 2017–2018 Pakistan Economic Survey, the overall literacy rate, including children 10 years old and above, is 58% [4].

**Table 27.1** Selected demographic indicators for country

| Year | 2014 | 2015 | 2016 |
|---|---|---|---|
| Total population (million) | 188.02 | 191.71 | 195.4 |
| Urban population (million) | 72.50 | 75.19 | 77.93 |
| Rural population (million) | 115.52 | 116.52 | 117.48 |
| Total fertility rate | 3.2 | 3.2 | 3.1 |
| Crude birth rate/1000 | 26.4 | 26.1 | 25.6 |
| Crude death rate/1000 | 6.90 | 6.80 | 6.70 |
| Population growth rate (%) | 1.95 | 1.92 | 1.89 |
| Life expectancy (year) | | | |
| Females | 66.9 | 67.3 | 67.7 |
| Males | 64.9 | 65.2 | 65.5 |


J. A. Moura-Neto et al. (eds.), *Nephrology Worldwide*, https://doi.org/10.1007/978-3-030-56890-0_27

The gross domestic product (GDP) per capita in Pakistan was last recorded at 1196.60 USD per annum in 2018 [5]. Pakistan, indexed 0.562, ranks 150th on the Human Development Index (HDI); only 31.2% of the people are formally employed, and skilled laborers make up 28.3% of the labor force [6].

In the past 15 years, there has been a 14% increase in the total healthcare infrastructure. According to the 2014–2015 Pakistan Economic Survey, there were 1167 hospitals, 5695 dispensaries, 5464 basic health units (BHU) subhealth centers, 733 maternity and child healthcare centers, 675 rural health centers, and 339 tuberculosis (TB) centers, comprising a total of 118,869 beds and a population per bed of 1613. There have been 184,711 registered doctors, 16,652 dentists, 94,766 nurses, 34,668 midwives, and 16,488 lady health workers. It is observed that the tertiary care units in Pakistan are overburdened [7].

A large proportion of people living in rural areas and urban slums are desperately poor with limited access to improved health care. Other sources of disparity include continuing class and gender bias, which puts females and people belonging to certain classes of the society at a disadvantage.

## Brief History of Nephrology in Pakistan

Nephrology as a separate discipline of medicine started in 1970 when the first nephrology facility was established at one of the largest health institutions of Pakistan, the Jinnah Postgraduate Medical Centre, Karachi [8]. Pakistan Society of Nephrology (PSN) came into existence on May 18, 1995, and launched its journal entitled *Pakistan Journal of Kidney Disease* (PJKD) in September 2017. Over almost five decades, nephrology has expanded countrywide, and, as of current statistics, there are 150 registered nephrologists, with many registered for postgraduate program in nephrology [9].

Renal replacement therapy (RRT) was started as intermittent peritoneal dialysis (IPD) in 1970, hemodialysis (HD) was started in 1972, and the first renal transplant was performed in 1979.

## Renal Diseases in Pakistan

Most data regarding disease burden estimates are center-based, and the lack of a central registry system results in poor unanimity regarding epidemiology of any disease in the country. Because of poor health infrastructure, many patients seek nephrology advice only when disease has already advanced to end stage, and finding out the exact cause of renal failure is close to impossible in many of such patients. Those who can either be seen earlier and/or provide a good medical history certainly lead to the assumption that diabetic nephropathy and hypertensive nephrosclerosis are major contributing factors to end-stage renal disease (ESRD). Other contributing causes could be renal stone disease, glomerular diseases, tubulointerstitial nephritis, polycystic kidney disease (PCKD), reflux nephropathy, renovascular disorders, and other irreversible renal failure causes, which could have been prevented with proper medical care [10, 11].

Kidney stone disease is one of top causes of obstructive nephropathy in Pakistan, affecting all age groups. Stones, if left untreated, especially when causing obstruction to urinary outflow, may cause ESRD [12].

## Acute Kidney Injury

The tropical countries are those between the tropics of Cancer and Capricorn; Pakistan lies in this region. A number of diseases are confined to this region, and physicians must be aware of these conditions, even when people have travelled to other parts. The causes of acute kidney injury (AKI) in tropical countries can be due to infections, animal and plant toxins, drugs, poisons, or obstetric complications along with some newly emerging and rare causes for AKI [13].

### Infections

Although any severe infection can cause AKI, common tropical infections are malaria, leptospirosis, salmonellosis, shigellosis, and melioidosis, whereas less common are clostridium, diphtheria, dengue, leprosy, and rickettsia. Reported infections causing AKI, malaria, and dengue remain the most frequent ones for Pakistan.

**Malaria** Malaria is a common tropical infection acquired through the dermal sting of an infected *Anopheles* mosquito. AKI caused by malaria can be mediated through several mechanisms. It may be due to parasitized red blood cells in circulation causing obstruction in microcirculation. Another factor is hypovolemic shock, which can result from hyperpyrexia, sweating, decreased fluid intake, vomiting, and, in some cases, diarrhea. Vascular endothelial changes can also activate platelet adhesions, thrombocytopenia, and disseminated intravascular coagulation. Rise in inflammatory cytokines particularly tumor necrosis factor α, interferon γ, interleukins 1,4,6,8, endothelial leukocyte adhesion molecules-1, and intracellular adhesion molecules-1 is well established [14–17].

Though AKI has been mostly reported with *P. falciparum* in the literature, it can result from *P.vivax* as well

[14, 17, 18]. In a large published series [17], it was reported that malaria contributes to 12% of total AKI, while 59% of malarial AKI are falciparum and 16% vivax, and some reported having dual infection with both species. The prognosis in malarial AKI reported in a large series of 671 cases in Pakistan [17] showed complete recovery in 65% and death during acute illness in 21% of patients. Hyperkalemia, deranged liver functions, and altered sensorium were reported as indicators of poor prognosis in terms of death in patients with falciparum malaria associated with AKI [17, 18].

**Dengue** Dengue is an important viral infection transmitted through mosquito bites. It is widely spread in tropics and subtropical countries. Reported incidence is 50–100 million new cases every year across the globe [19, 20]. The first case of dengue in Pakistan was reported in 1982 [21]. Dengue can affect various organs simultaneously or one at a time; involvement of liver, hematological, nervous, and respiratory system has been widely reported [22]. A spectrum of renal involvement reported with dengue infection ranges from proteinuria, glomerulonephritis (GN), IgA nephropathy, to AKI [23]. AKI is mainly associated with hemorrhagic fever and shock syndrome and may present as part of multi-organ failure. Transient disruption in the function of endothelial layer is characteristic of dengue infection, which eventually leads to multiple consequences [19]. A Pakistani study comprising 43 patients with dengue-associated AKI reported complete recovery in 37 (86%) and death during acute phase in 6 cases (14%) [24].

**Leptospirosis** Leptospirosis has been widely studied in many Asian countries except Pakistan. Therefore, limited Pakistani literature on serum-prevalence studies is available. In a published study, the prevalence of leptospirosis during different months of the year revealed its highest number of cases in March, April, and August [25]. In the literature search for leptospirosis-associated AKI in Pakistan, no published report was found. In addition, salmonellosis causing AKI in country is nonexistent in the literature.

## Toxins

Use of certain poisonous substances for self-harm, accidental, or professional exposure may result in AKI. Paraphenylene diamine (PPD), methanol, organophosphorus compounds, phenobarbitone, benzodiazepines, paraquat, copper sulfate, tartaric acid, datura, and rat killer are the most common substances reported to be associated with AKI in Pakistan. In a published study of 184 patients with AKI secondary to poisoning, 133 recovered, and 37 died during acute illness [26].

**Paraphenylene Diamine Poisoning** PPD is an organic compound, a derivative of analine, with the formula C6H4(NH2)2. Human exposure is primarily through hair dyes and fortified "henna" which is used for tattooing. Occupational exposure is through photocopying and printing inks, black rubber, lithography plates, etc. [27]. PPD can cause local symptoms, particularly contact dermatitis in sensitive cases, oropharyngeal edema; rhabdomyolysis and AKI have been reported after oral intake. PPD ingestion is followed by complex reactions, leading to formation of several intermediate oxidation compounds. However, the major product is Bondrowski's base, which is an allergen, mutagenic, and highly toxic [28]. Hepatotoxicity is believed to result from direct exposure to oxidized substances. The largest published case series in Pakistan of AKI secondary to PPD poisoning reports 100 patients affected with this poison. RRT was required in 97% of the cases. Complete renal recovery occurred in 77%, while 16% died during the acute phase of illness. Liver functions started improving in 1–2 weeks, and complete renal recovery was observed over 6 weeks (range 2–10) [29].

## Animal Toxins

**Snakebites** Snakes commonly found in this country are (a) Indian pythons, which are found in vegetation near rivers and lakes; (b) two subspecies of cobras, which are found in desert areas, especially in vegetation such as damp grassland, often found around villages or areas with some cultivation; (c) two subspecies of the saw-scaled viper, found in large numbers in dry desert areas, sandy areas, rocky areas, and scrub forest; (d) Russell's viper found around India-Pakistan border in the east and to the Indus Valley in the west; and (e) the Indian krait found in the coastal lowlands in the north and eastward to Waziristan and Quetta regions. Snake envenomation in human, which can be complicated with AKI, remains an important public health problem among rural and semiurban communities in Pakistan. Renal injury has been reported from saw-scaled viper, Russell's viper, Indian krait, and cobra [30, 31]. Like other developing countries, the majority of victims are initially treated by professional snakebite healers, snake charmers, and religious men. Deaths often occur before the patients reach the hospital. In a published study of 115 cases of AKI secondary to snakebite, complete renal recovery was reported in 51% of patients, while 13% of patients died during acute phase of illness. Thrombocytopenia and deranged liver enzymes were statistically significant factors found in the deceased population [32].

**Scorpion Stings** According to published reports, there are about 2000 species of scorpion existing all over the world, most populated in warm and dry tropical regions. Among these, approximately 25–40 species have toxins dangerous to human. More dangerous species have been reported from Iran, Indian subcontinent (which includes Pakistan), Turkey, and Middle Eastern countries. *Mesobuthus tumulus*, an Indian red scorpion, is the most lethal species in the region [33]. Toxicity of the venom is contributed by its proteolytic content and phospholipases A2; each venom contains 50–100 different polypeptides. The renal injury may be caused by pigment nephropathy (myoglobin or hemoglobin pigment), interstitial nephritis by direct toxin effect, rhabdomyolysis, intravascular hemolysis, or vasculitis [34]. AKI may occur as part of multi-organ failure in selected cases. The largest study published from Pakistan is based on a series of 18 patients with AKI after scorpion sting. Patients in this series belonged to Baluchistan, a province of Pakistan. RRT was required in all patients. Complete renal recovery occurred in 72%, while two patients died during acute phase of illness [35].

## Rhabdomyolysis

A series of 334 cases of AKI secondary to rhabdomyolysis has been registered in Pakistan over a period of 25 years, and the authors have reported changes in the causes of rhabdomyolysis. The prevalence of traumatic rhabdomyolysis (which is mainly related to road traffic accidents) remained unchanged throughout the study period, whereas nontraumatic exertional rhabdomyolysis showed decline during the last 5 years of the study, this group mainly included rhabdomyolysis in people who were forced to do prolonged exercise by law-enforcing agencies in most of cases, and the nontraumatic non-exertional rhabdomyolysis showed a dramatic increase due to marked increase of PPD poisoning during the last 5 years. This series has shown a remarkable number of cases who developed rhabdomyolysis after physical torture [36]. Rhabdomyolysis in patients after PPD poisoning have shown good recovery; 77% of patient revealed complete recovery in an average of 6 weeks time [29].

## Obstetrical

AKI, in association with pregnancy, invariably occurs as a result of potentially preventable causes. Availability of healthcare facilities varies widely in different parts of world, even in same region, neighboring countries, or different parts of same country, and can present a wide range of statistics in this regard. In developed countries, the incidence of pregnancy-related AKI fell from 22% in the 1950s to 1% in the 1990s [37]. Published reports from Pakistan revealed 11–36% of total AKI resulted from complicated obstetrics [38, 39].

The development of AKI in obstetric patients differs pathogenically in early or late part of pregnancy or postpartum period. In the first months of pregnancy, prerenal AKI may result from hyperemesis or excessive blood loss, with inevitable abortion, or as a result of urinary tract infection or induced abortion. During the last months of pregnancy, intrarenal AKI is more prevalent, with preeclampsia being the most commonly addressed condition – although pathogenesis is not yet clearly understood; placental and systemic endothelial activation both may play a role. Other causes include HELLP syndrome, thrombotic microangiopathy, acute fatty liver, pyelonephritis, and acute tubular necrosis. Excessive blood loss before or soon after childbirth remains a main contributing factor to ischemic tubular necrosis. While sepsis may cause AKI in multifactorial manner, intrarenal hemodynamic changes, infiltration of inflammatory cells in renal parenchyma, endothelial dysfunction, activation of mediators, intraglomerular thrombosis, and tubular obstruction with necrotic debris may all contribute to pathology [40]. A published study over a span of 25 years from a tertiary renal care center in Pakistan described an increase in the incidence of pregnancy-related AKI during the last 5 years of the study period [11].

# Chronic Kidney Disease in Pakistan

Pakistan is one of the two most populous countries in South Asia. According to published reports, the burden of noncommunicable diseases has increased in recent years, and the estimated number of noncommunicable diseases has contributed to around 40% of all deaths [41].

A population-based study published from the metropolitan city of Karachi, which used albuminuria along with serum creatinine for determination of CKD, revealed a kidney disease prevalence of 16.6%. This study looked for the relationship of CKD with age, gender, history of diabetes mellitus and hypertension, as well as smoking status. Researchers found that none of the potential risk factors was statistically significant for mild kidney disease. However, they found that increasing age, presence of diabetes and/or hypertension, and history of smoking were statistically significant with the moderate kidney disease [42].

Since diabetes and hypertension are important risk factors for the development of CKD, the prevalence of diabetes has been reported after performing a cross-sectional survey in all provinces of country. The total number of subjects examined in this survey was 5433, and the prevalence of diabetes in the urban versus the rural areas was 6.0% in men and 3.5% in women, against 6.9% in men and 2.5% in women, respectively [43].

The prevalence of hypertension was also evaluated by analyzing the National Health Survey of Pakistan in different ethnic groups, and it was found that hypertension was more prevalent in urban (22.7%) versus rural population (18.1%). Proteinuria, which is a marker of CKD, was also evaluated in the same population-based study that differentiated proteinuria in ethnic terms and reported that one ethnic group differed from the others. An interesting observation in this study was that the ethnic group that was more prevalent for hypertension was not equally prevalent for proteinuria [44].

Another community-based cross-sectional study performed in the metropolitan city of Karachi reported a crude prevalence of reduced eGFR of 5.3% and albuminuria of 9.4%. CKD was observed in 12.5% of adults over 40 year of age. The prevalence of CKD and reduced eGFR was higher in women than in men in this study [45].

In the only national registry source of reported causes of CKD, based primarily on available data from dialysis patients (and not including the largest dialysis center in the country), hypertension contributes with 39.78% of the cases, diabetic nephropathy 35.8%, chronic GN 13.4%, PCKD 4%, renal calculus disease 3.2%, and others/unknown 3.7% [46].

The Sindh Institute of Urology and Transplantation (SIUT) data published in 2002 reported diabetes mellitus and hypertension contributing equally with 19.67% and 19.45%, kidney stone disease 7.2%, glomerular disease 9.9%, autosomal PCKD 3.6%, tubule-interstitial diseases 2.7%, renovascular diseases 2.1%, and unknown in 26.31% [10].

Among patients with AKI secondary to GN, according to a published report, 19.49% developed CKD [47]. Similarly, a study on AKI secondary to tubule-interstitial nephritis reported that 14.83% of the patients developed CKD [48].

## Kidney Stone Disease in Country

As Pakistan lies in the Afro-Asian stone belt, there is always a concern about knowledge of the incidence or the prevalence of renal stone disease in the country. A survey done in 1931 in the region revealed a high incidence in the northern part, while south India had the lowest. The highest incidence was in the provinces of Sindh and Punjab; both of these are part of Pakistan after 1947 [49].

A SIUT study published in 2002, which included 18,490 patients with urolithiasis, reported a prevalence of 12%; and the stone composition was calcium oxalate 65%, uric acid and urate 20%, struvite 12%, and others 1%. In the same study, urinary metabolic analysis found hyperoxaluria in 52%, hyperphosphaturia in 12%, hyperuricosuria in 10%, hypocitraturia in 57%, and hypomagnesuria in 34% [50].

Improved technology has revolutionized the management of stones; the introduction of extracorporeal shock-wave lithotripsy, fiber-optic semirigid and flexible ureteroscopes, and narrow caliber endoscopes have expanded minimally invasive options in management of urolithiasis, and people developing ESRD reaching to nephrologists has certainly minimized over the last decades.

## Renal Replacement Therapy in Pakistan

Internationally, it has long been recognized that there is an association between a country's GDP and its dialysis treatment rate.

The first RRT program started with a peritoneal dialysis (PD) facility established at the Civil Hospital, Karachi, in 1970. Subsequently, dialysis facilities became available at hospitals attached to the various medical colleges across the country.

### Hemodialysis

HD was started at the Military Hospital in Rawalpindi in 1972. The Kidney Foundation was established in 1996 by the most senior nephrologist in the country in association with some industrialists and journalists. This foundation worked raising financial funds for RRT in the country. According to their published 2014 report, there were 107 dialysis centers in both public and private sectors, with 891 total available dialysis machines. The dialyzer reuse is practiced in 76 of 107 (71%) centers [46]. Incidentally, one of Pakistan's largest institutions, the SIUT in Karachi, was not included in the published report. It is the largest dialysis center in Pakistan and performed about 28,000 dialysis sessions each year in the late 1990s [51]; this number has enormously increased to 368,754 sessions per year in 2018, with an increase in number of dialysis machines to 368 at 6 different satellite centers of the same institution (unpublished data). According to dialysis centers published registry, dietitians are available for dialysis patients in 17.76%, social workers in 21.49%, erythropoietin prescribed at 54.86%, parenteral iron in 47.30%, and oral iron in 52.70% of the centers. Same report mentioned 59.24% patients getting HD twice/week, 16.55% thrice/week, and 24.21% infrequently/irregularly HD. Doctors are available in 95% of dialysis centers. Long-term HD patient survival >10 years is 1.5%. Among registered dialysis population, 63% are male and 37% females [46].

About 82% of HD patients are getting dialysis via permanent angio-access. There is no strict observation of number of dialysis patients under care of dialysis technician or nurse; it may vary from one to four to eight patients a representative from SIUT has presented at alocal conference Hepatitis conversion rate of 40 % in 2017 while another center from same city of Karachi presentated Hepatitis C conversion rate of 14%. All patients who get registered for HD are screened for hepatitis B, C, and HIV. Most of the dialysis centers have segregated machines or areas for hepatitis B-positive patients and have applied this policy for hepatitis C as well.

Seroconversion for hepatitis C is quite high in dialysis population, ranging from 15% to 40% at different centers (unpublished data). During last year, one dialysis center faced an outbreak of seroconversion for HIV, though no published data can be found on exact figures.

There is no unanimous reimbursement program for dialysis expenditure, but some local government bodies and some private firms do pay for their employees, partial or in full. Private hospital may charge between 3000 and 11,000 PKR per HD session, and reimbursement is not uniform; some bodies reimburse 100% of expenditure, while others do not.

## Peritoneal Dialysis

The first PD facility in Pakistan was established at the Civil Hospital, Karachi, in 1970. In the beginning, only IPD was carried out at most PD centers. CAPD reached Pakistan by 1998. This modality on one hand has advantages of not requiring dialysis machine, can be done at home, decrease need of hospital visits by patients, blood loss is negligible, provides to a great extent a liberal diet (especially, some restrictions regarding fluid and sodium intake), better blood pressure control, and can be done at remote areas with less health facilities after giving little training to patient or one of the family members. Despite the abovementioned advantages, CAPD could not flourish in the country for various reasons, the most important ones being its cost and sustained availability of CAPD solutions. Then, there is the competition with the established modality of HD; it was thought that many nephrologists running their own HD centers would not like their business to be affected [52].

Currently, IPD is practiced on a very limited scale at some hospitals, and CAPD is further limited. Across the country, only 45 CAPD patients (40 adult and 5 pediatric) are registered, with only one company supplying solution with a cost of 21,000 PKR/month for the PD solutions, while a Tenckhoff catheter costs 16,000 PKR (conversion rate in early September 2019 was 1 USD = 156.40 PKR). According to a published report by Philip et al., in Bangladesh, PD costs 1.2 times more than HD, while in Pakistan, it costs 2.7 times more [53]. The source of this information is unknown to the authors (Philip et al.), as our communication with the supplier of Fresenius International Company concluded that PD solutions, if available, cost less for a whole month than getting HD at any private sector facility in the country. Automated PD (APD) is nonexistent in the country.

## Renal Transplantation

The ever-increasing number of patients on maintenance dialysis therapy demanded the initiation of a renal transplant program in Pakistan. The first renal transplant in Pakistan was performed in Rawalpindi in 1979. Since then, the renal transplantation program has gone through various stages of development. At the urology department of civil hospital Karachi (which attained status of SIUT in 1992), transplant activity started in November 1985. During the initial years, transplant activity was very slow, performing less than ten transplants/year across the country. In those years, the neighboring country, India, was the hub of commercial transplants, and people used to travel there to get transplant done mostly with purchased organs and rarely taking their family members as organ donors. After legislation in 1994 in India [54], the transplant activity graph has suddenly risen in Pakistan. While SIUT kept strict sustenance to do transplant with living-related donors, commercial transplant activity increased many folds in the cities of Lahore and Rawalpindi, in the Punjab Province. SIUT started a campaign against organ trade and the promulgation of a law in 1994, which, after overcoming several hurdles, finally was approved as a law for transplantation of human organs and tissues in 2010. Nevertheless, from time to time, the press reports some illegal transplant going on in one of these two cities of Punjab or in province of Khyber Pakhtunkhwa (KP) [55–57].

Currently, at least nine centers are performing renal transplants; six of them are in the government sector. The number in the private sector is not exactly known, as not all of them are performing legal transplants with living-related donors.

SIUT alone is performing the largest numbers of transplants; from November 1985 until September 12, 2019, 6037 transplants were performed. Of these, only 38 were from deceased donors (8 from national deceased donors and the rest of the kidneys were supplied by Eurotransplant foundation, Netherlands). The remaining renal transplants were done from living-related donors. One-year graft survival rate at this center is 92% and at 5 years 80% [51].

A survey done in 2006 at small villages of Punjab, evaluating causes for kidney sale, found that these vendors are living below the poverty line; 66% of them were bonded labors and sold their organs to pay debts or fulfill basic living requirement [58].

## Pediatric Nephrology in Pakistan

Kidney disease is a global public health problem affecting over 750 million persons worldwide. The burden of kidney disease varies substantially across the world, as does its detection and treatment [59]. Pakistan ranks sixth among nations with largest population and fifth among countries with largest youth population. Sixty-three percent of our population is less than 25 years of age, 53% below 19 years, and 35% between 15 and 24 years [60].

Because of complex and costly nature of kidney disease care, its provision is tightly linked with the public policies and financial status of the countries. The current burden of neither CKD nor ESRD care can be entirely publicly financed, and CKD prevention efforts are limited. Collaboration between public and private sector has emerged in order to provide RRT. This partnership has existed for more than 40 years in the city of Karachi, between SIUT and the public sector [59]. SIUT has played a vital role in raising the awareness, at the primary care physician level, about the prevalence and incidence of kidney diseases in Pakistan.

As this awareness honed further, the primary care physicians and even the newly trained nephrologists began identifying a large number of cases in the pediatric population. By the early 2000s, nearly 30% of the patients attending the nephrology clinics at SIUT were in the pediatric age group. This prompted the institution to establish Pakistan's first pediatric nephrology unit in 2005. However, pediatric nephrology services in Pakistan were first offered at the National Institute of Child Health (NICH), Karachi, where pediatricians with an interest in nephrology began offering HD and PD to children presenting with ESRD.

The pattern and prevalence of biopsy-proven renal disease (BPRD) vary across geographic areas, socioeconomic conditions, ethnicity, and age. Although a few reports of BPRD have been published from Pakistan, the true pattern of renal disease is still largely unknown [61].

Mubarak et al. reported nephrotic syndrome with its clinical subtypes as the most common in his series accounting for 69.4% of the cases. AKI and nephritic syndrome were indications for biopsies in 19.7% and 6.5% of the cases, respectively. Systemic diseases involving kidney-like systemic lupus erythematosus and Henoch-Schonlein purpura are rare entities. Further breakdown of nephrotic syndrome revealed minimal change disease (MCD) as the predominant lesion in 29.4% of the biopsies. This is in keeping with several studies around the world, which showed that MCD is the most common lesion in children with BPRD. The next most frequent renal disease in this study was focal segmental glomerulosclerosis (FSGS), noted in 21.8% of the cases. Out of 158 cases of renal failure in children, renal biopsy showed crescentic GN as the most common cause 24.6%, followed by chronic sclerosing GN and postinfectious GN in 12.6% and 10.1%, respectively [62].

Pediatric kidney stones disease remains endemic in the developing nations like Pakistan, affecting children at ages less than 1 year to adolescence. The prevalence rate is high at 5–15% compared to 1–5% in developed countries [63].

The province of Sindh has one of the highest prevalence of stone disease in Pakistan. Multiple factors including hot humid climate, inadequate fluid intake, consanguineous marriages, and recurrent diarrhea in malnourished children predispose to occurrence of urinary tract stones [64]. This has resulted AKI and CKD in 14% and 20%, respectively. It is also responsible for ESRD in 20% of the children undergoing renal transplantation [65, 66].

Tresa V. described etiology, clinical profile, and short-term outcome of AKI in children from tertiary care centers in Pakistan and found that primary renal disease (intrinsic renal) was the most common cause of AKI in 63.8% followed by obstructive uropathy (postrenal) in 24.1% of the cases. Among primary renal disease, postinfectious GN was the most common entity followed by crescentic GN. However, urolithiasis was seen as the leading cause among obstructive uropathy [67].

RRT options available in Pakistan include PD, HD, and renal transplantation. However, the overwhelming majority of dialysis modality offered to patients is HD as most centers are not equipped to impart patient education and training for PD.

Because of the fact that the SIUT was one of the first public sector kidney hospital and the largest, it offers the wide spectrum of pediatric RRT to its patients who represent nearly 50% of the documented pediatric nephrology population of the country [68].

In all, there are about ten pediatric centers spread across the five major cities of Pakistan offering these services to the patients. There are three centers in the country that perform pediatric kidney transplantation.

Until recently aspiring physicians had to travel abroad to seek training in pediatric nephrology, but now five centers have been approved for the fellowship training in pediatric nephrology across Pakistan.

An overwhelming percentage of the pediatric population seeks RRT in the few public sector hospitals where it is made available. There is no government program of cost reimbursement, while it is pertinent to note that less than 1% of the population has health insurance [68].

The Pakistani pediatric nephrology group was established few years back and provides an effective platform for the pediatric nephrologist to interact and collaborate.

Pediatric nephrology in Pakistan has now been firmly established as a specialty, and an ever-increasing number of general pediatricians are seeking placement for this fellowship; however, the magnitude of the patient population far exceeds the available resources in all respects. There is a need to train more people and have more pediatric renal units available, especially in the smaller cities which are closer to rural areas where such diseases are rampant. There should also be a focus of the health authorities on the prevention aspect of these diseases in order to reduce the disease burden in the long term.

## Nephrology Practice in Pakistan

Nephrology is a rapidly growing specialty in Pakistan, and there are two types of postgraduate degrees awarded in this sub-specialty of medicine. One is M.D, which only some recognized institutions can award, and the candidates, after getting trained under supervision of certified nephrologist, go through extensive evaluations of theory and practical exam and writing of thesis which they have to defend at the time of the final evaluation. The other is FCPS, a fellowship degree awarded by a college for postgraduate doctors; the candidate has to take training at a recognized institution under supervision of certified nephrologist and have to go through theory and practical exam and write either a dissertation or publish two original papers in recognized journals. University hospitals or state-run hospitals are in the process of developing the nephrology specialty at each of these hospitals, similarly private hospitals want to install few dialysis machines and little set up of nephrology so that they can earn more. Therefore, every now and then, there are job advertisements for nephrologists. However, a budding nephrologist would be at a loss in the long term if joining some small private clinics and also private hospitals, as they do not pay much, and, then, the nephrologist also has to practice in other clinics. On the other hand, university-based hospitals always provide an opportunity to progress in learning as well as teaching at the same time. Dialysis nurses or trained technicians are in a better situation to find higher salary jobs at private clinics.

## Future Perspectives

We forecast that the global burden of kidney disease will continue to grow due to the increased demand for care as the population ages and prevalence of systemic diseases like diabetes and hypertension is also increasing, contributing to CKD. There is an unequal distribution of the ratio of nephrologists to patients throughout the country (more population residing in rural areas and more nephrologists and nephrology care based in main cities). This is a problem without a simple solution as choice of where to practice is influenced by additional factors aside from patient location. There should be state-run programs together with the nephrology community to promote interest and provide a robust nephrology workforce for years to come.

A well-designed future plan for a selected path to deal with CKD burden will require demands for country's healthcare system and burden on health budget. Without adequate preparation and planning, a progressive mismatch may occur between the kidney care services demand and the supply of a trained nephrology workforce. This may lead to a reduction in the quantity and quality of care.

There is also need for future effective training programs at the undergraduate and postgraduate level and adoption of novel recruitment strategies. Enhanced opportunities for research in the field of the most prevalent renal diseases in the country should be part of the implementation process. Cooperation at international level is desirable, and the International Society of Nephrology (ISN) is already offering different training and supportive programs at availing facilities at sister renal units abroad. Postgraduate in nephrology and opportunities to get trained at recognized renal units are real today; the only problem with these programs is that some of candidates do not return to the home country and thus desired effect not achieved.

One of pediatric nephrology center in city of Karachi is planning to start automated PD (APD) and CAPD in children, as children of less than 2 years of age are dying because of nonavailability of age-matched HD disposables in Pakistan.

## Interventional Nephrology

Nephrologists have to come across some interventions in routine practice, which includes renal ultrasonography, renal biopsy, PD catheter placement for IPD as well as for CAPD and APD, achievement of vascular access via temporary and tunneled catheters, vascular mapping, percutaneous balloon angioplasty, thrombectomy, and intravascular coil and stent insertion. In Pakistan, many of these procedures used to be done by nephrologists previously (the author has experience of doing these procedures along with creation of arteriovenous fistulas and placing Scribner's shunt for dialysis access in the early 1990s). Over recent years, many of these procedures have been taken over by radiologist and surgeons, even though it would be more advantageous for patients if the nephrologists perform these procedures, as they know their patient more than others. Recent data from various countries have shown that a nephrologist can be successfully trained as a competent interventionist [69].

## Deceased Organ Transplant

Deceased donor organ transplant has not yet taken off in the country; SIUT, being the largest transplant center, is fully committed to improving the practice.

There is dire need of making central registry for all CKD patients, along with central registry of all intensive care units (ICU) and trained staff in these ICUs. There is a need for well-trained transplant counselors who can approach the family of the potential donor diagnosed with brain death in any of the registered ICUs. There should be criteria, well agreed upon for the selection of recipient; and, then, this recipient list would be identified from the registry and processed for transplant, all of this in accordance with international standards of care and practice. Organ procurement comes next on the list, and staff would require training for performing the procedure. Further down is the step of transferring retrieved organs from one place to other.

In the country, the public is not very well aware of possibilities and details of organ donation and transplantation, even healthcare professionals lack knowledge about the subject. For increasing awareness among common men and healthcare professional, multiple steps were taken including use of print, electronic and social media, as well as organizing seminars for the latter group. However, much information and education remain to be done in this regard.

Religious leaders, from all religions practiced in the country, were approached and provided with knowledge of science about organ transplantation; many of them were convinced and promised to use this knowledge to help common men make organ donation decisions during life and after death.

## Conclusion

In conclusion, like other developing countries, Pakistan has very limited resources on budgeting and provision of healthcare facilities; furthermore, there is disparity in distribution of available resources. Some institutions have attracted the attention of philanthropists who provide funds and try to reach the poor population of the country to address their ailments resulting from renal diseases; to aid this cause, the government also provides some extra funding to such institutions. Lack of a central registry system is one of the primary obstacles to establishment of a deceased donor organ transplant program; other hindrances are undertrained ICU staffs, transplant coordinators, lack of proper ICU facilities, and poor understanding by healthcare professionals and society members regarding the issue. There is an increasing number of young postgraduates in both adult and pediatric nephrology, and, hopefully, this upcoming generation with more enthusiasm may expedite these shortcomings in country in the near future.

## References


1. World/Asia/Pakistan. https://www.worldatlas.com/as/pk/where-is-pakistan.html. Accessed on 4 May 2019.
2. Demographics of Pakistan. https://en.wikipedia.org/wiki/Demographics_of_Pakistan. Accessed 7 Feb 2019.
3. Population, labour force and employment. Chapter 12. http://www.finance.gov.pk/survey/chapters_16/12_Population.pdf. Accessed on 6 May 2019.
4. Alvi M. Pakistan's literacy rate stands 58 percent. Jeo News. https://www.thenews.com.pk/print/309542-pakistan-s-literacy-rate-stands-at-58pc. Accessed 7 Feb 2019.
5. Pakistan GDP per capita. https://tradingeconomics.com/pakistan/gdp-per-capita. Accessed 7 Feb 2019.
6. Ilyas F. Short roundup of health and infrastructure in Pakistan. 2000–2015. http://gallup.com.pk/wp-content/uploads/2016/09/Report-1-Short-Roundup-of-Health-Infrastructure-in-Pakistan1.pdf. Accessed 7 Feb 2019.
7. United Nations Development Program. Human development report 2006. http://hdr.undp.org/hdr2006. Accessed 30 July 2007.
8. Naqvi SAJ. Nephrology services in Pakistan. Nephrol Dial Transplant. 2000;15(6):769–71.
9. Pakistan Society of Nephrology. http://www.psn.com.pk/members.php. Accessed 7 Feb 2019.
10. Rizvi SAH, Manzoor K. Causes of chronic renal failure in Pakistan: a single large center experience. Saudi J Kidney Dis Transpl. 2002;13(3):376–9.
11. Naqvi R, Ahmed E, Sheikh R, Rizvi A. Obstetrical acute kidney injury: 25 years' experience from nephrology care unit in Pakistan. Open Access Library J. 2015;2:e1778. https://doi.org/10.4236/oalib.1101778.
12. Hussain M, Hashmi A, Rizvi SAH. Problems and prospects of neglected renal calculi in Pakistan. J Endourol Stone Dis. 2013;10(2):848–55.
13. Jha V, Parameswaran S. Community-acquired acute kidney injury in tropical countries. Nat Rev Nephrol. 2013;9(5):278–90.
14. Barsoum RS. Malarial acute renal failure. J Am Soc Nephrol. 2000;11:2147–54.
15. Mshana RN, Boulandi J, Mshana NM, Mayombo J, Mendome G. Cytokines in the pathogenesis of malaria: levels of IL-1_, IL-4, IL-6, TNF-_, and IFN-_ in plasma of healthy individuals and malaria patients in a holoendemic area. J Clin Lab Immunol. 1991;34:131–9.
16. Eiam-Ong S, Sitprija V. Falciparum malaria and kidney: a model of inflammation. Am J Kidney Dis. 1998;32(3):361–75.
17. Naqvi R, Akhtar F, Ahmed E, Sheikh R, Bhatti S, Haider A, Naqvi A, Rizvi A. Malarial acute kidney injury: 25 years experience from a center in an endemic region. Br J Med Med Res. 2016;12(6):1–6. Article no. BJMMR.21471. https://doi.org/10.9734/BJMMR/2016/21471.
18. Naqvi R. Plasmodium vivax causing acute kidney injury: a foe less addressed. Pak J Med Sci. 2015;31(6):1472–5. https://doi.org/10.12669/pjms.316.8859.
19. Simmons CP, Farrar JJ, Chau NV, Wills B. Current concepts: dengue. NEJM. 2012;366(15):1423–32.
20. Malavige GN, Fernando S, Fernando DJ, Seneviratne SL. Dengue viral infections. Postgrad Med J. 2004;80:588–601.
21. Hayes CG, Baqar S, Ahmed T. West Nile virus in Pakistan. Sero epidemiological studies in Punjab Province. Trans R Soc Trop Med Hyg. 1982;76:431–6.
22. Khalil MAM, Sarwar S, Chaudry MA, Maqbool B, Khalil Z, Tan J, Yaqub S, Hussain SA. Acute kidney injury in dengue virus infection. Clin Kidney J. 2012;5:390–4. https://doi.org/10.1093/ckj/sfs117.
23. Lizarraga KJ, Nayer A. Dengue-associated kidney disease. J Nephropathol. 2014;3(2):57–62. https://doi.org/10.12860/jnp.2014.13.
24. Naqvi R. Dengue infection causing acute kidney injury. Trop Med Surg. 2016;4:211. https://doi.org/10.4172/2329-9088.1000211.
25. Saleem MH, Khan MS, Durrani AZ, Ayesha Hassan A, Ijaz M, Ali MM. Leptospirosis: an emerging zoonosis in Pakistan. Pak J Zool. 2013;45(4):909–12.
26. Naqvi R. Acute kidney injury from different poisonous substances. World J Nephrol. 2017;6(3):162–7. https://doi.org/10.5527/wjn.v6.i3.162.
27. Hamdouk M, Abdelraheem M, Taha A, Cristina D, Ionel C, Alexandru C. The association between prolonged occupational exposure to paraphenylene-diamine (hair-dye) and renal impairment. Arab J Nephrol Transplant. 2011;4:19–23.
28. Nevo-Shor A, Abramovich E, Almog Y, Galante O. Laryngeal edema, rhabdomyolysis and acute renal failure following ingestion of 'black rock'. Isr Med Assoc J. 2013;15:519–20.
29. Naqvi R, Akhtar F, Farooq U, Ashraf S, Rizvi SAH. From diamonds to black stone; myth to reality: acute kidney injury with paraphenylene diamine poisoning. Nephrology. 2015;20:887–91.
30. Mahmood K, Naqvi IH, Talib A, Salkeen S, Abbasi B, Akhter T. Clinical course and outcome of snake envenomation at a hospital in Karachi. Singap Med J. 2010;51:300–5.

31. Chugh KS. Snake-bite-induced acute renal failure in India. Kidney Int. 1989;35:891–907.
32. Naqvi R. Snake-bite-induced acute kidney injury. J Coll Physicians Surg Pak. 2016;26(6):517–20.
33. Bawaskar HS, Bawaskar PH. Efficacy and safety of scorpion antivenom plus prazosin compared with prazosin alone for venomous scorpion (Mesobuthus tamulus) sting: randomised open label clinical trial. BMJ. 2010;341:c7136.
34. Viswanathan S, Prabhu C. Scorpion sting nephropathy. NDT Plus. 2011;4:376–82.
35. Naqvi R. Scorpion sting and acute kidney injury: case series from Pakistan. Br J Med Med Res. 2015;9(10):1–6.
36. Naqvi R, Akhtar F, Ahmed E, Naqvi A, Rizvi A. Acute kidney injury with rhabdomyolysis: 25 years experience from a tertiary care center. Open J Nephrol. 2015;5:67–74.
37. Krane NK. Acute renal failure in pregnancy. Nephrol Ther. 1992;12:115–25.
38. Ali A, Zafar S, Mehmood A. Obstetrical acute renal failure from frontier province: a three years prospective study. J Postgrad Med Inst. 2004;18:109–17.
39. Ansari MR, Laghari MS. Acute renal failure in pregnancy: one year observational study at Liaquat University Hospital, Hyderabad. J Pak Med Assoc. 2008;58:61–4.
40. Zarjou A, Agarwal A. Sepsis and acute kidney injury. J Am Soc Nephrol. 2011;22:999–1006. https://doi.org/10.1681/ASN.2010050484.
41. Jha V. Current status of end-stage renal disease care in India and Pakistan. Kidney Int Suppl. 2013;3:157–60. https://doi.org/10.1038/kisup.2013.3.
42. Alam A, Amanullah F, Ansari NB, Farrukh IL, Khan FS. Prevalence and risk factors of kidney disease in urban Karachi: baseline findings from a community cohort study. BMC Res Notes. 2014;7:179. http://www.biomedcentral.com/1756-0500/7/179-90.
43. Shera AS, Jawad F, Maqsood A. Prevalence of diabetes in Pakistan. Diabetes Res Clin Pract. 2007;76:219–22.
44. Jafar TH, Chaturvedi N, Gul A, Khan AQ, Schmid CH, Levey AS. Ethnic differences and determinants of proteinuria among South Asian subgroups in Pakistan. Kidney Int. 2003;64:1437–44.
45. Jessani S, Bux R, Jafar TH. Prevalence, determinants, and management of chronic kidney disease in Karachi, Pakistan – a community based cross-sectional study. BMC Nephrol. 2014;15:90–9. http://www.biomedcentral.com/1471-2369/15/90.
46. Dialysis Registry of Pakistan. 2014. http://www.kidneyfoundation.net.pk/. Accessed on 7 Feb 2019.
47. Naqvi R, Mubarak M, Ahmed E, Akhtar F, Bhatti S, Naqvi A, Rizvi A. Spectrum of glomerular diseases causing acute kidney injury; 25 years experience from a single center. J Renal Inj Prev. 2015;4(4):113–6. https://doi.org/10.12861/jrip.2015.24.
48. Naqvi R, Mubarak M, Ahmed E, Akhtar F, Naqvi A, Rizvi A. Acute tubulointerstitial nephritis/drug induced acute kidney injury; an experience from a single center in Pakistan. J Renal Inj Prev. 2016;5(1):17–20. https://doi.org/10.15171/jrip.2016.04.
49. McCarrison RA. Lecture on the causation of stone in India. Br Med J. 1931;4:1009–15.
50. Rizvi SAH, Naqvi SAA, Hussain Z, Hashmi A, Hussain M, Zafar MN, Mehdi H, Khalid R. The management of stone diseases. BJU Int. 2002;89(1):62–8.
51. Rizvi SAH, Naqvi SAA. Renal replacement therapy in Pakistan. Saudi J Kidney Dis Transpl. 1996;7(4):404–8.
52. Hussain R, Tufail M, Naqvi SAJ. Continuous ambulatory peritoneal dialysis (CAPD) as a model of renal replacement therapy (RRT) in children and adults Pakistan experience. Indian J Perit Dial. 2006;11:10–3.
53. Li PK, Chow KM. The cost barrier to peritoneal dialysis in the developing world—an Asian perspective. Perit Dial Int. 2001;21 Suppl 3:S307–13.
54. Shroff S. Legal and ethical aspects of organ donation and transplantation. Indian J Urol. 2009;25(3):348–55. https://doi.org/10.4103/0970-1591.56203.
55. Choudhury A. Police awaits enquiry report. Daily Dawn. 23 Oct 2010. https://www.dawn.com/news
56. Zafar MS. Kidney sale-purchase business in full swing in Punjab. Daily The News. 13 Aug 2011.
57. FIA busts illegal kidney transplant network in KP. Daily Dawn. 7th March 2019. https://www.dawn.com/news/1468080. Accessed 11 Sept 2019.
58. Naqvi SAA, Ali B, Mazhar F, Zafar MN, Rizvi SAH. A socioeconomic survey of kidney vendors in Pakistan. Transpl Int. 2007;20:934–9.
59. Crews DC. Burden, access and disparity in kidney disease. Pediatr Nephrol. 2019;34:541–8.
60. Mehnaz A. State of children in Pakistan-Confronting reality. JAMA. 2011;61(6):518–9.
61. Mubarak M. Pattern of renal disease observed in native renal biopsies in adults in single center in Pakistan. Nephrology. 2011;16:87–92.
62. Kazi JI. Pattern of pediatric renal diseases observed in native renal biopsies in Pakistan. J Nephrol. 2009;22(6):739–46.
63. Rizvi SAH. Pediatric urolithiasis. Developing nation perspectives. J Urol. 2002;168:1522–5.
64. Buck AC. The epidemiology, formation, composition and medical management of idiopathic stone disease. Curr Opin Urol. 1993;3(4):316–22.
65. Ramazan A. Pattern of renal disease in children. J Surg Pak. 2011;6:4–12.
66. Hussain M. Kidney stone disease: current concepts; causes and prevention. Dawn Advert Suppl. Thursday March 14, 2019.
67. Tresa V. Etiology, clinical profile and short-term outcome of acute kidney injury in children at tertiary care pediatric nephrology center in Pakistan. Ren Fail. 2017;39(1):26–31.
68. Chronic kidney disease in children and renal replacement therapies. Dawn Advert Suppl. Thursday March 10, 2016.
69. Rivera M, Quereda C. Diagnostic and interventional nephrology: an opportunity for Spanish nephrologists. Nefrologia. 2011;31(2):131–3.

# Nephrology in Saudi Arabia

# 28

Abdullah Al Sayyari, Soud Al Rasheed, Fayez Hejaili, and Faissal A. M. Shaheen

| | |
|---|---|
| Area[1] | 2,150,000 Km$^2$ |
| Population[1] | 34,218,169 (2019) |
| Capital | Riyadh |
| Three most populated cities | 1. Riyadh<br>2. Jeddah<br>3. Dammam |
| Official language | Arabic |
| Gross Domestic Product (GDP)[2] | 786.522 billion USD (2018) |
| GDP per capita[2] | 23,339 USD (2018) |
| Human Development Index (HDI)[3] | 0.853 (2018) |
| Official currency | Saudi Riyal |
| Total number of nephrologists | 295 |
| National society of nephrology[4] | Saudi Society of Nephrology & Transplantation www.ssn-sa.com |
| Incidence of End-Stage Renal disease[5] | 2017 – 233 pmp |
| Prevalence of End-Stage Renal disease[5] (on dialysis) | 2017 – 863.4 pmp |
| Total number of patients on dialysis[5] | 2017 – 19,659 |
| Number of patients on hemodialysis[5] | 2017 – 18,270 |
| Number of patients on peritoneal dialysis[5] | 2017 – 1389 |
| Number of renal transplantations per year[5] | 2017 – 921 |

[1] The General Authority for Statistics https://www.stats.gov.sa/en/5305) [accessed June 2019]
[2] Country Economy. https://countryeconomy.com/countries
[3] The World Bank. https://data.worldbank.org/country/saudi-arabia
[4] Human Development Report 2019 http://hdr.undp.org/sites/all/themes/hdr_theme/country-notes/SAU.pdf
[5] www.ssn-sa.com [accessed June 2019] Annual Report Saudi Center for Organ Transplanation www.scot.org.sa (accessed June 2019)

A. Al Sayyari · S. Al Rasheed · F. Hejaili
King Saud Bin Abdulaziz University for Health Sciences, Riyadh, Saudi Arabia
e-mail: RasheedS@NGHA.MED.SA

F. A. M. Shaheen (✉)
Suleiman Fakeeh Hospital, Jeddah, Saudi Arabia

## Introduction

The Kingdom of Saudi Arabia is a peninsula covering a large area of 2,150,000 Km$^2$. Its population is 34 million, of whom 39.6% are under the age of 18 years. The Arabian Sea in the South, the Arabian Gulf on the East, and Red Sea on the West. The capital city is Riyadh with the two main other cities being Jeddah on the Red Sea and Dammam on the Red Sea. Saudi Arabia is bordered by Jordan and Iraq to the north; Kuwait to the northeast; Qatar, Bahrain, and the United Arab Emirates to the east; Oman to the southeast; and Yemen to the south.

Saudi Arabia is the birthplace of Islam and encompasses the two most holy cities of Islam – Mecca and Medina, which attract millions of Moslem visitors every year as part of their religious obligations and rites. The Saudi population is rising at a rate of 4.4% a year and is becoming urbanized very rapidly.

The official currency is the Saudi Riyal, which is pegged to the US dollar so that the exchange rate remains constant at around 3.75 riyals per dollar. The Saudi political system is a monarchy but has a consultative parliament through which major policy decisions have to pass. Free health care is provided by the government to Saudi citizens with the cost paid largely by the Ministry of Health but shared by other governmental medical sectors.

Saudi Arabia is divided into 13 regions, each with its own regional capital. The regions are further subdivided into 118 governorates, which are further subdivided into sub-governorates or centers.

Saudi Arabia is the largest economy in the Arab world and is member of the G20 World Economic Group. Saudi Arabia is the world's largest exporter of petroleum and has the fifth-largest proven natural gas reserves.

The life expectancy in Saudi Arabia is 74.9 years according to World Bank data. It has a high prevalence of adult overweight and obesity, 69.7% and 35.5%, respectively. The infant mortality rate is 6 per 1000.



J. A. Moura-Neto et al. (eds.), *Nephrology Worldwide*, https://doi.org/10.1007/978-3-030-56890-0_28

## Epidemiology and Nature of Kidney Diseases in Saudi Arabia

The Kingdom of Saudi Arabia is a peninsula covering a large area of 2,150,000 $Km^2$. Its population is 33 million of whom 39.6% are under the age of 18 years and 30.4% of the total population are in the age range of 0–14 years [1]. This may be compared to the United Kingdom (UK), in which only 18.9% of the population is under 16 years old [2] and to Denmark in which only 16.4% of the population is below the age of 14 years [3]. Saudi Arabia has a high prevalence of consanguineous marriages; therefore, a high prevalence of kidney diseases inherited though recessive mutation inheritances is to be expected [4].

In 2017, it was reported that there were 18,270 patients on hemodialysis (HD), 1389 on peritoneal dialysis (PD), and 9810 patients being followed up with a functioning kidney transplantation (KT). The prevalence of Saudi patients on renal replacement therapies (RRT) is 1294.3 pmp with a breakdown of 802.4 pmp (HD), 61 pmp (PD). and 430.8 pmp (KT). The total RRT incidence is 273.4 pmp/year; and the breakdown by modality is 211.7 pmp/year (HD), 21.3 pmp/year (PD), and 40.5 pmp/year (KT). The KT incidence when broken down between deceased and living donors is of 6.4 pmp/year and 34.1 pmp/year, respectively.

The estimated prevalence of end-stage renal disease (ESRD) (dialysis dependence) among Saudi children is 59.6/million pediatric population. A prevalence of 51 pmp has been reported in Jordanian children [5] and around 65 pmp in Australia, Canada, Malaysia, and Western Europe [6].

The Kingdom of Saudi Arabia (KSA) has one of the highest prevalences of diabetes mellitus in the world, which has been rapidly rising over the years. It was reported to be 4.3% in 1987 (5.9% among females and 2.9% among males); in the same paper, obesity was observed in 41.2% of the diabetics and in 29.3% of the nondiabetics [7]. Since then, the prevalence of diabetes in the Saudi population has risen to 30% (34.1% in males and 27.6% in females), as reported by Alqurashi KA et al in 2011 [8]. The authors also reported a body mass index prevalence of ≥25 in 72.5% of the general population and of 85.7% among diabetics [8].

In the mid-1980s, the prevalence of diabetic nephropathy among the Saudi HD patient was reported to be 4% [9]. Now the prevalence ranges between 42.5% and 50% depending on the region of the country [10, 11]. In 1999, we reported that diabetic nephropathy accounted for 40.5% of incident ESRD patients [9]; and now it is approaching 50%.

In another KSA study, it was shown that the prevalence of diabetic nephropathy had increased from 2–6% in 1983 to 16–25% in 1999 (fourfold to eightfold rise). Similarly, the ESRD incidence due to diabetic nephropathy increased from 2% to 44% over the same period of time [12].

Saudis with diabetic nephropathy progress to ESRD faster than other ethnic groups. In a study in Saudis with biopsy-proven diabetic nephropathy, a mean baseline EDTA GFR of 44 ± 29 mL/min and a mean baseline serum creatinine of 165 umol/L, it was found that twenty patients (57%) required dialysis within 2 years of follow-up. Four patients (11%) died, and nine (26%) remained off dialysis. The factors associated with progression were found to be high baseline proteinuria, high levels of serum creatinine, histologic severity, lower baseline serum albumin, lower EDTA GFR, and higher BMI [13].

The substantial rise in the prevalence of diabetic nephropathy in KSA is associated with the obesity epidemic that has occurred, including in children. It is estimated that the energy intake (Kcal/day) among Saudis has increased from 86% of the recommended daily allowances (RDA) in 1961–1963 to 140% of RDA in 1995 and the protein intake has increased from 91% of RDA to 162% over the same period. The changes in dietary habits that occurred in 20 years in KSA took 137 years in Japan and 200 years in the United Kingdom [14].

The overall prevalence of overweight among Saudis is 38.3% in males and 27.6% in females [15]. More women (23.6%) than men (14.2%) are obese. The obesity rate in KSA is higher than that seen in the United States, Sweden, Italy, and Australia [16].

The prevalence of hypertension in KSA, as reported in 2007, was 26.1% in crude terms (28.6% in males and 23.9% for females) [17]. In a more recent paper, the overall prevalence was found to be 25.5% with only 44.7% of the affected population being aware that they are hypertensive and only 37.0% of them had the blood pressure controlled. Significant predictors of hypertension included male gender, urbanization, low education, low physical activity, obesity, diabetes, and hypercholesterolemia [18]. In another recent study among Saudi hypertensive persons, it was found that 41.4% had uncontrolled SBP and 34.8% had uncontrolled DBP [19].

There is only one paper that we are aware of that looked into the prevalence of chronic kidney disease (CKD) among the Saudi general population (mean age, 37.4 years). This study estimated CKD prevalence to be 5.7% using MDRD-3 equation and 5.3% using the CKD-EPI equation. CKD was significantly higher in the older age groups, with higher serum glucose, higher waist/hip ratio, and higher blood pressure [20].

Sickle cell disease (SCD) is prevalent in two areas of Saudi Arabia: the eastern and the southwestern regions. In patients from the eastern region, the disease is less severe, as it is associated with the Asian beta globin haplotype, whereas those in the southwestern region have the Benin haplotype [21].

In a study from the eastern region, the prevalence of proteinuria among the SCD population was estimated to be

8.4%, which is much lower than what has been reported in other SCD populations [22]. This is also consistent with the finding that only 1.17% of SCD patients from the eastern region developed ESRD. Furthermore, SCD patients who developed ESRD constituted only 1.44% of the ESRD population despite the high prevalence of SCD in this region. The prognosis of SCD patients developing ESRD and whether it differs from other SCD population has been studied. In this study the survival among SCD with ESRD patients did not differ from the other ESRD population in the same center, bearing in mind that the SCD group was younger than the general dialysis population (46.6 versus 60 years) [23].

Renal transplantation in KSA is carried out under the auspices of the Saudi Center for Organ Transplantation (SCOT). In 2017, a total of 921 kidneys were transplanted wherein 776 were from living donors and 145 from deceased donors. Since the start of the transplant program in 1979, a total of 8401 patients have been transplanted from living and 3108 from deceased donors.

The Saudi population is generally highly religious. It follows the teaching of Islam very closely. This has had an impact on the timeline and history of KT, which is discussed under the section on renal transplantation. Doctors looking after Muslim patients need also to know about the impact of fasting during the month of Ramadan on their patients with CKD, those on HD or PD, and those who have been transplanted; these issues are discussed at the end of the chapter.

While there are a number of causes of kidney failure in Saudi patients on dialysis, as reported in the registry of the SCOT [11], genetic and congenital anomalies of the urinary system are listed as the cause in only 2% and 1.6% of cases, respectively. However, we believe that this is an underestimation and many of the causes listed as "unknown" (7%) or hypertension (38%) may well be due to genetic factors. In one study done in 1080 HD patients from six cities in the Kingdom, it was observed that 21.5% have self-reported first-degree relatives with kidney disease, with no significant differences noted between regions or cities. Although there was higher prevalence in Jeddah patients than Riyadh patients, this did not reach a statistical significance. It is of note that there were significantly more patients with "unknown" or "hypertensive" diagnostic labels among the patients with family history of kidney disease than in the group without a family history (personal communication).

## Spectrum of Renal Biopsy Findings in Adults in Saudi Arabia

Among 1294 renal biopsies done in six large referral hospitals from different regions of KSA, 77.2% showed glomerulonephritis (GN); of these, 72.6% were primary GN. Focal and segmental glomerulosclerosis and membranoproliferative GN were the commonest types (21.3% and 20.7% respectively) of primary GN. Membranous GN and IgA nephropathy were found in 10.6% and 6.5%, respectively.

Lupus nephritis (LN) was the commonest form of secondary GN (57.0%) whereas amyloidosis was found in only 3.2% of the biopsies [24].

A recent study looked at changes in the pattern and spectrum of renal biopsy findings among Saudis over four 5-year-long eras, spanning the last 20 years. Focal segmental glomerulosclerosis remained the most common pathology with constant frequency throughout the four eras (23.6%, 19.8%, 24.1%, and 17.1%). IgA nephropathy prevalence increased progressively and membranoproliferative GN decreased significantly. LN remained the most common type of secondary GN [25]. Reports from the United States also show the dominance of FSGS among primary GN [26]. On the other hand, reports from China indicate the most common GN to be IgA nephropathy [27].

In a study of 99 Saudi patients over a 9-year period with biopsy-proven LN, 35.5% had nephrotic range proteinuria, 46.8% had eGFR < 60 ml/min/1.73 $m^2$, 65.5% had histological class IV, and the female to male ratio was 3.7:1. During follow-up, 28.2% required dialysis. The survival rates at 5, 10, and 15 years were 92%, 77%, and 77%, respectively [28].

Another study on crescentic GN among adult Saudi patients enrolled 72 cases. LN accounted for 49.3% of the cases, pauci-immune GN (PIGN) for 26.5%, other immune complex GN (ICGN) for 19% and post-infectious GN accounted for only 6.3%. The majority (85.7%) of the patients had renal impairment at presentation. By the end of the follow-up period of 26 months, 25.8% of the patients were requiring dialysis (16.7% in the LN group, 50% in PIGN and 25% in ICGN) and 21.7% had nephrotic range proteinuria. Half of the Saudi patients with crescentic GN were associated with LN, which is higher than that reported by others where PIGN was the more prevalent etiology [29].

## Acute Kidney Injury (AKI) in Adults

In a study of AKI from the Southern region of KSA covering a two-year period, 38.0% were community-acquired and 62.0% hospital-acquired AKI and it was determined that the incidence of AKI among the hospitalized patients was 0.6%. The spectrum of the causes of AKI was not different from previously reported in the developed world, except that snakebite and malaria contributed to 4.6% of the causes [30].

Snakebite and malaria are common health problems in the southern region of Saudi Arabia. Although it is a common problem, the true incidence of AKI following snakebite in the region is not known and few case reports have been published [31].

In one KSA study, AKI was seen in only 3% of cases of P. vivax malaria infection [32]. Almost similar findings were reported from Pakistan [33] whereas studies from India and Thailand reported much higher prevalences of AKI in 19 and 21% of patients, respectively [34, 35].

Severe forms of AKI were not observed in the malaria cases in KSA, as severe malaria leading to AKI is usually observed with heavy parasitemia or intravascular hemolysis with or without glucose-6-phosphate dehydrogenase deficiency [36].

Middle East respiratory syndrome coronavirus (MERS-CoV) was identified in Saudi Arabia in 2012 [37] and is postulated to be related to contact with camels. Many outbreaks have occurred since then. This infection is complicated by AKI in 40.9% of cases [38], and the occurrence of AKI is associated with a poor prognosis [38]. This compares to AKI occurring in only 5% during the SARS epidemics in Canada. The high prevalence of AKI among MERS-CoV patients may be related to preexisting comorbid conditions, such as diabetes, old age, and hypertension. The isolation of MERS-CoV from the urine of affected patients suggests the possibility of direct viral involvement of the kidneys [39].

The outbreak of Dengue fever was initially reported in Jeddah 2001. Since then, reports of outbreaks in Jeddah and Mecca in the Western Province of Saudi Arabia have been reported. The common symptoms are fever (100%), malaise (83%), musculoskeletal pain (81%), headache (75%), nausea (69), vomiting (65%), and abdominal pain (48%). 9.5% developed AKI [40].

## Aspects of Pediatric Nephrology in KSA

The KSA has a preponderance of young persons among its population. The prevalence of the age range 0–14 years among the Saudi population is 30.4% and the prevalence of those in the age range is 0–19 years is 39.1% [1]. This compares to the United Kingdom in which only 18.9% of the population was under 16 years old [2] and to Denmark in which only 16.4% of the population is below the age of 14 years [3].

Out of a total of 18,270 HD patients in KSA in 2017, 196 were under the age of 15 years (1.1%) and of a total of 1389 PD patients, 167 belonged to the pediatric age group (12%) [11]. The number of children on PD in KSA has not changed over the last 8 years [11]. The estimated prevalence of ESRD (dialysis dependence) among Saudi children is 59.6/million pediatric population. A prevalence of 51 pmp has been reported in Jordanian children [5]. The prevalence was reported to be around 65 pmp in Australia, Canada, Malaysia, and Western Europe [6].

SCOT – the organ procurement agency in Saudi Arabia – gives a higher priority for transplanting children such that 25% of standard deceased kidneys retrieved are offered to children although they contribute less than 2% of the total waiting list [11]. In 2016, 125 transplants from deceased donors were carried out in Saudi Arabia. Out of these, 88 (70%) were standard criteria donors and 37 (30%) were from expanded criteria donors. Out of the standard kidneys, twenty-one (23.9%) were given to children. The incidence of transplantation among Saudi children on dialysis can be estimated to be 5.9% per year and its incidence among the Saudi pediatric population under the age of 14 years is 3.4/million per year.

## Chronic Kidney Disease Among Saudi Children

A number of reports on the etiology of CKD among Saudi children confirm that the commonest causes are congenital malformation (50–64%) followed by heredofamilial causes in about 12–18% [41–43]. Similar findings were reported elsewhere. In a recent North American Pediatric Renal Trials and Collaborative Studies (NAPRTCS) report, congenital causes, including congenital anomalies of the kidney and urinary tract (CAKUT) (48%) and hereditary nephropathies (10%), were the most common causes whereas GN accounted for only 14% of cases [44, 45].

The rate of consanguinity among Saudi families exceeds 50% [46, 47]. This could explain the commonness of renal hereditary diseases, particularly those that are inherited in autosomal recessive fashion.

One study on 82 Saudi children with urinary tract infection (UTI) revealed that that Saudi children below the age of 7 years, who present with UTI, have a high incidence of vesicoureteral reflux and scarring (41%) [48], higher than what has been reported from elsewhere recently [49].

In a study of 85 Saudi children with urolithiasis, Al Rasheed et al. found that 10.6% had metabolic cause for their stone formation, 11.8% had a predisposing anatomical anomaly, and 17.6% presented with urinary tract infection [50].

## Spectrum of Renal Biopsy Findings in Children in Saudi Arabia

Most of the reported studies on the renal biopsy findings in Saudi children show that FSGS is the commonest histology type found. However, it should be noted that these reports emanated from tertiary care pediatric referral centres in KSA to which difficult cases would normally be referred and thus their findings may be selective and non-representative of the general trend.

In a study of 167 renal biopsies in Saudi children, Al Rasheed et al. found that nephrotic syndrome was the commonest indication for renal biopsy (in 77% of all cases); 23.3% showed minimal change, 24% showed mesangial proliferative glomerulonephritis, and 24% showed focal segmental glomerulosclerosis. The prevalences of congenital nephrotic syndrome and Alport's syndrome were higher than noted in the Western world (4.8% each). However, IgA nephropathy was less common, with no cases of IgA GN found. Only three biopsies revealed crescentic rapidly progressive GN, all of which were from children above 7 years of age [51].

In another study involving 36 renal biopsies, FSGS was found in 39%, IgM nephropathy and mesangioproliferative GN in 17% each, and minimal change disease and IgA nephropathy in 3% each [52]. In yet, another study involving 376 renal biopsies in children with GN, FSGS was found to be the most common (31.9%), followed by mesangioproliferative GN in 26.3%, minimal change disease in 14.6%, membranoproliferative GN in 8.0%, membranous GN in 4.8%, IgA nephropathy in 4.0%, post-infectious GN in 4.0%, Alport syndrome in 3.7%, and rapidly progressive GN in 2.7% [53].

Forty-nine Saudi families with 62 cases of nephrotic syndrome were studied for the frequency of inherited nephrotic syndrome by screening for mutations in NPHS1, NPHS2, LAMB2, PLCE1, CD2AP, MYO1E, WT1, PTPRO, and Nei endonuclease VIII-like 1 (NEIL1). Likely causative mutations were found in 51% of the families, the commonest genetic cause being a homozygous mutation in the NPHS2 gene in 22% of the families, followed by mutations in the NPHS1 gene 12%, PLCE1 gene in 8%, and MYO1E mutations in 6% of the families [54].

## Novel Hereditary Diseases with Tubular Dysfunction Described in Saudi Children

There have been some novel hereditary diseases with renal tubular components reported for the first time from Saudi Arabia. Among these is the syndrome of "marble brain disease" (osteopetrosis), manifested with renal tubular acidosis and cerebral calcification. Children suffering from this disease also have stunted growth and mental retardation. This syndrome has been shown to be linked to carbonic anhydrase II enzyme deficiency [55, 56].

In a study by Al Rasheed et al. carried out over a 10-year period, 28 Arab children with autosomal recessive osteopetrosis were seen in two hospitals in Riyadh, of whom 64% had associated renal tubular acidosis and 32% had malignant infantile osteopetrosis. Parental consanguinity was observed in 56% and 40% among patients with and without acidosis, respectively. Cerebral calcification and optic atrophy were more frequent in patients with acidosis [57, 58].

In another study, two novel mutations were identified in each of *AVPR2* and *AQP2* causing nephrogenic diabetes insipidus in Saudi families [59].

In a study of eight confirmed cases of cystinuria from five unrelated families, two new variants in the *SLC3A1* and *SLC9A7* genes were discovered. It is of note that 37.5% of these patients developed hypertension. Unlike other reports from the Mediterranean region, which report the most frequent mutation to be in the *SLC3A1* gene is M467T, three of the Saudi children with cystinuria (37.5%) from a single family were homozygous for the less common M467L mutation [60].

Familial hypomagnesaemia with hypercalciuria and nephrocalcinosis was described in seven KSA children from four different families. The presenting features were convulsions and carpo-pedal spasms, rickets, as well as recurrent UTIs and nephrocalcinosis in all patients. The renal function deteriorated in one patient progressing to ESRD after 4.4 years of follow-up. It was concluded that the clinical and biochemical findings were similar to previous reports, but with slower rate of kidney function deterioration [61].

## AKI in Children

We could find no reports on community or in-hospital AKI in Saudi children. However, the general impression is that the etiology and outcome in Saudi children do not differ greatly from what has been reported from the developed world with a prominence of volume depletion, sepsis, hemolytic uremic syndrome, and rapidly progressive GN [62].

In one pediatric study with biopsy-proven crescentic GN, a striking finding was that LN contributed 54.1% of the cases whereas in other reports, LN constituted less than 10% of the cases [63]. In an Indian pediatric report, LN contributed only 9.1% while post-infectious GN was the underlying etiology in 36.8% of the cases. Moreover, the report on Saudi children with crescentic GN observed a better renal outcome in the patients compared to the other reports; this is attributed to the less severe baseline renal impairment in that group [63–66].

There are a number of KSA Pediatric Intensive Care Units (PICU) AKI reports; in one report from Jeddah City, 102 cases of AKI were observed over a one-year period among admitted patients. These constituted 29% of all admissions to that PICU. Their mean age was 50.7 month and the underlying cause of AKI was sepsis in 34.3% [67]. Another study reported that 511 (37.4%) out of 1367 admitted to the PICU developed AKI, of whom 19.7% had severe AKI [68]. Their mean age was 47 months. The incidence of AKI in these PICU patients of 37.4% compares to 26.9% in a report involving a multicenter study of 32 PICUs [69]. In the Saudi study, it was found that even a small rise in the serum creatinine level was associated with increased mortality rate. This is similar to previous studies [70, 71]. Like in other studies, sepsis was found to be a major contributing factor for AKI in the Saudi study [72].

The causes of AKI among children differ between countries. The commonest causes in developed countries are sepsis, cardiac diseases, and inborn errors of metabolism [73–75]. The Saudi Arabian spectrum of AKI in the PICU setting is of similar pattern [68].

One study from Saudi Arabia looked into the use of CRRT in 96 critically ill children with a mean age of 6 years in the PICU. In two thirds of cases, the indication for CRRT was fluid overload followed by tumor lysis syndrome (18.8%) and metabolic encephalopathy (9.4%). Half of the patients who required CRRT died with the least mortality seen in primary renal disease (15.8%). This study found that the presence of fluid overload was associated with increased mortality. Similar finding was reported by Hayes et al. in 76 pediatric CRRT patients with an overall mortality 44.7% with sepsis and greater fluid overload being more common among patients who died [76].

## Hemodialysis

HD was started in in Riyadh Central Hospital in 1972 with two Travenol machines. Six months later another dialysis center was established in Jeddah. In 1975, two other units were established in Mecca and Medina.

According to Dr. Ayman Karkar, a prominent nephrologist from the eastern province of Saudi Arabia, the first HD unit in the area was established equipped with two Travenol machines in Dammam Central Hospital in 1974. In 1984, a large unit with 20 HD machines was established in the same city. This was followed, years later, by the establishment of more dialysis units in many areas all over the eastern region, including rural areas. In 1988, the medical services at the Arabian American Oil Company (ARAMCO) established its own HD unit. In 1996, additional space was granted and a PD unit was established next to the HD unit at Dammam Central Hospital (Ministry of Health).

In 2001, with a generous donation from the Kanoo family, Kanoo Kidney Center was established in Dammam Central Hospital (Ministry of Health) and is considered as a referral and training center. It trained more than 1300 nurses from all over the health sectors in Saudi Arabia.

The dialysis services in the eastern province were well developed due, at least in part, to the creation of the Directorate of Dialysis, which was tasked with the supervision of performance, clinical outcomes, education, and training (including weekly Journal Club meeting, monthly Nephrology Club and annual Nephrology, Dialysis and Transplantation Congress).

Until 5 years ago, the dialysis services in the Kingdom of Saudi Arabia were provided by three major medical sectors: the Ministry of Health (MOH), Governmental non-MOH sector (which cares for the employees of the Ministries of Defense, Interior, and the National Guard and their relatives), and the private sector. Over the last 5 years, a fourth important sector was added. This is the outsourcing sector, whereby a significant proportion of MOH stable dialysis patients were outsourced to be dialyzed in stand-alone centers run by major international dialysis provider companies, namely, DaVita and Diaverum. These companies won a 5-year tender and signed contracts to serve 5000 patients each. Both companies established additional dialysis clinics in different parts of KSA. More recently, these contracts were renewed with both companies for other 5 years.

Out of 10,203 patients on HD in the Kingdom in 2008, 65.9% were treated by the Ministry of Health (MOH) hospitals, 17.7% by non-MOH governmental hospitals, and 16.4% from the private sector [77]. By 2017, the number of patients on HD rose to 18,270 patients divided between the sectors as follows: 30.5% by MOH hospitals, 39.5% by non-MOH governmental hospitals, 16.8% by the private sector, and 13.2% by the dialysis provider companies (DaVita & Diaverum) [11]. Male gender contributes with 56% of all the dialysis population in Saudi Arabia.

The prevalence and incidence of ESRD increase sharply with age. The life expectancy in Saudi Arabia rose from an average life expectancy of 52 years in the 1950s to 74.8 years now [78]. With this, as well as the horrendous increase in the rate of obesity and diabetes in the Saudi population, a substantial rise in the ESRD incidence and prevalence is observed which is not the case in developed countries, in which these rates have declined or stabilized recently [79, 80].

In 2010, the incidence of ESRD among those over 65 years old was 893.7 pmp per year while they contributed only 3.2% of the total Saudi population [77]. Of all the patients on dialysis, 66.2% were over >45 years of age in 2008 and this has now risen to 70.5%. Of the HD patients, 68.5% are in the age range of 26–65 years, 0.27% are <10 years of age, and 9% are >75 years of age [11]. The other highly noticeable trend is the rise in the mean age of patients on dialysis. In the KSA, the mean age increased from 37.9 years in the early 1980s to 51.3 years by the end of the twentieth century [81]. By 2030, we estimate that the population over the age of 65 years will increase up to 13% in Saudi Arabia and that the number of ESRD in this age group will be four times what it is now.

The prevalence of HCV infection among Saudi HD patients was 68% in 1995 [82], dropping to 33% in 2010 [77] and to 10.7% in 2017 [11]. The decrease in prevalence is due to improved application of strict universal precautions by nurses. Some units in the Kingdom use geographical or temporal isolation of HCV positive patients. Nevertheless, there are still pockets of high prevalence of HCV particularly in the western and southern region, but even in these pockets, there has been a major reduction in HCV prevalence. It is worth mentioning that the number of patients with Hepatitis C has been continuously declining for the past 5 years with the current prevalence rate being 10%. Hepatitis B infections is well controlled with only 4% of HD patients being positive. There are only 18 HIV positive patients (0.1%).

Conventional hemodialysis is used in 89% of the HD patients. In some centers, however, such as those run by the Ministry of the National Guard centers as well as in the outsourced private centers (DaVita, Diaverum), the rate of hemodiafiltration (HDF) reaches 50% of the patients.

The most common vascular access is the arteriovenous fistula (AVF), being used by of 61% of HD population, followed by permanent dialysis catheter in 32%.

The target blood flow in HD is at least 350 ml/min, Kt/V of at least 1.3 and 12 h/week of dialysis. The target hemoglobin level is 11–12 g/dL.

It is estimated that the number of dialysis patients might reach 34,680 by 2030. At the current rate of reimbursement incurred by the Ministry of Health (MOH) for private dialysis management companies, the cost for dialysis by 2030 will be a staggering SR 7,022,700,000 annually (USD 1,872,720,000). This cost, of course, does not include expenses that result from the high hospitalization rates of dialysis patients (due mainly to cerebro-vascular disease, infection, and vascular access issues) as well as the cost of taking care of their multiple comorbidities, especially cardiovascular diseases.

The numbers of consultant and specialist nephrologists taking care of the dialysis patients in KSA are 295 and 457, respectively, and the number of nurses is 4693.

The prevalence of tuberculosis, a high proportion of which is extra-pulmonary [83], among Saudi HD patients has been reported to be 7%, which is twelve times more frequent than in the general population of KSA.

## Peritoneal Dialysis

PD was first introduced to Saudi Arabia by Professor Hassan Abuaisha in 1980, when he used intermittent peritoneal dialysis (IPD) to treat AKI at King Abdulaziz Hospital in Riyadh. In 1982, he introduced continuous ambulatory peritoneal dialysis (CAPD) at King Saud University–affiliated hospitals. We asked him to summarize his experience starting PD and he wrote the following:

"Saudi Arabia was one of the early starters of CAPD/APD compared to most countries worldwide. PD is perhaps the oldest modality of RRT in history, especially IPD. When I came to the KSA in 1976, I had a reasonably good experience with IPD based on our work on AKI [formerly known as acute renal failure (ARF)], in Sudan. I believed that IPD could save many lives threatened by AKI, but IPD never found a place in KSA because HD and KT were flourishing in the leading hospitals in the Kingdom in the 1980s.

"CAPD came first to existence worldwide in 1980s after the work of US and Canadian nephrologists/scientists in the late 1970s. The first congress on CAPD was held in Mexico in 1980, and I was fortunate to attend it. Here was a new approach to PD where you could use only 4–6 cycles of PD fluid (instead of 20 or so per 24-h as in IPD) and there was the fascinating concept of a permanent peritoneal access, which meant less infection episodes during PD. So, it was possible to treat ESRD using CAPD. The advantages for young children and patients living away from the major cities were convincing. However, almost all nephrologists working in the leading hospitals in KSA, especially the King-Faisal Hospital and Research Center (KFHRC) and the Military Hospital at Riyadh (mostly nephrologists from Europe and North America at that time), were not interested in CAPD. I once discussed the prospects of CAPD with an eminent British nephrologist and he told me: 'Frankly, to me, CAPD stands for Continuous Ambulatory *Purulent* Dialysis!' Well, to some extent he had a point then. The peritonitis rates were at best one episode every 6 months or so, those days. However, the situation has changed dramatically over time; currently, most guidelines do not accept peritonitis rates more frequent than an episode every 24 months, as adequate PD. In fact, nowadays peritonitis rates of as few as one episode every 5 years do not raise any eyebrows.

"When I came back from the conference at Mexico in 1980, I was enthusiastic about CAPD. So, I discussed the matter with Dr. Siraj Zagzoug, director of King-Abdelaziz University Hospital at Riyadh at that time. He listened carefully to my suggestions, looked at my detailed pictorial report, and decided to give it a try! Fortunately, the fund needed for the project was not a big obstacle. That was how CAPD was introduced to KSA (and in the whole region) for the first time and it became operational in 1982. Within a few years, automated peritoneal dialysis (APD) became a regular treatment, often preferred to the classical CAPD, in many hospitals across KSA. So, the Kingdom is a leading starter of regular PD compared to many countries worldwide.

"One of our very first patients was a boy only 1 year old at the time and we trained his mother to take care of his CAPD at home. After 2 years he was well enough to go for renal transplantation in the United States. We lost his follow-up, but 20 years later he showed up with an intention to get married, and I gladly accepted the invitation to attend his wedding ceremony. That is just a marker on the effectiveness of renal services on the survival of patients if well orchestrated."

At the present time, there are 37 centers in Saudi Arabia providing PD. There are 1389 patients, of whom 167 are children. The number of patients on PD has not changed substantially over the years. Continuous cycling peritoneal dialysis/automated peritoneal dialysis (CCPD/APD) modality is the commonest, being used in 71% of the patients followed by CAPD in 22% [11].

While the number of patients on HD rises in absolute numbers on annual basis, no such change in the number of patients on PD is seen. The prevalence of Saudi patients on PD is 61.0 pmp and the incidence is 21.3 pmp/year.

In a study covering a 5-year period about the experience on PD in a Saudi tertiary care center and published in 2011, the average age was reported to be 50.7 years with diabetes being the leading cause of ESRD. Among these patients. 38.9% were on CAPD and 61.1% APD. The peritonitis rate was one episode per 24.5 patient-months. The incidence of exit site infection was 0.214 per person-years. The commonest organisms causing peritonitis and exit site infection were Staphylococcus and Pseudomonas aeruginosa, respectively. At the end of the 5-year follow-up, 55.6% of the patients were still on PD, 20.6% were shifted to HD, and the overall mortality rate was 15.3% [84].

Another study looked into peritonitis rate among PD patients in the Saudi setting, with an overall peritonitis rate of one episode per 28.3 patient-months [85].

Tuberculous peritonitis has been reported to occur in 3.88% of all episodes of peritonitis among Saudi patients on PD [86]. This is higher than the one reported from India [87]. In a literature search on tuberculous peritonitis between January 1976 and January 1999, published in 2000, only 13 cases were reported from the United States [88].

A study comparing Saudi patients on HD and PD found that the quality of life (QoL) scores were significantly higher in PD patients in all domains and in the total QoL, with the exception of the score of physical QoL, which was higher in the HD patients [89].

In as survey of Saudi nephrologists, it was reported that most nephrologists were not satisfied with the rate of PD utilization among their patients. Many felt that 30% or more of their dialysis patients should be on PD. The responding nephrologist felt that the main the reason for underutilization was patient refusal (72%). The top reasons for patient refusal given by the nephrologists were "PD is not easy to perform at home" (79.8%) and "patients think HD is better" (73.7%). The nephrologists surveyed put forward the following suggestions to improve the utilization of PD in Saudi Arabia: (1) proper predialysis patients' education, (2) early referral, and (3) increase nephrologists' motivation [90]. They conducted another survey with 920 HD patients who had never been on PD in order to find out the reasons behind PD underutilization in KSA from the patients' perspectives. This study concluded that the main reason was that these patients had not received proper counseling and education about PD from their treating nephrologists at any time during the course of their disease [91].

## Kidney Transplantation

The organ transplantation history in Saudi Arabia went through a number of phases.

During the 1970s, Saudi patients were sent for KT to the United States when it was still possible for non-US citizens to receive deceased donor organs there. This phase allowed KSA transplant physicians early and close exposure to, the then new, immunosuppressive agents (cyclosporine and later tacrolimus).

The second phase involved the performance of living related transplantation within Saudi Arabia by a visiting team from St Thomas's Hospital, London, UK, who would perform a few transplants every few weeks. This phase spanned from 1979 to 1981, during which time Saudi transplant physicians and surgeons were being trained.

The third phase, besides continuing living related transplantation, incorporated obtaining deceased kidneys from Eurotransplant. This phase was of enormous benefit to us because it introduced us to the important business of organ procurement logistics and coordination. This initial phase of the Saudi experience with deceased kidney donation came through an agreement with Eurotransplant in 1981, by which it provided us with 64 deceased kidneys during 3 years, which for some reason were often suboptimal. However, this historical phase was useful to us in that it gave us a significant insight into deceased organ procurement logistics and coordination. This experience also led us to document in the medical literature, the utility of many of the then often discarded (marginal) kidneys with acceptable results, including those with exceptionally long ischemic times. A lot of those kidneys were what would now be labelled as "expanded pool" kidneys and thus were rejected by European centers as per clinical practice of the time, but we accepted them as we had an immense shortage of kidney organs. Such expanded pool kidneys are now routinely used in European and US centers. Among the kidneys we used, there were such as a half "horseshoe" kidney, one "third-hand" kidney [92], and kidneys with cold ischemic time as long as 72 h [93].

The fourth phase involved the use of kidneys from deceased donors procured locally. The very first deceased donor KT took place in December 1984 [94].

The fifth phase witnessed the establishment of the SCOT and the spread of KT across the country with the founding of ten renal transplantation centers serving all the regions of the country and the introduction by SCOT of multiorgan donation.

SCOT has a wide range of functions, including donation boosting from living and deceased donors, meticulous gathering of data on ESRD patients, and supervision of the ethical organ allocation. SCOT also carries out the important task of enabling the coordination between donor hospitals and transplant centers by providing coordinators, procuring teams, and assuring consent. SCOT has published a directory that regulates the practice of organ donation and transplantation in the KSA.

Since its inception, SCOT has been pivotal in developing and implementing strategies to increase awareness in both the medical community and the public with frequent school visits as well as in providing education for medical staff in ICUs and Emergency Departments.

Moreover, SCOT has developed strong collaborative links and communication with international bodies involved in organ donation and transplantation as well as contributing to international guidelines in these fields, becoming a model and prototype for an organ procurement organization in the Muslim world.

In order to organ donation and transplantation be a reality in KSA, the organ transplant medical community needed to have Fatwas (theological opinion) from the highest religious authorities that establishes the permissibility, in Islam, of performing transplantation using organs from brain-dead persons and equating brain death diagnosis as reflecting death. A decisive fatwa came about in 1982 (Decision No. 99, dated 25-8-1982), stating that according to Islamic Jurisprudence, it is permissible to perform deceased donor transplantation, which paved the way for us to start a cadaveric renal transplant program. Another landmark fatwa issued during the Islamic Jurisprudence Conference in 1986 in Amman opined that the diagnosis of brain death was permissible and can be used to diagnose an irreversible process. Another landmark fatwa issued in Saudi Arabia in 1988 allowed cessation of therapy, including ventilation, in hopeless cases.

There are 142 ICUs in the KSA, of which 74% participate in the brain death diagnosis and organ donation program. The active and willing involvement of these ICUs in close collaboration with SCOT has become a central component of organizing the KSA organ procurement during the past 30 years. By the end of 2015, a total of 11,220 possible deceased donors have been reported to SCOT.

Organ transplantation program in the Kingdom started in 1979 when the first kidney from a living donor was transplanted in Riyadh Military Hospital. By the end of 2017 a total of 11,509 kidneys were transplanted; 7838 were from living related donors, 3108 from deceased donors, and 563 from living unrelated donors.

In 2017, a total of 921 kidneys were transplanted; 776 from living and 145 from deceased donors. Among the 145 deceased kidneys, 26 were used for pediatric recipients and 119 for adults [11].

Out of the 145 deceased kidneys transplanted in KSA in 2017, 83% were from standard criteria donors and 17% from expanded criteria donors.

Kidney Donor Risk Index (KDRI) for locally deceased donors ranged between 0.73 and 2.58 with an average of 1.23. It is worth mentioning that 23 (31%) of the cases had a KDRI less than one, 38 (51%) were between (1.0 and 1.5), and 14 (18%) had a KDRI above 1.5.

The cold ischemia time (CIT) for locally transplanted deceased kidneys ranged between 2 h 30 min and 29 h 26 min with an average CIT of 10 h. In 75% of the cases, the deceased KT was done with a CIT of less than 12 h, in 22% transplantation was done within 12–24 h and in only 3% it was done within 24–29 h [11].

The standard maintenance immunosuppressive therapy consists of tacrolimus, prednisolone, and mycophenolate mofetil (MMF). Induction therapy for living-related transplantation is IL2 inhibitors and for deceased kidney donors is ATG. The therapy is paid by the government.

Some interesting observations arising from KT practice in Saudi Arabia are worth mentioning. For social reasons, pregnancy among Saudi post-transplant patients in the reproductive age group is manyfold commoner that in the West. This allowed for many publications on this topic [95, 96] reporting good outcomes for the mothers and babies [97–99], even after repeated pregnancies [100].

Reports on infections common in the region such as tuberculosis, non-typhoid salmonella and parasitic infections were also published [100, 101] as well as recommendations for appropriate cyclosporine dose adjustment when using rifampicin [102].

Kaposi sarcoma accounts for 75% of all post-transplantation malignancies in KSA and we had the opportunity to publish many papers on its natural history and treatment [103] and its involvement in children [104], the chest, [105] and the gastrointestinal tract [106]. A novel classification was developed for staging of post-transplantation Kaposi sarcoma, [107], its association with human herpesvirus 8 described [108], and the first report of its recurrence after reintroduction of immunosuppression also described [109].

## Fasting the Month of Ramadan and Kidney Disease

### Fasting in Post-transplant Patients

Fasting is one of five fundamental pillars of Islam [110, 111]. As such, it is obligatory for all adult Moslems to fast in the month of Ramadan [112]. There are clearly defined and specified exceptions to this rule, which allows for non-fasting [113]. Exceptions include the sick, travelers, debilitated elderly people, and pregnant and lactating women.

The Moslem Hejri calendar year is 11 days shorter than the Gregorian calendar. Therefore, Ramadan time moves throughout the four seasons and makes a full circle every 33 years. The time from sunrise to sunset and the ambient temperatures vary according the season that Ramadan falls under and the location in the world.

It is considered very sinful for an adult Moslem not to fast unless they come under one the categories exempted from fasting. It is, therefore, customary for transplanted patients to ask the advice of their doctors about the safety of fasting and feel that they are religiously released from the obligation to fast if a reliable doctor advises them against fasting. More KTs are being performed in Islamic countries and more Muslim transplanted patients living in non-Moslem countries [114, 115]. It is therefore important that doctors should have some reliable information on which they can reliably and honestly give advice to such patients.

The concern about fasting harming the transplanted patients is that volume depletion might lead to AKI that might lead to permanent damage [116, 117].

Another potential problem associated with fasting by sick patients has to do with drug compliance. In a study of 750 Ramadan fasting patients who were on prescribed drugs or diets for their conditions, 10% did not adhere to their medications and 19% did not adhere to their diets [118]. In another study of 81 fasting patients, 37 altered their drug dosage pattern, 35 missed doses, and four took all their medications as one single daily dose after breaking fast [119].

A number studies have investigated the effect of Ramadan fasting on kidney function in renal transplant patients. However, those were mostly single–center studies involving a small number of patients. Furthermore, they occurred at different times of the year with different durations between sunrise and sunset and at different daytime temperatures [120–127].

### Fasting and HD Patients

Intravenous fluids given during HD renders fasting invalid. Fasting is valid during non-dialysis days or if the HD session occurred after breaking of the fast (after sunset).

In one study, it was found that fasting HD patients were more likely to have higher interdialytic weight gain and potassium level and that was attributed to the increased intake of fluids and potassium-rich food after breaking the fast at sunset [128]. However in another study comparing fasting and non-fasting HD patients, no differences have been observed in relation to pre- and post-dialysis blood pressure, serum potassium, albumin, or weight gain. However, serum phosphorous was significantly higher in the fasting group as well as the rate of non-adherence to the dialysis sessions [129].

### Fasting and PD Patients

If fasting by a PD patient is to be religiously valid, the infusion of PD fluid should end before sunrise (the beginning of fast) and no further infusion is given until after the breaking of the fast (sunset).

The concern is that volume depletion would occur if their normal PD regimen is used without fluid intake for the 12–14 h of the fast. Moreover, following breaking the fast, there is usually an excessive consumption of fluid and potassium-rich juices and foods. To avoid these, Al Wakeel et al. suggested regimens aimed at reducing the dialysis workload in the evening and avoiding excessive removal of fluid during the daytime [130].

### Fasting and Predialysis CKD

In a study with 31 patients (14 stage III CKD, 12 stage IV and 5 stage V with a mean e-GFR of 29 ± 16.3 mL/min), all the patients tolerated fasting the whole month of Ramadan with weight reduction and lower blood pressure; and eGFR showed a significant improvement during the fast and the month after [131].

In another study, the GFR using DTPA dynamic renal scan was estimated as well and tubular cell damage by measuring the level of N-acetyl-B-D- glucosaminidase (NAG) in a fasting CKD group and fasting normal group before and after Ramadan. The change in GFR was not significantly different between the two groups. However, the percentage change in the urinary NAG was significantly higher in the CKD patients (236 versus −49.1, $p = 0.03$), suggesting that fasting Ramadan may have an injurious effect on the renal tubules in CKD patients [132].

## Nephrology Practice in Saudi Arabia

To work as a consultant nephrologist in Saudi Arabia, one needs to have trained in and passed a recognized and accredited Board in Internal Medicine (such as the Saudi Board in Internal Medicine which is a 4-year training program) followed by a Fellowship in Nephrology (such as the Saudi Fellowship in Nephrology which is a 2-year training program). Furthermore, a consultant must be registered and accredited to work as a consultant by the Saudi Council for Health Specialties (SCHS).

The salary scale for a consultant nephrologist differs from a medical sector to another but is in the region of USD 13,000–18,500/month plus free accommodation, leave travel and the children's tuition fees and free medical insurance for him/her and their dependents.

On average, the HD patient to nurse ratio is 1–3 and HD patient to consultant ratio is 1–100.

Most of the dialysis nurses are expatriate. Normally they are required to have a minimum of 2-year experience to be employed. The salary scale for dialysis nurses is really quite variable and could be anything between USD 1300 and 2100 month plus free accommodation and free medical cover.

In Saudi Arabia, there are 120 HD units, 37 PD centers, and 10 centers where renal transplantation is carried out. Most dialysis units have vascular access coordinator, social workers, renal dietitian, and, in some cases, a transplant coordinator.

The renal services are normally in charge of critical care nephrology where continuous renal replacement therapy (CRRT) is the normal mode of RRT in the ICUs. The ICU nurses are normally responsible for the CRRT.

Most tertiary care nephrology services are equipped with full laboratory support, renal pathology support, and with trained nephropathologists.

Many courses, workshops, and symposia on all aspects of nephrology are often organized in Saudi Arabia and nearby Dubai.

The capital city Riyadh is less than 2.5 h flight away to Dubai, Abu Dhabi, Bahrain, Doha, Amman and Cairo. If you have a working visa in Saudi Arabia, you will be able to visit most of these destinations without a visa.

Although the language of Saudi Arabia is Arabic, the day-to-day language used in hospitals and medical services is the English language. It is also the language of tuition in Saudi Medical schools. All doctors and nurses working in Saudi medical centers speak English. Translators are provided for non-Arabic-speaking doctors to communicate with the patient. It is also surprising that non-Arabic-speaking physicians do not learn sufficient Arabic to communicate with their patients.

## References


1. The General Authority for Statistics. https://www.stats.gov.sa/en/5305.
2. Office for National Statistics. https://www.ons.gov.uk/.
3. Denmark Age structure. https://www.indexmundi.com/denmark/age_structure.html.
4. Barbari A, Stephan A, Masri M, Karam A, Aoun S, El Nahas J, et al. Consanguinity-associated kidney diseases in Lebanon: an epidemiological study. Mol Immunol. 2003;39(17–18):1109–14.
5. Hamed RM. The spectrum of chronic renal failure among Jordanian children. J Nephrol. 2002;15:130–5.
6. Harambat J, Van Stralen KJ, Kim JJ, Tizard EJ. Epidemiology of chronic kidney disease in children. Pediatr Nephrol. 2012;27(3):363–73.
7. Fatani HH, Mira SA, El-Zubier AG. Prevalence of diabetes mellitus in rural Saudi Arabia. Diabetes Care. 1987;10(2):180–3.
8. Alqurashi KA, Aljabri KS, Bokhari SA. Prevalence of diabetes mellitus in a Saudi community. Ann Saudi Med. 2011;31(1):19.
9. Jondeby MS, De-Los Santos GG, Al-Ghamdi AM, Al-Hawas FA, Mousa DH, Al-Sulaiman MH, et al. Caring for hemodialysis patients in Saudi Arabia. Past, present and future. Saudi Med J. 2001;22:199–204.
10. Saleh FS, Naji MN, Eltayeb AA, Hejaili FF, Al Sayyari AA. Effect of thyroid function status in hemodialysis patients on erythropoietin resistance and interdialytic weight gain. Saudi J Kidney Dis Transpl. 2018;29(6):1274.
11. Annual report, Saudi Center of Organ Transplantation. scot.org.sa.
12. Al-Khader AA. Impact of diabetes in renal diseases in Saudi Arabia. Nephrol Dial Transplant. 2001;16(11):2132–5.
13. Al-Suleiman M, Kfoury H, Jondeby M, Burgos N, Al-Hayyan H, Al-Sayyari A. Progression of diabetic nephropathy in Saudi patients with type 2 diabetes mellitus. Endocrinologist. 2008;18:230–2.
14. Khan MA, Ai-Kanhar MA. Dietary energy and protein requirements for Saudi Arabia: a methodological approach. East Mediterr Health J. 1998;4(1):69.
15. AL-Qahtani AM. Prevalence and predictors of obesity and overweight among adults visiting primary care settings in the southwestern region, Saudi Arabia. Biomed Res Int. 2019;2019:1–5.
16. Al-Othaimeen AI, Al-Nozha M, Osman AK. Obesity: an emerging problem in Saudi Arabia. Analysis of data from the National Nutrition Survey. East Mediterr Health J. 2007;13(2):441.
17. Al-Nozha MM, Abdullah M, Arafah MR, Khalil MZ, Khan NB, Al-Mazrou YY, Al-Maatouq MA, Al-Marzouki K, Al-Khadra A, Nouh MS, Al-Harthi SS. Hypertension in saudi arabia. Saudi Med J. 2007;28(1):77.
18. Saeed AA, Al-Hamdan NA, Bahnassy AA, Abdalla AM, Abbas MAF, Abuzaid LZ. Prevalence, awareness, treatment, and control of hypertension among Saudi adult population: a national survey. Int J Hypertens. 2011;2011:174135.
19. Al Duraihim H, Alghamdi G, AlNemer M, Abdulaal AE, Al Sayyari A. Blood pressure control, lifestyle and disease awareness of Saudi hypertensive patients. Saudi J Kidney Dis Transpl. 2019;30:33–8.
20. Alsuwaida AO, Farag YMK, Al Sayyari AA, Mousa D, Alhejaili F, Al-Harbi A, et al. Epidemiology of chronic kidney disease in the Kingdom of Saudi Arabia (SEEK-Saudi investigators)—a pilot study. Saudi J Kidney Dis Transpl. 2010;21(6):1066–72.
21. Padmos MA, Roberts GT, Sackey K, et al. Two different forms of homozygous sickle cell disease occur in Saudi Arabia. Br J Haematol. 1991;79:93–8.
22. Alkhunaizi AM, Al-Khatti AA. Proteinuria in patients with sickle cell disease. Saudi J Kidney Dis Transpl. 2014;25:1038–41.
23. Alkhunaizi AM, Al-Khatti AA, Al-Mueilo SH, Amir A, Yousif B. End-stage renal disease in patients with sickle cell disease. Saudi J Kidney Dis Transpl. 2017;28:751.
24. Huraib S, Al Khader A, Shaheen F, Abu Aisha H, Souqiyyeh MZ, Al Mohana F, Soliman M, Al Wakeel J, Mitwalli A, Al Mohaya S, Said R, Abdulhaleem, Al Menawy L, Sohaibani M, Chan N. The spectrum of glomerulonephritis in Saudi Arabia: the results of the Saudi registry. Saudi J Kidney Dis Transpl. 2000;11:434–41.
25. AlFaadhel T, Alsuwaida A, Alsaad K, Almezaini L, Ahmed N, AlHamad MY, Bakheet A, Wadera J, Mokhtar G, Alsuwaida F, Siddiqui R. Prevalence and 20-year epidemiological trends of glomerular diseases in the adult Saudi population: a multicenter study. Ann Saudi Med. 2019;39(3):155–61.
26. Murugapandian S, Mansour I, Hudeeb M, Hamed K, Hammode E, Bijin B, et al. Epidemiology of glomerular disease in southern Arizona: review of 10-year renal biopsy data. Medicine (Baltimore). 2016;95(18):e3633.
27. Yang Y, Zhang Z, Zhuo L, Chen DP, Li WG. The spectrum of biopsy-proven glomerular disease in China: a systematic review. Chin Med J. 2018;131(6):731–5.
28. Durahim HA, Ghamdi GA, Seraya AA, Alkhiari R, Sayyari AA. Predictors of mortality and end stage renal disease in Saudi patients with lupus nephritis. Lupus. 2011;20(12):1329–35.
29. Oudah N, Al Duhailib Z, Alsaad K, Qurashi S, Ghamdi G, Flaiw A, Hejaili F, Farooqui M, Al Sayyari A. Glomerulonephritis with crescents among adult Saudi patients outcome and its predictors. Clin Exp Med. 2012;12(2):121–5.
30. Al-Homrany M. Epidemiology of acute renal failure in hospitalized patients: experience from southern Saudi Arabia. East Mediterr Health J. 2003;9(5/6):1061.
31. Al-Homrany M. Acute renal failure following snake bite: case report and review. Saudi J Kidney Dis Transpl. 1996;7(3):309.

32. Khan W, Zakai HA. Clinico-pathological studies of Plasmodium falciparum and Plasmodium vivax—malaria in India and Saudi Arabia. Acta Parasitologica. 2014;59(2):206–12.
33. Naqvi R, Ahmad E, Akhtar F, Naqvi A, Rizvi A. Outcome in severe acute renal failure associated with malaria. Nephrol Dial Transplant. 2003;18:1820–3.
34. Merchant S, Meshram R, Tamboli MM. Clinical manifestation and predictors of mortality in severe malaria in children. Sch J App Med Sci. 2016;4(6):1931–5.
35. Vannaphan S, Walters N, Saengnedsawang T, Tangpukdee N, Kham-In P, Klubprasit M, Wilairatana P, Looareesuwan S. Factors associated with acute renal failure in severe falciparum malaria pateints. Southeast Asian J Trop Med Public Health. 2010;41(5):1042.
36. Sitprija V. Nephropathy in falciparum malaria. Kidney Int. 1988;34:867–77.
37. Zaki AM, Van Boheemen S, Bestebroer TM, Osterhaus AD, Fouchier RA. Isolation of a novel coronavirus from a man with pneumonia in Saudi Arabia. N Engl J Med. 2012;367(19):1814–20.
38. Saad M, Omrani AS, Baig K, Bahloul A, Elzein F, Matin MA, Selim MA, Al Mutairi M, Al Nakhli D, Al Aidaroos AY, Al Sherbeeni N. Clinical aspects and outcomes of 70 patients with Middle East respiratory syndrome coronavirus infection: a single-center experience in Saudi Arabia. Int J Infect Dis. 2014;29:301–6.
39. Arabi YM, Arifi AA, Balkhy HH, Najm H, Aldawood AS, Ghabashi A, Hawa H, Alothman A, Khaldi A, Al Raiy B. Clinical course and outcomes of critically ill patients with Middle East respiratory syndrome coronavirus infection. Ann Intern Med. 2014;160(6):389–97.
40. Khan NA, Azhar EI, El-Fiky S, Madani HH, Abuljadial MA, Ashshi AM, Turkistani AM, Hamouh EA. Clinical profile and outcome of hospitalized patients during first outbreak of dengue in Makkah, Saudi Arabia. Acta Trop. 2008;105(1):39–44.
41. Mattoo TK, Al-Mohalhal S, Al-Sowailem AM, Al-Harbi M, Mahmood MA. Chronic renal failure in children in Saudi Arabia. Ann Saudi Med. 1990;10(5):496–9.
42. Kari J. Chronic renal failure in children in the western area of Saudi Arabia. Saudi J Kidney Dis Transpl. 2006;17(1):19–24.
43. Al Harbi N. Chronic renal failure in children in Asir region of Saudi Arabia. Saudi J Kidney Dis Transpl. 1997;8(3):294.
44. Ardissino G, Dacco V, Testa S, Bonaudo R, Claris-Appiani A, Taioli E, Marra G, Edefonti A, Sereni F. Epidemiology of chronic renal failure in children: data from the ItalKid project. Pediatrics. 2003;111(4 Pt 1):e382–7.
45. Warady BA, Chadha V. Chronic kidney disease in children: the global perspective. Pediatr Nephrol. 2007;22(12):1999–2009.
46. El-Hazmi MA, Al-Swailem AR, Warsy AS, Al-Swailem AM, Sulaimani R, Al-Meshari AA. Consanguinity among the Saudi Arabian population. J Med Genet. 1995;32(8):623–6.
47. El-Mouzan MI, Al-Salloum AA, Al-Herbish AS, Qurachi MM, Al-Omar AA. Regional variations in the prevalence of consanguinity in Saudi Arabia. Saudi Med J. 2007;28(12):1881–4.
48. Al-Ibrahim AA, Girdharilal RD, Jalal MC, Alghamdy AH, Ghazal YK. Urinary tract infection and Vesicoureteral reflux in Saudi children. Saudi J Kidney Dis Transpl. 2002;13:24–8.
49. Keren R, Shaikh N, Pohl H, Gravens-Mueller L, Ivanova A, Zaoutis L, Patel M, deBerardinis R, Parker A, Bhatnagar S, Haralam MA. Risk factors for recurrent urinary tract infection and renal scarring. Pediatrics. 2015;136(1):e13–21.
50. Al-Rasheed SA, El-Faqih SR, Husain I, Abdurrahman M, AlMugeirin MM. The aetiological and clinical pattern of childhood urolithiasis in Saudi Arabia. Int Urol Nephrol. 1995;27:349–55.
51. Al-Rasheed SA, Al-Mugeiren MM, Al-Salloum AA, Al-Sohaibani MO. Childhood renal diseases in Saudi Arabia. A clinicopathological study of 167 cases. Int Urol Nephrol. 1996;28(5):607–13.
52. Kari J. Pattern of steroid resistant nephrotic syndrome in children living in the kingdom of Saudi Arabia: a single center study. Saudi J Kidney Dis Transpl. 2009;20(5):854–7.
53. Al-Sabban E. Spectrum of glomerular disease among children in Saudi Arabia. Saudi J Kidney Dis Transpl. 1997;8(3):285.
54. Al-Hamed MH, Al-Sabban E, Al-Mojalli H, Al-Harbi N, Faqeih E, Al Shaya H, Alhasan K, Al-Hissi S, Rajab M, Edwards N, Al-Abbad A. A molecular genetic analysis of childhood nephrotic syndrome in a cohort of Saudi Arabian families. J Hum Genet. 2013;58(7):480.
55. Ohlsson A, Stark G, Sakati N. Marble brain disease: recessive osteopetrosis, renal tubular acidosis and cerebral calcification in three Saudi Arabian families. Dev Med Child Neurol. 1980;22:72–84.
56. Ohlsson A, Cumming WA, Paul A, Sly WS. Carbonic anhydrase II deficiency syndrome: recessive osteopetrosis with renal tubular acidosis and cerebral calcifi cation. Pediatrics. 1986;77:371–81.
57. Al-Rasheed SA, Al-Mohrij O, Al-Jurayyan N, Al-Herbish A, Al-Mugeiren M, Al-Salloum A, Al-Hussain M, El-Desouki M. Osteopetrosis in children. Int J Clin Pract. 1998;52(1):15–8.
58. Al-Rasheed SA Osteoporosis Textbook of clinical pediatrics ed. Elzouki A et al. Springer Science & Business Media; 2011.
59. Carroll P, Al-Mojalli H, Al-Abbad A, Al-Hassoun I, Al-Hamed M, Al-Amr R, et al. Novel mutations underlying nephrogenic diabetes insipidus in Arab families. Genet Med. 2006;8:443–7.
60. Obaid A, Nashabat M, Al Fakeeh K, Al Qahtani AT, Alfadhel M. Delineation of cystinuria in Saudi Arabia: a case series. BMC Nephrol. 2017;18(1):50.
61. Kari JA, Farouq M, Alshaya HO. Familial hypomagnesemia with hypercalciuria and nephrocalcinosis. Pediatr Nephrol. 2003;18:506–10.
62. Andreoli SP. Acute kidney injury in children. Pediatr Nephrol. 2009;24(2):253.
63. Alsaad K, Oudah N, Al Ameer A, Fakeeh K, Al Jomaih A, Al Sayyari A. Glomerulonephritis with crescents in children: etiology and predictors of renal outcome. International Scholarly Research Notices; Pediatr; 2011.
64. Srivastava RN, Moudgil A, Bagga A, Vasudev AS, Bhuyan UN, Sundraem KR. Crescentic glomerulonephritis in children: a review of 43 cases. Am J Nephrol. 1992;12(3):155–61.
65. Bagga A. Crescentic glomerulonephritis CH 34. In: Avner E, Harmon W, Niaudet P, Yoshikawa N, editors. Pediatric nephrology. 6th ed. Berlin, Heidelberg: Springer; 2009.
66. Shalaby M, Khathlan N, Safder O, Fadel F, Farag YM, Singh AK, Kari JA. Outcome of acute kidney injury in pediatric patients admitted to the intensive care unit. Clin Nephrol. 2014;82(12):379–86.
67. Kari JA, Alhasan KA, Shalaby MA, Khathlan N, Safdar OY, Al Rezgan SA, El DS, Albanna AS. Outcome of pediatric acute kidney injury: a multicenter prospective cohort study. Pediatr Nephrol. 2018;33:335–40.
68. Sanchez-Pinto LN, Goldstein SL, Schneider JB, Khemani RG. Association between progression and improvement of acute kidney injury and mortalityin critically ill children. Pediatr Crit Care Med. 2015;16:703–10.
69. Claure-Del GR, Bouchard J. Acid-base and electrolyte abnormalities duringrenal support for acute kidney injury: recognition and management. Blood Purif. 2012;34:186–93.
70. Miklaszewska M, Korohoda P, Sobczak A, Horbaczewska A, Filipiak A, Zachwieja K, Kobylarz K, Tkaczyk M, Drozdz D, Pietrzyk JA. Acute kidney injury in a single pediatric intensive care unit in Poland: a retrospectivestudy. Kidney Blood Press Res. 2014;39:28–39.
71. Rustagi RS, Arora K, Das RR, Pooni PA, Singh D. Incidence, risk factors and outcome of acute kidney injury in critically ill children—a developing country perspective. Paediatr Int Child H. 2017;37:35–41.

72. Bunchman TE, McBryde KD, Mottes TE, Gardner JJ, Maxvold NJ, Brophy PD. Pediatric acute renal failure: outcome by modality and disease. Pediatr Nephrol. 2001;16(12):1067–71.
73. Hui-Stickle S, Brewer ED, Goldstein SL. Pediatric ARF epidemiology at a tertiary care center from 1999 to 2001. Am J Kidney Dis. 2005;45(1):96101.
74. Symons JM, Chua AN, Somers MJ, Baum MA, Bunchman TE, Benfield MR, et al. Demographic characteristics of pediatric continuous renal replacement therapy: a report of the prospective pediatric continuous renal replacement therapy registry. Clin J Am Soc Nephrol. 2007;2(4):732–8.
75. Al-Ayed T, Siddiqui NU, Alturki A, Aljofan F. Outcome of continuous renal replacement therapy in critically ill children: a retrospective cohort study. Ann Saudi Med. 2018;38(4):260–8.
76. Hayes LW, Oster RA, Tofil NM, Tolwani AJ. Outcomes of critically ill children requiring continuous renal replacement therapy. Crit Care. 2009;24(3):394–400.
77. Al-Sayyari AA, Shaheen FA. End stage chronic kidney disease in Saudi Arabia. A rapidly changing scene. Saudi Med J. 2011;32(4):339–46.
78. https://www.worldlifeexpectancy.com/saudi-arabia-life-expectancy.
79. Grassmann A, Gioberge S, Moeller S, Brown G. ESRD patients in 2004: global overview of patient numbers, treatment modalities and associated trends. Nephrol Dial Transplant. 2005;20:2587–93.
80. Foley RN, Collins AJ. End-stage renal disease in the United States: an update from the United States renal data system. J Am Soc Nephrol. 2007;18:2644–8.
81. Shaheen FA, Al-Khader AA. Epidemiology and causes of end stage renal disease (ESRD). Saudi J Kidney Dis Transpl. 2005;16:277–81.
82. Huraib SO. Hepatitis C in dialysis patients. Saudi J Kidney Dis Transpl. 2003;14:442–50.
83. Malik GH, Al-Mohaya SA, Al-Harbi AS, Kechrid M, Azhari O, Shetia S, Tashkandy MA, Ahmad K, Bhat AW, Want MA, Subramanian PT. Spectrum of tuberculosis in dialysis patients in Saudi Arabia. Saudi J Kidney Dis Transpl. 2003;14(2):145.
84. Alwakeel JS, Alsuwaida A, Askar A, Memon N, Usama S, Alghonaim M, Feraz NA, Shah IH, Wilson H. Outcome and complications in peritoneal dialysis patients: a five-year single center experience. Saudi J Kidney Dis Transpl. 2011;22(2):245.
85. Alfayez SM, Alsaqoub SM, Qattan AY, Alghamdi MA, Elfeky DS, Alrowaie FA, Aljasser DS, Syed SB. Peritoneal dialysis related infections in a tertiary care hospital in Riyadh, Saudi Arabia. Saudi Med J. 2019;40(2):147.
86. Waness A, Al Shohaib S. Tuberculous peritonitis associated with peritoneal dialysis. Saudi J Kidney Dis Transpl. 2012;23(1):44.
87. Abraham G, Mathews M, Sekar L, Srikanth A, Sekar U, Soundarajan P. Tuberculous peritonitis in a cohort of continuous ambulatory peritoneal dialysis patients. Perit Dial Int. 2001;21(Suppl 3):S202–4.
88. Talwani R, Horvath JA. Tuberculous peritonitis in patients undergoing continuous ambulatory peritoneal dialysis: case report and review. Clin Infect Dis. 2000;31(1):70–5.
89. Bayoumi M. Life style modification toward improving quality of life and effects on caregivers' burden: development of new nursing theory. Ann Nurs Primary Care. 2018;1(1):1007.
90. Dahlan R, Qureshi M, Akeely F, Al Sayyari AA. Barriers to peritoneal dialysis in Saudi Arabia: nephrologists' perspectives. Perit Dial Int. 2016;36(5):564–6.
91. Dahlan RA, Alsuwaida AO, Farrash MS, Qureshi MA, Hejaili F, Al Sayyari AA. Let us listen to patients: underutilization of peritoneal dialysis from patients' perspectives. Perit Dial Int. 2017;37(5):574–6.
92. Al-Hasani MK, Saltissi D, Chang R, Van HG, Tegzess AM. Successful regrafting of an explanted transplant kidney. Transplantation. 1987;43(6):916–7.
93. Chang RW, Saltissi D, Al-Khader A, Abomelha M, Jawdat M. Survival of sub-optimal cadaver renal grafts with prolonged cold ischaemic times using cyclosporin. Nephrol Dial Transplant. 1987;1(4):246–50.
94. Al-Sayyari AA. The story of the first deceased donor kidney donation in Saudi Arabia – by a firsthand witness. Saudi J Kidney Dis Transpl. 2017;28:983–91.
95. Al-Khader AA, Absy M, alHasani MK, Joyce B, Sabbagh T. Successful pregnancy in renal transplant recipients treated with cyclosporine. Transplantation. 1988;45:987–8.
96. Shaheen FA, al-Sulaiman MH, al-Khader AA. Long-term nephrotoxicity after exposure to cyclosporine in utero. Transplantation. 1993;56:224–5.
97. Al-Khader AA, Al-Ghamdi G, Basri N, et al. Pregnancies in renal transplantrecipients—Withafocuson the maternal issues. Ann Transplant. 2004;9:62–4.
98. Al-Khader AA, Shaheen FA. Posttransplant complications encountered in renal transplantation in the Middle East. Transplant Proc. 2004;36:180–3.
99. Al-Khader AA, Basri N, AlGhamdi G, et al. Pregnancies in renal transplant recipients—with a focus on babies. Ann Transplant. 2004;9:65–7.
100. Owda AK, Abdalla AH, AlSulaiman MH, et al. No evidence of functional deterioration of renal graft after repeated pregnancies—a report on three women with 17 pregnancies. Nephrol Dial Transplant. 1998;13:1281–4.
101. al-Sulaiman MH, Dhar JM, alHasani MK, Haleem A, al-Khader A. Tuberculous interstitial nephritis after kidney transplantation. Transplantation. 1990;50:162–4.
102. Dhar JM, al-Khader AA, alSulaiman M, al-Hasani MK. Nontyphoid Salmonella in renal transplant recipients: a report of twenty cases and review of the literature. Q J Med. 1991;78:235–50.
103. Al-Sulaiman MH, Dlhar JM, al-Khader AA. Successful use of rifampcin in the treatment of tuberculosis in renal transplant patients immunosuppressed with cyclosporine. Transplantation. 1990;50:597–8.
104. Al-Sulaiman D, Mousa Z, Rassoul A, Abdallah M, Abdur Rehman AA, Al-Khader AA. Transplant-related Kaposi sarcoma in children. Nephrol Dial Transplant. 1994;9:443–5.
105. Gunawardena KA, al-Hasani MK, Haleem A, al-Suleiman M, alKhader AA. Pulmonary Kaposi's sarcoma in two recipients of renal transplants. Thorax. 1988;43:653–6.
106. Hanid MA, Suleiman M, Haleem A, al Karawi M, al Khader A. Gastrointestinal Kaposi's sarcoma in renal transplant patients. Q J Med. 1989;73:1143–9.
107. Al-Khader AA, Suleiman M, Al-Hasani M, Haleem A. Posttransplant Kaposi sarcoma: staging as a guide to therapy and prognosis. Nephron. 1988;48:165.
108. Qunibi W, Al-Furayh O, Almeshari K, et al. Serologic association of human herpesvirus eight with posttransplant Kaposi's sarcoma in Saudi Arabia. Transplantation. 1998;27:583–5.
109. al-Sulaiman MH, Mousa DH, Dhar JM, al-Khader AA. Does regressed posttransplantation Kaposi's sarcoma recur following reintroduction of immunosuppression? Am J Nephrol. 1992;12:384–6.
110. The Five Pillars of Islam. https://www.khanacademy.org/humanities/ap-art-history/cultures-religions-ap-arthistory/a/the-five-pillars-of-islam. Accessed 20 May 2019.
111. Pillars of Islam the Oxford Dictionary of Islam. http://www.oxfordislamicstudies.com/article/opr/t125/e1859. Accessed 20 May 2019.
112. The Holy Quran, Chapter of Al Baqarah (the Cow) verse 182.
113. Valid excuses for not fasting. https://www.islamweb.net/eramadan/articles/179261/valid-excuses-for-not-fasting. Accessed 20 May 2019.
114. Ghods AJ. Current status of organ transplant in Islamic countries. Exp Clin Transplant. 2015;13(1):13–7.

115. Shaheen FA, Al-Jondeby M, Kurpad R, Al-Khader AA. Social and cultural issues in organ transplantation in Islamic countries. Ann Transplant. 2004;9(2):11–3.
116. Cheah SH, Ch'Ng SL, Husain R, Duncan MT. Effects of fasting during Ramadan on urinary excretion in Malaysian Muslims. Br J Nutr. 1990;63(2):329–37.
117. Rapoport A, From GL, Husdan H. Metabolic studies in prolonged fasting: I. Inorganic metabolism and kidney function. Metabolism. 1965;14(1):31–46.
118. Yucecan NK. Some behavioural changes observed among fasting subjects, their nutritional habits and energy expenditure in Ramadan. Int J Food Sci Nutr. 2000;51(2):125–34.
119. Aslam M, Healy M. Compliance and drug therapy in fasting Moslem patients. J Clin Hosp Pharm. 1986;11:1–5.
120. Ghalib M, Qureshi J, Tamim H, Ghamdi G, Flaiw A, Hejaili F, et al. Does repeated Ramadan fasting adversely affect kidney function in renal transplant patients? Transplantation. 2008;85(1):141–4.
121. Said T, Nampoory MRN, Haleem MA, Nair MP, Johny KV, Samhan M, et al. Ramadan fast in kidney transplant recipients: a prospective comparative study. Transplant Proc. 2003;35(7):2614–6.
122. Einollahi B, Lessan-Pezeshki M, Pourfarziani V, Aghdam B, Rouzbeh J, Ghadiani MH, et al. Ramadan fasting in kidney transplant recipients with normal renal function and with mild-to-moderate renal dysfunction. Int Urol Nephrol. 2009;41(2):417–22.
123. Boobes Y, Bernieh B, Al Hakim MR. Fasting Ramadan in kidney transplant patients is safe. Saudi J Kidney Dis Transpl. 2009;20(2):198–200.
124. Hejaili F, Qurashi S, Binsalih S, Jaradt M, Al Sayyari A. Effect of repeated Ramadan fasting in the hottest months of the year on renal graft function. Nephrourol Mon. 2014;6(2):e14362.
125. Qurashi S, Tamimi A, Jaradat M, Al Sayyari A. Effect of fasting for Ramadan on kidney graft function during the hottest month of the year (August) in Riyadh, Saudi Arabia. Exp Clin Transplant. 2012;10(6):551–653.
126. Ibrahim IA, Hassan EA, Alkhan AM, Hussein MA, Alhabashi AF, Ali TZ, Shah YZ, Alahmadi IS, Abdelsalam MS, Rashwan ME, Abdulbaki A. Ramadan fasting in kidney transplant recipients: a single-centre retrospective study. J Transplant. 2018;2018:4890978.
127. Bouby N, Fernandes S. Mild dehydration, vasopressin and the kidney: animal and human studies. Eur J Clin Nutr. 2003;57(S2):S39.
128. Al-Khader AA, Al-Hasani MK, Dhar JM, Al-Sulaiman M. Effect of diet during Ramadan on patients on chronic haemodialysis. Saudi Med J. 1991;12(1):30–1.
129. Alshamsi S, Binsaleh F, Hejaili F, Karkar A, Moussa D, Raza H, Parbat P, Al Suwida A, Alobaili S, AlSehli R, Al Sayyari A. Changes in biochemical, hemodynamic, and dialysis adherence parameters in hemodialysis patients during Ramadan. Hemodial Int. 2016;20(2):27.
130. Al Wakeel J, Mitwalli AH, Alsuwaida A, Al Ghonaim M, Usama S, Hayat A, Shah IH. Recommendations for fasting in Ramadan for patients on peritoneal dialysis. Perit Dial Int. 2013;33(1):86–91.
131. Bernieh B, Al Hakim MR, Boobes Y, Abu Zidan FM. Fasting Ramadan in chronic kidney disease patients: clinical and biochemical effects. Saudi J Kidney Dis Transpl. 2010;21:898–902.
132. El-Wakil HS, Desoky I, Lotfy N, Adam AG. Fasting the month of Ramadan by Muslims: could it be injurious to their kidneys? Saudi J Kidney Dis Transpl. 2007;18:349–54.

# 29 Nephrology in Singapore

Damon Tan and Adrian Liew

| | |
|---|---|
| Area | 724.2 $km^2$ |
| Population[1] | 5.64 million (2018) |
| Capital | Singapore |
| Three most populated cities: | Not applicable (Singapore is an island city-state) |
| Official languages | English, Malay, Chinese, Tamil |
| Gross domestic product (GDP)[2] | 491.175 billion SGD |
| GDP per capita[2] | 87,108 SGD |
| Human development index (HDI)[2] | 0.932 (2017) |
| Official currency | Singapore Dollars (SGD) |
| Total number of nephrologists | 108 |
| National society of nephrology | Singapore Society of Nephrology |
| Incidence of end-stage renal disease[3] | 2017 – 324.5 pmp |
| Prevalence of end-stage renal disease[3] (including patients with a functioning kidney transplant) | 2017 – 2160.5 pmp |
| Total number of patients on dialysis[3] (all modalities) | 2016 – 6671<br>2017 – 7007 |
| Number of patients on haemodialysis[3] | 2016 – 5848<br>2017 – 6113 |
| Number of patients on peritoneal dialysis[3] | 2016 – 823<br>2017 – 894 |
| Number of renal transplantations per year[3] | 2016 – 95<br>2017 – 112 |

Table Reference:

1. Department of Statistics, Singapore. https://www.singstat.gov.sg. Accessed 30 June 2019
2. United Nations Development Programme. Human development reports. https://hdr.undp.org/en/countries/profiles/SGP. Accessed 30 June 2019
3. National Registry of Diseases Office. Singapore Renal Registry Annual Report 2017. https://www.nrdo.gov.sg/publications/kidney-failure. Accessed 1 Feb 2020

## Introduction

Singapore is a small densely populated island nation at the southern tip of the Malaysian Peninsula. It is a multi-racial and multi-religion community, with four major ethnic groups using English as the primary national language. Healthcare delivery had improved significantly since the country gained its independence in 1965, with life expectancy at birth increasing from 76.0 years in 1990 to 83.2 years in 2017 [1]. The public healthcare sector comprises seven tertiary level general hospitals, two specialized hospital looking after maternal/child health and mental health, respectively, and 18 primary care centres known as polyclinics. In addition, nine community hospitals provide subacute and intermediate care for patient requiring prolonged recovery. Polyclinics provide subsidized outpatient healthcare to about 25% of the population, with the remaining 75% being cared for by private general practitioners [2]. On the other hand, the private healthcare sector is supported by ten private hospitals, which provide both private inpatient and specialized outpatient care.

## Brief History of Nephrology in Singapore

The first renal unit was established at the site of the current Singapore General Hospital in 1961 by Professor Khoo Oon Teik, who is universally acknowledged to be the 'Founder of Nephrology in Singapore' [3]. During those times, only patients with acute kidney injury were offered dialysis, with the first patient receiving dialysis through the twin coil artificial kidney. It was not only until 1968 that the chronic haemodialysis programme took shape in Singapore [4]. Peritoneal dialysis, on the other hand, was only introduced in Singapore in 1980, with a formalized chronic peritoneal dialysis programme beginning later in 1986, while the first kidney transplant in Singapore was performed on 8 July 1970, from a deceased donor with a brain tumour [5]. This landmark surgery was deemed a success and paved the way for the country's first renal

D. Tan
Lee Kong Chian School of Medicine, Nanyang Technological University, Singapore, Singapore

A. Liew (✉)
The Kidney & Transplant Practice, Mount Elizabeth Novena Hospital, Singapore, Singapore



J. A. Moura-Neto et al. (eds.), *Nephrology Worldwide*, https://doi.org/10.1007/978-3-030-56890-0_29

transplantation programme which celebrated its 500th renal transplant in 1994.

With the advent of the chronic haemodialysis programme in 1968, it was realized that funds are required to assist needy patients who required long-term dialysis. A year later, on 7 April 1969, Professor Khoo formed and inaugurated the National Kidney Foundation of Singapore (NKF) [3], which held the first fundraising event for needy patients requiring dialysis through a film premiere in the same year. In 1972, the Singapore Society of Nephrology was then established to promote the development of nephrology in the country, with the first Asian Colloquium of Nephrology Conference organized in Singapore as a meeting of expert nephrologists in the region.

## Renal Diseases in Singapore

Kidney disease continues to impose a heavy burden on Singapore's healthcare system, with the country ranking 5th and 4th in the world for incidence and prevalence of treated end-stage renal disease (ESRD), respectively [6]. While data for ESRD is available, a formal registry for chronic kidney disease (CKD) has not been established in Singapore. Based on the National Health Survey in 2010 [2], the prevalence of CKD Stages 3–5 amongst residents aged 18–69 years was 2.3%, with males having a higher prevalence than females (2.8% versus 1.7%). The prevalence of CKD was also affected by age, increasing from 0.4% for those under 40 years to 2.0% between 40 and 54 years, and 6.8% amongst those aged 55–69 years. Furthermore, the prevalence of CKD was found to increase at an annual rate of 21.3% from 2007 to 2011 [7], amongst patients in the polyclinics, with majority being contributed by diabetic kidney disease.

Indeed, diabetic kidney disease has been the main cause of the ESRD burden in the country, with Singapore placing second amongst countries in the world having the highest incidence of treated ESRD due to diabetes [6]. This has alarmed the Singapore government sufficiently to declare a countrywide war on diabetes [8], with a national HALT-CKD programme implemented in 2017 to screen high-risk patients for CKD and to control CKD risk factors at the primary care level [9].

Notwithstanding the high incidence of diabetic kidney disease, glomerulonephritis (GN) remains an important cause of CKD and ESRD in Singapore. IgA nephropathy continues to be the most common pattern of biopsy-proven GN over the last four decades in the local setting, though its incidence has decreased from 1.8 in 100,000/year in the 1970s to 0.34 in 100,000/year in the current era [10]. In addition, there had been significant increases in the prevalence of focal segmental glomerulosclerosis in the last decade.

## Renal Replacement Therapy in Singapore

Healthcare financing in Singapore is anchored on the twin philosophies of individual responsibility and affordable healthcare for all, and it is disbursed through heavy government subsidies and the 3M framework (Fig. 29.1) – Medisave, Medishield Life and Medifund [11]. In the same way, fiscal support for renal replacement therapies (RRT) is built around these foundations of healthcare financing to help defray the high cost of dialysis treatment in Singapore. Patients with ESRD, depending on their financial situation, would be able to utilize:

(a) Government dialysis subsidies, which assist patients who are financially challenged, and are available at a tiered quantum based on their household per capita income. Patients with household income above a certain ceiling will not be able to enjoy these subsidies (Table 29.1).

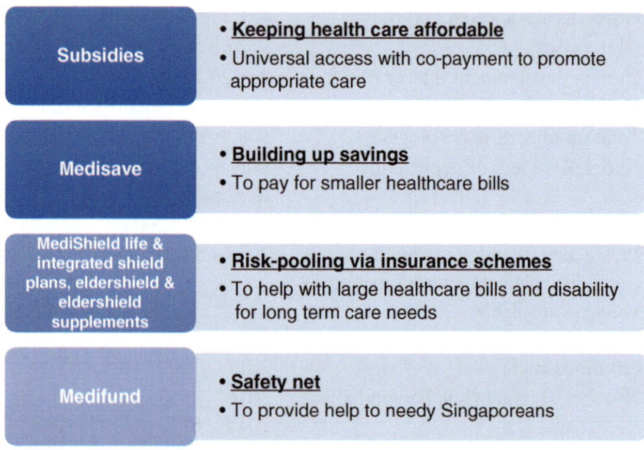


**Fig. 29.1** Framework of healthcare financing in Singapore

**Table 29.1** Monthly government subsidies for patients on haemodialysis or peritoneal dialysis

| Household per capita monthly income (SGD) | Community haemodialysis subsidies per month (SGD) | | Peritoneal dialysis subsidies per month (SGD) | |
|---|---|---|---|---|
| | Singapore citizens | Permanent residents | Singapore citizens | Permanent residents |
| $700 and below | $1160 | $927 | $1210 | $977 |
| $701 to $1100 | $813 | $650 | $863 | $700 |
| $1101 to $1600 | $581 | $465 | $631 | $515 |
| $1601 to $1800 | $476 | $382 | $526 | $432 |
| $1801 to $2600 | $337 | $268 | $387 | $318 |
| $2601 and above | $0 | $0 | $0 | $0 |

Reference: Ministry of Health [20]

(b) Medishield Life is a basic health insurance plan for all Singaporeans, which will provide coverage for dialysis but capped at SGD 1000 per month or 90% of the remaining cost of RRT after government subsidies, whichever is lower.
(c) Medisave is a compulsory personal saving plan, which, after the above assistance, could be used to offset the monthly cost of dialysis, up to a maximum of SGD 450 per month.
(d) Out-of-pocket payment after exhausting the above assistance programmes.
(e) Financial assistance from Voluntary Welfare Organizations (VWO) such as the NKF if the residual costs continue to be beyond the financial means of the patients.

Over the years, Singapore has seen a rapid rise in the incidence of ESRD patients treated with dialysis, from 165.3 per million population (pmp) in 1999 to 296.3 pmp in 2017 [12]. Notwithstanding the high incidence of diabetes mellitus and an ageing population, the greater availability and avenues for dialysis funding had ensured that no patient is ever denied RRT because of financial concerns. Therefore, the provision of substantial financial assistance from the above initiatives had removed high dialysis costs as a deterrent for RRT. Patients are less resistant in considering dialysis treatment, and physicians are less hesitant in promoting RRT, and both of these two perspectives had contributed to the rapid increase in ESRD patients being initiated on dialysis treatment in recent years.

## Haemodialysis

Haemodialysis remains the predominant RRT modality in Singapore, with 87.2% of the prevalent dialysis population undergoing long-term chronic haemodialysis in 2017, albeit a gradual decline in the percentage of incident ESRD patients being placed on this modality from 87.5% in 2008 to 78.0% in 2017 [12]. The significant growth in the ESRD population over the last decade has placed significant pressure to provide affordable dialysis treatment for all patients. This resulted in less discriminative financial subsidies against haemodialysis. Coupled with the greater familiarity with haemodialysis, inequitable levels of peritoneal dialysis expertise and a higher demand for dialysis therapies, this had resulted in a surge of patients being placed on haemodialysis towards the end of the last decade (Fig. 29.2).

Chronic haemodialysis in Singapore is a community-based programme, with patients undergoing dialysis treatment in satellite haemodialysis centres near to their place of residence. The majority of the patients (62.1%) are receiving haemodialysis therapies in dialysis centres managed by VWOs, with the remaining being treated mainly in private haemodialysis centres (36.2%) [12]. A small proportion (1.7%) of haemodialysis patients are managed in government hospitals, who are considered to require more intensive nursing care or have greater haemodynamic instability during dialysis. Consequently, as of August 2018, the NKF, which is the largest renal-related VWO in Singapore, operates 33 of the 100 licensed haemodialysis centres in the country.

All chronic haemodialysis centres in Singapore no longer reuse dialyser, with single-use dialyser being the norm for both patients with or without blood-borne virus infections (hepatitis B, hepatitis C and HIV). While convective therapies such as haemodiafiltration and haemofiltration are available in Singapore, the cost of these treatments is significantly higher and without additional reimbursement from the national insurance or government subsidy programmes. Consequently, their utility is rare and the prevalence of these

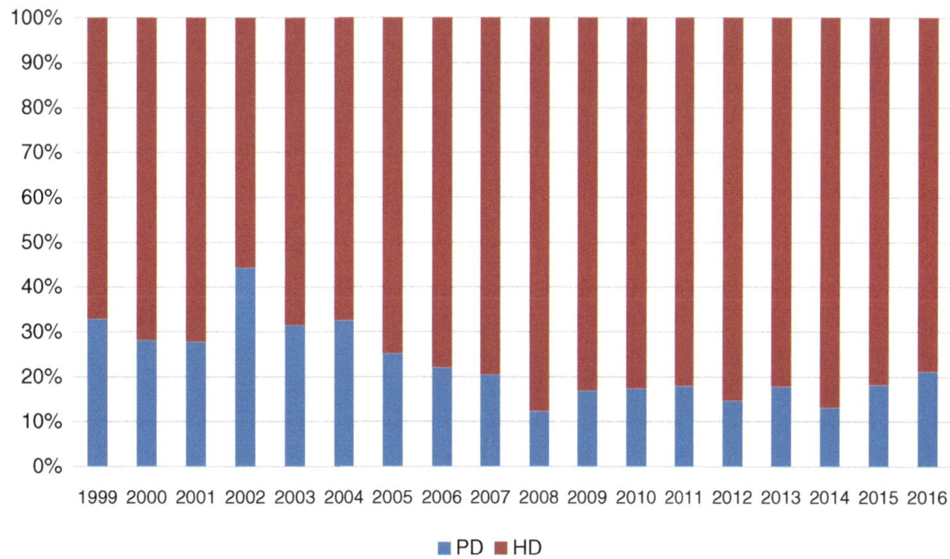


Fig. 29.2 Trends in the utilization of dialysis modality in Singapore

therapies is not systematically collected by the Singapore Renal Registry.

The 1-year, 5-year and 10-year reported survival rates of patients on definitive haemodialysis are 90.5%, 61.1% and 35.7%, respectively, with a median survival of 6.8 years [12]. There is no national registry pertaining specifically to haemodialysis; however, the NKF, which received the greater proportion of haemodialysis patients in the country, do report on clinical outcomes. While a high proportion of incident patients in the NKF (66.6%) were initiated with a tunnelled haemodialysis catheter without a pre-fashioned native vascular access, the majority eventually end up with a functioning arteriovenous fistula (AVF) or graft (AVG) [13]. Of the prevalent patients in the NKF programme, only 16.3% will be on long-term catheter-based haemodialysis [13].

## Peritoneal Dialysis

The high haemodialysis population in the last decade had resulted in significant stresses on healthcare resources, and the continued establishment of community haemodialysis centres in land-scarce Singapore is not sustainable to mitigate the dialysis demands in the long term. In a major review of dialysis provision in 2000, the Ministry of Health, Singapore, estimated that the direct cost of dialysis treatment and its associated services was in excess of SGD 90 million or about SGD 36,000 per patient per year [14]. In addition, it was also observed that despite the overall lower cost of peritoneal dialysis, there was a disproportionately higher number of patients receiving haemodialysis treatment.

Consequently, the Ministry of Health set a target in the 2000 review to increase the proportion of patients receiving peritoneal dialysis to 35% by 2005 and 40% by 2010 [14]. The levels of government subsidies for peritoneal dialysis were subsequently increased vis-à-vis haemodialysis, so that the direct out-of-pocket expenses for patients would be less for peritoneal dialysis. In tandem, educational initiatives were introduced to improve the public's and patients' awareness and understanding of peritoneal dialysis and resulted in a significant increase in the prevalence and incidence of patients on peritoneal dialysis to about 44.4% in 2002 (Fig. 29.2).

Unfortunately, the pressure to provide affordable dialysis to all patients in the mid-2000 removed the differential financial benefits towards peritoneal dialysis and the initial growth of peritoneal dialysis was not sustained, hovering below 20% of the dialysis population in the last 10 years. Recognizing the impetus to ensure a sustained provision of ESRD care and changes in the healthcare setting in this era, the Ministry of Health revisited the options of care delivery in this population again in 2015, and mapped out a strategy to increase the utilization of peritoneal dialysis in Singapore, which included the following:

**Table 29.2** Differences in survival of patients on haemodialysis and peritoneal dialysis, stratified by different time periods

| | 1999–2002 | | 2003–2007 | | 2008–2012 | | 2013–2017 | |
|---|---|---|---|---|---|---|---|---|
| | HD | PD | HD | PD | HD | PD | HD | PD |
| 1-year survival (%) | 91.5 | 84.3 | 89.2 | 87.5 | 90.0 | 90.2 | 91.6 | 92.4 |
| 5-year survival (%) | 62.4 | 32.2 | 59.0 | 37.9 | 60.5 | 45.7 | – | – |
| 10-year survival (%) | 40.1 | 16.3 | 33.7 | 20.2 | – | – | – | – |
| Median survival (years) | 7.6 | 3.2 | 6.5 | 3.7 | 6.6 | 4.5 | Not reached | |

(a) Peritoneal dialysis was accorded a slightly greater amount of financial subsidy from the government across all tiers of household per capita income (Table 29.1).
(b) Promoting the awareness and enhancing the community support for peritoneal dialysis by both the government healthcare and VWO sectors.
(c) Physician-integrated CKD programmes, with emphasis placed on peritoneal dialysis education, harmonization of dialysis counselling towards greater peritoneal dialysis focus and minimizing administrative hurdles towards peritoneal dialysis.

In terms of peritoneal dialysis outcomes, the Singapore Renal Registry reported 1-year, 5-year and 10-year survival rates on peritoneal dialysis to be 88.6%, 40.5% and 21.1%, respectively, with a median survival of 3.9 years [12]. While this appeared to be inferior to the survival of patients on haemodialysis, it may be a reflection of the differences in the casemix of patients and did not take into account the improvement in care and technology across different time periods. Indeed, when stratified across different time intervals, the survival of patients on peritoneal dialysis had improved significantly across the years, with even a suggestion that peritoneal dialysis may have a superior survival over haemodialysis in recent years (Table 29.2).

## Renal Transplantation

In 1987, the Human Organ Transplant Act (HOTA) was implemented in Singapore to improve organ transplant rates through deceased donation. Since then, the HOTA had undergone several revisions till the key iteration in 2009, where deceased donation was extended to include corneas, kidneys, liver and heart from all Singaporeans and permanent residents 21 years old and above, who do not have any mental disorders [15]. Deceased donation, therefore, became an opt-

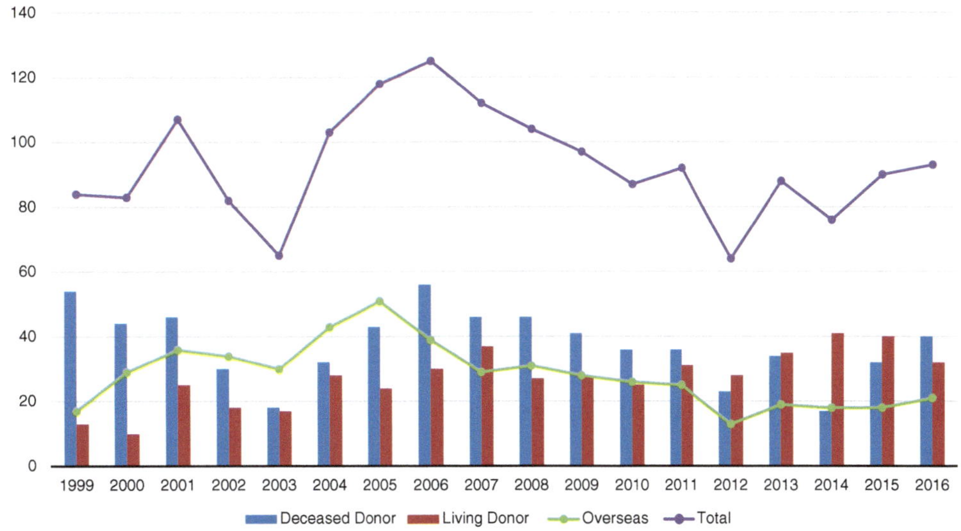


**Fig. 29.3** Number of incident kidney transplantations by donor characteristics

**Table 29.3** Graft and patient survival in Singapore 1999–2017, stratified by type of kidney transplantation

| | Graft survival | | | Patient survival | | |
|---|---|---|---|---|---|---|
| | Local living donor | Deceased donor | Overall | Local living donor | Deceased donor | Overall |
| 1-year survival (%) | 99.2 | 95.8 | 97.2 | 99.2 | 97.4 | 98.2 |
| 5-year survival (%) | 94.5 | 85.1 | 88.9 | 96.1 | 91.6 | 93.4 |
| 10-year survival (%) | 83.1 | 68.1 | 75.5 | 90.0 | 82.0 | 85.4 |
| Median survival (years) | Not reached | 16.2 | Not reached | Not reached | Not reached | Not reached |

out system across the nation, rather than through an unsolicited voluntary process.

Deceased donors remain the predominant source of kidneys for transplantation in Singapore, while efforts are made to increase the rate of living donation in the last few years (Fig. 29.3). Overseas transplantation, often through commercial means, used to be rampant at the start of this century; but with the concerted international efforts to abolish commercialized transplantation, the incidence of this group of transplant recipients had decreased significantly in the last decade [12].

Currently, all deceased donor renal transplantations are performed exclusively in two public hospitals, while living donor renal transplantation occurs in the same two public hospitals and three private sector healthcare institutions. Efforts have been made over the last two decades to improve the renal transplantation rates in Singapore, and some of these included nationwide educational efforts to promote living donation, preferential subsidies for immunosuppression medications post-transplantation and developing capabilities and infrastructure for ABO-incompatible renal transplantation and paired exchanges.

The outcomes of renal transplantation in Singapore are excellent, with 1-year, 5-year and 10-year graft survival being 97.2%, 88.9% and 75.5%, respectively [12], with patient survival noted to parallel similar exceptional trends (Table 29.3). Like in many countries, the outcomes of living donor renal transplantation surpassed that of deceased donor renal transplants (Table 29.3). A living donor care registry exists in Singapore, and outcomes of living donor after nephrectomies for transplantation are excellent. Over a 2-year period, while the eGFR of living donors decreased by 33.8% from baseline after kidney donation, the renal function recovered gradually to stabilize at 29.6% from baseline [16]. There were also no cases of ESRD or deaths amongst local living donors, when followed up for 24 months after kidney donation [16].

## Other Nephrology Services in Singapore

### Paediatric Nephrology

Paediatric nephrology services are provided by only two children hospitals in Singapore – the National University Hospital (NUH) and the Kandang Kerbau Women and Children Hospital (KKWCH). Both hospitals have capabilities for management of children with general nephrology conditions, critical care nephrology and continuous renal replacement therapy (CRRT), chronic haemodialysis and chronic peritoneal dialysis. Renal transplantation, both deceased donor and living donor, however, is only performed in the NUH.

### Acute Kidney Injury and Critical Care Nephrology

Critical care nephrology with capabilities for all forms of CRRT is available in all the acute public hospitals in Singapore and managed by nephrologists in collaboration with intensivists. There is, however, no registry data that exists for acute kidney injury or the casemix and outcomes of nephrology-related conditions in the intensive care setting. Information regarding this area is therefore limited.

## Nephrology Practice in Singapore

### Training

Nephrology training for physicians in Singapore is a 3-year training programme that occurs after 3 years of accredited internal medicine training and is administered only in three sponsoring institutions in the public sector healthcare institutions. The average annual intake of nephrology fellows hovers around two to three training candidates per institution per year. The training programme consists of structured rotations of 4–6 monthly blocks in core specialties of nephrology, including general nephrology, haemodialysis, peritoneal dialysis, renal transplantation, glomerulonephritis and critical care nephrology. Trainees are also assessed and evaluated on the six core competencies that are modelled after the Accreditation Council for Graduate Medical Education (ACGME) system [17] and include Practice-Based Learning and Improvement, Patient Care and Procedural Skills, System-Based Practice, Medical Knowledge, Interpersonal and Communication Skills and Professionalism. A summative assessment examination is conducted at the end of the 3-year training period, which upon passing the necessary requirements, the candidate will be accorded nephrology specialist privileges with the Singapore Specialist Accreditation Board.

Renal nursing training occurs mainly on the job, while a 1-year advanced diploma course in nephrology is available and administered by one of the polytechnics. However, attaining the diploma is not a prerequisite for nephrology nurse practice. Similarly, there are no formal postgraduate training programmes for renal pharmacists or renal dieticians to enter into these specialized allied health fields of nephrology practice.

### Hospital-Based Practice

Nephrologists in Singapore are mainly in hospital-based practice, with about 80% practising exclusively in the public institutions and the remaining 20% in the private sector. The daily duties are mainly clinical, comprising both inpatient and outpatient responsibilities, while a proportion of time may be devoted to undergraduate and postgraduate education, clinical research or administrative obligations. In addition, nephrologists may be required to review patients in community haemodialysis centres on a regular basis.

Currently, seven public sector hospitals provide renal care to all the subsidized patients in the country. All these hospitals have the capability to deliver all aspects of basic nephrology care, including renal biopsies, continuous renal replacement therapies (CRRT), critical care nephrology, acute and chronic haemodialysis and chronic peritoneal dialysis, while only two hospitals have been designated to have transplantation capabilities. Most, if not all, with some degree of variability, have multidisciplinary teams that include renal nurses, renal pharmacists, renal dieticians, medical social workers, dialysis or transplant counsellors and coordinators.

### Salaries of Nephrologists

In 2012 and 2014, the Ministry of Health underwent a major review of the salaries of doctors in the public healthcare institutions, with an aim to improve the retention of doctors in the public sector [18]. The new salary framework took into account the roles of doctors in the public sector in areas such as education and research, as well as market trends, so as to close the salary gap between the public and private sectors. While speculative, this could have been one of the successful reasons in reducing the exodus of nephrologists from the public institutions to the private sectors in recent years.

## Future Perspectives of Nephrology in Singapore

The burden of kidney diseases and dialysis poses a significant pressure on the healthcare system in Singapore, and the prospect of expanding haemodialysis centres in land-scarce Singapore is not sustainable in providing accessible RRT for all ESRD patients. Consequently, a strategic roadmap for mitigating the rising ESRD load was developed by the Ministry of Health and comprised five broad areas:

(a) Prevention, Early Intervention and Management of Kidney Diseases
(b) Peritoneal Dialysis Preferred Strategy
(c) Promotion of Living Donor Renal Transplantation
(d) Optimizing Haemodialysis Capabilities
(e) Advance Care Planning and Palliative Care Nephrology

## Prevention, Early Intervention and Management of Kidney Diseases

Given that diabetes mellitus and hypertension are the two leading causes of preventable ESRD in Singapore [12], it is important strategically to focus on upstream preventive measures to reduce the prevalence of ESRD. The HALT-CKD (Holistic Approach to Lowering and Tracking CKD) programme [9] is a national initiative that started in 2017, which systematically screens for CKD in patients with diabetes and hypertension in the primary care institutions. Key interventions are implemented in patients diagnosed with early stages of CKD, involving blood pressure and diabetic control, optimizing the doses of ACE inhibitors or angiotensin receptor blockers and lifestyle modifications. Patients are tracked longitudinally for compliance and response, with early referral to nephrology services for pre-emptive preparation for RRT at CKD Stage 3B. In its early stages of implementation, the HALT-CKD will be evaluated for its effectiveness in reducing the rate of ESRD in the country within the next 3–5 years.

## Peritoneal Dialysis Preferred Strategy

Peritoneal dialysis has been assessed to be more cost-effective and is a much more sustainable RRT modality in managing the ESRD load in Singapore. Taking into account the relatively lower current prevalence rate of ESRD patients on peritoneal dialysis, the aim is to increase the utilization of peritoneal dialysis in the country to 30% by the year 2025 [19]. To achieve this endeavour, the Ministry of Health in Singapore will progressively effect several initiatives, which include:

(a) Strengthening professional and patient education on peritoneal dialysis
(b) Providing adequate support for patients on peritoneal dialysis through assisted peritoneal dialysis programmes
(c) Enhancing community support for peritoneal dialysis patients, including home visits
(d) Having a more discriminative financial differential for out-of-pocket payment between both dialysis modalities, in favour of augmenting the subsidies towards peritoneal dialysis

## Promotion of Living Donor Renal Transplantation

With renal transplantation providing the best outcomes for patients with ESRD, efforts to increase living donor renal transplantation is a key strategy in improving the care of ESRD in Singapore. Public educational efforts will be augmented, to begin earlier at the schooling age. Initiatives to minimize inconvenience to potential living donors will be examined and implemented accordingly, to encourage living donation and remove administrative and financial obstacles to renal transplantation. Issues such as time off work, lack of insurance coverage and financial cost of pre-donation evaluation, surgery and post-surgical care are identified deterrents to living kidney donation and will be reviewed with the respective stakeholders to make the process less onerous.

## Optimizing Haemodialysis Capabilities

Expanding the number of haemodialysis centres is a challenge in land-scarce Singapore, and the nursing manpower required to support these centres will be limited. Therefore, instead of building more haemodialysis centres with the need to augment nursing manpower, the strategy would be to optimize the utilization of resources in existing centres such as promoting self-dialysis and nocturnal haemodialysis in these units. The Ministry is also exploring the feasibility of developing a home haemodialysis programme in Singapore.

## Advance Care Planning and Palliative Care Nephrology

Besides dialysis, conservative management is also an option for ESRD patients, particularly for those in poor condition, with multiple co-morbid illness or have haemodynamic instability, and who would not benefit from dialysis treatment. However, given the sensitive and emotional considerations for the patients and their caregivers, there is a need to provide more support and assurance to patients opting for conservative management in the decision-making process. In addition, there is a need to develop a robust palliative care framework for patients who have eventually decided on non-dialytic treatment for their ESRD condition, so that they do not feel abandoned during the last phase of their condition. The fraternity will work to align the advance care planning parameters for CKD and ESRD patients, so that the discussion can start earlier at CKD Stage 3 or 4. The Ministry is also currently working to ramp up the capacity for palliative care services in the home and inpatient settings, and to partner with home care providers to expand home palliative care services beyond oncology, so as to include patients with end-stage organ failure. With stronger palliative care and support available, the option of conservative management would be less intimidating to patients and their caregivers, as they would be more assured of receiving timely symptomatic treatment and emotional support in their end-of-life stages.

## Conclusion

Singapore continues to face challenges in providing care to patients with kidney diseases. Despite having the necessary infrastructure and healthcare resources currently to provide renal replacement therapies to the increasing ESRD population, dialysis alone is not a sustainable option in the long run. Prevention of ESRD and retarding the progression of CKD continues to be a key strategy in addressing the high ESRD disease burden, while decreasing the reliance on haemodialysis would be necessary to ensure appropriate access to care for all patients.

## References


1. United Nations Development Programme. Human development reports. https://hdr.undp.org/en/countries/profiles/SGP. Accessed 30 June 2019.
2. Ministry of Health, Singapore. National Health Survey 2010. https://www.moh.gov.sg/resources-statistics/reports/national-health-survey-2010. Accessed 30 June 2019.
3. Lee EJC, Chew CH. Dr Khoo Oon Teik (1921–2012). Ann Acad Med Singap. 2012;41:234–5.
4. Choong HL, Pwee HS, Woo KT, et al. Maintenance haemodialysis in Singapore. Singap Med J. 1991;32:133–8.
5. National Library Board, Singapore. First kidney transplant. https://eresources.nlb.gov.sg/infopedia/articles/SIP_1647_2010-02-19.html. Accessed 30 June 2019.
6. United States Renal Data System. USRDS 2018 annual data report. https://www.usrds.org/2018/download/v2_c11_IntComp_18_usrds.pdf. Accessed 30 June 2019.
7. Ang GY, Heng BH, Liew AST, et al. Quality of care of patients with chronic kidney disease in national healthcare group polyclinic from 2007 to 2011. Ann Acad Med Singap. 2013;42:632–9.
8. Ministry of Health, Singapore. War on diabetes. https://www.moh.gov.sg/wodcj. Accessed 30 June 2019.
9. Ministry of Health, Singapore. Speech by Mr Chan Heng Kee, Permanent Secretary, Ministry of Health, at the 3rd Kidney Care Conference 2019, 25 May 2019. https://www.moh.gov.sg/news-highlights/details/speech-by-mr-chan-heng-kee-permanent-secretary-ministry-of-health-at-the-3rd-kidney-care-conference-2019-25-may-2019. Accessed 30 June 2019.
10. Woo KT, Chan CM, Lim C, et al. Changes in primary glomerulonephritis in Singapore over four decades. Clin Nephrol. 2019;91:155–61.
11. Ministry of Health, Singapore. Healthcare schemes & subsidies. https://www.moh.gov.sg/cost-financing/healthcare-schemes-subsidies. Accessed 30 June 2019.
12. National Registry of Diseases Office. Singapore renal registry annual report 2017. https://www.nrdo.gov.sg/publications/kidney-failure. Accessed 1 Feb 2020.
13. The National Kidney Foundation Singapore. NKF Singapore haemodialysis programme clinical outcomes – annual report 2015–16. https://www.nkfs.org/images/clinical-outcomes-annual-report/NKF_HD_Clinical_Outcomes_Annual_Report_2015-16.pdf. Accessed 30 June 2019.
14. Tan CC, Chan CM, Ho CK, et al. Health economics of renal replacement therapy: perspectives from Singapore. Kidney Int Suppl. 2005;94:S19–22.
15. Attorney-General's Chambers, Singapore. Singapore Statutes Online. Human Organ Transplant Act (Chapter 131A). https://sso.agc.gov.sg/Act/HOTA1987. Accessed 30 June 2019.
16. Ho MZJ, Zheng H, Lee JJM, et al. Selection and short-term outcomes of living kidney donors in Singapore – an analysis of the donor care registry. Ann Acad Med Singap. 2017;46:424–32.
17. NEJM Knowledge+ Team. Exploring the ACGME core competencies (Part 1 of 7). https://knowledgeplus.nejm.org/blog/exploring-acgme-core-competencies/. Accessed 30 June 2019.
18. Today Online 13 March 2014. Senior doctors, dentists in public sector to get 9% pay rise. https://www.todayonline.com/singapore/senior-doctors-dentists-public-sector-get-9-pay-rise. Accessed 30 June 2019.
19. Zaobao Singapore 26 November 2017. Increasing peritoneal dialysis to 30% by 2025. https://www.zaobao.com.sg/znews/singapore/story20171126-813902. Accessed 30 June 2019.
20. Ministry of Health, Singapore. Subsidies for government-funded intermediate long-term care services. https://www.moh.gov.sg/cost-financing/healthcare-schemes-subsidies/subsidies-for-government-funded-intermediate-long-term-care-services. Accessed 30 June 2019.

# Nephrology in the Sultanate of Oman

# 30

Issa Al Salmi, Yaqoub Al-Maymmani, Mohammed Al-Riyami, Waleed Al-Rajhi, Ruqiya Al-Za'abi, Intisar Al-Alawi, Medhat Ali, Ehab Abul Raziq Mohammed, and Fatma Al Rahbi

## Abbreviations

| | |
|---|---|
| APD | Automated peritoneal dialysis |
| AV | Arteriovenous |
| AVF | Arteriovenous fistula |
| AVG | Arteriovenous graft |
| BMI | Body mass index |
| BP | Blood pressure |
| CAPD | Continuous ambulatory peritoneal dialysis |
| CGA | Cause, glomerular filtration rate [GFR] category, and albuminuria |
| CKD | Chronic kidney disease |
| CRF | Chronic renal failure |
| CVA | Cerebrovascular accident |
| CVC | Central venous cannula/catheter |
| CVD | Cardiovascular disease |
| DM | Diabetes mellitus |
| DN | Diabetic nephropathy |
| eGFR | Estimated glomerular filtration rate |
| ESRD | End-stage renal disease |
| FVC | Femoral venous cannula/catheter |
| GCC | Gulf Cooperation Countries |
| GFR | Glomerular filtration rate |
| GN | Glomerulonephritis |
| GNI | Gross National Income |
| HD | Hemodialysis |
| HRQoL | Health-related quality of life |
| HTN | Hypertension |
| JVC | Jugular venous cannula/catheter |
| KDOQI | Kidney Disease Outcomes Quality Initiative |
| KDQOL | Kidney disease and quality of life |
| KF | Kidney failure |
| KSA | Kingdom of Saudi Arabia |
| *M* | Mean |
| ME | Middle East |
| MOH | Ministry of Health |
| MR | Mortality rate |
| *N* | Number |
| NCDs | Non-communicable diseases |
| NKF | National Kidney Foundation |
| NRLD | Non-related living donor |
| NSAIDS | Non-steroidal anti-inflammatory drugs |
| OMJ | Oman Medical Journal |
| OMR | Omani Rial |
| *P* | P-Value |
| P.cath | Permicatheter |
| PD | Peritoneal dialysis |
| Pmp | Per million population |
| PRD | Primary renal diagnosis |
| QoL | Quality of life |
| RA | Renal Association |
| RCTs | Randomized control trials |
| RDCs | Renal dialysis centers |
| RRT | Renal replacement therapy |
| RT | Renal transplant |
| SCOT | Saudi Center for Organ Transplantation |
| SD | Standard deviation |
| SLE | Systematic lupus erythematous |
| SQU | Sultan Qaboos University |
| SQUH | Sultan Qaboos University Hospital |
| SQUML | Sultan Qaboos University Medical Library |
| SRR | Scottish Renal Registry |
| UAE | United Arab Emirates |
| UK | United Kingdom |

I. Al Salmi (✉) · Y. Al-Maymmani · M. Al-Riyami
E. A. R. Mohammed · F. Al Rahbi
The Renal Medicine Department, The Royal Hospital, Muscat, Oman

W. Al-Rajhi
College of Pharmacy and Nursing, Nizwa, Oman
e-mail: w.alrajhi@unizwa.edu.com

R. Al-Za'abi
Nurse Tutor, Muscat, Oman

I. Al-Alawi
The National Genetic Centre, The Royal Hospital, Muscat, Oman

M. Ali
The Renal Medicine Department, Nizwa Hospital, Nizwa, Oman


J. A. Moura-Neto et al. (eds.), *Nephrology Worldwide*, https://doi.org/10.1007/978-3-030-56890-0_30

| | |
|---|---|
| UKRR | United Kingdom Renal Registry |
| UN | United Nations |
| USA | United States of America |
| USRDS | The United States Renal Data System |
| WHO | World Health Organisation |

| | |
|---|---|
| Area | 309,500 $Km^2$ |
| Population[1] | 4,647,110 (2018) |
| Capital | Muscat (Mct) |
| Three most populated cities | 1. Bushar (299,238)<br>2. As Seeb (265,901)<br>3. Salalah (235,563) |
| Official language | Arabic |
| Gross domestic product (GDP)[2] | 79.277 billion USD (2018) |
| GDP per capita[2] | 16,415.157 USD (2018) |
| Human Development Index (HDI)[3] | 0.834 (2018) |
| Official currency | Oman Rial (OMR) |
| Total number of nephrologists | 110 |
| National society of nephrology | Oman Renal Failure Society |
| Incidence of end-stage renal disease | 2018 – 200 pmp |
| Prevalence of end-stage renal disease (on dialysis) | 2018 – 1150 pmp |
| Total number of patients on dialysis (all modalities) | 2018 – 2300<br>2019 – 2500 |
| Number of patients on hemodialysis | 2018 – 2056<br>2019 – 2201 |
| Number of patients on peritoneal dialysis | 2019 – adults 190, pediatric 37 |
| Number of renal transplantation per year | 2018 – 30 pmp<br>2019 – 25 pmp |
| Vascular access rate | AVF – 76%<br>AVG – 6%<br>Permcath – 16%<br>Temporary access – 2% |
| Mortality rate | 2018 – 8.1%<br>2019 – 10.8% |

1. National Center for Statistics and information. Population statistics. At URL https://www.ncsi.gov.om/Elibrary/LibraryContentDoc/bar_population2018_ea9a7a9b-65d1-4b2a-856e-093d4406209d.pdf
2. The World Bank. https://data.worldbank.org/country/oman?view=chart
3. United Nations Development Programme Human Development Reports. http://hdr.undp.org/en/countries/profiles/OMN

## Introduction

The Sultanate of Oman is in the south-eastern corner of the Arabian Peninsula. The total area of the Sultanate is around 309.500 square kilometers and the density is 16 per $Km^2$ [42 people per $mi^2$ [1]. The population of Oman according to the National Center for Statistic and Information was 4.65 million by the end of 2018, of which about 56% are Omani citizens [2], and with 1 million aged 14 years and below [2]. The Omani population is relatively young [median age, 29.3 years], of which 12% and 34% of the population are under 5 years and under 15 years, respectively, whereas only 3.8% are 60 years and above [2]. Oman population is equivalent to 0.06% of the total world population and 71.0% of the population is urban (3,551,726 people in 2019) [2]. The sex ratio is 102 males per 100 females; and the cingulate mean age at first marriage is 25 years for females and 28 years for males [3].

Since 1970, Oman has undergone rapid socioeconomic development along with demographic trends that have been positively reflected in all sectors, including the health service sector. Examples include a rise in life expectancy at birth and a decline in the frequency of infectious diseases. Free-of-charge health services are provided to all citizens by the Ministry of Health (MoH) with a total workforce of 56,152, including 9132 registered physicians, 19,938 nurses (372 are specialized in renal dialysis; 291 [78%] of them are Omanis), 2387 laboratory technicians, 1350 dentists, 2445 pharmacists, and 2020 assistant pharmacists [4]. According to the MoH 2017 annual report, for every 10,000 population, there are 20 doctors and 43.7 nurses in the country when compared to 9.0 doctors and 26.0 nurses in 1990. In 2017, the nurse–doctor ratio was 2.2, and medical officer–specialist ratio was 1.3 [4]. The MoH provides primary health care through 270 health care centers (including non-MoH), 76 hospitals, and 1215 private clinics and diagnostic health centers [5, 6].

In recent years, Oman has been facing a rapid change in the disease profile, from first-generation diseases such as infectious to non-communicable diseases, including cardiovascular diseases [CVD], diabetes mellitus [DM], chronic kidney disease [CKD], and cancer. In fact, the burden of non-communicable diseases has been a global public health concern, with chronic disease accounting for 61% of global deaths and 49% of the worldwide burden of disease. According to the World Health Organization (WHO), CKD is the sixth main cause of death in Oman, with a rate of 18.10 per 100,000 population (2.97% of total deaths) [7, 8]. Oman was ranked 51st among the top world countries in which CKD is a major cause of death [7]. In addition, 40% of inpatient and 55% of outpatient morbidity in 2005 was caused by chronic non-communicable diseases, compared to 36% and 43% in 1995. The prevalence of hypertension [defined as blood pressure ≥ 140/90 mm Hg] among individuals of both sexes aged ≥20 years has increased considerably, from 27% in 1995 to 32% in 2000 [6]. CKD is a global issue and is ranked among the top 25 causes of years of life lost due to premature mortality. In Oman, using this ranking system, CKD was ranked 11th in 2010, moving from its previous position of 22nd in 1990. Similarly, CKD was ranked 22nd within the top 25 causes of disability-adjusted life years in the Omani population [6]. Oman has witnessed significant development over the past 49 years, becoming one of the wealthy countries in the Arabian Gulf area [9, 10]. Health services have developed accordingly, including services for CKD patients. However, this dramatic enlargement in economic status has been accompanied by changes in the lifestyle of the Omanis which are presumed to contribute to increasing the incidence of end stage renal disease (ESRD) [10, 11]. This dramatic alteration in lifestyle has challenged the healthcare system in Oman to meet the increase in non-communicable diseases. The causes of renal failure are still mostly due to DM, hypertension, and chronic glomerulonephritis (GN); and many cases present at an advanced stage. DM is responsible for almost 50% of the causes of CKD on dialysis in this population [7, 10, 11].

The delivery of treatment for ESRD presents significant expenses and ethical challenges in all countries, including Oman. The national dialysis services in Oman have stretched between 1985 and 2019 to include an additional private-sector dialysis unit to meet the demands for dialysis treatment. Since the health services in Oman are provided by the national health system, the services for citizens with renal failure are fully paid for by the government [11]. Despite the expansion of dialysis services of hemodialysis (HD) and peritoneal dialysis (PD), kidney transplantation (KT) is limited within Oman, which could be a factor that may challenge the sustainability of the health services [3, 7, 10, 11].

## History of Nephrology in Oman

*Introduction* In the 1950s–1960s, nephrology care was launched in the modern world. After two to three decades, nephrology care was started in Muscat, the capital of Oman, in the early 1980s as a result of initial efforts from the MoH, and some non-Omani nephrologists pioneers who worked for the MoH of Oman at that time [12].

*Initial Nephrology Services* The first renal replacement therapy (RRT) care in Oman was PD for acute kidney injury (AKI) cases. The hospital-based modality was the only treatment of kidney disease at that time in Oman. This service started in April 1980 by Dr. AM AL Riyami who was a consultant in general internal medicine. General nephrology services were made available in Muscat between the years 1980–1983 [12]. The general nephrology services consisted of a nephrology Out-Patient Department (OPD), a hypertension referral clinic and a pediatric nephrology (out-patient clinic) on a weekly basis in Al-Nahda Hospital (an old hospital situated in Muscat, and which still exists). Between 1980 and 1983, PD was still the only conducted RRT in Oman, but only for AKI patients [7, 10, 11].

*Development of Nephrology and Dialysis Capacity* The first HD center opened on March 12, 1983, at the Al-Nahda Hospital with seven HD machines and serving 35 patients [9, 12]. The patients who were on HD outside the country in places such as Bombay, India were transported gradually to Oman to resume their dialysis in the Al-Nahda Renal Dialysis Center where the father of nephrology in Oman, Dr. Humood Al Marhuby, orchestrated their return back home. Al-Nahda Renal Dialysis Center took the role required at that time for teaching and training nephrology staff, this center being part of a program developed by the MoH at that time. This program was called Chronic Renal Failure Program (CRFP), and directed to treat Omani patients in their country, instead of taking them abroad for treatment [8, 11]. In 1986, the transplant program was started in cooperation with Oxford University (United Kingdom – UK), the patients and donors being sent to the UK for renal transplant. In 1986, the HD availability increased to thirteen beds. Moreover, a plan was made by the MoH to establish additional HD centers across the country, the outreach places of Oman [9, 10, 12].

In 1987, the Royal Hospital (a large tertiary teaching hospital where all specialties and subspecialties are offered for all the Omani's citizens) was inaugurated, with the Renal Center with six HD beds. Intermittent Peritoneal Dialysis (IPD) was also made available besides HD. In 1988, the first living related KT was performed at the Royal Hospital. In the same year, the first cadaveric renal transplant was accomplished at the Royal Hospital [7, 11].

Continuous ambulatory peritoneal dialysis (CAPD) was introduced in Oman in 1992, and the first patient was dialyzed in the Royal Hospital at Muscat. In 1993, the PD structured program was properly started in Oman [9, 10].

The first remote Renal Dialysis Center (RDC) outside the capital and the second in Oman started its service in the northern region of Oman in September 1991. On April 4, 1992, a third RDC was opened in the southern region of Oman. The central RDC (named Bushar) of the Royal Hospital was launched on January 29, 1998 in the capital of Oman, Muscat. This RDC is managed by a nephrology team led by a nephrologist and assisted by nephrology nurses. The creation and maintenance of the Oman's RRT register was a personal effort from Dr. Hamood Al-Marhubi who was the nephrologist in charge of the central RDC. The effort was continued after Dr. Hamood's retirement by Dr. Yaqoob Almaimani, who is the current nephrologist in charge of the central RDC. Credit should be given to these people for securely retrieving these fundamental data for all these years [10]. Dr. Hamoud Amur Ali Al Marbury joined MOH in 1973 and retired in December 2013 [10]. In 1982 after completing a nephrology training at the University of Vienna, he joined the nephrology services at Al-Nahdha Hospital. PD services of acute and hospital-based facility were the only treatment for ESRD available at that time. He devoted most of his life to improving the nephrology services in Oman. He has a big role in supporting and starting training Omani nurses in the specialty of nephrology, followed by renal dialysis specialty program launched at Oman Specialized Nursing Institute (it is renamed at present to be the Higher Institute of Health Specialties), which has helped to train Omani nurses in dealing with renal patients. He showed great interest in spreading and improving the awareness of kidney disease and its management among health care providers as well as the general population. One of the activities he established was "Think Kidney Symposium." He started the first kidney disease awareness campaign during the celebration of World Kidney Day in March 2008 along with a Walkathon, followed by yearly awareness campaign during Muscat festival.

The 2004 annual health report published by the Oman's MoH showed that Oman had 13 RDCs (Ministry of Health-MoH, 2004). These RDCs had a combined total of 113 HD stations and served 558 patients by the end of December 2003 (Ministry of Health – MoH, 2004). These HD centers increased gradually to 15 RDCs by the end of 2005 (Ministry of Health – MoH, 2006). The 15 RDCs had a combined total of 158 HD stations and treated 618 patients per annum. By 2008, the MoH was successfully running 17 RDCs that combined a total of 169 HD stations serving 737 patients on HD (Ministry of Health – MoH, 2009).

The Minister of Health, His Excellency Dr. Ahmed Al Saidi, appointed Dr. Issa Al Salmi, MD, BA, MB, Bch, BAO (Trinity College), FRCPI, MRCP (UK), FRCP, MIPH (AUS), PhD (AUS), FASN (USA), as the chairperson for the Committee for Improvement of Renal Service in the Sultanate of Oman, as per Ministerial decision number 92/2011. The committee consists of nephrologist clinicians, nurses, pharmacists, engineers, and administrative and support personnel to enable it to perform its tasks throughout the country.

By the end of 2015, the MoH owned 18 RDCs with 217 HD stations covering 1439 patients on dialysis per annum per total population (Ministry of Health – MoH, 2016). Between 2012 and 2015, the MoH did not increase the number of RDCs (Fig. 30.1), but increased the number of HD stations in some of the existing RDCs such as the central RDC, which started with 28 HD stations and increased to 42 HD stations by the end of 2015; also the MoH handed over 160 patients to a private contractor to run these patients' dialysis. At present, there are 24 HD centers around the country serving all dialysis patients in the country.

The standard HD prescription blood flow for a new patient first HD ranges from 150 to 300 ml/mint, and later on, it is increased to a range of 200–600 ml/mint. The frequency for most patients is three times/week for 3–4 h, but almost 10% have twice/week for 3–4 h. It is based on patients' general condition, vascular access flow, and blood pressure. The average dialysis facility setting consists of one nurse to 2–4

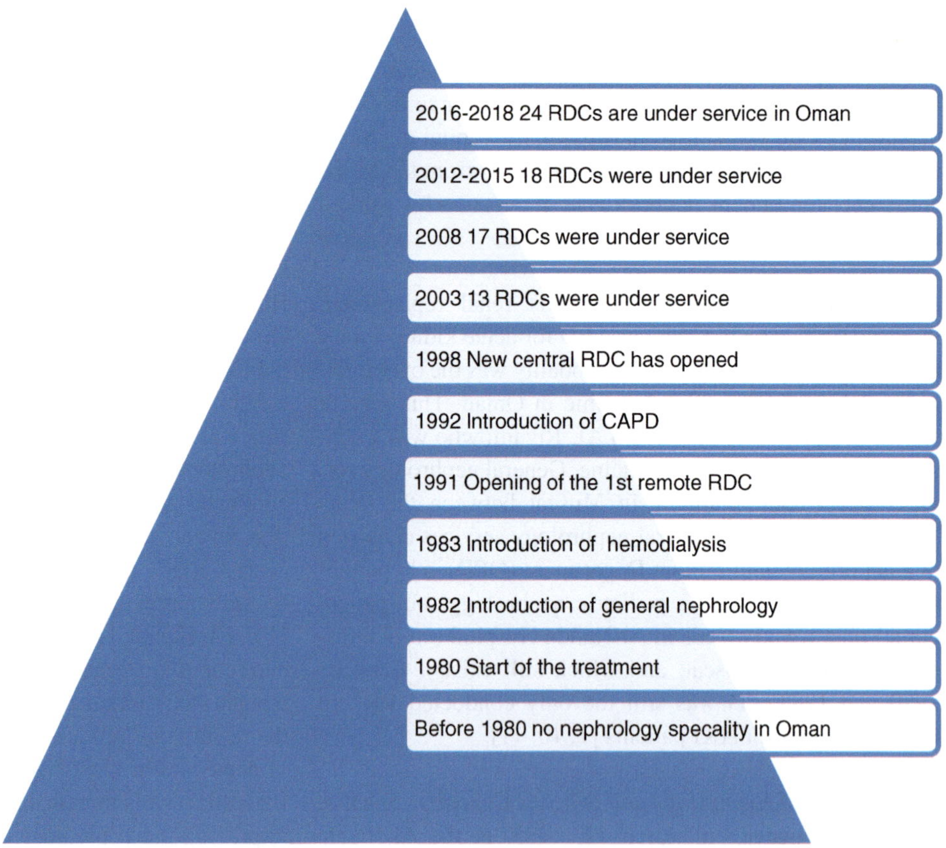


**Fig. 30.1** The increase in dialysis treatment capacity in Oman 1980–2018

patients and one nephrologist per maximum 50 patients. Each dialysis facility has a pharmacist, technicians, dieticians, non-medical helpers, and administrative personnel. In addition, in each region of the country the hospitals have social workers to help in providing certain logistics and funding for many patients across the country.We have HDF post dilution and it works only with high flux dialyzers, which are very expensive; they are not available most of the time, but mostly used for AKI.

*Nephrology Nursing Education Program* Renal dialysis specialty program was launched at Higher Institute of Health Specialties in 1997 and is one of the major accomplished nursing education programs to meet the demands of competent nurses in nephrology specialization. The main aim of this program is "to prepare post-basic nurses for specialist practice so that they will deliver high-quality care to those patients in need of this specialist care and to prepare qualified nephrology nurses to be able to work independently, efficiently and effectively". Three hundred forty-four nephrology nurses have graduated from this program and made significant career changes [Higher Institute of Health Specialties, 2017/2018; Higher Institute of Health Specialties, 2018]. Nephrology nursing involves both preventing diseases and assessing the health needs of patients and families where the often highly technological setting is contrasted with the caring, supportive, and educative environment, necessary for the care of those who are chronically ill. This postgraduate program consists of 30 credit hours which consists of ten [10] courses which are extended over three semesters. This program's curriculum "is designed with integrated theoretical and clinical courses that work interdependently to meet the program's requirements, along with the acquisition of advanced knowledge and skills as well as development of highly acceptable professional attitude and values" (Higher Institute of Health Specialties, 2017/2018; Higher Institute of Health Specialties, 2018). The program learning outcomes outlined to be achieved by the nephrology student nurses are the following:

1. Critical evaluation of service delivery to inform the optimizing of care within the national health care system at primary, secondary, and tertiary level
2. Professional understanding and accountability in the application of socio-cultural, legal, and ethical principles to achieve the delivery of optimum patient care within the nephrology care setting
3. Efficient utilization of leadership, knowledge of management strategies, and skills to promote enhanced levels of professional nursing practice in the nephrology setting
4. Analytical decision making in applying the principles of physiology to underpin practice
5. Critical evaluation of the concepts and principles of different diagnostic and treatment modalities for short- and long-term care
6. Efficient utilization of research in the practice through critical appraisal of existing evidence and evaluating practice outcomes
7. Critical evaluation of the bio-psychosocial scope of treatment and care of patients with kidney disease

© (Higher Institute of Health Specialties, 2017/2018; Higher Institute of Health Specialties, 2018).

## Renal Diseases in Oman

Today, the main cause of ESRD in many countries, including Oman, is DM as a consequence of the global obesity pandemic. In fact, DM is the most prevalent disease in the Middle East and North Africa (MENA) region among International Diabetes Federation (IDF) regions, with approximately 40 million adults [18–99 years] affected and 373,557 deaths due to diabetes [13]. In 2017, almost 370,104 adults (18–99 years) had DM in Oman, forming a national prevalence of 10.4% and age-adjusted comparative prevalence of 12.0% [13]. Thus, it is estimated that one in ten adults has DM in Oman [13]. A study of diabetes complications and associated conditions amongst Omani patients showed that 51% of the subjects were obese, 20% had coronary artery disease, 66% hypertension, 10% retinopathy, 15% micro-albuminuria, 31% overt diabetic nephropathy, and 9% neuropathy [6, 14].

Glomerular diseases are fundamental health concerns causing CKD in Arab countries, yet limited epidemiological data is available due to the lack of national renal biopsy registries in most of these countries. In Oman, the spectrum of glomerular diseases is similar to that of other Arab countries. Primary glomerular diseases are more frequent (69.1%) than secondary glomerular diseases (30.9%), and lupus glomerulonephritis (LN) is the main dominant pathology (30.4%) [15]. Focal segmental glomerulosclerosis (FSGS) is the most common primary glomerular disease followed by minimal change disease (MCD), whereas lupus nephritis (LN) is the most prevalent types of secondary glomerular diseases. In pediatrics (˂14 years), LN and membranous glomerulonephritis (MCD) are the most frequent glomerular diseases compared to LN in young adults (15–25 years) and MGN in patients of older age (≥25 years) [16]. Similar to other Arab countries, a few cases of immunoglobulin A (IgA) nephropathy are detected in Oman by renal biopsy [15].

Nephrolithiasis is defined by the formation of crystal aggregates in the urinary tract leading to kidney stones, while nephrocalcinosis is characterized by the deposition of calcium salts in the renal parenchyma. In Oman, kidney and urinary stones are common reasons for requesting medical consultation. Approximately 190 per 10,000 population are hospitalized annually for the treatment of calculus of the kidneys, ureters, and lower urinary tract, hence requiring frequent urological treatments [17]. A recent study evaluating the biochemical, metabolic, and radiological data of 255 patients with this disease revealed that hypertension, DM, urinary tract infection, obesity, and atrophic kidney are the most common comorbidities associated with nephrolithiasis and uric acid stone formation [17]. Stone analysis detected calcium oxalate as the most frequent composition (73%) in patients from Oman, which is similar to those reported in Kuwait, Iraq, the United States, and France [17]. Mostly, the probability of stone formation is high in the Middle East countries where environmental and sociocultural factors such as hot and humid climate and diets as well as genetic make-up are the primary contributors [17].

The incidence and prevalence of inherited diseases causing renal diseases are substantially more common in the Arab world than other regions, leading to significant mortality and morbidity, possibly associated with the high rate of consanguinity [18]. Similarly, inherited and congenital kidney disease may be essential causes of ESRD in the Omani population with high degrees of consanguinity [56.3%] [19]. A wide range of autosomal recessive diseases leading to CKD in childhood are common in Oman, causing a serious healthcare burden, including autosomal recessive polycystic kidney disease (ARPCKD) [19], congenital hepatic fibrosis and Caroli's disease [20], renal tubular acidosis and congenital nephrotic syndrome [19], ciliopathy syndromes [19], and primary hyperoxaluria [21]. Additionally, cystinuria is a rare autosomal recessive disease characterized by the formation of cysteine stones in kidneys, found more frequently in Oman and constituting 4% of adults' stones, opposed to the worldwide prevalence of 1% [17]. A recent study found that genetic kidney diseases comprise 5% of all causes of ESRD [7], which is in line with the estimated percentage of the Gulf Cooperation Countries (GCC) (4.43%) [22]. In Oman, patients with inherited kidney disease start RRT at a younger age (mean age, 29 years), being more prevalent in the pediatric and early age group (0–19 years: 46.8%, 20–44 years: 23.7%) when compared to the elderly patients (≥65 years: 3.6%) [7]. Autosomal dominant polycystic kidney disease (ADPKD) was the most prevalent genetic kidney disease causing ESRD amongst Omani [7].

Systemic lupus erythematosus (SLE) is a common chronic multi-systemic autoimmune disease which follows an aggressive course in many patients [23]. The SLE clinical disease spectrum of Omani patients appears to be consistent with that found in neighboring Middle East countries and Caucasian populations, upon which half of patients have renal involvement [23–27]. An epidemiological study of familial juvenile SLE revealed that mucocutaneous manifestations, arthritis, and nephritis are the most prevalent features in Omani and Saudi children, anticipating an autosomal mode of inheritance [24]. Furthermore, differences in the mean age of SLE onset has been observed in Omani children as they have an earlier age of onset (8.6 years) when compared to Saudi (12.1 years) and other Arabic countries, supporting the demand for more comprehensive multi-centers studies [24, 27]. In terms of organ involvement, a tribal and geographical variance among Omani SLE patients has been found, indicating both genetic and environmental effects [24, 26–28]. Moreover, geographical clustering of childhood onset SLE was recognized in the eastern region of Oman (Sharqiya region), accounting for 41% of the cases [25, 26]. Another recent study of 966 patients diagnosed at the Royal Hospital, from 2006 to 2014, revealed that SLE is more prevalent in Omani female (88.7%) and the overall mean age at presentations was 35.5 years [23]. Analysis of clinical presentation of SLE patients indicates that musculoskeletal manifestations such as arthralgia, myalgia, and arthritis are frequently seen in Omani patients [23].

## Chronic Kidney Disease Epidemiology in Oman

CKD is ranked as the eighth highest cause of all deaths in Oman in 2017, with an increasing percentage of 78% between 2007 and 2017, and it is the 10th cause of years of life lost (YLLs) due to premature mortality, with 77.7% increase between the same period (2007–2017) [3, 8]. In 2009, a preliminary survey carried out with nearly 40,000 persons aged 40 years or more all over Oman to evaluate non-communicable disease (NCDs) in the general population estimated that 70.9% of this population was obese, 14.4% had hypertension, 8% DM, and 9.9% CKD with an estimated glomerular filtration rate (eGFR) ≤ 60 ml/min/1.73m$^2$ [10, 11]. It also showed that 29% had mild renal failure (eGFR 60–90 ml/min/1.73 m$^2$), 9% moderate renal failure (eGFR between 30 and 59 ml/min/1.73 m$^2$), while 1% had severe renal failure (eGFR < 30 ml/min/1.73 m$^2$) [11]. Since a strong relationship exists between kidney disease and NCDs that are considered as risk factors for CKD including DM, hypertension, and obesity, it is essential to recognize CKD as a major NCD in Oman [10, 11]. In a recent study of 208 children aged 0–13 years with different CKD stages, who were followed at the Royal Hospital for over 12 years, a mean annual incidence rate of 24.0 per million child populations was reported [16]. A low number of those children (12.9%) presented in stage II, while 25% in stage III, 20.7% in stage IV and the majority (41.3%) in stage V at diagnosis [16]. These alarming figures of CKD prevalence in general population might still be underestimated since CKD is often silent or under recognition in the general population unlike the onset of ESRD, which is certainly recognized by the requirement of RRT.

The prevalence of ESRD patients receiving RRT in Oman at the end of 2013 was 655.8 per million population (pmp), with an incidence of 120 pmp [11]. The yearly prevalent counts of new patients treated for ESRD faced rapid increase; for example, it rose from 1535 in 2008 to 2851 in 2015, with a change in the prevalence rate from 463.5 to 670.1 pmp at the same period. In Oman, CKD is more prevalent in males than in females and the mean age of starting RRT is approximately 50 years [8–11], which is in line with Middle East countries. However, a remarkable difference is noted with the developed countries including the United State (US) and the United Kingdom where the median age is ≥61 years [8, 9]. Furthermore, a sharp rise in the incidence and prevalence of ESRD patients with ageing in Omani population has been noted, particularly after 45 years of age [11].

Nowadays, diabetic and hypertensive nephropathies are the two major causes of CKD in Oman, accounting for 46% and 19–22% of ESRD patients requesting RRT, respectively [10, 11]. DM is more prevalent among older patients [≥45 years] and its incidence has raised from 5.8% in 1983 to 46% in 2013 [10, 11]. Chronic GN is the third underlying cause of renal failure, accounting for 15–18% of ESRD patients [7, 8, 10, 11]. The alteration in the main cause of CKD from GN in 1983 to diabetic nephropathy in recent times is a reflection of satisfactory health care diagnoses system as well as alteration in the socioeconomic status and lifestyle of the population in Oman [11]. In general, diabetic and hypertension are considered as the major leading causes of kidney failure in many Arab countries including Egypt, Jordan, Kuwait, Saudi Arabia, Tunisia, UAE, and Qatar [11]. Rises in these chronic diseases may be associated with population growth and aging, deficiency of physical activities, obesity, and urbanism, which are themselves considered as dominant CKD risk factors [10, 11]. In recognition of these challenges, and with the expected increase of diabetes and hypertension in the developing countries during the next two decades, it is essential for health care providers in Oman to develop strategic health care actions that shift from care and treatment to prevention of these epidemics.

## Renal Replacement Therapy Scenario in Oman

ESRD is a serious and irreversible condition. Understanding the impact of ESRD and its treatment on an individual's quality of life (QoL) is important. There are limited studies that assess QoL and health-related QoL (HRQoL) in Arab Muslim patients, and Oman in particular. Thus, a large-scale cross-sectional study was conducted to assess the level and predictors of QoL/HRQoL among Omani patients [3]. Results revealed that, similar to ESRD patients worldwide, Omani patients have low levels of HRQoL, particularly on the physical and mental health components. These findings were consistent with results from three observational studies in ESRD patients and patients with other chronic conditions, such as osteoporosis. However, Omani patients rated their mental health components better when compared to physical health components. Families in Oman are more of an introverted type of families and looking after family members is considered as an obligation. It was not surprising that patients reported better level of social function compared to the other aspects of QoL [3]. Supportive social environment, friends, and family can improve patients' mental health and role functioning [3].

Omani patients on dialysis usually experience a burden of symptoms and complications associated with dialysis and ESRD; recent studies show that the life expectancy and bearing of the burden of disease and treatment among ESRD patients have increased. This seems encouraging because it perhaps reflects that the current standards and complex medical care provided to ESRD patients are effective and could be an influencing factor for better HRQoL. In fact, it may lend support to nephrology services within and outside Oman to further improve the care of patients with ESRD [3].

Fatigue and pain were significant among Omani ESRD patients, and this is consistent with the results of previous studies in ESRD patients. Fatigue and pain were the most significant burdensome symptoms that patients reported. It was found that about 50% of patients with ESRD experienced pain, using the McGill QoL Scale [3]. It is not surprising that these findings are important for a number of reasons: first, ESRD patients have numerous symptoms, many of which can be severe. Second, symptoms that are common in dialysis patients such as muscles cramps, drowsiness, or restless legs usually are not included in symptoms measures, which raises the possibility that symptom burden might be even higher than that observed in this study. Also, many ESRD patients found that physical symptoms accounted for one-third of the impairment in HRQoL [3].

Mood symptoms are commonly experienced by ESRD patients. Forty-one per cent of patients reported symptoms of anxiety and 43% reported depressive symptoms. Also, 25.9% patients had anxiety and 28% of patients had depressed symptoms, using the Hospital Anxiety Depression Scale (HADS) instrument [3]. However, the diagnosis of mood symptom in ESRD patients could be highly variable, from patients showing no symptom of the disease to patients who show severe symptoms. This is perhaps due to different concepts of depression and anxiety, which may vary from isolated symptoms to major depressive and anxiety disorder. Anxiety and depression may affect the patient with ESRD in many ways. Overall, patients with ESRD have higher morbidity and mortality caused by the chronicity of the disease. For this reason, early recognition of mood changes and establishment of specific intervention to this group of patients are necessary [3].

Lastly, the concept of spirituality must also be considered as a possible drive for providing the purpose of life for some individuals. It is a kind of connectedness and it describes a way of being that is characterized by certain identifiable values in regard to self, others, and life. Religiosity is often understood as an individual's involvement in a set of beliefs and social activities as a means of spiritual expression, and this may include adherence to religious practices and traditions, such as Christmas, fasting during Ramadan, or adhering to specific dietary regimens such as avoiding alcohol and being vegetarian. The interplay between the two concepts of spirituality and religiosity may affect how individuals live and may also affect their moral decisions. These consequently affect their day-to-day choices. In Islam, for instance, being religious is considered an essential element of happiness. Muslims perceive life satisfaction to be connected with Allah's or God's satisfaction through the dialogue and performance of worship, which results in the belief of having a pleasant and satisfied life [3].

## Peritoneal Dialysis in Oman

The outcome of PD has improved over the last years and is becoming equal to HD, even its survival being better in the first 2 years.

Despite the long distances to RDC and the delay in the creation of permanent vascular accesses for many patients, PD was only provided to sporadic cases initiated at the tertiary hospital in Muscat (Al-Nahda and the Royal Hospital). It started as an urgent start indication of dialysis, first at Al-Nahda Hospital in 1982, then at the Royal Hospital in 1987 [9]. First cases for chronic PD started at the Royal Hospital in 1992 [9]. In 2010, chronic PD service became available by the MoH and started at secondary hospitals mainly at Nizwa Hospital (a hospital situated at about the middle of Oman, 150 km far from the capital). Since then, the PD penetration has increased from 30 to 190 patients, representing 10% of the total Omani dialysis population, while it comprises 54% of the total dialysis population at Nizwa Hospital (90 PD out of total 166 dialysis patients). Set-up for PD services mainly at Nizwa and Royal Hospitals includes:

- Pre-dialysis clinic for counselling and preparation of stage 4/5 CKD to RRT and selection of modality
- Bedside PD catheter insertion under fluoroscopy guidance by nephrologist for most of the cases; and surgical by laparoscopic insertion, as backup for those failed cases by the nephrologist
- Protocol for early initiation during break-in period for patients who need dialysis to avoid insertion of CVC
- Training for patients and caregivers for PD and exit site dressing followed by home visit post training
- PD OPD attended by nephrologist and nurse staff expert in PD and training
- Monthly review of PD prescriptions for necessary adjustments as per clearance; UF and laboratory tests
- Periodic procedures and KPI:
  1. Retraining every 6 months and whenever necessary
  2. Transfer set exchange every 6 months and whenever necessary
  3. Kt/v [PD and urine] every 6 months and after prescription change
  4. PET every year

Out of the 190 PD patients in Oman, 17.5% are pediatric patients (defined as younger than 13 years old) and 18.5% adult patients (13 years old or older); both groups are being treated at the Royal Hospital. Meanwhile, 51.5% of adult PD patients are being followed at Nizwa Hospital and the remaining 30% are being treated at secondary hospitals in six different regions around Oman. The Royal Hospital, however, receives the patients from all the secondary hospitals for difficult cases and major complications, and even for initial catheter insertion and initial management. Thereafter, these patients are referred back to the secondary hospitals for further follow-up.

Eighty percent (80%) of our PD patients have selected PD as initial modality from pre-dialysis clinic, whereas 20% were transferred from HD (8% selected PD and 12% had vascular access failures – Fig. 30.2). Mean age is 50.3 years with nearly equal female to male ratio. Patients on PD for more than 5 and 3 years are 10% and 21%, respectively.

Seventy percent (70%) of PD patients are using APD and CCPD while 30% are on CAPD. PET showed equal percentages between low and high transport membrane. Sixty percent of CAPD patients are high/high average transporters, while 51% of APD patients are low/low average transporters. Ninety-one percent (91%) have Kt/v more than 1.8.

Peritonitis rate in 2018 was one episode/54 patient-months or 0.22 episode/year. Refractory peritonitis represented 21% of the total peritonitis episodes for these patients whereas 63% (7 out of 11 episodes) of them were managed successfully without HD by simultaneous insertion of a new PD catheter with the clearance of the infection. Four of the refractory episodes were due to fungal peritonitis that was noticed to happen after the use of broad spectrum of antibiotics and steroids. Therefore, we added prophylactic fluconazole in our protocol when these drugs are used, and until now no new episode has been detected.

All episodes of relapsing peritonitis are managed successfully without removal of peritoneal dialysis catheter (PDC), using Heparin-Antibiotic Lock of PDC throughout treatment.

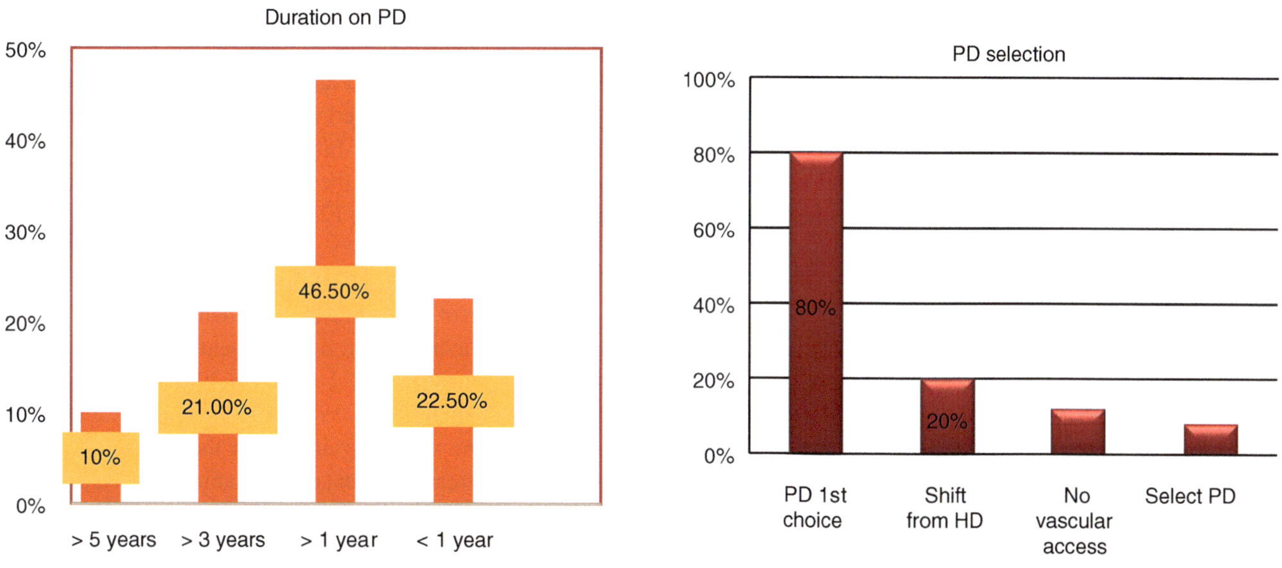


**Fig. 30.2** Duration and PD selection in Oman

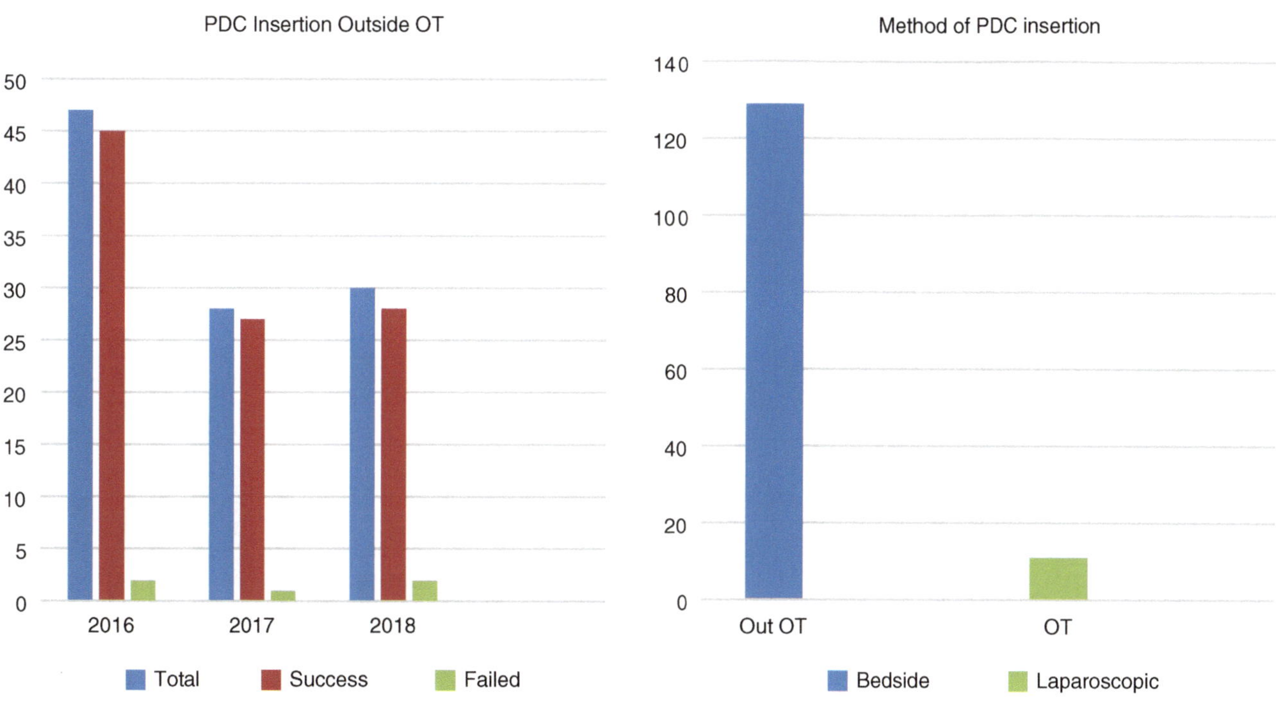


**Fig. 30.3** Peritoneal dialysis catheter (PDC) insertion outside operation theater (OT) and method of PDC insertion

Initially, PD catheter insertion was mainly in the operation theater (OT), either surgically or laparoscopically; but since 2016 the main approach is through percutaneous insertion under fluoroscopy guidance by nephrologist at Nizwa Hospital while those with previous surgeries or who failed bedside insertion are going for laparoscopic insertion in the OT (Fig. 30.3).

To avoid the use of CVC and their complications, if the patient needs dialysis during the break-in period, we initiate PD using APD with small volumes, frequent cycles, and long duration in supine position. Also, for patients with no permanent vascular access, we offer temporary PD until the creation, maturation, and use of vascular access, in order to avoid the use of CVC. We are encouraging temporary PD as CRRT therapy for critical area patients instead of HD (continuous or intermittent) and CVC. Both timed insertion of PDC and PD initiation during the break-in period result in a significant increase in the number of PD patients and reduction in the use of CVC and their complications.

The PD dropout is mainly due to death (42%), 28% shifted to HD (being 24% due to technique failure: mainly refractory peritonitis, and 4% due to patient's request), and 19% other causes. A positive dropout reason is KT representing 11% (Fig. 30.4).

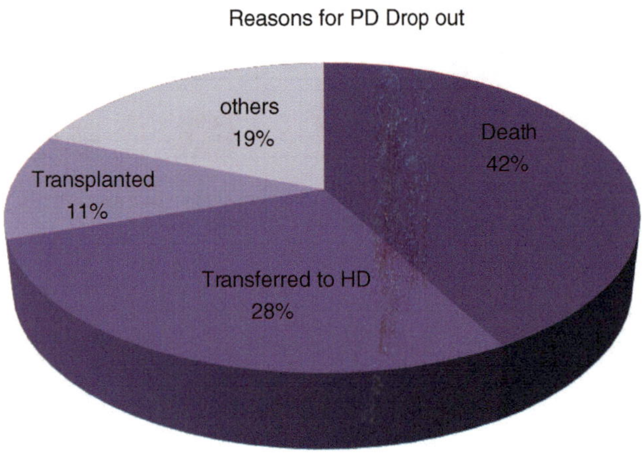


**Fig. 30.4** Reasons for PD treatment dropout

## Maintenance Hemodialysis in Oman

*Prevalence* Woods and Prabhakar (1985) reported 113 patients who were diagnosed with ESRD and started dialysis between March 1983 and July 1985 [12]. The mortality at that time was 17.7% (of the whole dialysis population in Oman including AKI) [10, 12].

The prevalence statistics from 1998 to 2015 showed an overall increase in HD treatment in Oman [7, 8, 10]. The HD subpopulation increased from 35 patients in 1983 to about 2056 patients in 2018 (31 December 2018). The available HD prevalence in the years 1983–2015 in Oman is illustrated in Fig. 30.5. The mean prevalence for the years 1983–2018 was 1090 HD-treated patients per annum. The overall trend showed an increase in HD treatment prevalence over the years with slight dips in years 2003, 2005, and 2006 (Fig. 30.5) [10]. Since 2007, the prevalence of ESRD on HD has been steadily increasing. For the past 3 years, the prevalence has increased to 1617 (2016), 1767 (2017), and 2056 patients on HD in 2018 [10].

It was possible to calculate the prevalence rate for HD treatment as the estimated census for Omani population and total population at risk was available for the years 1983 and

**Fig. 30.5** Prevalence of hemodialysis treatment in Oman (1983–2015)

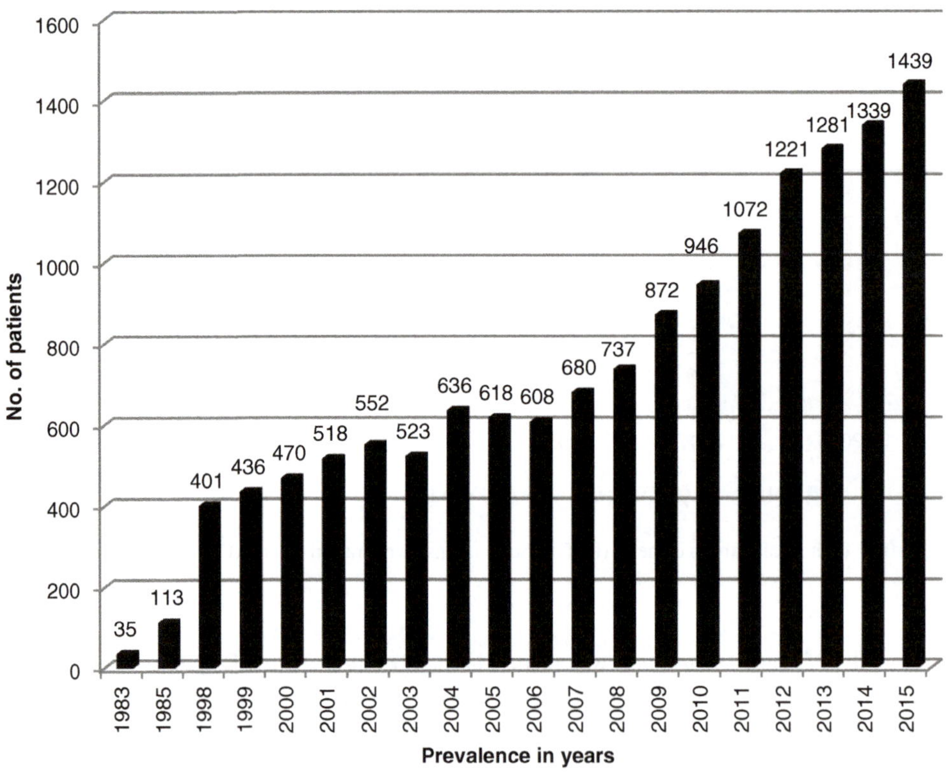

onward. However, the prevalence for the years 2003 and 2013 was selected and calculated to the last available census of 2018 (Table 30.1). This prevalence rate was calculated across the total population in order to observe the significant increase in prevalence rates [10].

*Incidence* Statistics of the ESRD incidence were available for the years 1983–2018. The new patients registered in 1983 were 34 patients, and in 2015 there were 230 patients per total population. The incidence of ESRD patients across the years until the end of 2015 per Oman is displayed in Fig. 30.6. The incidence reported by the end of the year 2018 was 400 patients per country per annum [10].

*Death Frequency and Causes* It is an important piece of information to report the causes of death of HD patients and all modalities as well. The causes of death for the three treatment modalities – HD, PD, and KT – have been recorded in Oman's RRT register at the central RDC for the years 1983–2010. There were seven causes of death identified as follows: CVD, cerebrovascular accidents (CVA), hemorrhage, hepatic causes, infection, malignancy, and other causes where other causes were either not listed or unknown causes secondary to not knowing the cause of death when death occurred, as most of these persons died at their homes. The causes of RRT population death in 2001–2010 are displayed in Fig. 30.7 [10].

**Table 30.1** Prevalence rates for hemodialysis-treated patients in certain years

| Year | Prevalence | Omani pop. | PR of Omani pop. |
|---|---|---|---|
| 2003 | 523 | 1,782,000 | 29.3/100,000 |
| 2013 | 1281 | 2,172,000 | 59/100,000 |
| 2018 | 2056 | 2,579,000 | 89.2/100,000 |

*Pop.* population, *PR* prevalence rate, *NOTE* the registry does not account for non-Omani who usually return home country for their RRT. Only a very small number of non-Omani continued to dialyze in private but not included in the registry

The overall statistics results for the causes of death over the years 1983–2010 are displayed in Table 30.2. Finally, the death causes for years 2011–2015 were reported precisely in total as 449 death causes and the top three causes were: unknown ($n = 148 = 33\%$), CVD ($n = 108 = 24\%$), and infection ($n = 107 = 23.8\%$) [10].

*The Cost* The total dialysis sessions increased from 45,113 dialysis sessions in 1998 to 191,638 dialysis treatments in 2015 across the whole of Oman, as reported by Oman's MoH (Fig. 30.8). The direct cost of a single dialysis session in the public sector was given by MoH as 49.8 Omani Rials (49.8 OMR = 129.4 USD). So, from these data, the cost of the dialysis sessions increased dramatically from 2,246,627 OMR (~5.8 million USD) in 1998 to 9,543,572 OMR (~25 million USD) in 2015 which is a 325% increase. In addition, in Oman, by law, we cannot reuse the dialyzer for more than one time. The cost for all years is displayed in Fig. 30.8 [10].

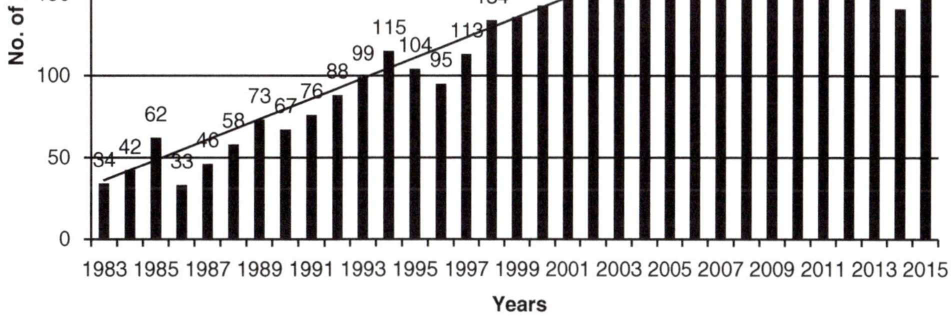


**Fig. 30.6** Incidence of ESRD in Oman [1983–2015]

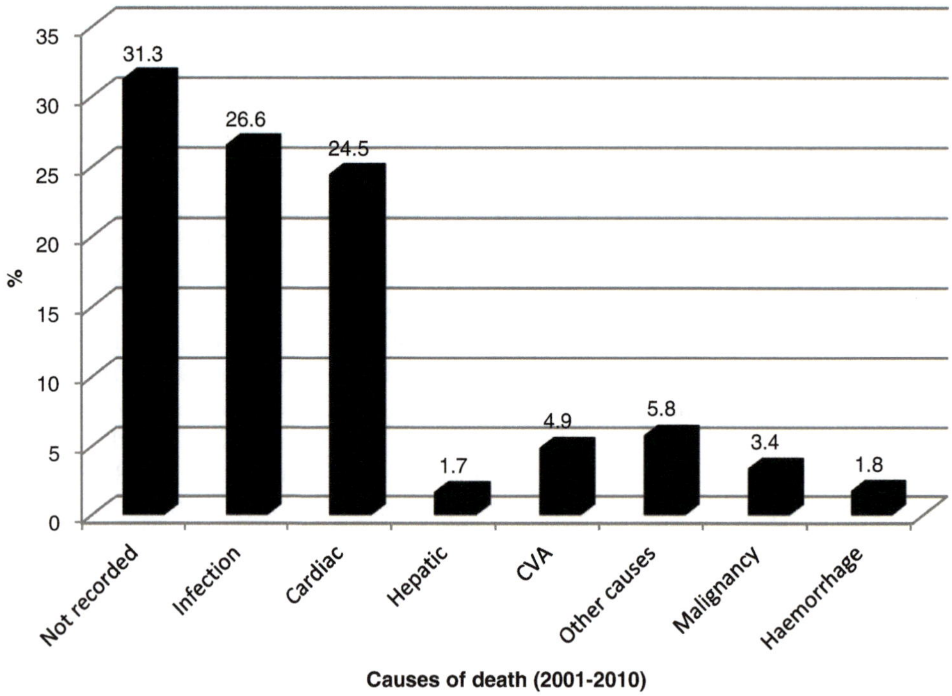


**Fig. 30.7** Causes of RRT population death (2001–2010)

**Table 30.2** Causes of RRT population death across genders

| | | HD patients *n* | | | RT patients *N* | | | PD patients *n* | | | All patients *n* | | |
|---|---|---|---|---|---|---|---|---|---|---|---|---|---|
| Period | Cause of death | M | F | T | M | F | T | M | F | T | M | F | T |
| 1983–1990 | Not recorded* | 28 | 29 | 57 | 2 | 6 | 8 | 0 | 1 | 1 | 30 | 36 | 66 |
| | Infection | 6 | 3 | 9 | 7 | 9 | 16 | 0 | 0 | 0 | 13 | 12 | 25 |
| | Cardiac | 10 | 8 | 18 | 2 | 3 | 5 | 0 | 1 | 1 | 12 | 12 | 24 |
| | Hepatic | 0 | 0 | 0 | 4 | 3 | 7 | 0 | 0 | 0 | 4 | 3 | 7 |
| | CVA* | 2 | 0 | 2 | 2 | 1 | 3 | 0 | 0 | 0 | 4 | 1 | 5 |
| | Other cause | 2 | 1 | 3 | 0 | 1 | 1 | 0 | 0 | 0 | 2 | 2 | 4 |
| | Malignancy | 0 | 0 | 0 | 2 | 1 | 3 | 0 | 0 | 0 | 2 | 1 | 3 |
| | Hemorrhage | 0 | 1 | 1 | 1 | 0 | 1 | 0 | 0 | 0 | 1 | 1 | 2 |
| | Total | 48 | 42 | 90 | 20 | 24 | 44 | 0 | 2 | 2 | 68 | 68 | 136 |
| 1991–2000 | Not recorded* | 64 | 83 | 147 | 11 | 8 | 19 | 1 | 0 | 1 | 76 | 91 | 167 |
| | Infection | 29 | 30 | 59 | 37 | 30 | 67 | 1 | 1 | 2 | 67 | 61 | 128 |
| | Cardiac | 47 | 24 | 71 | 9 | 3 | 12 | 0 | 0 | 0 | 56 | 27 | 83 |
| | Hepatic | 4 | 2 | 6 | 5 | 7 | 12 | 0 | 0 | 0 | 9 | 9 | 18 |
| | CVA* | 16 | 6 | 22 | 2 | 3 | 5 | 0 | 0 | 0 | 18 | 9 | 27 |
| | Other cause | 7 | 7 | 14 | 2 | 0 | 2 | 0 | 0 | 0 | 9 | 7 | 16 |
| | Malignancy | 4 | 7 | 11 | 5 | 2 | 7 | 0 | 0 | 0 | 9 | 9 | 18 |
| | Hemorrhage | 4 | 3 | 7 | 3 | 0 | 3 | 0 | 1 | 1 | 7 | 4 | 11 |
| | Total | 175 | 162 | 337 | 74 | 53 | 127 | 2 | 2 | 4 | 251 | 217 | 468 |
| 2001–2010 | Not recorded* | 136 | 122 | 258 | 8 | 12 | 20 | 4 | 2 | 6 | 148 | 136 | 284 |
| | Infection | 112 | 90 | 202 | 14 | 14 | 28 | 5 | 6 | 11 | 131 | 110 | 241 |
| | Cardiac | 102 | 102 | 204 | 11 | 5 | 16 | 0 | 2 | 2 | 113 | 109 | 222 |
| | Hepatic | 6 | 3 | 9 | 5 | 1 | 6 | 0 | 0 | 0 | 11 | 4 | 15 |
| | CVA* | 20 | 20 | 40 | 2 | 1 | 3 | 0 | 1 | 1 | 22 | 22 | 44 |
| | Other cause | 24 | 27 | 51 | 0 | 2 | 2 | 0 | 0 | 0 | 24 | 29 | 53 |
| | Malignancy | 15 | 8 | 23 | 4 | 4 | 8 | 0 | 0 | 0 | 19 | 12 | 31 |
| | Hemorrhage | 10 | 5 | 15 | 0 | 0 | 0 | 0 | 1 | 1 | 10 | 6 | 16 |
| | Total | 425 | 377 | 802 | 44 | 39 | 83 | 9 | 12 | 21 | 478 | 428 | 906 |
| | *Total* | 648 | 581 | *1229* | 138 | 116 | *254* | 11 | 16 | *27* | 797 | 713 | *1510* |

*M* males, *F* females, *T* total, *Not record* not recorded, *CVA* cerebrovascular accident
*<0.05

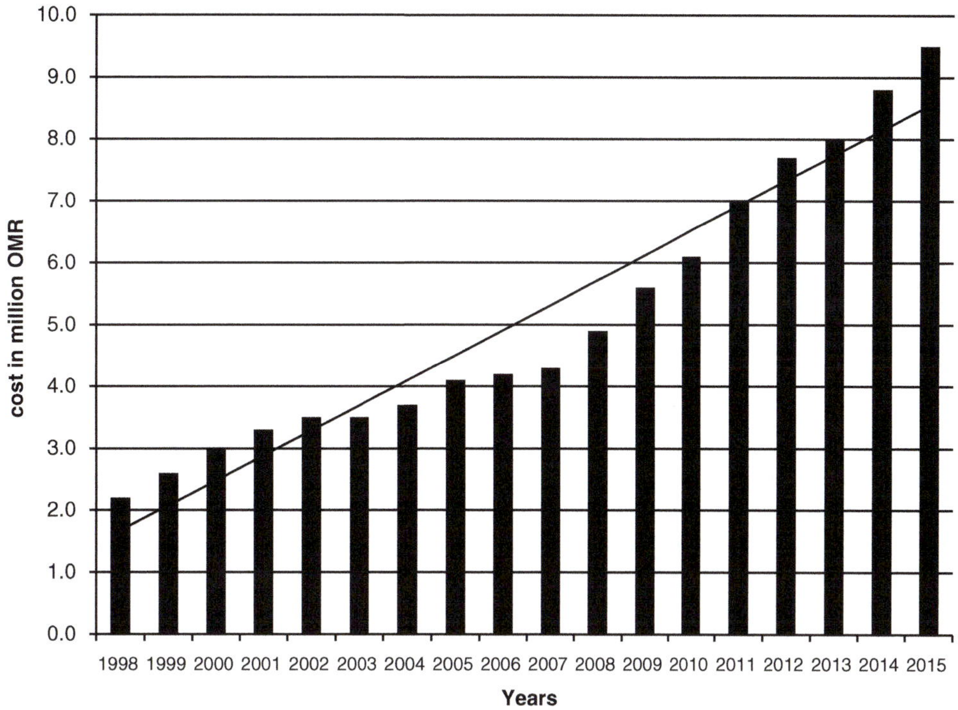


**Fig. 30.8** The cost of dialysis sessions per annum for Oman (1998–2015)

## Convective Therapies in Oman

*Developments of Continuous Renal Replacement Therapy (CRRT) in Oman* In 1977, Dr. Peter Kramer was the first to describe such type of therapy in the literature. It was named CAVH (continuous arterio-venous hemofiltration). The blood was moved from an artery to a vein through a hemofilter. Ultrafiltration rate was controlled by raising and lowering the drain bag.

At the Royal Hospital, the first form of RRT was introduced in 1991; it was not a very complex technique, but two large bore cannulas were inserted in both femoral veins and were run through a membrane, and ultrafiltration was done.

Since the early 1980s, a blood pump and a double-lumen catheter in a large vein have been used to provide a consistent blood flow, and thus ultrafiltration. This so-called Veno-Venous technique has been since then adopted and improved to become the standard in CRRT. In the 1990s, the first fully automatic machines were made and became immediately popular in intensive care settings.

The Royal Hospital embraced this therapy quite early, and the first proper CRRT was done in the adult ICU of the Royal Hospital in 1997, using double lumen catheter in femoral vein. This was done using earlier model of Fresenius machine, heparin as anticoagulation in most cases, but other means of anticoagulation, such as using prostacyclin (Flolan) or saline flush, were also used in patients who had heparin-related risks of bleeding.

In 2000, the Royal Hospital then started using CRRT machines from B. Braun, and most of the patients had continuous veno-venous hemofiltration (CVVH) as the preferred modality of CRRT technique. Most critically ill patients with hemodynamic instability admitted in Adult Intensive Care unit at the Royal Hospital who required renal support would get this treatment. This therapy was a combined initiative of Nephrology and Adult Intensive Care at that time.

In 2003, the Royal Hospital acquired state-of-the-art CRRT machines for adult ICU from Fresenius Medical, and started the program of CRRT in critically ill patients in ICU, with proper training of ICU nurses and doctors. This training module established at the Royal Hospital ICU has helped train the nurses to run this modality of therapy in adult ICU, independent of nephrology department involvement, considering that the resource utilization in the nephrology department were stretched beyond limits. From 2003 onward, most patients in ICU have had CVVHD modality as the preferred mode. It is worth noting that CRRT program in Sultan Qaboos University Hospital (SQUH) was established around the same time. The program ran successfully in adult ICU patients for the next 8–9 years, but there were challenges faced when patients were in DIC, had risk of bleeding due to heparin, or developed heparin-induced thrombocytopenia.

In 2011/2012, the Royal Hospital adopted the citrate-calcium method of regional anticoagulation, along with the

SQUH, for critically ill patients in ICU. Oman has been the first GCC country to take up this modality on records. As is the norm in the ICU, the nursing staff and doctors at Royal Hospital underwent extensive training before starting this modality in ICU patients. The staff are well trained to run CVVH and CVVHD in sick ICU patients, and recently CVVHDF has also been added to the treatment options, in patients where it is indicated.

Adult ICU at the Royal Hospital is a busy unit, and a snapshot of the ICU will suggest that at least 2–3 patients will be receiving CRRT treatment at a given time (30 CRRT days/month).

From 2015 to 2016 onward, most hospitals in the Sultanate of Oman are using CRRT modality of treatment in ICU patients who require renal support.

In pediatric intensive care unit, CRRT has been used since 2011, and since 2014, it has been incorporated as a proper training program for ICU nurses and doctors.

The Royal Hospital staff at adult ICU is also involved in training other staff (doctors and nurses) in CRRT. Adult ICU team has also conducted workshops on nephrology critical care for doctors and nurses in the country.

## Dialysis Reimbursement Policies in Oman

Our policy is that there is no reuse of dialysis catheters. All expenses are paid by the MoH, with no exception. Free-of-charge health services are provided to all citizens by the MoH. All types of renal dialysis are free-of-charge as well as if it is provided either by the national public system or by the private sector. Non-Omani ESRD are few cases and they are self-paid. The Oman's MoH has to endure a source of funding, which will support in achieving all the vision planned by 2050. This sustainability is very challenging since the income of Oman is diminishing because of the reduction in the oil prices in the international market. Renal care is also one of the health services that is struggling to sustain persistent fund to keep this important service running up to the golden standards and free of charge to enhance accessibility and equitability [10, 11].

## Acute Kidney Injury and Critical Care Nephrology in Oman

There are limited knowledge and studies about AKI in Oman; in one study done by Balushi F et al. to determine the incidence, etiology, and outcome of AKI at a teaching hospital in Oman (Unit of Nephrology, Department of Medicine, Sultan Qaboos University, Al-Khoud, Oman) from July 2006 to June 2007, they found that the incidence of AKI was 0.54% whereas the etiology of AKI was pre-renal (50.9%), obstructive (4.6%), and acute tubular necrosis (44.4%). RRT was required in 24.1% of the cases; 33.3% of the patients who developed AKI died during same hospital admission, 34.26% recovered to discharge with no renal impairment, and 1.85% recovered with dialysis dependence [29]. A prospective 2018 study by Al Majarfi et al. included all consecutive incident HD patients at the Royal Hospital, Muscat, Oman for a 1-year period from 2014 to 2015 showing that sepsis is the main cause of AKI, 17% of all patients initiating on HD, and it is leading cause of AKI in critical care and intensive units with high mortality rate, while contrast induced nephropathy (CIN) represent 2.5% of the patients of the same studies [30]. This Hospital-based study of initial HD session at a tertiary care found that 5% patients became dialysis independent and that 4.5% of patients died during their admission for initial HD [30].

There is a great need to establish AKI registry or data entry program to record the incidence of AKI at a national level. Also, more studies are needed to give clear input and more details about AKI and its causes and management issues. The MoH has started CKD and AKI classification as a must, whenever a patient is seen, and to be entered in the computerized system medical record, a national program that can be accessed everywhere from all MoH health centers of the.

## Pediatric Nephrology in Oman

In Oman, most children with renal disease are referred from all over the country to the pediatric nephrology center at the Royal Hospital. This center provides services to all pediatric patients with renal disease. All types of pediatric dialysis including PD and HD are provided. It is also the only pediatric KT center in Oman. Some children with renal disease are seen at SQUH, as it is the second pediatric nephrology center in the country. Ultimately, all children who need RRT, dialysis, or transplantation are referred to pediatric nephrology center at the Royal Hospital. The renal disorders commonly seen by the pediatric nephrology team at the Royal Hospital are described as follows.

*Congenital Anomalies of Kidney and Urinary Tract (CAKUT)* They are common in children and represent approximately 30% of all prenatal diagnosed malformations. Reported incidence in live and stillborn infants is 0.3–1.6 per 1000 children. CAKUT is one of the most common diseases encountered in our outpatient and inpatient daily work. These children can be diagnosed by antenatal scan or later as incidental finding during routine ultrasound of kidney and urinary tract, or these children may present with urinary tract infection or voiding dysfunction or with CKD. CAKUT is the most common etiology of CKD in our patients [52.9%], including obstructive uropathy, renal dysplasia/hypoplasia, vesico-ureteric reflux, and neurogenic bladder [7]. Children with CAKUT have lower progression rate to CKD compared to children who have GN, this observation being seen in our patients [7] as well as in other previous reports [16]. In 1996, a retrospective study about the frequency of posterior valve (PUV), done on Omani newborns, concluded that the frequency of PUV was higher when compared to previous reported and associated with increase consanguinity, but there was no clear pattern of inheritance [31].

*CKD* A retrospective study was conducted of all children followed at the Royal Hospital below the age of 13 years diagnosed with CKD stages 2–5. A total of 208 children were diagnosed with CKD from January 2004 to January 2016. The mean annual incidence rate was 24.0 (SD ± 5.6) per million. Sixty-three percent were males. The mean age at diagnosis was 3.6 ± 3.5 years (median 2.0) with 61% below the age of 3 years. Consanguinity was seen in 42%, and 31% had positive family history of renal disease. The most common etiology study was congenital CAKUT in 110 children (53%). Hereditary renal disease was seen in 66 children (32%), of which ARPCKD was the leading cause in 25 patients (12%). Chronic GN accounted for 8% of the cases [7, 16].

More than half of the children were hypertensive at the time of diagnosis, and 63.1% had anemia of chronic disease. The median follow-up period was 4 years, during which 116 children (57.9%) required dialysis. Fifty-seven children (27.4%) underwent KT, while thirty-six children (17.3%) died [32].

*Hereditary Renal Disease* Oman similar to other Middle East countries has a high incidence of consanguineous marriage, and this explains the higher incidence of hereditary renal disease in Omani children. In a recent report about CKD in Omani children, hereditary renal disease was the second most frequent etiology in our patients, including ARPCKD, primary hyperoxaluria type 1, familial focal segmental glomerulosclerosis, and congenital nephrotic syndrome [16, 21]. In a previous report from four different families with each family having more than one affected child, eighteen children were diagnosed to have primary hyperoxaluria with a median presentation at 7 months of age. The consanguinity rate in this study was 100%; and the most common mutation in the AGXT gene in these children was c.33–34ins [16, 21].

*RRT in ESRD Pediatric Population* PD was started for adult ESRD patients in 1980, while HD was introduced in 1983 for both adults and older children [7, 8, 16]. The first pediatric CAPD treatment in Oman was performed in 1994 at the Royal Hospital [8, 16]. This was a 17-month-old boy with ESRD secondary to Deny-Drash syndrome (WT1 mutation). In the pediatric nephrology center at the Royal Hospital all children who progress to ESRD are offered dialysis, except if the parents refuse dialysis and they consider that their child QoL is not going to improve if they are dialyzed. Another reason is if a child has had other organ failure preventing them to be treated with dialysis. In the past, most patients were on HD and only a small number on CAPD [16]. At present, most children requiring dialysis are offered PD because now there is a well-established pediatric PD program in Oman.

*KT: Living-Donor and Deceased Donor in ESRD Pediatric Population* The KT in Oman started in 1988 and it included both pediatric and adult. The first KT to an Omani child was performed in 1994. The kidney was retrieved from a 10-day-old preterm deceased donor baby. It was recorded to be the world's youngest cadaveric kidney transplantation [31].

Recently, we have reported on 70 Omani children who had KT between1994 and 2015 [31]. Twenty-seven from living donor, 42 living unrelated donor (commercial transplantation), and 1 deceased donor; the median age at transplantation was 9 years [31]. The most common etiology was CAKUT in 32.8% followed by hereditary renal disorders, familial nephrotic syndrome, and PCKD. About 50% of them were on HD before transplantation, 38% were on PD, and 14 had preemptive KT [7, 16]. The conclusion of this study indicated that children who underwent living related KT have a good outcome comparable to international results, whereas children who received living unrelated KT presented with a high risk for surgical complication and decreased graft and patient's survival.

In summary, we have more children with renal disorder secondary to hereditary nephropathies due to high consanguinity rates among the population. We have many children with stage V CKD but less than one third of them have been transplanted due to the unavailability of a deceased donor transplant program and shortage of donors. The need to establish a deceased donor program to increase the number of children going for kidney transplantation is demanded. Besides, more effort is needed on genetic counseling and prevention as well as more effort is also required to promote living organ donation.

## Renal Transplantation in Oman

In Oman, in the period of 1980–1988, there were no kidney transplantation centers. Oxford University in the United Kingdom was the primary center for KT of Omani ESRD patients, as donors and recipients were sent there as part of an agreement between the MoH and Oxford University [11, 12]. During the period 1983–1988, fifty-six patients received a living donor transplantation within the MoH-Oxford Program. However, all living unrelated donor (LURD) KT patients were going on their own to some Asian countries, like India. In addition, 20 patients underwent KT in the period from March 1983 to July 1985, of which 18 patients survived while two died because of graft rejection in LURD transplant recipients [12]. Before 2009, most ESRD patients who required KT were sent abroad with their potential donors a part of an official cooperative program and only a few patients had KT locally. Initially, a visiting transplant surgeon was performing the surgeries. Later, a local surgical team was created. Currently, patients that require dual liver kidney transplant are still being sent abroad as a liver transplant program is still in the process of establishment.

In 1988, Renal Transplantation Program in Oman was established as a cooperative scheme between SQUH and the MoH. It included both adult and pediatric and activated with both living related donor (LRD) and deceased donor (DD) transplants. However, transplantation from living unrelated donor was not and is still not performed in Oman, in order to avoid concealed commercialism, although some Omani patients have had such operations abroad and they are being followed up in the country. For living related kidney, transplant cases were performed at two biggest referral hospitals in Oman: the Royal Hospital and SQUH [16].

Dr. Daar was a pioneer in kidney transplantation in the Middle East countries. He is an outstanding Omani national in the field of surgery, who was born in Tanzania. In 1990, he moved to Middle East where he was involved in founding two new medical schools in UAE and Oman. In Oman, he was appointed professor of surgery at Sultan Qaboos University for one decade (1990–2001). He is a professor of public health sciences at the Dalla Lana Faculty of Public Health, University of Toronto, with a cross-appointment in the Department of Surgery. Abdullah Daar started KT programs in Oman in 1988. In the latter country, he was the founding professor of surgery at Sultan Qaboos University and the "transplantation culture" and set up an immunology service. In 1998, he performed the first deceased donor KT in Oman. The kidney was spontaneously donated by the family of an American expatriate. Also, while in Oman, Abdullah Daar performed a unique transplantation from a 33-week-gestation, i.e., preterm donor with brain death into a 17-month-old recipient boy who is alive and doing well more than 10 years later. This became the official world record for the youngest-ever deceased donor renal transplantation and has yet to be surpassed. The mother of the brain-damaged 33-week donor, a Dutch woman, sought the donation.

In 1993, Omani transplantation legislation was established, by which the only living related donors (LRD), by blood or marriage, were allowed. Omani legislation prohibits commercial transplantation. Accordingly, this law prohibits the transplant commercialism, allows deceased donor transplantation, and outlines the criteria for forming brain death.

The Royal Hospital webpage reported more than 800 patients with a functional graft and on regular follow-up with

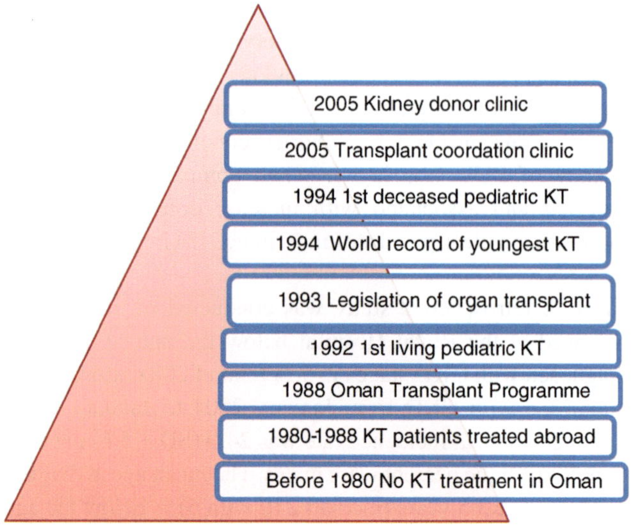


**Fig. 30.9** The major accomplishments in the field of renal transplantation in Oman

nephrology services in the Sultanate in 2014. By early 2019, we had almost 2000 patient with functioning graft.

The major achievements in KT took place in the year 2005. In this year, two vital units were established, which are the transplant coordination unit and the kidney donor clinic. These two units contributed significantly to the increase from the average of 6.5 transplants per annum to 12 by the end of 2005 and to 23 transplants by the end of 2009 (Fig. 30.9).

*Deceased Transplantation Program in Oman* The brain death concept is still distant in the Omani public. The meaning is that an individual is dead, according to medical definition, while the heart is still beating, causing a lot of confusion between the patient caregivers and the caring doctor. This misunderstanding of the concept of brain death avoids the use of these individuals as potential organ donors, which is a problem in an era where the need for organs exceeds their availability.

In Oman, despite the permission from religious and legal authorities to use organs from deceased donors, we are now practicing almost solely living related donor KTs. The public attitude toward donation is essential in all transplantation programs. Furthermore, a survey was carried out in 2010 to assess Omani populations' attitude toward organ transplantation showed great public acceptance of kidney donation during life and very low acceptance after death. However, religious and sociocultural factors have to be further investigated and regulations and laws have to be strengthened to further expand the facility and to prohibit organs commercialism action.

A common thread that binds all faiths of the world is that the saving of life overrides all objections, and no religion is against organ donation. Kingdom of Saudi Arabia (KSA) and Kuwait have successful KT programs, which might encourage the KT program in Oman to assume some variations to the present system in order to make the program more active. The MoH has provided all the resources for successful KT program in Oman such as the transplant coordination unit and kidney donor clinic.

Though Oman deceased donor transplants program was among the earlier programs in the Gulf region, it was not fully supportable, and the transplantation program turns now to be mainly living related donor transplants program. The major challenge causing the unsuitability of this program in Oman compared to the neighboring countries was the absence of resources. The brain death criteria have been accepted by civil authorities and religious authorities, but have not yet been accepted by the public at large, possibly due to poor awareness programs and media announcements.

Transplantation from deceased donors is still scarce in many Arab countries. In Oman, almost all transplantations depend on living related donors despite the permission from religious and legal authorities to the use of deceased donors.

*Limitations of DD Program and Ways of Improvement* A clear guideline related to the diagnosis of brain death and guidelines related to the withdrawal of life support in these patients is needed in the country. With high prevalence of non-communicable disease in the country, it is difficult to find living related to donate kidney or part of liver, and hence a good number of people travel overseas for commercial transplantation including kidney, pancreas, and liver. Despite proper settings with advanced equipment and well-trained clinicians being available, deceased program still stands still. However, the health systems across the country have failed to bridge the gap that exists between medical knowledge, legality of brain death, religious views, and the education of our community in this regard.

In order to resolve this, different institutions across the country need to come together to form a committee in order to deal with this important and critical subject. Secondly, there is a need to arrange and conduct a forum, including religious and legal authorities, to review and discuss organ donation status in the country and come to a consensus on policies and guidelines relating to the process of organ donation. Finally, it is essential to educate the public on sensitive issues such as this and increase their overall awareness of brain death as a medical condition [7, 8, 11]. Also, it goes without saying that the DD program needs a good network of donors' coordinators all over the country's ICUs departments.

In the same way, the absence of a kidney patients association is an important obstacle to the provision of patients with CKD and their relatives; a strong stand and voice to address various requirements and needs is needed. The government has failed to provide such a comfort zone or even permit its launch to serve an important public service to improve the care of people with ESRD.

*Juridical-Ethical and Socio-Cultural Framework* In Oman, the decision to donate organs is a crucial step in the process of transplantation. Moreover, Arab countries have poor transplant rates because of multiple factors, among them, low levels of infrastructure, inadequate trained professional staff, lack of a legal structure leading the brain death program, religious, cultural, and social constraints, patient anxiety, physician bias, commercial encouragements that favor dialysis, and geographical remoteness. The decision is based on personal or familial opinions that are strongly influenced by many factors, including education, socioeconomic status, religion, and cultural characteristics.

Up to date, however, the MoH has delivered all the resources for a successful KT program in Oman such as the transplant coordination unit and kidney donor clinic. The program was able to achieve the world record for the youngest donor in kidney transplantation, which shows that the program had the potential to accomplish a major number of KT surgeries. Furthermore, the United States Renal Data System (USRDS, 2015) has provided kidney transplantation statistics for Oman (18 pmp/2013 kidney transplants per annum) which is comparable with KSA (18.6 pmp/2013), Kuwait (16.6 pmp/2013 kidney transplants per annum), higher than Bahrain (6.7 pmp/2012), but less than Poland (29 kidney transplants per annum), and the United Kingdom (51 kidney transplants per annum). This concludes that there is no apparent problem within the Oman kidney transplantation program, but the main problem could be the lack in the number of donated kidneys as there is no sufficient living or deceased donors at present for Oman's CKD population [10].

## Organ Procurement and Transplantation Network Policies

For living related donors (LRD), the MOH are following such donor criteria as in Table 30.3.

In addition, Figs. 30.10 and 30.11 show the kidney recipient and donor work-up pathway that is followed for the kidney donors who are monitored in kidney donor clinic.

**Table 30.3** Donor criteria of LRD

| Kidney donor criteria | |
|---|---|
| 1. | Age $^{>}$ 18 |
| 2. | Recipient's relative |
| 3. | Willing to donate, not being coerced |
| 4. | In a good health, no major medical or psychiatric illness |
| 5. | Non-smoker, non-drug consumer, and non-alcoholic |
| 6. | BMI $^{<}$ 30 |
| 7. | ABO compatible |

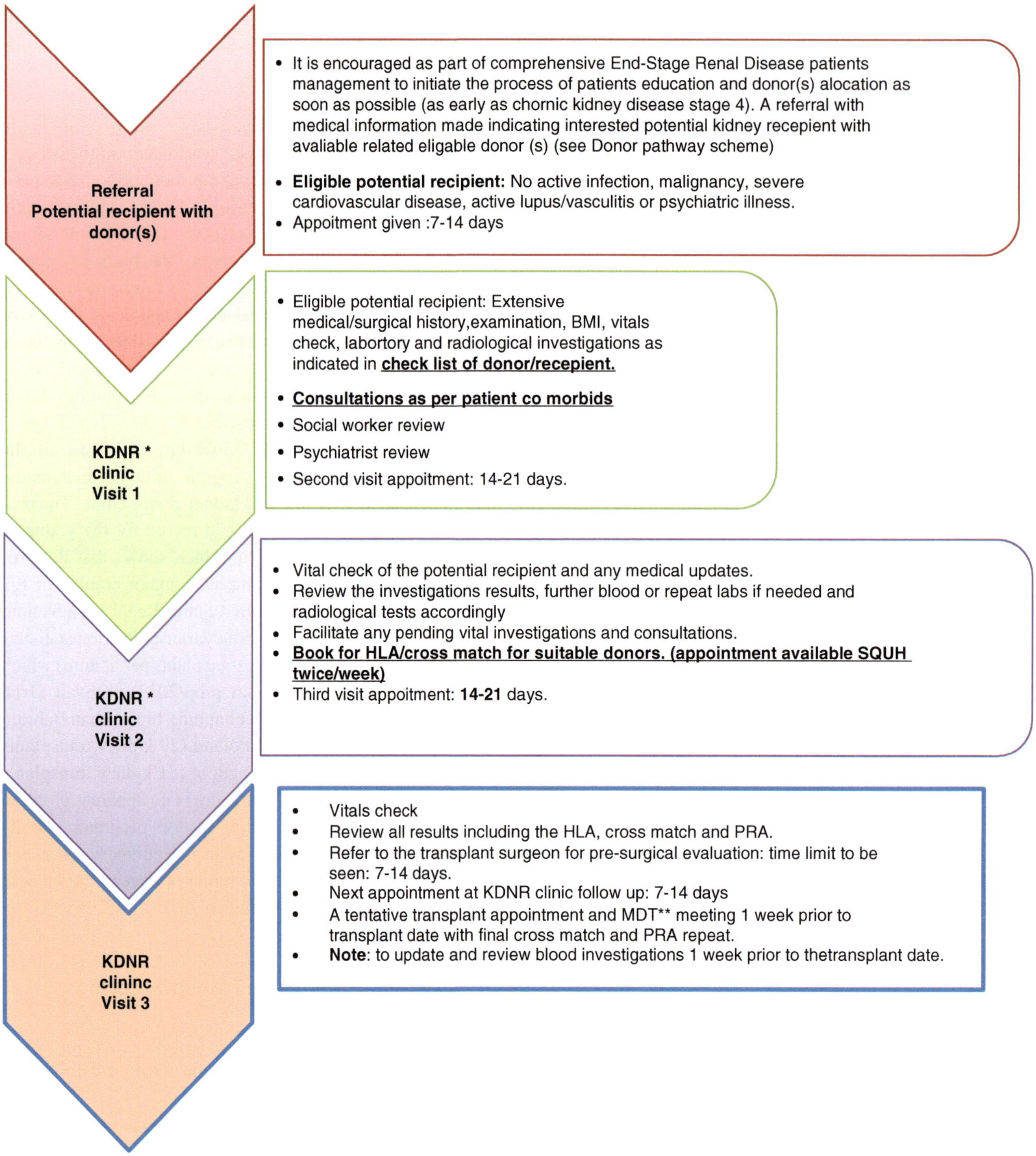


**Fig. 30.10** Kidney recipient work-up pathway. (Total maximum time limit: 60 days. *KDNR kidney donor clinic, **MDT multidiciplinary transplant teamNotes: Transplant coordinator to contact potential recipient to update and also follow up specially those missed appointments. Once transplant done, the recipient will be followed at the transplant clinic appointments)

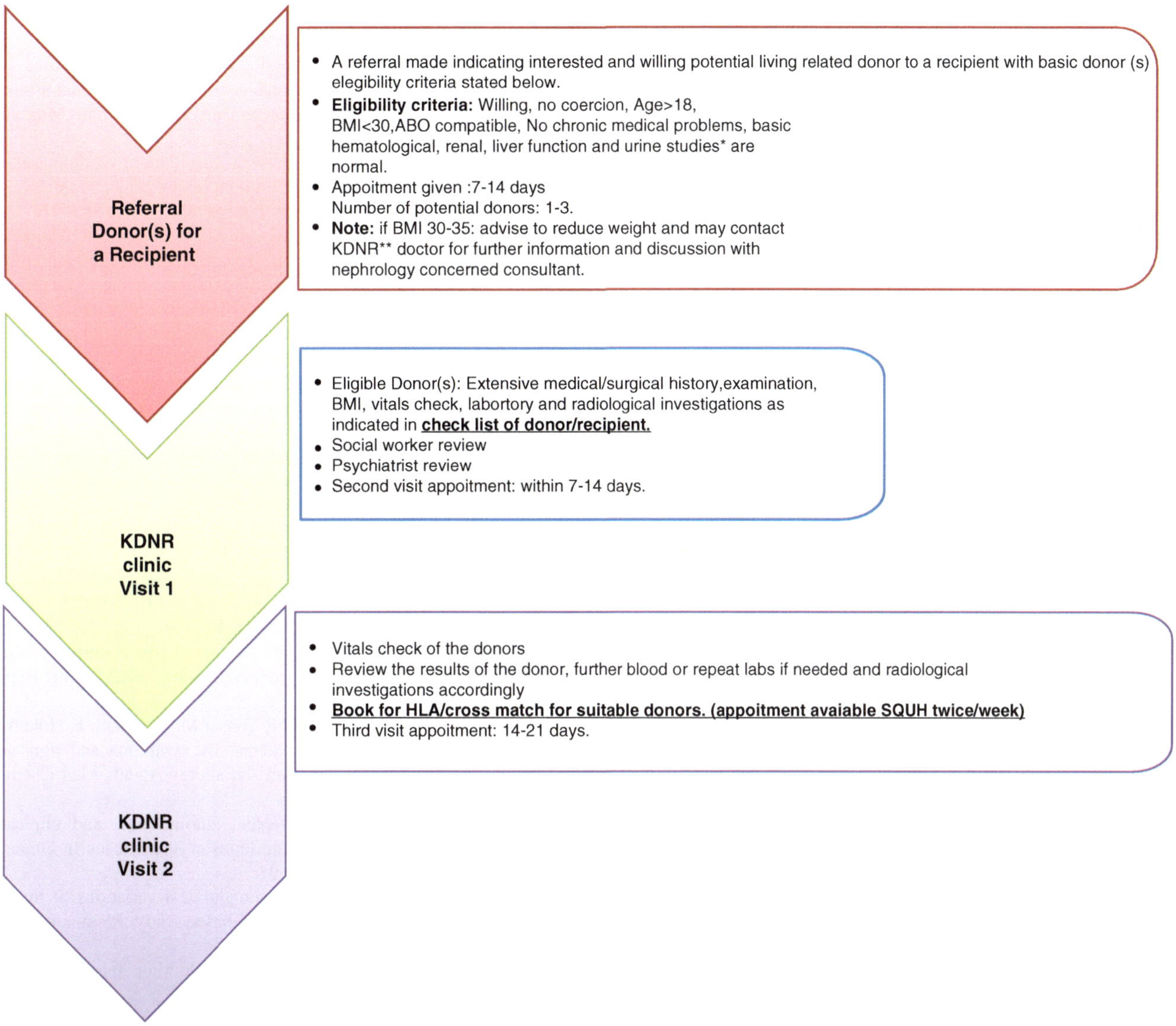


**Fig. 30.11** The donor pathway in the kidney donor clinic. (Total maximum time limit: 60 days. *Blood group, complete blood count, liver function test, urea, electrolytes, serum creatinine, eGFR, urin analysis, urine protein creatinine ratio, **KDNR kidney donor clinic, ***MDT multidiciplinary transplant team. Notes: Transplant coordinator to contact potential donors to update and also follow up specially those missed appointment. Once transplant done, donor will be followed in the KDNR clinic appointments regularly for 12–24 months)

## Nephrology Practice and Job Market

Nephrologist census (Omani x non-Omani): most nephrologist in Oman are non-Omani and mostly from Egypt and Indian Subcontinent countries. The job market is quite good with increasing demand for nephrologist with high turnover as they tend to move to another country/region once given a better offer. The senior consultant salary is almost 15,000 USD per-month tax free, but this could increase with participation in education and supervision of undergraduate and postgraduate student as well with other various non-clinical practices. Usually after the age of 60 years, non-citizens are given retirement and let go but still can work in private nephrology care.

Nephrology training was done entirely outside in North America, Europe, and Australia for Omani clinicians. However, recently, the Oman Medical Specialty Board have approved the nephrology fellowship program of at least 2 years post 4 years of Internal Medicine Training.

Renal nurses' census: Because of nephrology diploma in nursing, most of nurses are Omani but still many others from India and Philippines. The percentage varies from almost

30% to over 75% of nurses being Omani. Nurse's salaries vary from almost 3000 USD per month to almost over 10,000 USD per-month tax free.

The work in Oman is generally quite easy which start from 7:30 am until 2:30 pm, but nurses work in shifts similar to that in the United Kingdom. In general, there is no payment for overtime, and it is part of overall monthly salary. The weather is quite good, except in the summer, especially in Muscat where it is hot and humid. Social life is very good and many good places to spend weekend and holidays without any cost.

## References


1. World meters. 2019. Oman population. At https://www.worldometers.info/world-population/oman-population/. Accessed on 23 June 2019.
2. National Center for Statistics and information. Population statistics. At https://www.ncsi.gov.om/Elibrary/LibraryContentDoc/bar_population2018_ea9a7a9b-65d1-4b2a-856e-093d4406209d.pdf. Accessed on 23 June 2019.
3. Alrajhi W. Quality of life and health related quality of life in patients with ESRD: an Omani context. PhD thesis, University of Dundee, 2018.
4. Ministry of Health, Oman – MOH. 2018. Chapter four [Human resourcces for health]. In: Annual Health Report 2017. Muscat: Department of Health Information & Statistics. Available at https://www.moh.gov.om/documents/274609/2607839/%D8%A7%D9%84%D9%81%D8%B5%D9%84+%D8%A7%D9%84%D8%B1%D8%A7%D8%A8%D8%B9/a0f8759f-f029-31be-2d04-d57b9f-f107ab. Accessed on 23 June 2019.
5. National center for statistics and information. 2018. Health statistics 2017. Available at https://www.ncsi.gov.om/Elibrary/LibraryContentDoc/bar_Health%20Statistics%202017_64562188-d6ed-4050-913c-94dea305f03c.pdf. Accessed on 23 June 2019.
6. Al-Lawati JA, Mabry R, Mohammed AJ. Addressing the threat of chronic diseases in Oman. Prev Chronic Dis. 2008;5(3):A99.
7. Al Alawi I, Al Salmi I, Al Mawali A, Al Maimani Y, Sayer JA. End-stage kidney failure in Oman: an analysis of registry data with an emphasis on congenital and inherited renal diseases. Int J Nephrol. 2017; https://doi.org/10.1155/2017/6403985. Epub 2017 Jun 8.
8. Al Alawi IH, Al Salmi I, Al Mawali A, Sayer JA. Kidney disease in Oman: a view of the current and future landscapes. Iran J Kidney Dis. 2017;11(4):263–70.
9. Al-Marhuby H. Renal replacement therapy in sultanate of Oman. Saudi J Kidney Dis Transpl. 1998;9(4):459.
10. Al-Za'abi R. The Oman's treated chronic kidney failure population in years 1980 to 2015: an epidemiology research. PhD thesis, University of Glasgow, 2018. https://pdfs.semanticscholar.org/77e1/9ee718eeddc5e7085d40d281cad3120003f7.pdf.
11. Al Ismaili F, Al Salmi I, et al. Epidemiological transition of end-stage kidney disease in Oman. Kidney Int Rep. 2016;2(1):27–35. https://doi.org/10.1016/j.ekir.2016.09.001.
12. Woods H, Prabhakar N. Chronic renal failure program March 1983 to July 1985. Oman Med J. 1985;11(2):29.
13. International Diabetes Federation. IDF Diabetes Atlas [cited 2019 April]. Available from: http://www.diabetesatlas.org/.
14. Al-Sinani S, Al-Mamari A, Woodhouse N, Al-Shafie O, Amar F, et al. Complications and associated conditions among Omani type 2 diabetes patients at Sultan Qaboos University Hospital, Muscat, Oman. J Fam Med. 2014;1(3):6.
15. Alwahaibi NY, Alhabsi TA, Alrawahi SA. Pattern of glomerular diseases in Oman: a study based on light microscopy and immunofluorescence. Saudi J Kidney Dis Transpl. 2013;24(2):387–91.
16. Al Riyami M, Al Shehhi M, Al Riyami M, Al Selemi T, Al Mamary L, Al Kalbani N, Al Ghaithi B, Al Maskari A, Al SS. Epidemiology and outcome of CKD in Omani children. Kidney Int Rep. 2019;4(5):727–32. https://doi.org/10.1016/j.ekir.2019.02.014.
17. Al-Marhoon MS, et al. Urinary stone composition in Oman: with high incidence of cystinuria. Urolithiasis. 2015;43(3):207–11.
18. Tadmouri G, Nair P, Obeid T, Al Ali M, Al Khaja N, Hamamy H. Consanguinity and reproductive health among Arabs. Reprod Health. 2009;6(1):17.
19. Rajab A, Al Rashdi I, Al SQ. Genetic services and testing in the Sultanate of Oman. Sultanate of Oman steps into modern genetics. J Community Genet. 2013;4(3):391–7.
20. Al-Lawati TT. Fibropolycystic disease of the liver and kidney in Oman. Arab J Gastroenterol. 2013;14(4):173–5.
21. Al Riyami MS, et al. Primary hyperoxaluria type 1 in 18 children: genotyping and outcome. Int J Nephrol. 2015;2015:634175.
22. Hassanien A, Al-Shaikh F, Vamos E, Yadegarfar G, Majeed A. Epidemiology of end-stage renal disease in the countries of the Gulf cooperation council: a systematic review. JRSM Short Rep. 2012;3(6):38.
23. Metry A, Al Salmi I, Al Balushi F, Yousef M, Al Ismaili F, Hola A, Hannawi S. Systemic lupus erythematous: symptoms and signs at initial presentations. Antiinflamm Antiallergy Agents Med Chem. 2019;18:1.
24. Al-Maini MH, et al. Demographic, autoimmune, and clinical profiles of patients with systemic lupus erythematosus in Oman. Rheumatol Int. 2003;23(4):186–91.
25. Al Maini MH, et al. Tribal and geographical variations of lupus in the Sultanate of Oman: a hospital-based study. Rheumatol Int. 2002;21(4):141–5.
26. Abdwani R, et al. Epidemiology of juvenile idiopathic arthritis in Oman. Pediatr Rheumatol Online J. 2015;13:33.
27. Abdwani R, et al. Geographical clustering of juvenile onset systemic lupus Erythematosus within the Sultanate of Oman. Oman Med J. 2013;28(3):199–203.
28. Abdwani R, Rizvi SG, El-Nour I. Childhood systemic lupus erythematosus in Sultanate of Oman: demographics and clinical analysis. Lupus. 2008;17(7):683–6.
29. Balushi F, Khan S, Riyami D, Ghilaini M, Farooqui M. Acute kidney injury in a teaching hospital in Oman. Saudi J Kidney Dis Transpl. 2011;22(4):825–8.
30. Al Majarfi A, Al Salmi A, Metry AM, Al Ismaili F, Hola A, Hannawi S. Epidemiology of patients at initial treatment with hemodialysis. ARC J Nephrol. 2018;3(1):6–12.
31. Rajab A, Freeman NV, Patton M. The frequency of posterior urethral valves in Oman. Br J Urol. 1996;77(6):900–4.
32. Al Riyami M, Al Saidi M, Al Ghaithi B, Al Maskari A, Lala S, Mohsin N, Hirshikesan L, Al KN. Pediatric renal transplantation in Oman: a single-center experience. Oman Med J. 2018;33(1):7–14. https://doi.org/10.5001/omj.2018.03.

# Nephrology in Thailand

# 31

Kearkiat Praditpornsilpa, Kriang Tungsanga, Somchai Eiam-Ong, Khajohn Tiranathanagul, Nattachai Srisawat, Natavudh Townamchai, and Kamonwan Tangvoraphonkchai

| | |
|---|---|
| Area | 513,120 km$^2$ |
| Population[1] | 69.42 million (2018) |
| Capital | Bangkok |
| Three most populated cities: | Bangkok<br>Nonthaburi<br>Nakhon Ratchasima |
| Official language | Thai |
| Gross Domestic Product (GDP)[2] | $490,120 billion (2018) |
| GDP per capita[b] | $6590 (2018) |
| Human Development Index (HDI)[3] | 0.755 (2017) |
| Official currency | Baht |
| Total number of nephrologists | 871 (2018) |
| National society of nephrology | The Nephrology Society of Thailand (NST)<br>www.nephrothai.org |
| Incidence of end-stage renal disease[d] | 362.87 pmp |
| Prevalence of end-stage renal disease[4] (including patients with a functioning kidney transplant) | 1439.7 pmp |
| Total number of patients on dialysis[4] (all modalities) | 2015 – 78,348<br>2016 – 86,116 |
| Number of patients on hemodialysis[4] | 2015 – 54,104<br>2016 – 59,745 |
| Number of patients on peritoneal dialysis[4] | 2015 – 24,244<br>2016 – 26,371 |
| Number of renal transplantations per year[5] | 2017 – 709<br>2018 – 670 |

References
1. World population prospects – population division. population.un.org. United Nations Department of Economic and Social Affairs, Population Division. Retrieved November 9, 2019
2. Report for selected countries and subjects – Thailand. IMF. Retrieved 29 October 2018
3. Global 2016 human development report overview – English (PDF). New York: United Nations Development Programme (UNDP). 2017. pp. 22–24. Archived (PDF) from the original on 23 March 2017. Retrieved 22 March 2017
4. Annual report Thailand renal replacement therapy (preliminary 2016). The Nephrology Society of Thailand (NST). Retrieved 7 June 2019
5. Annual report 2018 organ transplantation in Thailand. Thai Transplant Society (TTS). Retrieved 22 January 2020

K. Praditpornsilpa · K. Tungsanga · S. Eiam-Ong
K. Tiranathanagul · N. Srisawat · N. Townamchai
Department of Medicine, Chulalongkorn University, Bangkok, Thailand

K. Tangvoraphonkchai (✉)
Mahasarakham University, Maha Sarakham, Thailand
e-mail: kamonwan.tangvoraphonkchai@nhs.net

## Introduction

Thailand is located at the center of the Southeast Asian Indochinese Peninsula and covers a total area of approximately 513,000 km$^2$, which is the 50th largest country in the world. Thailand is bordered to the north by Myanmar and Laos, to the east by Laos and Cambodia, to the south by the Gulf of Thailand and Malaysia, and to the west by the Andaman Sea and southern Myanmar. The country is divided into six regions: north, northeast, central, south, east, and west, comprising 76 provinces. The north and the northeast are highland, whereas the east and the south are coastal and islanded area. With different landscape and culture, Thailand has a variety of attractive landmarks such as jungle, sandy beaches, ancient ruins, temples, parks, and shopping malls. Bangkok is the capital city and one of the world's top tourist destinations, which is located at central region. Bangkok is also a center of technology, economics, education, industry, politics, and medical facilities. Nearly 8.3 million of population, Bangkok is the most crowded city in Thailand. The Thai royal family who is the spiritual centre of Thail people, resides in Bangkok. Instead of ruling the country and having political power, the major role of the Thai royal family is to support several social development projects and be a symbol of the kingdom.

Situated close to the equator, Thailand is an endemic area for a number of tropical diseases, such as melioidosis, leptospirosis, dengue, malaria, and tick-borne disease. However, the recent national health data showed noncommunicable illness such as cardiovascular disease, cancers and traffic accident contributed greater part of death toll in Thailand than infectious illness. It should be implied that despite the



J. A. Moura-Neto et al. (eds.), *Nephrology Worldwide*, https://doi.org/10.1007/978-3-030-56890-0_31

improvement of public health and infrastructure, the number of aging population is growing and result in increasing incidnce of noncommunicable disease.

## Brief History of Nephrology in Thailand

Modern nephrology in Thailand started in early 1960 when acute kidney injury (AKI) associated to Asiatic cholera with acute tubular necrosis and hypokalemic nephropathy was reported by Benyajati et al. [1]. The major advancement in studying tropical renal diseases, particularly AKI, has been subsequently carried out by Sitprija et al. [2, 3]. Tropical disease-associated AKI can be infectious and noninfectious related [4]. The leading causes of infections are leptospirosis, malaria, and dengue virus. Regarding noninfectious-related etiologies, snakebite, plant, and chemical toxins are common causes of AKI. Besides renal function reduction, various fluid and electrolyte disturbances are also common in tropical disease-associated AKI, including hyponatremia, hypernatremia, hypokalemia, hyperkalemia, hypocalcemia, hypercalcemia, hypophosphatemia, and hypomagnesemia. Of interest, stones, potassium depletion, and endemic distal renal tubular acidosis are highly prevalent in northeastern Thailand.

The Nephrology Society of Thailand (NST) was established by Benyajati et al. in March 1976, aiming to update current academic knowledge among the members, to convey the renal health knowledge to the public, to stimulate renal research activities of the country, and to train and produce kidney-related personnel. Regarding renal replacement therapy (RRT), hemodialysis (HD) was firstly utilized in 1964 as chronic intermittent HD in patients with end-stage renal disease (ESRD). Peritoneal dialysis (PD) was primarily used as intermittent PD (IPD) in 1968 and was subsequently employed as chronic PD in 1982. In 2008, the Thai government launched the "PD-first policy" to provide free PD as the first line of treatment for ESRD patients under the coverage of the National Health Security Office (NHSO), which takes care of approximately 70% of the Thai population [5]. The first case of kidney transplantation (KT) was successfully performed with a deceased donor in 1972 [6].

## Renal Disease in Thailand

Thailand is one of the tropical countries, the area of the earth located around the equator. Like other tropical countries, there are two settings of kidney diseases in Thailand. The first setting comprises renal disorders similarly reported in other countries such as AKI from ischemic and nephrotoxic factors, CKD from diabetes mellitus (DM) and hypertension (HT), and primary as well as secondary glomerulonephritis. The second setting, named tropical renal disease, includes kidney diseases, which are prevailing in the tropical countries and contribute certain roles in tropical disease-associated AKI.

SEA-AKI study, the cohort of 5476 patients across 17 ICU centers in Thailand, recently reported an incidence of AKI of 52.9% [7]. The highest AKI incidence by stage was stage 3, stage 2, and stage 1, respectively, contrasting to data from high-income countries, which showed stage 1, stage 2, and stage 3, respectively. This might be explained by the limitation of the number of ICU beds and the delayed AKI recognition in Thailand. Older age, female gender, admission to a regional hospital, medical ICU, high body mass index, primary diagnosis of cardiovascular-related disease and infectious disease, higher Acute Physiology and Chronic Health Evaluation II (APACHE II), nonrenal Sequential Organ Failure Assessment (SOFA) scores, underlying anemia, and use of vasopressors were all independent risk factors for AKI development.

As a middle-income country, the prevalence of predialysis CKD in Thailand was 17.5% [8]. This was greater than the global prevalence, which accounted for low-, middle-, and high-income nations all together. Consistent with global reports, CKD stage 3 and female gender had the highest prevalence (7.5% and 18.5%, respectively), and there was an upward trend with increasing age. The largest prevalence of CKD was located in the capital and nearby regions, in spite of better education and infrastructure systems. CKD prevalence was significantly associated with older age, DM, HT, hyperuricemia, female gender, history of using traditional medicines, and a history of kidney stones. Despite a considerably high prevalence, awareness of CKD in the Thai general population was only 1.9%. This was also illustrated by the prevalence of high salt intake of 73.4% and a mean total daily sodium intake of 3.4 g/day [9].

An 8-year follow-up observational study showed the incidence of CKD to be 28% and risk for CKD progression 23%. HT, DM, and low income were associated with new cases of CKD, whereas DM and hyperuricemia were related to CKD progression. The top five etiologies of dialysis prevalence and incidence reported from the Thai Renal Replacement Therapy registry (TRT registry) 2015 [10] were DM, HT, obstruction, presumed glomerulonephritis, and urate nephropathy. This set of etiologies had not changed since 2010. Biopsy-proven glomerulonephritis was ranked 8th, and the two most common pathology diagnoses were IgA nephropathy and focal segmental glomerulosclerosis.

According to the data, the Thai government has increased the concern over CKD and sequelae. The expansion of the elderly population raised even more concern of the CKD situation because of the increasing number of patients with DM and HT, which are both major CKD risk factors. Subsequently, the Thai government issued a policy to establish CKD clinics in all hospitals under the Ministry of Public Health, in order to provide an integrated community health service based on a chronic care model. The purpose of CKD clinics is to slow down CKD progression, prevent and minimize complications, and prepare for RRT, including treatment options education, access surgery, and transplant listing. Ideally, the structure of a Thai CKD clinic comprises one nephrologist, one CKD nurse manager, one dietitian or nutritionist, one pharmacist, one psychiatrist or psychologist, and one physical therapist and palliative care team.

The implementation of the CKD clinic is the continuum of noncommunicable disease (NCD) care, which has been organized since 2011. The operation of a NCD and CKD clinic is centrally regulated by the Bureau of Noncommunicable Diseases, which plays a pivotal role in setting clinical targets, measuring outcomes, providing incentives for any achievement, and analyzing and reporting data. The Provincial Public Health Offices are responsible for monitoring the performance of local CKD clinics, collecting data, and submitting to the Bureau of NonCommunicable Diseases. Additionally, village health volunteers (VHVs), who reside geographically within the patients' community, take part in health promotion by educating, monitoring, and delivering a variety of support.

A survey of CKD clinic implementation in 2017 [11] showed that 7.14% of hospitals did not set up a CKD service due to insufficient staff, space, and budget. A small portion (17.7%) of the CKD services operated as a part of a NCD clinic, whereas 82.3% ran the service separately. Most of the financial resources for CKD clinic operation came from individual hospital funding. Although the NHSO provided partial endorsement, financial constraint remained a major barrier. Moreover, a lack of healthcare professionals, especially nutritionists and dietitians, was a common issue among rural hospitals. Instead, dietary advice was commonly carried out by general or CKD nurses. Despite the overburdened service, CKD clinics have to perform data collection and submission as additional workloads. General or CKD nurses were usually responsible for data input, even though they had several other assignments. Because they were overloaded with work, most of hospitals had never analyzed or applied their data to clinical practice. As such, balancing between data collection and staff workload is a challenge for clinical directors and policymakers.

## Reimbursement of Nephrology in Thailand

Cost of CKD care in Thailand was partly reimbursed by the Thai National Health Care System which covers primary prevention for CKD at risk population, secondary prevention to delay CKD progression and RRT for ESRD [12]. Although the Thai National Health Care system provides financial risk protection and access to health services, there are discrepancy pathways for coverage of nephrology service by different reimbursement plans. As of 2019, three major health reimbursement programs have served Thailand's population of 68 million. The Civil Servant Medical Benefit Scheme (CSMBS) started by Royal Decree in 1980, for civil servants and their families, namely, spouse, parents, and children under 18 years of age, covers 4.4 million population. CSMBS reimbursement is tax based, is noncontributory, and is an open-end budget, which has no ceiling to include total CSMBS reimbursement. In other words, the government will pay for all health expenses for the civil servant and family. The Social Security Scheme was launched in 1990, covering formal sector private employees for non-work related sickness, maternity and invalidity including cash benefits and funeral grants. The scheme is financed by tripartite contributions from government, employers and employees, each of 1.5% of payroll (total of 4.5%). The Universal Health Coverage Scheme (UCS) was introduced in 2002 by the NHSO, which is theoretically available to all other Thai nationals covering most of the population (48 million population) besides Civil Servant Welfare System and Social Security System. UCS is tax based, noncontributory, closed-end budget as SSS, and overseen by the Ministry of Public Health that operates most of government health facilities. According to the World Bank, 99.5% of the population have health protection coverage under Thailand's overall healthcare system.

These three major health reimbursement programs (CSMBS, SSS, and UCS) are responsible for primary CKD prevention [13]. Thai population who has CKD risk factors such as old age, diabetes, hypertension etc is eligible for CKD screening regarding their health covereage schemes. For diabetes patients ,the reimbursement would cover blood test, glycemic control and some medication. The reimbursement also cover the cost of renal stone therapy which is the four most commonly known ESRD etiologies in Thailand. The primary CKD prevention screens Thai for an early intervention. The Thai SEEK study, an epidemiologic study from 2009, showed a total CKD burden of 17.5% of the Thai population, classified by CKD stages 1, 2, 3, 4, and 5 with 3.3%, 5.6%, 7.5%, 0.8%, and 0.3% of the Thai population, respectively [8]. For secondary prevention, CSMBS, SSS, and UCS endorse and reimburse interventions to delay renal progression by multidisciplinary team CKD in clinics providing care for early-stage CKD patients. CKD clinics in Thailand are usually formed with a number of staffs who response in different parts of CKD care included nephrologist, nurse, dietitian aiming to achieve national CKD goals which are centrally set and monitored by Bureau of Noncommunicable disease included percentage of ACEI? ARB prescription among CKD, incidnece of anemia/hyperphosphatemia/acidosis etc.

The privileges for RRT reimbursements are different among the three reimbursement schemes [14]. Before 1999, only civil servants and their families had the right to reimburse RRT via CSMBS. This privilege covered HD, PD, and KT. In 1999, about 9 years after the operation of SSS for social welfare and medical coverage, SSS decided to include HD, PD, and KT for the private working population. Although NSH's ideology is to narrow the gap of inequality of Thai population, this ambitious mission created a challenging issue at the begining: how Thailand, an upper-middle-income country determined by gross national product per capita and the World Bank, will financially survive with universal healthcare coverage policy? This debating agenda caused reluctance to include RRT at the initial rollout of UCS. In 2008, UCS decided to include RRT by PD as PD first for equality in access to dialysis for ESRD patients. Nephrologists, health economists, civil and professional societies, namely, the Nephrology Society of Thailand and the Thai Kidney Foundation, and patients' groups who are the major stakeholders advocated this policy as a turning point in ESRD care in Thailand. PD-first policy was a relief for health professionals by eliminating the scenario where ESRD patients could not have access to chronic dialysis and thereby died due to uremia caused by financial incapability. In the past, before PD 1st policy implementation, ESRD patients who could not afford hemodialysis, would be left untreat until die. Nephrologist faced with hard situation to inform patients and family that life-saving treatment required money, without money they could not survive. The PD 1st policy had been greatly relief this tension among Nephorlogist, patients and family [15].

PD-first policy in Thailand was based on the facts that PD is a home dialysis modality, logistic friendly, more economical than HD, and requiring fewer health professional staff especially dialysis nurses. Moreover, the clinical outcomes are comparable with HD, for example, patient survival and quality of life [16–18]. In addition, PD first does not require HD machine and water treatment setup and can be financially sustainable in upper-middle-income country more than HD. To alleviate the cost of PD solution procurement, central purchasing up front has been exercised for price negotiation with the industry. Similar purchasing strategies apply to the purchase of PD catheters. The centralized, transparent, and Mass PD solution purchase decreased the financial burden of the fiscal reimbursement RRT budget and made the closed-end budget estimation feasible and manageable. PD-first policy is designed to be flexible and allows HD reimbursement in case of PD contraindication. The PD contraindication criteria have been set up by consensus between the medical specialists and the payer. The committees at regional and national levels make the decision based on the consensus criteria. The full reimbursement is also allowed if the patients need dialysis mode switching to HD, guided by standard clinical criteria such as inadequacy of PD and technical failure. In 2017, the ratio of incident ESRD patients receiving PD to HD treatment in Thailand was 50:50.

Same as CSMBS and SSS, UCS fully reimburses KT. There are two types of kidney transplantation for ESRD with RRT ; living-related and cardeveric kidney transplants. The pre-emptive living-related KT (CKD4-5 without RRT) can also be done in Thailand. Term "living related" means donor and recipient should be legally approved for their biological relationship, also includes spouse with marriage certification. In addition, CSMBS, SSS, and UCS reimburse recombinant human erythropoietin (rHuEpo) for treatment of renal anemia for RRT patients. However, the dose of rHuEpo in SSS and UCS is strictly guided and has ceiling dosage limitation. Most of the reimbursed rHuEpo brands in UCS are biocopies of rHuEpo. Similar purchasing strategies by central purchasing up front also apply to biocopy to alleviate financial UCS budget. Cost of ESRD medication is also accounted for reimbursements. However, some medications are not covered. As such, patients have to copay or fully pay for particular drugs. The range of eligible medications for each scheme is diverse. Basically, CSMBS reimburses a wider range of medications than the other two schemes. High-cost drugs, for example, lanthanum carbonate and sevelamer, are only eligible for CSMBS. Most hospitals regulate the use of expensive drugs such as calcimimetic drug by authorizing committees or clinical directors to be responsible for prescription. Patients usually collect their prescription from hospitals. In some cases, patients can also collect some drugs from pharmacies.

Despite ongoing sustainable RRT reimbursement in Thailand since 2008, the reimbursement issues continue being a challenge. The next challenge for our reimbursement system includes the equility between three reimbursement programs. Generally, CSMBS covers more medical service and medication than UCS and SSS. For instance, CSMBS fully covers all RRT disrecard modalities, while UCS would cover only PD except patient is contraindicated to start with PD. Therefore, patients under UCS usually start RRT with PD disregard their preference, otherwise they need to pay by their own. Another issue is the accessibility of more complicated treatment in each area. With more complex disease, resource usually limits in Bangkok and central region. Reimbursement for complex disease such as lupus nepritis, vasculitis also limit especially for costly intervention or treatment. The current closed-end budget which limits a ceiling for reimbursement of the RRT amount per case and per treatment in SSS and UCS has been inadequate to cover more efficient dialysis for complicated patients such as convective mode hemodialysis, automated PD, more biocompatible PD fluid, desensitized treatment for kidney transplant recipients, etc. The reimbursement should proceed to cover the treatment for more complicated patients such as ABO-incompatible KT, KT in highly sensitized patients, automated PD for high transport peritoneal membrane, use of biocompatible PD fluids, home HD for younger patients, use of expensive monoclonal antibody for patients who need the treatment such as eculizumab, etc. The more medical benefits for Thai kidney patients should cover genetic testing for therapeutic guidance such as genetic glomerulopathy, kidney disease caused by complement mutation, etc.

## Renal Replacement Therapy in Thailand

### Acute Renal Replacement Therapy

In 2014, the national survey to explore the acute RRT practice in Thailand [19] showed a marked difference from those observed in resource-sufficient countries. Nephrologists had a major role (86.4%) in deciding the initiation and selection of RRT modality in Thailand. In this survey, intermittent hemodialysis (IHD) was the first preferable mode of RRT (72%) followed by continuous renal replacement therapy (CRRT, 12%), sustained low-efficiency dialysis (SLED, 10.0%), and PD (6.0%), which contrasted to previous studies where CRRT was the preferable mode. This noticed difference could be related to the lower cost of IHD and the availability of equipment. In SEA-AKI study [7], there were greater rates of RRT use in patients who were covered by Civil Servant Medical Benefit Scheme than other reimbursement schemes. Even though provincial hospitals had the highest rates of severe AKI (29%), they had the lowest rates of RRT (5.9%). In addition, patients treated in university hospitals were more likely to receive RRT than the general public hospitals, which include regional and provincial hospitals. These findings might reflect the limitations in healthcare budget and process of care.

The results from the Beginning and Ending Supportive Therapy for the Kidney (BEST Kidney) study [20] conducted among 53 centers from 23 countries showed that a range of costs were greater with CRRT, starting from 3629.8 USD/day with CRRT to 378.6 USD/day with IHD. The median difference in cost between CRRT and IHD was 289.60 USD (IQR 116.8–830.8) per day. In Thailand, the average cost of CRRT is 1000 USD/day, while the cost of IHD is only 100 USD/day. Focusing on the site of vascular access, the right internal jugular vein was the most common site of insertion (70.4%). The most common indication for CRRT was hemodynamic instability with the continuous veno-venous hemofiltration (CVVHF) as the most preferable mode of CRRT. From current evidence comparing different modalities of CRRT, there is no evidence that CVVHF (convection) is different from the continuous veno-venous hemodiafiltration (CVVHDF – convection plus diffusion) in terms of patient or renal outcomes. The preferred CRRT dose is 20–25 ml/kg/dose, which is in line with current evidence suggesting no additional benefit in using effluent rate in excess of 20 ml/kg/h [21].

### Chronic Renal Replacement Therapy

#### Hemodialysis and Hemodiafiltration

HD is the predominant RRT modality in Thailand and contributes with 63.02% (54,104) of the 85,848 patients on dialysis for the prevalence, whereas the incidence is 52.88% (11,038 out of 20,874 patients) according to the latest Thailand RRT report of 2015 data [10]. These percentages have been gradually reduced from more than 80% since 2008 when the "PD first" policy was introduced by the government under the universal coverage program. There are more than 600 HD centers distributed in the whole country of 76 provinces, and 24% of them are located in Bangkok. Most of the HD patients are fully or partially reimbursed for the HD treatment by the CSMBS, the SSS, or the UCS. The reimbursement is in the range of 1500–2000 bath (47–63 USD) per HD session. Only 18.2% is self-payment without reimbursement. The frequency of HD varies between twice and thrice weekly, an average of 2.5 ± 0.5 times/week. The factors that determine the frequency of HD include residual renal function, achievement of target spKt/Vurea according to the Nephrology Society of Thailand recommendation, and financial burden. The average HD time, blood, and dialysate flow rates are 4.0 ± 0.1 h, 313.6 ± 64.2 ml/min, and 524.4 ± 95.5 mL/min, respectively. The frequent or long in-center HD modalities are uncommonly prescribed. Self-cannulated home HD has been introduced to only a few patients. The most common vascular access type is AVF (65.2%), while the second and the last are permanent cuffed catheter (20.2%) and AV graft (AVG) (14.7%), respectively. High-flux dialyzers are more frequently prescribed than low-flux dialyzers. The super high-flux or medium cutoff dialyzers are just introduced to some patients. The majority of HD centers reuse dialyzers up to 10–20 times. Dialyzer cleaning and reprocessing are usually performed by HD nurses with manual method or, less commonly, using automatic reuse machine. The efficiency of reuse is appropriately evaluated by standard measurements. Measures of dialysis adequacy and nutritional status are performed regularly at least every 1–3 months and demonstrated to be spKt/V 1.7 ± 0.4, URR 74.7 ± 9.1%, nPCR 1.2 ± 1.0 g/kg/day, and serum albumin 3.7 ± 0.6 g/dL. In 2015, the prevalence of HD patients who had hepatitis B and C infection was 4% and 3.7%, respectively; there were also 161 patients with HIV infection. The head of each HD center is a nephrologist. The HD nurses have various roles in a HD center, not only patient care but also the daily monitoring of water treatment, preparing the dialysis circuit, and reuse process. One HD nurse usually is responsible for four stable chronic HD patients. The other support personnel such as HD technician and the water treatment engineer who could share the HD nurse workload are not formally available but they will be in the near future. There is a nonprofit organization that certifies, monitors, and recertifies the HD centers' quality in various aspects including organization, staffing, water treatment, machine, equipment, patient care, and patient outcomes. The national comprehensive dialysis registries have been established for a decade.

Hemodiafiltration (HDF) is the convective therapy that is available and increasing in popularity in Thailand. HDF is defined as a blood purification therapy combining diffusive and convective solute transport achieved by an effective convection volume of at least 20% of the total blood volume, using a high-flux membrane characterized by an ultrafiltration coefficient (KUF) greater than 20 mL/h/mmHg/m$^2$, and a sieving coefficient (S) for β2 microglobulin (β2M) of greater than 0.6 [22]. The HDF with internal fluid substitution technique called double high-flux HD was the first HDF modality that was introduced in the country in 2002. Double high-flux HD is set up using two high-flux dialyzers in the serial alignment. The restrictor is applied in the countercurrent dialysate pathway between the two dialyzers. The convection occurred in the first while the fluid substitution from fresh dialysis fluid took place in the second dialyzer. The original fixed restrictor design was improved by the new design adjustable C-clamp restrictor design leading to the capability to adjust the convective volume (Fig. 31.1). This new system was called convective-controlled double high-flux hemodiafiltration (CC-HDF). A previous study demonstrated that this technique was safe and provided comparable efficacy with the high-efficiency post-dilution online HDF [23].

Later, HDF with external fluid substitution called online HDF (online preparation of substitution fluid) was introduced in Thailand in 2003. The ultrapure grade of dialysis water was the requirement in the center that provided online HDF treatment. Two standard methods of fluid substitution in online HDF comprise post-dilution and pre-dilution modes. Pre-dilution was used in most of online HDF at the early era. After the survival benefit of high-efficiency post-dilution online HDF was published [24], some centers changed to post-dilution as the first choice. HDF treatment contributed only 1% of all HD treatments in 2010 but has been growing in modality share. A report from HDF centre demonstrated a 10-year survival outcome of 61.8%, and the mean survival time among patients who conducted high-efficiency online HDF [25]. Besides standard pre- and post-dilution techniques, mid- and mixed-dilution online HDF have been introduced in clinical practice to avoid the technical problem of post-dilution technique as well as reduced small solute clearance from hemodilution of pre-dilution technique [26, 27]. Despite the growth of online HDF utilization, there is no specific reimbursement item of this modality. Besides ESRD patients, online HDF is also utilized in septic AKI patients in order to enhance inflammatory cytokine removal, not only intermittent but also a prolonged intermittent fashion called SLED-f (sustained low-efficiency diafiltration) [28].

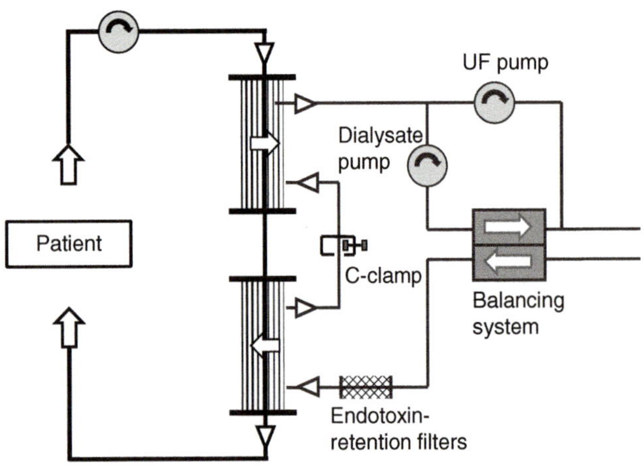


Fig. 31.1 Convective-controlled double high-flux hemodiafiltration (CC-HDF)

## Peritoneal Dialysis

Thailand is one of the few countries where "PD first" policy has been adopted. This policy has been implemented since 2008, 6 years after the inception of the UCS. There were, however, formerly two major health-funding schemes, the CSMBS for government employees and SSS for formal private employees, but a substantial portion of Thai people were left unsecured by any benefit. UCS was responsible for nearly 80% of the Thai population and covered the largest portion of CKD patients. As such, the majority of ESRD patients who demanded RRT were under UCS. Although both CSMBS and SSS have included RRT in their package, RRT was not initially offered by the UCS because of the expected huge expenses. In 2004, the NHSO, which is responsible for the UCS, examined the value for money of dialysis, included the costs of providing RRT in the UCS over 15 years, and carried out a public survey for RRT options [14]. This study showed that neither PD nor HD was cost effective, but PD offered better value than HD. Accordingly, PD-first policy was introduced for ESRD patients under UCS based on the facts that PD was cheaper than HD, required fewer staff, and could be performed by the patients at home with minimal infrastructure. After the implementation, almost 20,000 Thai patients have been able to access PD with comparable outcomes to international standards [29].

The objectives of PD-first policy are to achieve equality in access to RRT across the three health-funding schemes with acceptable outcomes, reduce catastrophic health expenditures incurred by patients on low incomes, and minimize the impact on overall national healthcare budget. This policy fully reimburses for ESRD patients who start with PD and partially reimburses for patients who opt to start with HD, before launching the PD-first policy. If patients opt to start RRT with HD after the launch of PD-first policy, they must take responsibility of all expenses related to HD such as HD treatment, vascular access creation, and repair. However, if there is any contraindication to PD based on criteria established by the Nephrology Society of Thailand, and decided upon by committees at regional and national levels, HD costs may be fully repaid. In addition, if a patient starts with PD but has to shift to HD later because of any medical or social problems related to the therapy, the costs would continue to be entirely reimbursed.

Pertaining to the cooperation between three main stakeholders, policymakers, kidney professionals, and civil society, PD-first policy has been successfully implemented. The NHSO plays an important role as a policymaker with the support from the Ministry of Public Health. The PD-advocating nephrologists take the lead on clinical guidance with backup from the Nephrology Society of Thailand. The group of human immune decficiency and cancer patiens provided endorsement to the kidney patient club to set up and assist the other two sectors. There are four key strategies behind policy implementation: cost containment, incentive schemes, expansion of PD centers, and establishing community support groups [30]. The Government Pharmaceutical Organization centrally purchases all PD supplies, resulting in price reduction and cost containment. Regarding incentive schemes, the NHSO initially paid PD units and staff to promote PD practice. The NHSO also set up PD education centers located nationwide to support clinical services, academic activities, and training programs in each region. Additionally, local kidney patient clubs collaborate with PD units to deliver both direct and indirect support depending on local policy.

In 2007, a year before the launch of PD-first program, the proportion of yearly incidence ratio between PD and HD patients of all health schemes was 8:145, and it increased to 141:168 by 2015 [10]. The number of PD training centers increased from 51 to 111 by 2011 [31]. The incidence of RRT cases and the number of PD centers doubled by 7 and 3 years, respectively, and the gap between PD and HD new cases was closer. It should be noted that UCS had the largest portion of PD cases (88%) and the proportion of PD was greater than HD by 60:40 in 2015 [30]. The 1- and 5-year survival rates were 82.6% and 54%, and the median time of patient survival was 70.1 months [32]. Factors associated with low patient survival rates were female gender, old age at the time of PD initiation, patients under the CSMBS, low education level, and DM [32]. The 1- and 5-year technique survival rates were 94.8% and 80.8%. The peritonitis rate was 1 episode/23 months [6]. Both patient survival and technique survival rates of 2013–2016 were better than 2008–2012 [32]; however, factors related to technique survival and peritonitis had never been reported. The growing number of ESRD patients who could access RRT and better survival rates indicated the successful adoption of the policy among Thai nephrologists, CKD clinics, public hospitals, the Thai government, and patients under UCS.

## Kidney Transplantation

The first KT in Thailand was successfully performed on March 3, 1972 [6]. However, transplant rate was very low in the first few decades due to the transplant team unfamiliarity with brain death diagnosis. In 1988, the Thai organ donation center was established under the supervision of the Thai Red Cross Society, which is a nonprofit organization, for transparently organizing the allocation system in Thailand. In 1989, the brain death criteria were published by the Thai Medical Council. From that time on, the number of KT in Thailand has been increasing yearly. Data from the recent KT registry showed that there were 670 patients transplanted in 2018, which 188 cases were living-related donor KT and 482 cases were deceased donor KT. There were 29 patients whose age was under 18 years old. So far, there have been 9520 kidney transplant patients in Thailand.

### Medical Expense

The medical expenses of Thai citizens are covered by one of the three funds. The first funding program that covers KT expenses and immunosuppression is the Civil Servant Medical Benefit. The Social Security Scheme and the Universal Health Coverage Scheme started covering KT expenses from 2004 and 2008, respectively. KT is the only RRT in Thailand with the expenses being covered by the government. All Thai people who undergo KT in government hospitals will be covered for all medical expenses during operation and posttransplantation follow-up. However, the expenses for pretransplant desensitization are not covered, but it is now under cost-benefit evaluation and should be covered in the next phase.

### Outcomes

In the 2000s, the proportion of incident KT cases was similar between deceased donors (DKT) and living-related donors (LKT). However, the proportion of DKT was dramatically increased to 70% in the last decade. This could be explained by the successful country policy for promoting organ donation and establishment of donor hospitals in the whole country. Patients are eligible for DKT waiting list only when they are being treated with HD or PD. Patients who already received DKT during 2018 have spent 62.5 months on dialysis, while LKT recipients spent 27.8 months waiting for a

KT. The donor for LKT must be blood relatives or spouses who have been married for at least 3 years or have sibling.

The major induction immunosuppressive drugs are anti-IL2 receptor antibody and anti-thymocyte globulin. The number of patients who have been transplanted without antibody induction has decreased, being only 15% in 2018. The maintenance regimen mainly consists of tacrolimus, mycophenolic acid, and prednisolone.

The 1-year, 5-year, and 10-year LKT allograft survival rates are 98.8%, 96.5%, and 85.6%, respectively, whereas the 1-year, 5-year, and 10-year DKT allograft survival rates are 95.5%, 85.5%, and 66.6%, respectively. The 1-year, 5-year, and 10-year LKT patient survival rates are 99.0%, 97.9%, and 92.2%, respectively, and the 1-year, 5-year, and 10-year DKT patient survival rates are 96.6%, 92.3%, and 80.6%, respectively (data from Thai Transplant Registry 2018).

### High Immunologic Risk Patient

In general, kidney transplantation has been performed based on kidney transplant usually performed on negative testing of CDC-AHG crossmatch and compatible ABO blood group. However, the ABO-incompatible KT program has been first started in Thailand in 2008 at King Chulalongkorn Memorial Hospital with excellent outcomes [33]. The HLA-incompatible transplantation (DSA positive/CDC-AHG negative) is generally performed in many transplant centers with individualized desensitization protocol. The methods for antibody removal are conventional plasmapheresis, double filtration plasmapheresis, and ABO immunoadsorption (Glycosorb®). Unfortunately, there is no IgG immunoadsorption available in Thailand. The paired kidney donation program is not yet performed in Thailand because the donor of LKT must be a relative of the recipient.

### Organ Procurement and Transplantation Network Policies

The Thai organ donation center is the only organization in Thailand responsible for organ sharing and allocation under the supervision of the Thai Red Cross Society. Transplantation in Thailand must be under the regulation of the Thai organ donation center and follow the Declaration of Istanbul. Every potential deceased donor must be reported to the Thai organ donation center. The organ retrieval teams come from all organ transplant hospital members. The scoring and allocation systems are published to the public on the website of the Thai organ donation center. Potential recipients who are eligible for DKT waitlist registration must be ESRD patients who are undergoing HD or PD. The regulation is the reason why preemptive KT can be only performed for LKT recipients. Panel reactive antibody (PRA) assay is usually tested by using phenotypic bead from commercial kit. While, calculated PRA (cPRA), was calculated based on HLA antibody identified by single antigen bead (SAB), in other words, this test is more quantitative than PRA assay. DKT recipients must have negative CDC-AHG and ABO blood group identical to donor. After establishment of the cPRA, virtual crossmatch will be utilized for our DKT waitlist.

## Human Resource in Nephrology Service in Thailand

The quest to prevent CKD, slower CKD progression and expand RRT facility need bot adequate number and qualification of human resource. The district hospital and sub-district health office are the major taskforces for primary CKD prevention. Typically, the district hospitals have 30-60 beds available and 3-5 physicians who are majority general practitioners, perform healthcare and coordination with sub-district health service. Minority of district hospitals have more than 120 beds and more physicians, that some of them are specialty such as surgeon, obstetrician and paediatrician. However, main mission of these hospital is community health services. Sub-district health office is operated by three public health officers or nurses and village health volunteers (VHVs) [34]. There are about 1 million VHVs in Thailand. They are volunteer villagers who have received formal practical training on public healthcare principles and are responsible for 10–12 households in the village. One typical Thai village has 50–100 households. VHVs also work as middlemen collect and share information between physicians and patients, and closely monitor health issues in certain areas.

CKD clinic in provincial hospitals and medical centers is the major taskforce for the delay in CKD progression. The CKD clinic is operated by internal medicine physician, nephrologist, nurse, and dietitian. The Thai Medical Council and the Royal College of Physicians of Thailand (RCPT) oversee the standard quality of HD centers. The requirement of manpower for HD unit is a strict compulsory requirement for HD unit accreditation. The accreditation links to the eligibility for the reimbursement. Nephrologist or internist or pediatrician who has been trained and certified for HD care by the RCPT is in charge and responsible for HD patients. A full-time trained and certified HD nurse is a must requirement for HD center in Thailand. The compulsory standard quality of HD center in Thailand also includes the ratio of HD nurse to dialysis patient of 1:4. The nurses assigned to care for HD patients must be a certified HD nurse or a nurse who has completed a formal HD training curriculum. The training curriculum has been overseen and regulated by the RCPT and the Thailand Nursing and Midwifery Council. Nurses who have completed the HD training curriculum are eligible for a certified diplomate of HD nurse.

All HD centers in Thailand require quality accreditation. The Medical Council of Thailand is a non-governmental organization that is resposible for regulate and control medical practice in Thailand, and develop outline for medical education. This organization also investigate for any complaint, mistake or misconduct related to medical practice. There are many sectors under Medical Council of Thailand, such as RCPT, Royal College of Surgeons of Thailand (RCST) and all medical schools in Thailand. Not only number and qualification of HD staffs, other issues include water quality, equipment, space, infectious control, patients' safety issues, and standard of care are also required for accreditation of HD unit. Also, HD center must register patients' data, treatment data, laboratory data, clinical outcome, and water treatment quality (bacteria cultures, contaminants, and endotoxin levels) to the TRT registry. The Nephrology Society of Thailand is responsible for TRT registry. Most of PD-first activities and PD patients are treated in public hospitals. Nephrologists and PD nurses are the main human resources. PD nurses are trained by PD nurse training curriculum or by in-house training. Other staffs include social worker and home healthcare team.

Becoming a nephrologist in Thailand requires a certification from the Royal College of Physicians of Thailand (RCPT). The Nephrology Society of Thailand (NST), working under the RCPT, mainly conducts nephrology board examination every year. The NST is also responsible for training programs and supervision of all training centers. Each training center is responsible for its own trainee selection. Eligible trainees should be licensed as physicians in Thailand, complete 3 or more years of board internal medicine training, and pass the examination. All trainees are required to spend 2 years in the general nephrology program, which includes theoretical and practical training on HD, PD, ESRD, AKI, critical care nephrology, renal transplantation, and clinical nephrology. All centers are available for hands-on training of temporary catheter insertion, and some centers offer PD catheter insertion program. The nephrology board examination is composed of MCQ, MEQ, OSCE, and long case examination. International certified nephrologist would need to pass this examination for permission to work legally as a nephrologist in Thailand. After finishing general nephrology program, some centers provide additional programs on transplantation and critical nephrology.

## Highlights of Nephrology in Thailand

It is very fortunate for Thailand that our royal family has been actively engaged in improving kidney care. Established in 1978, the Kidney Foundation of Thailand (KFT), previously presided over by Her Royal Highness Princess Galyani Vadhana, the Princess of Naradhiwas Rajanagarindra, has contributed enormously to the progress of nephrology and kidney patient care in the country. In addition to providing HD at a subsidized price, the KFT also provides financial support for procurement of dialysis machines and establishment of dialysis and transplantation services at rural hospitals, facilitating medical and nurse training in nephrology and dialysis, and facilitating kidney transplantation [35]. Currently, the KFT and a new nonprofit foundation, Bhumirajanagarindra Kidney Institute Foundation, are graciously presided over by Her Royal Highness Princess Maha Chakri Sirindhorn, the second daughter of the late King Bhumibol Adulyadej. With such enormous support from the royals, the ISN presented the ISN Special Recognition Award to HRH Princess Sirindhorn, in recognition of HRH extraordinary contribution to caring for CKD patients in 2016 (Figs. 31.2 and 31.3) [36].

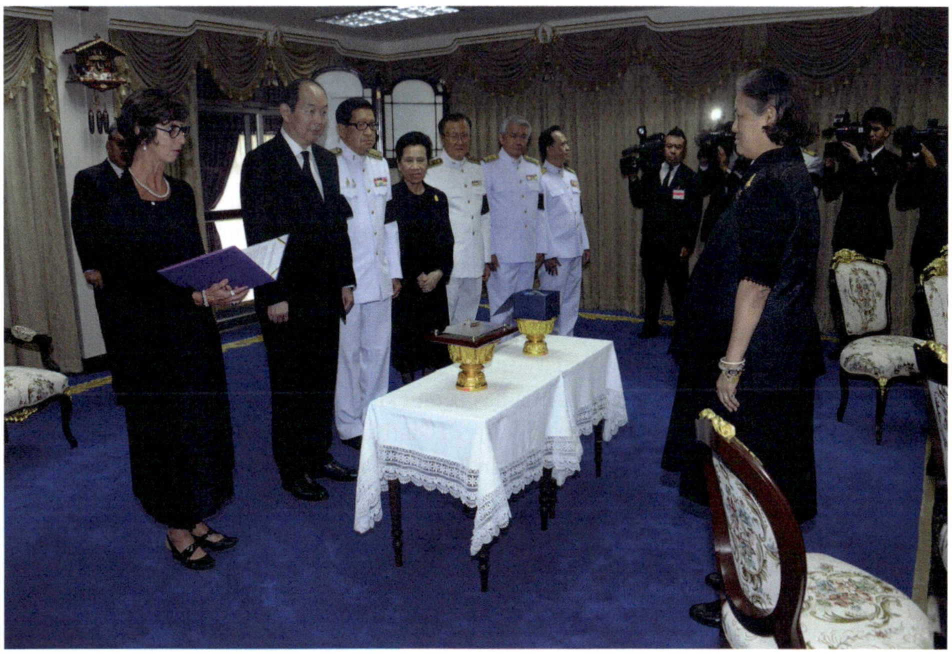

**Fig. 31.2** Prof. Adeera Levin (far left) and Prof. Masaomi Nangaku, President and Executive Council member of the International Society of Nephrology, presented the ISN Award to Her Royal Highness Princess Maha Chakri Sirindhorn at Chitralada Palace, Bangkok, on December 27, 2016. (The photo was graciously provided by Her Royal Highness Princess Maha Chakri Sirindhorn's Personal Affairs Division, Bureau of the Royal Household, the Royal Thai Government)

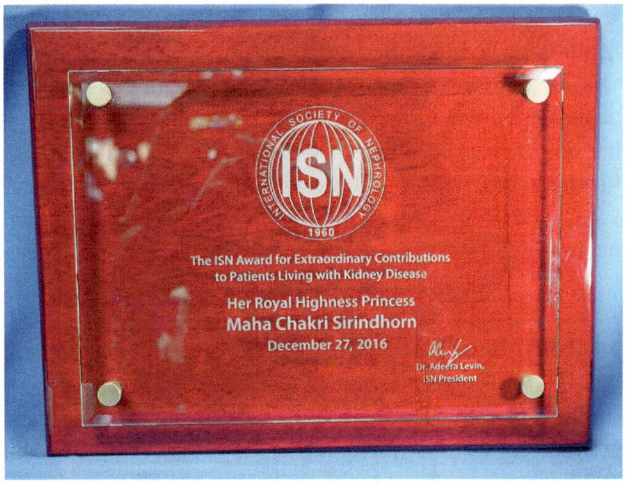


Fig. 31.3 The ISN Award for extraordinary contributions to patients living with kidney disease. (The photo was graciously provided by Her Royal Highness Princess Maha Chakri Sirindhorn's Personal Affairs Division, Bureau of the Royal Household, the Royal Thai Government)

Several major events have occurred since the establishment of modern nephrology in Thailand, more than half a century ago. The most important impact is the expanded government support for RRT under UCS in 2008 [13]. In the past, only patients who could afford dialysis, would receive treatment and survive. After establishment of PD 1st policy and UCS reimbursement program, each Thai have chance to access RRT without financial barrier [37]. Since then, the prevalence of RRT has increased almost threefold, and the penetration of PD almost sixfold within 7 years [10].

Hypokalemia is an electrolyte disorder that occurs in various diseases commonly observed in the northeastern of Thailand. These include sporadic form of hypokalemic periodic muscle paralysis [38], thyrotoxic periodic paralysis, distal renal tubular acidosis [39], hypokaliuric hypocitraturic nephrolithiasis [40], and sudden unexplained death syndrome [41]. Mutation of anion exchanger-1 gene was detected in patients with endemic distal renal tubular acidosis [42] and that of cardiac sodium channel gene (SCN5A) in those with sudden unexplained nocturnal death syndrome [42, 43]. However, causes of the other clinical entities have remained unclear. It is likely that dietary potassium deficiency among northeastern Thais might have played a significant role in these diseases [44].

Acute kidney injury (AKI) secondary to certain tropical diseases such as malaria and leptospirosis has been existing for decades and poses high mortality [45, 46]. Recently, the THAI-LEPTO score has been developed and validated in patients with acute leptospirosis [47]. This score is a simple and cheap point-of-care test for diagnosing acute severe leptospirosis. It would be useful and convenient for early detection of the infection in a resource-limited setting. Moreover, a multicenter network studying AKI in ICUs was set up in Thailand. More than 5000 cases with AKI have been enrolled from 17 centers across the country [7]. Half of the cases developed AKI and about one-third were categorized as severe. With this platform, it will be possible to identify risk factors of AKI, develop prognostic scoring model, or create algorithm for early intervention and timely treatment of leptospirosis and its complication.

An exponential rise in the number of patients with RRT after pronouncement of the PD-first policy mandates a huge demand for cheap rHuEpo. As for Thailand, biocopies of rHuEpo have been available since 1997. In the past, these products were approved and licensed through the generic small molecule chemical drug pathway. Therefore, there has been ever more than 20 biocopies product in Thai marget. rHuEpo is known to be associated with immunogenicity. The most serious event is pure red cell aplasia (PRCA) [48]. In Caucasian population, the rate of PRCA for alpha rHuEpo was 35.8 per 100,000 patient-year [49]. A study in Thailand showed that biocopies of rHuEpo could induce PRCA with an estimated risk of one out of 2608 patients [50]. Quality assessment of rHuEpo products biocopies in Thailand revealed that most of the biocopies tested were contaminated with high levels of protein aggregates, dimeric or trimeric forms of proteins, endotoxin, or host cell (rodent) proteins [51]. Besides heterogeneity in manufacturing processes of biologics, standard of cold-chain storage and logistics, routes of drug administration, or contamination with aggregates or foreign proteins as described, genetic susceptibility to immunogenicity of the biologics could have contributed to high incidence of PRCA in Thailand. Patients having human leukocyte antigen (HLA)-DRB1*09 are more likely to develop anti-rHuEpo-associated PRCA [52]. This HLA allele is more common in Asian population but rare in Caucasians. These findings raise concerns about the quality of manufacturing processes and safety of biocopied rHuEpo products available in Thailand. Currently, there has been much improvement in regulation of biological drug licensing which complies with the Western standard.

The number of patients with pre-dialysis CKD is also alarmingly high. More than 3 million Thais are having CKD stages 3–5 [8]. To tackle this problem, the Ministry of Public Health (MOPH), thanks to a unique primary healthcare structure of Thailand, has utilized a community-based approach to manage patients with DM, HT, and early CKD. A district hospital is the smallest unit of healthcare service where a multidisciplinary care team exists. At the village level, there is a sub-district health office, consisting of community nurses and public health officers, and VHVs who are responsible for primary healthcare of the villagers (10–12 households in the village per VHV). All over the country, there are nearly 10,000 sub-district health officers and more than 700,000 VHVs. To prove a concept whether these primary healthcare workers could be utilized to manage patients with CKD, a pilot controlled trial was conducted in two rural districts [53]. Patients with CKD stages 3 and 4 in one district were managed with the conventional way of practice, whereas those in the other district were managed by a multidisciplinary care team at a district hospital in combination with home visit by community nurses and VHVs. Educational materials, program training, and practice guideline checklist were provided to the healthcare team of the intervention group. At the end of a 2-year follow-up, patients with CKD in the intervention group had lower dietary salt and protein intake and lower rate of eGFR decline than the control group. This could be implied that community health workers led by general practitioners can be helpful in delaying CKD progression. With these promising results, CKD was pronounced as a goal in the National Health Strategic plan for the next two decades. Provincial and district hospitals nationwide are required to report to the MOPH certain key performance indicators related with CKD control. These include the percentage of patients with DM or HT being screened for CKD; the percentage of patients with DM or HT having adequate glycemic or blood pressure control, respectively; and the percentage of patients with CKD who receive angiotensin-converting enzyme inhibitors or angiotensin receptor blockades. Public hospitals also have to report the percentage of those who had rate of glomerular filtration rate decline less than −4 mL/min/year.

In conclusion, during the last half-century or more, nephrology in Thailand has been transformed from communicable disease-oriented to noncommunicable disease-oriented platform. Through unrelenting collaboration among all healthcare workers and public sectors involved, it is promising that, in the future, Thailand would be one of developing countries which succeeds in combating the problem of CKD progression and its complication.

## Future Perspective of Nephrology in Thailand

How to provide a more efficient CKD prevention is the core issue of the future perspective of nephrology in Thailand. The more efficient CKD prevention starts from an effective CKD screening program for population at risk of CKD, especially the Thai population [54]. From national data, there was an increasing trend of aging (over 60 years old) population in Thailand. Moreover, life expectancy was showed to be higher than in the past. It should be implied that there was a trend toward greater aging population in the future that would lead to more incidence of chronic illness. Apart from decision to suspend life with RRT, how to offer conservative or palliative care as an option for the aged ESRD population and should be systematically explored. The consensus for this issue should not depend only on financial burden but also consider the balance between the benefit of RRT and the suffering of the elderly population.

How to effectively delay CKD progression is another important future perspective. Currently, it can be fair to state that global nephrology progressively accumulates medical knowledge of how to delay CKD progression, and it is unquestionable that the ongoing basic research and clinical studies in nephrology will provide new novel or breakthrough treatment to delay CKD progression in the future. However, it is also a question of how to effectively implement the already known knowledge and current standard of care to delay CKD progression to cover most of the Thai patients. The strategy should not aim solely to prescribe more medications but should also focus on how to enhance CKD patients' health literacy. Health literacy is the degree to which individuals have the capacity to obtain, process, and understand basic health information and services needed to make appropriate health decisions [55]. In order to improve health literacy, there are a wide range of skills to be use included communication skill, critical analysis, numeracy skill and interaction skills. Apart from individual skills, other factors such as, culture, accessibility to technology and finacial status could also determine health literacy. The disruption of informative technology, health information, mobile application, wearable medical devices, and telemedicine will unquestionably facilitate health literacy to achieve better kidney health of Thai population in the future.

Besides KT, home dialysis should be an option for every ESRD patient. Home dialysis includes home HD and PD [56]. Although PD has already been established in Thailand, home HD has not yet been set up. Currently, in Thailand, home HD needs more user-friendly HD machine and home-based water treatment, price lowering strategy, and patient training for self-cannulation and self-HD machine operation. The combination of PD and home HD can be a more efficient dialysis option to preserve residual renal function, to maintain adequate middle-molecule uremic toxin clearance, and at the same time to preserve the peritoneal membrane to avoid future PD technical failure.

## Conclusion

Thailand is an endemic area of several tropical illnesses. Although tropical diseases and infectious-related disorders were formerly impacted, they have been gradually overshadowed by noncommunicable disease. The prevalence of pre-dialysis CKD in Thailand was greater than the global prevalence and became a current issue. This could be linked to the upward trend of dialysis patients and centers, which resulted in catastrophic national health expenditure. With the attempt to overcome this burden, the Thai government released several campaigns and issued policies to slow down CKD progression. The model of CKD clinic is a multidisciplinary approach, which has been implemented in all levels of public hospitals, in order to improve health promotion and increase access of healthcare even in remote areas. The introduction of new reimbursement program; UCS and the PD 1st policy, which mainly apply for majority of Thai population, are laudable initiatives and a bold attempt to approximate the gap between wealth and poor in access to health services. In order to avoid financial burden, any project aiming to decelerate CKD progression or providing economical RRT with comparable outcomes to international standard is set as priority.

## References

1. Benyajati C, Keoplug M, Beisel WR, Gangarosa EJ, Sprinz H, Sitprija V. Acute renal failure in Asiatic cholera: clinicopathologic correlations with acute tubular necrosis and hypokalemic nephropathy. Ann Intern Med. 1960;52:960–75.
2. Sitprija V, Indraprasit S, Pochanugool C, Benyajati C, Piyaratn P. Renal function in malaria. J Trop Med Hyg. 1966;69(10):242–6.
3. Sitprija V. Renal failure in tropical disease. J Med Assoc Thail. 1973;56(11):631–3.
4. Barsoum R, Fayad T, Praditpornsilpa K, Sitprija V. Chapter 63: tropical nephrology. In: Barsoum RS, Fayad T, Praditpornsilpa K, Sitprija V, editors. Schrier's diseases of the kidney. 9th ed. Philadelphia: Lippincott Williams & Wilkins; 2012. p. 2912.
5. Dhanakijcharoen P, Sirivongs D, Aruyapitipan S, Chuengsaman P, Lumpaopong A. The "PD first" policy in Thailand: three-years experiences (2008–2011). J Med Assoc Thail. 2011;94(Suppl 4):S153–61.
6. Benyajati C, Pochanugool C, Sitprija V, Suvannapha R, Bunyaratavej P, Satitpunwaycha P, et al. Early experience in renal transplantation in Thailand. J Med Assoc Thail. 1973;56(7):398–403.
7. Srisawat N, Kulvichit W, Mahamitra N, Hurst C, Praditpornsilpa K, Lumlertgul N, et al. The epidemiology and characteristics of acute kidney injury in the Southeast Asia intensive care unit: a prospective multicentre study. Nephrology Dialysis Transplantation 2020:35(10):1729–38.
8. Ingsathit A, Thakkinstian A, Chaiprasert A, Sangthawan P, Gojaseni P, Kiattisunthorn K, et al. Prevalence and risk factors of chronic kidney disease in the Thai adult population: Thai SEEK study. Nephrol Dial Transplant. 2010;25(5):1567–75.
9. Buranakitjaroen P, Phoojaroenchanachai M. The prevalence of high sodium intake among hypertensive patients at hypertension clinic, Siriraj Hospital. J Med Assoc Thail. 2013;96(Suppl 2):S1–8.
10. Thailand Renal Replacement Therapy Registry 2015 Report: The Nephrology Society of Thailand; [cited 2019 May 28]. Available from: http://www.nephrothai.org/images/Final_TRT_report_2015.
11. Taptagaporn S, Mongkonsomlit S, Kaewdok T, Wattanasoei S, Rakkapao N. Evaluation and lesson distilled on implementation of chronic kidney disease clinic, under policy of Ministry of Public Health. Nonthaburi: Health systems research institute; 2017. 187 p.
12. Treerutkuarkul A. Thailand: health care for all, at a price. Bull World Health Organ. 2010;88(2):84–5.
13. Tangcharoensathien V, Pitayarangsarit S, Patcharanarumol W, Prakongsai P, Sumalee H, Tosanguan J, et al. Promoting universal financial protection: how the Thai universal coverage scheme was designed to ensure equity. Health Res Pol Syst. 2013;11:25.
14. Teerawattananon Y, Mugford M, Tangcharoensathien V. Economic evaluation of palliative management versus peritoneal dialysis and hemodialysis for end-stage renal disease: evidence for coverage decisions in Thailand. Value Health. 2007;10(1):61–72.
15. Tantivess S, Werayingyong P, Chuengsaman P, Teerawattananon Y. Universal coverage of renal dialysis in Thailand: promise, progress, and prospects. BMJ. 2013;346:f462.
16. Chiu YW, Jiwakanon S, Lukowsky L, Duong U, Kalantar-Zadeh K, Mehrotra R. An update on the comparisons of mortality outcomes of hemodialysis and peritoneal dialysis patients. Semin Nephrol. 2011;31(2):152–8.
17. Liem YS, Bosch JL, Arends LR, Heijenbrok-Kal MH, Hunink MG. Quality of life assessed with the Medical Outcomes Study Short Form 36-Item Health Survey of patients on renal replacement therapy: a systematic review and meta-analysis. Value Health. 2007;10(5):390–7.
18. Mehrotra R, Chiu YW, Kalantar-Zadeh K, Bargman J, Vonesh E. Similar outcomes with hemodialysis and peritoneal dialysis in patients with end-stage renal disease. Arch Intern Med. 2011;171(2):110–8.
19. Srisawat N, Sintawichai N, Kulvichit W, Lumlertgul N, Sitticharoenchai P, Thamrongsat N, et al. Current practice of diagnosis and management of acute kidney injury in intensive care unit in resource limited settings. J Crit Care. 2018;46:44–9.
20. Srisawat N, Lawsin L, Uchino S, Bellomo R, Kellum JA, Investigators BK. Cost of acute renal replacement therapy in the intensive care unit: results from the beginning and ending supportive therapy for the kidney (BEST kidney) study. Crit Care. 2010;14(2):R46.
21. Vijayan A, Palevsky PM. Dosing of renal replacement therapy in acute kidney injury. Am J Kidney Dis. 2012;59(4):569–76.
22. Tattersall JE, Ward RA, group E. Online haemodiafiltration: definition, dose quantification and safety revisited. Nephrol Dial Transplant. 2013;28(3):542–50.
23. Tiranathanagul K, Yossundharakul C, Techawathanawanna N, Katavetin P, Hanvivatvong O, Praditpornsilp K, et al. Comparison of middle-molecule clearance between convective control double high-flux hemodiafiltration and on-line hemodiafiltration. Int J Artif Organs. 2007;30(12):1090–7.
24. Maduell F, Moreso F, Pons M, Ramos R, Mora-Macia J, Carreras J, et al. High-efficiency postdilution online hemodiafiltration reduces all-cause mortality in hemodialysis patients. J Am Soc Nephrol. 2013;24(3):487–97.
25. Tiranathanagul K, Susantitaphong P, Srisawat N, Mahatanan N, Tungsanga K, Praditpornsilpa K, et al. Ten-year survival of end-stage renal disease patients treated with high-efficiency online hemodiafiltration: a Cohort Study of a Center in South East Asia. Nephron. 2018;139(2):150–8.
26. Susantitaphong P, Tiranathanagul K, Hanvivatvong O, Homsin U, Wittayalertpanya S, Khemsri W, et al. A simple efficient technique of 'mid-dilution' on-line hemodiafiltration. Blood Purif. 2009;28(2):93–101.
27. Susantitaphong P, Tiranathanagul K, Katavetin P, Hanwiwatwong O, Wittayalertpanya S, Praditpornsilpa K, et al. Efficacy comparison between simple mixed-dilution and simple mid-dilution on-line hemodiafiltration techniques: a crossover study. Artif Organs. 2012;36(12):1059–65.
28. Tiranathanagul K, Tunpornchai J, Srisawat N, Susantitaphong P, Paditpornsilpa K, Eiam-Ong S. Enhancing cytokine clearances with sustained low-efficiency diafiltration (SLED-f) using high cut-off dialyzer in septic AKI patients: a randomized trial. J Med Assoc Thail. 2019;102(4):423–31.
29. Sakthong P, Kasemsup V. Health utility measured with EQ-5D in Thai patients undergoing peritoneal dialysis. Value Health. 2012;15(1 Suppl):S79–84.
30. Chuengsaman P, Kasemsup V. PD first policy: Thailand's response to the challenge of meeting the needs of patients with end-stage renal disease. Semin Nephrol. 2017;37(3):287–95.
31. Liu FX, Gao X, Inglese G, Chuengsaman P, Pecoits-Filho R, Yu A. A global overview of the impact of peritoneal dialysis first or favored policies: an opinion. Perit Dial Int. 2015;35(4):406–20.
32. Changsirikulchai S, Sriprach S, Thokanit NS, Janma J, Chuengsaman P, Sirivongs D. Survival analysis and associated fac-

tors in Thai patients on peritoneal dialysis under the PD-first policy. Perit Dial Int. 2018;38(3):172–8.
33. Avihingsanon Y, Townamchai N, Nivatvongs S, Ratchanon S, Praditpornsilpa K, Tiranathanagul K, et al. Living-donor kidney transplantation across ABO barriers: The first case in Thailand. Asian Biomed. 2010;3:525–9.
34. Kowitt SD, Emmerling D, Fisher EB, Tanasugarn C. Community health workers as agents of health promotion: analyzing Thailand's village health volunteer program. J Community Health. 2015;40(4):780–8.
35. Morad Z, Choong HL, Tungsanga K. Suhardjono. Funding renal replacement therapy in southeast Asia: building public-private partnerships in Singapore, Malaysia, Thailand, and Indonesia. Am J Kidney Dis. 2015;65(5):799–805.
36. ISN. CKD awareness in Thailand gets royal seal of approval 2017. Available from: https://www.theisn.org/component/k2/itemlist/user/83-addralevin.
37. Praditpornsilpa K, Lekhyananda S, Premasathian N, Kingwatanakul P, Lumpaopong A, Gojaseni P, et al. Prevalence trend of renal replacement therapy in Thailand: impact of health economics policy. J Med Assoc Thail. 2011;94(Suppl 4):S1–6.
38. Phakdeekitcharoen B, Ruangraksa C, Radinahamed P. Hypokalaemia and paralysis in the Thai population. Nephrol Dial Transplant. 2004;19(8):2013–8.
39. Nilwarangkur S, Nimmannit S, Chaovakul V, Susaengrat W, Ong-aj-Yooth S, Vasuvattakul S, et al. Endemic primary distal renal tubular acidosis in Thailand. Q J Med. 1990;74(275):289–301.
40. Tungsanga K, Tosukhowong P, Sriboonlue P, Sridama V, Prasongwatana V, Sitprija V. Hypokaliuric—hypocitraturic nephrolithiasis: a unique clinical entity of Northeast Thailand. In: Ryall R, Bais R, Marshall VR, Rofe AM, Smith LH, Walker VR, editors. Urolithiasis 2. Boston: Springer; 1994.
41. Tosukhowong P, Chotigasatit C, Tungsanga K, Sriboonlue P, Pansin P, Sitprija V. Hypokalemia, high erythrocyte Na+ and low erythrocyte Na,K-ATPase in relatives of patients dying from sudden unexplained death syndrome in north-east Thailand and in survivors from near-fatal attacks. Am J Nephrol. 1996;16(5):369–74.
42. Sritippayawan S, Sumboonnanonda A, Vasuvattakul S, Keskanokwong T, Sawasdee N, Paemanee A, et al. Novel compound heterozygous SLC4A1 mutations in Thai patients with autosomal recessive distal renal tubular acidosis. Am J Kidney Dis. 2004;44(1):64–70.
43. Pittiwararom R, Vongpaisarnsin K, Hoonwijit U. SCN5A gene exome sequencing profile in sudden unexplained nocturnal death syndrome in Thai population. Chula Med J. 2019;63:111–8.
44. Sriboonlue P, Prasongwatana V, Suwantrai S, Bovornpadungkitti S, Tungsanga K, Tosukhowong P. Nutritional potassium status of healthy adult males residing in the rural northeast Thailand. J Med Assoc Thail. 1998;81(3):223–32.
45. Sitprija V. Nephropathy in falciparum malaria. Kidney Int. 1988;34(6):867–77.
46. Sitprija V, Pipatanagul V, Mertowidjojo K, Boonpucknavig V, Boonpucknavig S. Pathogenesis of renal disease in leptospirosis: clinical and experimental studies. Kidney Int. 1980;17(6):827–36.
47. Sukmark T, Lumlertgul N, Peerapornratana S, Khositrangsikun K, Tungsanga K, Sitprija V, et al. Thai-Lepto-on-admission probability (THAI-LEPTO) score as an early tool for initial diagnosis of leptospirosis: result from Thai-Lepto AKI study group. PLoS Negl Trop Dis. 2018;12(3):e0006319.
48. Bennett CL, Luminari S, Nissenson AR, Tallman MS, Klinge SA, McWilliams N, et al. Pure red-cell aplasia and epoetin therapy. N Engl J Med. 2004;351(14):1403–8.
49. Macdougall IC, Casadevall N, Locatelli F, Combe C, London GM, Di Paolo S, et al. Incidence of erythropoietin antibody-mediated pure red cell aplasia: the prospective immunogenicity surveillance registry (PRIMS). Nephrol Dial Transplant. 2015;30(3):451–60.
50. Praditpornsilpa K, Tiranathanagul K, Kupatawintu P, Jootar S, Intragumtornchai T, Tungsanga K, et al. Biosimilar recombinant human erythropoietin induces the production of neutralizing antibodies. Kidney Int. 2011;80(1):88–92.
51. Halim LA, Brinks V, Jiskoot W, Romeijn S, Praditpornsilpa K, Assawamakin A, et al. How bio-questionable are the different recombinant human erythropoietin copy products in Thailand? Pharm Res. 2014;31(5):1210–8.
52. Praditpornsilpa K, Kupatawintu P, Mongkonsritagoon W, Supasyndh O, Jootar S, Intarakumthornchai T, et al. The association of anti-r-HuEpo-associated pure red cell aplasia with HLA-DRB1*09-DQB1*0309. Nephrol Dial Transplant. 2009;24(5):1545–9.
53. Jiamjariyapon T, Ingsathit A, Pongpirul K, Vipattawat K, Kanchanakorn S, Saetie A, et al. Effectiveness of integrated care on delaying progression of stage 3–4 chronic kidney disease in rural communities of Thailand (ESCORT study): a cluster randomized controlled trial. BMC Nephrol. 2017;18(1):83.
54. Beard JR, Officer A, de Carvalho IA, Sadana R, Pot AM, Michel JP, et al. The world report on ageing and health: a policy framework for healthy ageing. Lancet. 2016;387(10033):2145–54.
55. Taylor DM, Fraser S, Dudley C, Oniscu GC, Tomson C, Ravanan R, et al. Health literacy and patient outcomes in chronic kidney disease: a systematic review. Nephrol Dial Transplant. 2018;33(9):1545–58.
56. Morton RL, Snelling P, Webster AC, Rose J, Masterson R, Johnson DW, et al. Dialysis modality preference of patients with CKD and family caregivers: a discrete-choice study. Am J Kidney Dis. 2012;60(1):102–11.

# Nephrology in Turkey

# 32

Tevfik Ecder, Mustafa Arıcı, Kenan Ateş,
Oğuz Söylemezoğlu, Gültekin Süleymanlar,
and Aydın Türkmen

| | |
|---|---|
| Area[1] | 783,562 Km$^2$ |
| Population[1] | 82.9 million (2019) |
| Capital | Ankara |
| Three most populated cities | 1. Istanbul<br>2. Ankara<br>3. Izmir |
| Official language | Turkish |
| Gross domestic product (GDP)[2] | 852.7 billion USD (2017)<br>771.4 billion USD (2018) |
| GDP per capita[3] | 10,513.65 USD (2017)<br>9370.18 USD (2018) |
| Human Development Index (HDI)[4] | 0.806 (59th position, 2019) |
| Official currency | Turkish Lira |
| Total number of nephrologists[5] | 800 |
| National society of nephrology | Turkish Society of Nephrology<br>www.nefroloji.org.tr |
| Incidence of end-stage renal Disease[6] | 2018 – 149 pmp |
| Prevalence of end-stage renal Disease[6] | 2018 – 988 pmp |
| Total number of patients in dialysis (all modalities)[6] | 2017 – 61,981<br>2018 – 63,835 |
| Number of patients on hemodialysis[6] | 2017 – 58,635<br>2018 – 60,643 |
| Number of patients on peritoneal dialysis[6] | 2017 – 3346<br>2018 – 3192 |
| Number of renal transplants per year[6] | 2017. – 15,330<br>2018 – 17,220 |

1. Turkish Statistical Institute. Accessed in January 2020. Available in: www.turkstat.gov.tr
2. The World Bank. Accessed in January 2020. Available in: https://data.worldbank.org/country/turkey?view=chart
3. The World Bank. Accessed in January 2020. Available in: https://data.worldbank.org/indicator/NY.GDP.PCAP.CD?locations=TR
4. United Nations Development Programme. Human Development Reports. Access in January 2020. Available in: http://hdr.undp.org/en/countries/profiles/TUR
5. Turkish Society of Nephrology. Accessed in January 2020. Available in: www.nefroloji.org.tr
6. Süleymanlar G, Ateş K, Seyahi N. Registry of the Nephrology, Dialysis and Transplantation in Turkey. Registry 2018. Ministry of Health and Turkish Society of Nephrology Joint Report. Published by the Turkish Society of Nephrology. Ankara, 2019

## Introduction

The Republic of Turkey was founded in 1923 by Mustafa Kemal Atatürk after the collapse of the Ottoman Empire. Turkey occupies a unique geographic position, lying partly in Asia and partly in Europe. Throughout its history it has acted as a bridge between the two continents. The capital is Ankara, and its largest city and seaport is Istanbul. Table 32.1 summarizes the demographic characteristics of Turkey [1].

The political system in Turkey is a democratic parliamentary republic system, which is based on social justice and the rule of law in a secular constitution, allowing multiple politi-

T. Ecder (✉)
Demiroglu Bilim University Faculty of Medicine, Department of Internal Medicine, Division of Nephrology, Istanbul, Turkey
e-mail: tevfik.ecder@demiroglu.bilim.edu.tr

M. Arıcı
Hacettepe University Faculty of Medicine, Department of Nephrology, Ankara, Turkey
e-mail: marici@hacettepe.edu.tr

K. Ateş
Ankara University Faculty of Medicine, Department of Nephrology, Ankara, Turkey
e-mail: Kenan.Ates@medicine.ankara.edu.tr

O. Söylemezoğlu
Gazi University Faculty of Medicine, Department of Pediatric Nephrology, Ankara, Turkey

G. Süleymanlar
Akdeniz University Faculty of Medicine, Department of Nephrology, Antalya, Turkey

A. Türkmen
Istanbul University Faculty of Medicine, Department of Internal Medicine, Division of Nephrology, Istanbul, Turkey



J. A. Moura-Neto et al. (eds.), *Nephrology Worldwide*, https://doi.org/10.1007/978-3-030-56890-0_32

**Table 32.1** Demographic characteristics of Turkey

| | |
|---|---|
| Population | 82.9 million |
| Urban population | 72.2% |
| Population growth rate | 1.28% |
| Male/female | 49.31%/50.69% |
| Median age | 30.2 years |
| Life expectancy | 76.4 years (Males: 73.3 years, Females: 79.4 years) |

cal parties. Turkey is classified among the upper middle-income countries.

Chronic kidney disease (CKD) is a growing health problem worldwide that may lead to end-stage renal disease (ESRD) and cardiovascular complications [2, 3]. Despite improvements in patient care, CKD is still associated with high morbidity and mortality. According to the Chronic Renal Disease in Turkey (CREDIT) study, the prevalence of CKD in Turkey is 15.7% [4]. Moreover, this study showed that patients with CKD have high rates of cardiovascular risk factors with a high risk of morbidity and mortality.

The ESRD incidence and prevalence have been increasing gradually in Turkey during the last decades, as in many other countries; and the need for renal replacement therapy (RRT) has been met with an increasing number of dialysis centers and renal transplantations [5, 6].

## Brief History of Nephrology in Turkey

The first independent and registered department of nephrology was founded in Istanbul Medical Faculty by Dr. Kemal Onen in 1965, who 5 years later also founded the Turkish Society of Nephrology (TSN) [7].

Regular hemodialysis (HD) was first introduced in Turkey around 1965. The first successful renal transplantation in Turkey was performed from a living-related donor by Dr. Mehmet Haberal at the Hacettepe University Hospital in 1975. The same team carried out renal transplantation in 1978 from a deceased donor [8]. At present, renal transplantation is performed mainly in 75 centers by specialized transplantation surgeons. Regular HD is performed in 882 centers nationwide, and in the dialysis units, there is availability for almost anyone who needs dialysis [5].

TSN, as the major nongovernmental organization of nephrologists, is actively making a national ESRD care registry. TSN also prepares local, regional, and national continuous medical education activities, winter schools, or annual congresses for postgraduate education of nephrologists in Turkey. TSN is also organizing "nephrology board examinations" for Turkish nephrologists since 2008. Currently, TSN has 590 active members and also 7 branches with their own separate memberships in Istanbul, Izmir, Kayseri, Antalya, Bursa, Adana, and Ankara. Turkish Journal of Nephrology is a double-blind peer reviewed, open access, international online-only publication of the TSN. The journal is a quarterly publication, published on January, April, July, and October. The publication language of the journal is English.

## Renal Diseases in Turkey

### Chronic Kidney Disease

CKD is a growing public health problem that may lead to ESRD. It is also associated with an increased risk of cardiovascular complications. A Turkish population-based, national survey on the populations aged over 18 years, the so-called Chronic Renal Disease in Turkey (CREDIT) study was performed to determine the prevalence of CKD and to evaluate relationships between CKD and cardiovascular risk factors [4]. A cluster sampling technique was used to select the study participants. A sampling frame was defined as the 7 geographical regions of Turkey that included 81 cities. The study sample was comprised of 23 cities.

A total of 10,872 participants were included in the study. A low glomerular filtration rate (GFR) (<60 mL/min/1.73 m$^2$) was present in 5.2% of the subjects who were evaluated for GFR, while microalbuminuria and macroalbuminuria were observed in 10.2% and 2.0% of the subjects, respectively. The prevalence of CKD was estimated as 15.7% in the Turkish adult population. The prevalence rates for CKD stages 1, 2, 3, 4, and 5 were 5.4%, 5.2%, 4.7%, 0.3%, and 0.2%, respectively. The majority of the subjects with CKD were in stages 1–3. CKD was significantly more common among women than men (18.4% vs. 12.8%, $p < 0.001$). The prevalence of CKD also increased with increasing age of the subjects. The odds ratios of CKD ranged from 1.45 to 2.18 for every 10 years increase in age for subjects over 30 years. The prevalence of CKD was found to be 11.5% in the population aged <60 years, while it was as high as 38.3% in subjects aged 60 years or over. Stage 3 CKD was especially more common among subjects aged over 60 years (1.6% vs. 21.5%). CKD prevalence was slightly higher among subjects living in rural areas than in those in urban areas (16.8% vs. 15.2%). CKD prevalence was highest among subjects from the Marmara region (19.7%) followed by Southeastern Anatolia (18.6%), the Black Sea (16.1%), East Anatolia (14.2%), the Aegean (13.8%), Central Anatolia (12.6%), and the Mediterranean (11.7%) regions.

In the general population, the prevalence rates for hypertension, diabetes, dyslipidemia, obesity, and metabolic syndrome were 32.7%, 12.7%, 77.0%, 20.1%, and 32.3%, respectively. The prevalence of hypertension was higher in subjects with CKD than in those without CKD (56.3% and 31.0%). Similarly, the prevalence rates of diabetes (26.6% vs. 10.1%), dyslipidemia (83.4% vs. 75.8%), obesity (29.2% vs. 20.0%), and metabolic syndrome (46.0% vs. 29.8%) were significantly higher in subjects with CKD compared to subjects without CKD. Furthermore, the prevalence of these cardiovascular risk factors gradually increased in subjects having advanced stages of the disease. Thus, CKD was found to be strongly associated with these cardiovascular risk factors.

The prevalence of decreased GFR and microalbuminuria was higher in subjects having these risk factors, particularly in those having hypertension and diabetes. The prevalence of CKD among subjects with and without hypertension was 25.3% and 10.6%, respectively. Similarly, CKD was significantly more common in subjects with diabetes than in nondiabetic subjects (32.4% vs. 13.0%).

In conclusion, the CREDIT study has defined that CKD prevalence in Turkey is higher than in those of many industrialized Western countries. Associations between CKD and several cardiovascular risk factors emphasize that CKD is a major public health problem and a major predictor of overall morbidity and mortality.

A striking increase in prevalence of ESRD requiring RRT has been observed over the past 18 years (Fig. 32.1). The most common RRT modality is HD followed by kidney transplant (KT) and peritoneal dialysis (PD), respectively. Rates of diabetes mellitus and hypertension as causes of ESRD increased, whereas those of chronic glomerulonephritis and urologic disease decreased.

## Acute Kidney Injury

There is neither a national registry nor large cohort studies about acute kidney injury (AKI) in Turkey. However, its incidence and causes seem to be similar to those of high-income countries.

The nephrology community in Turkey was very successful in the management of patients with AKI due to crush syndrome after the Marmara earthquake, which hit the most densely populated area at the eastern end of the Marmara Sea in northwestern Turkey on August 17, 1999. The number of documented cases of AKI following this event exceeded all similar cases previously reported for any single earthquake [9]. A total of 639 patients (291 female and 348 male) with AKI due to crush syndrome were hospitalized in 35 hospitals [10]. Among these, 477 patients needed dialysis, and a total of 5137 HD sessions were performed to these patients. The mortality rates were 17.2 and 9.3% in dialyzed and nondialyzed patients, respectively. Findings significantly associated with mortality were sepsis, thrombocytopenia, disseminated intravascular coagulation, and acute respiratory distress syndrome, as well as abdominal and thoracic traumas.

## Renal Disease in Pediatric Population

The pediatric population aged 0–17 years is around 23 million and consists in 28.3% of the total population. Currently, there are 35 pediatric nephrology centers in Turkey, and all centers are based at the major pediatric teaching hospitals around the country, each providing comprehensive diagnos-

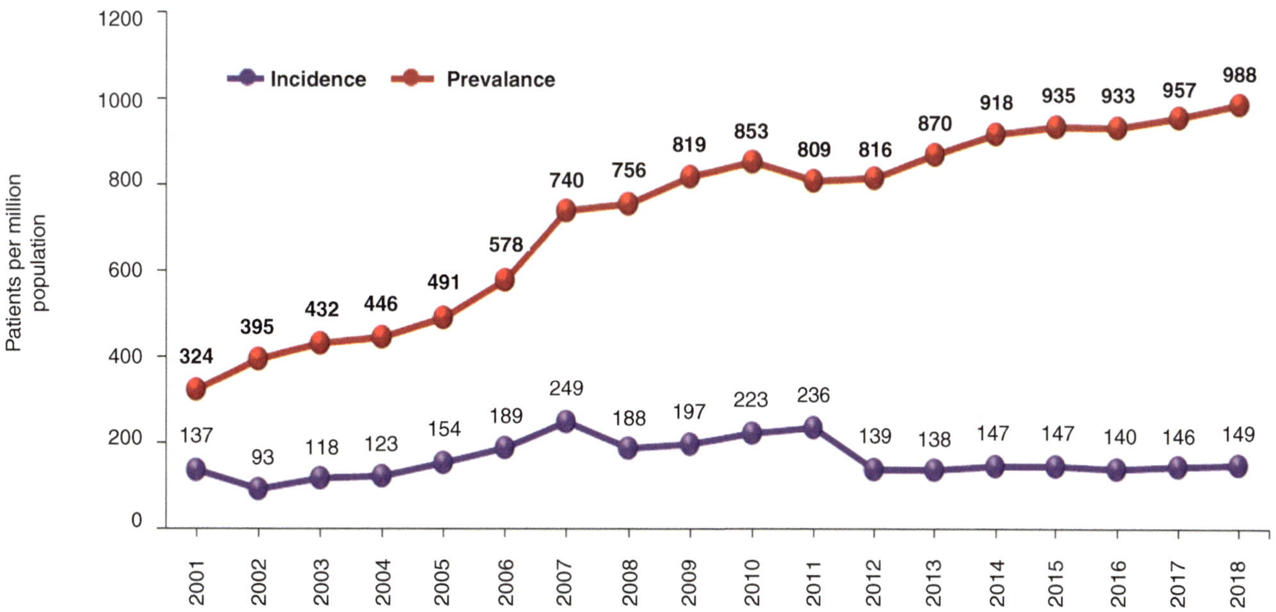


**Fig. 32.1** Incidence and prevalence of end-stage renal disease by years in Turkey

tic and therapeutic services for children with AKI and CKD, including acute and chronic dialysis. Sixteen of these centers also provide KT. Most centers have a team including 2–4 pediatric nephrologists.

The incidence rate of CKD is nearly of 10.9 (12.2 for boys and 9.7 for girls) pmp, considering the GFR levels below 75 ml/min/1.73 m$^2$ [6]. As for the underlying etiology of CKD, urological problems such as vesicoureteral reflux (18.5%), obstructive uropathy (10.7%), and neurogenic bladder (15.1%) are the leading underlying conditions causing CKD, with a total frequency of 44.3% [11]. The predominance of moderate to severe CKD (stage III–V) consists of 88% of the patients and reflects the late diagnosis and referral pattern. These diseases (urological conditions, tubule-interstitial diseases, hypoplasia, and dysplasia) are followed by cystic renal diseases and primary glomerulonephritis. There is also increasing recognition of familial and genetic forms of nephrotic syndrome causing renal failure, with the identification of podocin and other mutations in children in Turkey [12]. Postinfectious glomerulonephritis is still a problem in Turkey, but pediatric nephrology centers successfully manage the disease and prevent its progression. In a population-based CKD study, the frequencies of overweight and obese children were found to be 9.3 and 8.9%, and the mean eGFR was lower in patients with higher body mass [13].

Every year nearly 50–75 patients enter the PD program, which is delivered almost exclusively as continuous cycling PD (CCPD) using a number of platforms and utilized as the primary mode of dialysis in young children. Automated PD (APD) has been the modality of choice in recent years in most of the centers. One third of these patients have been under the age of 6. Growth retardation has been present in 73% of these patients, erythropoiesis-stimulating agent (ESA) usage around 69%, and peritonitis rate nearly 0.27 episode per patient year [5].

HD is the second preferred RRT for children and is mostly available in the larger centers. Chronic HD has been offered to older children or those deemed clinically unsuitable for PD. Only 10% of the HD patients are under the age of 5 years. In small children below the age of 3 years, vascular access is a major problem. Every year around 50 pediatric patients start HD treatment, and the growth retardation rate is present in 75% of these patients. Most of the HD patients present anemia and nearly 75% receive ESA treatment [5]. KT transplantation numbers are increasing in Turkey, and this also includes the pediatric population. In 2018, there were 331 pediatric transplantations, which consisted of 8% of all kidney transplants. Preemptive KT was performed in 24% of these patients. Transplantation was performed with kidneys from deceased donors in 35% of the patients, and this number is higher than in the adults. The immunosuppressive protocols include calcineurin inhibitors, mycophenolate mofetil, steroids, and induction therapy in mostly deceased donors KTs. The overall patient and graft survival is comparable with the Western countries [5]. One-year graft and survival are 94% and 97%, respectively.The total percentage of pediatric KT among all kidney transplant numbers is only 7.45%. There is a low transplantation rate especially under 5 years. The rate of transplantation in this group is 11% in Turkey and 23% in the USA. Pediatric transplantation should be increased in Turkey.

## Renal Replacement Therapy in Turkey

The incidence and prevalence of RRT for ESRD patients are increasing worldwide. Turkey, with a population of 83 million, has an ESRD prevalence of 988 per million of population (pmp) and incidence of 149 pmp as of 2018.

Turkey has one of the largest treated ESRD patient populations in Europe. A total of 81,055 patients with ESRD were being treated with one form of RRT by the end of 2018. The number of dialysis centers has grown to 882 with around 63,835 patients on chronic dialysis (60,643 regular HD patients and 3192 PD patients). KT is presently carried out in 75 centers all over the country.

Despite a stable trend in incidence in the last 18 years, there has been a threefold increase in prevalence. The number of KT centers increased to 75 from 24 over the last 16 years. A total of 28,210 KT have been performed over the last decade. The structural, legal, and economic arrangements have significantly increased the number of KT since 2008. However, the increase appears to be predominantly in living donor transplants. Mild decline in the relative rates of cadaveric renal transplants has been observed.

## Hemodialysis

HD is the most commonly used RRT in Turkey. A significant increase in the number of HD patients has been observed during the last two decades (Fig. 32.2). According to the 2018 TSN Annual Report, a total of 60,643 patients were having chronic HD treatment, comprising 74.8% of the ESRD population in Turkey. HD reimbursement in Turkey is significantly lower than in many other countries [14, 15]. The current reimbursement is 40 USD per session.

Although the convective therapies offer better patient outcomes in HD patients, the incidence of hemodiafiltration (HDF) is only 1.31% in Turkey [5, 16]. The major reason of this low rate is the low reimbursement paid for dialysis therapies. High-flux dialyzers were used in 46.3% of the prevalent HD patients as the end of 2018 [5]. The reuse of dialyzers is not performed at all in Turkey.

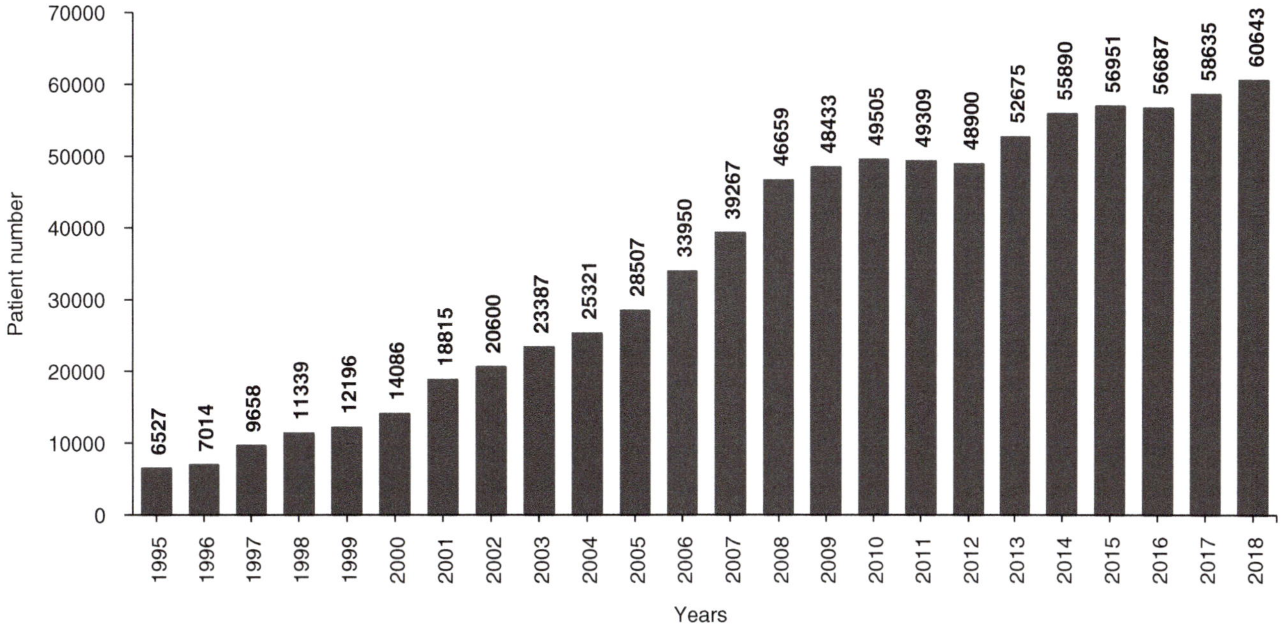


**Fig. 32.2** The number of hemodialysis patients by years in Turkey

The prevalence of patients with positive hepatitis serology decreased significantly during the last two decades. The prevalence of HD patients who are positive for hepatitis B is 2.6% and 3.5% for hepatitis C. The prevalence of patients who are positive for HIV is only 0.08%.

In 2013, the international Dialysis Outcomes and Practice Patterns Study (DOPPS), a prospective cohort study of HD practices, and outcomes of adult (18+ years of age) HD patients ongoing since 1996 initiated data collection of a nationally representative sample of 20 HD units in Turkey [17].

The characteristics of the Turkish patients included in the DOPPS study were compared with those of the patients in Europe, North America, and Japan. The patients in Turkey were younger (60.0 years) compared with patients in Europe (64.9 years), North America (61.7 years), and Japan (62.6 years). Body mass index was lower in patients in Turkey (25.3 kg/m$^2$) compared to patients in Europe (26.2 kg/m$^2$) and North America (28.5 kg/m$^2$). Median dialysis vintage was longer in Turkey (3.7 years) compared to Europe (3.4 years) and North America (2.7 years) but shorter than Japan (5.9 years).

According to the results of the DOPPS study in Turkey, diabetes was the most common ESRD cause (37%); arteriovenous fistula use was 83%; and mean single pool Kt/V was 1.61. Compared with other international regions, Turkey had the highest mean hemoglobin (11.5 g/dL), ferritin (771 ng/mL), and interdialytic weight gain (3.28%), while Turkey had the lowest mean systolic blood pressure (127 mmHg) and ESA prescription (57%). Turkish patients also reported the highest depression scores.

Although the dialysis population is becoming older in Turkey, it is still younger than the dialysis population of many Western countries and Japan. Diabetes is the most common cause of ESRD in Turkey and is substantially higher than that seen overall in European HD units in DOPPS. There is a continuous increase in the prevalence of diabetes in Turkey. According to the Turkish Epidemiology Survey of Diabetes, Hypertension, Obesity, and Endocrine Disease (TURDEP-II) study, the prevalence of diabetes in the adult general population is 16.5%, translating to 6.5 million adults with diabetes in Turkey [18]. These figures are alarming and underscore the urgent need for national programs to prevent diabetes and its complications.

Turkish HD patients have the highest prevalence of hypertension (32%) and lowest prevalence of glomerulonephritis (6%) as a primary cause of ESRD compared to other DOPPS regions. These figures may suggest that there is an overdiagnosis of primary hypertension among Turkish HD patients. It may be speculated that some patients with secondary hypertension due to glomerulonephritis who present at a late stage of their disease when a definite diagnosis with a kidney biopsy is not possible may have been diagnosed as primary hypertension.

## Peritoneal Dialysis

PD in Turkey was first applied in the late 1950s using PD solutions in bottles for patients with AKI. In 1968, these solutions were used in ESRD patients as intermittent PD treatment [19]. After the introduction of continuous ambulatory peritoneal dialysis (CAPD) by Moncrief and Popovich in 1976, this treatment was started to be applied as a chronic RRT modality from the mid-1980s in Turkey. However, the peritonitis rate was very high due to use of a non-disconnecting collapsible bag system with simple spike, and the technical survival was also very low.

At the beginning of the early 1990s when disconnecting delivery systems became available, the dropout declined and PD treatment became an effective RRT modality. In 1996, Eczacıbaşı-Baxter began to produce PD solutions in Turkey. In addition to CAPD treatment, APD was also introduced with imported machines (first PAC-Extra and then Home-choice) in 1997. These contributed to the rapid development of chronic PD. In 2000 icodextrin-based and amino acid-based PD solutions and in 2006 biocompatible PD solutions with neutral pH and low glucose degradation product were started to be used [20]. These novel PD solutions gave physicians the opportunity for individualization of PD prescription and also contributed to improving PD technique survival.

Interest in PD treatment increased after 1990, and the nephrology departments of many hospitals started to establish their own PD units. Also, some young nephrologists went to well-known international PD centers for training in PD. In 1998, the Turkish Multicenter Peritoneal Dialysis Study Group (TULIP) was established with the participation of 11 PD centers in different regions of Turkey [21]. The TULIP began to organize the regular training meetings in various regions of the country and initiated numerous multi-center scientific studies. This resulted in a substantial increase in the number of patients treated with PD and also provided new opportunities for multinational studies.

As shown in Fig. 32.3, throughout 1990–2000s the number of patients treated with PD in Turkey was continuously increasing and reached 6109 patients in 2008 [5]. During this period, the rate of PD penetration among dialysis patients increased from 4.4% to 11.7%. After the peak in 2008, unfortunately the number of PD patients began to decline gradually in Turkey. As of the end of 2018, there were only 3192 patients under PD treatment, and the PD penetration rate was decreased to 5.0% [5].

The decrease in PD rate may be due to several factors. The mortality and dropout rates may have contributed to the observed reduction in the number of PD patients. However, annual mortality and dropout rates in our PD population are not higher than expected. According to 2018 data, these rates are 8.9% and 12.0%, respectively [5]. Although the rate of KT in PD patients is higher than in HD patients, the absolute number of PD patients undergoing transplantation is relatively low (in 2018, 157 patients) [5]. The absence of any increase in the number of patients starting PD is probably the most important factor. The number of patients starting PD, which was 1559 in 2010, decreased to 886 in 2018 [5]. It may also be a factor that the annual cost per patient in PD is higher than HD in Turkey.

According to the 2018 TSN annual report, a total of 3192 PD patients (50.8% female and 49.2% male) at 139 centers are followed up in Turkey; 42.3% of these patients are in the 45–64 ages, and 22.7% are 65 years or older. The number of

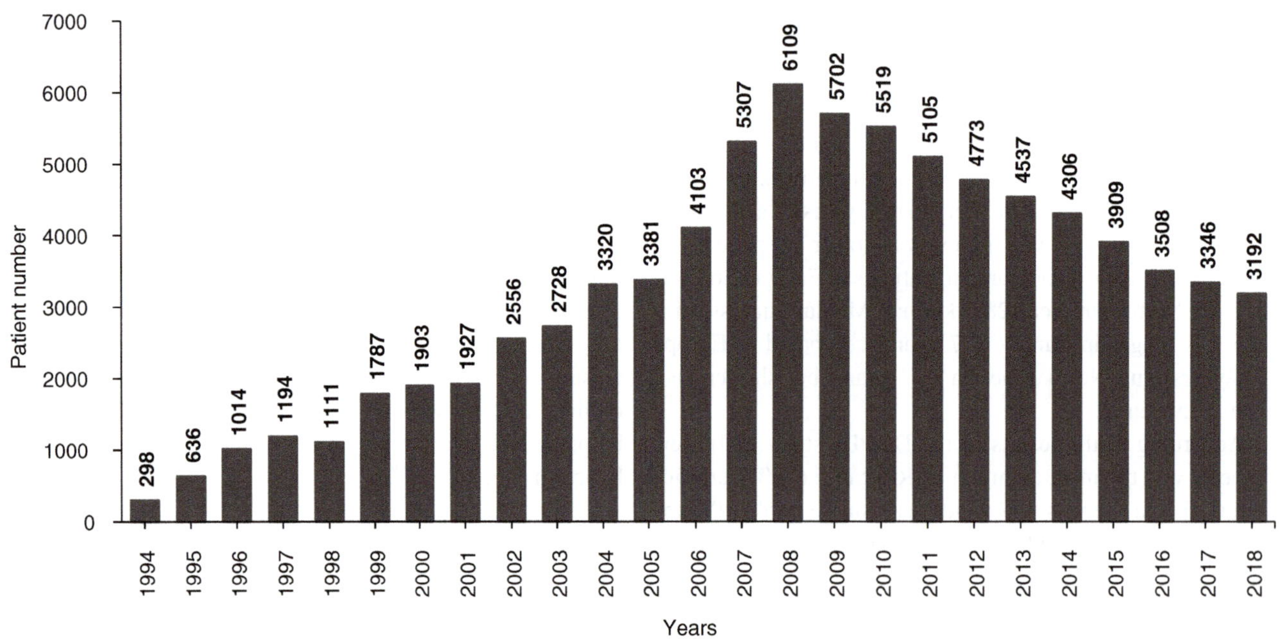


**Fig. 32.3** The number of peritoneal dialysis patients by years in Turkey

pediatric PD patients is 389 (12.3%). Overall, the PD patients are younger than HD patients. The duration of PD in the majority of patients (69.2%) is less than 5 years, and the rate of patients undergoing PD for more than 15 years is 1.0%. Hypertensive nephropathy and diabetic nephropathy are the most common etiologies of ESRD in incident PD patients (29.1% and 27.5%, respectively) [5].

CAPD is the most preferred PD modality in adult patients. As of the end of 2018, 67.0% of PD patients are on CAPD and 33.0% on APD. In pediatric patients, APD is more preferred than CAPD [5].

Today, PD solutions from Baxter, Fresenius, and Biopharma are available in Turkey. As of the end of 2018, biocompatible dialysis solutions with neutral pH and low glucose degradation products are used in more than 70% of PD patients. Approximately 63% of PD patients are using icodextrin-based PD solution in at least one exchange daily [5].

Clinical results are satisfactory with respect to peritonitis incidence, dialysis adequacy, renal anemia, and mineral metabolism. The incidence of peritonitis is one episode per 50 patient-months as of the end of 2018. The most common PD noninfectious complication is hernia (6.1%). Dialysis dose is adequate in the majority of the PD patients. Kt/V urea is over 1.7 in 89.2% of the patients. In 73.6% of the PD patients, arterial blood pressures are below 140/90 mmHg. Serum albumin level, which is an indicator of nutritional status, is above 3.5 g/dL in 74% of PD patients. The rate of active ESA usage in our PD population is 52.2%. This rate is significantly lower than in European countries and the USA. Despite the low ESA usage rate, hemoglobin level is greater than 10 g/dL in more than 80% of PD patients. Serum phosphorus level is lower than 5.5 mg/dL in 75% of PD patients. Approximately 82% of patients use phosphate-binding agents, and 69% of patients use PTH-suppressive drugs. Calcium acetate and oral vitamin D are the most preferred agents [5].

Dialysis and/or ultrafiltration failure seems to be the most important factor for switching to HD (46.1%); this is followed by PD-related infections (19.1%) and mechanical complications (18.0%). In 2018, cardiovascular diseases were the most common cause of death among PD patients, with a rate of 54.3%, followed by cerebrovascular events (12.9%) and infections (12.9%) [4]. The ranking of the most common causes of death remains similar to previous years [5].

An overview of the history and current situation of PD in Turkey has been presented here. As mentioned above, the quality of PD treatment in Turkey is very satisfactory. However, a decline in the number of patients undergoing PD after the peak in 2008 is noteworthy. In order to prevent this decrease in PD penetration rate, measures such as review of nephrology education programs, increase of postgraduate education activities, generalization of predialysis patient education programs, reducing the cost of PD treatment by increasing domestic PD solution production, and government incentives should be taken.

## Renal Transplantation

Renal transplantation is the treatment of choice among RRTs in Turkey. However, the rate of KT in all RRTs is only 21% [5]. The prevalence of CKD in Turkey is 15.7%, and approximately 70,000 of these patients are in stage 5 [4]. More kidneys (from deceased and living-related donors) are needed for transplantation; however, as in the rest of the world, the most important problem in Turkey is the shortage of organ supply.

The law of harvesting, storage, grafting, and transplantation of organs and tissues was enacted in 1979 before most of the European countries [7]. In 2001, the Ministry of Health established a national coordination center for organ transplantation, and the kidney allocation system was launched at 2008. The number of KT centers has gradually increased and reached 75. The major reason for this increase was the fact that in 2004, private universities and hospitals were allowed to perform KT. Ten of them are large centers and perform more than 100 kidney transplants per year.

The Netherlands, the USA, Jalisco state (Mexico), and Spain are the leading countries in the world regarding renal transplantation numbers pmp. Turkey is located in the middle of this list with the 38 renal transplantations pmp per year.

KT activities increased about four times between 2004 and 2018. However, the increase in cadaver donor numbers is not satisfactory. According to the TSN Registry, a total of 3871 renal transplantations were performed in 2018. Of these, only 859 (22.2%) were from deceased donors [5]. Over 2000 brain deaths were declared in the ICUs in Turkey in 2018; in spite of this, unfortunately only 25% of them were used. This is a multifactorial problem consisting of social, ethical, and religious issues.

Most living-related donations were done from relatives. The use of unrelated living donors has increased in recent years, up to 9.39% in 2018. Furthermore, the number of paired kidney donation has also increased, as paired kidney exchange programs are implemented within each center itself. Work is underway to develop the national paired kidney exchange program.

Inherently, most of the KT patients belong to the young and middle age groups. Transplantation operation may be risky for geriatric patients with comorbid problems like cardiovascular disease, malignancies, and infectious disease. Only 3.9% of KT in 2018 were performed in patients over 65 years of age [5].

HD is the first treatment modality in most of the transplant patients (52.0%) [5]. The rate of PD patients is 4.1%, and the rate of preemptive transplantation is 43.9%. The rapid increase in preemptive transplantations has been remarkable in recent years.

First-year graft and patient survivals are 95.8% and 97.8%, and the 5-year graft and patient survival rates are 87.6% and 94.5%, respectively. These rates show us satisfactory KT results in Turkey comparable to Western countries.

The mortality rate in all KT patients in 2018 was 2.96%; being 1.55% in living-related donor transplantations and 8.37% in deceased donor transplantations. The mortality rate in cadaveric transplantation is unacceptable, as it seems there have been some problems in cadaveric donation. The leading causes of mortality are infectious diseases and cardiovascular diseases; and we have been observing gradually decrease in mortality due to infections in the last few years.

There is a National Coordination System which is located in Ankara. There are many subunits attached to the National Coordination System, such as the National Coordination Center (NCC), the Regional Coordination Center, the Organ Transplant Centers, and HLA typing laboratories.

There is a national waiting list for all organ types, separately from the deceased donor transplantation. The donor hospital declares organs' availability and reports to the NCC. The NCC allocates the organs according to strict allocation rules and then distributes them to transplantation hospitals. Turkey is separated into nine different areas for the organ allocation. All of these nine areas are attached to the NCC.

It is well-known that the two important factors affecting success in KT are pathology and immunology support. There are some shortcomings in these two issues in Turkey. There are few pathologists involved specifically in transplant pathology. Experienced transplant pathologists are located in a few centers. It seems difficult for them to serve all patients in the whole country. Increasing the number of transplant pathologists should be one of the important goals. On the other hand, there are more than 40 tissue-typing and transplantation immunology laboratories. The problem with this issue is the lack of standardization. Only seven of these laboratories are European Federation for Immunogenetics (EFI) accredited. The number of laboratories open to international quality controls should be increased. After training in nephrology and urology/surgery, specialization training in transplant surgery and transplant nephrology has become a necessity.

For the next 10 years, cadaveric donation rates in Turkey should be increased. Moreover, both short- and long-term survivals in all transplantations should be prolonged. For this purpose, transplantation pathology and immunology should be supported and improved, and transplantation centers should be well controlled.

There has been a dramatic increase in the number of kidney transplantations performed during the last 5 years (Fig. 32.4). The low number of deceased donor KT still remains to be a major problem (Fig. 32.5). Patient and graft survival rates are comparable to those of Western countries. Main cause of death is related to infection, and the most common reasons for graft loss are death and chronic allograft nephropathy.

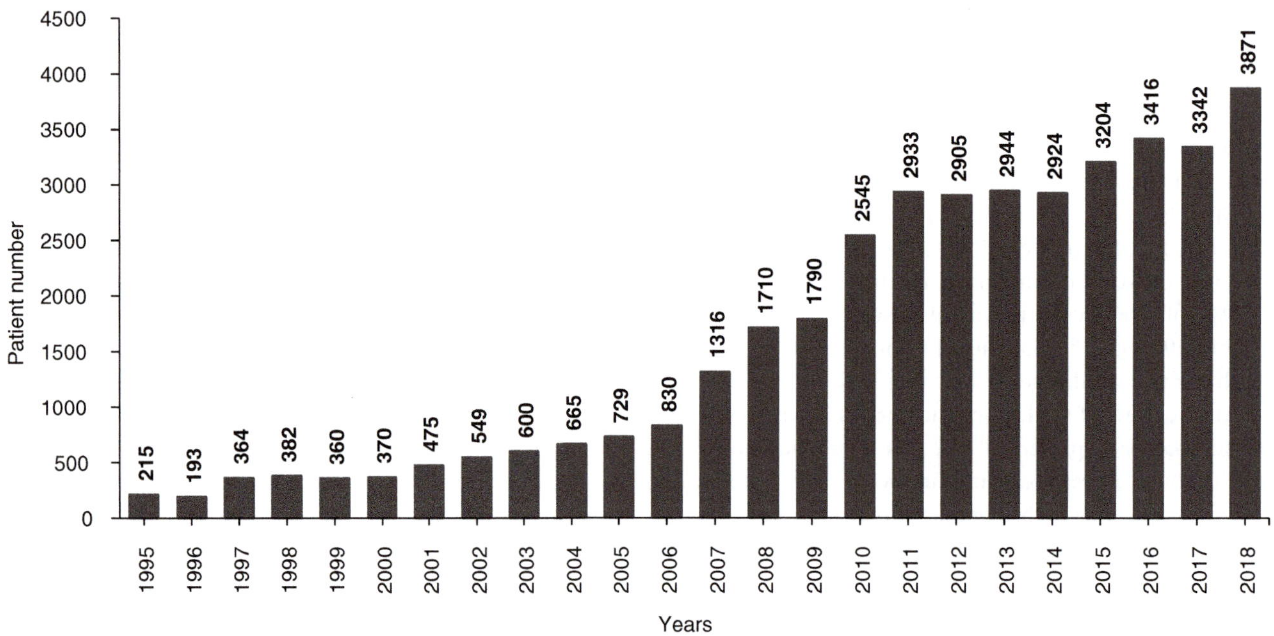


**Fig. 32.4** The number of kidney transplant recipients by years in Turkey

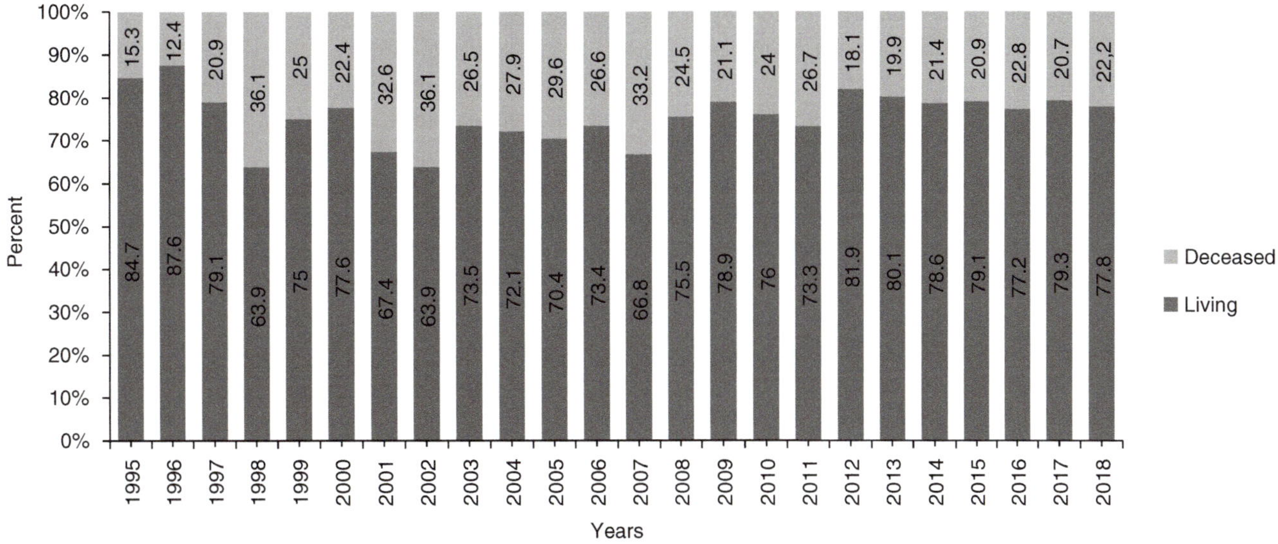


**Fig. 32.5** Donor source in incident transplant patients by years in Turkey

## Nephrology Practice in Turkey

There are approximately 600 adult and 200 pediatric nephrologists in Turkey. With these numbers, Turkey has one of the lowest ratios of nephrologists (10 pmp and 10 per 1000 ESRD patients) among European countries [22–24]. In Turkey, in order to qualify as a nephrologist, a physician should first get an internist specialization degree following a 4-year education; this education should be completed by submitting a medical thesis. Internists then enter a nationwide subspecialty examination. According to the scores they get, eligible candidates apply for fellowship to nephrology subspecialty centers. In Turkey, there are 58 centers who provide subspecialty education for nephrology fellowship [23]. Nephrology subspecialty education is 3 years. This education comprises a structured program, where trainees learn both basic and clinical principles of nephrology. During their education, all nephrology fellows should have at least 6 months of education and practice in HD, 3 months in PD, and 3 months in KT. The rest of the education consists of clinical practice in nephrology outpatient and inpatient clinics. During the training, nephrology fellows should learn certain abilities, such as performing percutaneous kidney biopsy and insertion of temporary or permanent dialysis catheters. Some centers have more interventional nephrology approaches, like insertion of a PD catheter or surgically creating an arteriovenous fistula.

Nephrologists usually work in secondary or tertiary centers. Almost all cities in Turkey have a nephrologist working either in state or university hospitals. Nephrologists in Turkey are responsible for taking care of all kidney patients not only in nephrology departments but also in all departments of the hospital. There are 75 renal transplantation centers in Turkey, and nephrologists have a pivotal role in patient recruitment, selection, and pre- and postoperative care of transplant patients. Nephrologists have a close connection with ICUs and share the responsibility with intensivists for the care of kidney patients (including continuous RRT) in ICUs.

There are 882 HD centers in Turkey [5]. The regulations of dialysis facilities are defined by the Ministry of Health. According to these regulations, at least one certified physician must be recruited for every 50 patients. In addition, there has to be at least one nurse or one dialysis technician for every five patients. Each dialysis facility should also recruit a renal dietitian.

Most HD patients (65% of the HD population) are dialyzed in private centers. Most private centers have a general practitioner or internist who is continuously taking care of patients. These HD practitioners receive a special certificate following 3–6 months of education for HD practice. HD certificate education is given by the nephrology training centers. Although certified HD practitioners cover the shortage of nephrologists, they frequently feel themselves on their own when they face serious problems (either technical or medical) in their units. Some private units are parts of big dialysis chains and have technical or medical backups, but this is not the case for many small for-profit private centers. As many centers have no close connections with a nephrology unit or a nephrologist, HD practitioners may have no or a few chances to receive support when needed. When a patient needs a referral to a nephrology center, there is not enough communication between the dialysis unit and nephrology center. These problems are affecting the quality of care and continuity of care, especially for dialysis patients with many comorbidities. All HD centers are regularly audited, by government officials for various parameters including patient safety and quality of care.

There are 120 PD centers in Turkey. Majority of these centers are public-funded centers, and nephrologists have a principal role in caring of PD patients. In academic settings, nephrologists provide consulting and ongoing care in outpatient and inpatient settings, perform basic science and clinical research in kidney diseases, and teach medical students and residents.

There is not a regular patient referral system from the primary care clinics to the nephrology centers in Turkey. However, there is general coverage for health expenditures, and all costs of kidney patients are being paid by the government. This enables kidney patients to have an easy access to nephrology clinics as soon as they are aware of their kidney problems. The Ministry of Health has prepared an action program to prevent and control kidney disease in 2014 [25]. This program has been prepared in collaboration with TSN. Currently, the Ministry of Health is preparing national guidelines for kidney patient care. Although there are efforts for multidisciplinary team work approaches, it is still in its infancy in Turkey.

As the nephrology workforce in Turkey is still inadequate, there is an intense workload on the nephrology health workers. This creates a general burnout within the nephrology community, but this also has a positive effect as there is an increased demand for nephrologists and, thereby, a larger job demand for nephrologists. Despite the increased demand, pay-per-performance amounts for nephrology procedures are not satisfactory, and salaries of nephrologists fall below several other disciplines. The average monthly salary of a nephrologist ranges from 1200 to 3000 USD according to the pay grade and place of work (public or private). The average salary of a renal nurse is between 500 and 800 USD according to the pay grade and place of work (public or private).

## Future Perspectives of Nephrology in Turkey

The prevalence of CKD is increasing in Turkey because of the increase in the number of patients with obesity, diabetes, and hypertension along with the aging of the population. The continuing rise in the prevalence of patients on RRT causes an enormous economic burden to the healthcare system. It is clear that this problem will continue to grow in the future. Therefore, the main aim should be the primary prevention for those who are at increased risk of CKD. Health policy should concentrate on education programs in order to increase the awareness of the disease, together with the lifestyle modifications, such as weight loss and cessation of smoking.

## Conclusion

CKD, which is an important public health problem in Turkey, is associated with increased risk of morbidity and mortality. The demographic and clinical characteristics of patients with CKD in Turkey are comparable to those of the Western countries. While the prevalence of patients who need RRT is increasing, the population is becoming older with the rise in the quality of care. However, this would worsen the economic burden of the CKD in the future. Therefore, the best long-term approach would be to target more efforts on the primary prevention of the disease.

**Conflict of Interest** The authors declare that they have no conflict of interest.

## References

1. Turkish Statistical Institute. Accessed in January 2020. Available in: www.turkstat.gov.tr.
2. Crews DC, Bello AK, Saadi G, for the World Kidney Day Steering Committee. Burden, access and disparities in kidney disease. Clin Kidney J. 2019;12:160–6.
3. Hallan SI, Matsushita K, Sang Y et al., for the CKD Prognosis Consortium. Age and association of kidney measures with mortality and end-stage renal disease JAMA. 2012;308:2349–60.
4. Süleymanlar G, Utaş C, Arınsoy T, Ateş K, Altun B, Altiparmak MR, et al. A population-based survey of chronic renal disease in Turkey - the CREDIT study. Nephrol Dial Transplant. 2011;26:1862–71.
5. Süleymanlar G, Ateş K, Seyahi N. Registry of the nephrology, dialysis and transplantation in Turkey. Registry 2018. Ministry of Health and Turkish Society of Nephrology Joint Report. Published by the Turkish Society of Nephrology. Ankara, 2019.
6. Süleymanlar G, Serdengecti K, Altiparmak MR, Jager K, Seyahi N, Erek E, on behalf of the Turkish Registry of Nephrology, Dialysis and transplantation. Trends in renal replacement therapy in Turkey, 1996-2008. Am J Kidney Dis. 2011;57:456–65.
7. Erek E, Süleymanlar G, Serdengecti K, and the Registry Group, Turkish Society of Nephrology. Nephrology, dialysis and transplantation in Turkey. Nephrol Dial Transplant. 2002;17:2087–93.
8. Haberal M. Transplantation in Turkey. Clin Transpl. 2013:175–80.
9. Erek E, Sever MS, Serdengecti K, et al. An overview of morbidity and mortality in patients with acute renal failure due to crush syndrome: the Marmara earthquake experience. Nephrol Dial Transplant. 2002;17(1):33–40.
10. Sever MS, Erek E, Vanholder R, et al. Renal replacement therapies in the aftermath of the catastrophic Marmara earthquake. Kidney Int. 2002;62(6):2264–71.
11. Bek K, Akaman S, Bilge I. Chronic kidney disease in Turkey. Pediatr Nephrol. 2009;24:797–806.
12. Ozaltın F. Primary coenzyme Q 10 (CoQ 10) deficiencies and related nephropathies. Pediatr Nephrol. 2014;29(6):961–9.
13. Soylemezoğlu O, Duzova A, Yalçınkaya F, Arinsoy T, Suleymanlar G. Chronic renal disease in children aged 5-18 years. A population based survey in Turkey, the CREDIT-C study. Nephrol Dial Transplant. 2012;27 Suppl 3:iii146–51.

14. Tatar M, Ergin G, Ecder T. Cost analysis of private hemodialysis centers in Turkey. Turk Nephrol Dial Transpl. 2013;22:270–82.
15. Vanholder R, Davenport A, Hannedouche T, Kooman J, Kribben A, Lameire N, et al. Reimbursement of dialysis: a comparison of seven countries. J Am Soc Nephrol. 2012;23:1291–8.
16. Ok E, Asci G, Toz H, Ok ES, Kircelli F, Yilmaz M, et al. Mortality and cardiovascular events in online haemodiafiltration (OL-HDF) compared with high-flux dialysis: results from the Turkish OL-HDF Study. Nephrol Dial Transplant. 2013;28(1):192–202.
17. Ecder T, Utaş C, Ateş K, Bieber B, Robinson BM, Pisoni RL, Suleymanlar G. The dialysis outcomes and practice patterns study (DOPPS) in Turkey. Hemodial Int. 2017;21(3):430–9.
18. Satman I, Omer B, Tutuncu Y, Kalaca S, Gedik S, Dinccag N, et al. Twelve-year trends in the prevalence and risk factors of diabetes and prediabetes in Turkish adults. Eur J Epidemiol. 2013;28:169–80.
19. San A. History of Turkish nephrology. Ankara: Anatolia Kidney Foundation Publication; 2002.
20. Utaş C. The development of PD in Turkey. Perit Dial Int. 2008;28:217–9.
21. Ersoy FF. The TULIP story. Perit Dial Int. 2008;28:220–3.
22. Sharif MU, Elsayed ME, Stack AG. The global nephrology workforce: emerging threats and potential solutions! Clin Kidney J. 2016;9(1):11–22.
23. Kidney Health for Life (KH4L). Chronic kidney disease multinational inventory. Accessed in January 2020. Available in https://www.theisn.org/all-articles/560-kidney-health-for-life-kh4l.
24. Bello AK, Levin A, Manns BJ, et al., for the Kidney Health for Life Initiative. Effective CKD care in European countries: challenges and opportunities for health policy. Am J Kidney Dis. 2015;65(1):15–25.
25. Türkiye Böbrek Hastalıkları Önleme ve Kontrol Programı 2014–2017. Accessed in January 2020. Available in https://sbu.saglik.gov.tr/Ekutuphane/Yayin/503.

# Nephrology in the United Arab Emirates

# 33

Mona Al-Rukhaimi, Zubaida Al Ismaili, and Ali Alobaidli

| | |
|---|---|
| Area[1] | 83,600 Km$^2$ |
| Population[1] | 9,682,088 (2019) |
| Capital | Abu Dhabi |
| Three most populated cities: | 1. Dubai (4,177,095)<br>2. Abu Dhabi (2,784,490)<br>3. Sharjah (2,374,132) |
| Official language | Arabic |
| Gross domestic product (GDP)[2] | 732.861 billion USD (2018) |
| GDP per capita[2] | 70,262 USD (2018) |
| Human Development Index (HDI)[2] | 0.863 (2018) |
| Official currency | UAE dirham (AED) |
| Total number of nephrologists[3] | 120 |
| National society of nephrology | Emirate Nephrology Society (EMAN)<br>www.ema.ae & www.eman-uae.com |
| Incidence of end-stage renal disease[3] | 2018 – 135 pmp |
| Prevalence of end-stage renal disease (on dialysis) | 2018 – 260 pmp |
| Total number of patients on dialysis[3] (all modalities) | 2017 – ~2400<br>2018 – ~2500 |
| Number of patients on hemodialysis[3] | 2017 – ~2300<br>2018 – ~2400 |
| Number of patients on peritoneal dialysis[3] | 2017 – ~100<br>2018 – ~100 |
| Number of renal transplantations per year[3] | 2017 – 36<br>2018 – 62 |

Table references:
1. www.worldometers.info
2. Human Development Indices and Indicators, 2018 statistical update
3. Data collected by the Emirate Nephrology Society

M. Al-Rukhaimi (✉)
Department of Medicine, Dubai Medical College, Dubai, United Arab Emirates

Z. Al Ismaili
Pediatric Institute, Sheikh Khalifa Medical City, Abu Dhabi, United Arab Emirates
e-mail: zuismaili@seha.ae

A. Alobaidli
Department of Medicine, Nephrology, Sheikh Khalifa Medical City, Abu Dhabi, United Arab Emirates
e-mail: aobaidli@seha.ae

## Introduction

The United Arab Emirates (UAE) is part of the Gulf Cooperation Council (GCC) for the Arab states of the Gulf region, and these countries are an integral part of the wider Arabic region. The GCC is composed of six countries including the UAE, the Kingdom of Saudi Arabia, Oman, Kuwait, Qatar, and the Kingdom of Bahrain. The GCC countries are located on the Arabian Peninsula that comprises an area of 2,673,108 km$^2$ and a population of approximately 56 million according to a 2018 estimate. A unified economic agreement between these countries was signed on November 11, 1981, in Abu Dhabi, the capital of the UAE.

On December 2, 1971, the UAE was established by unification of seven emirates. The Federation comprises seven emirates: the Abu Dhabi emirate, which is also the capital, and Dubai, which is the major commercial center. The other emirates are Sharjah, Ajman, Fujairah, Ras al-Khaimah, and Umm al-Quwain.

Prior to the establishment of the Federation, each of the emirates had its own separate independence. However, after the formation of the UAE, the Rulers agreed to draw up a provisional constitution specifying the powers that were to be allocated to the new federal institutions while maintaining substantial local government authority.

In 2018, the total population of the UAE was estimated to be 9.6 million, 1.4 million being Emirati citizens, and 8.2 million expatriates; 42.8% of the total population lives in Dubai, 29.0% in Abu Dhabi, and 24.7% in Sharjah.

The UAE vision is one that empowers women, embraces diversity, encourages innovation, and welcomes global engagement and is committed to encouraging values of inclusion and coexistence with a designated Ministry of Tolerance that implements programs fostering respect, peaceful coexistence, and mutual understanding among people in the UAE.

All GCC states have experienced unprecedented socioeconomic transformation that has led to higher standards of living, stable currencies, and low inflation rates. The local populations of the GCC countries are generally small, and,


J. A. Moura-Neto et al. (eds.), *Nephrology Worldwide*, https://doi.org/10.1007/978-3-030-56890-0_33

therefore, a high proportion of the work force consists of expatriates from other countries. The prevailing political and social system of these states has mostly been conservative and tribal in nature, with strong family and tribal ties, although over the years it has been witnessing modernization with global prospective as the majority of the population have immigrated from over 200 countries for living and work.

Oil and gas are the main resources of the GCC countries. However, they have begun aggressive plans of economic reforms toward diversifying their resources. The economy of the UAE is the second largest in the Middle East, with a gross domestic product of 732.861 billion USD (2018 estimates) and the most diversified economy in the GCC, although still significantly reliant on petroleum. The UAE has worked in the past two decades on building a strong semi-industrial base economy, providing the necessary infrastructure to be a tourist destination, a financial hub, as well as a center for trade and transit between Asia and Europe.

The UAE has made substantial investments in healthcare infrastructure and seen an incremental increase in healthcare spending, especially in recent years, with the introduction of mandatory health insurance and universal access to care since 2007 [1].

Mandatory health insurance introduction allowed further investment into the healthcare infrastructure with the private sector playing a greater role in both the delivery of the healthcare to the population and its financing. New sets of quality standards are being adopted, for both public and private healthcare delivery systems, with the aim to rank the providers relative to their outcomes and, accordingly, determine their reimbursements.

Currently, major academic medical centers from North America, Australia, and the European Union have partnered with both public and private institutions for healthcare provision. There are six medical schools and nursing and health science colleges spread across the UAE attracting undergraduate students from the UAE and abroad. In addition, an expansion of postgraduate training programs at academic teaching hospitals is ongoing.

Cardiovascular disease is the principal cause of death in the UAE, constituting 28% of total deaths; other major causes are accidents and injuries, malignancies, and congenital anomalies [2]. According to the World Health Organization data from 2014, 37.2% of adults in the UAE are clinically obese, with body mass index (BMI) scores of 30 or more. The overall improvement in healthcare services and public health of the UAE and other GCC countries have been impressive. The average life expectancy rose from 60.5 years in 1978 to 73 years in 2004 and currently is estimated to be at 78.5 years, whereas during the same period, infant mortality fell from 69 deaths per 1000 live births to 18. The average crude birth rate is 18.4% and the crude death rate is 2.9%. Those below 15 years of age comprise 19.7% of the total population, while those greater than 65 years of age comprise only 1.6% of the population [3, 4].

## Brief History of Nephrology in the UAE

The UAE independence happened in 1971 with a population estimated then, around 200,000 people. With the flow of the oil revenues, the country started to invest in healthcare and education. One of the oldest hospitals, opened in 1968, was the Abu Dhabi Central Hospital, and soon many health services were offered including outpatient renal services. Dr. Avinash Pingle, the nephrologist at the Central Hospital, was instrumental in setting up the first dialysis unit in the UAE and also for introducing nephrology as a specialty to the country. The Central Hospital in Abu Dhabi was the only center offering such services until 1980, receiving patients not only from the UAE but also from neighboring countries such as Oman and Bahrain. The first peritoneal dialysis (PD) program was initiated in 1976, and the first chronic hemodialysis (HD) program was established in 1977. The services were then extended to be available in each emirate of the country. Currently, there are 33 dialysis units in the country, of which 10 are operated by the private sector and the rest by the government.

Kidney transplantation was first started in 1985. The federal law that regulates organ and tissue transplant in the UAE was issued in 1993 and the Ministerial Decision on the implementation regulation of the law issued in 2010. All regulations in the UAE are committed to the Istanbul Declaration. The transplantation in the UAE has gone through several phases. The updating of the implementation procedures of the law, from accepting only living donation, to a recent acknowledgment of patients diagnosed with brain death as potential donors, has permitted the start of a national deceased multi-organ donation and transplantation program.

## Kidney Disease in the UAE

In the UAE, similar to other countries, chronic kidney disease (CKD) has become an increasingly significant clinical and public health issue. This is because during recent decades, the UAE has undergone significant rapid economic growth and modern infrastructure development, following the discovery of oil. This economic progress has clearly brought many social benefits and opportunities for the country, including an increase in life expectancy. On the other hand, rapid modernization and urbanization have contributed to a substantial increase of risk factors for many chronic diseases like CKD, hypertension (HTN), diabetes mellitus (DM), obesity, dyslipidemia, and smoking.

Information on the epidemiology of CKD and associated risk factors are in general limited in the UAE and GCC, when compared to Western countries. However, with the recent implementation of electronic medical records, more awareness of chronic diseases and their economic burdens, as well as implementation of population-based screenings due to health insurance requirements, led to a significant amount of data available. Accordingly, there has been an increasing number of research publications that addressed kidney disease in the UAE and the GCC with details on prevalence and incidence of risk factors and their public health implications [5–8].

Simultaneously, these data and public health challenges prompted the local health authorities and the Federal Ministry of Health (MoH) to significantly strengthen its health data systems to assess the baseline and measure the impact of targeted interventions. For example, the unique population-level screening (Weqaya) program for UAE Nationals living in Abu Dhabi, collecting every 3 years from the age of 18, has recruited more than 94% of the adults into a screening program for the rapid identification of those at risk and deployment of targeted interventions to control these risk factors. Similar changes to health policy and practices have led to raising awareness, behavioral change, and an empowerment of the community to enable individuals to make healthier choices [9–11].

According to a study of CKD epidemiology and referral patterns [12] conducted in Abu Dhabi, using the available screening population data combined with data from the unified electronic medical records (EMR) system, the dialysis prevalence in Abu Dhabi was estimated at around 370 per million population (pmp) with an annual growth of 12–15%. Among Emiratis, 4.6% of males and 2.8% of females had an eGFR between stage 3 and 5 CKD. Among expatriates, 4.2% of males and 3.2% of females had an eGFR between stage 3 and 5 CKD. The Dialysis Outcome and Practice Pattern Study (DOPPS) data [13], for which the UAE and the rest of GCC joined phase 5, indicated that diabetes is reported as the primary cause of end-stage renal disease (ESRD) for 41% of HD patients in the GCC compared to 43% in North America and 25% in Europe. Among the GCC countries, DM as the cause accounts for 39%, followed by HTN 34% in the UAE. In another study [14] performed by a single government center in Dubai, the data shows that DM as the cause of ESRD accounts for 57%. These studies and a few others [15] demonstrate the need to improve the identification and referral of CKD patients and the need to increase public and physician awareness of CKD.

## Renal Replacement Therapy in the UAE

### Hemodialysis

The first chronic HD program was established in Abu Dhabi in 1977, followed by the emirate of Dubai in 1980 and then the rest of the emirates. By the end of 2018, the total number of patients on HD was estimated to be around 2500, being 1200 in Abu Dhabi Emirate, 600 in Dubai, and the rest in the other emirates. As per data reference in the table for the year 2018, dialysis prevalence is estimated to be around 260 pmp and the dialysis incidence 130 pmp. Outsourcing of the dialysis services to private international companies has been established by the Emirate of Abu Dhabi for the last 5 years, through Abu Dhabi Health Authority and recently by the MoH in the emirates of Fujairah and Ras al-Khaimah.

All forms of therapies are available in the UAE. The typical HD prescription has a dialysate flow of 500 ml/min and blood flow rate that ranges between 250 and 350 depending on the patient weight and the vascular access. The conventional in-center 4-hour, thrice-weekly session is the standard in the UAE. Eleven percent of the patients are on hemodiafiltration (HDF) prescription. Dialyzer reuse is not allowed in the UAE. The main vascular access is arteriovenous fistula in 55% of the patient, followed by central dialysis catheter 41%, and 4% have graft [16].The annual mortality is estimated to be around 8.5% [13]. All the nephrologists in the UAE follow the international KDIGO/KDOQI guidelines in relation to dialysis adequacy or lab parameters. In addition, the Emirate Nephrology Society has created and distributed a flow chart to all dialysis units in the country regarding the management of CKD bone mineral disorder (CKD-MBD).

The dialysis services as well as all the ESRD drugs such as erythropoietin, phosphate binders, and others are fully covered by the government for the nationals and through insurance, self-payment, or charity for the UAE residents.

Home HD (HHD) was introduced in 2017 through the private sector and is sponsored by the government for the nationals. It has provided relief to geriatric and disabled patients, for whom going to the center three times per week posed a problem; nearly 147 patients in Abu Dhabi and Dubai are getting this service as of the end of 2019.

In addition, all forms of continuous renal replacement therapies (RRT) as well as plasmapheresis and the use of dialysis or hemoperfusion in the treatment of poisoning are available in the majority of intensive care units (ICU) in the country.

The dialysis units in the country, whether stand-alone or in-hospital, have to undergo a listening process and fulfill all the requirements as per government health authority roles and regulations, before establishment.

The average dialysis facility in the UAE will have nephrologists, dialysis nurses, a dietitian, and a social worker. Dialysis technicians are hardly appointed in the Emirates. There is no fixed ratio of staff to patient, but roughly it is around 1 doctor per 30–50 patients and 1 nurse per 4–6 patients on dialysis.

## Peritoneal Dialysis

The first PD program was established in 1976, and nowadays there are around 100 patients throughout the country on this modality, either in the form of continuous ambulatory peritoneal dialysis (CAPD) or automated peritoneal dialysis (APD). Few centers offer this type of therapy to the patients. As the number of patients leaving the program due to death, shift to HD, or transplantation was almost equal to the number of patients who were recruited to this type of therapy, the total number remains stable over the years. In fact, a once weekly multidisciplinary clinic consisting of a nephrologist, a dialysis nurse, and a dietitian has been created in one of the in-hospital dialysis center, called "renal school clinic" with the aim of teaching patients in CKD stage 4–5 about CKD and the available RRT and giving them the chance to meet with patient on HD and PD, so they can have informed choice about the modalities of therapy. Despite that, the number of patients who choose PD remains low.

## Renal Transplantation

Organ transplantation in many Middle East countries was influenced in the 1970s and 1980s by Islamic scholars' opinion (Fatwas) about brain death and the shortage of technical transplant expert teams to perform the procedures before initiating kidney transplantation.

A key fatwa in neighboring Saudi Arabia came about in 1982, which permitted deceased donor transplantation and paved the way to start a cadaveric renal program. Another progressive fatwa was issued, at the meeting of the Islamic Jurisprudence Conference in 1986 in Amman Jordan, declaring that the diagnosis of brain death was permissible and could be used to diagnose an irreversible process, and, soon after in 1988, another landmark fatwa was issued in Saudi Arabia allowing cessation of life-sustaining therapy, including ventilation, permitting wider practice of deceased donation, and transplantation in the Middle East [17].

Some of the landmarks of transplantation in the UAE were the first living-related kidney transplant performed by Dr. Abdallah Daar at Mafraq Hospital in Abu Dhabi in 1985 and the first two cadaveric transplants, from kidneys donated to the UAE from European Union, in 1989. This first phase lasted until 2002 with a total of 62 living-related kidney transplants and 2 cadaveric kidney transplants performed with a 5-year graft survival of 82%.This initial success drew patients from neighboring countries such as Sudan and Yemen to perform the procedure in the Emirates.

A presidential transplantation decree was issued in 1993, and a Federal National Transplant Committee was established soon after to work on needed bylaws and policies. The transplant program at Mafraq Hospital was not sustainable due to lack of availability of permanent teams and relocation of the existing experts. To meet increasing demands, many patients were getting support for transplantation in the United State of America and the European Union, as was the practice for most GCC countries. Some patients were also seeking commercial transplantation with poor outcomes. In December 2007, a steering committee from the Transplantation Society and the International Society of Nephrology (ISN) met in Dubai under the umbrella of the Emirate Nephrology Society to enhance the global efforts to address the growing problems of organ sales, transplant tourism, and trafficking in organ donors in the context of the global shortage of organs. The preparatory work of the steering committee was a key achievement for the transplant community leading to the Declaration of Istanbul on Organ Trafficking and Transplant Tourism, which helped many countries to start their ethical national living and deceased organ donation programs.

In 2008, phase two for the transplantation program in the UAE was initiated when Shaikh Khalifa Medical City – SKMC, part of the Abu Dhabi Health Services Company network, reestablished a kidney transplantation program in partnership with Cleveland Clinic Foundation. The program included living-related pediatric and adult kidney transplantation for all residents in the UAE at the government expense. By the end of 2016, 160 cases of living-related kidney transplants and 2 cases of cadaveric transplants donated to the UAE from Saudi Arabia had been performed.

The immunosuppression protocols follow the KDIGO guideline, where IL2R antibodies are used for induction in patients with low immunological risk who are going to be on CNI and MMF-/MPA-based regime. Those with high immunological risk will receive thymoglobulin induction. Steroid is used in the first 5 days and then usually stopped for patients with low immunological risk and immediate graft function and for those with increased cardiometabolic risk.

In 2017, phase three for transplantation started in the UAE with the new transplantation law signed by the president of the UAE, providing needed legal support for recognition of brain death as death and permitting the start of deceased donation. At the same time, there has been significant investment in the transplant programs, which led to start deceased organ donation including the start of the UAE's heart, lung, liver, and expansion of the transplant program with 14 deceased donations saving the lives of more than 40 transplant recipients by the end of 2018. To date there are four transplant programs, two in Abu Dhabi and two in Dubai. Three performing kidney to date there are four transplant programs, two in Abu Dhabi and two in Dubai all performing kidney transplant while the multiorgan transplant program is done only in Cleveland Clinic Abu Dhabi hospital.

There have been significant training programs for the ICU staff on organ donation protocols, and there have been many capacity building programs in collaboration with international centers such as the Donation and Transplantation Institute in Spain and others. There are plans underway to establish the UAE Organ Procurement Organization (OPO) to take organ donation to a more systematic approach in the coming period, and the federal and local health authorities are addressing the required resources needed.

Of note is that all the kidney transplantation procedures, plus medications that have been done, were either health insurance sponsored or covered by governmental mandated funds free of charge, with over 20 nationalities benefiting from the program with 1- and 3-year graft survival for adult age groups, 98% and 96%, respectively, and graft survival at 1- and 5-year for pediatric age group of 96.7% and 83.3%, respectively. These results are equivalent to data from many US and international programs [18].

## Pediatric Nephrology

The incidence of pediatric kidney diseases has been several times higher in the UAE compared to most of the Western countries, most likely due to the high rate of consanguinity [19, 20]. Unfortunately, there are almost no accurate data regarding the epidemiology so far. Some of the top hereditary diseases are congenital nephrotic syndrome, autosomal recessive polycystic kidney disease, and nephropathies [21]. On the other hand, we are seeing more CKD caused by secondary causes due to the increasing advancement in treating complex diseases like cardiac, malignant, and rheumatic diseases.

The first pediatric nephrology center in the UAE was established in Abu Dhabi (Central Hospital) in 1991, shortly followed by another center in the Emirate of Dubai (Dubai hospital) in 1993. Chronic dialysis services in the form of PD were introduced in both Abu Dhabi and Dubai in 1992 and 1996, respectively. HD was initially provided in the form of acute dialysis, but subsequently, chronic programs were established in 1995 and 1996 in Abu Dhabi and Dubai, respectively. Pediatric kidney transplantation was first established as a living-related program at Sheikh Khalifa Medical City (SKMC), Abu Dhabi, in 2010 followed by a deceased donor program in both Abu Dhabi (SKMC) and Dubai (Al Jalila Children hospital) in 2017 and 2018, respectively.

Currently there are four centers within the UAE providing almost the whole spectrum of pediatric nephrology care including all dialysis modalities, living and deceased kidney transplantation, plasma exchange, and special treatments for complex glomerulonephritis and hemolytic uremic syndrome.

The choice of the different RRT is mainly depending on the size of the patients, donor availability, and family comfort. In general, patients would be equally distributed between the two dialysis modalities, if kidney transplantation is not an option. However, PD is a more common option in infants and toddlers.

Kidney transplantation through transplant tourism is, unfortunately, very popular in children with ESRD, especially because the local deceased donor transplant program has only been established very recently. Studies have already shown that transplant tourism carries a higher rate of complications and shorter graft survival rate [22].

Access to the pediatric nephrology services varies according to the Emirate and the patient insurance and residency status. SKMC accepts all UAE nationals (Thiqa) children below the age of 16 years without any referrals. Abu Dhabi residents who are non-UAE nationals can be seen (with a referral), provided that they have coverage from their insurance company. Unfortunately, usually the insurance rejects to cover the cases, and they end up getting an activity-based mandate coverage, which is from the Abu Dhabi government. Dubai Hospital provides a free access for all UAE nationals. For the nonnationals, a valid insurance is required to get coverage except for chronic dialysis patients who can be covered through charitable bodies as far as they have Dubai residency.

## Acute Kidney Injury and Critical Care Nephrology

Acute kidney injury (AKI) is common worldwide and associated with significant morbidity, mortality, and resource utilization. Over the past two decades, there has been substantial progress in the field of AKI. In particular, work on consensus definition, epidemiology and database studies, AKI biomarkers, and the appropriate dosing of RRT has continued at a brisk pace.

In the UAE, unfortunately, there is no data registry for AKI. Available RRT for critical care nephrology include continuous therapies and conventional or prolonged intermittent HD, performed in wards or ICU. In one publication on 2004 regarding the experience of one tertiary hospital with AKI, it was found that out of all 81 patients admitted with or who developed AKI in the hospital over a 18-month period, 10% were direct admission to nephrology service with AKI, and 90% developed AKI in the hospital. Thirty percent were referred by oncology services and 15% by general medicine. Sepsis was the cause in 44% of the patients, followed by drug nephrotoxicity in 14% and obstructive uropathy in 9%. Sixty patients (74%) were managed conservatively, and 21 (26%) required RRT. Patients' survival for those managed on the ward was 71% compared to 33% for ICU patients. Renal survival was 83% for ward patients, compared to 48% for those in the ICU [23]. This single-center data is consistent with the international data in regard to sepsis being the leading cause of AKI, and patients who needed ICU treatment showed a worse prognosis for both patient and renal survival.

## Nephrology Practice in the UAE

There are mainly four health authorities in the country. The MoH covers all the Emirates, Abu Dhabi Health Authority covers the Emirate of Abu Dhabi, Dubai Health Authority covers the Emirate of Dubai, and Sharjah Health Authority covers the Emirate of Sharjah. All four authorities are working in harmony.

The UAE nephrologists are mainly North American or UK trained, but, in general, a physician has to hold a Bachelor of Medicine, Bachelor of Surgery, or, in Latin, *Medicine Baccalaureus Baccalaureus Chirurgiae* (abbreviated in many ways, e.g., MBBS, MBChB, MBBChir) or an equivalent qualification from an accredited institution with completion of adult or pediatric nephrology specialty qualification. Physicians with an accredited American Board of Adult or Pediatric Nephrology Certification, Pediatric Nephrology Certificate of the RCPSC, Certification by the College of Family Physicians Canada (CFPC), Certificate of Completion of Specialist Training (CCST), or Certificate of Completion of Training (CCT) from the UK will attain the title of Consultant Adult or Pediatric Nephrology without the experience requirements. All foreign doctors should speak English.

Subspecialty training is in general underdeveloped in the Emirates. The nephrology fellowship program was established in Sheikh Khalifa Medical City (SKMC) in Abu Dhabi in 2012. Requirement for enrollment includes Arab Board or Jordanian Board in Internal Medicine. The training duration is 2–3 years and includes rotations in general nephrology, dialysis, renal transplantation, pathology, and interventional radiology. There will be an annual assessment as well as an exit exam to be Arab Board in Nephrology certified. At the end of 2019, six fellows had graduated and four were in training.

The average monthly income for a nephrologist in the UAE ranges between 8000 and 27,000 USD, depending on their career ladder and for a dialysis nurse between 1600 and 3000 USD.

For other health professionals related to nephrology, e.g., nurses, dialysis technicians, dietitians, or intensivists, and for any job vacancy, the reader can refer to any of the following websites:

- Ministry of Health – www.mohap.gov.ae
- Abu Dhabi Health Authority – www.haad.ae
- Dubai Health Authority – www.dha.gov.ae
- Sharjah Health Authority – www.sha.gov.ae

## Highlights of Nephrology in UAE

The Emirates Nephrology Society was founded in 1996, under the umbrella of the Emirates Medical Association. Since its establishment, the society has been active in providing education to its membership and the greater region. It has developed close working relationships with a number of international and regional associations. It started with 15 members and now its membership exceeds 120 members.

The Emirates Medical Association Nephrology Society (EMAN) has an excellent track record of hosting successful events, working closely with international and regional associations on these projects. The president of the society was an ISN council member from 2011 to 2017 and an executive council member from 2015 to 2017.

In particular, the ISN-EMAN update course in Nephrology takes place every 3 years and has grown steadily since the first edition in 1998. In 2014, this was joined with the 12th Congress of the Arab Society of Nephrology and Renal Transplantation (ASNRT) and resulted in an event with over 600 delegates from 28 countries.

They were also the host of the third conference of the Pan-Arab Hypertension Society, which attracted over 1600 delegates. The 13th Middle East Society of Transplantation (MESOT) Congress combined with MESOT Transplant Games in 2012 welcomed over 1000 delegates to Abu Dhabi, a record attendance for the event. In addition the society has hosted for the first time in the Middle East region the International Society for Hemodialysis (ISHD) congress in Abu Dhabi in Dec 2018 and the International Society of Organ Donation and Procurement (ISODP) Congress in Dubai in Nov 2019. Moreovere, the society has won the bid for World Congress of Nephrology (WCN) March 2020 in Abu Dhabi however was cancelled due to Covid-19.

The society played a major role in collecting the data regarding the status of nephrology in the country, in leading the activities during World Kidney Day, and in conducting the first survey on organ donation public opinion.

Kidney health and nephrology are of particular interest for the UAE. The founder and much loved first president of the country, HH Sheikh Zayed Al Nahyan, received a kidney transplant in 2000. As a result, the UAE initiated the largest charity run in support of renal patients, research, training and public awareness programs, and the Zayed Charity Marathon, which is held annually in New York, Abu Dhabi, and Cairo.

The UAE has made significant progress in its healthcare system over the past 41 years. The healthcare sector continues to undergo major transformations to ensure that it is well integrated in order to meet international healthcare standards. Educational standards are rising rapidly in the UAE. Citizens and residents have taken advantage of higher education facilities, including establishment of postgraduate nephrology training, the Accreditation Council for Graduate Medical Education (ACGME) and the Arab Board Nephrology fellowship, throughout the country. Many foreign institutions, including American, British, and Australian universities, have established branches in the UAE.

## Future Perspectives of Nephrology in the UAE

The future challenges of nephrology in the UAE, as in many other countries, are to decrease the prevalence of CKD. Early detection and management of chronic diseases, such as DM and HTN, which are the main underlying causes for ESRD, will help in achieving this goal.

Indeed, there is always the need for promotion of a brain death diagnosis and deceased donation program, in order to achieve country's self-sufficiency through enhancing awareness, understanding, and acceptance from the public, patients, and healthcare professionals. In addition, the country's futuristic plan toward innovation, availability of G5 Internet, use of big data, and encouraging research could further help in disseminating knowledge and awareness.

## Conclusion

The UAE, even though being a young country, started offering complex renal services to the UAE and neighboring countries' patients since its establishment in 1971. While the country has made great strides, there is still much to be done in terms of disease registry, prevention, and achieving self-sufficiency in organ donation.

## References


1. Hamdi S, Shaban S, Mahate AA, Younis MZ. Health care reform and the development of health insurance plans: the case of the emirate of Abu Dhabi, UAE. J Health Care Finance. 2014;40(3):47–66.
2. United Arab Emirate/Institute for Health Metrics and Evaluation. www.healthdata.org.
3. Ram P. Management of Healthcare in the Gulf Cooperation Council (GCC) countries with special reference to Saudi Arabia. Int J Acad Res Bus Soc Sci. 2014;4(12)., ISSN:2222-6990.
4. Population by Emirate 1975-2005 (webpage on the internet). United Arab Emirates: National Bureau of Statistics.
5. Saadi H, Carruthers SG, Nagelkerke N, Al-Maskari F, Afandi B, Reed R, et al. Prevalence of diabetes mellitus and its complications in a population-based sample in Al Ain, United Arab Emirates. Diabetes Res Clin Pract. 2007;78:369–77. https://doi.org/10.1016/j.diabres.2007.04.008.
6. Alhyas L, McKay A, Balasanthiran A, Majeed A. Prevalences of overweight, obesity, hyperglycaemia, hypertension and dyslipidaemia in the Gulf: systematic review. JRSM Short Rep. 2011;2:55. https://doi.org/10.1258/shorts.2011.011019.
7. Sulaiman N, Elbadawi S, Hussein A, Abusnana S, Madani A, Mairghani M, Alawadi F, Sulaiman A, Zimmet P, Huse O, Shaw J, Peeters A. Prevelance of overweight and obesity in United Arab Emirates Expatriates: the UAE National Diabetes and Lifestyle Study. Diabetol Metab Syndr. 2017;9:88. https://doi.org/10.1186/s13o98-017-0287-0.
8. Razzak HA, Harbi A, Shelpai W, Qawas A. Prevalence and risk factors of cardiovascular disease in the United Arab Emirates. Hamdan Med J. 2018;11:105–11.
9. Hajat C, Harrison O, Shather Z. A profile and approach to chronic disease in Abu Dhabi. Glob Health. 2012;8:18. https://doi.org/10.1186/1744-8603-8-18.
10. Al-Shamsi S, Regmi D, Govender RD. Chronic kidney disease in patients at high risk of cardiovascular disease in the United Arab Emirates: a population-based study. PLoS One. 2018;13(6):e0199920. https://doi.org/10.1371/journal.pone.0199920.
11. Hajat C, Harrison O, Al Siksek Z. Weqaya: a population-wide cardiovascular screening program in Abu Dhabi, United Arab Emirates. Am J Public Health. 2012;102:909–14. https://doi.org/10.2105/AJPH.2011.300290.
12. Richards N, Hassan M, Saleh AK, Dastoor H, Bernieh B, Abouchacra S, et al. Epidemiology and referral patterns of patients with chronic kidney disease in the Emirate of Abu Dhabi. Saudi J Kidney Dis Transpl. 2015;26:1028–34. https://doi.org/10.4103/1319-2442.164600.
13. Alsahow A, Alrukhaimi M, Al Wakeel J, Alghamdi S, Alghareeb S, Alali F, Alsalmi I, Alhelal B, Bieber BA, Pisioni RL. Demographic and key clinical characteristic of hemodialysis patients from the Gulf Cooperation Counsil countries enrolled in the dialysis outcomes and practice patterns study phase 5 (2012–2015). Saudi J Kidney Dis Transpl. 2016;27(suppl):S12–23.
14. Alalawi F, Ahmed M, Alnour H, Noralla M, Alhadari A. Epidemiology of end-stage renal disease in Dubai: single-center data. Saudi J Kidney Dis Transpl. 2017;28:1119–25.
15. Al Shamsi S, Dhanhani AA, Sheek-Hussein MM, Bakoush O. Provision of care for chronic kidney disease by non-nephrologists in a developing nation: a national survey. BMJ Open. 2016;6:e010832. https://doi.org/10.1136/bmjopen-2015-010832.
16. AlYousef A, AlGhareeb S, Al Wakeel J, Al-Ghamdi SM, Bober BA, Hassan M, Al Maimani Y, Alkandari N, Ahmed HZ, Fawzy A, Pisoni RL, GCC-DOPPS 5 Study Group. Hemodialysis delivery, dialysis dose achievement, and vascular access types in hemodialysis patients from the Gulf Cooperation Council countries enrolled in the dialysis outcomes and practice patterns study phase 5 (2012-2015). Saudi J Kidney Dis Transp. 2016;27(6 Suppl 1):S42–50.
17. Al Sayyari AA. The history of renal transplantation in the Arab world. Am J Kidney Dis. 2008;51(6):1033–46.
18. Kumar G, ALIsmailli Z, Ilyas SH, Ayyash B, Tawfik E, Almasri O, Al Hadhrami H, Al Yafi Z, El Ghazali G, Alkhasawneh E. Good outcome of the single-center pediatric kidney transplant program in Abu Dhabi. Pediatr Transplant. 2019;00:e13566.

19. Algazali LI, Dawodu AH, Sabarinathan K, Varghese M. The profile of major congenital abnormalities in the United Arab Emirate (UAE) population. J Med Genet. 1995;32:7–13.
20. Al Talabani J, Shubbar AI, Mustafa KE. Major congenital malformations in United Arab Emirates (UAE): need for genetic counselling. Ann Hum Genet. 1998;62:411–8.
21. Abou-Chaaban M, Almurbatty B, Abdulmajid M. Spectrum of pediatric diseases in Dubai. Saudi J Kidney Dis Transpl. 1997;8(3):310–3.
22. Majid A, Alhalidi L, Ahmed BQ, Opelz G, Schaefer F. Outcomes of kidney transplant tourism in children: a single centre experience. Pediatr Nephrol. 2010;25:155–9.
23. Bernieh B, Al Hakim M, Boobes Y, Abuchacra S, Dastoor H. Pattern of acute renal failure in a tertiary hospital in the United Arab Emirates. Transplant Proc. 2004;36(6):1780–3.

# Part IV

# Europe

# Nephrology in Albania

# 34

Myftar Barbullushi, Alma Idrizi, Nevi Pasko, Erjola Likaj, Ariana Strakosha, Nereida Spahia, Ahmet Duraku, Saimir Seferi, Suela Mumajesi, Albana Gjyzari, Vilma Cadri, Matilda Imeraj, and Merita Rroji

| | |
|---|---|
| Area | 28,748 $Km^2$ |
| Population[1] | 2,862,427 |
| Capital | Tirana |
| Three most populated cities | 1. Durrës<br>2. Elbasan<br>3. Shkodër |
| Official language | Albanian |
| Gross domestic product (GDP)[2] | 15,059 million USD (2018) |
| GDP per capita[2] | 5239 USD (2018) |
| Human Development Index (HDI)[3] | 0.785 (2017) |
| Official currency | Albania Lek (ALL) |
| Total number of nephrologists | 110 |
| National society of nephrology | Albanian Society of Nephrology www.asn.al |
| Incidence of end-stage renal disease[4] | 2017 – 89.6 pmp |
| Prevalence of end-stage renal disease[5] | 2017 – 546.8 pmp |
| Total number of patients on dialysis (all modalities) | 2017 – 1259<br>2018 – 1260 |
| Number of patients on hemodialysis | 2017 – 1211<br>2018 – 1220 |
| Number of patients on peritoneal dialysis | 2017 – 48<br>2018 – 40 |
| Number of renal transplantations per year | 2017 – 24<br>2018 – 17 |

1. Institute of Statistics 2019
2. Albanian GDP – Gross Domestic Product Report 2018; https://countryeconomy.com/gdp/albania
3. Human Development Report for Albania 2018
4. ERA-EDTA Annual Registry data 2017 (unpublished data)
5. ERA-EDTA Annual Registry data 2016

## Introduction

The Republic of Albania is a country in Southeast Europe, on the Adriatic and Ionian Seas within the Mediterranean Sea. It shares land borders with Montenegro to the northwest, Kosovo to the northeast, North Macedonia to the east, Greece to the south, and a maritime border with Italy to the west.

Albania is fairly densely populated for a small country with 2.9 million inhabitants living in 11,100 square miles (28,748 $km^2$), with a population density of around 265 people per square mile. The very low fertility rate of just 1.49 children per woman, together with massive migration, has greatly affected the demographics of the country during the last decades. The declining growth rate in Albania is expected to continue in the coming years, with the rate becoming negative around the year 2027 and getting down to roughly −0.66% in 2050.

Tirana is the capital and largest city of the Republic of Albania. Albania is an ethnically homogeneous country, where the overwhelming majority of the population speaks Albanian, which is also the official language. It has two distinct dialects: Tosk, spoken in the south, and Gheg, spoken in the north. The country is a laic state, and therefore does not have an official religion. Religious tolerance is considered to be a fundamental value of the nation. According to Albania's 2011 census, 58.79% of the population are Muslim, while Christians account for 16.92% of the population. The official currency is LEK which is equals with 0.0081 Euro and 0.0090 USD.

The history of Albania forms a part of the history of Europe. During the classical times, Albania was home to several Illyrian tribes but also Thracian and Greek tribes, as well as several Greek colonies established on the Illyrian coast. In the third century BC, the area was annexed by Rome and became part of the Roman provinces of Dalmatia, Macedonia, and Moesia Superior. Afterward, the territory remained under Roman and Byzantine control until the Slavic migrations of the seventh century [1].

M. Barbullushi · A. Idrizi · N. Pasko · E. Likaj · A. Strakosha
N. Spahia · A. Duraku · S. Seferi · S. Mumajesi · A. Gjyzari
V. Cadri · M. Imeraj · M. Rroji (✉)
Service of Nephrology, University Hospital Center "Mother Teresa", Tirana, Albania


J. A. Moura-Neto et al. (eds.), *Nephrology Worldwide*, https://doi.org/10.1007/978-3-030-56890-0_34

In the Middle Ages, the Principality of Arbër and a Sicilian dependency known as the medieval Kingdom of Albania were established. Some areas became part of the Venetian and Serbian Empire but passed to the Ottoman Empire in the fifteenth century. It remained under Ottoman control as part of the province of Rumelia until 1912, when the first independent Albanian state was founded by an Albanian Declaration of Independence. A short-lived monarchical state known as the Principality of Albania (1914–1925) was succeeded by an even shorter-lived first Albanian Republic (1925–1928). Another monarchy, the Kingdom of Albania (1928–1939), replaced the republic. The country endured an occupation by Italy just before World War II.

After the collapse of the Axis powers, Albania became a communist state, the Socialist People's Republic of Albania, which for most of its duration was dominated by Enver Hoxha (died 1985). Hoxha's political heir Ramiz Alia oversaw the disintegration of the "Hoxhaist" state during the wider collapse of the Eastern Bloc in the later 1980s. The 1992 elections ended 47 years of communist rule [2]. The Socialist Republic was dissolved and the Republic of Albania was established. Albania is a parliamentary republic. Free-market reforms have opened the country to foreign investment, especially in the development of energy and transportation infrastructure. An amelioration of the economic and political conditions in the early years of the twenty-first century enabled Albania to become a full member of NATO in 2009, of the Organization for Security and Co-operation in Europe, of the Council of Europe, and of the World Trade Organization. Albania is one of the founding members of the Energy Community and Union for the Mediterranean. The country is applying to join the European Union. According to the World Bank classification, since 2009, Albania has been a country with medium income per capita. The last reported GDP is 15,059 million USD and the last reported GDP per capita 5239 USD [3].

## The Health System and Services

The Albanian health system is mainly public. The state provides the majority of services to the population in the domain of promotion, prevention, diagnosis, treatment, and rehabilitation. The private sector covers mostly pharmaceutical and dental services and some specialized diagnostic clinics and hospitals mainly concentrated in Tirana. The diagnostic and curative health services are organized in three levels: primary, secondary, and tertiary healthcare services. Public health services and promotion are provided in primary healthcare and supported and supervised by the Institute of Public Health and the Regional Directorates of Public Health.

In 2013, the Albanian government pledged to implement universal healthcare coverage and has since undertaken a series of steps toward the implementation of this model. During the past 3 years, significant results in improving health and medical services for the population were noted: Over one million citizens aged 35–70 are provided with an annual free checkup, achieving prevention and early diagnosis for chronic diseases. For the first time in public healthcare services, the services of the family doctor are free of charge for all citizens without distinguishing between the insured and the uninsured. Since 2014, the emergency service is operating during the tourist season; the hemodialysis (HD) service network once located only in Tirana was expanded to the main cities of the country, and the prices of drugs decreased by 30%. Health services in primary and hospital care are purchased by the Compulsory Health Insurance Fund. In 2015, by law, health insurance is compulsory for all economically active and non-active population. The Fund is funded by integrating the salary tax (3.4%) with the total budget revenues for the non-active population. Voluntary registration is provided for those not covered. Health insurance contributions increased from 23.02% in 2013 to 27% in 2015. Estimates put the current health expenditure for 2018 between 6% and 7% of the GDP or more than 1 billion USD, out of which almost 60% is paid privately [4].

## Brief History of Nephrology in Albania

Nephrology in Albania was under the Internal Medicine Service until 1985, and since that time it has been separated and now functions as an independent field.

Renal replacement therapy (RRT) in Albania started with the chronic HD program at the University Hospital Center "Mother Teresa" in 1985. The program was created mainly for the purpose of treating the head of the state Enver Hoxha, who suffered from advanced diabetic nephropathy. In spite of him never been treated with HD, the country had a great opportunity to offer HD to ESRD patients, but unfortunately, this remained embryonic for many years. Initially, there were only a few cases treated with acute kidney injury (AKI) due to septic abortions. After 1995, some acute patients were treated with peritoneal dialysis (PD). At that period, Albania was a country with an extremely poor economy, which meant that no more than just a few patients could be kept alive on RRT.

For more than two decades, the HD unit in the Department of Nephrology at the University Hospital Center in Tirana (in our days the University Hospital Center "Mother Teresa") was the only HD unit operating in the country, treating a total of 20 patients, for 4 hours, 3 times per week. All patients receiving chronic dialysis treatment were relatively young, less than 40 years old (mean age 29.8 ± 8.3 years old), and none of them was diabetic or had any significant comorbid illness. Patients over the age of 50 years, diabetic, and with comorbid disease were not accepted for dialysis; so, most

ESRD patients were managed conservatively. The reason for this very limited number of patients treated with HD was mostly economic rather than medical. New patients were admitted to the dialysis program only if one of the established patients died or received a transplant abroad (at this time there was also not a renal transplantation program in Albania). Only a few renal transplants were performed abroad at that time and were followed by nephrologists from the University Hospital Center of Tirana, helping to create the first experience with renal transplantation. Denial of dialysis to the patients was a desperate and painful situation especially for nephrologists [5–7].

In 1998, after the Kosovo War, the situation changed. The number of patients at the UHC "Mother Teresa" doubled, and a PD program of continuous ambulatory peritoneal dialysis (CAPD) for chronic patients was successfully initiated in 2003. In 2004, two other public dialysis centers were opened in Shkodra and Elbasan. The first living donor kidney transplant was performed in Albania in the private sector at the American Hospital in 2007 [8]. An immense "RRT gap" (the difference between the number of people receiving RRT and the number in need of it) highlighted the magnitude of the difficulties our country faced. Therefore, our first target was the expansion of RRT accessibility to reduce the RRT gap.

In 1996, Professor P. Zucchelli (Bologna), supported by the ISN (International Society of Nephrology), ERA-EDTA (European Renal Association), and Kuratorium Gesellschaft Nephrologie, led an effort to help nephrologists upgrade the field of nephrology in Eastern Europe, including Albania, the least known and perhaps most needy country in Eastern Europe at that time [9]. The goal of this mission was to obtain detailed information on the demography of renal disease and its treatment, the training of nephrologists in charge of patients with end-stage renal failure (ESRD) and renal disease in general, the academic life in Albania, and, finally, the scientific exchange of Albanian nephrologists with the nephrological community abroad.

The Albanian Society of Nephrology was founded in 1993 and had about 25 members at its inception. Currently, the Society numbers around 110 members. The Society organizes the annual meeting, as well as international and national continuous medical education (CME). Today, there are many ERA-EDTA and ISN members within the Albanian nephrological community, whereas it was impossible to have such a number of members in international societies two decades earlier.

The training of young nephrologists has been the most rewarding investment in Albania. From around 50 nephrologists in 1997, now there are about 110, and almost all cities in Albania are covered by nephrologists.

The focus of nephrology in recent years has been chronic kidney disease (CKD) and the increasing number of patients with ESRD.

## Renal Diseases in Albania

Chronic diseases present a significant challenge to the twenty-first century global health policy. Over the past years, an increase in the prevalence of RRT has been observed in almost all Western European countries, which is partly explained by the decreased mortality and mainly by the increased incidence rate of ESRD. Here it is important to underline the increased acceptance rate of diabetic and older patients. On the other hand, in developing nations, the epidemiological data remain poorly characterized for CKD due to few community-based studies, inconsistent assessments of kidney function, and no standardized or nonvalidated approaches. However, rapid urbanization coupled with changes in the environment, as well as numerous communicable and noncommunicable risk factors, indicate an already high prevalence of CKD that may be growing quickly. The growing prevalence of chronic diseases, such as CKD, has severe implications on health and economic output of these countries. The rapid rise of common risk factors, such as diabetes, hypertension, and obesity, especially among the poor, will result in even greater and more profound burdens that developing nations are not equipped to handle.

In the past, the epidemiological data on the incidence and prevalence of ESRD on a national scale in Albania have been largely unknown. The first study that tried to estimate the incidence of CKD in Albania was part of the PECO-93 project (Cooperation in science and technology between the European Union and the countries of Central and Eastern Europe and independent states of Soviet Union) initiative of the European Commission for the promotion of research collaboration between EU countries and ex-communist states to support these countries since the beginning of the reform process, in order to ease their transition toward a market economy [5]. The study was based on data collected by nephrologists in Tirana during a year, and the incidence of referred CKD and those accepted for RRT could be estimated. According to this study, in 1996, the annual incidence of CKD was approximately 116 patients per million per year, whereas 50–60 patients per million per year would be in ESRD and would need RRT. Around 77% of the CKD patients on the study were under the age of 40 and had no comorbidities [5]. Glomerulonephritis, the most common renal diagnosis, affected 26% of the patients. The exact incidence might have been higher because of screening difficulties, poor referrals, missed diagnoses, and lack of access to healthcare centers due to inadequate healthcare infrastructure. In the presence of a poorly resourced renal service in the immediately post communism era, the treatment with RRT was mainly provided to young people with no comorbidities.

For the first time in 2006, on the frame of INTERREG III Italy-Albania Program and in collaboration with the Regional Healthcare Agency of Puglia, a project was undertaken to establish a National CKD Registry in order to provide epidemiological information of patients undergoing RRT in Albania [10]. An electronic database of all patients receiving RRT (HD, PD, and renal transplant) was created, and all renal units following patients with ESRD submitted their data. The total RRT prevalence was estimated as 118.5 pmp, significantly lower than those reported in the national registries of Western Countries [11, 12]. According to the data of this observation, the number of patients receiving HD increased from 20 patients in 1996 to 86 pmp in 2007, demonstrating increased government support for the treatment of renal patients. Pyelonephritis was the main CKD diagnosis of patients on RRT (37.1%), followed by glomerulonephritis and adult polycystic kidney disease (ADPKD) with 16.4% and 6.7%, respectively. Diabetes type 1 and 2 were present only in 5.6% of the patients. Significantly, the mean age of patients receiving HD remained low (only 40.1% over 50 years old), and very few patients could afford renal transplant abroad. Until the end of 2007, 363 patients were on RRT, 60.6% in HD, 9.6% on PD, 26% were transplanted, and for 3.8% it was not reported the modality of RRT. HD and PD were the first RRT proposed for the majority of uremic patients in Albania [10].

The creation of a renal database under the INTERREG project was the first great experience and helped the implementation of the national renal registry. Since then, continuing active efforts have been made to collect data from all centers treating ESRD patients by HD, PD, and performing kidney transplantation. Each center registers new patients treated with RRT and provides demographic data, etiology of renal diseases, and outcomes information. Every year the data are sent to the national registry in the University Hospital Center in Tirana. Since 2011, Albania has been part of the ERA-EDTA ESRD registry [13, 14], and, since 2017, it has been part of the USRDS data system. In fact, the implementation of this database made possible the analysis of the evolution of CKD and the evaluation of epidemiological parameters in the population during recent years in our country.

Regarding the primary kidney disease as cause of ESRD in prevalent patients, tubule-interstitial diseases were the most common with 24.1% and 122.4 pmp, followed by diabetes mellitus with 15.9% and 80.4 pmp and glomerulonephritis (14.6% and 7.1 pmp) [15]. We do not have data on rare diseases, but we are trying to create a database, starting firstly with Fabry's disease diagnosing in dialysis patients. Chronic tubule-interstitial disease as a cause of CKD may be overestimated due to late referral and not clear diagnosis (Fig. 34.1), [13–19]. Due to the late patient referral to the specialist and only when the disease has progressed to its late stage, it is often difficult to establish the cause of ESRD. Although, it is important to underline that the unknown diagnosis, which have been relatively high around 27.6% in 2011, has shown a decreasing trend toward 14% in 2017. This is explained by a better follow-up of CKD patients and due to our continuous education program with primary care physicians. This program successfully started this year

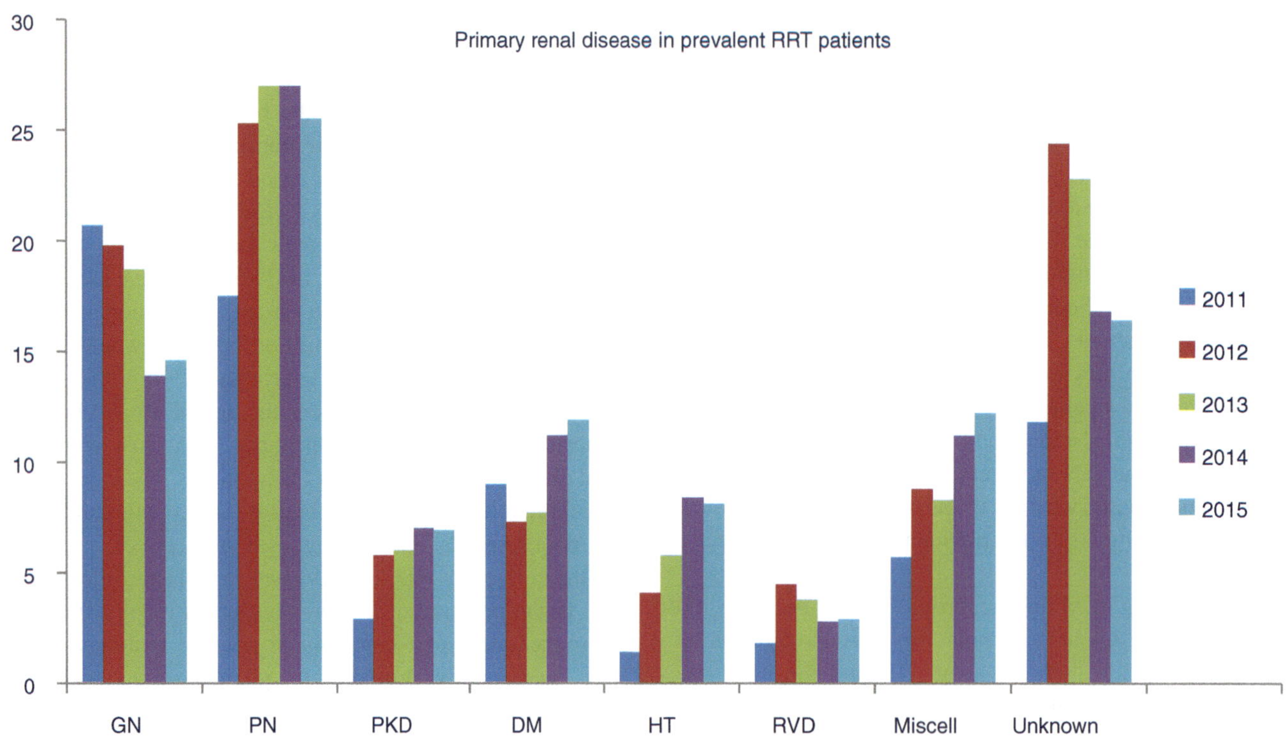


Fig. 34.1 Percentages by primary renal disease of prevalent RRT patients during 2011–2016

in Tirana with the topics: "Planned prevention for progression of CKD and its complications" and "Planned nephrology care." This was 5 days (5 hours each day) CME course, and after each presentation, the audience has to fill a questionnaire to evaluate the gained knowledge and to help the lectors to improve their presentations. We have planned to extend the program throughout the whole country.

Data about incidence, severity, and outcome of acute kidney injury (AKI) according to the KDIGO criteria has been only based on one reported retrospective cohort study. This study involved 382 adult patients (≥18 years) admitted in the cardio-surgical and polyvalent intensive care unit of the University Hospital Center "Mother Teresa," during 2007 (January–December); 46.1% of the patients met the KDIGO criteria for AKI during the study period. AKI patients were older, 60.5 ± 12 years vs non-AKI patients 52.2 ± 16 years; $p < 0.001$. RRT (HD) was needed in 1.6% patients. Complete recovery of renal function in the hospital worsened with the progression of KDIGO stage: stage I 71.3%, stage II 38.8%, and stage III 9.1%; $p < 0.001$. Mortality according to the groups was non-AKI patients 4.4%; stage I 12.8%; stage II 18.4%; and stage III 75.8%; $p < 0.001$ [20]. It is one of our foci to improve our recognition of AKI in Albania. AKI and CKD are closely linked and likely promote one another. As the number of AKI survivors increases, we need to better understand other clinically important outcomes after AKI and to identify those at highest risk and develop strategies to optimize their care.

## Renal Replacement Therapy in Albania

During the last decade, Albania has undergone profound political and economic changes. A greater government support has resulted in an increase in the number of patients receiving RRT, and after 2007, RRT, mainly HD, has been available for each patient with CKD, accompanied by a consistent growth of RRT.

Since 2007, the total number of patients receiving RRT constantly increased, and currently we have 1670 patients on RRT. This increase was especially due to the high rate of acceptance of patients on dialysis and increased number of patients that performed a kidney transplant in Albania. Over many years, the incidence of CKD patients who started RRT was observed to be higher in males compared to females. Based on published registry data in 2016, the incident rate was 104 pmp for males versus 57.6 pmp for females, and the overall incidence of RRT was 87 pmp (adjusted incidence). It is evident the number of incident patients is increasing steadily; during the last decade, this number increased from 76.5 pmp in 2011 to 88 pmp in 2016. Data about incident patients accepted for therapy at day 91 for each therapy are presented on Fig. 34.2 [13–19]. Although we had a slight increase in mean age of incident patients (from 47.6 years in 2011 to 52.6 years in 2016), it is still below the mean age in most Western European countries but similar to other developing countries [21, 22].

Regarding the cause of renal failure in the incident patients, the rates of patients with diabetes and hypertension have steadily increased in recent years, from 13.8% and 7.5% in 2011 to 20% and 12.2%, respectively, in 2017. However, we remain at the lowest level in Europe.

On December 2016, there were 1450 patients on RRT, 953 were men (50.6%) and 539 were female (47.9%). The adjusted (for age and sex) overall prevalence rate was 501 pmp: 622 pmp males and 373 pmp females. At the end of 2016, 1119 patients were on HD treatment; 47 patients (3.2%) received PD, while 251 patients (17.3%) had a functioning kidney transplant. According to data from renal registries, treatment modality rates have been relatively static over the last years, although a trend for increasing use of renal transplant has started to emerge in 2014–2016, while

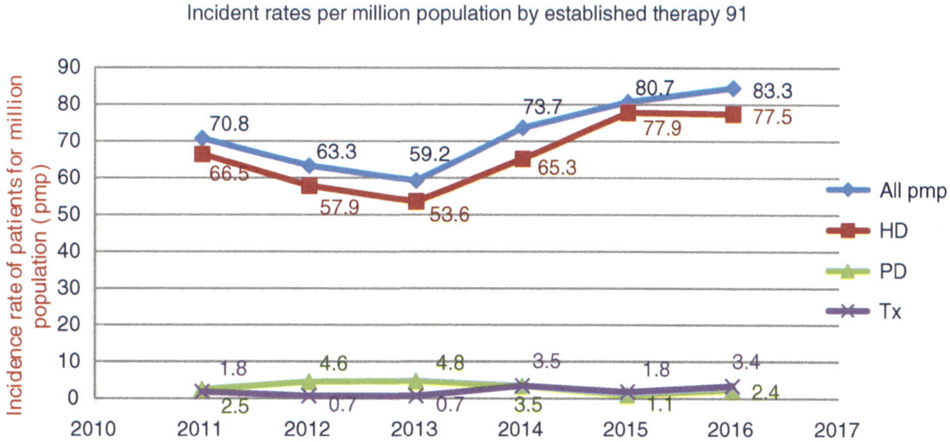


**Fig. 34.2** Incident rate of patients on RRT per million population. (Data 2011–2016)

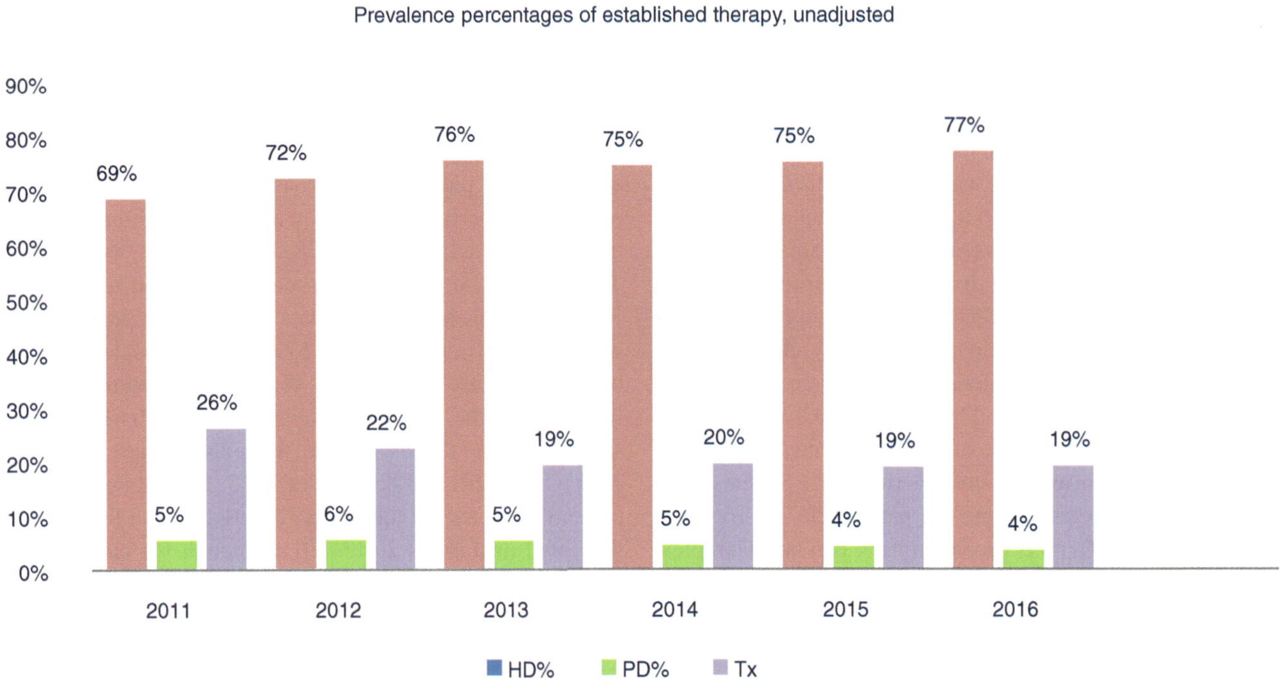


**Fig. 34.3** Prevalence percentage of established therapy from 2011 to 2016

the prevalence of patients with PD remained largely unchanged (from 15.4 pmp in 2011 to 16.4 pmp in 2016). Data on prevalent patients on RRT 2011–2016 are presented on Fig. 34.3 [13–19].

## Hemodialysis

HD is the main RRT in Albania, and the vast majority of patients, 94.9%, continue to start RRT with HD. An explanation for that would be the lack, until recently, of a program of appropriate education of CKD patients in the pre-dialysis stage, the late referral from the general practitioner, and the possibility to perform a kidney transplant only from relative living donors. In addition, we would say that a part of that reality would be explained by the private sector investments in in-center HD, which seems to be more profitable.

Currently, the number of patients treated with HD is around 1268 where 18.8% are diabetics. Based on registry data, the number of HD patients doubled from 2011 to 2016 (from 554 patients to 1119 patients) [13, 15]. Data on incidence and prevalence of patients on HD between 2011 and 2016 are presented in Figs. 34.2 and 34.3 [13–19]. Apart from public centers, private HD centers were opened, and, in 2015, we have the availability of private-public partnership (PPP) centers (PPP is one variety of partnerships, which has been largely used during the 5 last years in our country that can be established among public sector and private entities, aiming to use public infrastructure for offering private services).

Only 10% of patients are treated in public hospitals (two HD Unit, UHC "Mother Teresa," and Regional Hospital of Gjirokastra) and the others in the private sector (seven private centers and five PPP). All HD units in Albania have available only standard conventional bicarbonate-buffered HD with high-flux dialyzers. The reuse of dialyzers is not allowed in Albania. The average Qb (blood flow) prescribed in our centers in patients with AV fistula is 300 ml/min. Anticoagulation in HD mainly consists of a standard dose of heparin given as a bolus at the start of the dialysis treatment, with a mid-treatment dose to maintain suitable anticoagulation. In addition, low molecular weight (LMW) heparin products like dalteparin and tinzaparin are also in use. The mainly reimbursed regime of dialysis prescription is three sessions 3.5–4.5 hours per week. Occasionally, when it is evaluated for critical clinical condition, the patient could have four dialysis sessions per week, and in this case, the reimbursement is done based on the doctor prescription. In the UHC "Mother Teresa," we try to successfully apply incremental dialysis, and we are working through education programs to promote it. Hemodiafiltration, hemofiltration, and home HD are not available for chronic patients. The ratio of HD patients per nurse varies from 3.5 to 4.

Currently, dialysis for AKI is performed only at the UHC "Mother Teresa," but it can also be performed in main private hospitals according to individual payment. RRT options for

AKI include intermittent hemodialysis (IHD) in the dialysis unit and various forms of continuous renal replacement therapy (CRRT) in intensive care units (ICUs) using Prismaflex System (CVVHD, CVVHDF, CVVHF). Critical ill patients are treated mainly in ICUs where they are followed by an intensivist and nephrologist. For these patients, CRRT is available.

Since the beginning, HD treatment has been supported by the state. Currently, dialysis reimbursement is foreseen for all valid candidates in the context of offering the whole population free healthcare service, which has been a government program. The calculation of mean cost per session was firstly done in 2014 and is currently approximately 11,186 ALL (this is the value reimbursed by the Compulsory Health Insurance Fund for each dialysis session). In 2017, the value of reimbursement for vascular access was also calculated with the idea of starting dialysis in a planned manner, with permanent vascular access, and currently it is 10705ALL for AV fistula and 50.288 ALL for AV graft. Currently, among the dialysis patients, the percentage of AV fistulas, AV graft, long-term catheters, and temporary catheters is 71.8%, 3.6%, 11.1%, and 13.5%, respectively (unpublished data).

In the cost of the dialysis session, erythropoiesis-stimulating agents (ESA), intravenous iron, phosphate binders, or other medications such as antihypertensives are not included. However, they are also separately fully reimbursed (100%) for all chronic HD and PD patients based on these drugs' prescription protocols. The ESAs available are 2000 IU of epoetin alfa, 2000 IU of epoetin zeta, 2000 IU of epoetin βeta, and methoxy polyethylene glycol epoetin βeta in different doses. The main intravenous prescribed iron is iron sucrose, mainly used based on the results of ferritin and TSAT. Sevelamer carbonate is the only phosphate binder reimbursed, but neither form of Vit D nor calcimimetic is in the supported list of drugs.

We have had a high prevalence of hepatitis C in the dialysis units, reported 27% in 2013 and 25.4% in 2016 [23, 24]. One explanation might be the contribution of patients with long dialysis vintage, who have had a considerable number of blood transfusions prior to EASs' era [23]. The prevalence of hepatitis B in the general Albanian population is around 9.5% as Albania is considered an endemic country [25]. There are no infected patients with HIV in our dialysis units. We are trying to apply a strict policy for general infection control practices and follow-up monitoring to prevent transmission of hepatitis C and B. Implementation of infection control practice has already given excellent results translated into a very diminished incidence of hepatitis C and B in the last 3 years. Currently, the prevalence of hepatitis C is 15.7%, the prevalence of hepatitis B 5.2%, and the prevalence of coexistence of hepatitis C and B is around 1.9% (unpublished data).

Resources available for kidney care and opportunities for high-quality clinical practice for nephrologists are improving in Albania, although they are still lagging behind other regions of Europe.

## Peritoneal Dialysis

The PD program for treating chronic patients in Albania started in 2003 in the University Hospital Center "Mother Teresa," but it did not experience the same rate of expansion that HD has had. Being the only PD unit serving mainly patients with long distances from home to HD centers, it increased quickly, and this served to create a good experience for the staff and thereby to accept the concept of another RRT option. However, PD was not influenced by the ownership structure of dialysis facilities like HD and remained the only one in public university dialysis unit supported entirely with public funds. Nowadays the center has a well-organized CAPD program based on an "integrated care approach." Automated PD is not available. PD catheter is always inserted by a dedicated surgeon, having a very limited number of mechanical complications. In Albania, like most other European countries, there is a lack of manufacturing plants for CAPD fluids. Although the cost of PD was not officially calculated, it is around 85% of the HD cost and is totally supported by the hospital. There are one nephrologist and two nurses which care for all PD patients. The incidence and prevalence of CAPD based on the data of our national registry are presented in Figs. 34.2 and 34.3 [13–19]. The number of PD patients which have been treated in PD program for more than 3 months since 2005 is around 199 patients, 29.1% diabetics, mean age 53.3 ± 15.03 years old, and mean time in the therapy 32.39 ± 27.34 months. Around 7.5% of the PD patients have been transplanted, and 8.5% of patients have been transferred from HD to PD due to vascular access failure. Around 88.9% of patients have been on PD more than 1 year, 37.7% from 3 up to 5 years, and 19.8% have stayed on PD for more than 5 years. The annual mortality rate for 2018 was around 19.5%. The PD has been seen as an alternative for younger patients waiting in transplant list and for elderly patients with comorbidity (unpublished data).

CAPD patients and technique survival data in Albania are, at least, comparable to those reported by larger registries and by other centers recognized for their excellence in CAPD care. However, only conventional lactate-buffered glucose-based PD solutions (Dianeal PD4; 40 mmol/L lactate; pH 5.3 to 5.5 containing 1.36, 2.27, or 3.86% dextrose as appropriate; Baxter Healthcare PD solution) are in use, and icodextrin is not yet present. In an 8-year cohort study (2005–2013), the patient survival during the first year was 94.1% and in the second year 82.1% [26]. Cardiovascular mortality was the main cause of mortality in 53% of the cases. Higher comorbidity index, lower albumin levels, and lower residual renal function (RRF) were the main risk factors for worse survival. Technique survival was 92.3% during the first year, 79.5% and 69.6% in the second and fifth year, respectively, whereas the peritonitis rate was 1:43 patient months. There has not been found difference in technical survival between diabetics and nondiabetics patients. The number of peritonitis, high transport membrane type, and late referral were risk factors for low technical survival. Ultrafiltration failure followed by peritonitis was the main reason of transfer patients with more than 24 months in therapy to HD. Quality of life (QoL) was reported to be equal with that of HD, although PD performed better in some quality domains such as bodily pain, emotional functioning, and mental health [27].

The incremental approach of PD is a strategy that we are applying with patients that start PD in a planned way in order to preserve RRF and trying to improve the QoL of our patients. For 5 years, we have offered PD as an urgent-start method for CKD patients, mainly for patients being transferred from HD without vascular access supported by the surgeon for placement of PD catheter using the Seldinger technique. Patients have started PD after 48 hours in a continuous fashion, supported by the nurse until family training has been done. We found the strategy to be feasible and safe. The complication rate in our patients has been low and agrees with that of other reports in this field. In addition, we have had good results using PD for the treatment of CKD patient with congestive heart failure.

Although the PD program has stayed stable for more than a decade, the prevalence of PD in Albania is the lowest in comparison with other modalities. It is in the focus of the national program of the Albanian Society of Nephrology to increase the penetrance of PD in other dialysis centers. Good outcome results and the lower cost of therapy are two strong points that may help us in our initiative. Taking into account the advantages of each dialysis modality, it is the duty upon each nephrologist to adjust the requirements of each ESRD patient at certain times of his/her RRT life in order to achieve a better survival, a higher QoL, and a lower cost of the therapy. This is the complete concept of integrated care in RRT, which we need to spread also in other dialysis centers of our country.

## Renal Transplantation

Regarding kidney transplantation, the Albanian activity is limited to date to outpatient care of patients who have undergone a kidney transplant from living donors (in most cases) or from cadaveric donors performed abroad. The first living donor kidney transplant was performed in Albania in 2007 in the private sector, American Hospital [8]. In 2009 in collaboration with the transplant unit of the University of Bari was performed the first living transplantation in University Hospital Center "Mother Teresa," and there are also two private centers, American Hospital and Hygeia Hospital. Since then, more than 160 living donor kidney transplants have been performed in Albania, mainly in the private sector, but totally reimbursed by the government.

Currently, we are following approximately 360 transplanted patients. The prevalence is about 97 pmp, higher than a decade before, but still lower than the successful regional models. The number of new transplants performed on 2017 and 2018 was 24 and 17, respectively. About 70% of the patients are genetically related (Fig. 34.4) (unpublished data).

Mean donor age is 46.3 ± 10.1 years, and mean recipient age is 31.5 ± 19.2 years [unpublished data]. Renal transplantation from living donors is the main modality (about 90% of patients). The female gender is significantly more frequent

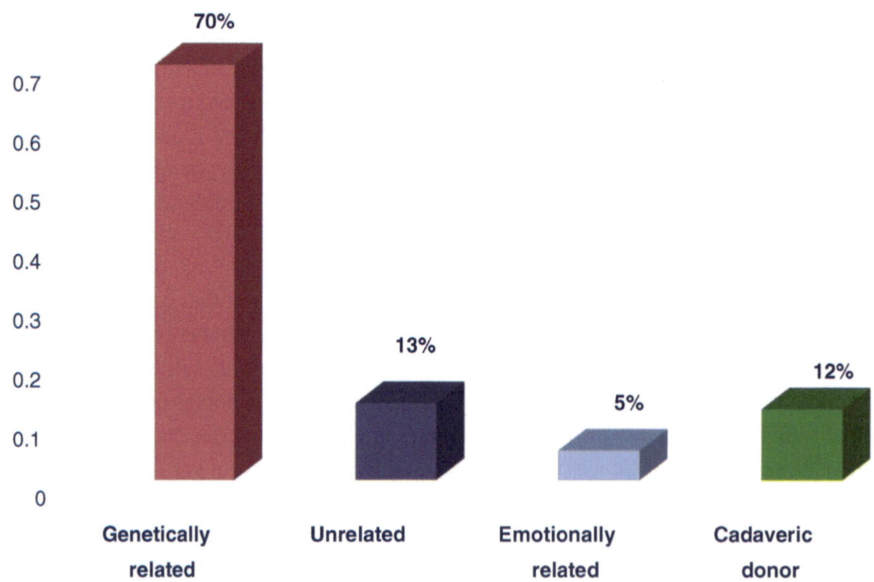


**Fig. 34.4** Donor-recipient relationship

among donors, which emphasizes the need for more gender equity as far as the altruistic willingness for organ donation is concerned. The posttransplant therapy is reimbursed by the State Health System for all the transplanted patients. Mainly immunosuppression schemes consist in tacrolimus, mycophenolate mofetil/Myfortic, and low dose of prednisone. A limited number of patients are on ciclosporin and everolimus.

Albania has only a living donor program, without any progress toward deceased donation in the last decade. The process of living kidney donation is coordinated by the National Transplant Center. Parents, children, siblings, relatives, spouses, or cousins of first generation may donate a kidney to a family member if they are matched. Transplantations from deceased donors are currently not carried out due to the lack of the infrastructure for performing it.

In comparison with those successful regional models, the observed deficiency can be attributed to the lack of proper organizational infrastructure, which lies within the absence of a competent authority or national transplant coordinator/body, and lack of regular public education, allocated funds for deceased donation, and transplant medicine, established registries, transplant waiting list management, and highly trained transplant coordinators [28, 29]. The number of kidney transplantations in Albania needs to be increased significantly by expanding it with paired exchange living donation and also by implementing an efficient deceased donor kidney transplantation program.

## Nephrology Practice in Albania

The Nephrology Care Service in Albania is organized as follows:

- 13 main public structures of nephrology and/or dialysis
- 7 satellite structures
- 11 private structures

The public system is organized as ambulatory nephrology care, secondary care organized in regional hospitals when nephrology is part of the Internal Medicine Service, and tertiary nephrology care which is the Department of Nephrology, Dialysis, Transplantation in the University Hospital Center "Mother Teresa" in Tirana.

The system needs to be better organized in order to be more effective so there is room for improvement. As the incidence of CKD escalates and the burden of kidney disease is so high for all countries, investing in preventive measures and educating the public and the medical community are necessary. Prevention and treatment of CKD in Albania are the responsibility of public facilities belonging to the national health system. Private facilities should also be organized through the Nephrology Society in order to be a better coordination between public and private, especially in the case like ours where 90% of patients in dialysis are treated in private and PPP structures. The Department of Nephrology at the University Hospital Center "Mother Teresa" has prepared a nephrology developing program for the period 2017–2021, with the aim to improve prevention, early referral, and treatment of CKD.

The mission of the Department of Nephrology, Dialysis, Transplant, at the University Hospital Center "Mother Teresa," is to diagnose and treat patients with kidney disease according to guidelines and protocols developed by the Department; to treat patients with acute and chronic dialysis (HD, PD); and to prepare patients for kidney transplant and follow-up after the surgery as well as training and education of the students and trainees of the Faculty of Medicine.

The main focus has been the implementation of the guidelines in the national nephrology care system. Based on the three main objectives of preventing, diagnosing, and treating CKD, the service is organized in units as follows:

- Clinical nephrology unit (including hypertension of diabetic nephropathy)
- Dialysis unit
- Transplant unit
- Patient unit
- Ultrasound unit
- CKD prevention and treatment unit (based on basic checkup examinations: complete urine, urea, creatinine) and CKD registry
- Unit of prevention and treatment of renal calculus and disorders of mineral metabolism
- Unit of glomerular pathologies (including renal biopsy)
- Unit of hereditary and rare diseases

Over the past several years, we have seen increased discussion of the clinical practice of nephrology, including utilization of ESA agents, agents for treatment of CKD-MBD, changing focus to CKD patients and their management, vascular access management, AKI, diabetes control, hypertension, cardiovascular events, etc. These interventions have posed a positive impact on the individual's and communities' health and a positive impact on the economy and constitute cost-effective interventions.

One important strategy in our national program is to increase the number of patients on stage 3 B referred from primary care physicians to nephrologists and decreasing the number of patients with late referral. We are doing it through an education program with primary care physicians.

Renal nurses are very important members of our medical team who care for patients in all stages of kidney disease, including the stage when it is necessary to replace renal function. Nephrology nursing encompasses the primary, secondary, and tertiary care of individuals with potential and progressive CKD, ESRD, AKI, and other healthcare conditions requiring nephrological intervention. Nephrology nursing involves both preventing disease and assessing the health needs of patients and families and education for RRT modalities. They are always trying to help patients to manage their life in dialysis. Their education consists in 3 years bachelor plus 2 years master degree. They actively participate in professional role development activities including continuing education, quality assessment and improvement, and the review and clinical application of research findings. In these days, we are facing with the emigration of high-qualified nurses to Western Europe countries.

## Future Perspectives of Nephrology in Albania

CKD is a growing public health problem in Albania. Our main strategy for the future of our society is CKD prevention and awareness of the population about renal diseases. Focused on that, in 2016, the National Program for Prevention of CKD was created in Albania with the objective of:

- Reduction of CKD risk factors in the general population
- Identification of individuals at increased risk for developing CKD
- Early CKD diagnosis and effective treatment to delay its progression
- Establishment of a CKD surveillance system at the primary healthcare level
- Good cooperation between primary care physicians and nephrologists to decrease late referral
- Improvement of PD program and extending it
- Improvement of living donation program
- Establishment of deceased donation program
- Creation of an integrated national nephrology network

Support by the government started the second part of the year 2016, screening for CKD patients a part of health screening for noncommunicable diseases to the age group of 35–70. In addition to laboratory tests such as blood glucose, lipids, hemogram, blood pressure measurement, urinalysis, and creatinine test were going to be included. Population screening for CKD is cost-effective in some studies when taking into account incident ESRD and fatal and nonfatal cardiovascular events. In addition, targeted screening for CKD in people with high blood pressure and diabetes mellitus is seen a more economically viable strategy. We considered screening a very important strategy, because the burden of kidney disease should be recognized and it should be prioritized alongside other highlighted noncommunicable diseases taking into consideration our health resources.

Besides, we saw that we need to prioritize the decrease of unknown diagnosis of CKD. We have started this year screening HD patients for Fabry disease, and nephrology is now part of the national screening including data and registry for rare diseases.

In addition to the effort from the professionals to improve the living donation program and prioritizing preemptive transplantation, the governmental support with allocated funds for deceased donation, updated legislation, and established national coordinating body is ultimately recognized as essential for the successful donation and transplantation.

We believe that an effective workforce is essential for delivery of high-quality CKD care. Based on that, the nephrology training programs were evaluated last year, and the nephrology training curriculum improved and extended from 3 to 4 years in order to align with current trends in technological advancement and development. In Albania, there is only one University Hospital Center training the new nephrologists. The trainees do not perform internal medicine before beginning the fellowship in nephrology. In addition, the self-directed study by the trainee has been emphasized, and competence to practice nephrology is presumed, in part, on the basis of adequate exposure to a program's curriculum.

Being part of multicentric studies across the region or internationally is one of the main goals of our Society of Nephrology in order to increase research activity of young generations and to increase the Albanian scientific reports.

However, the success of such strategies requires government support and health financing; we strongly believe that positive energy and willingness of our community will enable to fulfill all our goals.

## Conclusion

Nephrology in Albania has achieved great improvement in the last two decades. The possibility of treating every ESRD patient with RRT became a reality in the last decade, and this is considered our greatest success. Currently, we have a well-established living donor transplantation as well as PD program, which represent promising advances in both modalities. We believe that our national program for early detection and prevention of CKD progression and associated complications could help us in improving patient outcomes and reducing the impact of CKD on our limited healthcare resources. Advancing from the tradition of the old masters in our national nephrology, there is a young and energetic team of nephrologists throughout the Albanian territory who must achieve the goals.

## References


1. Elsie R. The early history of Albanian. 2012. www.elsie.de.
2. Albania | History, Geography, Customs, & Traditions. Britannica 2019. https://www.britannica.com.
3. Albanian GDP - Gross Domestic Product Report 2018; https://countryeconomy.com/gdp/albania.
4. Albanian National Health strategies 2016–2020. https://shendetesia.gov.al.
5. Khan IH, Thereska N, Barbullushi M, MacLeod AM. The epidemiology of chronic renal failure and provision of renal services in Albania. Nephrol Dial Transplant. 1996;11(9):1751–4.
6. Barbullushi M, Koroshi A, Tase M. Albanian contribution to the treatment of refugee renal patients from Kosovo. Nephrol Dial Transplant. 2000;15(8):1261.
7. Barbullushi M, Elezi Y, Idrizi A. Kosovo 2002: the epidemiology of renal disease and the impact of 1999 Kosovo war on end-stage renal disease patients. Nephrol Dial Transplant. 2002;17(12):2275–6.
8. Seikaly MG, Barbullushi M, Allabjeu K. A major milestone in the history of Albanian kidney transplant. International Albanian Transplant Team (IATT). Pediatr Transplant. 2008;12(4):402–6.
9. Zucchelli P. Report on a fact-finding mission on nephrology in Albania. Nephrol Dial Transplant. 1997;12:259–60.
10. Studio di prevalenza della nefropatia cronica in Albania. Programma di iniziativa comunitaria INTERREG III Italia-Albania. Final report 2009.
11. Moeller S, Gioberge S, Brown G. ESRD patients in 2001. Global overview of patient's treatment modalities and development trends. Nephrol Dial Transplant. 2002;17:2071–6.
12. Lameire N, Jager K, Biesen W, et al. Chronic kidney disease: a European perspective. Kidney Int. 2005;68:30–8.
13. Noordzij M, Kramer A, Abad Diez JM, et al. Renal replacement therapy in Europe: a summary of the 2011 ERA–EDTA Registry Annual Report. Clin Kidney J. 2014;7:227–38.
14. The European Renal Association – European Dialysis and Transplant Association (ERA-EDTA) Registry Annual Report 2011.
15. Kramer A, Pippias M, Noordzij M, et al. The European Renal Association – European Dialysis and Transplant Association (ERA-EDTA) Registry Annual Report 2016: a summary. Clin Kidney J. 2019: 1–19. https://doi.org/10.1093/ckj/sfz011.
16. The European Renal Association – European Dialysis and Transplant Association (ERA-EDTA) Registry Annual Report 2012.
17. The European Renal Association – European Dialysis and Transplant Association (ERA-EDTA) Registry Annual Report 2013.
18. The European Renal Association – European Dialysis and Transplant Association (ERA-EDTA) Registry Annual Report 2014.
19. The European Renal Association – European Dialysis and Transplant Association (ERA-EDTA) Registry Annual Report 2015.
20. Gjyzari A, Gjata M, Idrizi A, et al. MP292. Incidence, severity and outcome of acute Kidney Injury according to KDIG criteria between Intensive Care Unit patients. Nephrol Dial Transplant. 2017;3(23):iii533–4. https://doi.org/10.1093/ndt/gfx167.mp292.
21. Haghighi AN, Broumand B, D'Amico M, et al. The epidemiology of end-stage renal disease in Iran in an international perspective. Nephrol Dial Transplant. 2002;17(1):28–32.
22. Sakhuja V, Sud K. End-stage renal disease in India and Pakistan: burden of disease and management issues. Kidney Int. 2008;63:115–8.
23. Golemi D, Musta E, Riza F, Thereska N, Resuli B. Prevalence of hepatitis C virus (HCV) infection in haemodialysis units. Bull Med Sci. 2013;45(1):39–43.
24. Ulqinaku D, Basho M, Bino S, et al. Int J Ecosyst Ecol Sci. 2016;6(1):117–22.
25. Resuli B, Prifti S, Kraja B, et al. Epidemiology of hepatitis B virus infection in Albania. World J Gastroenterol. 2009;15(7):849–52. https://doi.org/10.3748/wjg.15.849.
26. Rroji M, Seferi S, Burazeri G, Thereska N. Patients and technique survival in patients on Chronic Ambulatory Peritoneal Dialysis. A eight-year longitudinal study. Nephrol Dial Transplant. 2014;29(3):223–32. https://doi.org/10.1093/ndt/gfu154.
27. Rroji M, Seferi S, Likaj E, Cadri V, Barbullushi M. Comparison of quality of life in patients undergoing haemodialysis and peritoneal dialysis. Nephrol Dial Transplant. 2018;33(1):516. https://doi.org/10.1093/ndt/gfy104.SP498.
28. Spasovski G, Busic M, Pipero P, Sarajlić L, Popović AS, Dzhaleva T, Codreanu I, Ratković MM, Popescu I, Lausević M, Avsec D, Raley L, Ekberg H, Ploeg R, Delmonico F. Current status of transplantation and organ donation in the Balkans – could it be improved through the South-eastern Europe Health Network (SEEHN) initiative? Nephrol Dial Transplant. 2012;27(4):1319–23.
29. Spasovski G, Busic M, Delmonico F. Improvement in kidney transplantation in the Balkans after the Istanbul Declaration: where do we stand today? Clin Kidney J. 2016;9(1):172–5.

# 35 Nephrology in Bulgaria

Evgueniy Stefanov Vazelov, Boris Iliev Bogov, Maria Simeonova Gaydarova, Marin Ivanov Georgiev, and Dimitar Lubomirov Roussinov

| | |
|---|---|
| Area | 111,000 km$^2$ |
| Population[1] | 7,000,039 (2018) |
| Capital | Sofia |
| Three most populated cities | 1. Sofia<br>2. Plovdiv<br>3. Varna |
| Official language | Bulgarian |
| Gross domestic product (GDP)[2] | 65.133 billion USD (2018) |
| GDP per capita[2] | 9272 USD (2018) |
| Human Development Index (HDI) | 0.816 (2018) |
| Official currency | Bulgarian lev (BGN) |
| Total number of nephrologists | 347 |
| National society of nephrology | Bulgarian Society of Nephrology (BSN)<br>www.bgnephrology.com |
| Incidence of end-stage renal disease[3] | 2018 – 160 pmp |
| Prevalence of end-stage renal disease[3] | 2018 – 630 pmp |
| Total number of patients on dialysis (all modalities)[3] | 2017 – 3863<br>2018 – 3893 |
| Number of patients on hemodialysis[3] | 2017 – 3627<br>2018 – 3655 |
| Number of patients on peritoneal dialysis[3] | 2017 – 136<br>2018 – 138 |
| Number of renal transplantations per year[4] | 2017 – 40<br>2018 – 25 |

Table references:

1. National Statistical Institute. Statistical data. *Demographic and social statistics*. Health. Available at http://www.nsi.bg/en/. Accessed (16.07.2019)
2. The World Bank. https://data.worldbank.org/country/bulgaria
3. Vazelov E. Dialysis treatment in Bulgaria in 2018. Academy "Nephrology" conference, Bansko 10-12.05.2019
4. Ministry of Health. Department "Education and qualification." Personal communication

## Introduction

The Republic of Bulgaria is situated in the Eastern European region. It is bordered by several Balkan countries – Greece and Turkey to the south and Serbia and Northern Macedonia to the west. River Danube is a natural border with Romania to the north, and the Black Sea forms the eastern boundary. The First Bulgarian Empire founded in AD 681 was one of the oldest European states and practically dominated most of the Balkan Peninsula for more than three centuries. During the reign of Simeon the Great, the territorial expansion of the state was most prominent. Bulgarian cultural influence over the Slavic nations by developing and spreading the Cyrillic script was also of paramount importance. In the early eleventh century, the Byzantine Empire conquered the Bulgarian Empire, until a successful Bulgarian revolt in 1185 established a Second Bulgarian Empire, which reached its zenith under the rule of King Ivan Asen II in the thirteenth century. After numerous exhausting wars and feudal strife, the Second Bulgarian Empire disintegrated in 1396, and its territories fell under Ottoman ruling for nearly five centuries. At present, it is a unitary parliamentary republic, which is a member of the European Union, NATO, and the Council of Europe. Economically it belongs to the group of upper middle-income countries, which has an impact on all areas of human activities, including medicine.

Nephrology in Bulgaria, as a narrow specialty in the field of internal diseases, emerged as such in the mid-1960s, and its regulation began in 1973. The initiation of applying dialysis methods for the treatment of chronic kidney disease, as well as in cases of acute kidney injury, dates back to 1958 and precedes the formation of nephrology as a specialty. The first kidney transplants were performed in 1968 (pediatric) and in 1969 (adult). At the end of 2018, the number of patients treated with hemodialysis and similar methods was 3655 and with peritoneal dialysis (APD and CAPD) was 130, and the number of renal transplant patients was 638.

E. S. Vazelov (✉) · B. I. Bogov · M. I. Georgiev
University Hospital "Alexandrovska" Sofia, Sofia Medical University, Sofia, Bulgaria

M. S. Gaydarova · D. L. Roussinov
University Pediatric Hospital Sofia, Sofia Medical University, Sofia, Bulgaria
e-mail: gaydarova@nephros.net



J. A. Moura-Neto et al. (eds.), *Nephrology Worldwide*, https://doi.org/10.1007/978-3-030-56890-0_35

The chapter describes the history of the development, current situation, and problems that need to be addressed in order to secure a better future for the specialty.

## Brief History of Nephrology in Bulgaria

Ancient medicine has left its traces in the lands inhabited by the Thracians and later by the Bulgarian tribes. Their knowledge and practice in times when standards, guidelines, and consensus conferences did not exist formed the ancient roots of sanitation and medicine in our lands. There are numerous archaeological artifacts showing skills in ancient town planning in regard to sanitation (waste pits and waste areas, proximity to fresh water in the form of lakes, rivers, springs) and in medicine (use of herbs and surgical procedures) [1, 2]. Mineral water from thermal springs was used as treatment of kidney stones, which can be considered the forerunner of nephrology [3].

In modern times, the first nephrology clinic in Bulgaria was founded in 1966 under the leadership of Prof. Georgi Magdrakov at the ISUL Sofia hospital under the name "IV Internal Clinic with Nephrology and Pulmonology" [4, 5]. Till that time, lectures in nephrology in the field of internal medicine training were taught in the Department of "Internal Medicine" of the Higher Medical Institute Sofia. After the retirement of the founder, the Clinic was headed consecutively by Prof. Atanas Maleev (1972–1973), Prof. Svetoslav Razboinikov (1973–1975), and Prof. Anjel Astrug (1978–1985). In addition to practical treatment of renal diseases, the 64-bed Clinic provided teaching, training, research, and postgraduate qualification. The first graduates of the main course in nephrology at the clinic in 1966 were Dr. Ivan Karastanev, Dr. George Toledov, Dr. Apostolova, and Dr. Boteva from Plovdiv, Dr. Nazarov from Rousse, Dr. Bratov from Burgas, Dr. Jeleva from Sliven, Dr. Angel Monov from Pleven, and Dr. Emilia Haritonova from Stara Zagora. After the establishment of the Medical Academy (MA) in 1972, Prof. Atanas Maleev, Assoc. Prof. Ignat Andreev, Dr. Georgi Stefanov, Dr. Mihail Bakardjiev, Dr. Shipkov, Dr. Tishkov, Dr. Gruev, Dr. Patev, Dr. Gochev, Dr. Mushomov, Dr. Stefanova (the last nine listed future-to-be professors and associate professors) as well as Dr. Gavrilov, Dr. Chukanov, Dr. Yoveva, Dr. Atanasova, Dr. Mutafova created the foundations of bulgarian nepkrology [6]. After the creation of the Medical Academy (MA), similar to other medical specialties, including nephrology, powerful clinical units were formed – initially centers, which later grew into institutes. In the area of kidney disease, the Scientific Institute of Nephrology, Urology, Hemodialysis and Transplantation (SINUHT) was established, including several specialized urological clinics and a two-part dialysis clinic. SINUHT initially united all nephrology units in two nephrological clinics – nephrology clinics I and II. Over time, some structural changes have been made leading to the establishment of two nephrology clinics at the Scientific Institute of Internal Diseases (SIID), led by Prof. Ivan Gruev and Prof. Nikolay Belovezhdov. The newly created nephrological units were aimed at initially training students and later testing new drugs for renal patients. The I and II nephrology clinics in SINUHT remained with their task of providing postgraduate qualification and continuing medical education for physicians. After the dissolution of the Medical Academy and the revival of the Sofia Medical University, the classical structures, departments, and clinics were reinstituted. Independent nephrology clinics at the Medical Universities in Plovdiv, Varna, and Pleven were led by Prof. D. Dimitrakov, Prof. D. Nenov, and Associate Prof. A. Monov. At the Thracian University in Stara Zagora and at the Medical Faculty in the Sofia University, nephrology teaching is held at the Department of Internal Medicine. In the district hospitals of Plovdiv, Rousse, Bourgas, Gabrovo, and Vratsa, there are also nephrological wards with experience and competent leaders [6, 7].

The impetus in the development of nephrology in Bulgaria was also partly due to acquiring the official status of a separate specialty from Internal Medicine, which took place in 1973 (Official Bulletin of the Ministry of Public Health No. 1, year XXIV, 1973). The first doctors who received this specialty certificate were Dr. Gena Stefanova, Dr. Dobrin Mushmov, Dr. Ivan Gruev, and Dr. Lyubomir Teodosiev – all of them have made important contributions to the development, training, and practice in Bulgaria [6].

The first pediatric nephrology clinic was established under the leadership of Associate Professor Angyozova in 1983, as a separate clinical center for the pediatricians, who were involved with the treatment of children with kidney problems and diseases. Three years later, in 1986, a specialized dialysis center headed by Associate Professor Adriana Anadoliyska started to function. The first renal biopsy in a child was performed in 1986; now it is a routine practice as part of the evaluation of patients with renal problems. In this same clinic, for the first time in Europe, treatment with recombinant erythropoietin for children with anemia, due to chronic kidney disease (CKD), was prescribed in 1989 [8]. For the first time in Bulgaria, treatment with recombinant growth hormone for children with CKD and growth retardation was implemented in 2000 [8]. The pediatric nephrology clinic with a functioning dialysis center, situated in the University Pediatric Hospital in Sofia, remains the only specialized clinic in this field in Bulgaria nowadays.

## Renal Diseases in Bulgaria

The whole population of the country and also the majority of the medical community live with the outdated belief that CKD are quite rare. According to the National Statistics Institute (NSI) data, the urinary and genital tract diseases were only 1.1% of the causes of death in 2005, and in 2006, they were even fewer – 1.05%. This percentage rises in the second decade – in 2018, out of a total of 108,526 deaths, 1539 were associated to diseases of the genitourinary system – 1.4% [9]. In general, the CKD incidence is underestimated, and this wrong assumption leads to erroneous planning of nephrological support in the country.

The first screening for adult CKD incidence was conducted in 2007, covering a total of 1982 people – 1366 women (68.9%) and 616 men (31.1%). Screened individuals up to 60 years old were 1600 (80.7%) and over this limit 382 (19.3%). The risk factors in the studied population were smoking 42%, hypercholesterolemia 22.4%, obesity (not graded) 49.8%, arterial hypertension (AH) 33.2%, and diabetes mellitus (DM) 7.8%. With estimated glomerular filtration rate (eGFR) above 90 ml/min, there were 1106 (55.8%); in the range 60–90 ml/min, 715 (36.1%); below 60 ml/min, 161 (8.1%); between 60 and 30 ml/min, 156 (7.85%); between 30 and 15 ml/min, 0.15%; and below 15 ml/min, 0.1% of the group. Microalbuminuria-positive tests showed an incidence of 27.2% (539), significantly higher (59.4% and 41.5%) in patients with DM and AH, respectively. For overweight people, the incidence of microalbuminuria was also higher than in the general population. For individuals over 60 years of age, the incidence of microalbuminuria was significantly higher than in the younger age, which was associated with the reduction in eGFR with age. In general, according to KDIGO definition, 514 individuals in this cohort (25.9%) have eGFR below 60 ml/min/1.73 $m^2$ and/or microalbuminuria/albuminuria, which shows a high incidence of CKD in the screening group [10].

In 2011, in order to early diagnose e-CKD patients, screening was conducted in randomly selected individuals in an outpatient setting, comparing data from electronic records (Internet) and other official sources for outpatient nephrology in a large Northeastern Bulgarian region. The data from the 2500 prospectively screened individuals included 1607 men and 893 women. The results showed that 7.36% of all patients had an eGFR below 60 ml/ min/1.73 $m^2$. Microalbuminuria was estimated in 8.16%; a total of 15.52% of the individuals met the KDIGO criteria for CKD [11].

Among males with CKD, DM incidence was 9.43%, AH 22.64%, and gout 10.37%. In female individuals with CKD, the results for DM 9.52% and AH 21.42% were very similar when compared to the male group; however, a lower percentage of individuals had abnormal uric acid results 7.14%. The conclusion of the study was that due to the lack of complaints in the initial CKD stages, it is rarely timely diagnosed if not targeted. An alarming finding was that about 90% of the patients after a first nephrological examination were included in dispensary and 30% required the onset of erythropoietin treatment [11].

Another pilot study conducted in 2017 [12] aimed at screening CKD in high-risk individuals and tried to establish a link between laboratory markers of CKD, AH, and DM and the number of risk factors. The screened individuals were 110 (70 female and 40 male) with a mean age 64.7 ± 14.2 years. The data showed a mean eGFR (MDRD) value for the group of 81.86 ± 25.88 ml/min, with only 40% of the patients with normal eGFR and 24% with eGFR under 60 ml/min or CKD. Arterial hypertension was ascertained in 67.3%, with only 24% of hypertensive patients achieving good control. Diabetes mellitus was found to be 21.8%, and obesity – 63.6%. Three of the risk factors (obesity, diabetes, and hypertension) were ascertained in 21 individuals of the screened cohort (19%), 2 risk factors (AH and obesity) were in 67 (60.9%), and 1 risk factor (hypertension or obesity) was in 7 (6.3%). Almost a third (32.9%) of the hypertensive individuals had an eGFR of less than 60 ml/min, whereas in the absence of hypertension, only 9.4% had eGFR below 60 ml/min [12].

Pediatric nephrologists, in the first decade of this century, carried out a screening of more than 5000 children from different parts in Bulgaria for renal malformations and other diseases with renal involvement, including Balkan endemic nephropathy (BEN) – 13.27%; different types of renal malformations in a study population of 6-month-old babies were ascertained [13].

Balkan endemic nephropathy, originally described in 1956, is a unique familial, chronic renal disease encountered with a high prevalence rate in Serbia, Bulgaria, Romania, Croatia, and Bosnia and Herzegovina [14]. The most prominent features of the disease are its endemic nature, long incubation period, familial clustering of the disease, and an unusually high incidence of associated upper urothelial cancer (UUC). There are no clear-cut data on BEN incidence and prevalence, since the studies carried out in different endemic areas yielded contradictory information. In spite of intermittent variations, the incidence of new cases has remained stable over time until the beginning of the new millennium [15]. However, it can be said that no more cases of Balkan endemic nephropathy have been reported in Bulgaria for more than 18–20 years. Although largely discussed in several previous decades, this endemic disease is not mentioned as a cause of CKD stage 5, not only in Bulgaria but also in other neighboring countries [16].

The implementation of the government program concerning the expatriation of all people from disease-endemic areas to other parts of the country played a huge role. It has been estimated that almost 100,000 people are at risk of BEN, whereas 25,000 have the disease. The clinical signs and symptoms of BEN are non-specific and often remain unrecognized for years. There are no pathognomonic diagnostic features of BEN, but the set of epidemiological, clinical, and biochemical data along with the pattern of pathologic injury in the absence of any other renal diseases are highly suggestive of this entity. Although the etiology has been extensively studied, fostering the publication of various hypotheses, only one of them has provided conclusive evidence related to the etiology of BEN. Studies conducted over the past decade have provided particularly strong arguments that BEN and UUC are caused by chronic poisoning with aristolochic acids (AAs). In light of these later studies, one can raise the question whether AAs could be responsible for previously and currently widespread unrecognized global renal disease and UUC.

The familial pattern of BEN suggests a multifactorial nature of the etiology of this disease, which potentially includes genetic predisposition of individuals suffering from BEN [17]. Indeed, combined effects of genetic and environmental factors might lead to the development of BEN, determining its clinical and epidemiological characteristics and disease progression. This hypothesis was investigated among various Bulgarian families, where family members suffered from BEN and included 4077 persons from 417 affected families [18]. The authors concluded that all patients with BEN belonged to families. Interestingly, even residents from non-endemic villages who were identified to be members of BEN families who had migrated from the places they were born (i.e., villages in BEN areas) were diagnosed to suffer from BEN. Moreover, in this study, epidemiological characteristics of the BEN disease indicated the involvement of genetic disorders, in which the proportion of the affected offspring was associated with the number of parents affected by BEN [18]. Accordingly, the risk of developing BEN was much greater in first-degree relatives than second-degree relatives and was considerable weaker in distant relatives.

To resolve additional genetic factors that influence the development of BEN, cytogenetic investigations were carried out. These studies aimed to investigate the impact of chromosomal abnormalities on the occurrence of BEN and the frequent association with cancer [15, 17]. It was shown that in healthy relatives of BEN patients born in non-endemic areas, a specific BEN-associated locus exists in 3q2 [19]. Alterations in 3q25 could also dictate genetic susceptibility for the development of BEN in relatives of patients having BEN [17]. More recently, next-generation sequencing (i.e., exome sequencing) demonstrated three mutant genes associated with the process of angiogenesis: *CELA1* (the gene of chymotrypsin like elastase-1), *HSPG2* (the gene of heparan sulfate proteoglycan 2), and *KCNK5* (the gene of potassium channel subfamily K member 5) [20]. Therefore, the authors suggested that abnormal angiogenesis may be important in the molecular pathogenesis of BEN [20].

Epigenetic modifications may also influence the development of BEN. In a case-control study, differentially methylated regions were identified which showed hypomethylation of the promoters of genes *HDAC11* (the gene of histone deacetylase 11), *IL-17RA* (the gene of 17 receptor, alpha subunit), and *SECG61* (the gene of protein translocase complex, SecE/Sec61-gamma subunit) [21]. This suggests that dysregulation of genes involved in immunological responses could be a mechanism in BEN pathogenesis.

In spite of all the above, weed control for *A. clematitis* plants alone would not be sufficient to reduce the incidence of BEN and aristolochic acid nephropathy. Systematic studies of AA levels in soil, surface water, food crops, and foodstuffs are needed to identify high-risk areas. In addition, it is imperative to develop water treatment methods and soil treatment methods and give priority to land and water recovery. Last but not least, local authorities must act in a timely manner to educate and inform their people about the existence of these completely unexpected toxic substances in their food and drinking water and the environment.

To summarize these several studies and also others, which are not discussed in this chapter, renal pathology in the country does not greatly differ from regional and global [16].

## Renal Replacement Therapy in Bulgaria

### Hemodialysis

In Bulgaria, at the end of the 1950s, with the active participation of urologists, Professor Dr. Anton Chervenakov and Professor Dr. Nikola Atanasov started the application of hemodialysis (HD) as a method of extracorporeal blood purification for urologic patients, where the underlying disease became complicated with acute kidney injury (AKI).

The first HD procedure was conducted in 1958 in the urological clinic of the university postgraduate teaching hospital "ISUL" by Dr. Mihail Karapandov with one of the two imported German-made dialysis devices "Nefra II," which were allocated to the "Alexandrovska" hospital and to the ISUL. The following year Dr. Emanuil Patev joined the team at the Urology Clinic and later became the first Head of the HD Department in the same clinic, at the end of 1961 [4].

The staff included two doctors, Dr. Petkov and Dr. Mutafova, two nurses, and a technician. Initially, there were cases of AKI, mostly in women with septic abortion leading to AKI. Subsequently, Dr. Emanuil Patev, who is the founder of HD treatment in Bulgaria, described his previous activity and presented a doctoral thesis on AKI, which was also the first one in the field of nephrology in Bulgaria [4, 22].

Later, Professor Dr. Georgi Stefanov and Associate Professor Dr. Mihail Bakardzhiev outlined the perspectives in the treatment of AKI. Other good connoisseurs of AKI were Dr. Todor Todorov from the dialysis center in the National Institute for Emergency Medicine "Pirogov" and Associate Professor Dr. Angel Monov in the university hospital in Pleven [6].

A conclusion can be drawn from all these facts, that the application of dialysis methods in Bulgaria preceded the start of university education in "nephrology" as a separate specialty in the domain of "internal medicine." A study of the incidence of CKD leading to end-stage renal disease (ESRD) conducted by Professor Dr. Anjel Astrug together with the Department of Science at the Ministry of Health has objectively identified the need for dialysis treatment available to the patients across the country. The first dialysis centers outside of Sofia were established – in Vratza (an area known for the high prevalence of Balkan endemic nephropathy) and consecutively in the following university hospitals, Varna, Plovdiv, and Pleven, in 1974 [4, 7].

Between 1975 and 1979, in-hospital dialysis centers were opened in Gabrovo, Burgas, Rousse, and Stara Zagora as well as in the Institute of Emergency Medicine "Pirogov." Over the years they have been developing specialists who have left a lasting trace in the Bulgarian nephrology – Professor Dr. Dimitar Dimitrakov, Professor Dr. Dimitar Nenov, Associate Professor Dr. Angel Monov, Dr. Hristo Genov, Dr. Rumen Bratov, and Dr. Velislav Anastasov. Since 1980, 32 new dialysis centers have been created in Bulgaria.

The organization of dialysis structures in all former district towns was followed by the opening of centers in regional hospitals. Altogether, 22 dialysis centers were opened between 1983 and 1986, bringing their total number to 65. In Sofia, during the same period, specialized centers were opened at several Institutes of the Medical Academy – for diabetic patients (at the Institute of Endocrinology, Gerontology and Geriatrics), infectious diseases (at the Institute of Infectious and Parasitic Diseases), and a pediatric dialysis center at the Pediatric Institute [6].

In order to achieve operational and scientific management of the entire dialysis network, a Coordination Center was established at the Medical Academy. It became a training base for all dialysis staff in the country for the management of HD and vascular access.

The main task of the Coordination Center was for a period of 5 years to develop 50 new centers in the country to cover all patients in need of HD treatment. The Coordination Center has grown with a limited care subsidiary in today's Hospital "Tsaritsa Giovanna - ISUL" and two holiday centers in the resorts of Albena and Sunny Beach. New units were opened at the Coordination Center: Surgical, Resuscitation, Computer, Technical, and Rehabilitation. At this center, a unique model was created for the first time in the world [4].

It is characterized by physicians and specialists with a different focus, united by an idea – dialysis treatment – internists, surgeons, nephrologists, cardiologists, neurologists, psychologists, physiotherapists, laboratory specialists, chemists, biologists, electrical engineers, and computer specialists. From the foundation until 2000, the head of the center was Professor Dr. Zdravko Kiryakov.

A specialized pediatric dialysis unit was established in April 1986 at the Department of Pediatric Nephrology, Scientific Institute of Pediatrics, Sofia. It is still the only pediatric dialysis unit in Bulgaria and is dedicated to serve all children with AKI and stage 1–5 CKD from all over the country. Patients with stage 1–4 CKD are consulted on regular basis with conservative treatment, including erythropoietin-stimulating agents and growth hormone therapy, monitored, and updated if necessary. HD and PD (CAPD and APD) are used for the treatment of children with AKI and stage 5 CKD. In a 30-year period ending in 2016, 697 children were treated in the pediatric dialysis unit – 235 of them with AKI. Moreover, during the same period, 92 children were transplanted.

HD is the predominant modality of treatment of CKD in the country with 97% of the total dialysis population being treated with HD. At the end of 2018, there were 80 dialysis centers in Bulgaria – 60 in state-owned or municipal-owned multiprofile hospitals and the remaining 20 in private multiprofile hospitals or free-standing dialysis centers. At the end of the year, 3655 patients were treated by HD in the country with approximately 4% (143 patients) on hemodiafiltration (HDF). The usual dialysis prescription is thrice weekly for 4 hours, but overweight patients usually are on extended HD sessions (up to 5 hours), or an additional fourth dialysis is scheduled. The largest center in the country is the Varna Medical University "St. Marina" Hospital, where 195 patients are treated with HD and, together with those on PD, the total number of dialysis patients exceeds 200. There are 8 centers treating more than 100 patients in the country.

The number of new patients starting dialysis treatment in 2018 was 1091 or about 158 per million population (pmp). Renal diseases leading to ESRD in these patients were diabetic nephropathy, 26.9%; hypertensive nephrosclerosis, 15.4%; chronic glomerulonephritis, 13.2%; renal vascular disease, 10.6%; chronic pyelonephritis, 7.8%; and others. The number of patients with diabetes mellitus is 765 or 20.9% of the total HD population, thus lower than reported from Western Europe, the United States, and most developed countries in Asia, but similar to other countries in the same region [16].

Two hundred and one patients (5.5%) had positive HBsAg, and 162 (4.4%) of the HD group were HCV antibody positive [23]. There is no official prevalence data for HIV-positive patients on HD.

The total number of deaths for the year 2018 was 945, with 197 cases in the first 90 days of treatment and 748 cases after this period. This is also one of the reasons for the sustained increasing trend in the HD population (around 1%), which can be observed in the last 3 years. A total of 1431 patients with AKI (postoperative cases in surgical and ICU wards and inpatients in therapeutic departments and clinics) were treated with HD and HDF in the past year. A total of 10,875 procedures were carried out in this cohort or an average of about 6 HD sessions per case. The lethality was 28.9% and the total number who died – 414 [23].

## Peritoneal Dialysis

Parallel to the treatment of acute and chronic renal failure by hemodialysis, use of PD also started in the mid-1960s. Prof. Dr. Ivan Gruev in cooperation with the following nephrologists Associate Professor Dr. Mihail Bakardzhiev and Associate Professor Dr. Emanuil Patev and doctors from other specialties (pediatricians, surgeons, microbiologists, laboratory doctors) started the use of intermittent peritoneal dialysis (IPD) [24]. Different aspects of IPD treatment predominantly in AKI but also ESRD patients have been studied – infections, method-related protein losses, and indication for specific patient groups [25, 26]. Consequently, the experience gained and the scientific findings reported enabled Professor Gruev to present a doctoral thesis in 1970 "Study on certain problems of peritoneal dialysis."

The introduction of long-term ambulatory peritoneal dialysis (CAPD) treatment in Bulgaria took place in the spring of 1984 in the Alexandrovska university hospital by a team headed by Professor Zdravko Kiryakov [27]. Due to a number of objective as well as subjective reasons, the number of patients treated with this method remained comparatively small until the mid-1990s. Subsequently, several nephrologists were sent to short- and medium-term specializations in different European countries and the United States to qualify for setting up CAPD treatment programs in several hospitals [28]. This resulted in significant increase in the number of patients on PD. A particularly important practical achievement is the massive use of the method in pediatric nephrology, where the method also has important advantages over HD. In 1993 treatment with CAPD in the pediatric ESRD patients was initiated, and in 2003 again for the first time in Bulgaria, treatment with APD in children with stage 5 CKD was performed. During the same year, PET test was started as a gold standard of individualization of the dialysis program. Between 2004 and 2006, the use of glucose-free solutions (Extraneal, Nutrineal) was also launched to expand the therapeutic options. During the last decade, APD has expanded its position, and in 2018, over one third of the patients on PD have the medical and social advantages of this method. In the last 10 years, the financing of PD has been changed, and medical insurance authorities pay a "day treatment package," which has stabilized the interest of the nephrology community in the use of the method. However, there are some obstacles for wider use of this method: the reimbursement of the surgical placement of the peritoneal catheter is not adequate, so the start of the method is hindered. Apart from this country-specific reason, there are several other drawbacks also typical for the whole Balkan region, such as the method being unpopular throughout patients and medical staff, small surface area of the countries, and hence nearness to a hemodialysis center and private sector investments in in-center HD facilities [16].

## Renal Transplantation

The concept of organ replacement and especially kidney transplantation (KT) inspired Bulgarian urology and nephrology community as early as 1963–1964. The Urological team, composed by Dr. Nikola Atanassov, Dr. Kiril Nikolov, and Dr. Hristo Koumanov from the Department of Urology at "Alexandrovska" University Hospital, started experimental surgery in rats and dogs exercising the suturing of vessels. The program succeeded in performing 42 kidney transplantations in dogs. In 1965, a fellowship at the Department of Urology-Kidney Transplantation Unit in Szeged, Hungary, was executed by Dr. Koumanov, as a final preparation before starting the kidney transplantation program in Bulgaria.

The first transplantation in Bulgaria was performed in a child on 14.12.1968 at the Department of Urology in the Institute for Emergency Medicine "Pirogov" by Professor Nikolai Minkov. Both kidneys were taken and transplanted with the ureters implanted on the skin. Unfortunately, the kidneys failed to produce urine. The first successful cadaver kidney transplantation was performed on 01.02.1969 at the Department of Urology in "Alexandrovska" University Hospital by Dr. Lambev, Dr. Nikola Atanasov, and Dr. Hristo Koumanov [29].

Although the first pediatric renal transplant in Bulgaria was performed more than 50 years ago, there is a tendency for the problem to be neglected by authorities, since currently there is no such activity. During the years, there were periods with relative increase in the number of pediatric renal transplants, but in general the rate was far from needed, and a lot of patients received renal transplants abroad. From 2004 to 2010, a joint Bulgarian-French program for development of pediatric renal transplantation was functioning to secure appropriate training for doctors and nurses. Under this program six pediatric renal transplantations were done with very good results. However, it was stopped by the Executive Agency "Medical Supervision" in 2010, and no more pediatric renal transplantations were performed in the country since then. Nevertheless, a lot of patients received a graft abroad – in the European Union (EU) or neighboring countries. All of them are followed thereafter at the pediatric dialysis unit.

Between 1969 and 1994, the legislation for organ donation allowed only taking organs from deceased donors. In 1994, the program for living-related donor renal transplantation was initiated with the changes in legislation allowing a kidney to be taken from a living donor. The program, however, had the limitations that only first-degree relatives such as parent, brother, and sister were considered potential donors. From 1994 to 1998, the program expanded, and 128 transplantations from living donors were performed.

There are two working programs for kidney transplantation right now – deceased and living donor. According to unpublished data (personal communication), 1-year graft survival is 80% and 10-year 58%. Reimbursement is secured by the Ministry of Health (MoH) and not by the National Health Insurance Fund (NHIF). It is 20,000 BGN (10,225 Euro) for the KT, up to 10,000 BGN (5112 Euro) for complications related to the operation and hospital stay, and 5000 BGN (2556 Euro) in case removal of the transplanted kidney is required. Cellcept and Advagraf are most widely used drugs in the immunosuppression schemes, and their reimbursement is also covered by the MH. Drug levels are individually monitored in a laboratory. The administration, regulation, waiting-list actualization, all documentation, coordination, and reimbursement are procured by the MoH and the Executive Agency "Medical Supervision" for transplantation, which are the administrative organs by the existing legislation.

There are 33 donor centers appointed by the Ministry of Health across the country as well as 3 centers for kidney transplantation. All expenses concerning donor identification, donor conditioning, kidney explantation, transplantation, follow-up, and complications are reimbursed by the MoH. The reimbursement rate is not attractive for the staff and not sufficient for the hospitals to cover all expenses, and most of the time, they generate financial negative results. The acting reimbursement policy logically leads to relatively low number of donor situations and transplantation accordingly. For example, in 2019 a total of 36 kidney transplantations (23 deceased and 13 living donor) were done which is 5 pmp. Compared to the number of kidney transplantations in Europe which ranges from 3 in Ukraine to 97 in Spain's Catalonia, this rate is very low [30]. Since the first one, approximately 1500 kidney transplantations have been performed. The precise number for the period between 1973 and 2009 was 972 (Fig. 35.1) and for the period between 2014 and 2019 was 243 kidney transplants.

Meanwhile, the appointed donor centers and transplantation units are well equipped, and the staff is well trained and experienced to perform far bigger number of transplantations. With respect to this, a considerable effort and social discussions have been initiated during the last years for implementation of a more effective kidney transplantation program.

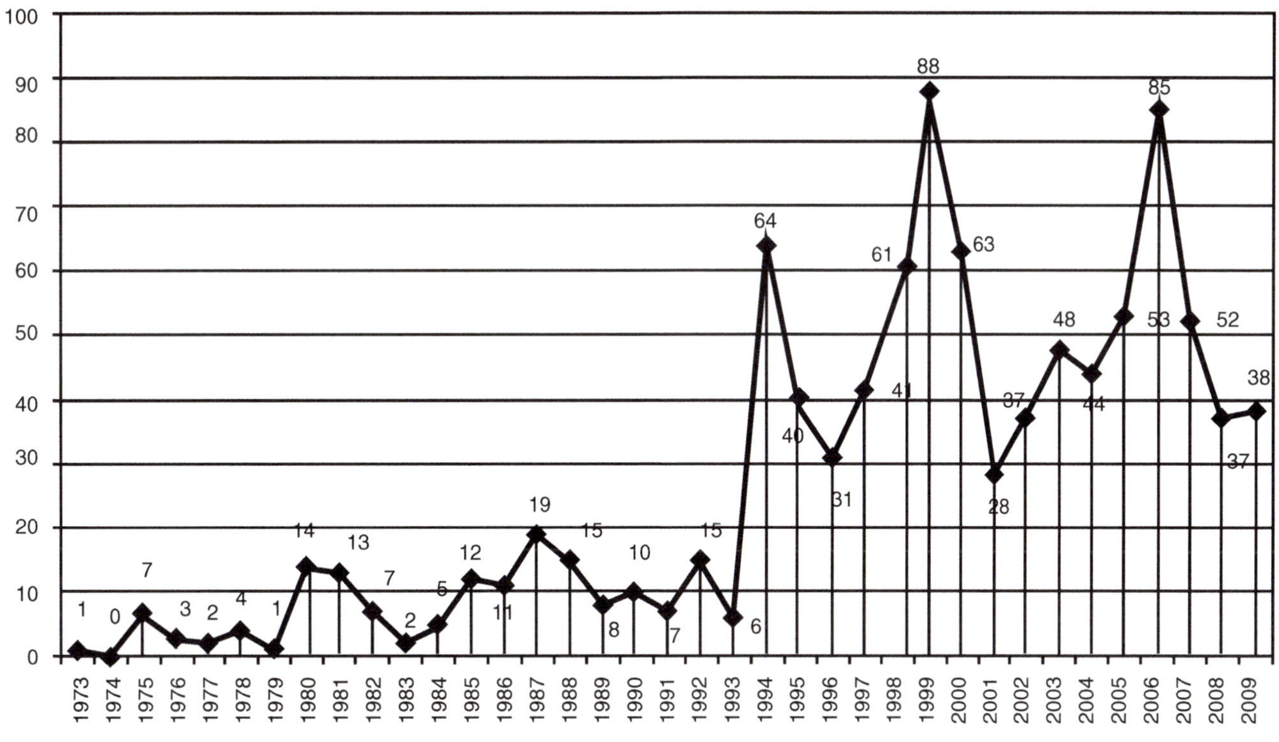


**Fig. 35.1** Total number of renal transplants by year (1973–2009)

## Nephrology Practice in Bulgaria

Prior to 2007 (Bulgaria's inclusion to the European Union), the specialty "nephrology" was acquired after receiving a specialty in "internal medicine." Specialization lasting 5 years in clinics and wards designated by the MoH for training bases was required as prerequisite to take the exam. After acquiring a specialty in "internal medicine" and in order to pass the exam and receive a specialty in "nephrology," additional specialization was required for 2 years in clinics and departments designated by the MoH as training basis in "nephrology." Thus, the training and acquisition of this specialty lasted, at least, 7 years.

After 2007, as a result of changes largely influenced by the idea of aligning specialization requirements with those in the European Union, nephrology became a first specialty, and no prior acquisition of an internal diseases specialty has been required. The amendment came into force with the adoption of Ordinance No. 34 of the Ministry of Health (Official Gazette No. 7/23.01.2007), which defined a training period of 4 years, which also includes 12 months of training in "internal diseases."

During the remaining 36 months, the training requires 24 months of clinical nephrology, 12 months of dialysis and kidney transplantation, and colloquiums. Over the next 12 years after its promulgation, the regulation has undergone several changes in terms of certain requirements and funding of training. From the beginning of its application until now, 117 nephrologists have acquired the specialty, and to date, the number of specializing fellows is 89. The overall number of certified nephrologists in the country is 347, but an uncertain number of them have retired. There is a tendency of aging, and the number of practicing nephrologists over 60 years of age is already 145, which can be analyzed as a negative trend (Ministry of Health, Department , 2019, Education and qualification, personal communication).

Pediatric nephrology was recognized as a subspecialty in Bulgaria in 2005. The training is 2 years as a second specialty after "pediatrics" and is under a common European syllabus. There are 21 pediatric nephrologists currently in Bulgaria, 4 of them retired, but some still practicing.

Nephrology in general is practiced in three kinds of medical establishments – outpatient clinics, hospital wards/clinics, and dialysis centers. The latter are predominantly part of hospitals (public, municipal, or private), but there are also free-standing dialysis structures. The ratio of public/private dialysis facilities is 3/1 as the number of the private has reached the figure of 20 out of a total of 80. "Home dialysis" and "limited care" programs do not exist in the country, and thus patient's choice of treatment methods is limited. Most dialysis facilities offer night shifts, which helps working patients keep their employment.

In all medical specialties, hospital admissions of health-insured persons are reimbursed by the National Health Insurance Fund through "clinical pathways" serving as algorithm for the order, volume, and to a certain extent quality of medical services, but also as a financial instrument. Nephrology wards/clinics are dependent on the quantity of patients admitted, since their number and the evaluation of the "clinical pathway" under which they are hospitalized form their financial status.

In 2017, the total number of hospital admissions for "diseases of genitourinary system" (Chapter XIV, block N00-N99 according to ICD-10) was 161,389, which formed 6.9% of the total of 2,258,579 hospitalizations in the country. There is also the assumption that in this chapter a large number of urological admissions are included. The real presence of strictly nephrology hospitalizations was close to one third of this total or 54,569 – approximately 2.3% – of hospital admissions [31, 32]. The largest number of nephrology admissions is for acute and chronic exacerbated pyelonephritis with 32,327 cases in 28,968 individuals, followed by already specified chronic glomerulonephritis – 10,218 admissions of 6055 patients. The hospitalizations for newly discovered glomerular diseases were 2134 of 1950 individuals. The number of hospital admissions for CKD (stages 1–5) was 4723 in 3742 patients and in AKI (conservatively or dialysis treated) 3167 in 3072 individuals [32].

Since 2012, financing of dialysis is procured also by the NHIF on the basis of annual contracts – appendix 18C for ambulatory procedures and appendix 19A for clinical procedures [31]. All HD disposables, PD solutions, all medications used to treat acute complications throughout the procedure and also for the treatment of chronic complications (anemia, CKD-MBD) and transport are included in the reimbursement which is as follows:

- Ambulatory procedure 1 (Apr. No. 1) "Chronic hemodialysis" is paid 170 Bulgarian lev (BGN) which is equivalent to 87 Euro.
- Apr. No. 2 ("Peritoneal dialysis with apparatus") – 130 BGN (66 Euro)/package/day.
- Apr. No. 3 ("Peritoneal dialysis without apparatus") – 93 BGN (47 Euro)/package/day.
- Clinical Procedure 1 (CPr. No. 01) "Dialysis treatment in acute conditions" – 170 BGN (87 Euro).

The total number of HD sessions performed for the whole 2018 was 575,938 with 565,153 in chronic HD patients (Apr. No 1) and 10,875 in CPr. No 1 [23]. The number of nursing staff has dramatically decreased in the country in the last 30 years from approximately 80,000 to a little bit more than 32,000, which is a tendency that has not bypassed renal nurses also [32]. Their number is still higher compared to neighboring countries in the region [16], but the trend of aging without adequate substitution with new graduates must be considered as a potential threat. There are no staff renal dietitians to provide the necessary dietary counseling to the patients on dialysis, and their responsibilities are to a certain extent taken by nephrologists, fellows, and nurses.

## Future Perspectives of Nephrology in Bulgaria

The issue of the financial valuation of dialysis activities is not persistently discussed at meetings between representatives of the NHIF, the Bulgarian Doctors Union (BDU), and the nephrological community. The price set for the most commonly used APr. 1 "Chronic hemodialysis" (including both labor and consumables, expensive drugs, and transport to and from the dialysis structure) has not changed in the last 5 years before 2020, when it was increased by 18%.

Even though, it is inadequately low in Bulgaria compared to even neighboring countries in the region with similar economic indicators – for example, in Northern Macedonia, it is about 7% higher; in Romania, about 35% higher; and in Greece, Croatia, and Slovenia, at an even higher price. The neglect of the objective, need to increase the price, leads to an inability to accumulate funds for periodic updating of the equipment and adequate remuneration of the staff. For this reason, the shortage of medical staff is increasingly felt, which is also affecting the quality of the activity. The single estimate of 170 BGN (87 Euro) equated to conventional HD also holds back the development of more modern methods such as HDF. The lack of a positive solution – an increase in the price – will deepen the demotivation of the staff and will generally create a tendency for the country to lag behind in this medical activity. There is a recent change in HD price, effective from the beginning of 2020 – from 144 BGN to 170 BGN for a dialysis session (PD payment is unchanged), but even though it is still lower compared to neighboring countries.

Surprisingly, low evaluation of dialysis activities does not stop private initiative to open new dialysis facilities. In a period of 12 years, 20 dialysis structures have started to function receiving accreditation by the MoH and contracts with the NHIF. The highest number of privately owned dialysis facilities is in the largest towns of the country – Sofia and Plovdiv – with three dialysis centers each. In smaller regional towns, opening of new private establishments is usually hindered by lack of adequately trained medical staff. This, on the other hand, can stimulate increased interest of starting fellowship in nephrology and qualification for renal nurses.

Concerning kidney transplantation, it is obvious that the greatest challenge is to overcome the low number of donors and the long waiting list – 1151 patients on dialysis program. The statistics is showing that in 22% of all identified donors, the relatives refused to give consent for donor donation, which is obligatory by the law, and this additionally decreases the number of cadavers.

Changes of the law for deceased donor donation as well as new rules for reimbursement are on the way. New perspectives are given as well as to the legislation and regulations regimen for living donor donation and including the possibilities for direct donation of biologically unrelated person and paired donation chains.

A closer collaboration program is initiated with the Health Commission of the European Parliament for financial aid allowing for modernization of sanitary aviation used for transport during donor situations. Since April 2019 Bulgaria started a program for joining Eurotransplant.

A problem which needs urgent attention is kidney transplantation in children as in Bulgaria there is no formal program active at present. With the initiative of the Ministry of Health for organizing National Pediatric Center, such a program is strongly considered and will be the mainstay of pediatric kidney transplantation in Bulgaria. Another unsolved problem in pediatric nephrology is the treatment and access to expensive medications, still not registered in the NHIF, which are not reimbursed.

In the "National Program for Nephrology and Dialysis Treatment 2001–2005," approved by the Council of Ministers at the end of 2000, there was a regulation stating that a full-scale national registry should be functioning by the end of the year 2004. Unfortunately, this program was not properly funded and also not extended into the period that followed, which had a negative impact on the overall development of nephrology as a specialty.

In general, lack of application of electronic health card as universal document is still a problem in Bulgaria, which, if settled, will improve registration and financial accountancy not only in nephrology.

## Conclusion

Early prevention and diagnosis of kidney disease is a problem that must be addressed as a matter of priority in accordance with the well-known slogan of the World Kidney Day 2007: "CKD: Common, Harmful, and Treatable" [33]. Medically and financially, it is much more cost-effective when an illness is treated in an early stage, which reduces costs and increases life expectancy.

Nephrology has a long history of development in Bulgaria. The level described in this chapter should not be taken for granted, as it can undergo changes in both positive and negative directions. The projected demographic crisis related to the aging of the population, as well as its decline, which is manifesting in Bulgaria in a particularly severe form, initially changes the needs for health services. Healthcare is a conservative system where changes are difficult to implement and also is a sector that requires huge financial resources. Funding of the system is an issue that has always sparked much discussion, but both in Bulgaria and globally, nephrology, in particular the treatment of CKD patients, is one of the most expensive medical activities. In this sense, the wider development of "home methods" such as peritoneal dialysis and efforts to expand transplant activity are fully justified in the country.

Staffing is also an issue that will become deeper and deeper, which is why an active policy is needed to retain and train healthcare personnel to meet the needs of the system. There is a great danger that some of the specialties that are not considered attractive, including nephrology, will be left without sufficient staff resources.

## References


1. Apostolov M. History of medicine. Sofia: Medicine and Physical Education Publishers; 1977. 176 p. (In Bulgarian).
2. Pamukova R, Radev E, Vizeva M. Why Thracians were the most long-lived people in antiquity? Trakia J Sci. 2018;16(1):97–104.
3. Nenov D, Nenov V, Lazarov G, et al. Treatment of renal stones in Bulgaria in ancient times ("Hissarya" baths). Am J Nephrol. 1999;19:163–4.
4. Kiryakov Z. History of nephrology, hemodialysis and transplantation in the Republic of Bulgaria. Nephrol, Hemodial and Transpl. 2006;3:5–10. (In Bulgarian)
5. Paskalev E. Clinical Center of Nephrology. In: Georgiev M, editor. 100 years Medical Faculty 1917–2017. Sofia: "St. Georgi Pobedonosets" Ltd.; 2017, ISBN 978-619-7283-13-6; 290-4. (In Bulgarian).
6. Kiryakov Z, Antonov S, Vazelov E, et al. History of nephrology, hemodialysis and transplantation in the Republic of Bulgaria. Asclepius. 2007;1:39–45. (In Bulgarian).
7. Vazelov E. History of dialysis treatment in Bulgaria. In: Paskalev E, editor. Nephrology. Sofia: Bulgarresurs Publishers; 2015. p. 701–3. ISBN 978-954-8885-18-8. (In Bulgarian).
8. Anadoliyska A, Roussinov D, Miteva P. ESRD in Childhood - 10 years of experience in children's dialysis center in Bulgaria. Pediatrics. 1996;3:16–8. (In Bulgarian).
9. National Statistical Institute. Statistical data. *Demographic and social statistics*. Health. Available at: http://www.nsi.bg/en/. Accessed 16 July 2019.
10. Krivoshiev S, Kraev Z, Todorov V, et al. Curr Nephrol. 2007;3–4:3–9. (In Bulgarian).
11. Madzhova V. Opportunities for early diagnosis of chronic outpatient kidney disease. Gen Med. 2011;3:4–6. (In Bulgarian).
12. Lyubomirova M, Georgieva I, Ivanov G, et al. Chronic kidney disease screening - when, how, why ? Mod Med. 2018;2:3–10. (In Bulgarian).
13. Boueva A, Marinova S, Miteva P, et al. The incidence of kidney anomalies among Bulgarian children. 45-th Annual Scientific Meeting of the European Society for Paediatric Nephrology, 6–8 September, 2012, Krakow, Poland (poster presentation).
14. Tanchev Y, Evstatiev Z, Dorossiev D, et al. Studies on the nephritides in the District of Vratza. Savremenna Medicina. 1956;7:14–29. (In Bulgarian).
15. Nenov VD, Nenov DS. Balkan nephropathy: a disorder of renal embryogenesis? Am J Nephrol. 2002;22:260–5.
16. Spasovski G, Rroji M, Vazelov E, et al. Nephrology in the Eastern and Central European region: challenges and opportunities. Kidney Int. 2019;96:287–90.
17. Toncheva D, Dimitrov T. Genetic predisposition to Balkan endemic nephropathy. Nephron. 1996;4:564–9.
18. Toncheva D, Dimitrov T, Stojanova S. Etiology of Balkan endemic nephropathy: a multifactorial disease? Eur J Epidemiol. 1998;4:389–94.
19. Stefanovic V, Toncheva D, Atanasova S, Polenakovic M. Etiology of Balkan endemic nephropathy and associated urothelial cancer. Am J Nephrol. 2006;1:1–11.
20. Toncheva D, Mihailova-Hristova M, Vazharova R, et al. NGS nominated CELA1, HSPG2, and KCNK5 as candidate genes for predisposition to Balkan endemic nephropathy. J Biomed Biotechnol. 2014;(7):920723. https://doi.org/10.1155/2014/920723.
21. Staneva R, Rukova B, Hadjidekova S, et al. Whole genome methylation array analysis reveals new aspects in Balkan endemic nephropathy etiology. BMC Nephrol. 2013;14:225. https://doi.org/10.1186/1471-2369-14-225.
22. Patev E. Acute kidney failure. 2nd revised edition; Medicine and Physical Education Publishers, Sofia; 1981; 198 p. (In Bulgarian).
23. Vazelov E. Dialysis treatment in Bulgaria in 2018. Academy "Nephrology" conference, Bansko 10-12.05.2019. (In Bulgarian).
24. Viktorov I, Gruev I, Patrashkov T. Peritoneal dialysis in clinical practice. Mil Med Iss. 1968;5:51–6. (In Bulgarian).
25. Gruev I, Karakasheva V. Protein losses in peritoneal dialysis. Internal Dis. 1969;4:441–4. (In Bulgarian).
26. Gruev I. Peritoneal dialysis in pediatrics. Pediatrics. 1968;5:462–6. (In Bulgarian).
27. Kiryakov Z, Kraev Z, Stanchev I, et al. Contemporary ambulatory peritoneal dialysis (KAPD) - first results in CKD treatment. Surgery. 1985;6:106–9. (In Bulgarian).
28. Vazelov E, Krivoshiev S, Antonov S, et al. End-stage renal disease and peritoneal dialysis in Bulgaria. Perit Dial Int. 2004;6:512–7.
29. Koumanov H. 50 years of kidney transplantation in Bulgaria. URONET. 2019;1:2–4. (In Bulgarian).
30. ERA-EDTA Registry Annual Report 2016: 30–31. https://era-edta-reg.org/files/annualreports/pdf/AnnRep2016.pdf. Accessed 16 July 2019.
31. National Health Insurance Fund. Annual Report 2017. https://www.nhif.bg/page/1763. Accessed 16 July 2019.
32. National Statistical Institute. *Zdraveopazvane 2018* accessed: 16 July 2019. https://www.nsi.bg/sites/default/files/files/publications/Zdraveopazvane_2018.pdf.
33. Levey AS, Andreoli SP, DuBose T, et al. CKD: common, harmful, and treatable—World Kidney Day 2007. Am J Kidney Dis. 2007;2:175–9.

# Nephrology in Croatia

# 36

Petar Kes and Sanjin Rački

## Abbreviations

| | |
|---|---|
| AIDS | Acquired immunodeficiency syndrome |
| AKI | Acute kidney injury |
| APD | Automated peritoneal dialysis |
| AVF | Arteriovenous fistula |
| CAC | Central venous catheter |
| CAPD | Continuous ambulatory peritoneal dialysis |
| CEE | Central and Eastern Europe |
| CEPD | Continuous equilibration peritoneal dialysis |
| CHIF | Croatian Health Insurance Fund |
| CISI | Croatian Institute for Social Insurance |
| CKD | Chronic kidney disease |
| CRRT | Continuous renal replacement therapy |
| CSNDT | Croatian Society of Nephrology, Dialysis and Transplantation |
| CVD | Cardiovascular disease |
| DALI | Direct adsorption of lipoproteins |
| ECMO | Extracorporeal membrane oxygenation |
| EN | Endemic (Balkan) nephropathy |
| EPS | Encapsulating peritoneal sclerosis |
| ESRD | End-stage renal disease |
| EU | European Union |
| GFR | Glomerular filtration rate |
| HELP | Heparin-induced extracorporeal LDL precipitation |
| HD | Hemodialysis |
| HDF | Hemodiafiltration |
| HF | Hemofiltration |
| ICU | Intensive care unit |
| KT | Kidney transplantation |
| MOF | Multiple-organ failure |
| PD | Peritoneal dialysis |
| pmcp | Per million child population |
| pmp | Per million population |
| RRF | Renal residual function |
| RRT | Renal replacement therapy |
| SFRY | Socialist Federal Republic of Yugoslavia |
| TA | Therapeutic apheresis |
| UF | Ultrafiltration |
| UHC | University Hospital Centre |
| VA | Vascular access |

| | |
|---|---|
| Area[1] | 56,594 km$^2$ |
| Population[2] | 4,284,889 (2011) |
| Capital | Zagreb |
| Three most populated cities: | (1) Zagreb<br>(2) Split<br>(3) Rijeka |
| Official language | Croatian |
| Gross domestic product (GDP)[3] | 60.81 billion USD (2018) |
| GDP per capita[4] | 15,870.30 USD (2018) |
| Human Development Index (HDI)[5] | 0.831 (2017) |
| Official currency | Croatian kuna (HRK) |
| Total number of nephrologists | 100 |
| National society of nephrology | Croatian Society for Nephrology, Dialysis and Transplantation www.hdndt.org |
| Incidence of End-Stage Renal Disease[6] | 2016 – 166 pmp |
| Prevalence of End-Stage Renal Disease[7] (including patients with a functioning kidney transplant) | 2016 – 1082 pmp |
| Total number of patients on dialysis (all modalities)[6] | 2015 – 2207<br>2016 – 2429 |
| Number of patients on hemodialysis[6] | 2015 – 2051<br>2016 – 2252 |
| Number of patients on peritoneal dialysis[6] | 2015 – 156<br>2016 – 177 |
| Number of renal transplantations per year[7, 8] | 2017 – 170<br>2018 – 183 |

P. Kes (✉)
School of Medicine, University of Zagreb, and Academy of Medical Sciences of Croatia, Zagreb, Croatia

S. Rački
Department of Nephrology, Dialysis and Transplantation, Rijeka University Hospital Centre, and School of Medicine, University of Rijeka, Rijeka, Croatia


J. A. Moura-Neto et al. (eds.), *Nephrology Worldwide*, https://doi.org/10.1007/978-3-030-56890-0_36

1. https://bs.wikipedia.org/wiki/Hrvatska
2. https://hr.wikipedia.org/wiki/Stanovni%C5%A1tvo_Hrvatske
3. https://tradingeconomics.com/croatia/gdp
4. https://tradingeconomics.com/croatia/gdp-per-capita
5. http://hdr.undp.org/en/countries/profiles/HRV
6. Croatian Registry of Renal Replacement Therapy – Annual Reports for the years 2015 and 2016. https://www.hdndt.org/registar/hrvatski-registar-nadomjestanja-bubrezne-funkcije.html
7. https://zdravlje.gov.hr/UserDocsImages/dokumenti/Tekstovi%20razni/Rezultati%20Nacionalnog%20transplantacijskog%20programa%202017_hr.pdf
8. https://zdravlje.gov.hr/UserDocsImages//dokumenti/Tekstovi%20razni//PRELIMINARNO%20IZVJE%C5%A0%C4%86E%202018%20za%20web.pdf

## Introduction

Until 1991, Croatia was a constitutional republic in the Socialist Federal Republic of Yugoslavia (SFRY) and was covered by a unique health system based on mutual solidarity. Nephrology in the SFRY was, as in other countries, a young branch of internal medicine whose development started in the 1960s by introducing renal replacement therapy (RRT) in everyday clinical practice. Initially, dialysis treatment was intended exclusively for patients with acute kidney injury (AKI), so that dialysis centers were gradually opened in hospitals over the next few years. Ten years later, the first successful kidney transplantation (KT) was performed [1]. In SFRY, nephrology developed slower than in developed European countries, yet more advanced than in Central and Eastern Europe (CEE) countries that were directly influenced by the Soviet Union.

The independence of Croatia was a process that started with changes in the political system and constitutional changes in 1990, which transformed the Socialist Republic of Croatia into the Republic of Croatia. The country officially declared independence in June 1991, along with dissolution of its association with SFRY. The Croatian independence was internationally recognized in January 1992. Unfortunately, the separation of the Republic of Croatia from the former SFRY was not conducted in a peaceful way. The Croatian War of Independence started in 1991, escalated to the sieges of Vukovar and Dubrovnik and fighting altogether, until the ceasefire on January 3, 1992, and significant reduction of violence. The war ended in August 1995 with Croatia victory. During the war in Croatia, there was a halt in the development of nephrology, especially KT. Because of the war escalation in 1991, some dialysis units as well as some hospitals were completely destroyed. Within a few days, many dialysis-treated end-stage renal disease (ESRD) patients were forced to flee from their hometowns. The patients were transferred to Zagreb, the capital of Croatia, and other towns far from the frontline, to help them find accommodations and facilities for their treatments. Most of the patients were evacuated to safe areas without their medical records. This proved to be a serious problem, along with putting strain on dialysis units that had inadequate space in hospitals and suffered shortage of medical staff and lack of dialysis equipment and drugs (e.g., erythropoietin) [2]. Despite these problems, all patients (including those that escaped from Bosnia and Herzegovina due to the war) received necessary treatment and care, thanks to the immense efforts invested by the medical staff. Not a single patient died due to not being admitted to a dialysis unit or receiving treatment [3]. Owing to humanitarian aid from all over the world, the treatment of all patients was possible.

The war in Croatia had temporarily stopped advancement of nephrology (with a particularly negative effect on KT), but after the establishment of peace and revival of the economy, the situation improved considerably.

## A Brief History of Nephrology in Croatia

In the Republic of Croatia, nephrology began to develop as a separate part of internal medicine in 1950, first at Rebro Clinical Hospital (now Zagreb University Hospital Centre, Zagreb UHC) and, soon afterwards, at the other clinical centers, followed by general hospitals all over the country. In addition to specialized hospital departments, nephrology has expanded by the establishment of polyclinical departments for appropriate and rational treatment of patients with primary and secondary (e.g., due to arterial hypertension and diabetes mellitus) urinary tract diseases. The kidney disease diagnosis was improved in 1959 by introducing percutaneous kidney biopsies. In clinical practice, first in departmental makeshift laboratory (in which doctors performed simple tests and microscopic examination of urine) and later in hospital laboratories, it became possible to perform basic and functional nephrology tests [4]. Collaboration with doctors of other specialties was ensured. Such a model of polyclinical care for kidney patients was accepted at a scientific meeting of nephrologists in Dubrovnik, for the whole former SFRY, in 1981. The rapid advancement of imaging diagnostics (radiological examinations, computerized tomography, magnetic resonance imaging, ultrasound) and functional analysis (radioisotope tests, renal clearances) has contributed to the important advancement of nephrology in the world, as well as in Croatia.

Since a large number of urinary tract diseases can occur early in life, pediatricians have been actively involved in nephrology. At the Zagreb UHC, a pediatric nephrology department was established as early as 1957, and later similar departments were established in other hospitals [4].

The use of dialysis in patients with AKI or ESRD made great progress in the development of nephrology. After successful experimental dialysis in nine dogs, the first hemodialysis (HD) in a uremic patient was performed on June 17, 1962, at the Sušak Hospital Surgery Department. It was an acute dialysis that lasted for 6 hours and led by Professor Jerko Zec [5]. In the early period, only these acute dialyses were performed. After the adoption of the so-called Quinton-Scribner AV shunt for arteriovenous connection in 1956, it became possible to perform the first Croatian multi-session chronic dialysis in a patient suffering from ESRD. The procedure was led by Professor Jerko Zec. Only 44 dialysis centers provided chronic dialysis in Europe at the time. After these pioneering efforts and later valuable experience, the Sušak Hospital dialysis team trained hundreds of physicians and other medical staff for new dialysis centers all over the country [5].

On June 3, 1948, at Zagreb UHC, Professor Laslo Kallai presented the first successful treatment of an AKI patient with peritoneal dialysis (PD) using a sterile solution drainage method through two intraperitoneal catheters and without the use of a machine. Glucose was used as the osmotic agent [6]. After that, PD was carried out sporadically in AKI patients until 1981, when it began to be used in patients with ESRD [7].

The first KT in Croatia was performed in Rijeka on January 30, 1971. The removal from the living donor (the patient's mother) was done by Vjerislav Peterković, while Professor Vinko Frančišković performed transplantation, after several years of practice on dogs and pigs [1]. The first KT from a deceased donor was also performed at the Sušak Hospital (now Rijeka UHC) on May 15, 1972 [1, 8, 9].

In the 1970s, the Sušak Hospital in Rijeka was a well-known educational center for transplant surgery in SFRY. A multidisciplinary approach to patients with transplanted kidney and those treated with dialysis has made it possible to determine their working ability, as well as the successful treatment of concomitant cardiac, gastroenterological, neurological, and other comorbidities. Particular attention has been paid to the problem of pregnancy in patients with transplanted kidney. The first methods of tissue typing were introduced at the Institute for Transfusion Medicine under the guidance of Professor Ksenija Vujaklija-Stipanović. The first interventions with the conventional ultrasound in the diagnostics of transplanted kidneys appeared in the second half of the 1970s (1976) with sonographic description of the acute "crisis" of kidney transplant rejection (Professor Željko Fučkar). On December 21, 1993, the surgical transplant team of the Department of Surgery and Department of Urology, Rijeka UHC, including Miomir Zelić MD, Professor Petar Orlić, and Professor Miljenko Uravić, performed the first simultaneous pancreas and kidney transplantation in Croatia [10].

KT at the Department of Urology, Zagreb UHC, started in 1973, headed by Professor Ljubomir Čečuk. In the first procedures, dialysis doctors led by Professor Ante Smetiško and Tissue Typing Center headed by Academician Andrija Kaštelan were involved [8]. In the last 20 years, Professors Zvonimir Mareković, Josip Pasini, Željko Kaštelan, and their multidisciplinary team from the Department of Urology, Zagreb UHC, have performed most KTs in Croatia.

At the beginning of the twenty-first century, KT was active in two transplant centers in Zagreb (Zagreb UHC – location Rebro and Merkur University Hospital) and one in Rijeka (Rijeka UHC). The transplant center Merkur University Hospital was established in 1998 with liver transplantation, followed by kidney and pancreas transplantation in 2003. The latest transplant center in Croatia was established in Osijek UHC in 2007 [8].

Many nephrologists have been involved in the development of KT. For the purpose of harmonization of all procedures related to KT, the board of the Croatian Society of Nephrology, Dialysis and Transplantation (CSNDT) supported the initiative of Professor Petar Kes and approved the creation of Croatian KT guidelines at the annual general meeting held in Zagreb on December 5, 2003. The status of patients on the waiting list for KT was revised, being the basis for the formation of a modern waiting list, which is necessary for inclusion in international associations [8]. The multidisciplinary approach to nephrology, and in particular to KT, is reflected in systematic education of physicians and other medical staff through numerous postgraduate courses. In 2014, Professor Petar Kes, Professor Nikolina Bašić-Jukić, and Professor Sanjin Rački founded the Croatian Transplantation School, which is held every year.

While Croatia was part of the former SFRY, there was the Society of Nephrology and Dialysis Society as two separate nonprofit organizations. Upon establishment of the independent Republic of Croatia, these two societies were united in the CSNDT under the auspices of the Croatian Medical Association. The primary objectives of CSNDT as the head professional association of physicians treating patients with renal disease include continuous professional development of its members through postgraduate courses in the field of nephrology, dialysis and KT, interactive symposia, seminars and workshops, as well as development of professional guidelines.

Even before the foundation of specialization in nephrology, under the auspices of CSNDT and School of Medicine, University of Zagreb, there was an ongoing postgraduate education in nephrology, dialysis, and transplantation (Dialysis Postgraduate Course and International Nephrology School) and later Croatian School of Kidney Transplantation, as well as training for doctors and nurses within the Pliva Institute for Dialysis, entitled Nephrology Weekend and Dialysis Practice. The founders and leaders of these training courses were Professors Petar Kes and Dragan Ljutić, later joined by Professors Sanjin Rački and Nikolina Bašić Jukić.

For better understanding of the needs of patients and to improve cooperation, courses and symposia were also organized for general practitioners and even patients in order to clarify the nature of their illness and treatment methods to improve their quality of life. Because of the increasing number of chronic patients and development of medicine, in 2001 CSNDT initiated the establishment of the Registry of Renal Diseases to collect important information on patients and their treatment.

Active participation in education, taking exams at the end of each course, and 10 years of work at nephrology department/dialysis were the main elements for the respective residency completed by acquiring the title of nephrologist (until then there was no residency in nephrology).

Currently, there is specialization in nephrology, which includes residency in internal medicine (22 months), nephrology (33 months), postgraduate study in nephrology (3 months), and Specialty Certificate Exam in Nephrology.

## Renal Diseases in Croatia

### Chronic Kidney Disease

In Croatia, the number of people with chronic kidney disease (CKD) is increasing. It is estimated that around 350,000 people (especially those older than 65) suffer from CKD or have a high risk to be affected. The most common causes of CKD are diabetes mellitus (mainly type 2) and arterial hypertension, followed by chronic glomerulonephritis, chronic pyelonephritis, and polycystic kidney disease. The number of patients with CKD in stages 1–4 can only be assumed. The RRT Registry, founded by the CSNDT in 2001, provides accurate data on patients undergoing RRT by dialysis or transplantation. According to these data, the prevalence of patients on RRT is constantly increasing; the percentage of males and females is approximately 52% and 48%, respectively; and the median age of patients starting RRT is 67.4 years (65% of the patients are aged >65). In the past 18 years, the most common cause of ESRD was diabetes mellitus (33%), followed by arterial hypertension (22%), chronic pyelonephritis (12%), chronic glomerulonephritis (12%), polycystic kidney disease (7%), chronic interstitial nephritis (4%), and endemic nephropathy (1%). Other diseases were recorded in 7% of patients, while the cause of the disease was unknown in 2% of ESRD patients. The 5-year survival of chronic dialysis and transplant patients in Croatia was 54.3% with annual mortality rate of 11.7% (highest in HD patients). According to 2018 data, the most common causes of morbidity and mortality continue to be cardiovascular disease (CVD) and stroke (57%), followed by infections (16%) and malignancies (12%).

The cost of ESRD patient management is very high. As currently there is no drug capable of halting the progression of kidney damage in CKD, attention is focused on early detection of renal disease, screening of CKD patients, specific therapy, slowing down progression, and treatment of complications and comorbidities. The role of general practitioners and patient compliance in the decision of the modality of RRT, as well as continuous education of nephrologists and public awareness of renal disease, is underlined.

The median number of pediatric nephrologists per million child population (pmcp) in Croatia is 8.6, and there are also 14 pmcp of general pediatricians with interest/activity in pediatric nephrology [11]. The incidence of CKD is around 8 per million children population, and prevalence is around 24 per million population. Findings and disorders increasing the risk of CKD development in children and adolescents are hereditary diseases including polycystic kidney disease, dysplasia or hypoplasia of the kidney, low birth weight, AKI, obstructive uropathy, vesicoureteral reflux with recurrent urinary tract infections, acute nephritic or nephrotic syndrome, hemolytic-uremic syndrome, vasculitis, and diabetes mellitus. Progression to ESRD needs consultations and continuation of treatment by pediatric nephrologists involved in dialysis and transplantation. There are defined algorithms for evaluation and treatment of children with AKI and CKD [12]. Due availability and application of all RRT methods require appropriate equipments, defined algorithms, and educated medical staff. The best-equipped pediatric nephrology department is located at the Zagreb UHC where pediatricians working in a ward, established 30 years ago, can care for children with acute and chronic kidney disease (including AKI and CKD/ESRD), prepare children for kidney transplantation, and monitor them after transplantation. KT from living relatives, diseased donors, and pre-emptive transplantation are practiced [13].

### Acute Kidney Injury

The prevalence of AKI in Croatia has increased in the last two decades. Recent hospital studies report AKI in up to 8.7% of admissions, particularly in patients treated at intensive care units (ICUs). Overall in-hospital AKI patients' mortality rate is around 20% but is significantly higher (up to 60%) in patients treated with dialysis in ICU (especially if the multiorgan failure has developed) [14]. The increased prevalence likely reflects an aging population burdened with multiple comorbidities. The etiologic factors include prerenal injury contributing to reduced renal perfusion, drug nephrotoxicity, diagnostic procedures requiring intravenous contrast, complex surgery, hospital-acquired infections, and sepsis. Treatment of the most severe patients is performed in the ICU by an intensivist and a nephrologist. In most hospitals, especially UHCs and specialized hospitals (e.g., for cardiac or transplant surgery), it is possible to compensate for the acute loss of renal function by the most acceptable RRT method (e.g., PD, HD, CRRT, or hybrid dialysis) [15].

The incidence of AKI in children aged ≤18 years in whom RRT methods are used is 12–14 per million children population/year. Acute PD (continuous equilibration peritoneal dialysis, CEPD) was more frequently used in the past, especially in newborns, infants, and small children, whereas acute HD was used in older children. Since 2002, continuous renal replacement therapy (CRRT) methods of RRT have been preferred, especially in ICU. Knowing the indications, association with multiple-organ failure (MOF) and possible complications of AKI is of utmost importance.

## Balkan Endemic Nephropathy

Endemic (Balkan) nephropathy (EN) is a chronic tubule-interstitial nephritis affecting residents of rural villages located in valleys near tributaries of the Danube River in Croatia, Bosnia, Bulgaria, Romania, and Serbia. The significant epidemiologic features of EN include its focal occurrence in certain farming villages, with unaffected villages located in close proximity; a familial but not an inherited pattern of the disease, frequently affecting members of the same household; occurrence only in individuals older than 18; occurrence in <10% of households in endemic villages; and strong association with upper urinary tract urothelial cancer [16]. A variety of environmental factors have been explored during the past 50 years, but the results of recent studies are fully consistent with the hypothesis that chronic dietary exposure to aristolochic acid is the cause of EN [17].

## Renal Replacement Therapy in Croatia

### Hemodialysis

From the early years of HD treatment up to date, great progress has been made in Croatia, which is based primarily on HD devices and equipment technological advancement, as well as medicines for patients with AKI or ESRD. Today, there are 45 dialysis centers in Croatia (of which eight are private), and dialysis treatment is available for all AKI and ESRD patients. Modern dialysis devices with volumetric ultrafiltration (UF), profiling of dialysis solutions, ultrapure dialysis fluid preparation with special filters (e.g., DIASAFE® *plus*), modern online HDF system, dialysis dose calculation, blood temperature monitoring, and a number of safety sensors are used.

Dialysis water preparation devices are supplied with, at least, reverse osmosis, and four dialysis centers produce ultrapure water. In some dialysis centers, it is possible to produce a dialysis solution according to the specific needs of the patients (e.g., with different calcium concentration). The standards for water quality for dialysis are in accordance with the EU guidelines.

A well-functioning vascular access (VA) is a mainstay to perform an efficient HD procedure. In Croatia, we are using four types of permanent VA: native arteriovenous fistulas (AVF) (63%), central venous catheters (CVC) (20%), arteriovenous grafts (1%), and ports (1%). In about 15% of ESRD patients, chronic HD is initiated by temporary CAC. The preferable locations for CVC insertion are the internal jugular and femoral veins. The subclavian vein is considered the third choice because of the high risk of thrombosis and later vein stenosis. Proper VA maintenance requires integration of different professionals to create a VA team (nephrologist, vascular surgeon, urologist, members of the dialysis staff, radiologist, and infectious disease consultant) [18, 19]. They should provide their experience in order to give the best options to uremic patients and the best care for their VA.

Despite lack of evidence from randomized controlled trials about the optimal time to start RRT, there has been a trend, which has leveled off since 2010, in Croatia towards earlier initiation of dialysis at higher levels of kidney function (especially in the pediatric population). This means that dialysis may be initiated if difficult-to-control symptoms of CKD or ESRD (e.g., metabolic acidosis, hyperkalemia, hypocalcemia, hyperphosphatemia, hypertension, fluid overload symptoms, renal osteodystrophy, nausea/vomiting, loss of appetite, malnutrition, growth impairment, etc.) or the degree of disability in daily life manifest during conservative medical management even if GFR >15 mL/min/1.73 $m^2$ [20, 21]. Conventional HD remains the most common treatment for ESRD in Croatia and is usually performed for 3–5 hours, 3 days per week. It should result in a weekly clearance, eKt/V, of more than 1.2 (for children and patients with high comorbidity 1.4). In the standard HD, blood and dialysate flow rates are between 250 and 400 ml/min (depending on patients' vascular access) and 500 and 800 ml/min, respectively. Unfractionated heparin and low-molecular-weight heparin are most commonly used as anticoagulant agents. It's our experience that compared to low flux dialysis, high flux dialysis, and convective therapies, such as hemofiltration (HF) and hemodiafiltration (HDF) provide higher clearance of larger solutes, removal of which might improve cardiovascular outcomes [22]. About 20% of patients with ESRD are treated with post-dilution HDF.

Eighteen years ago, in a prospective study on a cohort of 37 chronic HD patients, the method of automated capillary dialyzer reprocessing with peracetic acid, as a cleansing and sterilizing agent, was found to be a safe, effective, and money-saving method [23, 24]. However, the reuse of dialyzers did not enter into everyday clinical practice in Croatia.

Since the establishment of the Croatian Registry to replace renal function, the 91-day mortality rate from the start of HD treatment is between 10.7% and 13.4% [25].

The standards of treatment for renal anemia, bone disease, and dietary advice are in accordance with the EU guidelines. The prevalence of hepatitis B and C among dialysis patients is about 1% and 4%, respectively, and there are four patients with acquired immunodeficiency syndrome (AIDS) (two on HD and KT, each). Patients with hepatitis B and C and AIDS are dialyzed separately from the other patients. General population vaccination against hepatitis B is a common procedure, and modern Exviera® (dasabuvir) and Viekirax® (ombitasvir/paritaprevir/ritonavir) drugs are available for dialysis patients with hepatitis C [26].

Nephrologists are mostly responsible for the treatment of AKI patients. However, critically ill AKI patients are treated in ICUs under the supervision of an intensivist and a nephrologist. In most hospital settings, methods such as PD, HD, CRRT (all procedures), and sporadically hybrid dialysis are used. In case of indication, in clinical institutions it is possible to combine CRRT and extracorporeal membrane oxygenation (ECMO) treatment, improvise single-pass albumin dialysis, or lately use artificial liver support systems (Plasma Separation and Adsorption System /Prometheus System/ or Molecular Adsorbent Recirculating System /MARS/). All of the above methods are used in the treatment of adults and children with AKI (special clinical hospital for children). Therapeutic apheresis (TA) (mostly membrane and at Zagreb UHC also centrifugal) is performed by nephrologists [27]. Sometimes we combine CRRT and TA. In two UHCs, patients with refractory hyperlipidemia may be treated with the methods of direct adsorption of lipoproteins (DALI) or heparin-induced extracorporeal LDL precipitation (HELP).

Croatian nephrologists use adapted European guidelines for the organization and work in dialysis centers, prevention, and management of acute or chronic kidney disease.

The conditions for work in dialysis centers are determined by the rulebook on minimum conditions in view of space, employees, and medical-technical equipment for performance of health activities [28]. Doctors working in dialysis centers must be specialists of internal medicine and/or nephrologists or pediatricians with dialysis training. The provisions are as follows: (1) one doctor of medicine for 30 patients on chronic HD in clinical settings, (2) one doctor for 40 patients on chronic HD at dialysis centers in general hospitals and at PD, (3) one doctor for 50 HD patients in outpatient dialysis centers, (4) one bachelor of nursing specialist in HD for up to four patients at hospital dialysis centers, (5) one bachelor of nursing specialist in the field of HD for up to five patients in outpatient dialysis centers, and (6) one bachelor of nursing specialist in HD at ten patients on PD.

The Croatian Health Insurance Fund (CHIF) covers the cost of treatment with all types of extracorporeal RRT, TA, lipoprotein apheresis, and artificial liver. The annual cost of classic bicarbonate HD is 160,000 HRK (21,600 €), while online HDF costs 172,000 HRK (23,200 €).

## Peritoneal Dialysis

The number of patients treated with continuous ambulatory peritoneal dialysis (CAPD) and later with automated peritoneal dialysis (APD) has increased gradually, in parallel with technological advancement. New developments in preventing the causes of technique failure, including measures to prevent serious peritonitis episodes, and new biocompatible PD solutions with neutral (Balance) or physiological (Physioneal, Bicavera) pH, together with the advantages of some types of catheters and implantation techniques (e.g., peritoneoscopic implantation), as well as systematic education of patients and their family members, have encouraged us to apply PD more frequently in treating patients with AKI (especially children) and ESRD.

However, in Croatia, PD has always been (although not justified) the second method of choice for RRT. In the last two decades, the percentage of patients treated with this method has been between 2.8% and 7%. APD is used in 25% of patients. Peritoneoscopic implantation is the preferred method of catheter placement for PD. New biocompatible dialysis solutions are mainly used. There is an organized systematic training of patients for independent performance of PD. Today, the rate of peritonitis is low, i.e., one episode per 40–55 patient-month. The mean annual mortality rate is 8.6%, which is significantly lower than the mortality of patients treated with HD (12.6%) [29]. Due to previous poor experience with encapsulating peritoneal sclerosis (EPS) [30], treatment of PD patients is limited to up to 4 years.

Since the establishment of the Croatian Registry to replace renal function, the 91-day mortality rate from the start of PD treatment is between 5.6% and 8.6% [25].

The CHIF covers the cost of PD treatment. If CAPD is performed with solutions containing low-glucose degradation products, buffered with either lactate, bicarbonate, or both, and if the use of an amino acid-containing or 7.5% icodextrin-containing solution is indicated, the annual cost of treatment is about 150,000 HRK (20,300 €). Annual APD treatment costs 180,000 HRK (24,300 €).

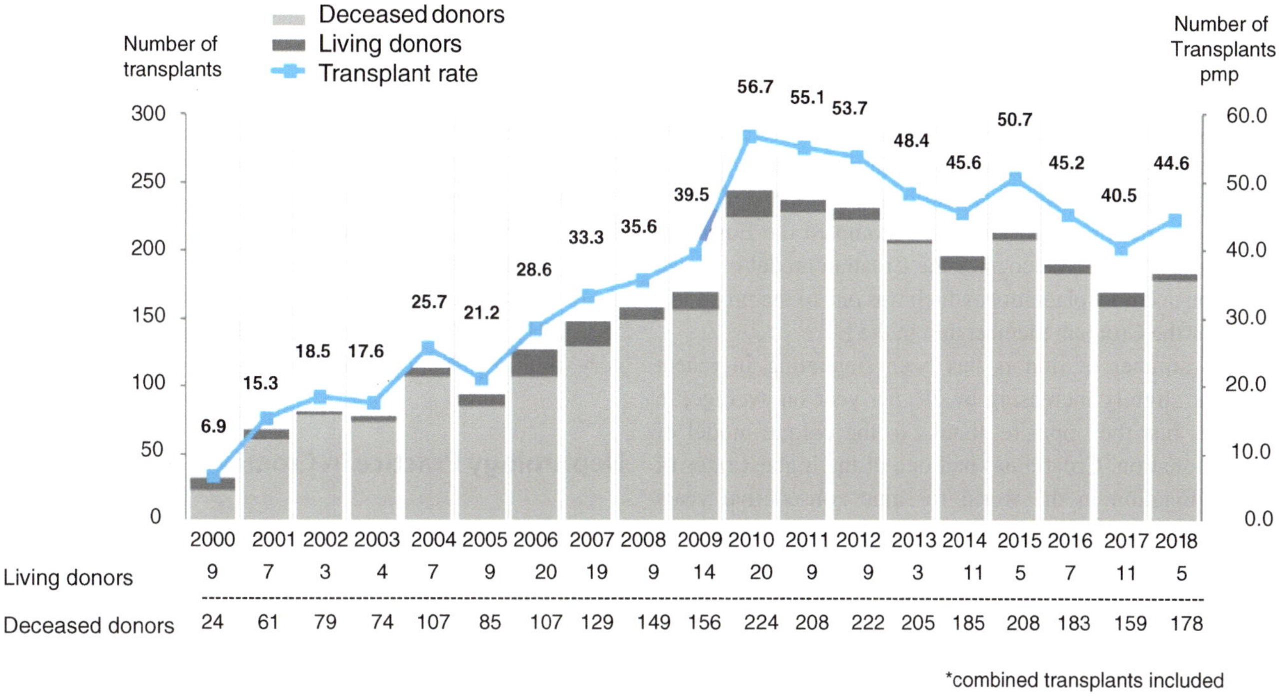


**Fig. 36.1** Kidney transplants in Croatia (2000–2018)

## Kidney Transplantation

Two decades ago, Croatia was lagging far behind other European countries with a low donation rate (2.7 donors pmp in 2000) and consequently with a small number of KTs. The persistent efforts to organize and gradually improve the national organ transplant program in Croatia have resulted in a steadily growing donor rate, which reached its highest level in 2015, with 37.9 donors pmp (Fig. 36.1). The transplant program is mostly based on deceased donors. There is a very low percentage of kidney-living donors (8.3% in the last 10 years), predominantly recipients' relatives (79.5%). Altruistic living kidney donation from unrelated individuals is allowed, but not encouraged. A sustained increase in organ donation rate was one of the preconditions for the Croatian full membership in the Eurotransplant (ET) in 2007 (at that time as the only one outside the EU). Today, the ET network consists of Austria, Belgium, Croatia, Germany, Hungary, Luxembourg, The Netherlands, and Slovenia, serving a total population of around 136 million people. ET membership has provided a larger donor pool and makes it easier to achieve better match between available donor organs and patients on the waiting list, thereby improving both short-term and long-term outcomes of transplantation. Owing to special ranking on the waiting list, children, high-immunized and high-urgency patients, have a better chance to receive an organ relatively quickly.

The key factors that have contributed to the development of a successful model for organ donation and KT in Croatia in the past two decades were the following [31, 32]: (1) legal regulation for deceased donation based on a presumed consent, which means that body parts may be used for transplantation only, if the deceased person did not make any written statement to be against organ donation [33, 34]. A non-donor registry has been implemented and maintained by the Croatian Ministry of Health; (2) appointment of the national transplant coordinator (since 2003, Mirela Bušić, MD), together with eight transplant coordinators attending a 24-hour duty desk at the Ministry of Health and 32 transplant coordinators at the hospitals. Both groups are joined in the national coordination network; (3) proactive approach and early identification of all potential donors, improvement and implementation of standardized protocols for optimal donor management; (4) improvements in the screening of candidates for KT, careful pretransplant patient evaluation, and waiting list management; (5) implementation of a new financial model with donor hospital reimbursement, as compensation for the lack of financial resources, inadequate salaries, and shortage of health personnel; (6) long-term positive promotion of organ donation in all public media, encouraged by the National Ministry of Health, professional societies of the Croatian Medical Association (primarily CSNDT), Croatian Medical Chamber, patient associations, and positive attitude of the authorities of religious communities, have improved public awareness of organ donation; and (7) the significant increase in the organ donation rate prompted the European health community to recognize the Croatian model of organ donation and transplantation, which was one of the preconditions for the Croatian membership in the ET.

The number of donors has been stagnating in recent years or slightly increasing by 2% per year on average, in Europe. Just the opposite, thanks to the unique model of organ donation, Croatia has had one of the highest rates of organ donation in the world for nine consecutive years (>30 pmp). In 2010, there was a record increase in the number of donors (64.9%) and total number of solid organ transplants (57%). At the same time, Croatia reported the highest deceased and living donors' KT rate (56.7 pmp) up to that date. The positive trend has stabilized at 48 pmp between 2011 and 2018 (range 39.7–55.2 pmp). Compared to 2017, the number of donated and transplanted organs increased by 19% and 11%, respectively, in 2018. A successful donor program with a record rate of 41 and 37 pmp performed organ donors was equally successfully followed by solid organ transplantation programs (183 kidneys, 133 liver, 37 heart, and 3 pancreas) with a total transplant rate higher than 86 pmp [35].

Thanks to good organization and increasing number of donors, a "senior program" was established in Croatia before joining the ET (2004) [36], while experience with combined organ transplantation (kidney and pancreas) was sporadic. Following the ET approach, combined organ transplantation (kidney en bloc, kidney + pancreas, kidney + liver, and kidney + heart) is routinely done in Croatia, and pre-emptive kidney transplantation has started. The active waiting list in Croatia was reduced by 85.6% between 2000 and 2014. In the last 4 years, there have been between 124 and 206 patients on the waiting list. The waiting time for the kidney transplant has been reduced from 12 years (2007) to less than 12 months. In the meantime, the average age of transplanted patients (but also deceased donors) has increased, and so did the number of patients with second transplant. Due to better prevention and treatment conditions, the number of transplant patients with hepatitis B or C decreased, and the first patients with AIDS were transplanted.

Croatia is an example that middle-income countries may follow the results of organ transplantation from developed countries only if there is consensus of the professional community and health policy on transplantation as a national, public health interest. Today, Croatia belongs to the category of countries with the most effective transplantation system in the world.

The financial model according to which donor preparation and organ transplantation are paid as a separate item of the state budget was implemented in Croatia in 2006. Depending on the complexity and type of transplant procedure, the price paid by CHIF ranges from 70,000 to 220,000 HRK (9500–29,700 €). For the preparation and realization of donors, the hospital receives an additional asset of 40,000–55,000 HRK (5400–7400 €), depending on the donor category (multiorgans, organ, and/or tissue) [31].

## Nephrology Practice in Croatia

Renal medicine has experienced unprecedented growth over the past 30 years, driven in part by the rising number of ESRD patients requiring dialysis and/or KT. Solid evidence for the increased numbers of patients requiring RRT is the development of multiple new renal units both in teaching hospitals and district general hospitals. Today, nephrology encompasses a wide range of clinical treatments for AKI, CKD, and ESRD, as well as the prevention and treatment of numerous complications of CKD, selection and preparation of KT patients, as well as care for patients after transplantation [37]. Training in nephrology follows the Croatian-agreed renal medicine curriculum (which is in accordance with the education program in the European Union) and is competency-based. During this period, the specialist trainee will rotate between the sub-disciplines of nephrology including KT, dialysis, and general nephrology. Procedural skills in placing ultrasound-guided central venous catheters for dialysis, native and transplant kidney biopsy, as well as the acquisition of knowledge for performing HD, PD, and APD, CRRT and TA methods are a mandatory component of training. During specialization, future nephrologists have to acquire due knowledge of kidney diseases and their interaction with other organ systems. Some nephrology trainees, and particularly those with special interest in AKI, have combined renal medicine and intensive care medicine training and forge a career in the interface areas between critical care and nephrology [15].

The renal workforce plays a pivotal role in kidney care delivery and includes primarily nephrologists, and nephrology-oriented nurses, who hold different levels of responsibility. Nephrology nurses work closely with patients who require ongoing care or life-sustaining treatment. Using dialysis, KT, and other treatment methods, nephrology nurses manage illnesses such as CKD and ESRD [7, 8]. Nurses working in the ICU where patients are treated for

AKI (which is often part of MOF) must be familiar with the technology of various dialysis treatments (CRRT, hybrid dialysis) and other extracorporeal treatments (albumin dialysis, hemoperfusion) [15, 38–40]. Their work directly impacts the quality of life and end-of-life care of renal patients.

Financial compensation plays an increasing role in choosing nephrology specialty training. Today, the average salary of a nephrologists and renal nurses is between 11,100 and 14,800 HRK (1500 and 800 €) and 6000 HRK (800 €), respectively. It is commonly believed that other internists (e.g., cardiologist, gastroenterologist) may achieve better earnings. Furthermore, salaries of nephrologists but also of nephrology nurses are significantly better in developed countries of the European Union, which is why nephrology medical staff are increasingly leaving Croatia.

## Highlight of Nephrology in Croatia

The tragic events that occurred in Croatia in mid-October 2001 resulted in unexpected deaths of 23 patients on chronic HD in a single week. Five patients died during HD, and another 18 patients died within several hours after HD had been completed. The clinical presentation was characterized by acute onset of illness with various degrees of chest tightness, progressive dyspnea, and cardiac arrest. Standard resuscitation measures, including mechanical respiratory assistance and inotropic agents, were unsuccessful. The warning of sudden deaths among ESRD patients treated with HD in six dialysis centers prompted us to organize an emergency medical council composed of nephrologists and epidemiologists. Epidemiological information was crucial to understand the events. It was found that HD injuries occurred simultaneously in several dialysis units with somewhat different dialysis practice. However, all patients that died were dialyzed by the Althane series single-use dialyzer (Baxter/Plivadial P-15/lot 2001F075 and P-18/lot 2001B17R). During the inquiry (October 13, 2001), all dialysis units were informed of suspicion regarding incriminated dialyzers and the necessity of their withdrawal from use. There were no additional deaths of HD patients after withdrawal of the incriminated dialyzers [41].

Considering the epidemiological and clinical facts, followed by subsequent animal experimental results, the cause of patient deaths was discovered. The causal agent was the performance test liquid (PF5070) used in the dialyzer manufacturing process to detect leaks in the bundle fibers. This test fluid was not removed properly after dialyzer assembly. The intravenous passage of PF5070 test fluid at the time of dialysis priming emulsified patient blood, thus creating microbubble aggregates that subsequently plugged pulmonary capillaries, created patchy lung infarction, and eventually led to severe hypoxemia with lethal outcome [42].

The quick and accurate conclusions made on the basis of epidemiological information allowed us to rescue the lives of many other patients in Croatian dialysis centers (they had a stock of "deadly" dialyzers) and probably in other countries as well. Furthermore, we helped explain sudden patient deaths during HD in Spain (later in August 2001) and in the meantime in the USA, Italy, Germany, Taiwan, and Colombia.

Undoubtedly, KT is the greatest success of Croatian nephrology, as described in a separate section. The example of Croatia shows that development of surgical transplant techniques, long-term transplant tradition, or existence of national transplant organizations is not, by themselves and individually, a guarantee for a successful transplant system, if they are not accompanied by a set of appropriate legal, financial, and primarily organizational measures. Today, there are several successful transplant organizational models, among which the Croatian model has established itself because of the results achieved. The specificity of our model is characterized by successful integration elements of good "European" medical practice and organizational solutions of developed European countries (e.g., Spanish model of transplant coordinators and ET allocation system) in the context of the political system and socioeconomic capabilities of your own health system. The Croatian model has been internationally recognized as very successful and suitable for implementation in other similar countries. Because of that, following the South-Eastern Europe Health Network meeting in 2001, Croatia became a pioneer in legislative changes and set an example for the Eastern and Central European region. Croatia remains the role model for the region with the most successfully providing support for development of deceased organ donation and transplant programs under the guidance of the Regional Health Development Centre on Organ Donation and Transplant Medicine [43].

## Future Perspectives of Nephrology in Croatia

Today, both in Croatia and the world, ever more patients are suffering from AKI, CKD, or ESRD. It is therefore important to detect patients at an early stage of the disease and treat them appropriately.

Because of the significant improvement in PD technology, individualization of dialysis treatment, preservation of renal residual function (RRF) (better than HD) that leads to longer ESRD patient survival, improvement in the quality of life (with lower treatment costs), and short waiting times for kidney transplant, it is advantageous to start with PD as the first dialysis method.

In Croatia, HD treatment is performed at a relatively high level. It is important to continue with improving working conditions in dialysis centers and continually renewing dialysis devices.

KT is at an enviable level and everything needs to be done to keep it so. The current educational framework in Croatia encourages students to pursue nephrology. In order to stimulate the interest of the students in their later specialization in nephrology, it is necessary to redesign educational styles and to emphasize the case-based application of theoretical and physiological principles within the internal medicine curriculum. It is also important to increase educational responsibilities of the nephrologists during medical student internship and encouraging nephrology mentorship for medical students.

Nephrology staff should be provided with better working conditions and appropriate wages, so that they would not go abroad after their expensive education.

## References


1. Primc D, Muzur A, Dorčić R, Markić D. New contributions to the study of the life and work of Vinko Frančisković (1919-1984), pioneer of Croatian cardiothoracic and transplantation surgery. Acta Med Hist Adriat. 2017;15(Suppl. 1):119–28.
2. Pavlović D, Kes P, Janković N, Čala S. Treating patients in war-torn Croatia. Nephrol News Issues. 1994;2(4):14.
3. Kes P, Ratković-Gusić I, Orlić-Čunović D, Rupčić V, Štefović-Fuchs A, Prša M. [Comparison of efficacy of hemodialysis treatment of domestic and exiled patients with uremia]. Acta Clin Croat 1992;31:243–52. (in Croatian).
4. Klancir S. [Nephrology]. In: Živković R, Oberiter V, Vrhovac B, editors. [The history of the internist profession in Croatia]. Zagreb: Academy of Medical Sciences of Croatia; 1998. p. 37–45. (in Croatian).
5. Zgrablić M. On the occasion of the 45th anniversary since the first-ever Croatian dialysis performed in Rijeka in 1962. Acta Med Hist Adriat. 2007;5(2):299–310.
6. Kallai L. [Anuria is cured by washing the peritoneum]. Lijec Vjesn. 1948;70(12):450–1. (in Croatian).
7. Furić Čunko V, Bašić Jukić N, Jakić M. [History of peritoneal dialysis]. In: Bašić-Jukić N, Rački S, editors. [Peritoneal Dialysis]. Zagreb: Medicinska naklada; 2017. p. 1–8. (in Croatian).
8. Kaštelan Ž, Bašić Jukić N, Furić-Čunko V. [History of Transplantation]. In: Bašić Jukić N, Kaštelan Ž, editors. [Kidney transplantation]. Zagreb: Medicinska naklada; 2016. p. 1–12. (in Croatian).
9. Kes P, Rački S, Bašić JN. Kidney donation and transplantation. Acta Med Croatica. 2012;66(1):151–2.
10. Fučkar Ž, Markić D, Španjol J, Valenčić M. [History of kidney transplantation in Sušak]. Acta Med Croatica. 2011;65(2):323–9.
11. Croatian Bureau of Statistic. Population estimate of Republic of Croatia, 2018. https://www.dzs.hr/Hrv_Eng/publication/2019/07-01-03_01_2019.htm - 2018 stanovništvo Accessed 20 Feb 2020.
12. Puretić Z. [Diagnostic and therapeutic algorithms in acute and chronic renal failure in children]. Paediatr Croat. 2008;52(Suppl 1):165–74.
13. Puretić Z, Bubić-Filipi L, Pasini J. Therapy with kidney transplantation in children in Croatia. Period Biol. 2010;112(1):62.
14. Kes P, Bašić-Jukić N. Acute kidney injury in the intensive care unit. Bosn J Basic Med Sci. 2010;10(Suppl 1):8–12.
15. Kes P. [Acute Kidney Injury]. Zagreb: Medicinska naklada; 2019. p. 1–1130. (in Croatian).
16. Jelaković B, Nikolić J, Radovanović Z, Nortier J, Cosyns JP, Grollman AP, et al. Consensus statement on screening, diagnosis, classification and treatment of endemic (Balkan) nephropathy. Nephrol Dial Transplant. 2014;29(11):2020–7.
17. Grollman AP, Jelaković B. Role of environmental toxins in endemic (Balkan) nephropathy. J Am Soc Nephrol. 2007;18(11):2817–23.
18. Rački S, Jelić Pranjić I, Devčić B. [Vascular access for hemodialysis in patients with acute kidney injury]. In: Kes P, editor. Acute kidney injury. Zagreb: Medicinska naklada; 2019. p. 818–35. (in Croatian).
19. Rački S, Orlić L, Maleta I, Živčić-Ćosić S. [Chronic kidney disease]. In: Fučkar Ž, editor. Urology. Faculty of Medicine, University of Rijeka; 2013. p. 287–306.
20. National Kidney Foundation. KDOQI clinical practice guideline for hemodialysis adequacy: 2015 update. Am J Kidney Dis. 2015;66(5):884–930.
21. Gotta V, Dao K, Rodieux F, Buclin T, Livio F, Pfister M. Guidance to develop individual dose recommendations for patients on chronic hemodialysis. Expert Rev Clin Pharmacol. 2017;10(7):737–52.
22. Mesaroš Devčić I, Bubić I, Rački S. [Online hemodiafiltration – new standard in the dialysis treatment?]. Med Flum. 2010;46(4):489–97. (in Croatian).
23. Kes P, Reiner Ž, Ratković-Gusić I. Dialyzer reprocessing with peroxyacetic acid as a sole cleansing and sterilizing agent. Acta Med Croatica. 1997;51(2):87–93.
24. Kes P, Reiner Ž, Starčević B, Ratković-Gusić I. Influence of erythropoietin treatment on dialyzer reuse. Blood Purif. 1997;15(2):77–83.
25. Croatian Society of Nephrology, Dialysis and Transplantation of Croatian Medical Association: The CSNDT register. https://www.hdndt.org/registar-nadomjestanja-bubrezne-funkcije.
26. Kes P, Slaviček J. [Hepatitis C virus and progressive kidney disease. Guidelines for detection, judgment, treatment, prevention of infection spread in hemodialysis units, treatment with infected patients, candidates for kidney transplantation, and treatment with patients suspected of having kidney disease associated with HCV infection]. Acta Med Croatica. 2013;67(4):361–6. (in Croatian).
27. Kes P, Janssens ME, Bašić-Jukić N, Kljak M. A randomized crossover study comparing membrane and centrifugal therapeutic plasma exchange procedures. Transfusion. 2016;56(12):3065–72.
28. [Regulations on minimum conditions concerning spaces, workers and medical.technical equipment for the performance of health activities]. Narodne novine, 61/11 i 128/12) (in Croatian). http://hkzr.hr/hr/wp-content/uploads/2012/02/Pravilnik-o-minimalnim-uvjetima-u-pogledu-prostora-radnika-i-medicinsko-tehni%C4%8Dke-opreme-za-obavljanje-zdravstvene-djelatnosti.pdf. Accessed 20 Feb 2020.
29. Rebić D, Matovinović MS, Rašić S, Kes P, Hamzić-Mehmedbašić A. The effect of preserved residual renal function on left ventricular structure in non-anuric peritoneal dialysis patients. Kidney Blood Press Res. 2015;40:500–8.
30. Bašić-Jukić N, Jurić I, Kes P. Encapsulating peritoneal sclerosis in a CAPD patient. BANTAO J. 2011;9(2):94.
31. Bušić M. [Organ donation and transplantation medicine in Croatia]. Medix. 2011;17(92/93):144–8.
32. Živčić-Ćosić S, Bušić M, Župan Ž, Pelčić G, Anušić Juričić M, Jurčić Ž, et al. Development of the Croatian model of organ donation and transplantation. Croat Med J. 2013;54:65–70.
33. [Law on changes and amendments to the act of procurement and transplantation of human body parts for treatment purposes]. *Narodne novine* 50/88; Dec 13, 1988. (in Croatian).

34. [Act on explanation and transplantation of human body parts for medical treatment purposes]. *Narodne novine* 177/04; Dec 15, 2004. (in Croatian).
35. Branger P, Undine Samuel. Annual Report 2018 – Eurotransplant International Foundation. CIP-Gegevens Koninklijke Bibliotheek, Den Haag 2018, pp. 1–104.
36. Bašić-Jukić N, Furić-Čunko V, Kes P, Bubić-Filipi L, Pasini J, Hudolin T, Jurić I. Outcome after renal transplantation in a "senior" program: the Croatian experience. Transplant Proc. 2008;40(10):3418–21.
37. Kes P. [What do we know about chronic kidney disease at the beginning of the 21st century]. Acta Med. Croatica. 2014;68(1):75–77. (in Croatian).
38. Premužić V, Bašić-Jukić N, Jelaković B, Kes P. Continuous veno-venous hemofiltration improves survival of the patients with congestive heart failure and cardiorenal syndrome compared to slow continuous ultrafiltration. Ther Apher Dial. 2017;21(3):279–86.
39. Premužić V, Bašić-Jukić N, Jelaković B, Kes P. Differences in CVVH vs. CVVHDF in the management of sepsis-induced acute kidney injury in critically ill patients. J Artif Org. 2017;20(4):326–34.
40. Bačak-Kocman I, Bašić-Jukić N, Lovčić V, Prkačin I, Miličić D, Kes P. Renal replacement therapy in cardiology wards: changing trends in a transitional country. Therap Apher Dial. 2012;16(2):163–8.
41. Gašparović V, Ostojić R, Gjenero-Margan I, Kes P. Sudden deaths in chronic renal failure patients on haemodialysis in Croatia. Croat Med J. 2001;42(6):606–10.
42. Canaud B, On behalf of the European Experts Panel. Performance liquid test as a cause for sudden deaths of dialysis patients: perfluorohydrocarbon, a previously unrecognized hazard for dialysis patients. Nephrol Dial Transplant. 2002;17(4):545–8.
43. Spasovski G, Bušić M, Delmonaco F. Improvement in kidney transplantation in the Balkans after the Istanbul declaration: where do we stand today? Clin Kidney J. 2016;9(1):172–5.

# Nephrology in the Czech Republic

# 37

Ivan Rychlík, Vladimír Tesař, Sylvie Dusilová Sulková, and Ondřej Viklický

*General Table.* General information about the Czech Republic

| | |
|---|---|
| Area[1] | 78,867 Km$^2$ |
| Population[2] | 10,649,800 (2019) |
| Capital | Prague |
| Three most populated cities | 1. Prague<br>2. Brno<br>3. Ostrava |
| Official language | Czech |
| Gross domestic product (GDP)[3] | 244,110,000,000 USD (2018) |
| GDP per capita[3] | 23,344 USD (2018) |
| Human Development Index (HDI)[4] | 0.888 (2017) |
| Official currency | Czech crown (CZK) |
| Total number of nephrologists[5] | 254 |
| National society of nephrology | Czech Society of Nephrology<br>www.nefrol.cz |
| Incidence of end-stage renal disease[5] | 2018 – 238 pmp |
| Prevalence of end-stage renal disease[5] (including patients with a functioning kidney transplant) | 2018 – 1151 pmp |
| Total number of patients on dialysis[5](all modalities) | 2017 – 6768 (638 pmp)<br>2018 – 6990 (656 pmp) |
| Number of patients on hemodialysis[5] | 2017 – 6373 (600 pmp)<br>2018 – 6631 (622 pmp) |
| Number of patients on peritoneal dialysis[5] | 2017 – 395 (37 pmp)<br>2018 – 359 (34 pmp) |
| Number of renal transplantations per year | 2017 – 469 (44 pmp)<br>2018 – 508 (48 pmp) |

Table References:

1. Czechia. In: World Fact Book. CIA. 2020. https://www.cia.gov/library/publications/the-world-factbook/geos/ez.html. Accessed May 21 2020
2. Počet obyvatel v obcích - k 1.1.2019. Czech Statistical Office. 2019. https://www.czso.cz/csu/czso/pocet-obyvatel-v-obcich-za0wri436p. Accessed May 21 2020
3. Czech Republic - Economic Indicators. Trading economics. 2020. https://tradingeconomics.com/czech-republic/indicators. Accessed May 21 2020
4. Czechia. United Nations Development Programme. 2020. http://hdr.undp.org/en/countries/profiles/CZE. Accessed May 21 2020
5. Národní data. Registr dialyzovaných pacientů. 2020. http://www.nefro.cz/o-rdp/rrt-data-v-čr/národn%C3%AD-data/. Accessed May 21 2020

## Introduction

The Czech Republic, officially also Czechia, was established in 1993 after a peaceful "divorce" of the previous Czech and Slovak Federative Republic (Czechoslovakia). It is a landlocked country located in Central Europe bordering four countries. The Czech Republic is a demographically stable country with 10,649,800 inhabitants in 2019. The information in the General Table summarizes key data concerning the Czech Republic [1–5].

The official currency is the Czech Crown (CZK), introduced in 1993 after the abovementioned separation of Czechoslovakia. Czech Republic is a member state of the European Union (although not a member of the eurozone, thus, the Euro is not the official currency) and North Atlantic Treaty Organization (NATO). The Czech gross domestic product was 244,110 million USD in 2018 [3]. The Czech economy is export-oriented with a large share of industry, especially automotive, and its biggest trading partner is neighboring Germany.

I. Rychlík (✉)
Czech Society of Nephrology (CSN), Prague, Czech Republic

Department of Medicine, Third Faculty of Medicine, Charles University and Faculty Hospital Kralovské Vinohrady, Prague, Czech Republic

V. Tesař
Czech Society of Nephrology (CSN), Prague, Czech Republic

Department of Nephrology, , First Faculty of Medicine, Charles University and General Faculty Hospital, Prague, Czech Republic

S. D. Sulková
Czech Society of Nephrology (CSN), Prague, Czech Republic

Hemodialysis Center, University Hospital, Hradec Králové, Czech Republic

O. Viklický
Czech Society of Nephrology (CSN), Prague, Czech Republic

Nephrology Department, Institute for Clinical and Experimental Medicine, Prague, Czech Republic



J. A. Moura-Neto et al. (eds.), *Nephrology Worldwide*, https://doi.org/10.1007/978-3-030-56890-0_37

The Czech Republic is a unitary state with a parliamentary democratic regime. The head of government is a prime minister. The Czech president does not have strong executive powers, although his informal role and moral authority are historically high. Administratively, there are 13 regions and the capital city of Prague, which have no legislative autonomy. There are 6253 municipalities and the 5 most populated are Prague, Brno, Ostrava, Pilsen, and Liberec [6]. The population is highly urbanized with approximately 73.5% urban dwellers [7]. The official language is Czech, which developed throughout centuries and finally codified in the nineteenth century.

Czech history is rich, dating back to the Dark Middle Ages, but its "golden era" was in High Middle Ages when Prague belonged among the cultural and also political cores of the Holy Roman Empire. In the second half of the fourteenth century, the Bohemian king Charles IV was also the Roman Emperor. Moreover, he established the Charles University in Prague which was the first university north of the Alps. The modern history is connected with the national movement in the nineteenth century which strived for political autonomy within the Habsburg empire in the beginning, later for full independence. Czechoslovakia was established an independent country in 1918 as one of the successor states of Austria-Hungary.

Yet the democratic so-called First Republic was highly developed and it had important Western allies (mainly France, UK), it did not prevail for a long time for it was seized by the Nazi Germany in 1939, Slovakia having separated from the rest of the state. After the World War II, Czechoslovakia was re-established but hardly as an independent country; it was under a strong USSR influence, participating in the introduction of a pro-Moscowian regime, which shortly after switched to an authoritarian communist rule. In 1989, the Czechoslovak Socialist Republic went through a so-called Velvet Revolution which led to the fall of the communist regime and the country regaining its independence. However, the nationalistic tendencies in Slovakia gradually led to the peaceful split of the federation, and in 1993, two successor states – the Czech Republic and Slovakia – came into existence. The Czech Republic entered NATO in 1999 and the European Union (EU) in 2004, finalizing its Euro-Atlantic integrational ambitions.

Healthcare in the Czech Republic was switched into a system of healthcare including insurance companies in 1990. All residents are currently members of the healthcare insurance system, being insured by one of the seven insurance companies. Healthcare providers are either public or private ones. Renal replacement therapy (RRT) is provided and fully covered for all patients. While transplantations are mostly performed by public entities, about two-thirds of chronic dialysis treatment are provided by corporate providers.

## Brief History of Nephrology in the Czech Republic

The origins of the Czech (or Czechoslovak) Society of Nephrology date back to the 1950–1960s and are closely connected with the activities of its founders – Jan Brod, Otto Schück, Josef Erben, Karel Opatrný, Jiří Jirka, and Mirko Chytil. The seminal person of Czech nephrology was undoubtedly Jan Brod (1912–1985) [8]. After graduation, he worked in the laboratory of Prof. Eppinger in Vienna in 1938, after World War II with Prof. Pickering in London and in the laboratory of the famous renal physiologist Homer Smith in the United States. He returned to Prague, Charles University, in 1947 and brought back the lifelong interest for renal physiology, pathophysiology, and the role of the kidney in the regulation of blood pressure. He founded the first nephrology-oriented division in Czechoslovakia. In 1951, he became director of the Institute for the Disorders of Circulation in Prague. He actively participated in the "Prague Spring" in 1968, and after the Soviet invasion to Czechoslovakia, he emigrated to West Germany where he continued his research and educational activities at the University of Hannover until his death. Jan Brod was a man with a high international reputation. In 1962, he was the President of the 2nd Congress of the ISN held in Prague. The scientific activity of Jan Brod focused on the role of the kidney in hypertension, but he was also interested in the treatment of nephrotic syndrome with cytotoxic drugs, acute glomerulonephritis, and pyelonephritis. He also introduced the renal biopsy in 1960 [9]. In 1973, his monograph *The Kidney* [10] was one of the most successful textbooks of nephrology of the time, at least in Europe. Renal physiology and clearance studies remained the main interest of another important Czech nephrologist Otto Schück. His monograph *Examination of Kidney Function* [11] remains probably the best textbook concerning the application of clearance methods in clinical nephrology.

The first hemodialysis (HD) to be performed in Prague was by Mirko Chytil and Severin Daum with a modified Alwall artificial kidney in the First Medical Faculty, Charles University in 1955 [12]. The young lady treated for suicide sublimate intoxication survived. At that time, Prague was the only place behind the "iron curtain" where the artificial kidney was available and patients from neighboring "socialistic" countries were transported to Prague by helicopter to be dialyzed. Chronic dialysis was also introduced in this department in the early 1960s which was soon followed by further dialysis units in Pilsen, headed by Karel Opatrný, and in Hradec Králové, headed by Josef Erben. The latter was a graduate fellow of Prof W. J. Kolff (Cleveland) where he learned how to perform dialysis and transplantation. In 1968, when he returned to Hradec Králové, Erben developed a Czechoslovak prototype of the so-called Hradec Králové dialysis system with central tubing of dialysate solution and six centrally simultaneously controlled dialysis monitors. Furthermore, in 1969, he published his experience with subclavian vein cannulation in chronic hemodialysis patients [13] which is generally considered to be the first report on this topic worldwide.

The nephrological section of the Czech Society of Internal Medicine was also formed by Brod, Chytil, Jirka, and others in 1958. It was the predecessor of the later Czechoslovak Society of Nephrology [12].

In the 1970s–1980s, dialysis devices were imported from Western countries (mostly Gambro AK-10 monitors). The interesting fact is that three different dialysis units (UL-2, Rena, Chiradis) were consecutively developed in Czechoslovakia during the 1970s, but they were not used widely. However, coil dialyzers were made in Czechoslovakia, sometimes literally "produced" by doctors at centers who made dialysis catheters and some other equipment by themselves. The production of dialysis central venous catheters was entrusted to the most careful ones: the first step was to carefully heat the razor-cut section of a scarce non-wettable plastic "tubing" imported from capitalist Sweden and centrally authorized by the Ministry of Health. After shaping the "tip" of the catheter, it was necessary to make the side holes to ensure that the surface remained non-wettable. There was a single-imported "spike," whose blade was maintained by grinding on sanitary tiles. Thus, the main problem of dialysis treatment was neither technology nor human factor but the permanently insufficient capacity of the centers. Technology has existed in the world but only in a ridiculously small amount in Czechoslovakia. Dialysis nephrology was not among the priorities of power structures. The important and internationally renowned person in this time was Albert Válek, who founded the largest dialysis unit in Prague, Strahov, and contributed to the promotion of dialysis methods and care for patients with end-stage renal disease (ESRD). He also contributed to the introduction of continuous ambulatory peritoneal dialysis (CAPD) in Czechoslovakia. In 1980, he organized the EDTA Congress and in 1988 the ESAO Congress in Prague. Home HD was carried out in the early 1980s, although temporarily and only in two to three centers. The sole reason was the effort to expand the dialysis capacity. Meanwhile, the same goal led to a large spread of "self-care" methods and even the application of peritoneal dialysis (PD) in unfavorable conditions. In Czechoslovakia in the 1980s, little progress was made in the field of nephrology, for example, in 1989 only about 50 patients pmp were dialyzed in only 23 dialysis units in the entire country of 15.3 million inhabitants in that time, and patients with systemic diseases affecting the kidney (including diabetes) and persons older than 50 years were excluded from the chronic dialysis program. All dialysis devices were imported, and domestically made coil dialyzers were prevalent. Single-imported hollow fiber dialyzers would be so rare that they would be reused (sterilizing agent would be acetic acid) repeatedly, up to more than ten times. Furthermore, the first experience with hemodiafiltration (HDF) using replacement solution in bags was also obtained in the mid-1980s, at that time as a part of aluminum intoxication treatment together with Desferal among other things [12].

The initiation of PD dates back to the mid-1970s. It was associated with two to three sites where, due to the critical lack of HD capacity, this method was introduced as having poor outcomes but still possible treatment option. The critical problem was not only the primary unfamiliarity with the method but also the technical problems and conditions. While relatively modern imported devices were available for HD, almost nothing was available for PD. Only PD catheters would be imported. The dialysis bags were completely unavailable. The only option was to use the solution in glass bottles. The solution for these centers was prepared by a magistral in friendly pharmacies, dissolving the salts in boiled sterile water. Overall results were poor. The main treatment and patient survival limitation would be peritonitis. Its occurrence used to be on the daily basis (the bottle solution was continually contaminated with air). The only positive thing was to gain experience; rarely it was possible to "bridge" the waiting period for HD [12].

Early attempts of kidney transplantation began in Hradec Králové as early as 1961; however, in 1966, the first successful living donor kidney transplantation was performed at the Institute for Clinical and Experimental Medicine (IKEM) in Prague with the important contribution of Jiří Jirka [12]. This was the beginning of the regular and expanding transplantation program in this institute, succeeded by further transplantation centers in Pilsen, Hradec Králové, Olomouc, Brno, and Ostrava. Jiří Jirka was also the first one who attempted to introduce the manual peritoneal dialysis program.

During the 1970s, two of the most prominent Czech nephropathologists – Josef Stejskal and Pavel Rossmann – advanced their career and became internationally known. Stejskal was focused on the topic of changes of the glomerular basal membrane [14] and Rossmann on rejection of kidney transplant [15].

The 1990s were characteristic with the dynamic development of renal treatment, especially dialysis. For instance, the number of dialyzed patients increased threefold. The significant modernization of medical appliances was an important feature of this period. Likewise, the research in dialysis started to be more important, and it was devoted the most to the topic of biocompatibility and coagulation (Karel Opatrný Jr), dialysis adequacy (František Lopot), renal bone disease (Sylvie Dusilová Sulková), but also conservative treatment (Vladimír Teplan). Moreover, other important nonphysicians dedicated their professional life to dialysis, among them František Lopot, clinical bioengineer, and Jitka Pancířová, renal nurse, who both were long-term presidents of EDTNA/ERCA.

In the 1990s, the Czech Society of Nephrology (CSN) broadened its activities and increased the number of its members. The society reorganized the National Dialysis Patients Register and introduced the Czech Registry of Renal Biopsies, and a new journal dedicated to nephrology (*Aktuality v nefrologii*) was founded. Furthermore, enhancement of the quality of nephrology education (theory and practice) was conveyed to the young generation of dialysis physicians. The CSN accommodated the centers with professional and organizational help, even the leaders came to assist centers where experienced doctors were missing. The CSN Junior Nephrologists Club was established and became an important and popular tool in nephrology education as well as a place to meet young colleagues from the entire country [12].

The development after 2000 has been characterized with stabilization of RRT, even more significantly after the Czech Republic entered the EU. On the other hand, the negative aspect of this period has been an outflux of medical personnel (physicians and nurses as well) abroad; the destination countries have been mostly Germany and Austria due to significantly better financial conditions.

Nevertheless, the total number of nephrology experts has increased during the last three decades. Besides nephrological, educational, and scientific activities developing significantly in Czechia, Prague has repeatedly been a venue of numerous European medical congresses – the ERA-EDTA hosted again its Congress in Prague in 2011. Many international educational meetings organized by the ERA-EDTA and the ISN as well as other medical societies focused on nephrology took place in Prague. New generations of Czech nephrologists have been highly involved in international cooperation (mostly under the umbrella of the ERA-EDTA) – Ivan Rychlík, Vladimír Tesař, and Ondřej Viklický among them. Despite the long-lasting history and the successes of the Czech nephrology, at the present time, nephrology has lacked the attention and interest of young colleagues, who otherwise would continue in the nephrological tradition, due to the high competition with other medical specialities.

## Renal Diseases in the Czech Republic

### Chronic Kidney Disease

Epidemiology of chronic kidney disease (CKD) in the Czech Republic is not significantly different from Western European countries, and Czech Republic belongs among the countries with the highest incidence and prevalence of RRT [16]. The most common cause of end-stage renal failure (ESRD) is diabetic kidney disease (more than 30% of all patients), followed by vascular disease (probably as combination of hypertensive nephrosclerosis and ischemic nephropathy); the proportion of ESRD caused by glomerular diseases is relatively stable and does not surpass 10–15%. Almost 8% of patients treated by RRT have developed ESRD due to autosomal dominant polycystic kidney disease, the most frequent inherited kidney disease in Czechia.

Among primary glomerulonephritides (based on the data from the Czech Registry of Renal Biopsies, running since 1994 and currently collecting more than 15,000 native renal biopsy records), the most frequent is IgA nephropathy (37%), followed by membranous nephropathy (13%) and focal segmental glomerulosclerosis (12%), among secondary glomerulonephritides, lupus nephritis (22%), and ANCA-associated vasculitis (19%) [17, 18]. There is no endemic renal disease in the Czech Republic, but because of very good screening and diagnostics of inherited metabolic disease, Czech Republic is among the countries with the highest number of patients with Fabry disease treated with chronic enzyme replacement therapy [19].

### Predialysis Care

Predialysis care is for a long time a routine part of outpatient dialysis preparation, particularly based on a local dialysis unit catchment area. A relatively new activity applied by insurance companies is the financial bonification of patient preparation to be enrolled preemptively to a kidney transplant waiting list, which is still rare. On the other hand, one very significant problem is late arrivals to predialysis care, which reaches about 20–40% of the patients entering RRT [20]. Long-term systematic hepatitis B vaccination practically eradicated this disease among the dialysis population. The same is true for recently applied hepatitis C antiviral therapy, fully reimbursed, which has resulted in almost null prevalence of HCV among dialysis patients. In 2018, the prevalence of HBV-DNA positivity was confirmed in about 0.3% patients and HBsAg positivity in about 0.6%. HCV-RNA positivity was confirmed in 0.1% and anti-HCV positivity in about 1.0%. HIV rate in HD population is not publicly available. A long-lasting problem is the limited capacity of vascular surgeons for early creation of arteriovenous fistulas, which is further enhanced by aging, high diabetes prevalence, and significant polymorbidity. This dismal situation results in increasing the number of patients entering chronic dialysis treatment with central venous catheters [5]. In the end of 1990s, the routine use of human recombinant erythropoietin (rHuEPO) started for predialysis patients and later. Other modern drugs like non-calcium-containing phosphate binders, vitamin D analogues, etc. were also introduced.

Since 2009, the CSN has also been running the Registry of Predialysis Patients (RIP) [5]; data are collected on voluntary basis from all predialysis patients treated in nephrology/dialysis units, cooperating with the registry of dialysis patients (RDP). The inclusion criteria are s-creatinine level >300 μmol/l for males and 250 for females and systematic outpatients management for CKD. Besides basic entry data (age, gender, height, weight, PRD – primary renal disease), further laboratory and therapy data are reported quarterly using an electronic database. In total, 5104 patients were reported in a 10-year period (2009–2018) from 71% of all dialysis units in the country, with male prevalence of 53% and median follow-up of 24 months. The most frequent PRDs were diabetic kidney disease 26%, glomerulonephritis 15%, ischemic nephropathy 12%, tubulointerstitial nephritis 9%, and inherited kidney diseases 3.5%, while the prevalence of unspecified contracted small kidney was quite high reaching 31%. Concerning drug treatment: 31% used ketoanalogues; 27% phosphate binders; 38% ACE-i; 26% ARB; 82% diuretics; 17% were treated with erythropoiesis-stimulating agents (ESA) with a mean dosage of 4547 IU; and 60% used vitamin D (all forms). Concerning follow-up, 44% entered RRT, 6% underwent transplantation (after starting RRT), and 18% died before entering RRT.

### Acute Kidney Injury and Critical Care Nephrology

Patients with acute kidney injury (AKI) are treated together by nephrologists and intensivists (particularly when they need to be admitted to the intensive care unit). There are no exact data on the epidemiology of AKI in the Czech population, but incidence and prevalence of AKI among hospitalized patients and its outcome may hardly be much different from that recently reported from Germany [21]. With the increasing number of diagnostic and therapeutic interventions, there is an increasing proportion of AKI associated with revascularizations and cardiovascular surgery, although sepsis definitely remains the leading cause of AKI in the hospital setting.

## Renal Replacement Therapy in the Czech Republic

RRT for ESRD in Czechia encompasses HD and PD modalities, as well as both living and deceased donor transplantations. The majority of prevalent patients either are undergoing HD or already transplanted. Of note, about two-thirds of dialysis patients are treated by online HDF which is fully reimbursed.

In 2018, the prevalence of patients in dialysis was 6990, and further 5204 were followed after kidney transplantation (Fig. 37.1). Most of the data presented herein is from the Czech Society of Nephrology's registry of dialysis patients (RDP) [5], which was converted to a fully electronic reporting system in 2004 and currently covers all dialysis centers in Czechia.

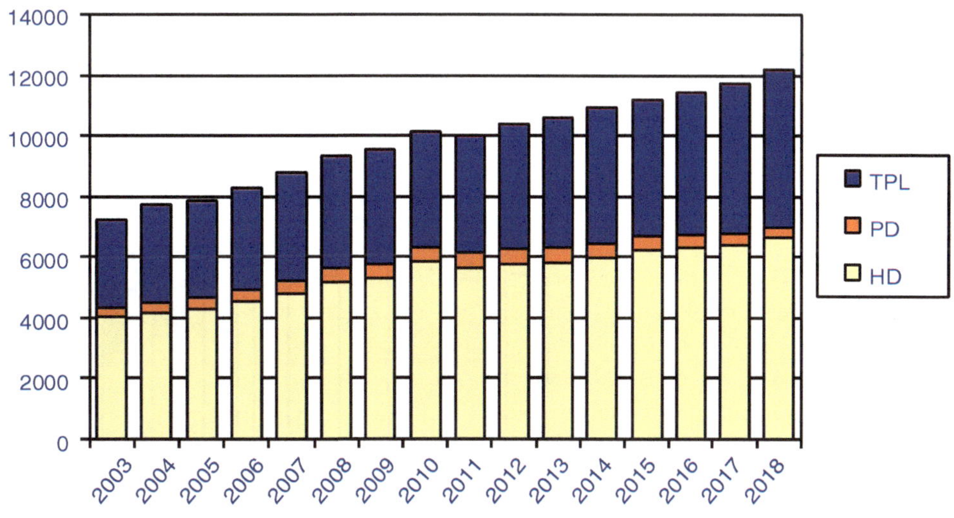


**Fig. 37.1** Prevalence number of patients in RRT according to treatment method in the Czech Republic (2003–2018) [5]. Abbreviations: *TPL* transplantation, *PD* peritoneal dialysis, *HD* hemodialysis

## Hemodialysis

Since the early 1990s, HD capacity has largely and rapidly developed, and the high quality of the equipment has been maintained, the number of centers rose to a hundred in a few years, and structural changes took place in the former exclusively state sector (establishment of new – both state and non-state – centers). HDF with online preparation of substitution solution has been for many years not only available but also a preferred method of extracorporeal treatment of chronic renal failure. Currently at least half of the centers use this method exclusively [5], and about 74% of all patients are treated with this method. Other convective methods have not been used so often (Fig. 37.2).

Erythropoietin or ESA products have been available since 1988, albeit at first in limited amounts, but today without any restrictions and fully covered by health insurance, i.e., without patient's financial contribution. Moreover, the complete dialysis care and even transportation to/from dialysis treatment is being covered by health insurance. After 2010, several new drugs have been introduced, which are currently used, e.g., calcium non-containing phosphate finder, analogues of vitamin D, etc. In addition, some new technological procedures have been implemented – e.g., bioimpedance hydration measurement (BCM, body composition monitor) [22].

Currently, there are more than 115 dialysis centers in the Czech Republic, often with 20 or more dialysis beds, run in 3 shifts regime. About one-third is nonprofit (public sites), and two-thirds are private dominated by Fresenius Medical Care and B. Braun. The standard schedule is 4–5 hours per session (96% of all patients; mean duration 4.34 hours) three times a week (89%), while other regimes are relatively minor (<4 hours 3.5%, >5 hours 0.7%), twice a week 10.3%, and others 0.7%.

No official HDF prescriptions exist, but the most common targets are blood flow ≥350 ml/min, convective volume >21.0 L/session, and online post-dilution HDF is used the most. Polysulfone membranes are the most commonly used, and reuse of dialyzers is not allowed.

With regard to vascular access – the prevalence of native AV fistulas is approximately 70%, grafts 5%, and long-term catheters 25%, but a lot of patients (about 50%) enter chronic dialysis with a temporary catheter. Monitoring of AVF function by the thermodilution method is widely applied among most of dialysis centers, and it is fully reimbursed.

The cumulative survival (Kaplan-Meier) of dialysis patients is given in Fig. 37.3. One-year survival rate is above 80%, 5-year survival rate reaches up to 52%, and about 7.5% of patients are transplanted each year. Although the difference between survival of diabetic and nondiabetic patients is unequivocal, higher survival of nondiabetics becomes significant after 2.5 years after initiation of treatment.

Detailed basic epidemiology data are given in the General Table.

## Peritoneal Dialysis

After the Velvet Revolution in 1989, there was a dramatic turnaround due to the increase of imported real PD solution bags. The pioneering centers in the method soon achieved great success. At the same time, they shared valuable experience with newly established centers. Throughout years, the number of PD patients increased up to 8%, but currently, approximately 5.1% of all dialysis patients are in the PD program in the Czech Republic [5]. The low utilization of this method relates certainly to the very dense network of HD centers (with free transport) and perhaps a certain habit of "dependency." In the vast majority of the sites, the method of dialysis treatment preferred by the patient is chosen. Prague-IKEM, Prague-VFN, and Pilsen-FN are the largest and most

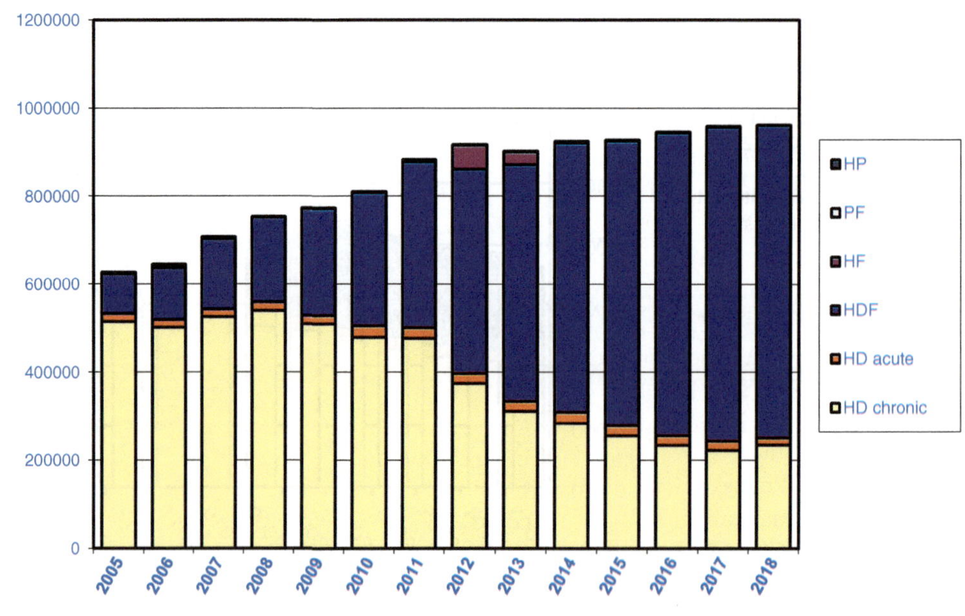


**Fig. 37.2** Number of extracorporeal procedures in 2018 [5]. Abbreviations: *HP* hemoperfusion, *PF* plasmapheresis, *HF* hemofiltration, *HDF* hemodiafiltration, *HD* hemodialysis

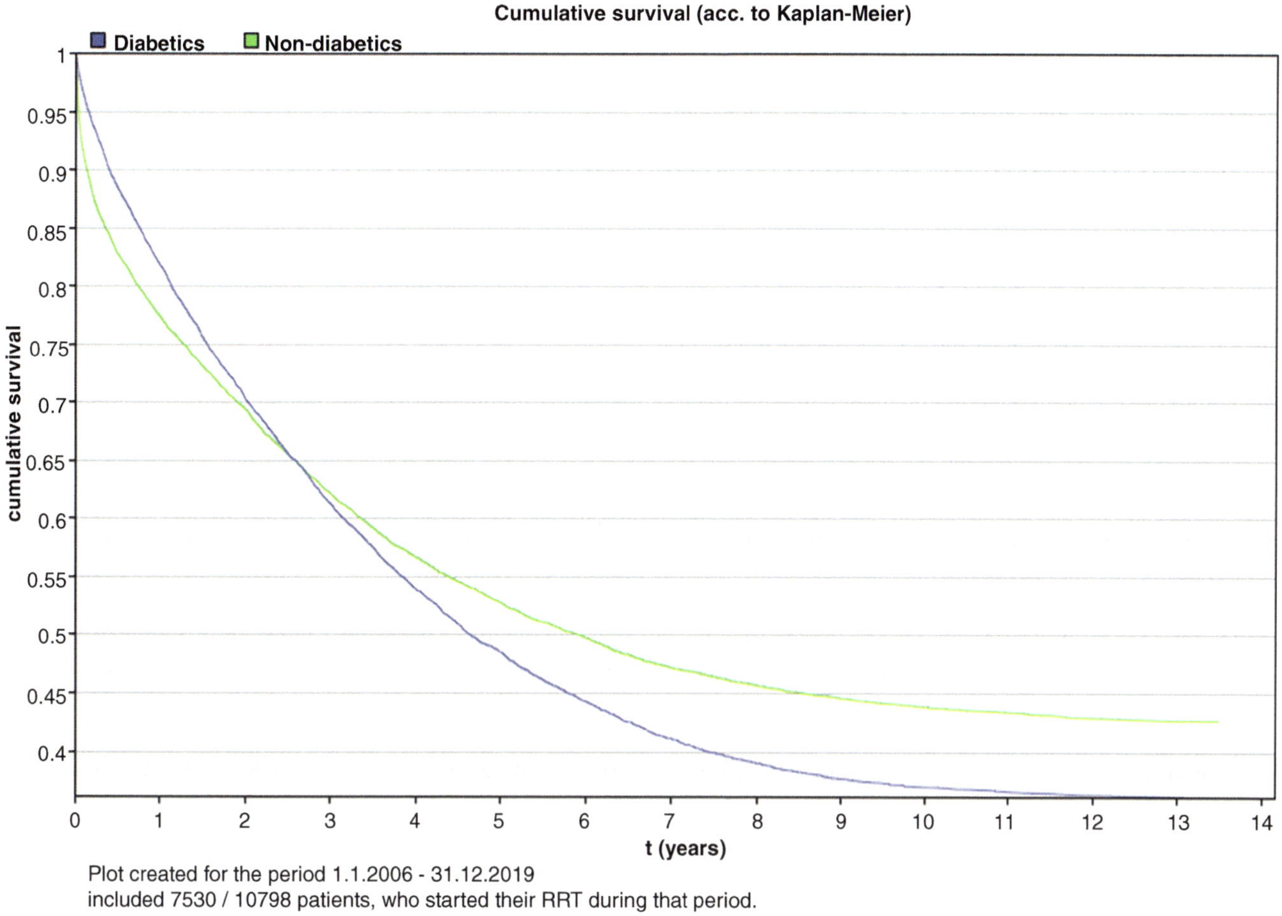


**Fig. 37.3** Survival of diabetics (N=7530) vs. nondiabetics (N=10798) (Kaplan-Meier) in Czechia [5]

**Table 37.1** Number of kidney transplantations in the Czech Republic in 2018

| | PRAHA - IKEM | PRAHA -MOTOL (Pediatric) | PILSEN | HRADEC KRALOVE | BRNO | OLOMOUC | OSTRAVA | *Total CZ* | *Total CZ/pmp* |
|---|---|---|---|---|---|---|---|---|---|
| DD kidney | 221 | 15 | 31 | 35 | 78 | 32 | 49 | *461* | ***43,5*** |
| LD kidney | 35 | 1 | 2 | 1 | 4 | 2 | 2 | *47* | ***4,4*** |

Abbreviations: *DD* deceased donor, *LD* living donor

experienced centers at present. Automated PD (APD) (cycler) takes approximately half of the patients, and other new technologies have been implemented throughout the last two decades [23]. In 2018, the peritonitis rate was 13.4% (48 cases in 37 patients out of 359).

## Renal Transplantation

### Organization of Transplantations in the Czech Republic

There are seven transplant programs in the country (IKEM Prague, Motol Prague, Brno, Hradec Králové, Pilsen, Olomouc, and Ostrava). Each transplant program has an assigned region with donor hospitals (Table 37.1). The transplant legislation is covered by the Transplantation Act from 2002. Presumed consent to donate organs is anticipated unless registered with the determination to donate an organ after death. The Czech Transplantation Coordinating Center was established in 2003 by the Czech Ministry of Health, and it operates under its direct supervision facilitating organ donations and transplantations, including the management of transplant registries, the coordination of procurements, and transplantations. Traditionally, the Czech Republic has been successful in facilitating deceased donor program with 25 brain dead donors pmp in recent years [24]. The first DCD (donor after circulatory death) kidney procurement was performed in Pilsen, and until now the DCD program is running in four centers; however a total number of retrieved DCD organs remain low. All transplant programs in the Czech Republic are fully reimbursed and included long-term immunosuppression.

## Kidney Transplantation

All seven transplant centers in the country perform kidney transplants with the highest volumes being performed at IKEM for adult and Motol for pediatric transplants (Table 37.1). The first-year graft survival rate is 95%. Median time to transplant from the initiation of dialysis oscillates about 700 days, and in some centers with a small number of patients on the waiting list, the time to transplant after listing is very short. Preemptive kidney transplantation (prior to initiation of dialysis) represents one-third of living donor programs, while it is rarer in deceased donor programs. All registered immunosuppressant drugs are available, while the combination of tacrolimus, mycophenolate mofetil, and steroids is currently used in all patients initially. Induction protocols include either rATG or basiliximab according to immunological risk, but more specific desensitization protocols are applied in patients with donor-specific antibodies.

Incompatible pairs are mostly referred to IKEM for either ABO incompatible transplants (desensitization protocol with rituximab and specific immunoabsorption established in 2011) or kidney paired donation which was initiated as early as 2003 and established as a program since 2012 with over 70 paired live donor transplants performed since then. Recently, IKEM initiated cooperation with Vienna, Austria, that resulted in a successful kidney swap between sensitized HLA incompatible pairs [25], and an altruistic donor-initiated binational chain with bridging donors has been ongoing. HLA incompatible live donor kidney transplants are only rarely accepted and treated with a desensitization protocol based on rituximab, apheresis, and IVIG. For deceased donors, the Luminex MFI threshold for kidney acceptance in a sensitized recipient varies among centers with a threshold <5000 at IKEM. Currently, more than 5200 kidney transplants are followed in the country [5].

## Nephrology Practice in the Czech Republic

The number of dialyzed patients has increased to almost 660 pmp and the number of dialysis units to more than 115, and there is now no limitation in access to chronic HD. The Czech Republic belongs to those countries with one of the highest annual rates of renal transplantation in Europe nowadays, with 48 transplanted patients pmp. Unfortunately, some problems have prevailed, and others have emerged. PD is still underdeveloped in the Czech Republic, i.e., only about 5.1% of dialyzed patients are treated by PD. The dialysis population in the Czech Republic is becoming older and older, with 74% of patients treated by HD being 60 years and over. Diabetic nephropathy now represents 33% of all causes of ESRD treated by HD, and the prevalence of DM among HD patients reaches 46%, mostly type 2 DM.

All types of RRT (HD, HDF, PD, transplantation) are fully reimbursed. The approximate coverage per each session is the following (in USD): HD 150, HDF 250, home hemodialysis 160, CAPD 75, and APD 180.

An interesting feature is the RRT financial bonification system, which was recently introduced to the reimbursement system in order to stimulate physicians and their sites to provide high-quality treatment [5]. It takes into account the quality of treatment data which the dialysis sites provide to the registries. To get the bonification, it requires that providers must follow international guidelines to ensure the quality of treatment. Moreover, the CSN is the main authority assessing the quality, and the healthcare companies respect its expert opinion and allocate the bonification accordingly.

Technical, spatial, and material requirements of a dialysis center are regulated by law. Similarly, the obligations concerning personnel are set: 1 full time nephrologists supervising maximally 12 beds and 1 nurse up to 5 dialysis beds. In 2018, 1884 employees worked in dialysis centers in total – 254 nephrologists (191 of them were board certified/75%) (Fig. 37.4) and 1347 dialysis nurses (824 fully certified /61%) with an average of 736 sessions per nurse. One hundred and sixty-nine orderlies and 114 dialysis technicians and administrators provided required support. Some dialysis units also involve renal dietitians and psychologists, but these are usually not employed full time. Training institutions are firstly accredited and then periodically inspected by the Ministry of Education. The curriculum requires 4 and 1/2 years of supervised training. During the first 2 years, the training consists mostly of internal medicine and 2 and 1/2 additional years of nephrology. During the second part of the education, a training center should provide a complete overview of nephrology including theoretical and practical training at least on HD, PD, ESRD, AKI, critical care nephrology, renal transplantation, and clinical nephrology.

It is a prerequisite for the head physician to have full qualification, i.e., state certificate (Ministry of Health) and medical chamber certificate, both in the field of nephrology. Each year, about 10–15 nephrologists are certified passing the state exam [26]. The medical staff must be permanently present at the dialysis site during treatment.

All centers currently have high standards of treatment and are regularly inspected. Mutual communication is at a very good level and is channeled by the Czech Society of Nephrology, which also organizes and guarantees professional and educational events (but it is not the only provider and guarantor of education).

While formerly many of the dialysis nephrologists themselves created vascular arteriovenous fistulas and even

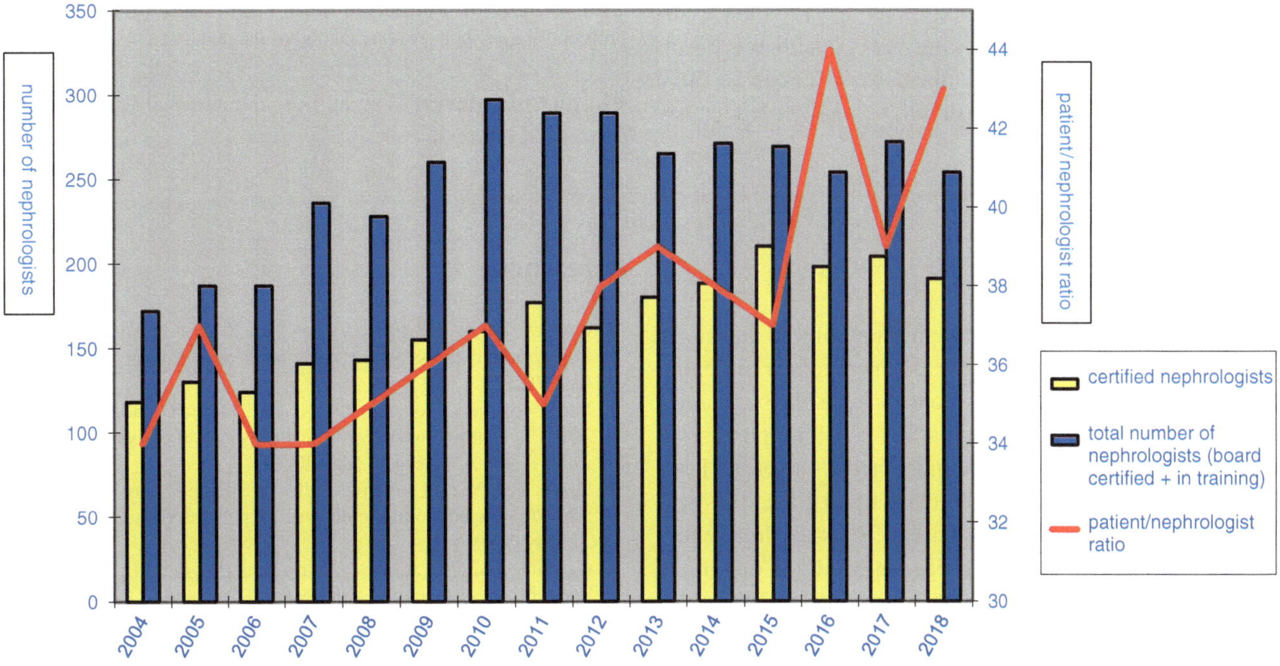


**Fig. 37.4** Number of physicians-nephrologists in 2018 [5]

"made" some dialysis equipment as described above, nowadays they have no competency to do so, nor are they forced by lack of them. On the other hand, completely top-quality equipment is available in the market. Further, the introduction of central temporary and long-term central venous catheters remains fully in the management of dialysis nephrologists.

Recently, the conservative approach overlapping with palliative medicine has become a legitimate part of especially dialysis nephrology.

The entire nephrological dialysis community works closely with transplantologists. In large numbers, patients are already prepared for inclusion in the waiting list for transplantation in the predialysis period [5]. The established "rule" is joint seminars and various business meetings, conferences, and congresses.

Concerning clinical nephrology, two university-based departments of nephrology and several divisions of nephrology located mostly in regional capital cities operate in the country. They provide full clinical nephrology services and consultation, including renal biopsy. However, like in other EU countries, there is a lack of experienced nephropathologists.

Concerning pediatric nephrology, one large Charles University-based center in Prague serves for kidney transplant for the whole country. Similarly as in adults, several pediatric nephrology units are located in regional capital cities. However, pediatric nephrologists are unified under the umbrella of the Pediatric Medical Society.

## Nephrology Job Market

In the early 1990s, there was a tremendous increase of the newly opened dialysis units and strong pressure on the qualification of new nephrologists and renal nurses to care for the increasing number of patients treated with RRT, and, as a result, the number of practicing nephrologists soared [27]. Currently, most of this strong generation approach retirement, and they will probably not be sufficiently replaced by newly qualified nephrologists. As in other countries, nephrology does not belong among the most attractive branches of internal medicine, definitely because of relatively limited progress concerning new treatments for the renal patients and inappropriate concentration of nephrology on RRT resulting in the loss of what previously was (and should remain) a part of nephrology (e.g., AKI, hypertension, electrolyte, and acid base disorders) in favor of intensivists or cardiologists. To attract young physicians to nephrology, our specialty is to be presented as a discipline with many overlaps with other branches of internal medicine (cardiology, diabetology, immunology, rheumatology, osteology, intensive medicine, etc.), and more attention should be paid to the recent progress in the treatment of glomerular and inherited kidney disease and renal transplantation and importance of procedural skills for the practicing nephrologist [28]. The average monthly salary (including overnight shifts and bank holiday bonuses) of a Czech physician is about 3400 USD, and nurses earn 1870 USD on average [29]. There are no nephrology-specific data available. As women prevail also among newly qualified nephrologists (61% of 466 CSN members were female in 2017 [18]), much greater attention should be paid to gender pay gap [30].

## Conclusion

The Czechoslovak and Czech nephrology played an important role in history and development of nephrology in Central Eastern Europe. The 1950s are considered as the beginnings of the discipline. Czechoslovakia had a special position at the socialist times when it was undoubtedly one of the leading countries in the field within the Eastern Bloc. This was demonstrated by the fact that the first HD was already performed in Prague as early as 1955. Jan Brod was one of the "founding fathers" of not only the Czechoslovak but also world nephrology, at those times.

Despite serious limitations of the local communist regime and lack of material and appliances in the nephrological healthcare, acute and chronic HD and transplantation were developing; therefore, after the collapse of the regime, there was a solid ground for further development. Hence, the era after 1989 can be definitely considered as further expansion of the Czechoslovak and after 1993 Czech nephrological care and its advancement.

The Czech Society of Nephrology belongs among the profoundly active ones. Its highest success is represented in several registries. The National Registry of Patients on Dialysis, which was established in 2006, currently contains 100% of data from all the dialysis centers in the Czech Republic. The Czech Registry of Renal Biopsies, founded in 1993, has more than 15,000 entries. The Registry of Predialysis Patients was established in 2009, and it covers half of the sites managing predialysis patients.

The Czech Republic is specific with the high rate of incidence of ESRD within the EU. For unclear reasons, but probably because of high prevalence of type 2 diabetes, obesity, and ischemic renal disease, there is a high volume of patients in RRT. The high number of kidney-transplanted patients belongs among the unique local features. Also, the bonification reimbursement system organized by the public healthcare insurance companies motivating dialysis units, which was recently introduced, represents an interesting means of how to foster the link between the healthcare providers, medical experts, general knowledge, patient well-being, and financing of costly treatment like the RRT.

The Czech Society of Nephrology would like not only to follow the great tradition of nephrology in the country but also to maintain European standards in both clinical nephrology and other modes of RRT.

**Acknowledgment** The authors would like to thank Vít Borčany who profoundly contributed to finalization of the manuscript.

**Conflict of Interest** The authors declare that they have no conflict of interest.

## References

1. Czechia. In: World Fact Book. CIA. 2020. https://www.cia.gov/library/publications/the-world-factbook/geos/ez.html. Accessed 21 May 2020.
2. Počet obyvatel v obcích - k 1.1.2019. Czech Statistical Office. 2019. https://www.czso.cz/csu/czso/pocet-obyvatel-v-obcich-za0wri436p. Accessed 21 May 2020.
3. Czech Republic - Economic Indicators. Trading economics. 2020. https://tradingeconomics.com/czech-republic/indicators. Accessed 21 May 2020.
4. Czechia. United Nations Development Programme. 2020. http://hdr.undp.org/en/countries/profiles/CZE. Accessed 21 May 2020.
5. Národní data. Registr dialyzovaných pacientů. 2020. http://www.nefro.cz/o-rdp/rrt-data-v-čr/národn%C3%AD-data/. Accessed 21 May 2020.
6. Počet obcí, částí obcí, základních sídelních jednotek a katastrálních území a úhrnné hodnoty podle krajů, okresů a správních obvodů obcí s rozšířenou působností. Czech Statistical Office. 2019. https://www.czso.cz/documents/10180/20567175/93833271.pdf/883077e4-0060-438a-9b29-f23607742a29?version=1.0. Accessed 21 May 2020.
7. Czech Republic: Urbanization from 2008 to 2018. Statista. https://www.statista.com/statistics/455811/urbanization-in-czech-republic/. Accessed 21 May 2020.
8. Rychlík I, Matoušovic K. Contribution of Jan Brod to nephrology. Kidney Blood Press Res. 2011;34:299–302.
9. Matoušovic K, Martínek V, Špatenka J, et al. Význam biopsie ledviny v současné nefrologie. Prakt Lék. 1999;79:194.
10. Brod J. The kidney. London: Butterworths; 1973.
11. Schück O. Funkční vyšetřování ledvin. Praha: Avicenum; 1979.
12. Matoušovic K, Rychlík I, Dusilová SS. Hereditatis petitio české nefrologie. Praha: Tigis; 2009.
13. Erben J, Kvasnička J, Baštecký J, Vortel J. Experience with subclavian vein cannulation in haemodialysis. Proc EDTA. 1969;6:59.
14. Stejskal J, Pirani CL, Okada M, et al. Discontinuities (gaps) of the glomerular capillary wall and basement membrane in renal diseases. Lab Investig. 1973;28:149.
15. Rossmann P, Matoušovic K, Jirka J. Renal allograft biopsy: image, interpretation, interventions. Praha: Academia; 1997.
16. Pippias M, Kramer A, Noordzij M, et al. The European Renal Association – European dialysis and transplant association registry annual report 2014: a summary. Clin Kidney J. 2017;10:154–69.
17. Maixnerová D, Jancová E, Skibova J, et al. Nationwide biopsy survey of renal diseases in the Czech Republic during the years 1993-2011. J Nephrol. 2015;28:39–49.
18. Czech Society of Nephrology. 2020. https://www.nefrol.cz. Accessed 21 May 2020. (official website of the Czech Society of Nephrology).
19. Merta M, Reiterová J, Ledvinová J, et al. A nationwide blood spot screening study for Fabry disease in the Czech Republic haemodialysis patients population. Nephrol Dial Transplant. 2007;22:179–86.
20. Smržová J, Urbánek T, Dvořák M, et al. What is the quality of predialysis healthcare in the Czech Republic? Kidney Blood Press Res. 2012;35:417–24. https://doi.org/10.1159/000336176.

21. Khadzhynov D, Schmidt D, Hardt J, et al. The incidence of acute kidney injury and associated hospital mortality. Dtsch Arztebl Int. 2019;116:397–404.
22. Dusilová SS. Hemodialýza. 2nd ed. Praha: Maxdorf Jessenius; 2007.
23. Bednářová V. Peritoneální dialýza. 2nd ed. Praha: Maxdorf Jessenius; 2007.
24. Koordinační středisko transplantací. 2020. https://kst.cz/. Accessed 21 May 2020.
25. Böhmig GA, Fronek J, Slavcev A, et al. Czech-Austrian kidney paired donation: first European cross-border living donor kidney exchange. Transpl Int. 2017;30:638–9. https://doi.org/10.1111/tri.12945.
26. Ministerstvo zdravotnictví ČR. 2020. https://www.mzcr.cz. (official website of the Ministry of Health of the Czech Republic). Accessed 21 May 2020.
27. Spasovski G, Rroji M, Vazelov E, et al. Nephrology in the Eastern and Central European region: challenges and opportunities. Kidney Int. 2019;96:287–90.
28. Norby SM. Requirement for procedural skills in nephrology training programs: framing the conversation. Clin J Am Soc Nephrol. 2018;13:1096–8.
29. Lékařům 84 tisíc korun měsíčně a sestrám polovinu. Platy se vyrovnaly průměru EU. Aktuálně.cz. https://zpravy.aktualne.cz/ekonomika/lekarum-84-tisic-korun-mesicne-a-sestram-polovinu-platy-se-v/r~08d70e086feb11e9ab10ac1f6b220ee8/. Accessed 21 May 2020.
30. Stevens KI, Soler MJ, Bruchfeld A, Mallamaci F. Paving the way towards gender equality: how are we faring in nephrology? Nephrol Dial Transplant. 2019. pii: gfz165. https://doi.org/10.1093/gfz165.

# Nephrology in Denmark

# 38

James Heaf, Nicolas Carlson, Johan V. Povlsen, Søren Schwartz Sørensen, and Per Wittenhagen

| | |
|---|---|
| Area | 42,933 Km$^2$ |
| Population[1] | 5,797,446 (2018) |
| Capital | Copenhagen |
| Three most populated cities: | 1. Copenhagen<br>2. Aarhus<br>3. Odense |
| Official language | Danish |
| Gross domestic product (GDP)[1] | 355.675 billion USD (2018) |
| GDP per capita[1] | 61,350.348 USD (2018) |
| Human Development Index (HDI)[2] | 0.930 (2018) |
| Official currency | Danish krone (DKK) |
| Total number of nephrologists | 120 |
| National society of nephrology | Danish Society of Nephrology<br>www.nephrology.dk |
| Incidence of end-stage renal disease[3] | 2017 – 124 pmp<br>2018 – 113 pmp |
| Prevalence of end-stage renal disease[3] (including patients with a functioning kidney transplant) | 2018 – 957 pmp<br>2019 – 960 pmp |
| Total number of patients on dialysis[3] (all modalities) | 2018 – 2608<br>2019 – 2605 |
| Number of patients on haemodialysis[3] | 2018 – 2067<br>2019 – 2064 |
| Number of patients on peritoneal dialysis[3] | 2017– 557<br>2018 – 541 |
| Number of renal transplantations per year[3] | 2017 – 250<br>2018 – 245 |

Notes

1. The prevalence figures for 2018 are as per 1.1.2018 and 2019 1.1.2019

Table references:

1. The World Bank. Accessed in March, 2020. Available in: https://data.worldbank.org/country/denmark?view=chart
2. United Nations Development Program. Human Development Reports. Accessed in March, 2020. Available in: http://hdr.undp.org/sites/all/themes/hdr_theme/country-notes/DNK.pdf
3. Danish Nephrology Registry (DNR) Annual Report, accessible on www.nephrology.dk

## Introduction

The Kingdom of Denmark is a small country in Scandinavia in Northwest Europe. The unified Kingdom of Denmark emerged in the eighth century. It was Christianized in 965 and converted to Lutheranism in 1536. During the Middle Ages, the country included Norway, southern Sweden, Iceland and parts of northern Germany but now consists only of mainland Denmark and the self-governing areas of Greenland and the Faroe islands. The country became a democratic constitutional monarch in 1849, and universal suffrage was introduced in 1908. The government relies on the support of a single-chamber parliament with 179 representatives elected approximately every 4 years by proportional representation. Denmark joined the NATO alliance in 1949 and the European Economic Community (now the European Union) in 1973.

The population is homogenous with 87% of the population of Danish descent. Nearly all have Danish as their primary language, but a large proportion are proficient in English. While the birth rate is low, the population continues to grow due to net immigration and increased longevity.

The economy was originally predominantly agricultural, but since 1945 the industrial and service sectors have expanded rapidly. It is based on free market capitalism, with regular negotiations between employers and unions to determine wage and working conditions. The level of unionization is high.

J. Heaf (✉)
Department of Medicine, Zealand University Hospital, Roskilde, Denmark
e-mail: heaf@dadlnet.dk

N. Carlson
Department of Nehrology, Righshospitalet, Copenhagen, Denmark

J. V. Povlsen
Department of Nephrology, Aarhus University Hospital, Aarhus, Denmark

S. S. Sørensen · P. Wittenhagen
H.C. Andersen's Children's Hospital, Odense University Hospital, Odense, Denmark


J. A. Moura-Neto et al. (eds.), *Nephrology Worldwide*, https://doi.org/10.1007/978-3-030-56890-0_38

The country is characterized by an extensive welfare state, with free healthcare, education, generous pensions, paid maternity and paternity leave, unemployment insurance and social welfare benefits. As a corollary, it has one of the highest overall tax rates in the world. Progressive income tax rates and cash transfers result in a low income inequality.

Denmark is one of the most socially developed countries in the world and rates highly in terms of income, health, education, environmental performance, civil liberties, social mobility and personal happiness. It has the lowest corruption index in the world.

## Healthcare in Denmark

The Danish healthcare system is universal and based on the principles of free and equal access to healthcare for all citizens. The healthcare system offers high-quality services, the majority of which are financed by general taxes [1]. The state holds the overall regulatory and supervisory functions, while five administrative regions are responsible for the hospitals and the general practitioners. All hospital treatment is free, and many specialist nephrological medicines, e.g. erythropoietin-stimulating agents, alfacalcidol, phosphate binders and immunosuppressive agents, are supplied free of charge. Other medicines are subsidized. Departmental budgets are determined by the hospital administration on an ad hoc basis. Budgets based on service rendered, using a disease-related group (DRG) system, are occasionally used.

Nephrology care is mainly supplied by 15 hospital-based nephrology departments, but the care of patients with non-specific stable chronic kidney disease (CKD) stage 1–3 is often delegated to the general practitioners. Dialysis treatment is also provided by several satellite centres administrated by the nephrology departments. Private nephrology care is virtually non-existent.

Renal transplantation is performed at three centres: Aarhus University Hospital, Odense University Hospital and Rigshospitalet in Copenhagen. Multiorgan transplantations are only performed at Rigshospitalet. The post-operative care is restricted to the transplantation departments for the first 3–12 months, after which the patients are returned to their local nephrology department.

Most Danish nephrologists are members of the scientific organization Danish Society of Nephrology (www.nephrology.dk).

## Brief History of Nephrology in Denmark

In common with most other countries, nephrology as an independent specialty appeared during the 1950s. The world's first paper on the results of renal biopsy was published by Paul Iversen and Claus Brun in 1951 [2]. Jørn Hess Thaysen from Rigshospitalet performed the first dialysis for patients with acute kidney injury (AKI) in 1955 and introduced maintenance haemodialysis (HD) for patients with end-stage renal disease (ESRD) in 1963. He was a cofounder of the European Dialysis and Transplant Association (EDTA) in 1964 and its president from 1975–1978. The first renal transplantation was performed by Ole Fjeldborg at Aarhus Kommunehospital in 1964. Renal care was primarily limited to a few specialist departments, but the rapid expansion of the dialysis population during the 1990s led to the establishment of 15 nephrology departments distributed throughout the country.

Hospital intermittent peritoneal dialysis (PD), using on-site preparation of PD fluid, has been performed since the 1960s. A common regime involved placement of a stiff PD catheter under local anaesthesia once a week followed by 60 litres of PD in a hospital bed during the following 24 hours. Continuous ambulatory PD (CAPD) was introduced in 1980 and automated PD (APD) in 1990. Due to its social advantages, and its particular value for the treatment of patients with fast peritoneal transport status, APD became very popular, encompassing 70% of all PD patients in 2008. Since then, CAPD has experienced a renaissance, and APD prevalence has fallen to 50%. This is probably due to the increasingly popular "gentle start" CAPD, where patients with significant residual renal function are initially treated with two bags of CAPD per day. The Danish Society of Nephrology was founded in 1969 and the Danish Nephrology Registry (DNR) in 1990 [3]. It registers clinical and biochemical data for all patients treated with transplantation since 1964 and all patients treated with dialysis since 1990. It forms the basis of national treatment quality indices, administered by the regional health authorities (Fig. 38.1).

## Renal Diseases in Denmark

Little information is available concerning the incidence and prevalence of CKD in Denmark. The Stockholm SCREAM project, which probably has a similar population [4], demonstrated a prevalence of 6%, corresponding to an incidence of 0.1–0.15%/year. The estimated number of patients with CKD in Denmark is thus 340,000, and the incidence is 7000/year. However, many of these patients will be undiagnosed, and most will be unknown to the nephrological centres. For this reason, the incidence and prevalence of specific diseases are unknown. The incidence of biopsy-proven glomerulonephritis (GN) is 50 patients per million population (pmp) [5]. Common incident diagnoses for patients with ESRD are diabetic nephropathy (25%), unknown (22%), hypertensive nephropathy (13%), GN (10%), polycystic disease (8%) and

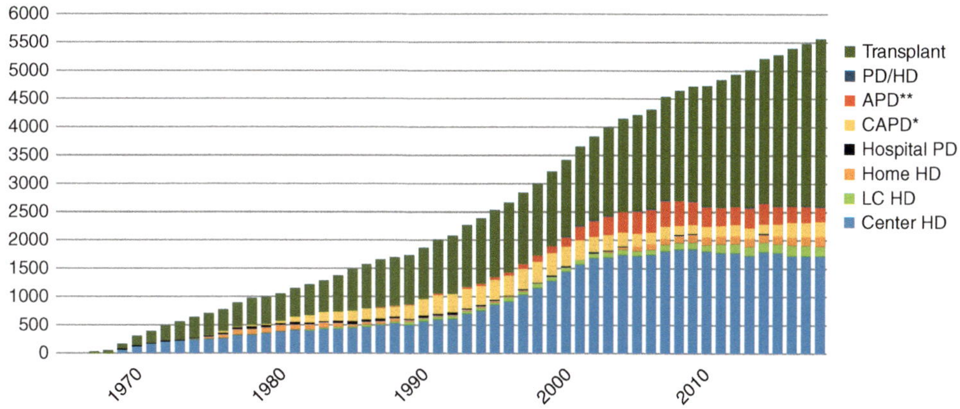


**Fig. 38.1** ESRD prevalence in Denmark 1964–2018. *Including home IPD until 1984. **Including home IPD after 1984

chronic interstitial nephropathy (8%). Apart from the occasional case of acute haemorrhagic interstitial nephritis secondary to rodent hantavirus infection, there are no specific regional renal diseases; sporadic episodes are particularly found in the south of Funen. The incidence of ESRD among the elderly has fallen since 2000, specially among patients aged 60–69 years where it has fallen from 400 to 240 pmp [6]. This may be associated with the fact that Denmark initiated uraemia prophylaxis programmes early [7, 8]. The prevalence of dialysis patients has been stable since 2005, while the number of transplanted patients continues to rise, from 2137 in 2010 to 2892 (503 pmp) in 2018 [3].

## Renal Replacement Therapy in Denmark

### Acute Kidney Disease

A total of 25 hospitals across Denmark provide nationwide coverage with regard to acute dialysis treatment. As such, management of patients requiring acute dialysis for AKI and critical care nephrology is a shared responsibility of intensive care specialists at 41 of 43 intensive care units (ICUs) and consulting nephrologists at 13 of 14 nephrology departments [9, 10]. Management of non-dialysis-requiring AKI is primarily a responsibility of internal medicine departments at all Danish hospitals; however nephrology departments consult and provide assistance as required. All patients with non-responsive AKI are commonly transferred to nephrology departments for specialized diagnostic work-up.

The burden of non-dialysis-requiring AKI in Denmark remains uncertain; however, AKI is estimated to be present in approximately one in every five patients hospitalized [11]. Conversely, the incident rate of dialysis-requiring AKI has been observed to have increased substantially throughout the early 2000s, with stabilization at an incident rate of approximately 350–400 per million since 2007 [12]. Notably, continuous growth has been restricted to elderly populations – plausibly due to an expanding indication for treatment in elderly patients – with incident rate of acute dialysis AKI currently estimated to exceed 1.500 per million in patients older than 75 years.

Continuous renal replacement therapies (CRRTs) were implemented into common clinical practice in Denmark throughout the late 1990s [13]. Currently, the CRRTs, i.e. standard therapies including continuous veno-venous hemofiltration (CVVHF), HD and haemodiafiltration (HDF), remain the predominant modalities provided in Danish ICUs, with HD commonly only initiated in a collaboration with consulting nephrologists. In comparison, most nephrology departments provide acute dialysis care using standard HD, and acute PD for treatment of AKI remains rare. Overall, the care for patients with dialysis-requiring AKI admitted to ICUs is commonly a shared responsibility between intensive care specialists and consulting nephrologists. Placement of acute vascular access is nearly always performed by intensive care specialists. Furthermore, consequent to the introduction of CRRTs, the decision and initial management pertaining to acute RRT in critical illness has shifted from the nephrology departments to ICUs. However, a majority of patients transfer to nephrology departments following stabilization of non-renal organ failures. The prevalence of acute dialysis in AKI in Danish ICUs is in the region of 6.5%, with unspecified, i.e. acute and chronic dialysis care provided in approximately 2000 out of 30,000 admissions in 2018 and acute dialysis in AKI provided to approximately 1000 patients [10]. In addition, nephrology departments in Denmark provide acute dialysis treatment in approximately 900 patients annually [12].

Patients receiving acute dialysis for AKI remain predominantly male (>60%) and older than 60 years. Comorbidity is abundant, with pre-existing CKD, cardiovascular disease and diabetes particularly common. Notably, the burden of pre-existing comorbidities is comparably smaller in patients treated in critical care compared to patients treated at nephrology departments.

The initial growth and subsequent stabilization of incident rates of acute dialysis in AKI observed in Denmark have coincided with growth and dissemination in the availability of CRRTs across ICUs in Denmark. As noted, the number of hospitals providing acute dialysis treatment has increased throughout the past two decades; currently, acute dialysis is provided at 25 hospitals across Denmark. As such, growth in incidence rates of acute dialysis for AKI has, plausibly and effectively, been driven by an increased application of acute dialysis treatment – specifically CRRT– in patients admitted to ICU, while employment and incidence rate of acute dialysis for AKI in nephrology departments remains unchanged [14]. Current incidence rates of acute dialysis in ICUs and nephrology departments are estimated to be approximately 4.500 and 1000 per million admissions, respectively.

The influence of increased capacity has also led to a decrease in the time from hospital admission to initiation of treatment in both patients treated in ICUs and nephrology departments. Currently, the median interval from admission to initiation of treatment is <4 days, with treatment duration decreasing to <15 days and only a small proportion of patients (2–4%) continuing dialysis treatment in an outpatient setting.

Acute dialysis treatment in Denmark has increasingly been observed to be associated with concomitant other organ failure, i.e. circulatory and respiratory failure, possibly due to the growing employment of acute dialysis treatment within the context of critical care and the increasing use of CRRTs. Concurrent mechanical ventilation and circulatory support is observed in >70% and >25% of patients initiating acute dialysis in the ICU, respectively [12], corresponding to incident rates of 1 per 1000 in patients with circulatory failure and 2 per 1000 in patients with respiratory failure [14]. Similarly, the incidence of acute dialysis for AKI in sepsis and following major surgery has also grown to a current estimate of approximately 5 per 10,000 and 1 per 10,000, respectively (Fig. 38.2).

## Chronic Dialysis

Peritoneal dialysis and haemodialysis are provided by 15 specialist nephrology departments and their satellite units. The HD unit size is 70–280 patients, with very small units in Greenland and the island of Bornholm. The PD unit size is 10–80.

The overall dialysis mortality is 15%/year. Mortality (censored for transplantation) during the first year is 22% for patients starting on HD and 12% for PD. The median survival is HD 3.1 years and PD 4.1 years. Uncensored median survival rates are 3.6 and 5.7 years, respectively. Twenty-three per cent of dialysis patients have been on continuous dialysis for more than 5 years.

The overall estimated annual costs of the various modalities are as follows (approximate figures in Euro): Centre HD 50,000, Home HD 30,000, CAPD 17,000, APD 24,000 and assisted APD 40,000.

## Haemodialysis

Most dialysis patients (72%) are treated by HD, mainly dialysed at one of the 15 nephrology departments or their satellite dialysis units. Seven per cent (7%) of HD patients are treated with limited care HD, where nursing assistance is available, but the patient performs most of the dialysis procedures.

The first home HD (HHD) patient started treatment in 1971; it rapidly became a very popular modality, comprising 19% of all dialysis patients in 1980. After the introduction of CAPD and APD, numbers fell, and the modality had almost disappeared in 2000. Since then the modality has experienced a renaissance, probably due to the excellent long-term results of the treatment. Currently, 8% are treated with HHD, mainly using dialysis machines installed free of charge in the

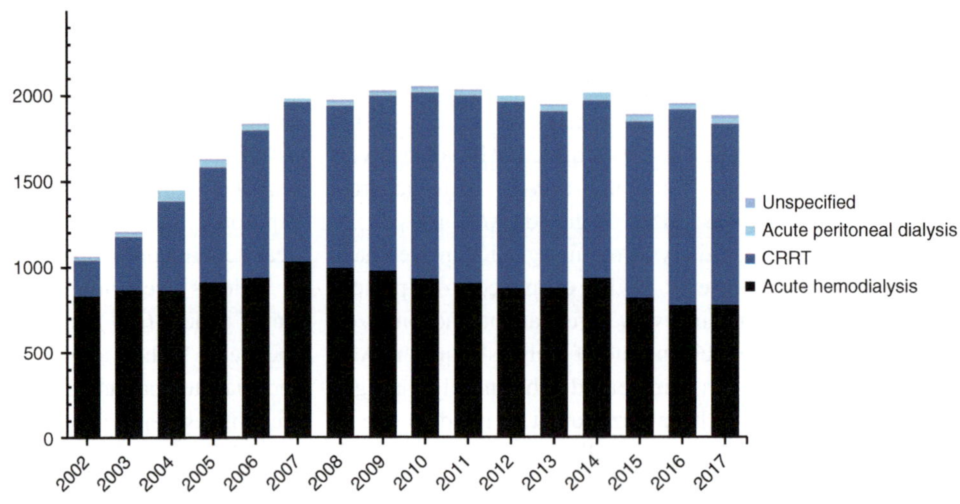


Fig. 38.2 Prevalence of dialysis treatment for acute kidney injury in Denmark 2002–2017

patient's home. This group includes a small number of patients who are treated with self-care dialysis, where the patient dialyses him- or herself without nursing support, using dialysis machines installed in stand-alone buildings. Some patients use a portable home dialysis machine (NxStage ®). Dialysis frequency for HHD patients varies from four to six times/week. These patients mainly start as limited care HD patients and are discharged to home therapy after 3–6 months training. Two centres in Denmark, which both have a "Home HD first" policy, have HHD prevalence rates of 14%.

Centre HD patients are usually dialysed for 3–5 hours (usually 4) three times per week. Twice weekly HD is sometimes used for patients with considerable residual renal function (RRF) and four times weekly for patients with unacceptable uraemia control. All patients use highly purified water and high flux dialysers. Filter reuse does not occur. Dialysate flow rate is 500 ml/min, and blood flow is 200–400 ml/min, the goal being 300 ml/min. Details concerning the use of haemodiafiltration are not available, but the use of ultrapure dialysate means that the treatment is available for all patients.

Dialysis patients are seen regularly by physicians, usually every 4–8 weeks, and otherwise as necessary. There is one dialysis nurse for every 2.5–3 patients. Dialysis technicians are not used, except for machine maintenance. There are no national rules concerning employee to patient ratios. Inpatient treatment is usually available at the same hospital, with a requirement of 7 beds/100 dialysis patients.

Arteriovenous fistula (AVF) is the preferred method of vascular access, and most centres have a "fistula first" policy, exceptions being made for elderly patients with poor cardiovascular status, where permanent tunneled jugular catheters may be preferred. AVF placement is performed at a number of vascular surgery departments, usually on an outpatient basis. The dialysis access at first dialysis is AVF 30%, permanent tunnelled catheter 15%, temporary tunnelled catheter 13% and temporary non-tunnelled catheter 42%.

The commonest dialysis machines are supplied by the Fresenius and Baxter companies. The regional authorities release regular tenders for the provision of new dialysis machines.

## Peritoneal Dialysis

The PD prevalence in Denmark remains relatively stable and high, with approximately 21% of the total dialysis population being managed on PD. Of these, 84% are autonomous PD patients taking care of their own dialysis treatment at home, while 16% are managed on assisted PD, where professional nursing assistance in the home is provided for disabled patients. Approximately half of patients are treated by APD and half by CAPD. The APD prevalence was 70% in 2008 but has since fallen. One possible explanation is the increasing popularity of "gentle start" CAPD, where patients with significant RRF start CAPD with a dose of only 2 L once or twice daily. Switch to APD or full-dose CAPD is only made when urea Kt/V or creatinine clearance fall below recommended levels due to falling RRF or if intractable electrolyte or clinical problems arise.

Several factors contribute to the high PD prevalence: the existence of "PD first" policies in many departments, the use of PD for unplanned dialysis initiation, the possibility of assisted PD in the home and the existence of multidisciplinary pre-dialysis outpatient teams.

### Pre-dialysis Clinics

These outpatient clinics usually consist of specialist physicians, nurses and dieticians; some also have social workers attached. They provide timely information about dialysis and transplantation, when the estimated glomerular filtration rate (eGFR) falls below 15–20 ml/min. All patients are offered a free, informed choice of dialysis modalities, including the possibility of conservative treatment, which may be relevant for elderly, sick patients. Early information permits the possibility of pre-emptive transplantation (8% of all ESKD patients) and allows timely placement of dialysis access, in particular AVFs and PD catheters. An important number (40%) of the patients are, a priori, judged unsuitable for home therapy either due to somatic, mental or (for PD) abdominal reasons. Patients with a choice of modality usually choose home-based therapies, primarily PD, due to its attractively low effects on social life, and the possibly of travel. PD catheter placement is usually done locally. There is some variation in technique. Many centres use the Seldinger technique, sometimes with ultrasonic guidance, while others use a laparoscopic technique or laparotomy. In some centres, the patient is admitted for 24 hours for observation. PD training is usually done 3 weeks after operation.

Outpatient PD physician and nurse consultations are made every 4–6 weeks.

### Unplanned Initiation of PD

Only approximately 15% of incident dialysis patients in Denmark are referred late. Despite this, dialysis is initiated in an unplanned way in 35% of the incident patients [10]. Previously, unplanned dialysis initiation was almost entirely based on HD using a temporary catheter for VA, despite the associated increase in mortality, need for hospitalization and risk of potentially lethal bloodstream infections, venous thrombosis and venous stenosis. Once started on HD, such "crash landers" are less likely to be transferred to a home-based dialysis modality later on. Accordingly, programmes for unplanned initiation of PD immediately after PD catheter implantation were established in Denmark 20 years ago [15–18].

For the late referred patient without any previous nephrological care, education or preparation and with urgent need for initiation of dialysis within hours or days, the decision of a future dialysis modality is obviously very difficult. This is particularly evident for patients with advanced age, a heavy burden of comorbidity and severe uremic intoxication as additional factors. However, even in this scenario, it has been shown that it is possible to give unbiased dialysis information to the patients and relatives, thereby giving them a real choice of dialysis modality selection. The desire for independence, a feeling of confidence and a home-based treatment are often decisive for the patient's final choice.

The original programme for unplanned initiation on PD was developed in Aarhus and has been described previously [15–18]. Briefly, the patients are started on APD in the supine position right after PD catheter implantation using a standard prescription for 12 hours overnight treatment with a reduced dwell volume and pre-programmed cyclers to make it easy. Patients are instructed to stay in bed to avoid increased intraperitoneal pressure and associated risk of leakage. A low tidal volume (50%) is used to reduce the risk of alarms during the first nights of treatment and is gradually increased to 75–85% during the first week. It is also important to remember bowel preparation to avoid constipation. After 1–2 weeks of treatment, patients are converted to an individualized programme for APD or CAPD. During the stay in hospital, the patients are trained for PD by expert PD nurses, or if they need assistance, the assistants are trained to visit and help the patients at home after discharge.

Published data have constantly shown that urgent start on PD with a break-in period of less than 2 weeks may be associated with a minor increased risk of mechanical complications but apparently no detrimental effect on patient survival, peritonitis-free survival or PD technique survival compared with elective start on PD. Recently, unplanned initiation of PD has been recommended in the latest update of ISPD guidelines for creating and maintaining optimal peritoneal dialysis access in adult patients [19]. In the urgent setting, the choice of modality has to be balanced between the potential for increased risk of mechanical complications related to urgent start on PD and the increased risk of bloodstream infections and central venous stenosis and thrombosis known to be associated with urgent start on haemodialysis using a central venous catheter [19].

### Assisted PD (AssPD)

Elderly are the largest and fastest growing group of patients with ESRD. Due to advanced age and a heavy burden of comorbidity, they are usually not candidates for kidney transplantation and are less likely to be offered a home-based dialysis modality, as old age is associated with more contraindications to PD. Some of these contraindications are non-modifiable conditions (e.g. multiple previous abdominal surgery with adhesion formation, large hernias, frequent diverticulosis or severe obesity), but the majority of physical disabilities (e.g. hemiparesis, impaired vision and hearing, decreased manual dexterity and strength) and psychosocial problems (e.g. cognitive problems, depression, noncompliance, social isolation and dependency on help) are barriers that can be overcome provided that proper support and assistance are offered to the patients at home. In addition, compared to HD, PD at home may offer several advantages that may be particularly important for patients with advanced age and severe comorbidity. The most important are the avoidance of transportation to the dialysis center, of VA for HD with its associated risk of bacteraemia and access failure, of hemodynamic instability during HD sessions and of post-treatment fatigue. Accordingly, programmes for AssPD were established in Denmark 20 years ago [17, 18, 20].

Usually professional public paid community nurses or nursing home staff are trained as assistants. A small team of assistants is trained for every patient. Professional nurses usually need remarkably short training. They are trained not only to set up the cycler and to connect and disconnect the patient, but also to take care of the exit site, dressings and fixation of the PD catheter, and to carefully observe the patient for infectious or mechanical complications, optimal fluid balance and nutritional status. Finally, they are trained to order PD fluids and other relevant equipment to carry out the treatment. Importantly, the dialysis units involved in AssPD must offer a 24-hour-a-day, 7-day-a-week telephone backup to support the patients on AssPD, their relatives and the assistants.

Both AssCAPD and AssAPD are offered, but AssAPD is often preferred because the assistant only has to visit the patient twice daily: A longer visit in the morning to disconnect the patient from the cycler, set up the cycler for the next night and take care of the patient, the exit site, possible complications and the logistics related to the treatment followed by a short visit in the evening to connect the patient to the cycler again. AssPD will usually be permanent, but for some patients, the need for assistance may gradually be reduced as the patient gains more knowledge, experience and confidence with the treatment.

AssPD patients have the same PD technique survival rate as conventional PD patients but may have an inferior patient- and peritonitis-free survival rate [17].

## Renal Transplantation

The Danish renal transplant programme started in 1964. All renal transplantations in Denmark are carried out under the auspices of the public health system. Presently,

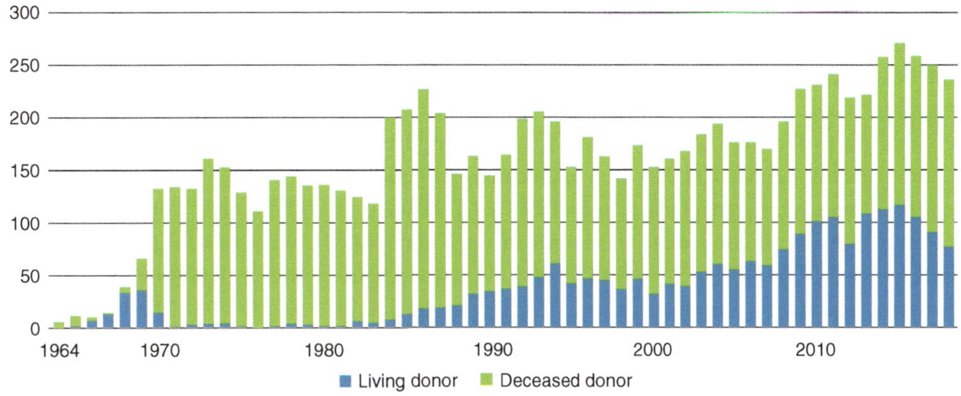


**Fig. 38.3** Transplantation activity in Denmark 1964–2018

there are three centres for renal transplantation placed at the university hospitals in Aarhus, Copenhagen and Odense, respectively. All three centres have programmes for adult living as well as deceased donor renal transplantation, whereas paediatric renal transplantations are only performed in Copenhagen and Odense. Simultaneous multiorgan transplantations, i.e. the kidney combined with the liver, lung or pancreas, are only performed in Copenhagen. All three centres have programmes for ABO-incompatible renal transplantation, acceptable mismatch programmes for highly immunized patients and paired donor exchange for living donor renal transplantation when appropriate.

Immunosuppression for renal transplantation with standard immunological risk is induction with basiliximab and maintenance with tacrolimus and mycophenolate mofetil, with or without prednisolone according to local centre practice.

Procurement of kidneys from deceased donors and work-up of living donors are taken care of by each individual centre in their own area of referral.

All Danish centres are members of the organ exchange organization Scandiatransplant together with the transplant centres from Estonia, Finland, Iceland, Norway and Sweden. Exchange of procured deceased donor kidneys through Scandiatransplant is based on a strict payback principle meaning that the individual centre is responsible for optimizing procurement in their area of referral as there is no net flow of kidneys between centres.

As the Danish health system is primarily public and non-commercial, renal transplantation is free of charge for the patients. All immunosuppressive medication is supplied by the hospitals. This also applies when the patients are discharged after the initial stay and are followed in the outpatient clinics at the renal transplant centres and when the patients are referred back to their local nephrology centre for follow-up. Follow-up of renal transplant patients is performed by the centres for nephrology at the public hospitals.

All living donors that donate to a Danish citizen are offered full compensation for loss of income and other expenses directly related to the donation or work-up. This also applies to donors that are residents from other countries as long as the recipient is a Danish resident.

On a national basis, the total renal transplant rate for 2016 was 44.9 pmp (26.4 for deceased donors) and 43.7 in 2017 (27.9 for deceased donors). In 2016, 41% of renal transplantations were with a living donor, and in 2017 it was 36%. Thus, Denmark is characterized by a relatively low rate of transplantation from deceased donors and a relatively high rate from living donors, as compared with other European countries.

Quality control for outcomes of renal transplantation for the three Danish centres is performed using mandatory reporting to the Danish Nephrology Registry. This publishes centre-specific data and comparisons, as well as aggregated Danish data for renal transplantation, in a yearly report [3] (http://nephrology.dk/dnsl/). Waiting list and transplantation statistics for all individual Scandiatransplant centres can be found on http://www.scandiatransplant.org/data/scandiatransplant-figures.

For living donor transplants, the 1- and 5-year patient survival rates are 99% and 93%, and graft survival rates are 98% and 90%. For deceased donors, the figures are 98% and 88% and 97% and 78%, respectively (Fig. 38.3).

## Paediatric Nephrology

### History

The history of paediatric care in Denmark dates back to 1850 with the opening of the first children's hospital in Denmark. It was a privately funded hospital in Rigensgade, Copenhagen, attended by one of the most famous physicians at that time Professor Harald Hirschsprung (1830–1916), who is often considered as the founder of paediatrics in Denmark [21]. Palliative care was the only treatment for children with severe CKD until dialysis and kidney transplantation became available in the 1960s.

### Renal Diseases and Incidence

The incidence of ESRD in Denmark has been stable within the last 8 years (2010–2017) at approximately 1 per 100,000 children. There seems to be a decline in the incidence, when comparing to the period 2000–2009, where the figure was approximately 1.5 per 100,000. The main causes of ESRD in children who were transplanted from 1994 to 2009 were as follows: 52% with congenital anomalies of the kidney and urinary tract (CAKUT), 15% with GN and 5% with steroid-resistant nephrotic syndrome (SRNS) [22]. These aetiologies are similar to the NAPRTCS registry reporting CAKUT in 49% of the children with ESRD [23]. The age of children with ESRD has been slightly decreasing from a median age of 13.3 years in the 1980s to 12.4 years from 2010–2018. In Denmark, prenatal ultrasonography is offered to all pregnancies, and approximately 98% are screened for congenital anomalies including CAKUT.

### Dialysis

Records of the first dialysis of a child in Denmark are inaccurate, with one source reporting PD in a 17-year-old girl with GN at Odense Hospital in 1969. Today paediatric dialysis is offered at three centres (Copenhagen, Odense and Aarhus) with PD as the preferred modality.

### Transplantation

After kidney transplantation evolved in paediatrics during the 1950s, the first kidney transplantation in Denmark was performed in 1969 at Odense Hospital (today Odense University Hospital), where a 17-year-old patient received a deceased donor transplant. Three years later in 1972, the first kidney transplant in a smaller child of 4 years was performed again at Odense Hospital. In total 443 children have been transplanted from 1969 until 2018. Since 1980, the rate of paediatric kidney transplantation has been very stable at approximately ten transplantations per year.

### Paediatric Nephrology Care Centres

Specialized treatment for paediatric nephrology is located at three locations in Denmark: Aarhus University Hospital, Copenhagen University Hospital and Odense University Hospital. All three hospitals offer dialysis for children, whereas only the hospitals in Copenhagen and Odense offer paediatric kidney transplantation.

## Nephrology Practice in Denmark

Virtually all nephrology professionals work in the public sector and are employed by one the county's five administrative regions. Professional qualifications acquired in European Union (EU) countries for professionals who wish to work in Denmark are accepted, while qualifications outside the EU will be subjected to a specific individual evaluation. All clinical posts require proficiency in Danish or similarly Scandinavian language (e.g. Norwegian or Swedish). Free language courses for immigrants are available. The normal working week is 37 hours, including evening, night and weekend duties. Many nurses and dieticians work part-time, while this is rare for physicians. The work environment is characterized by a non-hierarchical structure with relaxed interpersonal relationships. Five-week holiday entitlement is standard. The income figures shown here (in Danish kroner – DKK – per month) are only approximate and will depend upon qualifications, work schedules, etc. In January 2020, 1.00 DKK was worth 0.15 US dollar and 0.13 Euro. All positions have a pension plan. Marginal income tax rates are relatively high, 45–61% depending on income, but as a corollary, the government offers free primary, secondary and tertiary education, free healthcare and a comprehensive social support system.

### Physicians

A 6-year education is followed by 12-month clinical preregistration training. Nephrology specialist qualification requires a further 5-year training, consisting of postings at two to three nephrology departments, supplemented by specialist courses. There are no examinations, but completion of a detailed theoretical and practical syllabus is continuously assessed. Working hours are shorter than international norms, particularly for junior doctors, where overtime requirements are relatively rare. Nearly all doctors, including consultants, are expected to participate in duty rotas. University consultants are expected to participate in research and educational activities. Professors often combine their research activities (including supervision of PhD students) with clinical work.

Monthly income (in DKK): junior doctor 30,000; senior registrar 40,000; specialist nephrologist 55,000; consultant 63,000; and professor 70,000. There are no fee-for-service contracts.

### Nurses

A 3.5-year education is followed by specialist nephrology training for 3–12 months, depending upon clinical responsibility. There is no specialist examination. Nurses in outpatient and dialysis clinics will usually specialize in haemodialysis or peritoneal dialysis. All nurses working in inpatient wards and haemodialysis clinics and even many in outpatient clinics are expected to participate in duty rotas. Monthly income (in DKK) is 33,000.

## Dieticians

Most hospital dieticians will care for many categories of patients other than nephrological. The training lasts 2 years. Monthly income (in DKK) is 30,000.

## Highlights of Nephrology in Denmark

Noteworthy hallmarks of nephrology in Denmark include:

1. Home dialysis. Denmark has the highest prevalence of home dialysis in Europe: 28% of all dialysis patients (21% PD, 7% home HD). This is a result of deliberate policy decisions by many nephrology departments, since home dialysis is considered to result in better health outcomes, an improved social life and better rehabilitation. Treatment is also associated with substantial savings. Many areas also practice assisted PD, whereby professional assistance for disabled patients is provided in the home. Denmark was an early initiator of unplanned initiation of PD, which may also have contributed to the high PD prevalence.
2. Denmark was an early adopter of uraemia and diabetic nephropathy prophylaxis [7, 8]. This has probably resulted in a falling incidence of ESRD since 2000 and a stabilization of the dialysis population, despite increases in the obese and diabetic population. Denmark is thus a member of the small group of countries characterized by a high gross national product (GNP) but a low, and falling, ESRD incidence [24].
3. Detailed clinical and biochemical data on all ESRD have been registered in the DNR since 1990 [25] and form the basis for national quality assessment goals. The registry is >99% complete. Anonymized individual patient data are exported to the ERA-EDTA registry each year.
4. The country has a high scientific research activity, particularly in the field of diabetic nephropathy. The existence of the DNR and many other national databases permits linkage via patient national identity number resulting in the publication of many epidemiological articles.

## Future Perspectives of Nephrology in Denmark

The political, administrative, epidemiological and therapeutic environment in Denmark is stable, and only minor changes are expected in the future. The ESRD prevalence is expected to stabilize around 6000 patients (1050 pmp) within the next 10 years. The Danish Society of Nephrology plans the creation of a CKD registry in order to improve treatment quality for CKD patients not being treated with dialysis or transplantation, but these plans are at an early stage.

## Conclusion

Nephrological healthcare in Denmark is comparable to the best international standards. This is probably due to a high GDP, high professional standards and universal, free healthcare. The situation of nephrology in Denmark may be of interest for physicians in other countries, due to a number of special characteristics. Healthcare professionals enjoy a pleasant working environment.

## References


1. Healthcare in Denmark - an overview. Danish Ministry of Health. 2017. https://www.sum.dk/English/~/media/Filer%20-%20Publikationer_i_pdf/2016/Healthcare-in-dk-16-dec/Healthcare-english-V16-dec.ashx.
2. Iversen P, Brun C. Aspiration biopsy of the kidney. Am J Med. 1951;11:324–30.
3. Danish Society of Nephrology annual report 2017. www.nephrology.dk; 2018.
4. Gasparini A, Evans M, Coresh J, et al. Prevalence and recognition of chronic kidney disease in Stockholm healthcare. Nephrol Dial Transplant. 2016;31:2086–94.
5. Sørensen SS, Heaf JJ, Hansen A. Increased incidence and improved prognosis of glomerulonephritis in adults: a national 30 year study. Copenhagen: ERA-EDTA Congress; 2018.
6. Heaf JG, Wehberg S. Reduced incidence of end stage renal disease among the elderly in Denmark: an observational study. BMC Nephrol. 2012;13:131.
7. Kamper AL, Strandgaard S, Leyssac PP. Effect of enalapril on the progression of chronic renal failure. A randomized controlled trial. Am J Hypertens. 1992;5:423–30.
8. Gaede P, Vedel P, Parving HH, Pedersen O. Intensified multifactorial intervention in patients with type 2 diabetes mellitus and microalbuminuria: the Steno type 2 randomised study. Lancet. 1999;353:617–22.
9. Carlson N, Hommel K, Olesen JB, et al. Trends in one-year outcomes of dialysis-requiring acute kidney injury in Denmark 2005–2012: a population-based nationwide study. PLoS One. 2016;11:e0159944.
10. Dansk Intensiv Database. Årsrapport 2017/2018. 2018. https://www.sundhed.dk/content/cms/12/4712_did_aarsrapport_2018.pdf.
11. Susantitaphong P, Cruz DN, Cerda J, et al. World incidence of AKI: a meta-analysis. Clin J Am Soc Nephrol. 2013;8:1482–93.
12. Carlson N, Hommel K, Olesen JB, et al. Dialysis-requiring acute kidney injury in Denmark 2000–2012: time trends of incidence and prevalence of risk factors-a nationwide study. PLoS One. 2016;11:e0148809.
13. Toft P, Felding M, Tonnesen EK. Continuous venovenous hemodiafiltration in critically ill patients with acute renal failure. Ugeskr Laeger. 2000;162:2868–71.

14. Carlson N. Dialysis-requiring acute kidney injury in Denmark: epidemiological studies. Copenhagen: Faculty of Health Sciences, University of Copenhagen; 2019.
15. Povlsen JV, Ivarsen P. How to start the late referred ESRD patient urgently on chronic APD. Nephrol Dial Transplant. 2006;21(Suppl 2):ii56–9.
16. Ivarsen P, Povlsen JV. Can peritoneal dialysis be applied for unplanned initiation of chronic dialysis? Nephrol Dial Transplant. 2014;29:2201–6.
17. Povlsen JV, Ivarsen P. Assisted peritoneal dialysis: also for the late referred elderly patient. Perit Dial Int. 2008;28:461–7.
18. Povlsen JV, Sorensen AB, Ivarsen P. Unplanned start on peritoneal dialysis right after PD catheter implantation for older people with end-stage renal disease. Perit Dial Int. 2015;35:622–4.
19. Crabtree JH, Shrestha BM, Chow KM, et al. Creating and maintaining optimal peritoneal dialysis access in the adult patient: 2019 update. Perit Dial Int. 2019;39:414–36.
20. Bechade C, Lobbedez T, Ivarsen P, Povlsen JV. Assisted peritoneal dialysis for older people with end-stage renal disease: the French and Danish experience. Perit Dial Int. 2015;35:663–6.
21. Ibsen KK. Børnelægeri 100 år. publ Nordtryk, Frederikshavn, Denmark; 2008. p 1–304.
22. Wittenhagen P, Thiesson HC, Baudier F, Pedersen EB, Neland M. Long-term experience of steroid-free pediatric renal transplantation: effects on graft function, body mass index, and longitudinal growth. Pediatr Transplant. 2014;18:35–41.
23. Becherucci F, Roperto RM, Materassi M, Romagnani P. Chronic kidney disease in children. Clin Kidney J. 2016;9:583–91.
24. Heaf J. Current trends in European renal epidemiology. Clin Kidney J. 2017;10:149–53.
25. Heaf J. The Danish nephrology registry. Clin Epidemiol. 2016;8:621–7.

# Nephrology in France

# 39

Bernard Canaud and Gabriel Choukroun

| | |
|---|---|
| Area | 633,186 km$^2$ |
| Population | 66.6 million (2016) |
| Capital | Paris |
| Three most populated cities | 1. Paris<br>2. Marseille<br>3. Lyon |
| Official language | French |
| Geographic | France Mainland is located in Western Europe<br>French Overseas consist of 12 territories |
| Annual gross domestic product (GDP) | 2.591 trillion USD (2017)<br>2.780 trillion USD (2018) |
| GDP per capita | 9928.56 USD (2017)<br>8959.02 USD (2018) |
| Human Development Index (HDI) | 0.891 (26 rank, 2018) |
| Official currency | Euro (€, EUR) |
| Total number of nephrologists | 1657 (2017) |
| National society of nephrology | Société Francophone de Néphrologie Dialyse et Transplantation (SFNDT)<br>https://www.sfndt.org/ |
| Incidence of end-stage renal disease[1,2] | 2016 – 165 pmp<br>2017 – 172 pmp |
| Prevalence of end-stage renal disease[2] | 2017 – Mainland 1271 pmp<br>2017 – Overseas 2031 pmp |
| Total number of end-stage renal disease patients treated (dialysis and transplant) | 2017 – 87,275<br>47,985 (dialysis) – 39,288 (transplant) |
| Total number of patients on dialysis (all modalities)[1,2] | 2016 – 46,872<br>2017 – 47,985 |
| Number of patients on hemodialysis[1,2] | 2016 – 43,919<br>2017 – 44,962 |
| Number of patients on peritoneal dialysis [1,2] | 2016 – 2953<br>2017 – 3023 |
| Number of renal transplantations per year[1,2] | 2016 – 3176<br>2017 – 3782 |

## Introduction

### Identity Card of France

Much of France is located in Western Europe. This part is usually referred to as Metropolitan France or Mainland France (without Corsica). Mainland France is bordered by the English Channel in the northwest, the Pacific Ocean on the west coast, Belgium and Luxembourg in the north, Germany and the Alps in the east, the Pyrenees mountains in the southwest, and the Mediterranean Sea in the southeast. France has borders with Belgium and Luxembourg in the north, Germany and Switzerland in the east, Italy in the southeast, and Spain in the southwest. France covers a surface area of 633,186 km$^2$ including Corsica and overseas territories and is populated by 66.6 million inhabitants. French is the official language, and Euro (EUR, €) is the current currency. France is a founding member of the European Union and is a member of the UN Security Council, NATO, ESCE, G8, and G20. National holiday is July 14.

The most populated cities are, by decreasing order, Paris, 2,254,262; Marseille, 855,393; Lyon, 500,715; Toulouse, 458,298; Nice, 342,295; Nantes, 292,718; Strasbourg, 275,718; Bordeaux, 243,626; and Lille, 231,491 inhabitants [1, 2].

[1] https://www.agence-biomedecine.fr/IMG/pdf/rapportrein2016.pdf

[2] https://www.agence-biomedecine.fr/IMG/pdf/rapportrein2017.pdf

B. Canaud (✉)
Montpellier University, School of Medicine, Montpellier, France

Global Medical Office, Fresenius Medical Care, Bad Homburg, Germany
e-mail: Bernard.Canaud@fmc-ag.com

G. Choukroun
Internal Medicine, Dialysis and Transplantation Department, CHU Amiens-Picardie, Amiens, France

Society Francophone of Nephrology, Dialysis and Transplantation (SFNDT), CHABANIERE, France
e-mail: choukroun.gabriel@chu-amiens.fr


J. A. Moura-Neto et al. (eds.), *Nephrology Worldwide*, https://doi.org/10.1007/978-3-030-56890-0_39

## State Organization

France is a Constitutional Republic which was proclaimed after the French Revolution and the abolition of the monarchy on 22 September 1792. French Republics refer to a succession of republics, there have been five republics in the history of France, and the Fifth Republic started in 1958 under the leadership of General de Gaulle. The President of the Republic is elected by direct universal suffrage for 5 years. The legal age to vote is 18. Nationals of member states of the European Union can vote in municipal and European elections. The government consists of the Prime Minister, appointed by the President of the Republic, and ministers, deputy ministers, and secretaries of state, appointed by the President of the Republic on the proposal of the Prime Minister. Under the direction of the Prime Minister, the government determines and conducts the policy of the nation.

The state is represented in the regions and in the departments by prefects, who have authority over the decentralized state services. Parliament makes and votes laws and controls the government. It is bicameral: the National Assembly is made up of 577 deputies elected for 5 years by direct universal suffrage and Senate of 343 senators elected for 6 years by indirect universal suffrage. In case of disagreement between the two chambers, the National Assembly decides definitively.

## Territorial Organization

France is made up of several types of local authorities: region, department, and commune (or municipality) (Fig. 39.1). There are 13 regions with specific competencies (leader for the establishment of the regional economic development scheme, high school management, vocational train-

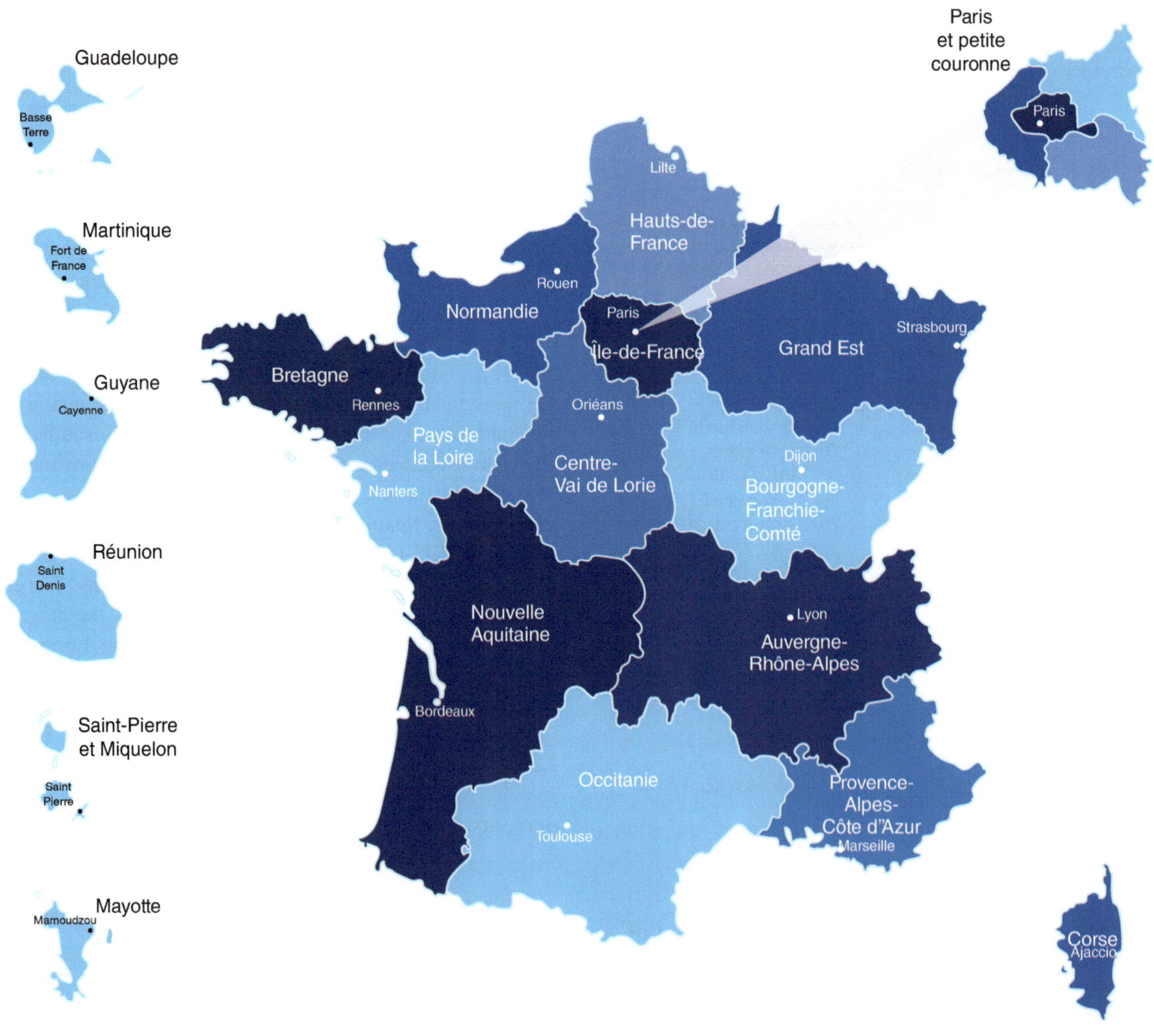


**Fig. 39.1** Territorial organization

ing, apprenticeship and orientation, economic development, management of European structural funds, management of structuring equipment (e.g., ports, airports), environment and energy transition, land use planning, housing, culture, and sport). There are 101 departments (including 5 overseas) with specific competencies (social action management and assistance, maintenance of departmental roads, management of colleges, territory development, cultural and sporting action). There are 35,416 towns on mainland France and 100 overseas with specific competencies (social action, social assistance management, management of departmental roads, civil status, management of primary school's planning, culture, sports equipment's, road maintenance, protection of public order).

The regional, departmental, and municipal councilors are elected by direct universal suffrage for a period of 6 years. They, respectively, elect the president of the Regional Council, the president of the Departmental Council, and the mayor. Municipalities can be grouped into community of municipalities or agglomeration. Since 2014, agglomeration communities can be grouped together in metropolitan areas to jointly manage economic policy, transport networks, as well as university and research resources and innovation.

There are five overseas territorial collectivities: Saint Pierre and Miquelon, the Wallis and Futuna Islands, French Polynesia, Saint Barthélemy, and Saint Martin. Each has a specific organization and skills [3].

## Climate

The climate in mainland France is temperate, with fairly marked regional differences. Temperatures are relatively mild, and rainfall is distributed throughout the year. Regional variations are due to latitude and the greater or lesser proximity to the sea or the mountain. On the French coasts, the temperature variations are less than in the rest of the country, but the rainfall is higher.

## History of Nephrology in France

Nephrology is a relatively young medical discipline that emerged in the 1960s when first attempts of renal replacement therapy of end-stage renal disease, formerly end-stage renal failure, were experimented clinically by pioneering doctors [4–6]. In the international context, but particularly in the French one, nephrology discipline has emerged and pulled out from internal medicine and metabolic and endocrine disease department and earlier was identified as a new specialty to satisfy end-stage renal disease patient needs with stammering therapeutic tools (dialysis, transplantation) and huge potential perspectives. The term "nephrology" was coined and promoted by some visionary kidney doctors called "fathers of nephrology" (e.g., John P Merrill, Jean Hamburger) to define the scope of this new medical discipline [7]. It was then further disseminated worldwide through the first international meeting on chronic renal failure settled in Evian in 1960 [8]. The success and enthusiasm sparked by this first meeting of kidney disease experts (Fig. 39.2) gave birth to the International Society of Nephrology that carried out the torch and led the fight against end-stage renal disease, a devastating and ever-fatal disease [9].

Interestingly and in a purely factual way, French nephrology has largely contributed to the development and the influence of this discipline through its own national specific actions and wide international collaboration. It is well recognized that French nephrology has contributed to the develop-

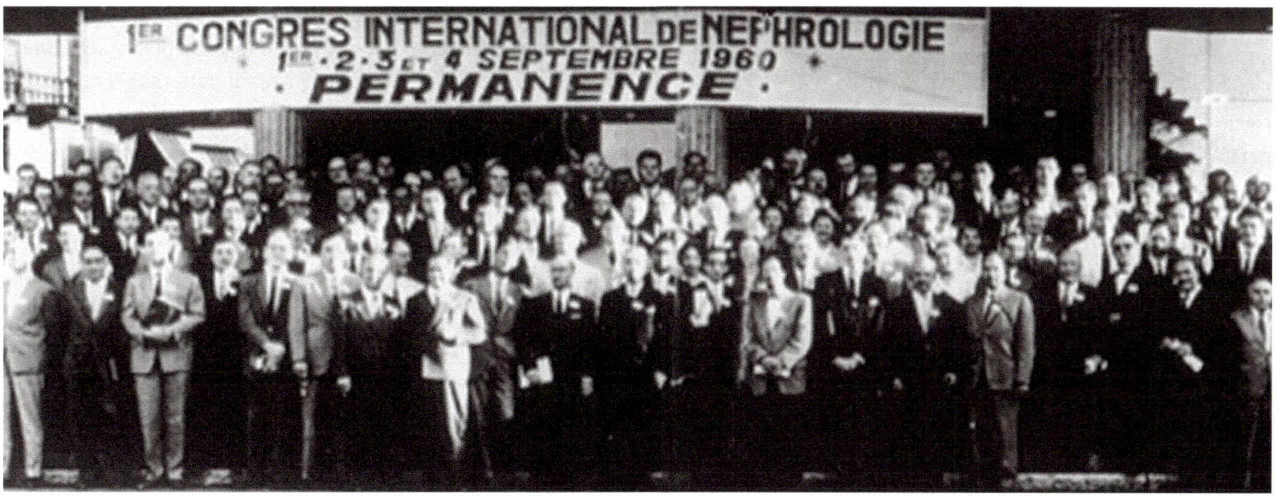


**Fig. 39.2** First meeting of the International Society of Nephrology, Evian, France (Sept. 1–4, 1960)

ment of the main chapters of our discipline through basic and clinical research, management of acute and chronic kidney injury, training and education program, conferences, and meetings. French nephrology is proud to leave such an important imprint on this complex, fascinating, and multifaceted discipline.

It is certainly not our intention to praise the merits of French nephrology in this paragraph, but simply to recognize and value the contribution of some of our mentors and masters in this fight against chronic kidney disease. The French Society of Renal Pathology was created first in 1949 by J Hamburger and transformed later (1959) into the French Society of Nephrology [8]. French nephrology has contributed significantly to the development of various chapters of our discipline with famous names who will remain forever. As duty of memory and recognition, we will only mention few items with leadership names and affiliation school.

1. Hydroelectrolytic disorders (Hamburger J, Richet G, and Ardaillou R)
2. Classification of renal pathology allowed by renal biopsies and histological analyses (Hamburger J, Morel-Maroger L, Gubler MC, Noel LH)
3. Understanding of genetic kidney disease and identification of immune disease-mediated glomerulonephritis (Grundfeld JP, Mery JP, Ronco P)
4. Development of kidney transplantation (Hamburger J, Traeger J, Kreis H, Soulilou JP, Legendre Ch) facilitated by tissue typing (Dausset J) and immunosuppressive protocols (Legendre Ch)
5. Innovative in the field of renal replacement dialysis (highly permeable membrane (AN69, Hospal), ultrafiltration controller (Hospal), water and sterile dialysate (Mion Ch, Canaud B), hemofiltration and online hemodiafiltration (Canaud B, Mion Ch, Shaldon S), dialysis modalities but also home therapy as well as peritoneal dialysis (Mirouze J, Mion Ch, Man NK, Mignon F, Jacob Cl, Laurent G, Charra B, Petitclerc Th, Canaud B))
6. Hypertension management (Corvol P, Menard J)
7. Complications of long-term dialysis patients (Chanard J, Drueke T)
8. Bone metabolic diseases (Fournier A, Drueke T)
9. Management of acute renal failure (Kleinknecht DJ, Canaud B)
10. Nutritional assessment and management (Fouque D)

## Renal Disease in France

### Nephrology Training

#### Organization of Medical Studies and Specialization in Nephrology

Medical studies are an exception in the French university landscape. They do not operate according to the European LMD (License-Master-Doctorate) plan, and their singularity also lies in the alternation between the acquisition of theoretical knowledge and practical hospital training. A schematic presentation of nephrology training is presented in Fig. 39.3. Initial training lasts from 10 to 11 years. The specialization in nephrology only occurs at the end of the medical course (sixth year of the medical course) and lasts from 5 years. The National Classification Examination (ECN) was introduced in 2009 as the only way for entering in medical specialization replacing the internship competition medicine dated from 1802 [10]. This ECN exam allows the candidate to choose the specialty discipline (e.g., nephrology) according to his ranking but also the university in which he can specialize. Nephrology fellowship training program is organized under responsibility of medicine training and research units (UFR) as part of universities and university hospitals (CHU) in partnership with regional hospitals (CHR). The preparation of the specialized diploma in nephrology (DES) is the responsibility of an inter-regional committee led by a regional coordinator in charge of the organization of theoretical and practical courses and evaluating their results. The teaching plan includes general elements (methodological, epidemiological, and clinical research, ethics) and specific elements (physiology and physiopathology; renal, genetic, and immunological; exploration; regulation of the composition of the internal environment and hydroelectrolytic disorders; acid-base balance; description of nephropathies including glomerulonephritis, congenital and hereditary nephropathies, vascular nephropathies, hypertension, chronic renal disease, and acute kidney disease; renal replacement therapy by dialysis and transplantation; management of the course of care of renal patients). Theoretical teaching is provided locally and regionally based on quarterly seminars and nationally in the form of bi-annual seminars by the University College of Nephrology Teachers (CUEN) [11]. The practical training of the resident is based on internship stays in university hospitals or contracted services. It consists of ten semesters of which at least five must

**Fig. 39.3** Nephrology training and professional development

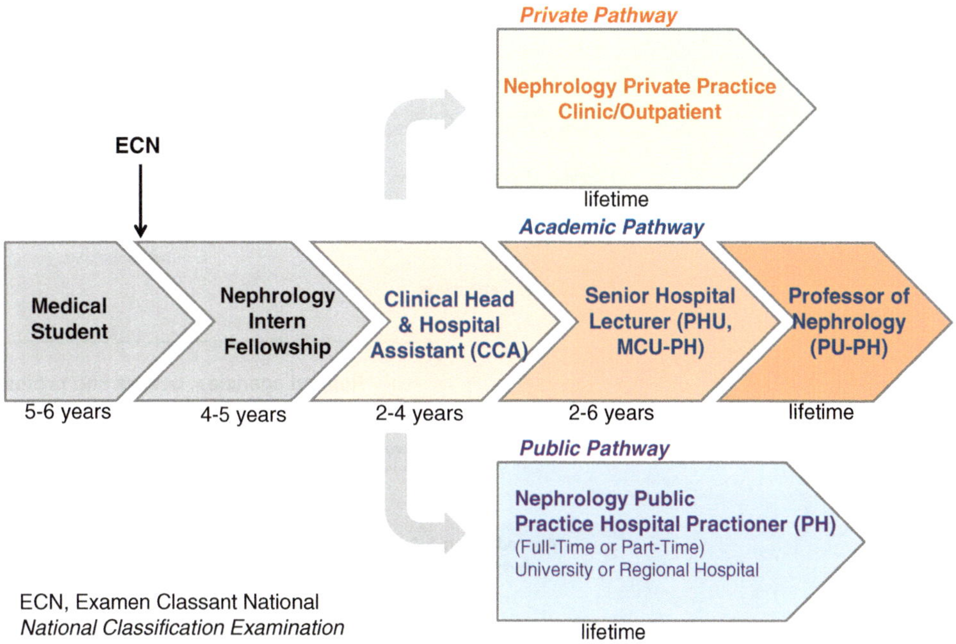


be in nephrology services, the others being performed in accredited services (e.g., resuscitation, internal medicine, functional exploration). During this time, the intern in nephrology carries out the medical functions under the responsibility of the head of department or director of unit or laboratory. He participates and contributes to the clinical care of hospitalized patients, teaching, or research activity under the responsibility of the head of the department. He is then regularly exposed to the problems of exploration and diagnosis, treatment, and overall care of kidney patients. He contributes according to his level of acquisition and his skills to the basic acts of so-called interventional nephrology (e.g., kidney biopsy, venipuncture, placement of nutrition or dialysis catheters, Doppler ultrasound exploration, management of dialysis session). The duration of each internship is one semester. The choice of interns is made by seniority of validated functions and according to the ranking in their discipline. At the end of the ten semesters of internship, the delivery of the diploma of nephrology specialist is validated by the inter-regional commission which is based on the validation of all the required internships, attested by a log of internship or failing by cards validation of achievements, by a written report on a clinical or fundamental research work performed during his internship or failing that by one or several publications. Prior to his specialized diploma in nephrology (DES), the intern must have supported his medical thesis on a personal scientific work or in the form of a synthesis of the scientific work that the candidate will have achieved during his hospital journey. At the end of this initial training, the intern will be able to apply for a 2-year position as a Clinical Head and Hospital Assistant (CCA, post-internship) in which he will be able to deepen his knowledge with dual university and hospital responsibilities. Along this journey, the young kidney doctor is encouraged to broaden his competence and scientific expertise through complementary master's degrees (1 and 2) but also to continue his research in the form of postdoctoral thesis (postdoc) to prepare for a university career.

## Nephrology Certification and Accreditation

Medical doctor's degree in medicine and specialization in nephrology must be certified and registered to the National Council of Physicians (CNOM), a notified body led by peers that guarantees skills, professional independency, and medical ethics [12]. Nephrology skills and training must be continuously updated throughout the professional career of the practitioner. This is part of a personal continuing professional development (CPD) program acquired through

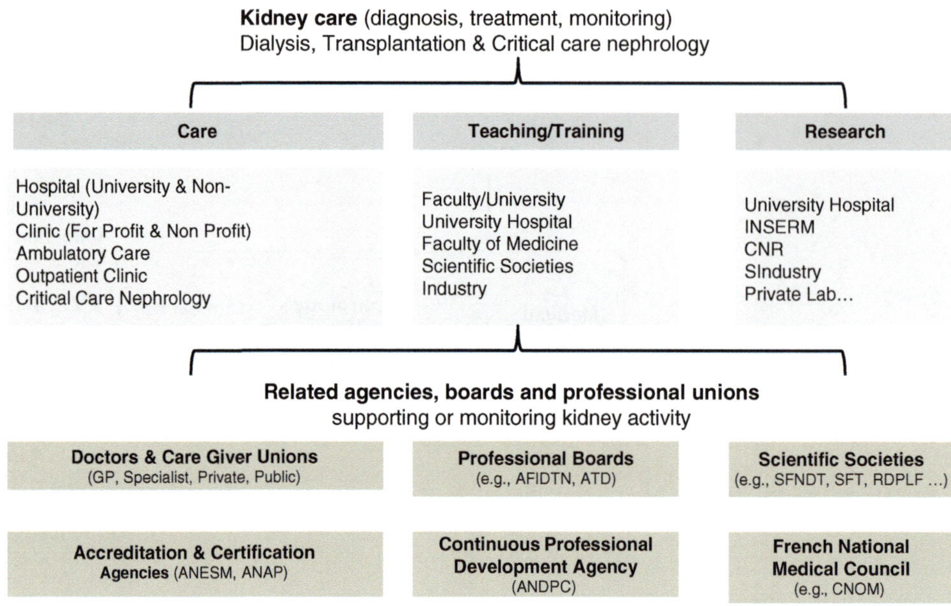


**Fig. 39.4** Nephrology activity and related agencies or boards

scientific meetings or symposia, or specific accredited training sessions, resulting in the acquisition of continuous medical education credits [13]. This procedure required to keep nephrologist's certification is certified by an independent organism [14]. Nephrologist activities as well as monitoring boards and certifying bodies are summarized in Fig. 39.4.

The Francophone Society of Nephrology, Dialysis, and Transplantation (SFNDT) brings together most nephrologists practicing in France and French speaking outside [15]. It represents the professional link and especially the educational and scientific relay necessary for the vitality and continuous updating of the nephrological community. The SFNDT has its own peer-reviewed journal entitled *Néphrologie & Thérapeutique*, editing research studies and reviewing articles in both French and English [16]. Other scientific societies adjacent to the discipline also contribute to this dynamic; they include but are not limited to the following: the Francophone Society of Transplantation (SFT) [17], the Francophone Society of Intensive Care and Resuscitation (SRLF) [18], the Francophone Registry of Peritoneal Dialysis and Home Hemodialysis (RDPLF-HDD) [19], the Francophone Society of Vascular Access (SFAV) [20], the Pediatric Society of Nephrology (SNP) [21], and the Francophone Society of Clinical Nutrition and Metabolism (SFNCM) [22].

Continuing education of caregivers (e.g., nurses, technician) of nephrology, dialysis, and transplant services is also very important. It is ensured by internal and specific professional training cycles in each of the healthcare structures (e.g., continuing education program) but also by companies or associations with national or international educational aims (e.g., Association Française des Infirmier(e)s de Dialyse, Néphrologie et Transplantation (AFIDTN) [23]). Similarly, pharmacists in health facilities in which nephrology activity is developed are grouped together through specific professional associations (e.g., Association of Home Dialysis Pharmacists (APDD) [24]). Also, dialysis technicians have developed a specific association (e.g., Association of Dialysis Technicians, ATD [25]). Networking activity at the country and the international level of these various societies and/or associations ensures the cohesion of the different health actors involved in renal care and helps to update knowledge in these different areas and to guarantee the best practices in renal patient care.

## Nephrology Practices - Nephrologist Demography – Workforce – Training and Certification

### Nephrologist Demography

The number of nephrologists increases almost linearly from the years 1990 until 2017 with a net annual gross rate of 3.5% as presented in Fig. 39.5. In 2013, as an example presented in Fig. 39.6, the net balance was 2.7% out of a total of 1491 active nephrologists.

In 2016, the number of nephrologists was 1672 (57% male and 43% female) with a mean age of 48.0 years (male 51 and female 44) (Fig. 39.7). Repartition of nephrology practices is presented in Fig. 39.8. Note that nephrology practice relies almost exclusively on healthcare facility. As shown, hospital based represents the majority (59%), fol-

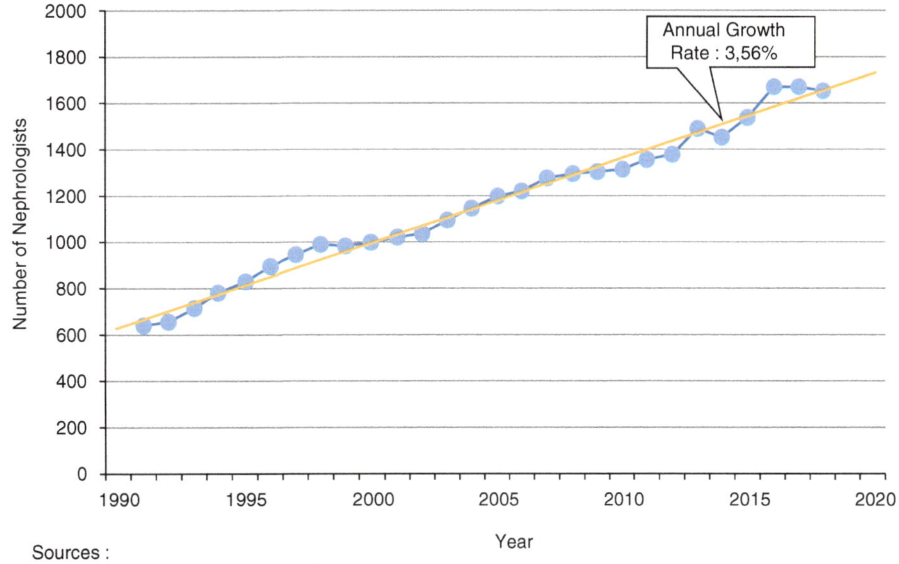


Sources :
http://www.data.drees.sante.gouv.fr
http://www.conseil-national.medecin.fr/

**Fig. 39.5** Demography of nephrologists

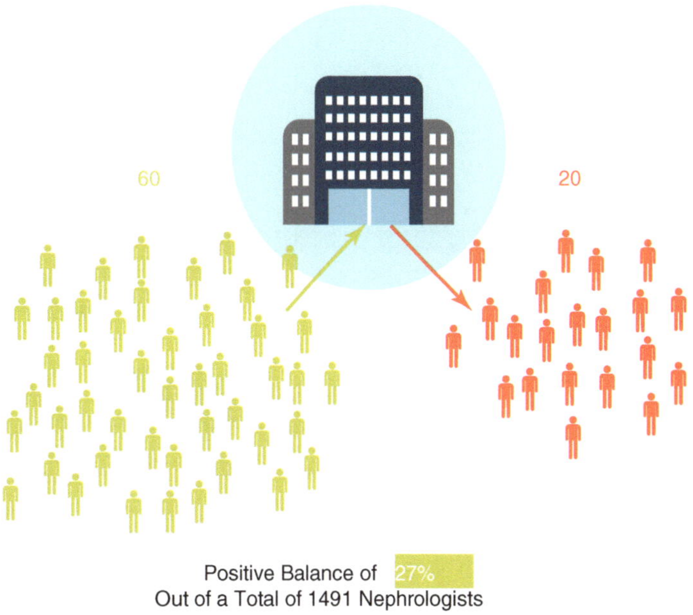


* New registered to French National Medical Council (CNOM)/Retirted

Sources :
http://www.data.drees.sante.gouv.fr
http://www.conseil-national.medecin.fr/

**Fig. 39.6** Incoming/outgoing ratio of nephrologists (fluxes of nephrologists) in 2013

lowed by private clinical based (20%) and then by mixed practice (11%) and non-hospital based including non-profit association care facility (10%). The gross median income per nephrologist depending on their mode of exercise, vintage, and type of activity may be estimated between 80,000 and 250,000€ per year.

Focusing on academic hospital, a schematic representation of the current number of teaching nephrologists is given in Fig. 39.9.

## Geographical Distribution

In France, the national average density was 2.30 nephrologists per 100,000 inhabitants in 2016 as presented in Fig. 39.10a [26]. Forecast evolution of nephrology task force by 2030 is presented in Fig. 39.10b. However, as shown in Fig. 39.11, the number of nephrologists varies tremendously according to the region in France, with den-

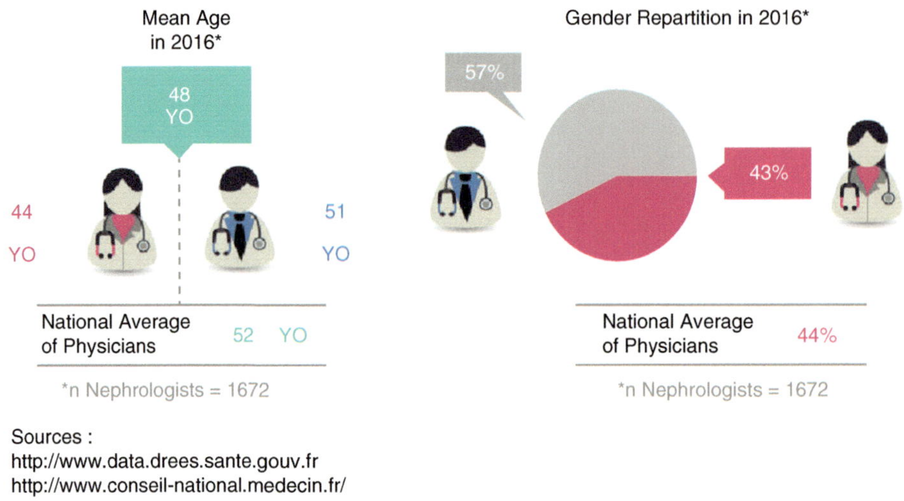


**Fig. 39.7** Profile of nephrologists in France in 2016

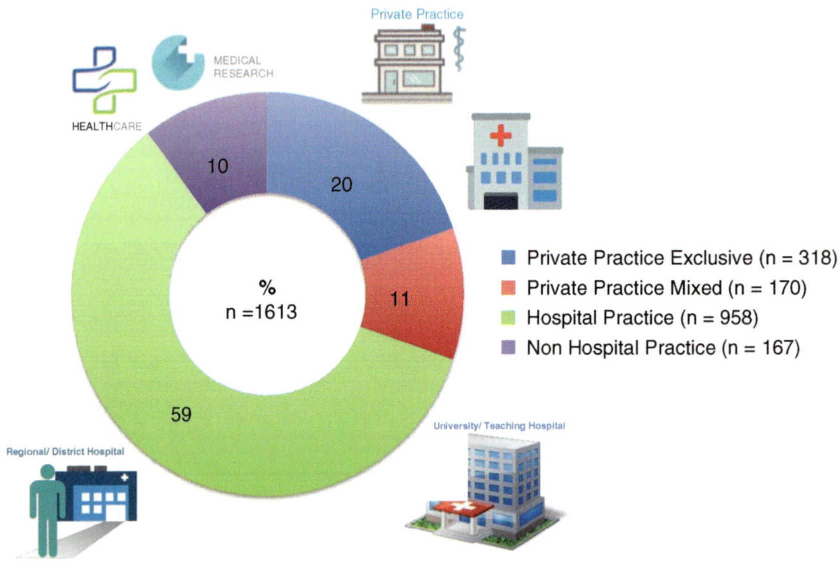


**Fig. 39.8** Distribution of nephrology practices in 2015

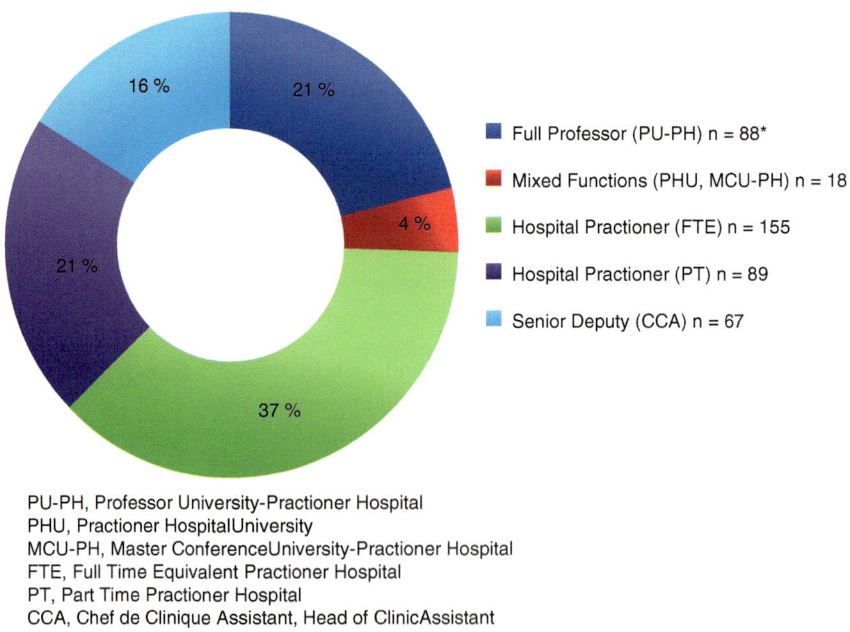


**Fig. 39.9** Distribution of nephrologists in University Teaching Hospitals (CHU)

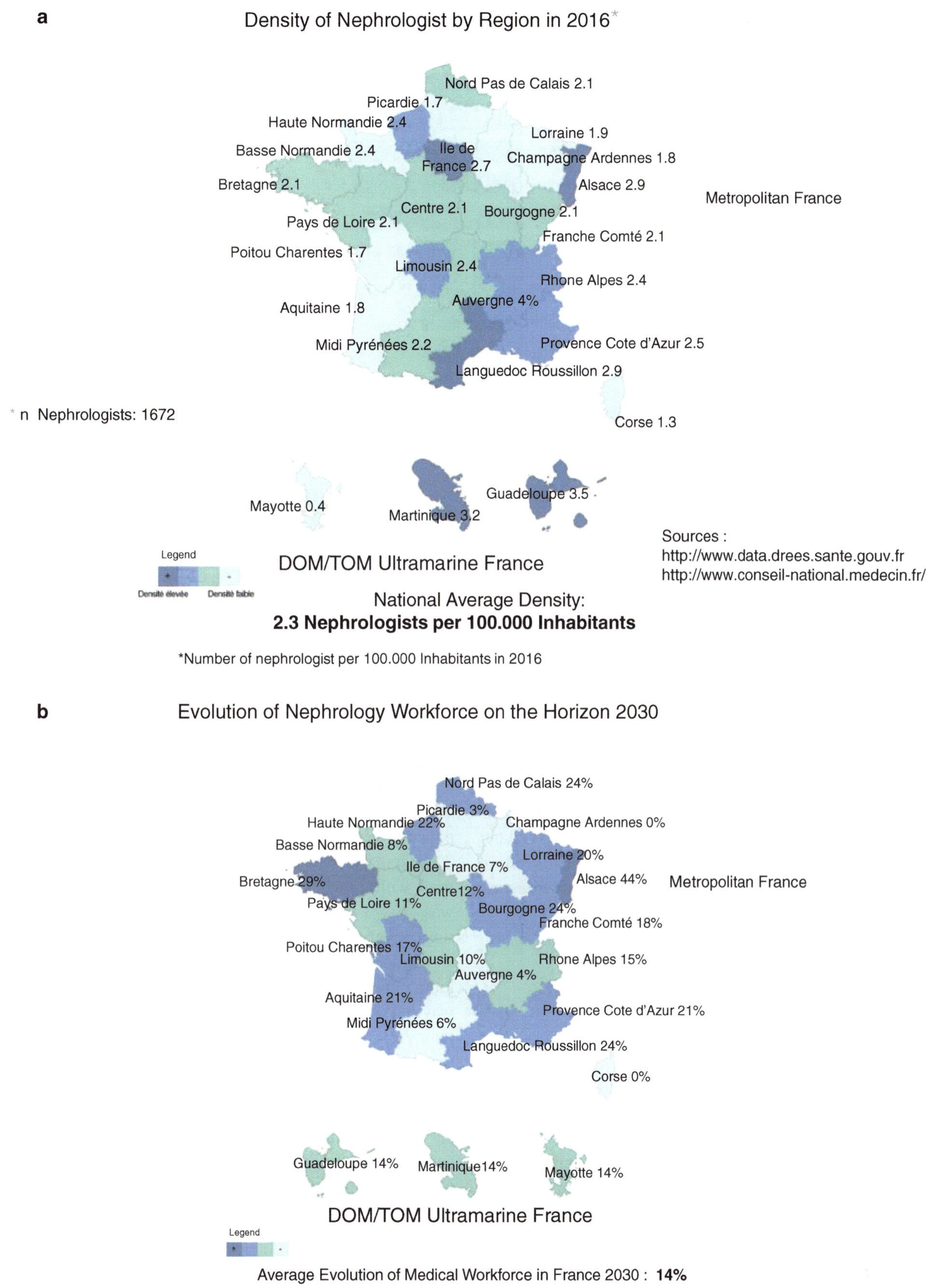


**Fig. 39.10** (**a**) Density of nephrologist by region in 2016. (**b**) Evolution of Nephrology Workforce on the Horizon 2030

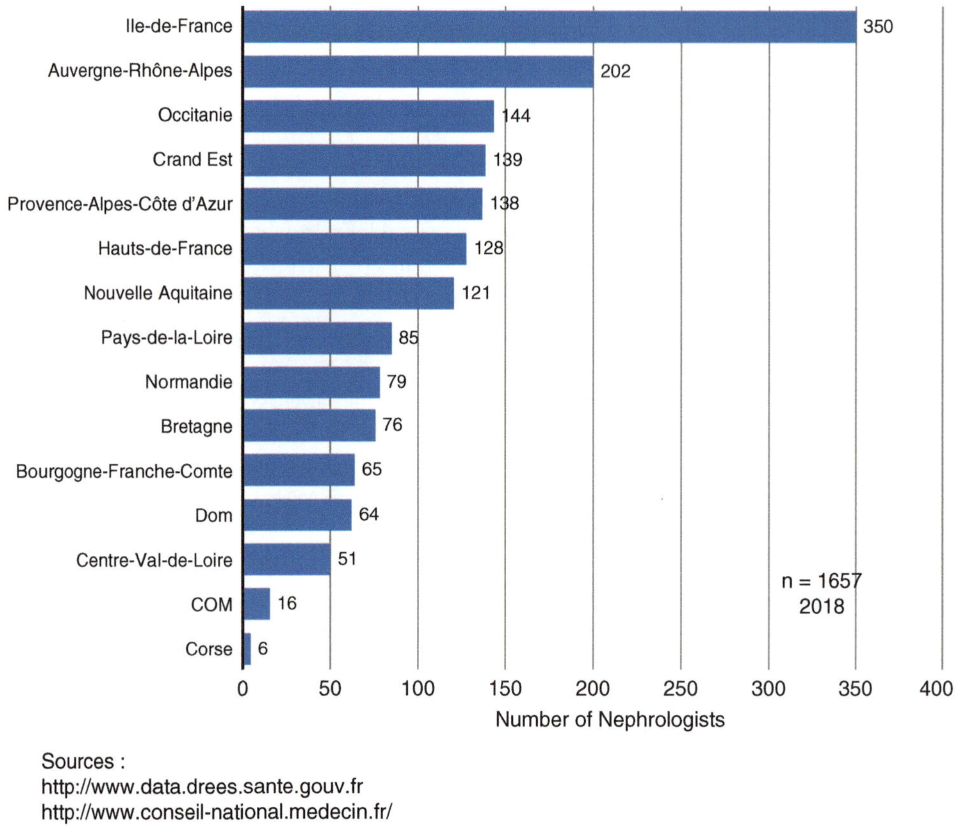


**Fig. 39.11** Number of nephrologists by region in 2018

sities varying from 1.3 (Corse) to 2.9 (Alsace, Languedoc). Using 2016 prevalence data of treated patients from the Biomedicine Agency ($n$ = 46,872 dialysis patients; $n$ = 37,811 transplant patients) and considering number of nephrologists ($n$ = 1672), one can easily calculate that each nephrologist was treating about 50 patients on ESRD. Indeed, this raw calculation ratio of work load per nephrologist does not account for the 3–5 million of inhabitants bearing significant chronic kidney disease (eGFR < 60 ml/min).

## Academic Nephrology: Teaching, Training, and Mentoring

### Nephrology Activity

In terms of nephrology activity, the most visible problem is the management of end-stage kidney disease patients. The prevalence has been gradually increasing over the last few years particularly in the oldest groups (over 75 and 85 years) which has for corollary of increasing frequency of comorbidities.

Flowchart of incoming and outgoing ESRD patients treated in France for the year 2017 is presented in Fig. 39.12. As shown, incidence of new patients starting renal replacement therapy was 172 pmp, prevalence of patients on maintenance therapy was 1294 pmp, renal transplant rate was 56 pmp, and mortality rate was 10.1%. All together 47,985 patients were on maintenance dialysis with a mean age of 71 years, while 39,288 patients were bearing a functional graft with a mean age of 58 years. Annual gross mortality was 16.3% and 2.3% in dialysis and transplantation, respectively.

Clinical nephrology is another important activity of the kidney specialist that should not be neglected since this is the way to detect and to manage more effectively kidney problems, to cure disease, to delay progression, or to prevent occurrence of associated complications. Based on abnormal serum creatinine value (>130 µmmol/l or eGFR < 60 ml/min), it has been estimated that 3–5 million French inhabitants are suffering from chronic kidney disease. This is not accounting for high-risk kidney patients such as patients with proteinuria, diabetics, and hypertensive or arteriopathic patients.

Fig. 39.12 Incoming/outgoing end-stage kidney disease patients in 2017. Repartition between dialysis and transplant patients

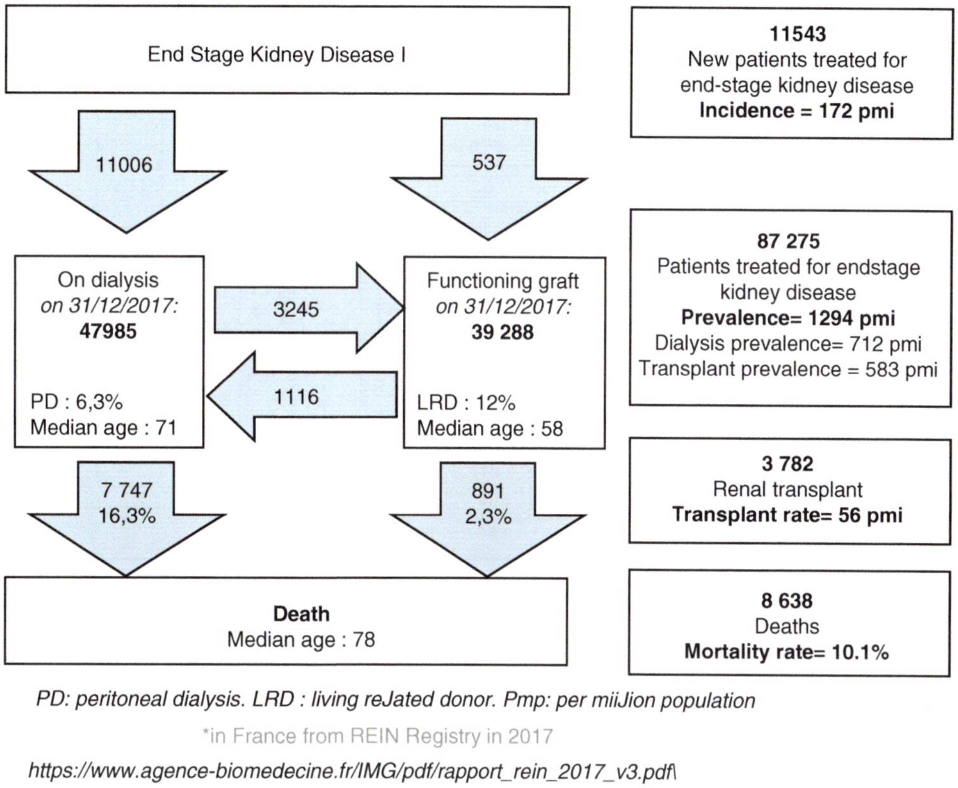


## Attractiveness of Nephrology

Unlike global and Western trend [27], French nephrology has become a quite attractive discipline for trainees and interns. It has been ranked among the first medical specialty selected from interns over the last few years for its attractiveness [28].

Diversity of activities (e.g., clinical nephrology, dialysis, transplantation, laboratory) is one of its positive aspects, but also the image of the discipline has been changed, thanks to the University College of Nephrology Teachers (CUEN), dynamism of university nephrology departments and scientific societies, and development and creation of various clubs and platforms where trainees and young nephrologists can meet and exchange.

Recent changes in intern fellowship program rules have permitted to increase significantly the number of fellows in nephrology training. Eighty positions in nephrology are open annually meaning that 320–360 interns are in training over the 4–5-year training period. Considering the potential of this new working force, one may consider that nephrology needs will be covered adequately for the next few years [29].

## Chronic Kidney Disease Management and Renal Replacement Therapy for ESRD in France

### Healthcare Regulation of Kidney Disease Care

The French health system is extremely regulated. The therapeutic management of chronic kidney disease is no exception to this rule. The treatment of kidney diseases relies on a mixed system provided by public (university and non-university hospitals) and private health institutions (hospitals or private clinics for profit and/or non-profit). This public-private networking system which ensures a tight health network of the national territory, allows complementary coverage to the nearest patients, and meets the same regulatory requirements has been reinforced in July 2009 by a new healthcare regulatory law (e.g., hospital, patient, health, and territories [30]). Specific setting for kidney care in France is presented in Fig. 39.13. Depending on chronic kidney disease stage, management differs but should follow the same rules and best clinical practices whatever the care is provided by private or public practitioners.

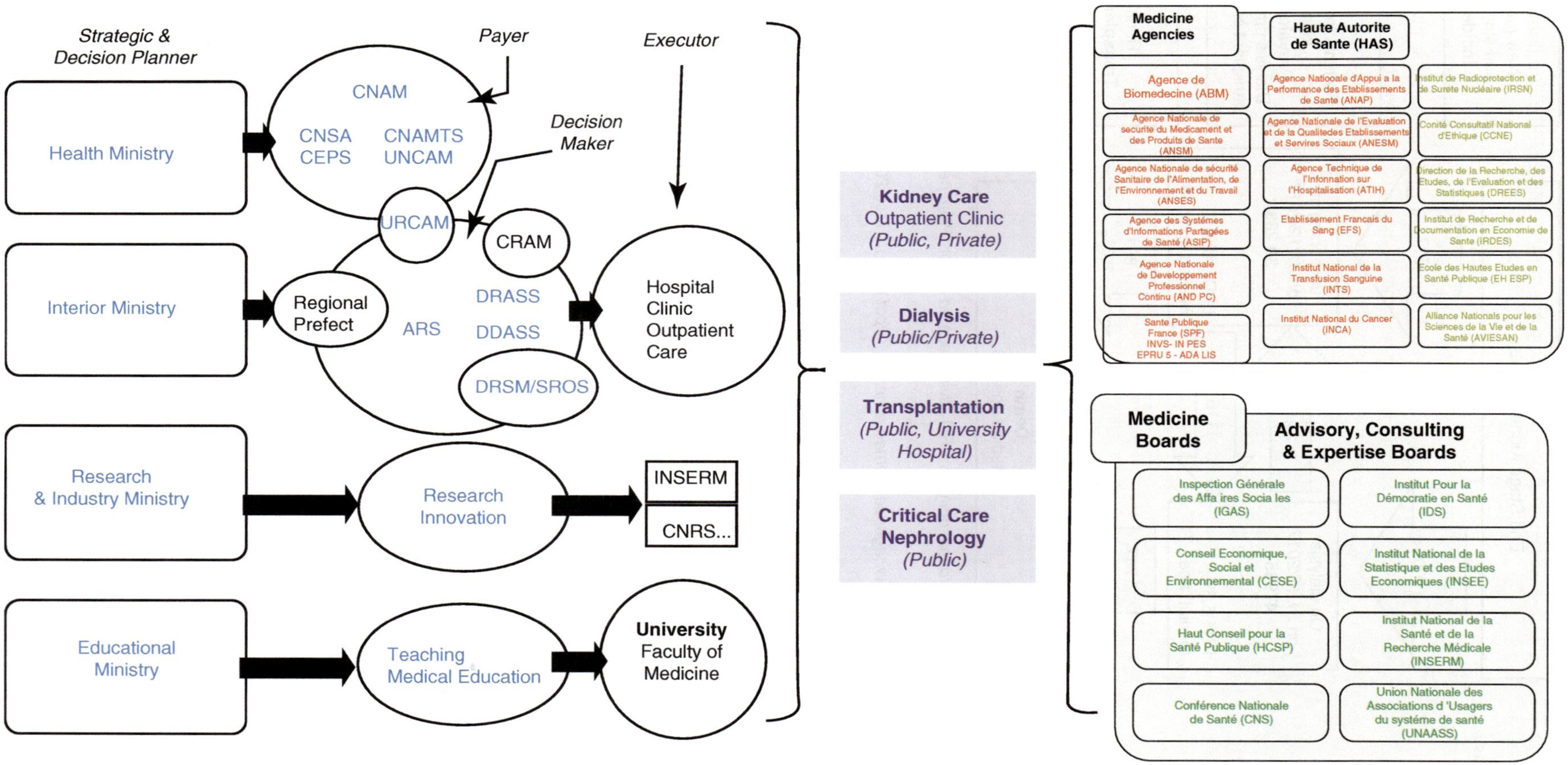


**Fig. 39.13** Kidney care in the context of French healthcare system

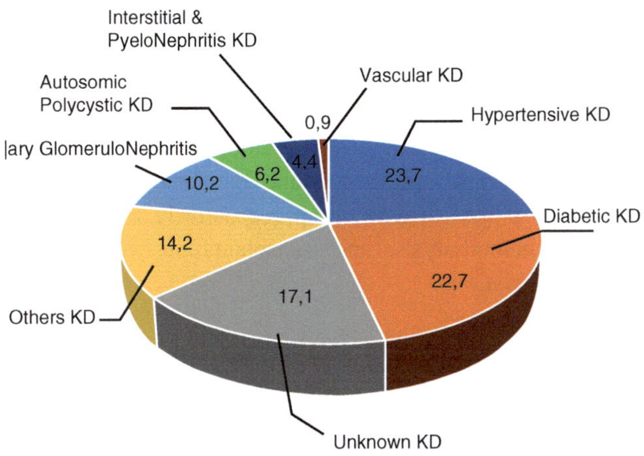


**Fig. 39.14** Primary underlying kidney disease among end-stage kidney disease patients in France in 2017

| France | |
|---|---|
| Legal Entity Care Provider | N (%) |
| Public | 151 ( 49.0) |
| Private For-Profit | 85 (27.6) |
| Private Non Profit (Association) | 72 (23.4) |
| Total | 308 (100) |
| Facility Provider | N (%) |
| CHU-CHR | 45 (14.6) |
| CH | 104 (33.8) |
| Private Clinic/Hospital (MCO) | 58 (18.8) |
| Dialysis Providers | 71 (23.1) |
| Others | 30 (9. 7) |
| Total | 308 (100) |
| Incenter, Medicalized & Self Care Unitst | 308 (100) |
| HD Stations | 4620 |
| N Dialysis Station per Unit (M±SD) | 14.8±7.9 |
| Home HD Stations | 800 |
| Total HD Stations | 4928 |

**Fig. 39.15** Hemodialysis facilities and dialysis stations

## Chronic Kidney Disease Management

Chronic kidney disease (CKD) management relies exclusively on referent nephrologist in collaboration with other specialists (e.g., diabetologist, cardiologist). It is based on outpatient clinic and ambulatory care with periodical consultations, clinical assessment, lab test, or imaging monitoring with medicine prescription. All related costs incurring to CKD patient monitoring and treatment are covered by the universal social security insurance system under the regime of the long-lasting disease (ALD30) as defined later on.

### Epidemiology of Kidney Disease in France

The total number of patients with kidney disease is difficult to estimate since we don't have a national registry recording CKD disease but also because we know that the disease remains silent till it reaches a very advanced stage (CKD3B). According to current estimates, the number of subjects with asymptomatic kidney disease is said to represent approximately 10% of the French population, the invisible part of the iceberg. It ranks chronic kidney disease in the "top list" of public health challenges, and screening for the disease should be routinely performed in high-risk subjects (hypertension, diabetes) and in the population aged over 60.

The current main primary causes of kidney disease are hypertension and diabetes. This is summarized in Fig. 39.14. Hypertensive kidney disease is the main cause of ESRD accounting for 24% of new cases. It is associated with narrowing of the kidney's small arteries (nephroangiosclerosis) with a reduction in vascularization leading to chronic ischemic kidney disease. Hypertensive nephropathy is frequently merged with vascular disease sharing a common pathophysiologic mechanism accounting for 1%. Diabetic kidney disease is the second leading cause of ESRD in developed countries. It represented 23% of new cases of ESRD in France in 2017. Primary glomerulonephritis, which represented the majority of kidney disease in the 1990s, now only affects 11% of patients. Pyelonephritis accounts for 4.3% of new cases of renal failure. Autosomic polycystic kidney disease is the most commonly hereditary disease observed with about 6.2% of new cases. Other causes or unknown origin of kidney diseases represented about one third of new cases.

### End-Stage Renal Disease Management

End-stage renal disease (ESRD) patient may benefit from dialysis care when necessary. It is at the discretion of the nephrologist to decide when and how to start renal replacement therapy. In all cases, the nephrologist must follow the recommendations and best clinical practices in use. He must present and explain all therapeutic modalities (e.g., in-center hemodialysis, home therapy, preemptive transplant) with their benefits and risks. The choice must be shared with patient and/or relatives and traced in the medical file. When renal replacement therapy has been indicated, the patient is then referred to the dialysis care provider habilitated to provide the adequate therapeutic option.

The dialysis units are part of health facilities and are thus managed by public, private, or associative healthcare providers (Fig. 39.15). Technical operating conditions of dialysis units have been redefined by law and known as "2002 September decrees" [31]. They apply to all renal care providers. These decrees specify the technical platforms and quotas of minimum caregivers to ensure safety and care quality to patients:

1. The hemodialysis center (CHD) mainly supports patients whose health conditions (e.g., comorbidity, handicaps) require the permanent presence of doctor. It specifies also the number of patients per nephrologist as well as the number of nurses and/or caregivers per series of patients treated. The center must be located geographically within

a healthcare facility with full hospital beds and emergency and continuous care services. The hemodialysis center has, on its own or by agreement, the services of a laboratory and imaging unit. The number of patients treated per day and per dialysis station is limited to 3.

2. Medicalized dialysis units (UDMs) mainly host patients who do not require a continuous medical presence during the session. The maximum number of patients treated per machine and per day is 3. The permanent presence of at least one nurse for every four patients per session is necessary. The medical team, without being physically present, must be able to intervene during the session, within times compatible with the imperative of security. The visit of the nephrologist is provided one to three times a week.
3. Auto-dialysis units or self-care dialysis (UADs) offer simple or assisted auto-dialysis: (a). The basic UAD is intended for autonomous patients who can provide themselves their own treatment. The permanent presence of a nurse is necessary to help patients when needed (one nurse for every eight patients). A personal and not sharable dialysis machine is assigned to each patient to provide more flexibility and wide range of treatment time schedule. (b). The assisted UAD is offered to semi-autonomous patients who require the assistance of a nurse to perform certain actions (e.g., arteriovenous fistula puncture). The maximum number of patients treated in this case is 2 per shift and per day. The unit has a permanent nurse for six treated patients and possibly other caregivers. The visit of the nephrologist, during the session, is provided at least once a quarter in simple UAD and at least once a month in assisted UAD. In addition, an external consultation must be carried out at least once a quarter.
4. Home hemodialysis (HDD) is offered to autonomous patients capable of performing all the necessary actions for their treatment, in the presence of a person from his entourage who can assist him.
5. Peritoneal dialysis (PD) is also offered to autonomous patients wishing to treat themselves at home. In these cases, the care operator is responsible for their training, monitoring, and logistical support. A specialized nurse must be able to provide a 24/24 and 7/7 operational support. In all cases, so-called "out-of-center" dialysis units and the operators responsible for these units must have, on their own or by convention, fallback protocols with specialized care structures capable of ensuring immediate care in case of complications and/or medical emergencies.

## Renal Replacement Therapy Health Trajectories and Figures

On December 31, 2017, 87,275 patients were receiving a renal replacement therapy in France, 55% on dialysis and 45% living with a functional renal transplant [32]. The overall crude prevalence was 1294 pmp. It was 1.7 higher in males. Prevalence was subject to regional variations with eight regions (four overseas) above the national rate. Renal transplant share varied from less than 40% in three regions to more than 50% in five regions and from 13% to 29% in overseas regions. The overall sex- and age-standardized prevalence was 45, 667, and 583 pmp, respectively, for peritoneal dialysis, hemodialysis, and transplantation, with marked regional variations.

## Hemodialysis Epidemiology, Practices, and Outcomes

In 2017, 11,006 new ESRD patients started renal replacement therapy by dialysis [32]. The overall incidence of renal replacement therapy (RRT) was 172 pmp (dialysis, 164 pmp; preemptive transplantation, 8 pmp). Median age at RRT initiation is 71 years. Those patients present a high rate of comorbidities especially diabetes (47% of the new patients) and cardiovascular diseases (57% of the new patients) that is increasing with aging. The first treatment option remains in center's hemodialysis. RRT started in emergency in 30% of the patients. The hemoglobin level at RRT start seems to be an interesting indicator of good management and follow-up since 60% of patients presenting an underprovided follow-up have a hemoglobin level under 10 g/dL, whereas only 40% of patients with an appropriate follow-up presented such a condition. On December 31, 2017, 47,985 prevalent ESRD patients including overseas territories were maintained on dialysis (hemodialysis 44,970 and peritoneal dialysis 3015). The overall prevalence of RRT in hemodialysis is 667 pmp and 45 pmp in peritoneal dialysis. Interestingly, the prevalence of hemodialysis patients in overseas territories is almost twice as compared to France mainland (hemodialysis 1902 pmp versus 636 pmp). It is interesting noting that elderly over 65 years account for 66% of the patients undergoing dialysis (median age: 71 years, stable since 2012). These patients present a high rate of comorbidity especially diabetes (43% of patients, increasing since 2012) and cardiovascular comorbidities (60% of patients) that increases with the patient's age.

Total number of dialysis facilities and dialysis stations is presented in Fig. 39.15. Home hemodialysis treatment tends to slightly increase with a share of 0.9% of dialysis patients with about 450 patients, mainly linked to the development of daily hemodialysis with availability of more friendly dialysis machines and delivery systems.

Vascular access used in 80% of patients is an arteriovenous fistula (AVF), while a tunneled central venous catheter is used in the remaining 20% of patients. Three sessions per week is the standard treatment in 94% of patients; two sessions or less per week concerns only 3.6% of patients reflecting either start of the RRT program or end-of-life patient management. Two percent of patients are on daily dialysis (>4 sessions per week).

The duration of the sessions is 4 hours in 71% of patients, between 3 and 4 hours for 19%, more than 4 hours for 8%, and less than 3 hours for 2%. Long dialysis longer than 6 hours is performed in 0.7% of patients.

Hemodialyzers are made of high-flux synthetic membranes in 90% of cases with a median surface of 1.80 $m^2$. The reuse of dialyzers and/or disposable dialysis material equipment is prohibited in France since 1995.

Hemodiafiltration is used in 35% of patients with differences ranging from 0% to 76% depending on the region but increasing steadily. The online method is almost the only substitution method with a median substitution volume of 21 liters per session in post-dilution mode.

Systemic anticoagulation is performed in almost 80% of cases with low molecular weight heparin, and the rest uses unfragmented heparin or another modality as needed.

The median electrolytic composition in mmol/liter of the bicarbonate dialysate is as follows: Na 138, K 2.0, HCO3 35, Ca 1.5, Mg 0.5, and acetate (80%) or citrate (20%) as acidifier.

The median Kt/V for patients having three hemodialysis sessions per week varies from 1.4 to 1.5 depending on the measurement method. The percentage of patients with an equilibrated Kt/V ($_{eq}$Kt/V) greater than 1.2 corresponding to the targets of adequate minimum dialysis according to the recommendations varies from 72% to 89% depending on the method. The percentage of patients with a Kt/V greater than 1.2 is higher in patients over 75 years of age. It is logically more important in patients with an AVF than in patients with a catheter.

Note that in all cases, there are strong regional disparities reflecting specific needs and more specific practices relating to patients with a specific medical profile or local adapted practices.

The length of renal replacement therapy in prevalent dialysis patients in 2017 had a median of 3.2 years. Dialysis vintage varies significantly from one region to another from 2.7 years in Corsica to 4.5 in La Reunion. Forty-eight percent of all patients have a total treatment duration of 2 years or less. This distribution is a reflection of patients treated exclusively by dialysis whatever the reasons are (e.g., hyperimmunized, high-risk) and regional transplant activity. Among patients treated for more than 20 years, 86% received a kidney transplant at least once [32].

In 2017, the prevalence of chronic carriers of viruses HBV, HCV, and HIV in 2017 was 0.7%, 1.0%, and 0.8%, respectively, with a significant decrease trend over the past decade. Among the 80 patients with HIV virus, 28 are at the AIDS stage, and 39% of these patients are treated in Île-de-France. Note that patients with chronic virus contamination are much more important in overseas territories with a prevalence for HBV, HCV, and HIV of 1.3%, 1.1%, and 1.1%, respectively [32]. It is forecasted that prevalence of HCV further decreases with access and generalization of anti-HCV treatment [33].

In 2017, overall patient survival rate of incident hemodialysis patients ($n$ = 53,971) equipped with an arteriovenous access at initiation starting in the period 2002–2017, at 1, 3, 5, and 10 years, was as follows: 89.4% (89.1–89.6), 72.0% (71.6–72.4), 57.1% (56.6–57.6), and 35.2% (34.6–35.8), respectively. Survival rate probability in diabetic, cardiac, and elderly patients is 10–20% lower and 5–10% better in younger and no comorbid patients.

## Peritoneal Dialysis Epidemiology, Practices, and Outcomes

On December 31, 2017, overall prevalent use of peritoneal dialysis modality was 3015, predominantly in France mainland with 2873 patients accounting for 95.2% of total share. The overall prevalence of peritoneal dialysis remains stable over time with a share of 6.2% of dialysis patients. Peritoneal dialysis represents the main home therapy option relying on continuous ambulatory peritoneal dialysis (CAPD) or automated peritoneal dialysis (APD) with a share of 3,7% and 2,5%, respectively [32].

Peritoneal dialysis is exclusively performed at home, either as self-care modality (about 40%) or as assisted-care modality (about 60%), mainly with CAPD requiring external nurse home intervention [34]. Peritoneal dialysis solutions are multiple, and prescription relies on various associations including icodextrin-based solution for long-dwell exchange in almost 80% of patients. Median exchange volume in CAPD is 6.2 liter/day (0.5–12) and in APD is 10.0 liter/day (2.0–18.0) based on six exchanges per week.

Even if the number of patients treated by PD increases (+3% per year), the relative share trend tends to decline by 2% per year between 2009 and 2017. For example, when analyzing patients' movement and turnover through the year 2017 ($n$ = 2970), 61% were still on PD, and 39% had left the modality, mainly by death (18%), by transfer to hemodialysis (11%), or by transplantation (9%). Outgoing flows are the highest of all modalities, reflecting a lower technical survival and a greater turnover of prevalent patients. The two main exit modes, renal transplant and death, illustrate patients' heterogeneity treated by PD and local policy of PD use.

## Kidney Transplantation Epidemiology, Practices, and Outcomes

Kidney transplantation is a highly recommended therapeutic option for patients with ESRD patients who can fit with this procedure [35]. Among all candidates for kidney transplant on the waiting list in 2017, 3782 kidney transplantations have been performed with 16% from a living donor and 15% having a second transplant. However, the state of shortage has worsened, and 18,793 were candidates for a kidney transplant in 2017 [32]. The probability of first wait-listing was of 5.6% at the start of dialysis (preemptive registrations), 16% at 12, 26% at 36, and 29% at 60 months. The probability of being registered was strongly related to age, diabetes, and region. Patient older than 60 had a very poor access to the waiting list, whatever their diabetes status was. Probability of first wait-listing was much lower (46% at 60 months) in type 2 diabetic, 40–59-year-old patients. Among patients less than 60 years old, the probability of being registered was 14% at the start of dialysis, 41% at 12 months, 64% at 36 months, and 70% at 60 months (median dialysis duration: 17 months). The percentage of patients back to dialysis after a transplant failure is slightly increasing in 2017. They were 1116 in 2017 and represented 9% of the cohort of the patients who started dialysis.

It must always be proposed, and a pre-transplant feasibility assessment must be carried out by the referent regional transplant team. It is important to note that kidney transplantation is the exclusive competence of accredited academic hospitals and under the different plans and laws governing organ transplantation [36, 37]. Today, 48 kidney transplant centers are accredited over all French territory (metropolitan and ultramarine) to perform all related procedures (pre-transplant, transplant, and post-transplant monitoring and management) to kidney transplant. The pre-transplant assessment consists in checking overall clinical condition, vital risk factors (e.g., cardiovascular history and status, oncological history), specific risks (e.g., blood group, HLA tissue typing, immunological status, viral risk), and anatomical problems (e.g., abdominal, pelvic, and peripheral artery network, vascular calcification). At the end of this assessment, the feasibility of the transplantation is retained or not. A registration on the national waiting list for cadaveric kidney transplant is then performed to the Biomedicine Agency (ABM). Patient, referring physicians, and stakeholders are then informed of the registration on the waiting list. Management of available kidney is then managed at the national level by the ABM according to relatively complex allocation criteria (e.g., compatibility levels, seniority, priority criteria, etc.) established by a national committee of experts. Kidney transplant allocation choices are made from a proprietary software (Cristal, ABM) that ensures best matching between donor and recipients selection criteria to ensure best outcome to transplant, but also to guarantee transparency and equity in the distribution of available organs. When living kidney donor transplantation is envisaged, the protocol is mainly managed by regional transplant team after registration to the ABM. In addition to patient recipient assessment, a precise checkup (e.g., tissue typing and compatibility, kidney function, vital risk, psychology stability) is performed to the family and/or living related donor candidate. Further possibilities were developed to expand kidney transplant capacity (e.g., paired or living donor exchange, desensitization in hyperimmunized patients, kidney harvesting in dead donors), but that will not be covered in this chapter.

Immunosuppression (IS) is administered to kidney transplant patients to prevent rejection episodes and loss of the renal allograft [38]. All transplant centers rely on an induction therapy with either interleukin-2 receptor antibodies or anti-thymocyte globulin and a maintenance therapy consisting in triple immunosuppression. The most frequently used substances for maintenance IS are glucocorticoids, antimetabolites (mycophenolate… mycophenolic acid), mTOR inhibitors (mTORi), calcineurin inhibitors (CNI), and the co-stimulation blocker belatacept. In France, best practice guidelines recommend a triple combination consisting of CNIs, antimetabolites, and corticosteroids as standard of care for 6–12 months, then after followed by tapering IS mostly relying on double combination aiming to suppress steroids. CNIs are considered as cornerstone of IS. Tacrolimus represents in most case the first choice as the mainstream of IS despite its strong diabetogenic propensity. Patient-focused IS protocol depends on patient age and status, organ functions (heart, kidney, liver), and laboratory data. Modification of IS may also result from initial patient response (e.g., acute rejection, side effects, poor tolerance) or high-risk patients (e.g., hyperimmunized, retransplant, solid cancer history, identified risk, virus carrier) or local practices contributing to clinical research. Post-transplantation diabetes mellitus represents a frequent complication that affects about one third of kidney transplant patients and needs IS adaptation. Opportunistic infections (cytomegalovirus and pneumocystis) and post-transplantation lymphoproliferative disorders (PTLD) are less frequently reported and best managed by prophylaxis, IS reduction, and targeted therapies.

Among all candidates for kidney transplant on the waiting list in 2017, 3782 transplantations were performed in majority from deceased-donor kidney transplants. Transplant from living related kidney donors represented 16% of patients, and 15% of cases corresponded re-transplantation (e.g., second or third transplant). Shortage of kidneys has worsened, and 18,793 were candidates for a kidney transplant in 2017. The percentage of patients back to dialysis after a transplant failure had increased in 2017. They were 1116 in 2017 and represented 9% of the cohort of the patients who started dialysis.

The probability of first wait-listing was of 5.6% at the start of dialysis (preemptive transplantation), 16% at 12, 26% at 36, and 29% at 60 months. The probability of being registered was strongly related to age, diabetes, and region. Patient older than 60 had a very poor access to the waiting list, whatever their diabetes status was. Probability of first wait-listing was much lower (46% at 60 months) in type 2 diabetic patients. Among patients less than 60 years old, the probability of being registered was 14% at the start of dialysis, 41% at 12 months, 64% at 36 months, and 70% at 60 months (median dialysis duration: 17 months).

According to annual Biomedicine Agency report, kidney graft survival probability shows significant outcome improvement according to transplant cohorts till 2006–2008: 1986–1990, 1991–1995, 1996–2000, 2001–2005, and 2006–2008 with 1-year survivals of 83,7%, 86,3%, 91,0%, 92,2%, and 92,6%. However, most recent 2009–2011 and 2012–2015 cohorts showed a slight decrease in 1-year survival to 91.7% and 91.6%. This change is likely due to the significant increase in elderly donors and the aging of recipient. These figures are to be compared with median survival of kidney graft which is 14 years [32].

In 2017, 891 deaths were recorded out of 38,226 patient-years at risk of dying with a functional graft. The annual mortality rate is very low (1–2%) until the age of 50 and then increases slightly. Transplant patients have a much lower mortality probability than those on dialysis patients. In 2017, for 1000 patients aged between 60 and 69 years, 115 versus 27 died in dialysis and kidney transplantation, respectively.

The study of temporal variations since 2012 demonstrated a +3% increase in standardized prevalence of ESRD patients with a functional transplant vs. +2% increase for dialysis, resulting in a decreasing gap between dialysis and transplantation prevalence, due to an increase number of renal transplant and a longer survival of transplanted patients.

## Renal Replacement Therapy in Pediatric End-Stage Renal Disease Patients

In this chapter we provide a brief summary of pediatric end-stage renal disease (ESRD) management regarding demographics, treatment modalities, and outcomes in France [32].

In 2017, 126 infants and adolescents (<20 years) were started on renal replacement therapy. The incidence of ESRD among patients under 20 years old was 7,7 pmh. The prevalence remained stable at 56,5 pmp. The first causes of ESRD are hereditary nephropathies and uropathies and renal hypodysplasia. Initial treatment was hemodialysis for 55% and peritoneal dialysis for 25% that is mainly used in younger children. In 2017, 26 preemptive transplantations were performed accounting for 21% of new patients. The probability of first wait-listing was of 18% at the start of dialysis (preemptive registration), 68% at 12, 83% at 24, and 93% at 60 months. The probability of first renal transplantation was of 20% at the start of renal replacement therapy (preemptive transplantation), 50% at 12, 71% at 24, and 89% at 60 months. Finally, survival analyses confirmed that younger children (under 4 years old) have the highest risk of death (91% survival rate at 5 years vs. 97% in patients over 4 years old) and that the treatment of choice is renal transplantation since it increases the expected remaining lifetime by about 20 years depending on the considered age compared to a patient that would stay on dialysis all his life.

In 2017, 923 young patients under the age of 20 residing in France received replacement therapy. The crude prevalence of ESRD treated in this age group is 56.5 pmh under 20 years of age with an increase according to age, varying from 19 pmh for children under 5–115 for 18–19 years old. The median age of these children and adolescents is 14.4 years, and 60% are boys. Kidney transplantation is the most frequently used treatment modality (76%). The share of transplants with living donors is 16%. Note that the priority in pediatrics to access a graft allows access to the transplant much faster than for adults. HD is used in 17% of children and adolescents and peritoneal dialysis in 7%. However, the distribution of treatment methods is age-dependent with frequent use of peritoneal dialysis in children under 4 years of age (37%).

## Acute Kidney Injury Management and Renal Replacement Therapy

In France, intensive care units (ICU) are shared among various departments (e.g., anesthesiology, resuscitation) and/or specialties (e.g., nephrology, cardiology, gastroenterology, surgery). Management and treatment of AKI is therefore shared among these departments according to patient pathway and severity of AKI. In France, about 950 public hospitals including university and general hospitals, 700 mixed public-private hospitals, and about 1000 private hospitals are distributed on mainland France. Among them, around 400 ICU are located in 320 institutions, representing approximately 4700 beds. The number of beds in private hospitals is around 12%. ICUs are polyvalent (50%), surgical (20%), or medical (12%) and admit around 150,000 patients per year. Non-kidney ICU teams manage AKI patients in relation with nephrologist experts [39].

The ICU is governed by Law Decrees (2002-466; 2003-45; 2006-72) framing the practices. The architecture of ICUs should include three areas: reception, hospitalization, and technical. The ICU team includes physicians, nurses, physiotherapist, and psychologist. The head of ICU is a physician certified in ICU and concerned specialty (e.g., nephrology, cardiology). Intensivists and/or ICU specialists should be in-house 24/7. A junior can be in-house on-call under the supervision of a senior on-call at-home. There is no ratio defining the number of intensivists by bed, but generally, at daytime, about four full-time seniors are required for ten beds. Regarding the nurse team, each unit includes a chief-nurse. The Law Decree imposes a ratio of 2 nurses for 5 patients and 1 nurse-assistant for 4 patients. The nurses are responsible for drug administration, parenteral nutrition, organ support (e.g., lung, renal, cardiac), quality of care, and prescription under the responsibility of physicians. Renal replacement therapy (e.g., intermittent of continuous option) is performed by certified and trained nurses under the supervision of physicians.

The cost of hospitalization is covered by the national social security agency. In routine, there is no interaction about hospitalization fees between patient's relatives and the medical team. Each public ICU belongs to an administrative entity including several departments, based on thematic or geographical features. A financial statement is presented at least once a year at the level of those entities. The staff resource represents 43% of total costs. For each ICU stay, the hospitals receive a lump sum, making it difficult to determine the specific cost of an individual stay.

By definition, ICU admission is based on the presence of at least two organ failures with a risk of death. The patients with a single organ failure are directed to specialty acute care units, and those stable with potential organ failure are admitted to intermediate care units. The mortality rates range from 15% to 25%, and 21% of patients discharged alive does not survive at 1 year [40]. Best clinical practices are framed by national guidelines, mainly produced by Société Francaise d'Anesthésie et de Réanimation and Société de Réanimation de Langue Francaise (SFAR-SRLF) and published in ACCPM [41].

End of life is framed by the Claeys-Leonetti Law of February 2, 2016. This Law aims at protecting the end-of-life patient against stubbornly and unreasonable cares. A right to a deep and continuous sedation until death for patients whose prognosis for survival is committed at short term was introduced. The decision to withhold or withdraw care must be consensual and reported in the patient's file. This decision is shared with the relatives, albeit being under the responsibility of the physician in charge. A procedure for advance directives has also been implemented, but their use remains marginal in the French ICUs [42].

Acute kidney injury (AKI) is highly prevalent among hospitalized patients translating a further aggravation of patient condition. Stage 3 acute kidney injury requiring dialysis (AKI3D) is associated with poor outcomes. AKI management in stage 1–2 AKI patients is ensured in nephrology ward and/or acute kidney care units, while stage 3 AKI requiring dialysis with or without additional organ support (e.g., lung, shock, sepsis, heart) are currently managed in intensive care units (ICU) under the supervision of intensivists and/or nephrologists depending on the local organization.

Epidemiologic features, patient medical profile, AKI context, and prognosis of AKI3D in France have been recently summarized in a large retrospective study in mainland France [43]. All hospitalizations for AKI3D from 2009 to 2014 were extracted from the comprehensive French hospital discharge database, which provides de-identified data with demographic and medical information about the admission diagnosis, underlying comorbidities, procedures performed, and complications. Over the study period, AKI3D increased from 475 (95% CI, 468–482) to 512 per million population (95% CI, 505–519) and all age groups particularly in elderly. AKI3D was twice as high in men as women. Median age was 68 years. The most common comorbidities were cardio-cerebrovascular diseases (64.8%), pulmonary disease (42.2%), CKD (33.8%), and diabetes (26.0%); all of these except CKD increased significantly over time. Heart failure (17.2%), sepsis (17.0%), AKI on CKD (13.0%), digestive diseases (10.7%), and shock (6.6%) were the most frequent principal diagnoses associated with AKI. The proportion of patients with at least one ICU stay and continuous renal replacement therapy increased from 80.3% to 83.9% and from 56.9% to 61.8%, respectively. In-hospital mortality was high but stable (47%) and higher in patients with an ICU stay.

In conclusion, the French ICU practice caring for severe AKI3D patients is surrounded by a tight legal frame. Public funding to hospital (university, tertiary) or clinic (private) through the national social security agency is the only source of income for ICU based on a lump sum based on a daily rate negotiated yearly with regional health agency (ARS).

## Healthcare Coverage and Cost of ESRD Patient Management

### Health Coverage for Kidney Disease Management

Kidney disease and chronic renal failure are listed as #19 out of the 30 long-lasting diseases (ALD30) and considered as "exonerating" disease totally covered by the universal national health insurance system (CNAM[3] and regional branches CRAM[4]) [44]. When a new kidney disease patient is diagnosed, family doctor and nephrologist must report and document the clinical case to the CRAM medical office for being recognized and covered by social security system. These rights will appear on patient's electronic card (Vital Card). In addition, this process opens the rights for the patient to be treated and to benefit from full coverage for all costs incurring from his kidney disease.

French healthcare system with a focus on chronic kidney disease management is schematically presented in Fig. 39.13. Regional health agencies (ARS) were created in 2010 to ensure healthcare regulation. They are responsible for CKD management as well as other diseases and/or all regional population health problems [45]. This includes periodic and regular update for adapting care offering infrastructure to patient population needs (e.g., dialysis unit creation and/or geo-

[3]CNAM, Caisse Nationale Assurance Maladie.

[4]CRAM, Caisse Régionale Assurance Maladie.

**Fig. 39.16** Average monthly cost of renal replacement therapy by modality for prevalent stable patient

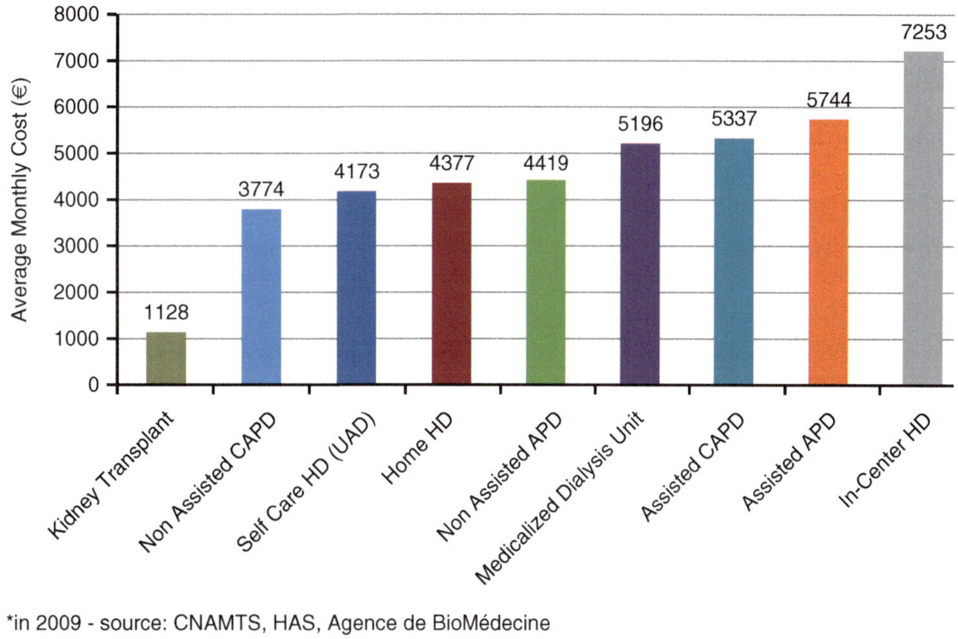


graphical distribution, number of dialysis stations by clinic and hospital, accredited units for organ transplantation or harvesting, number of kidney transplant), but also to allocate budget and promote new and/or innovative actions for kidney disease management (e.g., kidney network regrouping various competences and specialties for facilitating kidney disease management). This is part of a 5-year contract involving nephrologists and all care providers (e.g., public, private, and non-profit association) that is used by ARS[5] for establishing regional plan of end-stage kidney care supply (SROS[6]) [46].

The medical fees and expenses related to the treatment or monitoring of CKD are paid directly to the doctors (e.g., private or public) or to the care providers (e.g., pharmacist, laboratory, radiology, etc.). Thanks to personal electronic card (Vital Card), each patient may benefit from health insurance funding for CKD care. In other words, that means that CKD patient does not advance money for his care. This remains true across all kidney disease stages including dialysis and transplantation.

## Cost of End-Stage Renal Disease Management

During chronic kidney disease phase and outpatient clinic, cost is mainly related to consultations, lab test, imaging, and medicine prescription.

[5]ARS, Agence Régionale de Santé.

[6]SROS, Schéma Regional Organisation des Soins.

During renal replacement therapy phase, treatment cost includes dialysis reimbursement fees, use of disposable material, intradialytic medications (e.g., EPO, iron), and physician fees but also, during the interdialytic period, medicine prescription, specialized consultations, lab test, and imaging tests when needed. Renal replacement fees are based on dialysis facilities type (e.g., in-center, private or public, university) and location (e.g., home, self-care, hospital, clinic) but not on the modality itself. In other words, hemodialysis or hemodiafiltration received the same reimbursement fees. It is of interest to note that transportation to the dialysis unit is also reimbursed by the CRAM.

During renal transplantation and initial phase (first year), treatment cost includes surgical act, hospitalization, and immunomodulator treatment. After stabilization of kidney transplant patient (over the first year), the cost is mainly related to immunosuppressive therapy, patient monitoring, and management of side effects of transplantation and/or immunosuppressive therapy.

In all cases, treatment cost of ESRD patients whatever is the modality is very expensive. As shown in Fig. 39.16, a comparison of monthly total cost per patient is presented across different renal replacement options after patient stabilization (over first year) [47, 48]. As shown on this graph, in-center hemodialysis represents the most expensive renal replacement option, while the kidney transplant is the cheapest one. It is also interesting to note that home therapy, from either continuous ambulatory peritoneal dialysis (CAPD) or home hemodialysis, offers interesting and relatively cheaper treatment option compared to in-center hemodialysis.

Furthermore, if one considers the impact of renal replacement therapy on quality of life and recognizes that transplant and home therapy preserve best patient perception, it becomes clear that these two modalities have the best added value for ESRD patient care (improving outcome and reducing cost).

## New Perspectives

Kidney disease and chronic renal failure have become a public health problem and of major concern in France over the last few years, due to their prevalence, cost, and burden on patients and society [49]. As such, the management of kidney disease is a priority of the French health authorities. Several lines of thought are developed by the health authorities in partnership with the actors in the field to provide an answer to this problem. We will only mention here the main avenues explored to remedy this worrying situation.

In the short term, ways of improvement could be quickly put in place, but this will only be possible through a common will and consent of authorities and health actors to act in concert to:

1. Sensitize the general population and the non-medical specialized body to the burden of renal diseases in order to have preventive actions concerning food (salt), the way of life (physical activity, tobacco), added risks (self-medication), or better management of renal tropism (hypertension, diabetes)
2. Strengthen the training of junior doctors (interns) and, more generally, all healthcare providers to ensure better management of patients and, above all, ensure soft transition within the various therapeutic modalities
3. Improve the efficiency of care through better management of the patient trajectory through few actions:
   (a) Detect kidney disease earlier and better manage it to slow progression to kidney failure and prevent complications.
   (b) Promote therapeutic alternatives to in center-dialysis aiming at empowering patients and/or treating them in less medicalized structures (self-care units or home treatment) to reduce cost and improve outcome. In that sense new technology will help by developing personal and smart dialysis machine.
   (c) Increase the number of kidney transplants from either cadaver donor kidneys or live donors with truly incentive measures.
4. Develop or use new information and communication technologies to improve the quality of results and personalize treatment using big data and artificial intelligence such as:
   (a) Develop risk predictive models that facilitate therapeutic choices
   (b) Develop models of help and decision support for treatment
5. Review the model of care and its funding in order to evolve toward payment for performance and results and no longer for activity

In the longer term, other more innovative therapeutic approaches need to be explored. They can only be put into practice after clinical validation and delays that are difficult to define. These areas are evolving very rapidly and can arrive more quickly in the market than expected. This is the case of research topics such as regenerative medicine (renal repair by stem cells), wearable or implantable artificial kidney (nanotechnology), bioartificial organs (kidney organoids, recellularized kidney scaffold), and xenotransplantation with personalized organ that are currently explored in various research centers through France.

## References


1. France identity card and economic facts. https://www.oecd.org/fr/sites/edugeneralconference2008/informationsgeneralessurlafranceetparis.htm. Accessed on 26 Dec 2019.
2. https://countryeconomy.com/gdp/france. Accessed on 26 Dec 2019.
3. http://www.gouvernement.fr/action/les-metropoles. Accessed on 26 Dec 2019.
4. Merrill JP. Biography. https://www.asn-online.org/foundation/bio-merrill.aspx.
5. Merrill JP. The artificial kidney. N Engl J Med. 1952;246:17–27.
6. Eknoyan G. Nephrology: as it was then, but is not now. Am J Kidney Dis. 2017;69(1):129–35.
7. Nephrology. Wikipedia. https://en.wikipedia.org/wiki/Nephrology. Accessed on 26 Dec 2019.
8. Richet G. Clinical nephrology in the European French-speaking countries from 1945 to 1960: a physiopathological tradition. Nephrol Ther. 2009;5(3):210–3.
9. Diamandopoulos A. A timeline of the history of nephrology. http://www.era-edta.org/history/A_Timeline_of_the_History_of_Nephrology.pdf. Accessed on 26 Dec 2019.
10. Examen Classant National (ECN) – introduction. https://www.has-sante.fr/jcms/c_735114/fr/examen-classant-national-ecn-introduction. Accessed on 26 Dec 2019.
11. Collège Universitaire des Enseignants en Néphrologie (CUEN). http://cuen.fr/. Accessed on 26 Dec 2019.
12. Conseil National de l'Ordre des Médecins (CNOM). https://www.conseil-national.medecin.fr/. Accessed on 26 Dec 2019.
13. Moulin B, Frimat L. Avec la Commission de pédagogie et formation continue de la Société de néphrologie et les présidents de Commission. What's new in continuing medical education in nephrology in France? Nephrol Ther. 2014;10(2):71–3.
14. Association pour la Pédagogie et la Formation Continue en Néphrologie (APFCN). https://www.societe.com/societe/association-pour-la-pedagogie-et-la-formation-continue-en-nephrologie-829802297.html.
15. Société Francophone de Néphrologie, Dialyse & Transplantation. http://www.sfndt.org/sn/index.php.
16. Néphrologie et Thérapeutique. EM Consulte. Elsevier. https://www.em-consulte.com/revue/NEPHRO/presentation/nephrologie-therapeutique. Accessed on 26 Dec 2019.

17. Société Francophone de Transplantation. https://www.transplantation-francophone.org/. Accessed on 26 Dec 2019.
18. Société de Réanimation de Langue Française (SRLF). https://www.srlf.org/.
19. Registre de Dialyse Péritonéale de Langue Française et de Hémodialyse à Domicile. (RDPLF-HDD). https://www.rdplf.org/. Accessed on 26 Dec 2019.
20. Société Francophone de l'Abord Vasculaire (SFAV). http://www.sfav.org/. Accessed on 26 Dec 2019.
21. Société de Néphrologie Pédiatrique (SNP). https://snp-web.wixsite.com/site-snp. Accessed on 26 Dec 2019.
22. Société Francophone Nutrition Clinique et Métabolisme (SFNCM). https://www.sfncm.org/. Accessed on 26 Dec 2019.
23. Association Française des Infirmier(e)s de Dialyse, Néphrologie et Transplantation (AFIDTN). https://www.afidtn.com/.
24. Association des Pharmaciens de Dialyse à Domicile (APDD). https://www.apdd.org/. Accessed on 26 Dec 2019.
25. Association des Techniciens de Dialyse. http://www.dialyse.asso.fr/. Accessed on 26 Dec 2019.
26. Data sources. http://www.data.drees.sante.gouv.fr; http://www.conseil-national.medecin.fr/. Accessed on 26 Dec 2019.
27. Rondeau E, Luyckx VA, Anders HJ, Eckardt KU, Florquin S, Marti HP, Ølgaard K, Harden P, members of the Western Europe Regional Board, International Society of Nephrology. Challenges and opportunities for nephrology in Western Europe. Kidney Int. 2019;95(5):1037–40.
28. Brasme R, Larceneux F, Delion A, Aubert O, Bertocchio JP. French teaching in nephrology: what is the residents' feeling? Results from the first national survey. Nephrol Ther. 2017;13(6):485–94.
29. Les internes en médecine. Effectifs et répartition 2010–2014. https://solidarites-sante.gouv.fr/IMG/pdf/Rapport_2010-2011_Tome_1_Les_Internes_en_medecine-_Effectifs_et_repartition_2010-2014.pdf. Accessed on 26 Dec 2019.
30. LOI n° 2009-879 du 21 juillet 2009 portant réforme de l'hôpital et relative aux patients, à la santé et aux territoires. https://www.legifrance.gouv.fr/affichTexte.do?cidTexte=JORFTEXT000020879475&categorieLien=id. Accessed on 26 Dec 2019.
31. Décret n° 2002-1198 du 23 septembre 2002 relatif aux conditions techniques de fonctionnement des établissements de santé qui exercent l'activité de traitement de l'insuffisance rénale chronique par la pratique de l'épuration extrarénale et modifiant le code de la santé publique. https://solidarites-sante.gouv.fr/fichiers/bo/2002/02-39/a0393147.htm, https://www.legifrance.gouv.fr/affichTexte.do?cidTexte=JORFTEXT000000780502&categorieLien=id. Accessed on 26 Dec 2019, https://www.legifrance.gouv.fr/affichTexte.do?cidTexte=JORFTEXT000000232864&categorieLien=id. Accessed on 26 Dec 2019.
32. REIN annual report 2017. https://www.agence-biomedecine.fr/IMG/pdf/rapportrein2017.pdf. Accessed on 26 Dec 2019.
33. Isnard Bagnis C, Couchoud C, Bowens M, et al. Epidemiology update for hepatitis C virus and hepatitis B virus in end-stage renal disease in France. Liver Int. 2017;37(6):820–6.
34. Béchade C, Lobbedez T, Ivarsen P, Povlsen JV. Assisted peritoneal dialysis for older people with end-stage renal disease: the French and Danish experience. Perit Dial Int. 2015;35(6):663–6.
35. La greffe d'organes en 7 fiches pratiques. Vademecum Agence de Biomédecine. https://www.agence-biomedecine.fr/IMG/pdf/fiches_vademecum_vdef.pdf. Accessed on 26 Dec 2019.
36. Le plan greffe 2012–2016. Agence de la BioMédecine. https://www.agence-biomedecine.fr/IMG/pdf/2012_plan_greffe_vdef2.pdf. Accessed on 26 Dec 2019.
37. Plan 2017–2021 pour la greffe d'organes et de tissus. https://solidarites-sante.gouv.fr/IMG/pdf/plan_2017-2021_pour_la_greffe_d_organes_et_de_tissus.pdf. Accessed on 26 Dec 2019.
38. Hertig A, Rondeau E. Immunomodulation dans la greffe rénale: ce qui a changé en 20 ans. Réanimation. 2006;15(4):253–8.
39. Leone M, Constantin JM, Dahyot-Fizelier C, et al. French intensive care unit organisation. Anaesth Crit Care Pain Med. 2018;37(6):625–7.
40. Gayat E, Cariou A, Deye N, et al. Determinants of long-term outcome in ICU survivors: results from the FROG-ICU study. Crit Care. 2018;22(1):8.
41. Lefrant JY, Lorne E, Asehnoune K, Ausset S, Beaulieu P, Biais M, et al. Determining the editorial policy of Anaesthesia Critical Care and Pain Medicine (ACCPM). Anaesth Crit Care Pain Med. 2018;37:299–301.
42. Ledorze M, Veber B. le Comité éthique de la société Française d'anesthésie et de réanimation. Therapeutics limitation and discontinuation: impact of Claeys Leonetti law and of changes in the medical ethic code on anesthesiology and intensive care practices. Anesteziol Reanimatol. 2017;3:394–8.
43. Garnier F, Couchoud C, Landais P, Moranne O. Increased incidence of acute kidney injury requiring dialysis in metropolitan France. PLoS One. 2019;14(2):e0211541.
44. Liste des ALD 30 Liste des 30 affections de longue durée (ALD 30) qui donnent lieu à exonération du ticket modérateur (article d-322-1 du Code de Santé Publique). http://www.fondshs.fr/Media/Default/Images/Ressources-Allocations/Liste_des_ALD_30.pdf. Accessed on 26 Dec 2019.
45. Agence Régionale de Santé. https://www.ars.sante.fr/quest-ce-quune-agence-regionale-de-sante.
46. Enquête nationale schéma régional d'organisation sanitaire de l'insuffisance rénale chronique terminale (SROS/IRCT) - juin 2003 - Volet structure. https://www.ameli.fr/fileadmin/user_upload/documents/volet_structure.pdf. Accessed on 26 Dec 2019.
47. Benain JP, Faller B, Briat C, Jacquelinet C, Brami M, Aoustin M, Dubois JP, Rieu P, Behaghel C, Duru G. Cost of dialysis in France. Nephrol Ther. 2007;3(3):96–106.
48. Blotière PO, Tuppin P, Weill A, Ricordeau P, Allemand H. The cost of dialysis and kidney transplantation in France in 2007, impact of an increase of peritoneal dialysis and transplantation. Nephrol Ther. 2010;6(4):240–7.
49. Baudelot C, Combe C. Système de santé et maladie rénale chronique: réflexions, débats et propositions. http://www.sciencespo.fr/chaire-sante/content/systeme-de-sante-et-maladie-renale-chronique-reflexions-debats-et-propositions. Accessed on 26 Dec 2019.

# Nephrology in Greece

# 40

Christos Iatrou, Vasileios Zavvos, Ploumis Passadakis, Smaragdi Marinaki, Andromachi Mitsioni, and Ioannis Boletis

| | |
|---|---|
| Area[1] | 131,957 Km$^2$ |
| Population[2] | 10,816,286 (2011) |
| Capital | Athens |
| Three most populated cities | 1. Athens<br>2. Thessaloniki<br>3. Patras |
| Official language | Greek |
| Gross domestic product (GDP)[3] | 218.032 billion USD (2018) |
| GDP per capita[4] | 20,324 USD (2018) |
| Human Development Index (HDI)[5] | 0.872 (32rd, 2018) |
| Official currency | Euro |
| Total number of nephrologists[6] | 578 |
| National society of nephrology | Hellenic Society of Nephrology<br>www.ene.gr |
| Incidence of end-stage renal disease[7] | 2016 – 261 pmp (unadjusted) |
| Prevalence of end-stage renal disease[7]<br>(including patients with a functioning kidney transplant) | 2016 – 1359 pmp (unadjusted) |
| Total number of patients on dialysis[8]<br>(all modalities) | 2017 – 11,585<br>2018 – 12,055 |
| Number of patients on hemodialysis[8] | 2017 – 10,868<br>2018 – 11,333 |
| Number of patients on peritoneal dialysis[8] | 2017 – 717<br>2018 – 722 |
| Number of renal transplantations per year[8] | 2017 – 176<br>2018 – 141 |

1. Central Intelligence Agency. The World Factbook. Accessed 10 January 2020. Available in: https://www.cia.gov/library/publications/the-world-factbook/geos/gr.html
2. Hellenic Statistical Authority, 2011 census. Available in: https://www.statistics.gr/el/statistics/-/publication/SAM03/2011
3. The World Bank. Accessed 10 January 2020. Available in: https://data.worldbank.org/country/greece?view=chart
4. The World Bank. Accessed 10 January 2020. Available in: https://data.worldbank.org/indicator/NY.GDP.PCAP.CD?locations=GR
5. United Nations Development Program. Human Development Reports. Accessed 10 January 2020. Available in: http://hdr.undp.org/en/countries/profiles/GRC
6. Unpublished data derived from The Hellenic Society of Nephrology
7. ERA-EDTA Registry: ERA-EDTA Registry Annual Report 2016. Amsterdam UMC, location AMC, Department of Medical Informatics, Amsterdam, the Netherlands, 2018. Available in: www.era-edta-reg.org
8. Unpublished data derived from the "Board of Registry and Control of Renal Replacement Therapy"

## Introduction

Greece, officially Hellenic Republic, is a country located in Southeastern Europe. It shares land borders with Albania to the northwest, Northern Macedonia and Bulgaria to the north, Turkey to the northeast, and an extensive sea border with Turkey to the east. Greece's main geographical feature is an extensively mountainous (80% of land area) and peninsular mainland surrounded by a vast number of islands and

C. Iatrou (✉) · V. Zavvos
Center for Diagnosis, Treatment and Research on Kidney Diseases, Hygeia Hospital, Athens, Greece
e-mail: ciatroug@otenet.gr

P. Passadakis
Department of Nephrology, University Hospital of Alexandroupolis, Democritus University of Thrace Medical School, Alexandroupolis, Greece
e-mail: ploumis@med.duth.gr

S. Marinaki · I. Boletis
Department of Nephrology & Renal Transplant Unit, Laiko General Hospital, University of Athens Medical School, Athens, Greece
e-mail: laikneph@laiko.gr

A. Mitsioni
Department of Nephrology, Children's Hospital "P. & A. Kyriakou", Athens, Greece


J. A. Moura-Neto et al. (eds.), *Nephrology Worldwide*, https://doi.org/10.1007/978-3-030-56890-0_40

islets (between 1,000 and 6,000 depending on definition), of which 114 are inhabited and where 15% of the population resides.

Located in a strategic position at the crossroads of Europe, Asia, Africa, the Mediterranean Sea and the Black Sea, Greece has been inhabited since the remote past. One of the oldest and most important civilizations in world history (Ancient Greece) flourished in the area during the ancient times, with paramount contributions to Western philosophy, politics (democracy), science, and arts. For these reasons, scholars often consider it as the cradle of Western civilization. In modern times, Greece gained its independence from the Ottoman Empire in 1830, but during the nineteenth and twentieth centuries (until 1950), it was shaped through a series of wars and periods of political turmoil. Greece has been politically stable since 1974, with the establishment of a unitary parliamentary republic and the definitive abolition of monarchy. The Greeks are a homogeneous nation, the majority of Christian Orthodox religion, and the official language is the modern Greek language which, if seen in a continuum with its medieval and ancient versions, is one of the oldest languages on earth.

Greece is a developed country and a high-income, service-based economy. Merchant marine/shipping and tourism are important contributors to national domestic product. It is a member of the European Union and the official currency is the Euro. It is also a member of North Atlantic Treaty Organization (NATO). Since 2018, Greece is recovering from a decade-long severe economic and debt crisis, for which the country needed to implement strict fiscal stabilization programs to avoid default.

The Greek public health system, called National Health System (ESY in Greek), offers universal healthcare coverage, free at the point of delivery. The system is mixed, i.e., funded by both the national budget and public insurance funds and involves a mixture of public and private (contracted) providers. There is also a very developed private healthcare sector and a growing private insurance market. In the aftermath of Greece's economic crisis, the public healthcare system is currently at a breaking point, challenged by underfunding, staff shortages, and chronic insufficiencies in management and planning, combined with an aging population and an increased proportion of out-of-pocket expenditure.

## Short History of Nephrology in Greece

About 150 years ago, the great French physiologist Claude Bernard (1813–1878) acknowledged the mission and importance of the kidneys for our lives, thanks to the homeostatic regulation and maintenance of the "internal milieu" [1]. Much earlier, since 1681, Swiss physician Johann Jakob Wepfer had correlated chronic renal failure with polyuria and then with necrosis of atrophic kidneys in a patient with a 3-year history of polyuria who had died of cerebral hemorrhage [2]. Despite these early observations, nephrology started developing much later and was recognized as a specialty during the second half of the twentieth century. In Greece, the development of nephrology has generally followed a similar timescale as in most Western European countries, albeit with some delay. Today, nephrology and renal replacement therapy (RRT) are fully developed in Greece and in accordance with the internationally accepted standards of care, yet there are areas in need of significant improvements, and these should be the target of future policies.

Most would agree that the history of nephrology in Greece began in the late 1940s, when physicians E. Panagiotopoulos and D. Valtis successfully applied acute peritoneal dialysis (PD) at Laiko Hospital in Thessaloniki to treat a 25-year-old female patient with anuric acute kidney injury (AKI) following septic abortion, using improvised catheters and solution. They only managed to perform two 12-hour-long sessions of treatment due to outflow problems, and the patient passed away a few days later [3]. A few years later, in 1952, K. Tountas performed the first kidney transplantations in laboratory animals in the experimental operating theater, which he had organized at the Laiko Hospital in Athens [4]. In 1957, K. Tountas (then associate professor of surgery) and K. Kyriakou also performed the first hemodialysis (HD) session, using a twin-coil-Travenol artificial kidney, in a patient with barbiturate poisoning at the General Hospital of Nikaia-Piraeus.

Hippokratis Yatzidis, a founding member of EDTA, previously known as "West Europe Dialysis Association," was the first Greek physician to be specialized in nephrology (along with internal medicine and cardiology) at Hippokrateion Hospital in Athens. From 1955 to 1959, he worked at the Claude Bernard Association (ACB) research center in Paris, France, supervised by Professor Jean Hamburger. Upon his return to Greece in 1959, he was appointed as Associate Professor of Medicine at the University of Athens and formed a group of keen physicians, interested in various aspects of the emerging field of nephrology, based at Hippokrateion Hospital. Drs. Dimitrios Oreopoulos, Sonia Voudiklari, Georgios Psimmenos, Antonis Katirtzoglou, and Antonis Tzamaloukas, among others, were members of that group. Professor Yatzidis' vision was to establish a University Nephrology Center with experts in every special discipline of nephrology. For this purpose, he encouraged and helped his young collaborators to get fellowships in state-of-the-art nephrology centers in the USA, France, and the UK. The pioneering nephrology team had also set up its own biochemical laboratory and library. In 1959, the Department of Artificial Kidney at Hippokrateion Hospital of Athens was equipped with its first artificial kidney, a Kill-board dialysis machine with Dasco monitor, and Yatzidis' group focused on treating hospitalized patients with AKI from across the country. Meanwhile, the group had started publishing their first results and experience with artificial kidney [5].

Besides his efforts to treat patients usually presenting with AKI, Professor Yatzidis expanded his research interests towards the development of an activated charcoal column, which would remove uremic toxins and other poisons from the blood (hemoperfusion). This innovative invention earned him with international reputation, and the group presented their first results at the 1st EDTA-ERA Congress in Amsterdam in 1964. Meanwhile, since 1961, only a year after the first development of arteriovenous (AV) shunt in Seattle, USA, the group was competent in developing AV shunts made of Teflon (PTFE) and in surgically placing them intra-arterially and intravenously at the patients' carpal area for long-term use. In 1968, 2 years after the creation of the first AV fistula by Brescia MJ, Cimino JE et al., Yatzidis' group created their first AV fistula for patients on chronic hemodialysis and published their experience in the *New England Journal of Medicine* [5–8].

During the same period, in Thessaloniki, Professors K. Tountas and D. Valtis were treating patients with AKI with HD, using twin-coil Travenol artificial kidney, at the "AHEPA" Hospital. Prof. D. Valtis had received postgraduate training in Glasgow, Scotland, and in 1968, he organized the first HD unit at the "AHEPA Hospital." The following year, Dr. M. Papadimitriou began the HD program for patients with chronic kidney disease (CKD) using Kill-board dialysis machines.

In 1968, Professor Tountas also performed the first human kidney transplantation in Greece, which was the sixth such operation in Europe [4, 5].

In Athens, Professor S. Papastamatis, after returning from London, sent the nurse A. Zapraidou to receive training in HD, and in March 1969, they started the HD unit at the General State Hospital of Athens, together with Dr. D. Protogerou. That same year, another HD unit began to operate at the Laiko Hospital, led by Dr. A. Billis. Its main purpose was to support the hospital's expanding kidney transplantation program. The unit was initially equipped with a Dasco dialysis machine (Italy) and next year with a new Dasco Cal RP model [5].

During the early 1970s, several other HD units began to operate in Athens (at the Hellenic Red Cross Hospital, Hippokrateion Hospital and Evangelismos Hospital – to name a few), led by physicians who had returned to Greece after receiving postgraduate training in nephrology and dialysis abroad. Furthermore, due to the increasing population of end-stage renal disease (ESRD) patients, HD units started to develop at private hospitals as well, in Athens and Thessaloniki [5]. By 1976, HD units were operating only in Athens, Thessaloniki and Chania, Crete. Hence, ESRD patients only had two options: either to move permanently to one of these cities or to travel to Athens or Thessaloniki three times a week in order to receive dialysis. To solve this problem, S. Marketos, who was the general secretary of the Ministry of Social Services and a member of the Hellenic Society of Nephrology (HSN), suggested the gradual development of HD units at all district hospitals across the country. Due to the shortage of nephrologists at that time, these units were led by specialists in internal medicine, who had completed a 2-month intensive training course in hemodialysis [5].

On December 1, 1976, nephrology was recognized in Greece as a distinctive medical specialty, related to internal medicine or pediatrics, and the specialty curriculum and requirements for acquiring it were determined (Presidential Decree 882, Official Gazette of the Greek Republic 323/issue A/1.12.1976) [5].

Following this, the Ministry of Health soon acknowledged the importance and the rapidly increasing demand for dialysis services for patients with ESRD across the country, and to support the development of new HD units, the Hospitals of Athens and Thessaloniki started providing intensive educational courses in nephrology and dialysis nursing.

In July 1976, the "Panhellenic Union of patients with nephropathies undergoing HD or Transplantation" was established.

The first Department of Nephrology was established in July 1978 at the 7th "Therapeutirio" (infirmary) of the Social Insurance Institution (IKA in Greek - one of the country's major insurance funds) and was directed by Dr. V. Hadjiconstantinou. The same year, another Nephrology Department was founded at Evaggelismos Hospital, directed by Dr. A. Billis. In 1979, a new Nephrology Department was launched at B' Hospital of the Social Insurance Institute (Panaghia) in Thessaloniki, directed by Dr. G. Vagionas. An outbreak of dialysis dementia observed in 1978 and attributed to aluminum toxicity led the HSN to issue guidance stating that all HD units should install water treatment systems including softening, deionization, and reverse osmosis [5].

The following year, 1979–1980, Dr. K. Sombolos was the first in Greece to use isolated (vacuum) ultrafiltration, to treat overhydrated uremic patients in the HD unit of Laiko Hospital in Athens, and in 1983 he was also the first to use a subclavian catheter (Vygon single lumen) for HD in a hospitalized patient. Dr. Sombolos also applied continuous arteriovenous hemofiltration (CAVH) (a method developed by Kramer in 1977) for the first time in Greece, in March 1985 at the Papanikolaou Hospital in Thessaloniki [5].

Since 1990, the legislation was enriched and improved with a number of laws and presidential decrees [Presidential Decree 247 (Official Gazette of the Greek Republic 93/issue A/21.06.1991), Presidential Decree 517 (Official Gazette of the Greek Republic 202/issue A/24.12.1991), Presidential Decree 225 (Official Gazette of the Greek Republic 194/issue A/07.09.2000), Presidential Decree 235 (Official Gazette of the Greek Republic 199/issue A/14.09.2000), Law 4093 (Official Gazette of the Greek Republic 222/issue A/12.11.2012, article 67), Law 4316 (Official Gazette of the Greek Republic 270/issue A/24.12.2014, article 57)] that allowed the development of nephrology at a satisfactory pace. As of 2019, there are 26 Nephrology Departments, 33 PD units all based in public hospitals, and 181 HD units, evenly distributed between the public and the private sector [5, 9].

## Pediatric Nephrology in Greece

Until 1975, pediatric nephrology was not developed in Greece, and there was a complete lack of pediatricians with experience in dialysis. Thus, infants and children with AKI hospitalized in the pediatric hospitals of Athens were initially consulted and treated with acute PD, by Dr. A. Billis' group (one of the first to use acute PD in Greece since the late 1960s), based at the neighboring Laiko Hospital. It was after 1975 that the first pediatricians with training in nephrology assumed responsibility, thus relieving that burden on adult-oriented physicians [5].

The first pediatric HD session was performed in 1978, in an 11-year old boy at the University Pediatric Department of "P. & A. Kyriakou" Children's Hospital in Athens, using a parallel plate dialyzer and a radio-cephalic AV fistula in the elbow. It was performed by Drs. P. Zeis and C. Sinaniotis and by the nurse P. Tsougia, who had previous experience in pediatric dialysis from her nursing practice in London. Drs. P. Zeis and C. Sinaniotis (along with Dr. Ch. Bakopoulos from the Pediatric Department of "Agia Sofia" University Children's Hospital in Athens) are considered as the pioneers in the field of pediatric nephrology in Greece, and all were active members of the HSN [5]. In 1982, they also founded the first chronic HD unit for children, equipped with three dialysis machines. The unit was affiliated to the University Pediatric Department of "P. & A. Kyriakou" Children's Hospital. In addition, Dr. C. Stefanidis returned in 1982 after his long-term training in Canada under supervision by Professor D. Oreopoulos and established a CAPD program for children, using plastic bags for the first time in Greece. Dr. C. Stefanidis gradually became an expert in peritoneal dialysis in Europe [5].

In 1987, Dr. I. Sotiriou who had received full training in pediatric nephrology in France established the first pediatric nephrology unit in Northern Greece at the Hippokrateion University Hospital and initiated a PD program [5]. As of today, there are two Departments of Pediatric Nephrology in Greece (one in Athens and one in Thessaloniki, both hosting pediatric HD and PD units), as well as pediatric nephrology outpatient clinics operating within the Departments of Pediatrics in most University Hospitals.

## The Hellenic Society of Nephrology

The Hellenic Society of Nephrology (HSN) was founded in April 1970, by 22 founding members, and its first scientific meeting was held in Thessaloniki in June 1970. The 1st Panhellenic Congress of Nephrology was held in Thessaloniki in March 1980, and the following year (June 1981), the ISN's 8th International Congress of Nephrology was held in Athens [5].

In 1984, the HSN council offered its first scholarship to nephrologist G. Papadakis for a 1-year postgraduate training in Frankfurt, Germany. Since then, the HSN has given the opportunity to numerous of its members to receive scholarships for specific postgraduate training in well-known centers both in Europe and in the USA [5]. In 1984, an ad hoc committee formed by the HSN performed the first study to estimate the needs for renal replacement therapy (RRT) infrastructure and staff, for the developing National Health System (founded a year earlier, in 1983). The committee suggested the development of 370 hospital beds dedicated to nephrology, 418 artificial kidney machines, and 16 CAPD units, in order to meet current demand. They also suggested the appointment of 123 nephrologists at consultant level, including 26 clinical directors [5]. The same year, the HSN started offering training seminars in nephrology for nurses. By 1987, the HSN had 117 registered members.

In 1989, the Hellenic Nephrology journal started to be published and is published quarterly ever since. The HSN is hosting two scientific meetings per year and the biennial Panhellenic Congress of Nephrology, helping the dissemination of new developments in nephrology in the Greek community of nephrologists. It also provides auspices to a number of regional and local scientific meetings related to nephrology, organized by other stakeholders. It has also issued guidance for the diagnosis and management of kidney diseases and for RRT and hosts yearly training courses for nephrology trainees. As of 2019, there are 578 active members registered with the HSN (by professional address), 74 emeritus members, and 92 trainees (data provided by the HSN).

## The Greek Renal Registry

The first aggregated figures of Greek patients who underwent chronic HD from 1967 to 1972 were presented in 1973 during the 1st Balkan Meeting on Renal Diseases, held in Thessaloniki. Since 1975, several reports recording all patients on chronic HD and PD and kidney transplant recipients for the years 1967–1979 and 1980–1987 were presented at national meetings [5]. In 1983, there was a collaboration between the HSN and the Ministry of Health, in order to create an electronic registry for patients with kidney diseases. After a decree by the Ministry of Health in 1985, the "Board of Registry, Coordination and Control of RRT (YSE)" was ordained. The registry is currently based at G. Gennimatas General Hospital in Athens and participates in the ERA-EDTA Registry's activities, providing annual reports.

## Renal Diseases in Greece

Unfortunately, there is no registry of patients with CKD stages 1–5 (before RRT initiation); neither are there any large-scale epidemiological studies on CKD. Therefore, accurate data on the incidence and prevalence of the disease are not available. However, according to the data presented in the recently published Atlas of the International Society of Nephrology, the prevalence of CKD in Greece is estimated to be about 12%, equivalent to the rest of Europe [10].

For the same reasons, there are no data available on AKI either; therefore, the incidence, prevalence, causes, and severity of AKI in Greece remain unknown.

In contrast, there are accurate data for patients with ESRD undergoing RRT, systematically collected by the Greek renal registry (Board of Registry, Coordination and Control of RRT). According to the latest ERA-EDTA registry report, published in 2018 with data from 2016, the incidence of ESRD in Greece, adjusted for age and sex, was 210 per million population (pmp) (6th highest in Europe) and the adjusted prevalence 1,141 patients pmp (5th highest in Europe). As far as it concerns the causes of ESRD, glomerulonephritis was the cause in 17.2% of patients, pyelonephritis in 6.1%, polycystic kidney disease in 8%, diabetes mellitus in 19.1%, hypertension in 9.4%, renovascular disease in 1.3%, and miscellaneous causes in 9.8%. However, the cause was unknown in 29.2% of patients, which is a quite high rate [11]. A possible explanation for this finding might be that in Greece many patients with kidney disease are referred to nephrologists late in the course of CKD; thus, they are frequently not subjected to kidney biopsy and the cause of CKD remains undetermined.

Incidence and prevalence of RRT have increased since the 1980s, when systematic recording began, and their course is shown in Figs. 40.1 and 40.2. This increase might be attributed to the following causes: (1) high prevalence of obesity (37.4% of Greeks are overweight and 34.9% are obese according to a recent study, while Greece is among the European countries with the highest childhood obesity rates), (2) high percentage of hypertensive patients (today, hypertension concerns over 40% of adults and over 80% of the elderly, while it is estimated that at least 40% of hypertensive patients are not treated and only 15% of the total hypertensive population achieve good blood pressure control with drug therapy), (3) the existence of a large number of diabetic patients (in a recent study, total prevalence of diabetes mellitus in Greece is 7%, in adults is 8.2%, and in persons >75 years old is 30.3%), (4) aging of the population, and (5) initiation of HD irrespective of age and comorbidities, while at the same time the option of conservative management of ESRD and/or palliative care, even for patients with very low life expectancy, is not widely accepted [12–16].

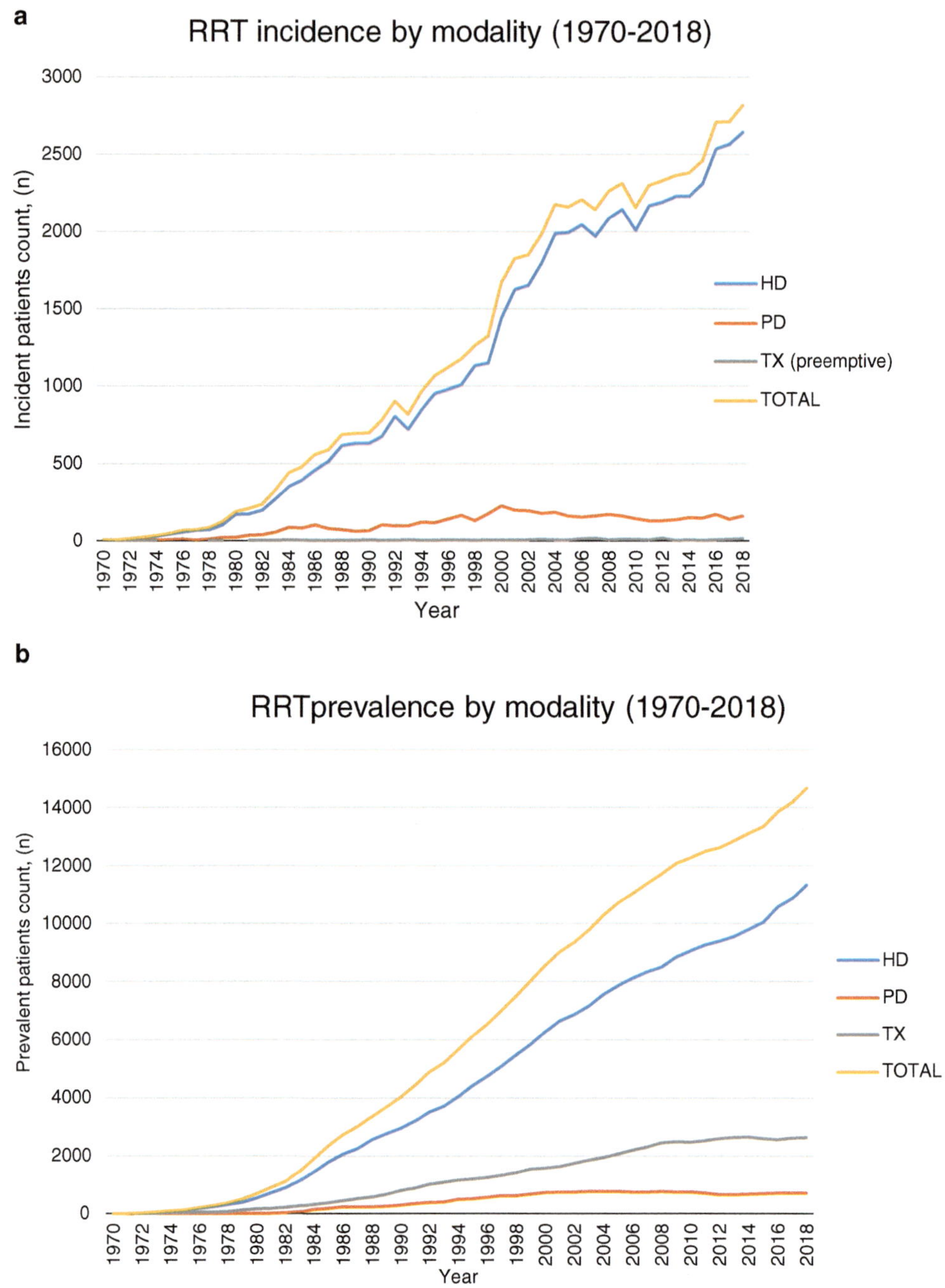


**Fig. 40.1** Incident (**a**) and prevalent (**b**) counts of renal replacement therapy (RRT) in Greece, by modality (1970–2018)

## Renal Replacement Therapy in Greece

### Hemodialysis

The development of HD in Greece has been shaped and is regulated by the following presidential decrees:

1. Presidential Decree 247 (Official Gazette of the Greek Republic 93/issue A/21.06.1991).
2. Presidential Decree 517 (Official Gazette of the Greek Republic 202/issue A/24.12.1991).
3. Presidential Decree 225 (Official Gazette of the Greek Republic 194/issue A/07.09.2000).
4. Presidential Decree 235 (Official Gazette of the Greek Republic 199/issue A/14.09.2000).

The first two of these laws have defined the conditions, requirements, and modus operandi for HD units operating at public and private hospitals and the next two for private HD units operating as individual facilities. In the official state nomenclature, the former are referred to as "Artificial Kidney Units" and the latter as "Chronic HD units." It is required

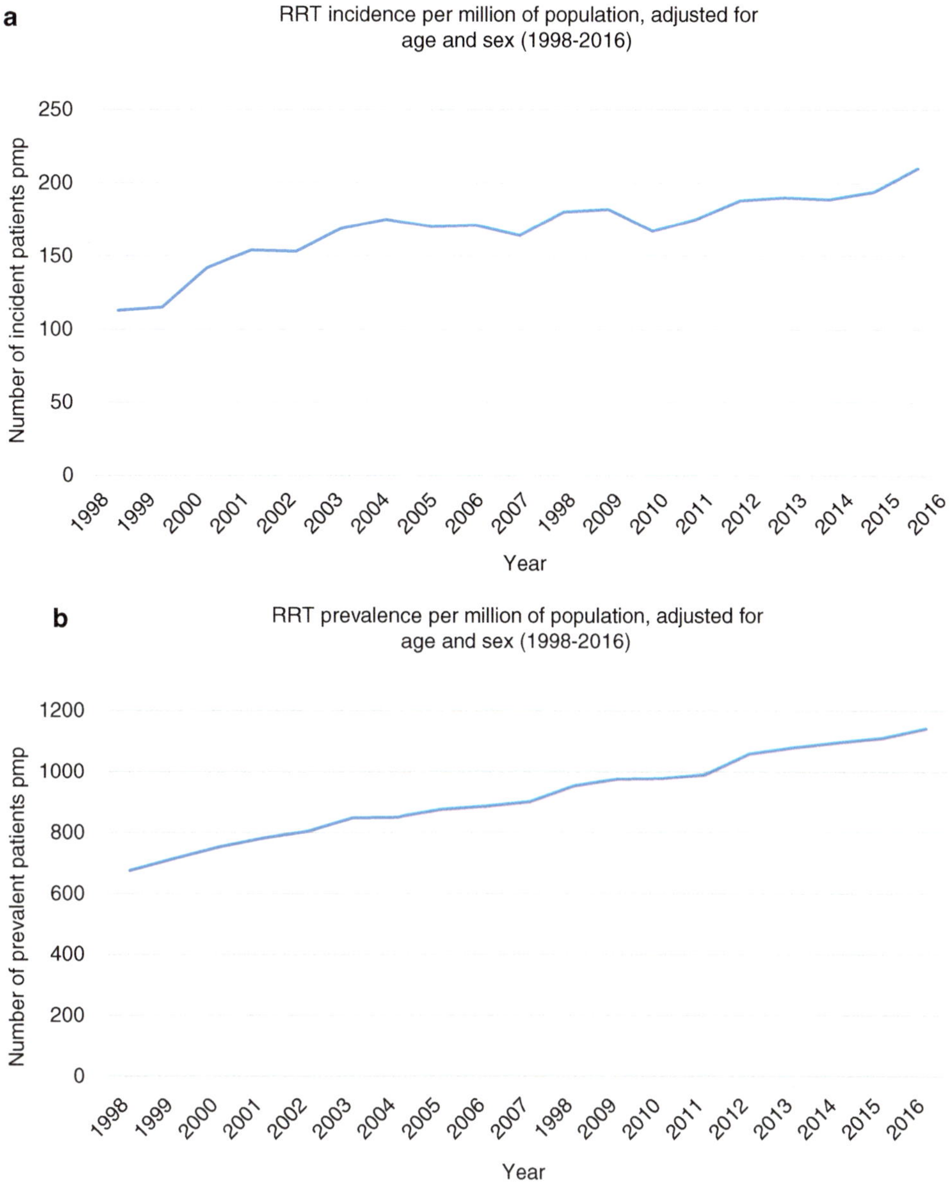


**Fig. 40.2** Incidence (**a**) and prevalence (**b**) of renal replacement therapy (RRT) in Greece, per million of population, adjusted for age and sex (1998–2016)

that all chronic HD units be scientifically linked to the nearest public hospital where there is a Department of Nephrology or a HD unit.

As previously mentioned, as of 2019 there are 181 HD units (94 in public hospitals, 34 in private hospitals, as well as 53 chronic HD units), dispersed throughout the country, even on small islands; thus, most patients undergoing HD do not need to move away from their homes permanently. According to recent data derived from the Greek renal registry, there are currently about 11,300 patients on HD, of whom 37% are treated in public HD units and 63% in private HD units (22% in private hospitals and 43% in chronic HD units).

There are 3,860 dialysis machines operating (50.7% in public hospitals and 49.3% in the private sector). According to the existing legislation, the number of dialysis machines in each HD unit can range between 5 (minimum) and 45 (maximum). Home HD is not developed and is not reimbursed.

A typical HD regimen consists of three 4-hour sessions per week, with blood flow rates >300 ml/min. Hemodiafiltration (HDF) is widely used, usually in post-dilutional mode, but it is required by law that the percentage of patients on HDF per dialysis unit cannot exceed 40%. Incremental dialysis in the form of two sessions per week or three sessions of <4-hour duration for patients with significant residual renal function is applied by some units, but the number of patients on such regimens is unknown. It is estimated that 1–1.5% of patients are dialyzing four times per week, as this requires an application process to allow reimbursement of the additional dialysis sessions. Dialyzer reuse is not allowed by law.

Regarding vascular access, a recent survey performed on a sample of 1,248 patients (representing approximately 11% of total HD population) revealed that 58.2% of patients commence dialysis with a central venous catheter (CVC), 33.2% with an arteriovenous fistula (AVF), and 8.6% with an arteriovenous graft (AVG), while functional vascular access at the time of the survey was AVF in 53.3%, CVC in 34.7%, and AVG in 12.1% of patients [17].

Approximately 3–4% of the HD population are hepatitis C positive, while less than 1% are positive for hepatitis B and human immunodeficiency virus (HIV). These figures are estimated based on unprocessed data derived from the electronic prescription platform as they are not routinely collected by the Greek renal registry. Mortality rates have remained stable for the last 5 years, with an average annual crude mortality rate of 196.6 deaths/1,000 patient-years (unpublished data derived from the Greek renal registry).

Treatment with HD is free for all patients who need it, as it is fully reimbursed by the insurance system, independent of whether the patient is treated in a public or private HD unit. Patients without insurance and patients on social protection plans still have access to treatment, but only in public hospitals. The same applies for their medications, i.e., they are fully reimbursed by the insurance system. In addition, there are a number of pension and tax benefits for ESRD patients.

The reimbursement price of each HD session is fixed and is different for conventional HD and online hemodiafiltration (HDF), with an average session price of about 140 euros for chronic HD units and 125 euros for all other HD units (Official Gazette of the Greek Republic 423/B/27.3.2007 and 807/B/22.5.2007). The price difference is justified by the fact that chronic HD units have significantly higher operating costs than hospital-based HD units. Chronic HD units operate in independent, purpose-built facilities – hence the investment costs are higher – and the staff-to-patient ratio is strictly determined by law. Moreover, these units need exclusive ambulance services, secretariat, etc. The price per HD session reimbursed includes all materials and consumables required to perform the session (including heparin) except for the dialyzer, lines, and fistula needles. The latter are also reimbursed, but according to current prices determined by the Price Observatory of the Greek Health Procurement Committee, a directorate of the Ministry of Health.

The average yearly cost for HD/patient is estimated to be €35–37,000 euros including travel expenses. It is estimated that the total cost of HD and hospitalizations of approximately 11,000 HD patients absorbs about 3% of the Greek health budget.

As previously stated, there is complete lack of epidemiological data regarding patients with AKI. Reimbursement of continuous renal replacement therapy (CRRT) amounts to 100 euros/day (including all materials and consumables required to perform the session (plus heparin) except for the dialyzer, the lines and the central venous catheter). This price is independent of the CRRT modality used (Official Gazette of the Greek Republic 807/issue B/22.5.2007).

## Peritoneal Dialysis

In the years following its first application, acute PD started to be used in selected patients with AKI. Its use expanded during the early 1960s, first at the "AHEPA" Hospital in Thessaloniki by the groups led by Prof. D. Valtis and Dr. G. Tsourouktsoglou, respectively, and later in Athens' "Alexandra" Hospital led by Dr. N. Papadogiannakis and "Vasileus Pavlos" Hospital (today Laiko Hospital), led by Dr. A. Billis. Since the early 1970s, its use was generalized and the groups in Thessaloniki started using PD to treat a few patients with ESRD. However, their efforts were hampered by the primitive PD apparatus available and by high rates of peritonitis [18]. As a result, according to anecdotal evidence, only a handful of patients remained prevalent on PD until 1980 (unpublished data from the Greek renal registry).

CAPD was introduced in the early 1980s, only a few years following its first use in the USA and Canada. This resulted in the establishment, from 1981 onwards, of long-term CAPD programs for patients with ESRD in Thessaloniki and Athens. In Thessaloniki, the first such programs were those at the "Hippokrateion" General Hospital led by Prof. M. Papadimitriou, "Agios Dimitrios" Hospital led by Dr. A. Dimitriadis, and "AHEPA" Hospital led by Dr. N. Dombros. In Athens, the first CAPD programs were those at the "Hippokrateion" General Hospital led by Dr. A. Katirtzoglou and Laiko Hospital, led by Dr. A. Agrafiotis [18]. The number of PD units increased steadily throughout the 1980s. However, for many years PD was not viewed as a first-line therapy for ESRD patients, and patient selection was usually done by negative criteria, i.e., most patients were offered PD if they were not fit for HD. For this reason, mortality in PD in Greece was initially much higher than in HD [19]. Automated peritoneal dialysis (APD) was also introduced in the mid-1980s, but for many years it was only available for very few patients. For example, in 1999 there were only 13 prevalent patients on APD. Its use expanded during the following decade, and in 2009 prevalent APD patients outnumbered CAPD patients for the first time (data derived from the Greek renal registry), while today approximately 2/3 of prevalent patients are on APD [11].

An important role in the development of PD in Greece has to be attributed to the presence of Prof. D. Oreopoulos, one of the world's pioneers in PD, in Toronto, Canada, since the early 1970s. Prof. D. Oreopoulos, already known as one of the pioneers in nephrology in Greece through his participation in H. Yatzidis' group, served as a beacon for Greek nephrologists, not only by inspiring nephrologists to engage with PD but also by training a number of leading Greek nephrologists in PD in Toronto Western Hospital.

After the expansion of PD programs observed during the 1980s and 1990s, PD incidence and prevalence in Greece remain stagnated during the last 15 years. On average, 150 new patients have started renal replacement therapy with PD each year, and 730 patients remain prevalent (with the exception of a peak 783 prevalent patients in 2004). However, due to the disproportionately large expansion of HD over the same period, the share of PD in RRT in Greece has been steadily decreasing over the last 20 years (Fig. 40.1). According to the most recent available data, there were 164 incident (5.8%) and 722 prevalent (4.9%) PD patients in 2018 (unpublished data derived from the Greek renal registry).

As of May 2019, there are 33 active PD units scattered around the country, 2 of which are based in pediatric departments [9]. All PD units are currently based in public hospitals (i.e., hospitals of the National Health System, or University Hospitals). There are no units developed in the private sector. The conditions and requirements for the establishment and operation of PD units are described in the Presidential Decree 517 (Official Gazette of the Greek Republic 202/issue A/1991).

The number of prevalent PD patients is about 720, including 24 pediatric patients. Use of PD is higher in Northern compared to Southern Greece. Although PD units are evenly distributed (16 vs 17, respectively), 60% of prevalent PD patients are treated by the units located in Northern Greece, despite the fact that approximately 40% of the population resides in Northern Greece and 36% of nephrologists are employed there (unpublished data derived from the HSN). Possible explanations might be the lower density of HD units or larger driving distances to the nearest HD unit, given that the density of HD units is highest in Athens. Accordingly, although 35% of the population lives in Athens' metropolitan area where approximately 40% of nephrologists are employed, the percentage of prevalent PD patients treated is only 18%. However, to our knowledge there is no available study on this issue.

Patients' training in PD is done either by the unit's PD nurses or, in some cases, by trainers provided by the industry. Assisted PD is a common practice, usually performed by spouses or other family members. Some PD units offer the option of in-center intermittent PD for very frail patients, in cases where home assistance is not available. Due to a widespread shortage of nursing staff in the National Health System, there are currently no PD units able to perform home visits and patients need to rely exclusively on family members for assistance.

PD costs are fully reimbursed by the insurance system; thus, treatment and ESRD-related medications are free for patients, as for HD. A recent study on the comparative costs for HD and PD revealed that the direct cost of PD is higher than of HD for the insurance system. This difference may be offset by the fact that PD units have lower operating costs, but if PD in public hospitals is compared to HD delivered by the private sector, then PD is a more expensive option [20]. The full, real-world costs including both direct and indirect costs, though, have not been studied systematically.

Given the lack of epidemiological data apart from those collected by the Greek renal registry, a promising effort to create a national PD registry with the aim to systematically collect and process data on PD in Greece has commenced since 2017. A national-level audit on peritonitis rates performed recently, as part of this developing registry, revealed a rate of 0.25 episodes per patient-year [21]. Mortality rates have remained stable for the last 5 years, with an average annual crude mortality rate of 167.6 deaths/1,000 patient-years (unpublished data derived from the Greek renal registry).

## Renal Transplantation

The first kidney transplant in Greece was performed on July 9, 1968, at the AHEPA Hospital in Thessaloniki, from a deceased donor. Two years later, on September 1, 1970, in Thessaloniki once more, the first kidney transplant from a living donor became a reality. In Athens, the first transplants were performed at the Laiko Hospital on March 8, 1971, from a deceased donor and on January 24, 1972, from a living donor, respectively.

Throughout the 1970s, kidney transplants were sparse and were mostly viewed as another surgical procedure rather than as a therapy for ESRD. In the 1980s, the first structured transplant units were established: one at the Laiko Hospital in Athens in 1983 and the other at the Hippokrateion Hospital in Thessaloniki in 1986. However, kidney transplants were still regarded as a primarily surgical procedure; thus, these first units were organized and supervised by surgeons, with nephrologists playing a consulting role.

In the meantime, the necessary legislation for the growth and function of transplant units was starting to form. The first law regarding transplantation was voted by the Greek parliament in 1978 (Law 821, Official Gazette of the Greek Republic173/14.10.1978), to be joined by the second in 1983 (Law 1383, Official Gazette of the Greek Republic 106/issue A/5.8.1983). In 1996, the "Uniformed System of Enrolment and Selection of Patients and Allocation of Renal Transplants" was formed, following another ministry mandate (Y4d/8874 Official Gazette of the Greek Republic 973/issue A/25.10.1996). In 1999, following a novel law (Law 2737,

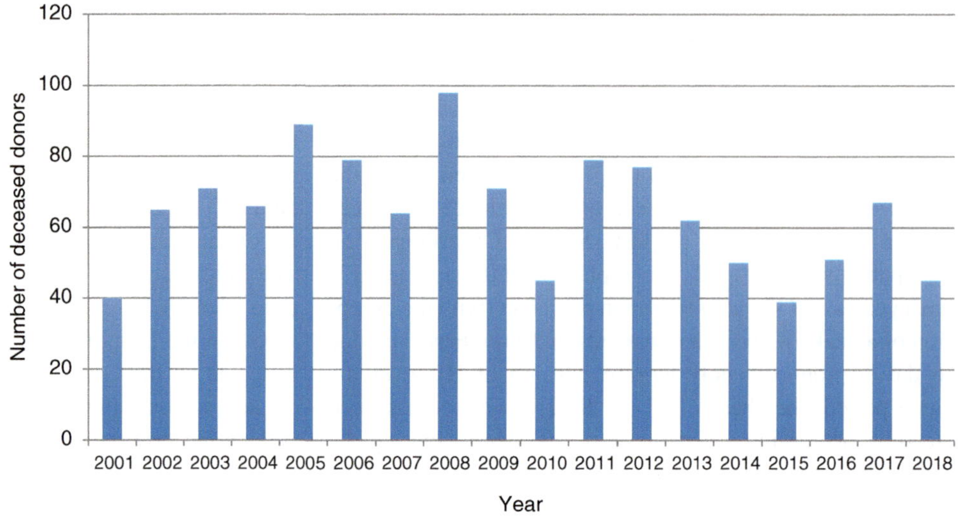


**Fig. 40.3** Deceased kidney donors in Greece (2001–2018)

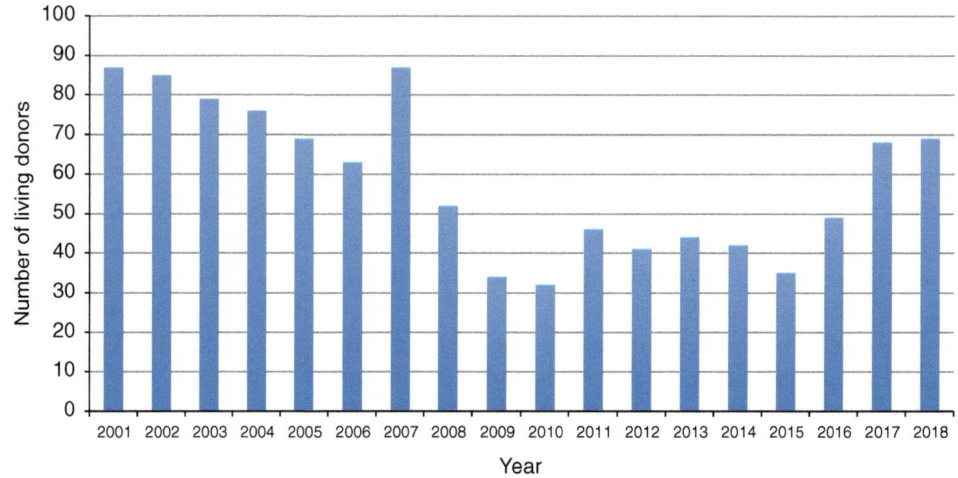


**Fig. 40.4** Living kidney donors in Greece (2001–2018)

Official Gazette of the Greek Republic 174/issue A/27.8.1999), the transplantation system was reformed in conjunction with the laws of the European Union and the Council of Europe. During 2001 it became fully compatible with the European and International regulations, and the National Organization of Transplantation (founded in 1999) started to act as a competent authority. Ever since, the Greek transplantation legislation has been reconstituted to follow the newest guidance provided by the aforementioned authorities.

Therefore, organ harvesting from potential brain dead donors is performed unless the deceased had expressed his/her opposition towards organ donation (opt out) and on the condition that the close family of the departed provide their consent. As for the eligible transplant candidates, they are enrolled in a National Registry, and the allocation of the renal grafts is based on a point system taking into account mainly the time a patient has been on RRT, as well as the HLA histocompatibility. Kidney donation from a living donor directly to a patient is only permitted when they are relatives or have a strong personal and emotional relationship. However, when such a direct donation is not possible for medical reasons, there is a provision for a kidney-paired donation. Alternatively, the living donor can donate via the National Registry, and their patient-couple is promoted onto the top of the waiting list.

There are currently five Renal Transplant Units in Greece. Among these, 2,427 kidney transplants have been performed at the Laiko Hospital in Athens since its official establishment in 1983 until the end of 2018. At the Hippokrateion Hospital in Thessaloniki, 1,790 kidney transplants have taken place since 1987, while at Evaggelismos Hospital in Athens, 700 kidney transplants have been performed since 1991. At the University Hospital of Patras since 1997, there have been 262 kidney transplants, and at the University Hospital of Ioannina, there have been 36 since 2011 (unpublished data derived from the National Organization of Transplantation). Kidney transplants from deceased compared to living donors per year from 2001 to 2018 are depicted in Figs. 40.3 and 40.4.

The main immunosuppression regimen currently in use is the combination of steroids, mycophenolic acid (either in the form of mycophenolate mofetil or sodium), and tacrolimus. At the induction stage, the anti-CD25 monoclonal antibody basiliximab is added to the aforementioned triple therapy. For certain indications, the antithymocyte globulin is preferred instead of basiliximab, avoiding tacrolimus at the initiation phase. During the maintenance stage, depending on the transplantation course and certain characteristics of the patient and/or graft, steroids could be withdrawn and either mycophenolic acid or tacrolimus could be substituted for by everolimus. Renal transplantation is fully reimbursed by the national insurance scheme through a fixed price for the procedure. Extra expenses, if needed, are covered by the hospital budget. Immunosuppressive treatment and all other medications needed by renal transplant recipients are also fully reimbursed by the insurance system.

Since 2005, much attention has been aimed at renal transplants of hypersensitized patients, resulting in 212 such transplants so far. Prior to implementing a cohesive program, very few of those patients were able to find a compatible donor kidney, while now their transplant rates have surpassed the corresponding figures for non-hypersensitized patients. Likewise, since 2005, a program for blood group incompatible transplants has commenced at Laiko Hospital, resulting in 60 ABO incompatible kidney transplants so far [22]. At the same hospital, a kidney exchange program has been in place since 2017, prompting four such transplants. Prior to setting up this program, the first transatlantic living paired kidney transplantation occurred between a couple from Laiko Hospital and a non-directed anonymous donor from Ohio, USA. The first step took place on December 15, 2001, in the USA when the Greek patient received a kidney transplant from that donor and 4 months later on April 19, 2012, his wife donated a kidney to a diabetic patient in Pennsylvania, USA, thus completing a seven-person transplantation chain. In an effort to expand further our kidney exchange program, Greece has recently been included in the South Alliance for Transplant initiative, an international agreement involving Spain, Italy, France, and Portugal, aiming to increase the pool of potential donor-recipient pairs. In addition, Greece also participates in the European Network for Collaboration on Kidney Exchange Programmes (ENCKEP) action, funded by the European Union's COST program.

Looking over the history of renal transplants in Greece, their development was not delayed, if the prosperity of the country is taken into account and the Greek governments have been fairly quick to lay the groundwork for the legislation that would allow these to grow. However, for about 20 years, renal transplants in Greece were sporadic and treated as surgical territory rather than an organized, multidisciplinary team treatment option for patients with ESRD. Another 10 years had to pass before the country fully adopted the European and International laws in the operation of the transplantation schedule as well as that of the existing Renal Transplant Units. Regrettably, this was not coupled with the necessary policies aimed towards the growth of donation. As a result, organ donation in Greece in the last 3 years amounts to a mean of 5 deceased donors pmp, a significant deficit compared to the European mean of 18 deceased donors pmp. The respective numbers of living donors at the same time interval are 6.1 and 10.8 pmp [23]. The causes of this shortcoming are beyond the purpose of this chapter, but there lie the current true needs of kidney transplantation in Greece.

## Nephrology Practice in Greece

Thirty-three years ago, Nephrology was recognized in Greece as a distinctive specialty related to internal medicine or pediatrics, with Presidential Decree 882 (Official Gazette of the Greek Republic 323/A/1.12.1976). That law also determined the conditions for acquiring the specialty (it was required that one had acquired the specialty of internal medicine or pediatrics after 3 years of training in internal medicine or pediatrics, respectively, and passing the relevant exams and had received a 2-year training in nephrology). Following this, a number of other laws were gradually introduced, defining both the specialty of nephrology as a core medical specialty and the requirements for its acquisition. These laws have been published in the following government newsletters:

1. Official Gazette of the Greek Republic 217/issue A/23.12.1985
2. Official Gazette of the Greek Republic 236/issue A/1994
3. Official Gazette of the Greek Republic 258/issue A/20.91995
4. Official Gazette of the Greek Republic 314/issue B/15.12.2014
5. Official Gazette of the Greek Republic 4138/issue B/20.9.2018
6. Official Gazette of the Greek Republic 2271/issue B/11.6.2019

At present, in order to become a specialist in nephrology in Greece, the trainee is required to complete a 2-year training in internal medicine, followed by 4-year training in nephrology (of which at least 18 months in clinical nephrology, 6 months in HD, 4 months in PD, 3–6 months in transplantation, 3 months in outpatient clinics; the remaining time can be used to train the student in different disciplines of the department, at the discretion of his/her clinical director).

After completion of training, the candidate has to pass the specialty certificate examinations, in order to register as a specialist.

Following specialist registration, a nephrologist can work in private practice, in the national health system, or in university posts, as well as in private nephrology departments and HD units. HD units (both of the public and the private sector) can also employ nurses after at least 6 months of training in HD, as well as physicians of other specialties (cardiologists, psychiatrists, etc.) as consultants, as well as renal dietitians. There are strictly defined nurse-to-patient and nephrologist-to-patient ratios for dialysis units of the private sector. For the aforementioned "chronic HD units," the minimum requirement is 1 nurse for 4 patients and 1 nephrologist (in addition to the medical director) for 40 patients with minimum 2 nephrologists per unit (Presidential Decree 225 (Official Gazette of the Greek Republic 194/issue A/07.09.2000)). Accordingly, for the aforementioned "Artificial Kidney Units" (operating within private hospitals), the nurse-to-patient ratio is 1:5, and the minimum requirement for nephrologists is one nephrologist as a medical director and one more physician for every ten patients. However, apart from the medical director, the remaining physicians can be nephrologists or alternatively internists or cardiologists with at least 3-month training in a Nephrology Department (Law 4600/2019/Official Gazette of the Greek Republic 43/issue A/09.03.2019). In public hospitals, the staff-to-patient ratio is not strictly defined by law, but for nurses the rule of thumb is to maintain the same ratio as in the private sector, while the number of nephrologists depends on the hospital's establishment plan and whether the hospital hosts a fully developed Nephrology Department or only a dialysis unit.

As of 2019, the number of registered nephrologists in the registry of the Hellenic Society of Nephrology is 578 (57 pmp), but a considerable number are now working abroad (UK, Germany, etc.), following the well-known economic crisis of 2008. Of those remaining in the country, about 50% work in nephrology departments of the National Health System and universities and 50% work in the private sector (mainly "chronic HD units"). It should be noted that, due to reduced appointments in the public sector during the last 15 years, most junior nephrologists are employed in the private sector and mainly in "chronic HD units." The number of these units across Greece is increasing relatively rapidly during the last few years, due to the current shortages of medical and nursing staff in public hospitals and the failure of public HD units to operate at full capacity. The salary of a junior nephrologist in public hospitals and private HD units is about the same and is close to 2,000 euros/month, after taxes and contributions (net income).

Given that the reimbursement price per HD session is almost equivalent for the public and the private sector, the increasing number of private HD units does not increase the state expenses and health budget. On the contrary, the state theoretically benefits from the reduction of operating costs for public HD units. The increase in private HD units, along with the funding and staffing problems of public hospitals and the relative increase in the number of incident HD patients, was accompanied by the movement of a number of HD patients towards the private sector. On the other hand, the actual reimbursement of HD session in the private HD units has been considerably reduced (by about 30%), following the introduction of a series of financial measures, as a result of the country's economic crisis and the implementation of fiscal stabilization programs. Such measures were (a) the introduction by the Ministry of Health of closed budgets by category of benefits for both the public and private sector, (b) the establishment of a compulsory refund rate per HD session for the private HD units (due to their mandatory interconnection with a public hospital – called interconnection fee), (c) a mandatory rebate per HD session for those units, and (d) clawback on their total annual revenue in case the pre-specified budget for reimbursement is exceeded. This reduction in reimbursement may lead to a gradual reduction of the services provided to the patients or may impact the quality of services, with unpredictable long-term consequences.

## Future Perspectives

A realistic future outlook of nephrology in Greece, should take into consideration two facts: first, that the prevalent ESRD population is still growing (Figs. 40.1, 40.2, and 40.5) and thus the demand for dialysis and transplant services is expected to increase further and, second, that the country's financial status demands careful planning of any policies, with strict cost control. In our opinion, there are four areas where improvements are needed and in which the country might benefit from investing.

The top priority should be an effort to increase transplant rates, in order to reduce the long waiting times for a transplant. To achieve this, a multifaceted approach is needed, targeting an increase in deceased and living donation on one hand (to overcome the severe deficit described previously) but also the adequate staffing and funding of the transplant units, as well as an increase in the availability of critical care beds (another crucial sector for organ donation where the country lags behind).

A second area needing improvement is nephrology-related research. Although the large nephrology departments systematically participate in large clinical trials (mainly industry-led), there is a need to promote investigator-led research. In addition, there is lack of epidemiology studies on kidney diseases (e.g., CKD, AKI, etc.), which are also important in order to be able to design policies tailored to the true needs. Basic research is also underdeveloped, but financial constraints may hinder large investments. To improve

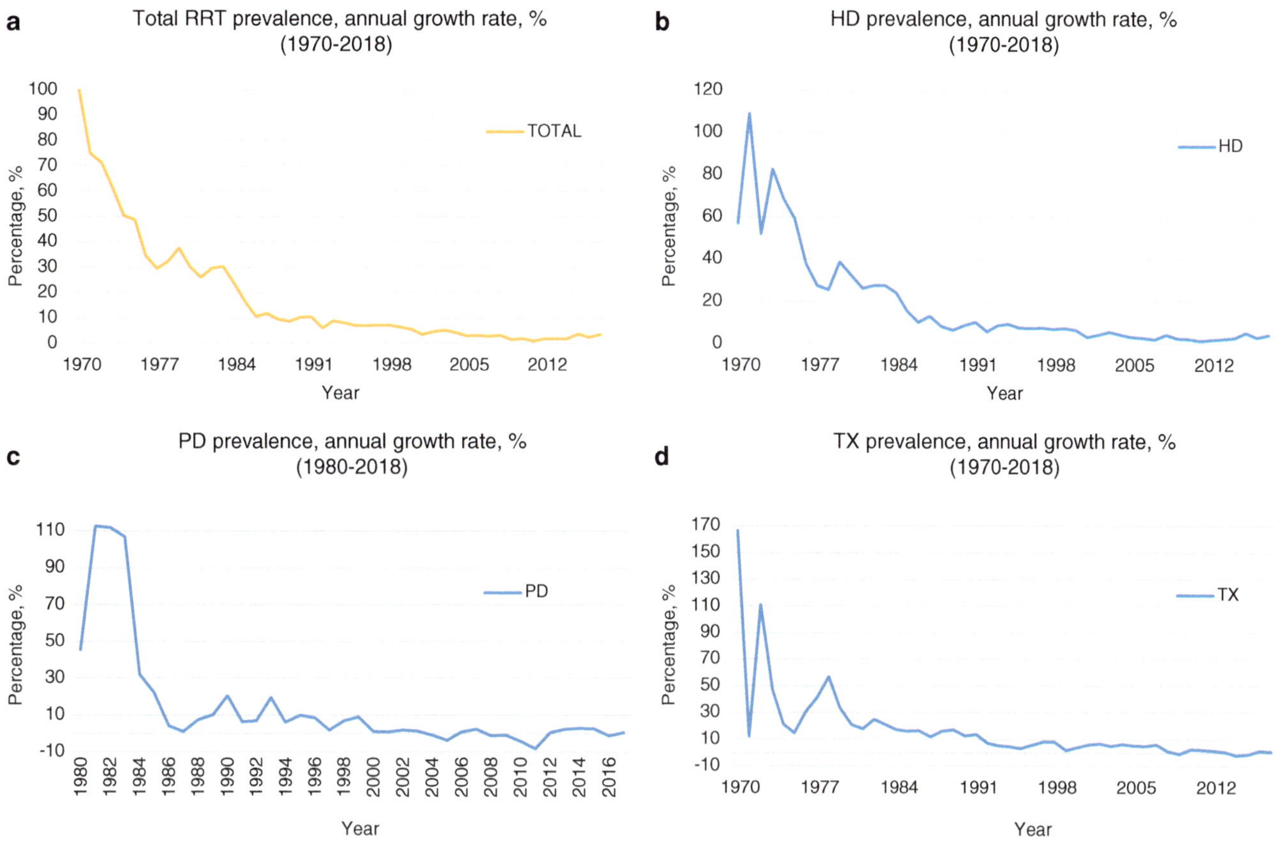


**Fig. 40.5** Annual growth rate of renal replacement therapy (RRT) prevalence in Greece, total (**a**) and by modality (**b**, **c**, and **d**) (1970–2018)

the current situation, there should be an effort to enhance international collaborations and participation in large, multiethnic schemes, as well as to seek international financial resources and grants through carefully designed research proposals. There is also a need to improve collaborations between the departments and universities in Greece, as due to the small population, the development of multicenter studies is the only way to produce powerful results. Finally, there is a need to support the renal registry with funding and staff, in order to improve its capabilities and expand its activity.

There is certainly some room for further development of PD, due to Greece's insular and mountainous terrain, which results in some areas being remote and difficult to access, especially during winter. Despite the expansion of HD units, which has made access to HD easier than ever before, there are still patients who need to drive long distances or travel to nearby islands in order to have dialysis, and these could be a target for PD development. However, PD is quite expensive for the insurance system, and any developments in this direction should be coupled by an effort to reduce PD costs.

The fourth area where further development is feasible is that of medical tourism. There are currently HD units located in touristic areas (e.g., Crete), but in our opinion dialysis-related tourism has a great potential. To achieve this however, the development of services of the private sector (HD units) is not sufficient. The public sector services in these areas need to improve as well (district hospitals, ambulance services, public HD units, etc.), in order to be able to support a potential seasonal growth of the dialysis population. For this reason, targeted policies and investment plans are needed, as well as a constructive collaboration between the health authorities and the business sector.

As for HD, recent policies in the direction of cost control might have a negative impact on the quantity and quality of the services provided, and in some cases they might affect the sustainability of services, while at the same time the capacity and facilities of the public HD sector are not able to cover demand. For this reason, careful consideration of policies is needed, in order to achieve reasonable cost reductions, without negatively affecting the quality of services.

## Conclusions

The development of nephrology in Greece started in the 1950s and has generally followed the developments in other European countries. Nephrology services expanded greatly since the 1980s, and today all disciplines of nephrology are fully developed. There is lack of epidemiological data on CKD and AKI, but there are data for patients on RRT. Incidence and prevalence of ESRD are among the highest in Europe, and prevalence is still growing. The number of patients on RRT including transplant recipients approaches 15,000, the vast majority of which are treated with HD. There is a developed private sector in HD services, and approximately 2/3 of patients receive HD in the private sector. However, all RRT treatments are free (fully reimbursed by the insurance system) for patients. As for PD, it is not widely used, but there is some potential for development, especially for patients who live in remote and difficult to access areas. Transplant rates are below the European average, and there is an urgent need to increase transplants. Regarding nephrology practice, the specialty of nephrology can be acquired after 6 years of postgraduate medical training. Appointments in the public sector are very few, and most nephrologists are employed by the private sector. The salaries for nephrology specialists are quite low compared to European countries, but satisfactory compared to the average salaries in Greece.

As far as it concerns the future, the top priority should be to achieve an increase in transplant rates. Besides that, there is a need to further develop nephrology-related research and a potential for the development of dialysis-related medical tourism. Financial constraints following the country's economic crisis are the major limiting factor for the future developments in nephrology; thus, careful and insightful planning involving all stakeholders is required.

## References

1. Bernard C. Leçons sur les phénomènes de la vie commune aux animaux et aux végétaux. Hachette Livre BNF; 2013.
2. Klemperer P, Federn W. The dilemma of Johann Jacob Wepfer: the history of the contracted kidney. Bull Hist Med. 1959;33(1):50–66.
3. Panagiotopoulos E, Valtis D. Observations from the application of peritoneal dialysis in cases of acute uremia. Arch Med Sci. 1950;6:301.
4. Medical Society of Thessaloniki: Tountas Konstantinos. Years 1967, 1968. http://www.ieth.gr/index.php/2012-11-19-15-46-55/2013-04-26-09-39-45/120-o-o-1967-1968. Accessed 10 Jan 2020.
5. Vafiadis S. The Hellenic Society of Nephrology: commemorative volume 1970–1990. Available in: https://www.ene.gr/DOCUMENTS/PDF/AT_1970_1990.pdf.
6. Yatzidis H. A convenient haemoperfusion micro-apparatus over charcoal for the treatment of endogenous and exogenous intoxications. Its use as an effective artificial kidney. Proc Eur Dial Transplant Assoc. 1964;1:83–7.
7. Yatzidis H, Oreopoulos D, Triantaphyllidis D, Voudiclari S, Tsaparas N, Gavras C, Stavroulaki A. Treatment of severe barbiturate poisoning. Lancet. 1965;2(7405):216–7. https://doi.org/10.1016/s0140-6736(65)90698-7.
8. Yatzidis H, Triantaphyllidis D, Kassioumis A. Ulceration of the toes associated with arteriovenous fistula. New Engl J Med. 1969;281(23):1307–8.
9. Hellenic Society of Nephrology. https://www.ene.gr/. Accessed 25 Nov 2019.
10. Global Kidney Health Atlas. International Society of Nephrology. 2017. https://www.theisn.org/global-atlas. Accessed 25 Nov 2019.
11. ERA-EDTA Registry Annual Report 2016. ERA-EDTA registry. 2018. http://www.era-edta-reg.org. Accessed 10 Dec 2019.
12. Hellenic Association of Geriatrics and Gerontology. http://gerontology.gr/2015/07/10/δημογραφικά-στοιχεία/. Accessed 10 Jan 2020.
13. Spinelli A, Buoncristiano M, Kovacs VA, Yngve A, Spiroski I, Obreja G, et al. Prevalence of severe obesity among primary school children in 21 European countries. Obes Facts. 2019;12(2):244–58. https://doi.org/10.1159/000500436.
14. Liatis S, Dafoulas GE, Kani C, Politi A, Litsa P, Sfikakis PP, Makrilakis K. The prevalence and treatment patterns of diabetes in the Greek population based on real-world data from the nation-wide prescription database. Diabetes Res Clin Pract. 2016;118:162–7. https://doi.org/10.1016/j.diabres.2016.06.018.
15. Hellenic Health Foundation. HYDRIA Project. Programme and targeted action on the diet and health of the Greek population: development and implementation of methodology and documentation. 2017. http://www.hhf-greece.gr/hydria-nhns.gr/images/hydria-results-eng.pdf. Accessed 10 Jan 2020.
16. Panagiotakos DB, Pitsavos CH, Chrysohoou C, Skoumas J, Papadimitriou L, Stefanadis C, Toutouzas PK. Status and management of hypertension in Greece: role of the adoption of a Mediterranean diet: the Attica study. J Hypertens. 2003;21(8):1483–9.
17. Papachristou E, Iatrou C, Papasotiriou M, pagoni A, Vakianis P, Kaplanis N, et al. Vascular access in adult hemodialysis patients in Greece: conclusions through a cross-sectional analysis. Nephrol Dial Transplant. 2016;31.(Suppl. 1:i259–73. https://doi.org/10.1093/ndt/gfw173.22.
18. Papadimitriou M, Hatzikonstantinou V. The journey of nephrology in Greece (originally in Greek). Edited by the Hellenic Society of Nephrology; 2015.
19. Tsakiris D, Hatzikonstantinou V, Sompolos K. Annual Report of the National Registry of patients on renal replacement therapy in Greece, 1996 (originally in Greek). Hellenic Society of Nephrology, 52nd Scientific meeting, Thessaloniki; 1996.
20. Koukou MG, Smyrniotis VE, Arkadopoulos NF, Grapsa EI. PD vs HD in post-economic crisis Greece—differences in patient characteristics and estimation of therapy cost. Perit Dial Int. 2017;37(5):568–73. https://doi.org/10.3747/pdi.2016.00292.
21. Pavlakou P, Balafa O, Dounousi E, Andrikos A, Tsirpanlis G, Perakis C, et al. Incidence and risk factors of peritonitis in peritoneal dialysis patients in Greece (originally in Greek). Hellenic Society of Nephrology, 20th Panhellenic Congress of Nephrology, Athens; 2018.
22. Melexopoulou C, Marinaki S, Liapis G, Skalioti C, Gavalaki M, Zavos G, Boletis JN. Excellent long-term patient and renal allograft survival after ABO-incompatible kidney transplantation: experience of one centre. World J Transplant. 2015;5(4):329–37. https://doi.org/10.5500/wjt.v5.i4.329.
23. National Organization of Transplantations. Available at: https://www.eom.gr.

# Nephrology in Italy

# 41

Antonio Bellasi, Biagio Di Iorio, Marco Franchin, Matteo Tozzi, Carlo Alfieri, Piergiorgio Messa, Claudio Ronco, and Luca Di Lullo

| | |
|---|---|
| Area[1] | 301,340 Km$^2$ |
| Population[1] | 60,431,283 (2018) |
| Capital[1] | Rome |
| Three most populated cities[1] | 1.Rome (2,318,895)<br>2.Milan (1,236,837)<br>3.Naples (959,470) |
| Official language[1] | Italian |
| Gross Domestic Product (GDP) [1] | 2.075 trillion USD (2018) |
| GDP per capita[1] | 35,391.7 USD (2018) |
| Human Development Index (HDI)[1] | 0.880 (2017) |
| Official currency[1] | Euro (€, EUR) |
| Total number of nephrologists[2] | 2718 |
| National society of nephrology | Società Italiana di Nefrologia (SIN) www.sinitaly.org<br>Società Italiana di Nefrologia Pediatrica (SINePe) https://www.sinepe.it/<br>Società Italiana di Cardio-Nefrologia (SIN CAR) http://www.sincar-italy.org/<br>Associazione Italiana di Cardio-Nefrologia (AICN) https://www.associazionecardionefro.it/ |
| Incidence of End-Stage Renal Disease[3] | 2015–154 pmp |
| Prevalence of End-Stage Renal Disease (on dialysis)[3] | 2015–770 pmp |
| Total number of patients on dialysis (all modalities) [3] | 2015–46,474 |
| Number of patients on hemodialysis [3] | 2015–42,068 (90.6%) |
| Number of patients on peritoneal dialysis [3] | 2015–4405 (9.4%) |
| Number of renal transplantations per year [4] | 2017–2244 (Deceased Donor 1934 – Living Donor 310)<br>2018–2117 (Deceased Donor 1831 – Living Donor 287) |

[1]https://en.wikipedia.org/wiki/Italy
[2]Quintaliani G, et al., *[Census of the renal and dialysis units by Italian Society of Nephrology: nephrologist's workload for renal patient assistance in Italy (2014–2015)]*. G Ital Nefrol, 2016. 33(5)
[3]The Italian Registry of Dialysis and Transplantation. https://ridt.sinitaly.org/
[4]Official data from Italian National Transplant Center

The authors declare that they have no conflict of interest.
In: Nephrology Worldwide. Moura Neto JA, Divino-Filho JC, Ronco C (eds).
Springer Nature Switzerland AG, 2020

A. Bellasi (✉)
Department of Research, Innovation, Brand Reputation, Ospedale di Bergamo, ASST Papa Giovanni XXIII, Bergamo (BG), Italy
e-mail: abellasi@asst-pg23.it

B. Di Iorio
Department of Nephrology and Dialysis AORN San Giuseppe Moscati, Avellino (AV), Italy

M. Franchin · M. Tozzi
Vascular Surgery Unit, Department of Medicine and Surgery, University of Insubria School of Medicine, ASST Settelaghi University Teaching Hospital, Varese (VA), Italy

C. Alfieri
Nephrology, Dialysis and Renal Transplantation, Fondazione IRCCS Ca Granda Ospedale Maggiore Policlinico, Milan, Italy

Department of Clinical Sciences and Community Health, University of Milan, Milan, Italy

P. Messa
Nephrology, Dialysis and Renal Transplantation, Fondazione IRCCS Ca Granda Ospedale Maggiore Policlinico, Milan, Italy

Department of Clinical Sciences and Community Health, University of Milan, Milan, Italy

Incoming president of the Italian Society of Nephrology (SIN), Rome (RM), Italy
e-mail: piergiorgio.messa@policlinico.mi.it

C. Ronco
DIMED - University of Padova, Department Nephrology Dialysis & Transplantation, International Renal Research Institute (IRRIV), San Bortolo Hospital, Vicenza, Italy
e-mail: cronco@goldnet.it

L. Di Lullo
Department of Nephrology and Dialysis, "L. Parodi – Delfino" Hospital, Colleferro (RM), Italy


J. A. Moura-Neto et al. (eds.), *Nephrology Worldwide*, https://doi.org/10.1007/978-3-030-56890-0_41

## Introduction

The Republic of Italy, globally known as Italy, is a country located in the south-central Europe. Italy, often described as a country shaped like a boot, occupies a peninsula that deeps into the Mediterranean Sea. In particular, Italy is bordered by the Adriatic Sea, Tyrrhenian Sea, Ionian Sea, and the Mediterranean Sea. To the North, Italy shares a border with France, Switzerland, Austria and Slovenia. The Italian population accounts for roughly 60 millions inhabitants (equivalent to 0.78% of the total world population) with a higher prevalence of females than males (in 2018 there were in Italy roughly 29.4 million males and approximately 31 million females) [1]. Based on recent elaboration of the United Nations data, it is expected to decline throughout the twenty-first century in consideration of a current death rate significantly exceeding the birth rate (a decrease of 124,427 people between year 2017 and 2018 was documented). However, the migratory flux may impact this trend in the future since Italy's foreign residents are outpacing the country's population growth with a foreign population that grew by 7.4% in 2012, compared to a "national" population growth of just 0.5% [1].

The official currency is Euro introduced in 2002 and symbolized as €. In November 2019, € 1.00 was worth 1.1 US dollar, 0.85 UK pound, 120.63 Japanese Yen, and 7.75 Chinese Yuan. The Italian gross domestic product (GDP) was USD 2.075 trillion in 2018, which makes Italy the eighth largest economy in the world [1].

The Italian political regime is a democratic parliamentary republic with a multi-party system. Italy has been a democratic republic since June second 1946, when the monarchy was abolished by popular referendum and a constituent assembly elected to draft a constitution, which was promulgated on 1 January 1948 [1].

The Italian capital is located in Rome. The country is divided in 20 regions (the first-level constituent entities of the Italian Republic), and although each region has some degree of administrative, political, legislative, and financial autonomy, there are cultural, geographical (climate, vegetation), and economic similarities among the regions. Among the 20 regions, 5 have a broader amount of autonomy (autonomous regions with special statute), but each region is an autonomous entity with defined powers. The autonomous regions with special statute (Sardinia, Sicily, Trentino-Alto Adige/Sudtirol, Aosta Valley, and Friuli-Venezia Giulia) benefit of a broader amount of autonomy, depending on their specific statute, in order to take into account cultural differences and protect linguistic minorities. Moreover, after the Second World War, the government wanted to prevent their secession from Italy [1].

With the exception of the Aosta Valley, each region is divided into a number of provinces (institutional bodies of second level), and the provinces are in turn divided into 7918 municipalities (in Italian, Comuni), the basic constituent entity of Italy. There are currently 103 institutional bodies of second level in Italy, including 80 active provinces, 2 autonomous provinces, 6 free municipal consortia, 14 metropolitan cities, and Aosta Valley Region. The densities of Comuni varies by province and region according to geographical and political needs [1].

Although Italian is the official language spoken in Italy, there are approximately 34 native living spoken languages and related dialects in Italy, most of which are Romance languages. Standard Italian is a direct descendant of Tuscan, the dialect spoken in Tuscany. However, 12 additional languages are officially recognized as linguistic minorities in Italy: Albanian, Catalan, Greek, Slovene, Croatian, French, Franco-Provencal, Friulian, Ladin, Occitan, and Sardinian. Of these, bilingualism is legally granted to German, Slovene, and French, enacted in the Regions of Trentino Alto-Adige, Friuli Venezia Giulia, and Aosta Valley, respectively [1].

Since 1978, healthcare is a constitutional right in Italy. Indeed, in this year the government established the SSN (Servizio Sanitario Nazionale) including universal coverage and tax funding [2]. SSN is provided to all Italian citizens and residents by a mixed public-private system. The SSN is organized under the Ministry of Health and is administered on a regional basis. Although SSN guarantees universal and "free" access to healthcare, there are criticisms regarding undercoverage, long wait times, and the quality of healthcare assistance [2]. Furthermore, according to the Italian National Outcomes Programme, a significant variation in quality and outcomes of care by regions is noticeable, and there is evidence of patient movement, generally from South to North, probably driven, at least in part, by a search for better quality.

## Brief History of Nephrology in Italy

Although Nephrology can be identified as a "novel" discipline, renal diseases studies hold an ancient history. Indeed, in 1827 Richard Bright first employed the term "nephrology" while describing the association between proteinuria and renal disease [3]. In the following decades, kidney diseases concern increased together with the development of knowledge in internal medicine. Only after the Second World War, together with the birth of dedicated renal scientific associations such as "Societé de Pathologie Renale" (France, 1949), "Renal Association" (England, 1950), and "Società Italiana di Nefrologia" (Italy, 1957), Nephrology disseminated in the medical community [3].

While the first renal medicine journal was published in Italy in 1954 (Minerva Nefrologica, ancestor of the now published Giornale Italiano di Nefrologia), the Italian Society of Nephrology (SIN) was founded in Parma only 3 years later on April 28 1957 by Prof. Luigi Migone (Parma) and Prof.

Gabriele Monasterio (Pisa) [3, 4]. Aside from the development of the scientific community, there are a few milestones that changed the history of renal disease development in Italy.

In 1947, Aminta Fieschi asked to produce an artificial kidney (manufactured by Cavallo Inc.) quite similar to Kolff dialyser [4]. In 1951, Emico Fiaschi performed the first renal biopsy at Institute of Clinical Medicine of Pisa University. Carmelo Giordano (1963) and Sergio Giovannetti (1964) developed the first prescriptions of low – protein based diet to optimize protein intake in uremic patients [5, 6]. In 1964, Sergio Giovannetti (together with Quirino Maggiore) published a paper on the Lancet, in which they recommended to avoid the prescription of a high protein intake, by removing non – essential amino acids from patients' diet [7].

In 1966, the first renal transplant was performed by Paride Stefanini, and 1 year later, in 1967, Antonio Vercellone, in Turin, scheduled the first treatment of a chronic hemodialysis (HD) program. A few years later, home HD and outpatient HD programs were, respectively, established in 1971 and 1973 [4].

In 1976, Pietro Confortini, Edmond Malan, and Girolamo Sirchia founded the first Italian Inter-regional Referral Centre for Kidney Transplantation (then called "North Italian Transplant Program" (NITp)) [6].

In the late 1970s, Italy experienced an increase in peritoneal dialysis (PD) activity especially in Brescia (with Rosario Maiorca), Vicenza (Giuseppe La Greca) and Perugia (Umberto Buoncristiani) [4].

In 1974, only two academic chairs were active (in Bari with Alberto Amerio and Naples with Carmelo Giordano). However, in the same year Giuseppe Maschio, an academic nephrologist, became Director of a non-academic Nephrology Unit in Verona. Shortly later, Verona managerial model was successfully replicated in Bologna with Vittorio Bonomini, Turin with Antonio Vercellone, Brescia with Rosario Maiorca, Ancona with Vittorio Mioli, and Modena with Alberto Albertazzi triggering the constitution of a Nephrology movement that led Italian Nephrology to the first tier in the world [4].

The Italian Society of Pediatric Nephrology was established in November 10 1984 based on the experience of the Study Group of the Italian Society of Nephrology founded in Vicenza in 1975 and promoted by some Pediatric Nephrologic Units set in Genova (Rosanna Gusmano), Torino (Rosanna Coppo) and Rome (Gianfranco Rizzoni) [4].

Among Italian pioneers, it's mandatory to include Giuseppe Remuzzi (Bergamo), main investigator of several clinical and experimental studies concerning the efficacy of ACE – inhibitors in delaying progression of chronic kidney disease (CKD) toward end-stage renal disease (ESRD) and immune tolerance to protect and encourage renal transplantation. Similarly, other pioneers of Italian Nephrology deserve mention: Claudio Ponticelli (Milan, Policlinico) for his studies on immunotherapies for primary glomerulonephritis and graft survival; Giuseppe D'Amico (Milan, San Carlo) who was the chairman of first meeting on updates in Nephrology; Francesco Locatelli (Lecco) opinion leader for anemia and its treatment; Francesco Paolo Schena (Bari) who founded the biggest immunohistopathology Italian study group and winner of over 100 research grants; Vittorio Emanuele Andreucci (Napoli) pioneer of kidney transplantation in southern Italy; Natale Gaspare De Santo (Napoli) for his studies on hydro – electrolytic metabolism and acid – base imbalance; Mario Timio (Foligno), father of Cardionephrology; Vittorio Bonomini, full professor of Nephrology at Sant'Orsola Hospital (Bologna) [4].

Italian Nephrology has given great impulse to knowledge during the last decades because Pioneers have been followed by other Nephrologists with overlapping scientific qualities and ambitions [4]. Since the early 1980s, a nephrologic spring has spread from North to South of Italy. In this context some investigators deserve mention for their contributions in various field of Nephrology: Carmine Zoccali (Reggio Calabria) for his clinical studies on hypertension and cardiovascular disease epidemiology in CKD patients; Loreto Gesualdo (Bari) and for his holistic and multidisciplinary approach to the world of Nephrology (last but not least his research on gut microbioma), and Diego Brancaccio, Mario Cozzolino, and Piergiorgio Messa (Milano - S. Paolo and Policlinico) for their findings on CKD – MBD and Polycystic Kidney Disease; Dario Roccatello (Torino) for his involvement in renal immunopathology and rare diseases; Sergio Stefoni and Gaetano La Manna (Bologna, S. Orsola) and Antonio Santoro (Bologna Malpighi) for their contribution to dialysis and transplantation; Lorenzo Calò (Padova) a world opinion leader for Bartter and Gitelman's syndromes; Giovambattista Capasso (Naples) for his endeavor in renal physiology and rare diseases; Giuseppe Conte for his studies on CKD epidemiology and nutrition in CKD; Carmine Pecoraro (Naples) for his contribution in the field of Pediatric Nephrology; Barsotti and Cupisti (Pisa) opinion leaders in nutrition in CKD; and Vincenzo Cambi (Parma) for his contribution in the field of hemodialysis and his studies on short dialysis. A significant number of Italian Nephrologists also provided a great impulse to dialysis techniques and likely contributed to the development in Mirandola, a little town near to Bologna, of the largest in the world, aggregated site of dialysis manufacturers, the so-called Dialysis Valley clinical laboratory [4].

## Renal Diseases in Italy

While data on CKD etiology are scarce, data on epidemiology in adults are nicely captured by a relatively recent study promoted by the Istituto Superiore di Sanità (ISS), the leading technical-scientific body of the Italian National Health Service which performs research, trials, control, counseling, documentation, and training for public health. Indeed, the aim of this epidemiological study named *Cardiovascular risk profile in Renal patients of the Italian Health Examination Survey (CARHES)* was to estimate the prevalence of a whole spectrum of CKD and associated cardiovascular (CV) risk factors in a nationally representative sample from the general adult population in Italy [8].

The survey lasted from April 2008 to December 2012 [8]. Procedures were planned according to the recommendations of the European Health Risk Monitoring– Feasibility of European HES projects (available at www.ktl.fi/fehes/) and the WHO MONICA (Multinational MONItoring of trends and determinants in CArdiovascular disease) project. According to the project methodology, a pre-planned sample size of 220 men and 220 women (in the age range of 35–79 years) per 1.5 million residents in each Italian region, was randomly selected from the resident list. Of importance, no additional restriction was applied to the list of residents to overcome a potential referral bias, a common issue of epidemiological studies [8].

According to the reported study results, the overall CKD prevalence was estimated at 7.05 (95% Confidence Interval: 6.48–7.65), affecting about 2,180,542 (1,075,354 men and 1,105,187 women) adult persons (age 35–79 years) in Italy [8]. Early stages of disease (according to the KDIGO classification) account for most of the estimated CKD population (overall estimated prevalence: 4.16% vs 2.89% for CKD stages 1–2 and CKD stages G3a–5, respectively). Of note, persons with Stage G3b–5 (i.e., estimated GFR <45 mL/min/1.73 m$^2$) represented only about 0.78% of the whole population in Italy and about the 11% of the whole CKD population. Similarly, proteinuria (assessed as albumin to creatinine ratio – ACR) of more than 30 mg/g was detected in 4.77% of subjects. Of these, 84.3% and 15.7% of proteinuric subjects presented moderate (ACR 30–299 mg/g) and severe (ACR $\geq$ 300 mg/g), respectively. Of note, concomitant presence of reduced eGFR and high albuminuria was relatively rare. Indeed, among subjects with eGFR <60 mL/min/1.73 m$^2$, moderate and severe albuminuria were present in about 17.0% and 6.7%, respectively [8].

While no geographic influence was noted [CKD prevalence was comparable in North (7.0%; 95% CI 6.1–7.9), Center (5.6%; 95% CI 4.3–7.0) and South (7.8%; 95% CI 6.8–8.8) of Italy], a higher prevalence of early – albuminuric – stages in males was observed. However, this gender difference disappeared in the more advanced stages of disease, G3a–5 [8]. As expected, CKD prevalence increased across age strata, from 2.7% at age 35–49 years to 17.0% at 70–79 years [8].

When compared with non-CKD subjects, reduced renal function was associated with higher prevalence of hypertension, diabetes, obesity, anemia, CV disease, and low education level. Similarly, dislipidemia and higher fasting glucose were also noted among CKD patients. Multivariable adjusted regression models suggested that age, hypertension, obesity, and presence of CV disease were independent predictors of low eGFR, while diabetes and smoking were more strictly related to albuminuria [8].

Although CKD was prevalent, awareness of the condition was poor. Indeed, only one person out of ten with CKD was aware of their condition. Awareness slightly increased to 18.4% in those subjects with eGFR <60 mL/min/1.73 m$^2$, suggesting that this condition often is not suspected until very late stages [8].

Since there is not a CKD registry in Italy, CKD etiology is not well established, and these data are reported only by few Italian regions. According to what has been reported by the "*Osservatiorio Regionale sulla Malattia Renale Cronica*" in Piemonte Region (North west of Italy), about one out of each four (25%) patients reach end-stage renal disease (ESRD) without a CKD diagnosis [9]. A substantial portion of these subjects are late referral or old and frail patients, not suitable for invasive investigation such as renal biopsy. Among those with established diagnosis, vascular diseases (25%) and diabetes (18%) are the most prevalent causes of CKD. Glomerular disease (12%), genetic diseases (11%), chronic pyelonephritis (8%), and other systemic diseases with renal involvement (1%) are other causes of chronic renal dysfunction [9].

## Acute Kidney Injury in Italy

Regarding acute kidney injury (AKI), the few available studies show a picture that bears similarities to that of countries with the same socioeconomic profile. In the 5-year period from 2007 to 2012 [10], the incidence rate of AKI in need of dialysis (AKI-D) treatment almost doubled and increased from 209 to 410 pmp cases. Notably, about one third were Intensive Care Units (ICUs) patients and the rest were dispersed in different medical wards [10]. Indeed, parallel to the increase in the number of cases requiring renal replacement therapies (RRT) in the ICUs, there is an increase in the number of non-critical patients developing AKI-D admitted to non-specialist departments. In the time window from year 2007 through 2012, the ratio of patients with AKI-D admitted in the Nephrology vs non-Nephrology wards went from a 1:1 in 2007 to 1:2.4 in the 2012, suggesting that this is a general trend [10].The main reason for this evident increase in the incidence of AKI over time (also in need of RRT) likely lies in the increased number of hospitalizations in subjects at risk for the presence of comorbidities and conditions that can be complicated with AKI [11]. Indeed, there is a known increase in hospitalizations in people with CKD, diabetes, heart failure, sepsis, neoplastic disease, and acute heart attack, often associated with old age. In these patients, compared to the past, there is also a greater use of invasive cardiological procedures, cardiac surgery, vascular surgery, and major surgery which can more frequently be associated with acute deterioration of renal function [11]. Besides the increased consumption of resources, AKI epidemiology questions the standard organization of hospitals and calls for newer approaches to provide the optimal care to patients with acute deterioration of renal function.

## Renal Replacement Therapy in Italy

RRT for ESRD in Italy encompasses HD and PD modalities, as well as both living and deceased donor transplantation. The majority of prevalent patients are either undergoing HD or already transplanted. Most of the data presented herein is from the The Italian Registry of Dialysis and Transplantation (RIDT), an annual voluntary survey. Despite its national scope and informative results, there are potential biases due to its self-reported nature and incomplete coverage [12].

The RIDT collects RRT data (i.e., dialysis and transplantation) in Italy, and, in spite of some incomplete data, it represents the best source for any epidemiological and statistical RRT information in Italy [12]. Indeed, data collection and storage started more than 15 years ago. At first, information was collected in the form of aggregated data. However, soon after the registry inception, it was decided to collect disaggregated data, to improve data completeness and allow in-depth statistical analysis [12]. However, data collection was interrupted between year 2012 and year 2016 due to some issues raised by the National Authority on Data Protection, and it was subsequently resumed in an aggregate form to comply with National and Regional Privacy Data Protection regulations [12]. Due to the interruption, data collection is not homogeneous across all Italian regions and/or macro-region. Currently only six regions (Calabria, Emilia Romagna, Friuli Venezia Giulia, Liguria, Sicilia, and Veneto) provide data with higher degree of completeness while other Regions provide incomplete data. Nevertheless, the 2013 and the 2015 RIDT reports covered about 86% and 96% of the whole Italian population receiving RRT [12].

Available reports of the RIDT describe incidence and prevalence of RRT patients (HD, PD, and transplantation) according to five classes of patient age (1–24, 25–44, 45–64, 65–74 and ≥ 75 years) and overall unadjusted mortality data, due to data incompleteness. Statistical inference on treatment effects adjusted for potential confounders is provided only for those regions that provide complete data [12].

## Incidence of Renal Replacement Therapy in Italy

Overall, RRT incidence has slowly declined in the recent past. Indeed, according to the 2011 and 2015 reports, it is estimated that every year the number of new cases decreased from 168 to 154 per million subjects. Nevertheless, between 8000 and 9000 people in Italy have started RRT treatment over the last three years (Fig. 41.1) [12]. Although the reasons are not elucidated, RRT incidence significantly differs among Italian regions. A graded increase in RRT incidence across the country is observed with the highest rate of RRT in the Southern and Western Regions of Italy (RRT incidence: 100 and 237 per million subjects, in Alto Adige and Marche, respectively)(Fig. 41.2) [12].

Factors such as age, comorbidities, as well as differences in practices may account to some of these findings. Age represents the main determinant for RRT with an increased risk

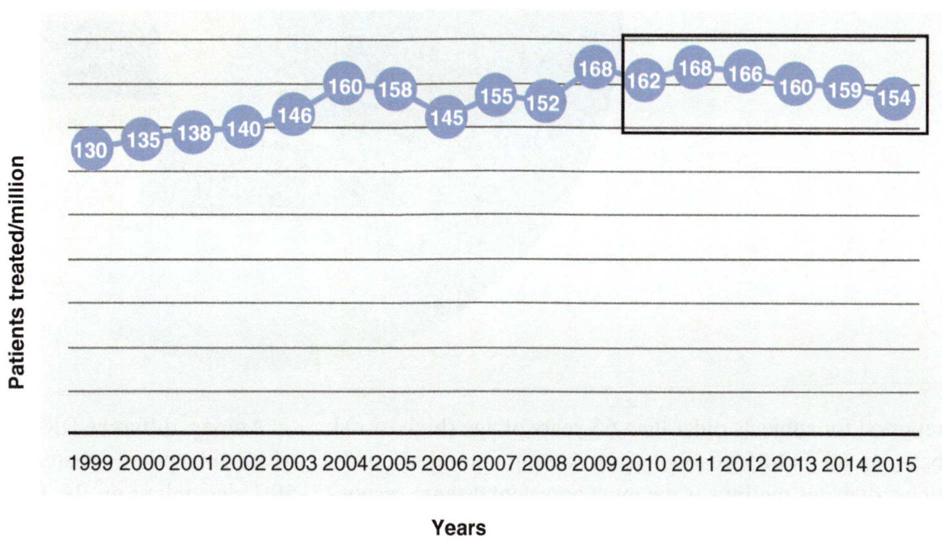


Fig. 41.1 Dialysis incidence in Italy. (Data from the Italian Registry of Dialysis and Transplantation (RIDT) [12])

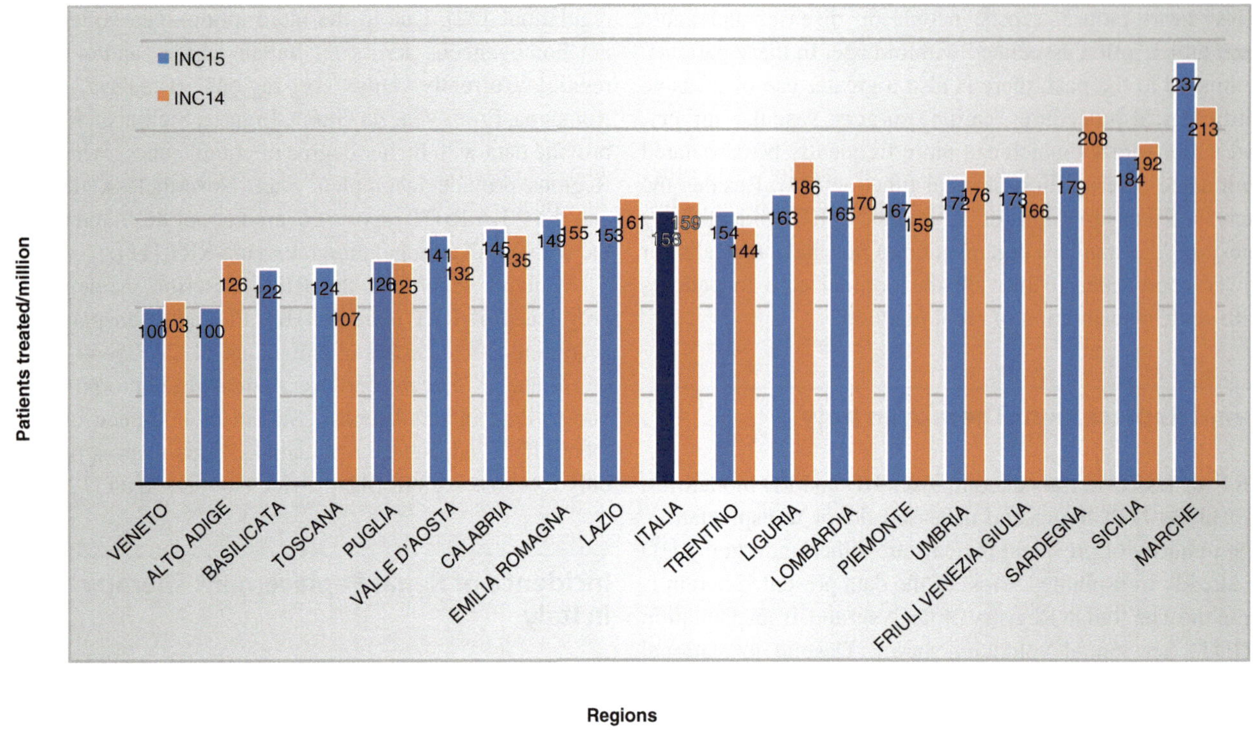


**Fig. 41.2** Dialysis incidence in Italy (Regional data) between year 2014 and 2015. (Data from The Italian Registry of Dialysis and Transplantation (RIDT) [12])

**Fig. 41.3** Etiopathogenesis of end-stage renal disease in Italy (2015 data). (Data from The Italian Registry of Dialysis and Transplantation (RIDT) [12]. GN glomerulonephritis, PN pyelonephritis, PKD polycystic kidney disease, DM diabetes mellitus, HT hypertension, RVD renovascular-disease, Misc miscellaneous, Unk unknown)

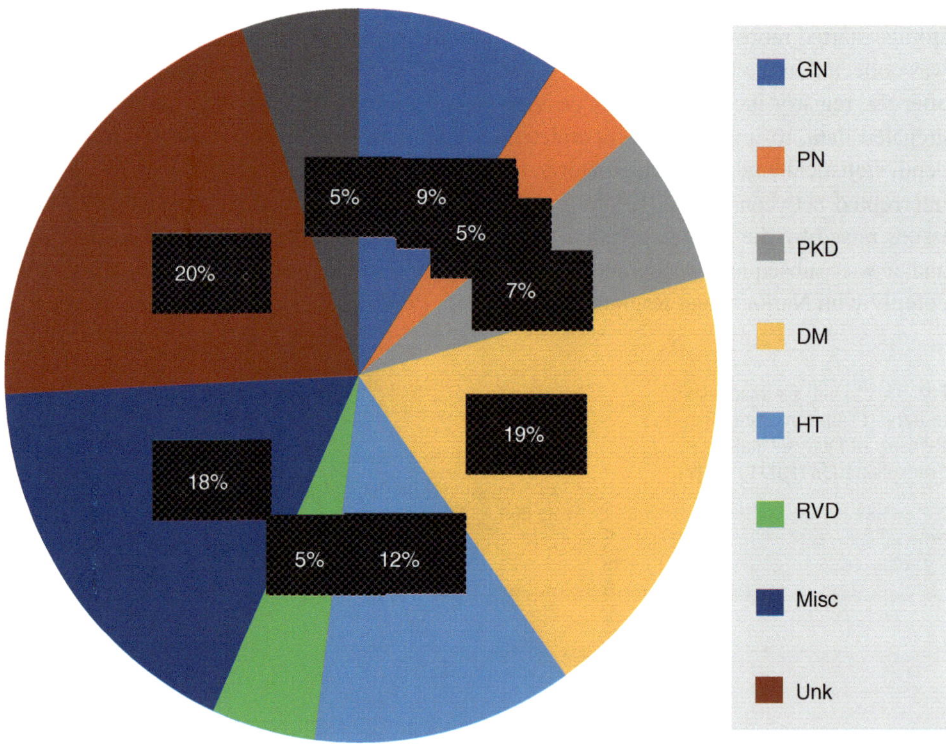


reported for subjects older than 65 years of age (highest risk between 80 and 85 years of age). Among comorbid conditions, diabetes mellitus is the most prevalent disease responsible for RRT (20%), followed by glomerulonephritis (10%) and polycystic kidney disease (7%) (Fig. 41.3) [12].

Among different RRTs, HD represents the first line of treatment option, whereas PD utilization ranges from 1 to 50% depending on the Italian region local policies (in two Regions, namely Veneto and Trentino, PD incidence is higher than of HD treatment [12].

## Prevalence of Renal Replacement Therapy in Italy

RRT prevalence is stable and has not changed substantially over the last 10 years, likely due to the decrease in the incidence trend (Fig. 41.4) [12]. However, while the overall RRT prevalence is similar across Regions, a significant regional variability in the use and prevalence of different types of RRT is reported (Fig. 41.5). Also some difference in the case-mix of the subjects receiving RRT is observed reflecting local demographic and clinical practice patterns. Indeed, higher transplantation rates is associated with lower use of dialysis, suggesting some degree of geographic heterogeneity in the access to transplantation [12]. Age distribution is also quite different among Italian regions and a higher prevalence of patients aged over 75 years in South than in North of Italy is reported (Fig. 41.6). Whether demographic differences may account for some of this variability, clinical practice patterns are also a potential explanation.

According to the 2015 Registry data report [12], about 42,000 and 4000 (8.6% of the population receiving dialysis) subjects are treated with HD and PD, respectively. Of interest, while HD is performed in every Nephrology Unit, significant differences in the use of PD among single centers, even in the same region, have been reported [12]. Cultural issues and dialysis reimbursement schemes explain the overall little attention paid to PD in Italy.

Hemodialysis is provided by both public as well as private dialysis centers. While dialyzer reuse is not permitted in Italy, large dialysis providers have invested in Italy. Data on the private center penetrance however depends on the Italian region, and data are not available for a comprehensive description of this trend. The large majority of HD patients are treated in-center facilities (71%) and only about one patient out of three receives dialysis either in a spoke center (29%) or at home (0.8%) [12]. Overall, convective (~50%) and diffusive (~50%) modalities are equally distributed in Italy, although the regional prevalence of convective treatments ranges from 22% to 54% [12].

While HD is the most prevalent RRT modality, vascular access is often placed and managed by vascular surgeons [13]. According to the Dialysis Outcomes and Practice Patterns (DOPPS) study [14, 15], a general increase in the use of central venous catheter (CVC) at expense of native arteriovenous fistula (nAVF) for HD is present in Italy. In fact, in the time window of the DOPPS study [14, 15], it was demonstrated a reduction in the prevalence of nAVF from 90% to 83% from 1996 to 2004, associated to a stable number of prosthetic vascular accesses (around 4–5%) and a parallel increase in the use of CVC. Of note, the increased use of CVC is not limited to elderly or patients with high degree of comorbidity. In fact, with reference to non-diabetics patients from 18 to 70 years old, the prevalence of CVC increased three fold in Italy, Germany, and France in comparison to the USA. Furthermore, little less than half of the incident dialysis patients started HD with a temporary CVC (40%). Additionally, only 56% of them received a permanent access during the following 180 days [14, 15].

Late patient referral, wrong fistula planning, or inappropriate facilities are plausible explanations for these figures

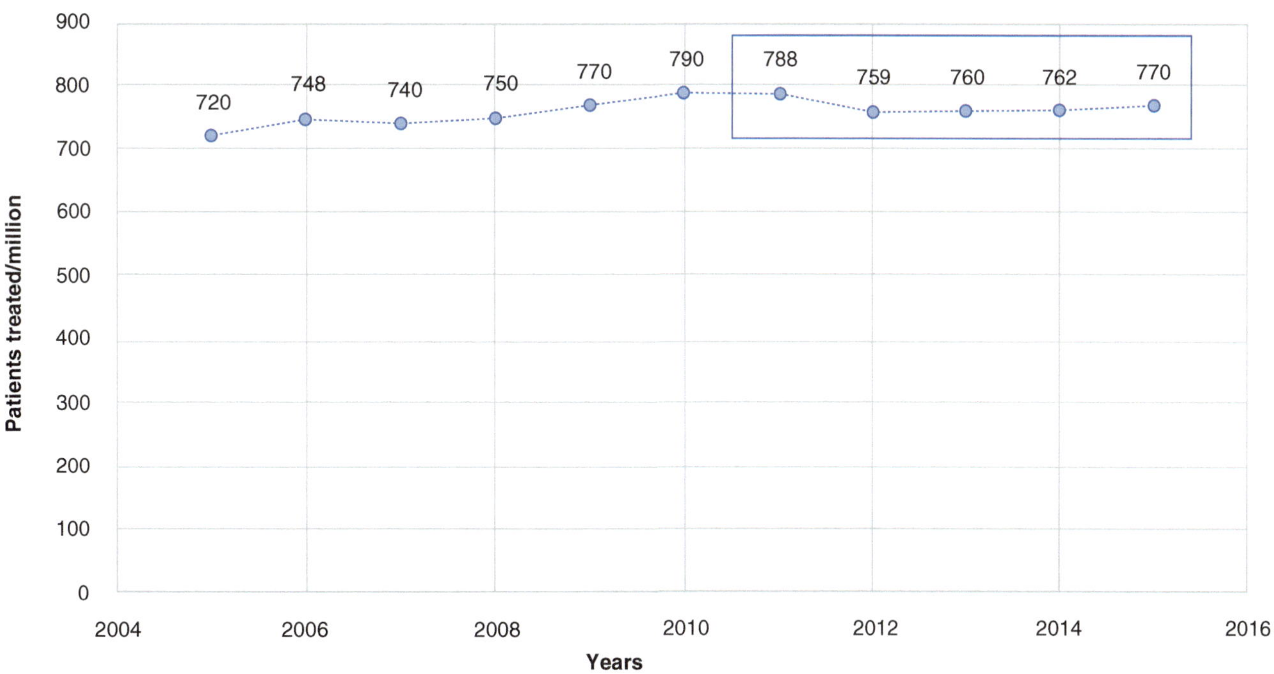


Fig. 41.4 Dialysis prevalence in Italy (Regional data). (Data from The Italian Registry of Dialysis and Transplantation (RIDT) [12])

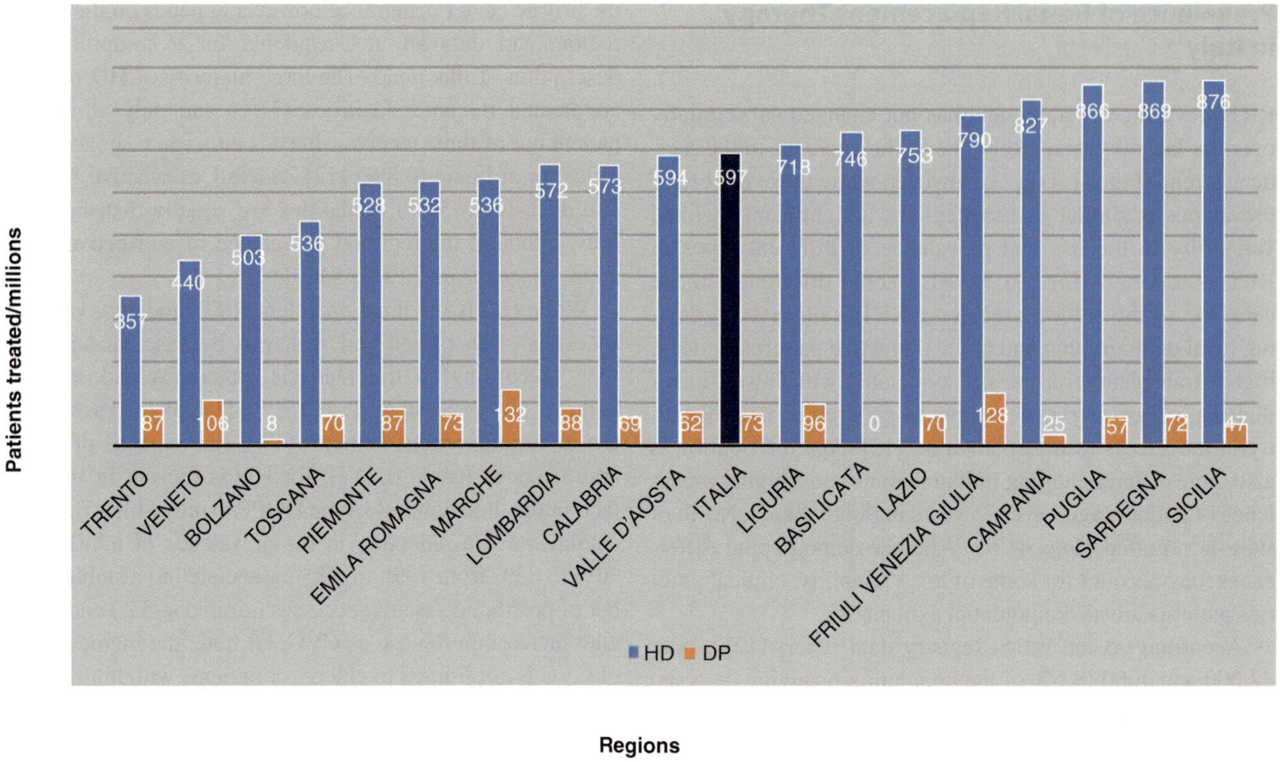


**Fig. 41.5** Dialysis prevalence in Italy (Regional data): hemodialysis (HD) vs peritoneal dialysis (PD). (Data from The Italian Registry of Dialysis and Transplantation (RIDT) [12])

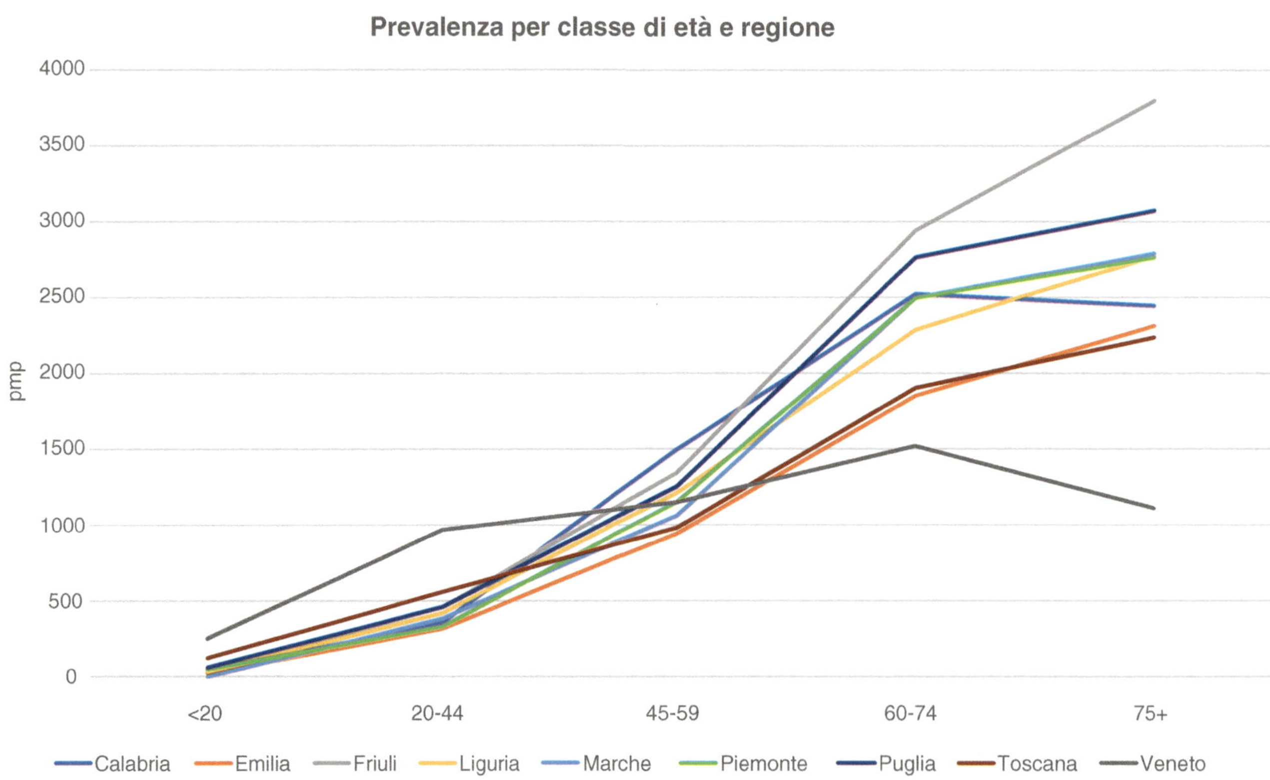


**Fig. 41.6** Age prevalence among dialysis patients according to the Italian region. Data from The Italian Registry of Dialysis and Transplantation (RIDT) [12]

[16]. Only 31.5% of the incident HD patients starting RRT through CVC receive a nephrology evaluation during the 4 months (60% of these within 30 days) prior to dialysis initiation, preventing a correct nAF planning. Additionally, among incident dialysis patients, none was considered for graft implantation and early cannulation as alternative to CVC. One potential explanation lies with the fact that in Italy 85% of vascular access (VA) are managed by nephrologists operating in facilities not suitable for complex VA creation. Accordingly, the average number of surgeons with appropriate skills for VA creation is less than 1 per center (1.6 per 100 patients), and Italy has on average only only 5–6 days/week surgeon accessibility, one of the lowest reported by DOPPS [14, 15].

## Mortality of Renal Replacement Therapy in Italy

Between year 2011 and 2015, the overall mortality rate of patients receiving dialysis was 16.8/100 patients/year [12]. However, this estimate decreased to about 10/100 patients/year when renal transplantation is considered. Although the reasons are not clear and registry data cannot provide with conclusive explanations, an inter-regional variability in mortality rate of RRT is reported. Whether differences in the case-mix or in clinical practice (such as access to transplantation) account for the variability in mortality rate deserve further and ad hoc investigations [12].

## Renal Transplantation

Despite the intense efforts devoted to developing novel approaches such as kidney regeneration and restoration to cure chronic kidney disease (CKD), renal transplantation (RTx) is currently the best RRT for CKD patients [17]. Consolidated data have in fact demonstrated that RTx increases quality of life and is associated with a reduced CV risk as well as increased survival of CKD patients as well as cost-savings [17, 18]. Also, a recent pharmacoeconomic analysis conducted in Italy reported a mid-term economic benefit for RTx compared to dialysis. According to the investigators, the estimated overall 3-year cost burden per patient receiving RTx or dialysis approaches 95,000 and 123,000 euros, respectively. Of note, 55.2% of RTx costs are related to the hospitalization at the the time of transplantation while the rest is due to the post-RTx follow up, making RTx a cost-effective strategy for ESRD after 3 years [18].

An optimal transplantation program with a fair organ allocation system and no social or cultural privileges implies the presence of a good transplant network, regulated by normative rules, able to cover and manage the entire area of the country. In addition, to be effective, the network should provide with a thorough evaluation of donors and recipients as well as allow for a fruitful collaboration between nephrologists and renal surgeons at the moment of RTx and during its follow-up.

In Italy, the RTx network organization has improved in the recent years, with the aim to optimize the deceased donor (DD) RTx network and promote living donor (LD) as well as cross-over (CO) donations. Transplant centers need to network and meet established standard criteria for accreditation, operation, and reimbursement of dialysis and transplant activities according to regional as well as national laws.

The network is structured in four different levels of coordination: (i) local; (ii) regional; (iii) inter-regional; and (iv) national (Fig. 41.7) [19]. The local coordination (LC) is composed of physicians (anesthesiologists, nephrologist, etc.) that have the role of identifying and communicating to the regional coordination level any potential DD. LC is also responsible for all the procedures correlated to the kidney withdrawal and transplantation. The regional coordination (RC) level is composed by 19 centers (one for each Italian region). Each regional center is responsible, for the coordination of all transplant activities for the geographic area of competence, including management of the RTx waiting list and organ allocation to transplant centers, according to the inter-regional coordination (IR-C) network policies. To expand organ availability, three different inter-regional coordination (IR-C) networks are currently present in Italy:

(i) Associazione Interregionale Trapianti (AIRT), composed by Piedmont, Valle d'Aosta, Tuscany, Emilia Romagna, Puglia, and autonomous province of Bolzano
(ii) North Italian Transplant program (NITp), composed by Friuli, Liguria, Lombardy, Marche, Veneto and autonomous province of Trento
(iii) Organizzazione del Centro Sud Trapianti (OCST): composed by the Abruzzi, Basilicata, Calabria, Campania, Lazio, Molise, Sardinia, Sicily and Umbria

IR-C has a crucial role in the RTx process. In fact, aside from collecting donor and patient data before and after RTx, IR-C manages the waiting lists, assigns organs to recipients according to specific pre-formed parameters, and is responsible for immunological screening and typing of donors and recipients as well as responsible for the donor-recipient compatibility assessment. IR-C is also responsible for the organ transport coordination and receives constant reports about RC activities. Finally, IR-C supervises the transplant process of the "urgent potential recipients," such as the hyperimmune patients or patients with limited dialysis access.

Finally, the Ministry of Health (MoH) through the National Transplant Center (Centro Nazionale Trapianti – CNT) supervises the national kidney procurement, transplant activities, and the status of the RTx waiting list. CNT functions are detailed in the art 8. of law 91/94 including the pro-

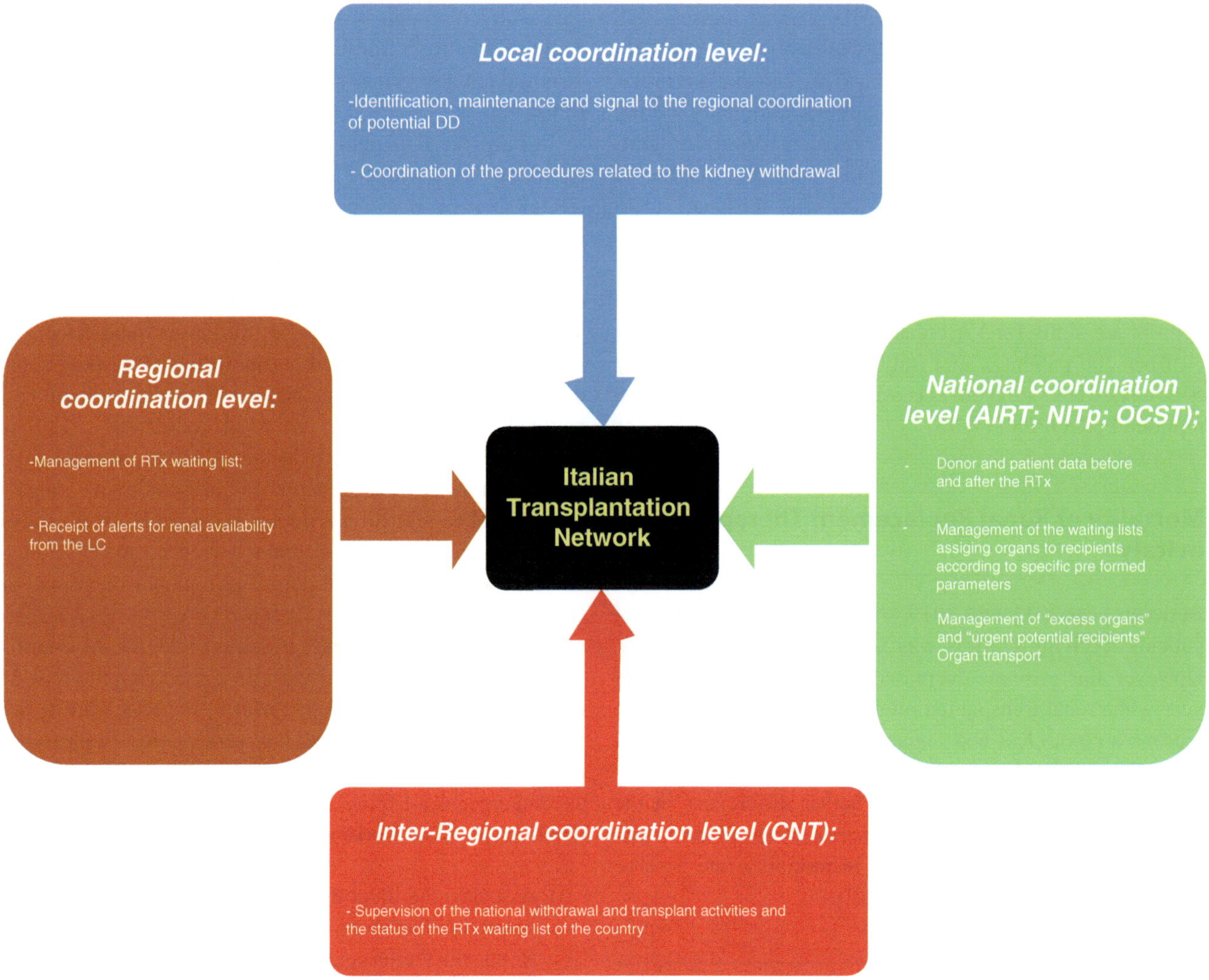


**Fig. 41.7** Principal activities of the different levels of coordination of the Italian Transplant Network. Footnotes: RTx renal transplantation, DD Deceased donor, LC local coordination level, AIRT Associazione Interregionale Trapianti, NITp Nord Italian Transplant program, OCST Organizzazione del Centro Sud Trapianti, CNT Centro Nazionale Trapianti

posal and monitoring of the implementation of specific laws related to improve the RTx procedures [20].

## Critical Care Nephrology in Italy

In the setting of critical care nephrology, available RRT modality options include conventional HD, prolonged intermittent hemodialysis (PIRRT), PD, and continuous therapies, performed in wards or ICU. Unlike RRT in ESRD, data about RRT in AKI is scarce. Nevertheless, it has been reported that the incidence of AKI needing RRT in Italy has almost doubled in recent years moving from 209 cases pmp in 2007 to about 410 cases pmp in 2012 [10, 11]. Of interest, about one third of cases are admitted to the ICU and only about one in four patients of those not treated in ICU are admitted to the Nephrology ward. While this provides evidence of a complicated scenario, it also suggests the organizational struggle to provide adequate care to AKI patients in Italy [14, 15].

## Pediatric Nephrology

Only five hospitals (located in Genoa, Milan, Padua, Rome, and Turin) in Italy have a department of Pediatric Nephrology in which kidney transplant is provided to pediatric patients with ESRD, while other 20 hospitals spread out in the Country offer a Pediatric Nephrology and Dialysis service. While only few centers provided pediatric nephrology care, a scientific society called Società Italiana di Nefrologia Pediatrica (SINePe) was founded in 1982 to aggregate all physicians and researchers involved in pediatric patients care. SINePe promotes the progress of clinical and experimental studies in Pediatric Nephrology, the scientific training of young researchers, as well as the dissemination of knowledge and teaching in the field of Pediatric Nephrology. SINePe encourages an active collaboration with the Ministry of Health as well as national societies, particularly with the Italian Society of Nephrology and the Italian Society of Pediatrics and international societies interested to foster Pediatric Nephrology in Italy.

## Nephrology Practice in Italy

Nephrology as a career is a relatively recent medical specialty in Italy, having become particularly popular from the 1970s to 1980s [3, 4], when professionals from other specialties migrated to nephrology attracted by its scientific research and technological advances, including dialysis and transplantation. To practice Nephrology in Italy, a 4-year post-graduate training (medical residency) is required. Training institutions are first accredited and then, periodically inspected by the Ministry of Education. This pathway requires 4 years of supervised training, 60 hours per week in average. The first year is to be spent in Internal Medicine and then, three additional years in Nephrology. During these three final years, the training center should provide a complete overview of nephrology, which includes theoretical and practical training at least on HD, PD, ESRD, AKI, critical care nephrology, renal transplantation, and clinical nephrology. Some centers offer additional supervised training in interventional nephrology or pediatric nephrology.

According to the 2012 SIN survey, there were about 2717 (50% are woman) practicing nephrologists in Italy, and 40% of them are older than 60 years of age [21, 22]. The distribution of nephrologists in different Regions of Italy is heterogeneous, ranging from 26 nephrologists pmp in Trentino Alto Adige to 90 nephrologist pmp in Sardinia. Nephrology service is offered both in public (332 hospitals) as well as private (283 hospitals) institutions. As a recent trend, multinational dialysis providers are developing strategic partnerships with hospital networks to provide inpatient RRT without the participation of the local nephrologist [21, 22]. In terms of reimbursement, the average monthly salary of an ordinary Italian nephrologist ranges from USD 3000 to 5000 per month. Although salary is regulated at national level, some geographic variability may apply [21, 22].

Nephrology practice in Italy allows a wide range of options, such as basic and clinical research, dialysis, transplantation, public health and epidemiology, management, palliative care, critical care, interventional nephrology, pharmaceutical industry, education, etc. In addition, it requires a multiprofessional team and the interactivity with other specialists for a comprehensive care of the patient. The specialty has a comprehensive theoretical foundation, including physiology, pathophysiology, hydro-electrolytic and basic acid disorders, complex cases, rare diseases, and a plethora of areas that captivate the young physician. However, the technology and therapeutic possibilities often experienced in high-end hospitals or university benches do not reproduce on a day-to-day basis, causing some frustration.

## Highlights of Nephrology in Italy

### Renal Transplantation in Italy

As mentioned above, despite all the difficulties involved, Italy has an efficacious public transplantation program, with a fair organ allocation system and no social or cultural privileges. However, the number of RTx per year is still far below the growing demands of the country.

### World Kidney Day in Italy

In order to disseminate among the population all aspects related to kidney disease through informational and educational materials, the SIN and the Italian Kidney Foundation (FIR - Fondazione Italiana del Rene) coordinate the World Kidney Day activities in Italy. Activities take place in all regions and cities of the country.

### The Italian Nephrological Community

The Italian nephrological community has always been active and committed to the promotion of nephrological knowledge. Over the years, some realities have assumed an international importance such as the International Renal Research Institute of Vicenza (IRRIV) which, in addition to standing out for its research programs, offers courses and training opportunities to students from all over the world.

## Future Perspectives of Nephrology in Italy

As in other countries, a current challenge for Nephrology in Italy is to increase the interest among medical graduates and to increase the number of physicians admitted to the post-graduate training program. The shortage of nephrologists in the country will increase in the next years due to a fairly old workforce and the early retirement programs recently introduced in Italy. Another challenging and urgent point is the need to increase the use of PD throughout the country and promote home dialysis programs to increase patient care and reduce the cost burden of dialysis. In these regards, specific strategies within the government and the SIN should be designed to establish the culture of PD and home dialysis, making these modalities valid options to all patients requiring RRT. Similarly, programs to increase organ donation and to implement pre-emptive kidney transplantation are needed to provide the many patients in the waiting list with the best care available for ESRD. Finally, new technologies such as telemedicine and artificial intelligence have showed some promising results to early renal disease detection as well as personalize care. Future efforts should be devoted to further elucidate if these technologies can be implemented on large scale and are cost-effective. Finally, creation or implementation of National Registries would offer an opportunity to access more extensive data on CKD epidemiology, treatment, as well as ESRD care and the possibility to standardize clinical practice on the national territory with implementation of common guidelines and outcome monitoring. The best example to be followed is represented by the Spanish experience [23]. In fact, the accurate analysis of regional registries permitted to obtain new advanced guidelines on ESRD care based on five indicators of quality: (1) percentage of patients receiving HD with native or prosthetic VA (standard 75%); (2) prevalence of native fistulas (standard 80%); (3) annual fistula thrombosis rate (standard 25%); (4) annual prosthetic vascular access thrombosis rate (standard 50%); and (5) prevalence of tunnelled CVC (standard <10% with infection rate < 10% within the first 3 months, and < 50% annually).

## Conclusion

Despite its young age, Nephrology in Italy is well organized as a medical specialty and society, and it has shown advances over the past years. The publicly funded healthcare system promotes universal access to healthcare for the entire population, which includes primary care and RRT including renal transplantation. Italy has also shown great engagement year after year through its World Kidney Day celebrations, helping to spread the word about the importance of early detection and CKD prevention throughout the country.

There are challenges and unsolved issues ahead that will need to be faced by the Nephrology community in Italy. The number of patients on chronic dialysis is steadily rising, while the number of nephrologists is decreasing, challenging the national health care system to find different organizational model to adequately treat all renal patients. An effort toward PD and home dialysis program is much wanted to provide state-of-the-art care and reduce the cost burden of RRT. Similarly, public-to-private partnerships are also becoming more popular. While these solutions may offer some economical advantages in the short term, a long-term evaluation is still required in order to conclude on the efficacy of these models. Finally, future and ad hoc efforts are required to test the cost-effectiveness of new technologies such as telemedicine or artificial intelligence to improve early detection and personalized care of renal patients.

## References


1. https://en.wikipedia.org/wiki/Italy.
2. https://en.wikipedia.org/wiki/Healthcare_in_Italy.
3. Eknoyan G. Why the history of nephrology? G Ital Nefrol. 2016;33:1.
4. Fogazzi GB, Schena FP. Persone e fatti della Nefrologia Italiana (1957–2007), vol. 2007. Milano: Wictig Editore; 2007.
5. De Santo NG, et al. Carmelo Giordano (1930-2016): uremia therapy by low protein alimentation and sorbents. G Ital Nefrol. 2018;35(Suppl 70):29–37.
6. Di Iorio B, et al. The Giordano-Giovannetti diet. J Nephrol. 2013;26(Suppl 22):143–52.
7. Giovannetti S, Maggiore Q, Low A. Nitrogen diet with proteins of high biological value for severe chronic uraemia. Lancet. 1964;1(7341):1000–3.
8. De Nicola L, et al. Prevalence and cardiovascular risk profile of chronic kidney disease in Italy: results of the 2008-12 National Health Examination Survey. Nephrol Dial Transplant. 2015;30(5):806–14.
9. https://www.regione.piemonte.it/web/temi/sanita/strumenti-operativi/malattia-cronica-renale-on-line-report-2017.
10. Fagugli RM, et al. Six-year single-center survey on AKI requiring renal replacement therapy: epidemiology and health care organization aspects. J Nephrol. 2015;28(3):339–49.
11. Fagugli RM, et al. Acute Kidney Injury: the nephrology plus value and competence and a good organization can ameliorate the prognosis. G Ital Nefrol. 2016;33:4.
12. The Italian Registry of Dialysis and Transplantation. https://ridt.sinitaly.org/
13. Fila B, et al. Quality assessment of vascular access procedures for hemodialysis: a position paper of the Vascular Access Society based on the analysis of existing guidelines. J Vasc Access. 2019:1129729819848624.
14. Asano M, et al. Vascular access care and treatment practices associated with outcomes of arteriovenous fistula: international comparisons from the Dialysis Outcomes and Practice Patterns Study. Nephron Clin Pract. 2013;124(1–2):23–30.
15. Pisoni RL, et al. Facility hemodialysis vascular access use and mortality in countries participating in DOPPS: an instrumental variable analysis. Am J Kidney Dis. 2009;53(3):475–91.
16. Ravani P, et al. Examining the association between hemodialysis access type and mortality: the role of access complications. Clin J Am Soc Nephrol. 2017;12(6):955–64.
17. Abecassis M, et al. Kidney transplantation as primary therapy for end-stage renal disease: a National Kidney Foundation/Kidney Disease Outcomes Quality Initiative (NKF/KDOQITM) conference. Clin J Am Soc Nephrol. 2008;3(2):471–80.
18. Axelrod DA, et al. An economic assessment of contemporary kidney transplant practice. Am J Transplant. 2018;18(5):1168–76.
19. Curtoni ES. Le reti collaborative per i trapianti. Annali istituto superiore di sanità. 2000;36(2):151–62.
20. Articolo 8 Legge 1° aprile 1999, n. 91 "Disposizioni in materia di prelievi e di trapianti di organi e di tessuti" pubblicata nella Gazzetta Ufficiale n. 87 del 15 aprile 1999.
21. Quintaliani G, et al. Census of the renal and dialysis units by Italian Society of Nephrology: structure and organization for renal patient assistance in Italy (2014-2015). G Ital Nefrol. 2016;33:5.
22. Quintaliani G, et al. Census of the renal and dialysis units by Italian Society of Nephrology: nephrologist's workload for renal patient assistance in Italy (2014-2015). G Ital Nefrol. 2016;33:5.
23. Ibeas J, et al. Spanish clinical guidelines on vascular access for haemodialysis. Nefrologia. 2017;37(Suppl 1):1–191.

# Nephrology in Ireland

42

Liam Plant

| | |
|---|---|
| Area[1] | 70,273 Km$^2$ |
| Population[2] | 4,921,500 (2019) |
| Capital | Dublin |
| Three most populated Cities & Suburbs [3] | Dublin 1,173,179 (FUA 1,830,000)<br>Cork 208,669 (FUA 410,000)<br>Limerick 94,192 (FUA 160,000) |
| Functional Urban Areas (FUA)[4] | |
| Official languages | English, Irish (Gaelic) |
| Gross Domestic Product (GDP)[1] | 382.49 billion current USD (2018) |
| GDP per capita [1] | 78,750 current USD (2018) |
| Human Development Index (HDI)[5] | 0.938 (4th position) (2017) |
| Official currency | Euro (€) |
| Total number of nephrologists[6] | 50 Consultant practitioners (2019)<br>≈30 whole time equivalents to Nephrology |
| National society of nephrology | Irish Nephrology Society www.nephrology.ie |
| Incidence of End-Stage Renal Disease (ESRD)[7] | 2013–88 pmp |
| Prevalence of End-Stage Renal Disease (ESRD)[7] | 2018–957 pmp |
| Number of ESRD patients on dialysis (all modalities)[7] | 2018–2124<br>*of whom* 16 are paediatric patients |
| Number of ESRD patients on Centre/Satellite-based haemodialysis/ haemodiafiltration[7] | 2018–1873<br>*of whom* 10 are paediatric patients |
| Number of ESRD patients on Home-based haemodialysis or peritoneal dialysis (APD/CAPD) [7] | 2018–251<br>*of whom* 6 are paediatric patients<br>*of whom* 55 are on Home Haemodialysis |
| Number of ESRD patients with a functioning kidney transplant [7] | 2018–2528<br>*of whom* 64 are paediatric patients |
| Number of renal transplants performed 2009–2018 [7,8] | 1708 (167 in 2018)<br>*of which* 338 were from Living Donors |

[1]The World Bank Group. Accessed in October 2019. Available from: https://databank.worldbank.org/views/reports/reportwidget.aspx?Report_Name=CountryProfile&Id=b450fd57&tbar=y&dd=y&inf=n&zm=n&country=IRL

[2]Central Statistics Office. Accessed in October 2019. Available from: https://www.cso.ie/en/releasesandpublications/er/pme/populationandmigrationestimatesapril2019/

[3]Central Statistics Office. Accessed in October 2019. Available from: https://www.cso.ie/en/media/csoie/newsevents/documents/census2016summaryresultspart1/Census2016SummaryPart1.pdf

[4]OECD Functional urban areas. Version: January 2019. Accessed in October 2019. Available from: http://www.oecd.org/cfe/regional-policy/Ireland.pdf

[5]United Nations Development Programme. Human Development Reports. Accessed in October 2019. Available from: http://hdr.undp.org/sites/default/files/2018_human_development_statistical_update.pdf

[6]Irish Nephrology Society (INS) Membership data. Personal communication from President of INS. October 2019.

[7]Health Service Executive National Renal Office. Programme Documents and Resources. Accessed in October 2019. Available from: https://www.hse.ie/eng/about/who/cspd/ncps/renal/resources/

[8]Organ Donation Transplant Ireland Annual Report 2018. Accessed in October 2019. Available from: https://www.hse.ie/eng/about/who/acute-hospitals-division/organ-donation-transplant-ireland/publications/organ-donation-and-transplant-annual-report-2018.pdf

## Introduction to Health and Healthcare in Ireland

The Republic of Ireland is situated in northwestern Europe, occupying five-sixths of the island of Ireland. It shares a 490 km land border with Northern Ireland, which is one of the constituent nations of the United Kingdom of Great Britain and Northern Ireland. Ireland is a unitary parliamentary republic with a written constitution and is a member of the European Union (EU), the Council of Europe, the

The author declares that he has no conflict of interest.

L. Plant (✉)
Department of Renal Medicine, Cork University Hospital and University College Cork, Cork, Ireland

Irish Nephrology Society (INS), Cork, Ireland
e-mail: william.plant@ucc.ie


J. A. Moura-Neto et al. (eds.), *Nephrology Worldwide*, https://doi.org/10.1007/978-3-030-56890-0_42

Organisation for Economic Cooperation and Development (OECD) and the United Nations (UN). The table summarises the main information of Ireland [1–8]. It is a small but prosperous state, ranking amongst the top 10 countries of the world for such indices as gross domestic product (GDP)/gross national income (GNI) per capita [1], human development index (HDI) [5] and human capital index (HCI) [9].

The overall responsibility for the creation and assessment of healthcare policy lies with the government, exercised through the Department of Health [10]. Healthcare reforms in 2005 led to the establishment of a single body – the Health Service Executive (HSE) – that is responsible for providing healthcare and social services to all of Ireland [10].

Following the presentation of the Sláintecare Report [11] by the Oireachtas Committee on the Future of Healthcare, and its acceptance by Government in May 2017, there began a process to implement the vision thereof. The Sláintecare vision is to achieve a universal single-tier health and social care system where everyone has equal access to services based on need, and not ability to pay. Over time, everyone will be entitled to a comprehensive range of primary, acute, and social care services. Sláintecare's aims are to improve patient and service user experience; improve clinician experience; lower costs; and achieve better outcomes.

Almost two thirds of the population (63.4%) reside in urban areas [12]. The median age of the population was 37.1 years in 2017 [12]. One in five (20.8%) was aged <15 years, and 13.9% were aged >64 years [12]. More than 10% (11.6%) (535,475) of the population were non-Irish nationals born in some 200 different countries [2]. Of these, two groups – those born in Poland and in the United Kingdom – accounted for over 225,000 persons [2].

In 2017, Ireland experienced a birth rate of 12.9/1000 population; a death rate of 9.6/1000 population; and a net migration rate of 4.0/1000 population [12]. Life expectancy at birth was 79.9 years for men and 83.6 years for women [12].

In 2017, health expenditure in Ireland amounted to €21.1 billion [13]. This equates to 7.2% of GDP or 11.7% of GNI [13]. Health expenditure had risen by 12.8% since 2012 [13]. The majority of health expenditure (73.3%) came from direct government funding; 14.4% was funded by health insurance and other private sources; 12.3% came from household out-of-pocket expenditure [13].

The largest proportion (37.2%) of expenditure occurred within hospitals, 18% in long-term residential facilities, and 20% was directed to ambulatory healthcare providers, predominantly general practitioners [13]. Curative and rehabilitative care services provided by hospitals amounted to over one-third of all spending, of which 63% was on in-patient services [13]. Expenditure on pharmaceuticals and other medical non-durables amounted to 13% of the total [13].

At 2.9 per thousand population, Ireland had a low number of practising doctors compared with an EU average of 3.6 in 2015 [14]. By contrast, there were 11.9 nurses per thousand population, compared with an EU average of 8.4 [14]. The number of hospital beds was half that of the EU average at 2.6 per 1000 population [14].

Entitlement to health services is primarily based on residency and means, rather than on payment of tax or pay-related social insurance [15]. Any person, regardless of nationality, who is accepted by the HSE as ordinarily resident in Ireland has eligibility to health services [15]. There are two types of eligibility: full eligibility for those qualified to hold a medical card and limited eligibility for those not qualified. Eligibility for a medical card is established on the basis of age and economic means. Those eligible have charge-free access to general practitioner (GP) services; prescribed drugs and medicines (subject to a modest prescribing charge); public hospital services; dental, optic and aural services; maternity and infant care services; and community and social services [15]. In 2017 [12], 33% of the population held a medical card. A further 10.2% held a doctor visit card allowing charge-free GP visits, but not charge-free prescription medications or exemption from hospital charges [12].

For those not so eligible, GP services incur out-of-pocket charges (which may qualify for taxation relief); prescription medications must be purchased (but charges are capped at €124 per month with a drugs payment scheme, of which 26.3% of the population avails [11]); public hospital outpatient consultations are charge-free, but inpatient care attracts a fee of €80 per day, subject to a maximum of €800 per year; self-referral to an emergency department may also incur a fee [12].

Less than half (42.8%) of the population hold some form of private health insurance, largely to cover inpatient charges, inpatient private consultant charges and some diagnostic test charges, in private hospitals or as private patients in public hospitals [12].

Some 5.5% of the population qualify for a long-term illness card, which allows charge-free access to medications appropriate to designated illnesses, such as diabetes mellitus [12]. Notably, renal diseases are not designated illnesses for this scheme.

## Brief History of Nephrology in Ireland

The beginnings of nephrology as a separate clinical discipline in Ireland may be traced back to the late 1950s [16]. In keeping with new thinking and new technologies then current in Europe with regard to the treatment of renal failure, a multidisciplinary team of doctors established the first Artificial Kidney – Renal Unit in the Charitable Infirmary, Jervis Street, Dublin. Those involved were Dr. Arthur P. Barry (Consultant Obstetrician and Gynaecologist), Dr. Gerard Doyle (Consultant Pathologist), Dr. William F. O'Dwyer (Senior Consultant Physician), Mr. Anthony Walsh (Consultant Urologist) and Dr. Joseph A. Woodcock (Consultant Anaesthetist), who became the first Medical Director of the Unit [16].

A Kolff twin-coil dialyzing unit [17] – the first of its kind in Ireland – was purchased. Staff visited the Artificial Kidney Unit at Leeds General Infirmary, where Dr. Frank Parsons had performed his first dialysis treatment on 30 September 1956. The first haemodialysis treatment (for AKI) in Dublin was performed in May 1958. There followed treatments for many patients, initially all with AKI adjudged to have a reasonable prospect of recovery and many with obstetric AKI [18, 19].

It was not until November 1964 that a programme for regular haemodialysis treatment for end-stage renal disease (ESRD) was established – lack of a sufficient number of machines to be allocated to long-term treatments (the unit possessed only two machines) and difficulty with maintaining long-term vascular access being notable barriers to this [16, 20]. The creation of native vessel arteriovenous fistulae from December 1966 represented a significant improvement in dialysis delivery [21].

In 1963, the first kidney transplant was performed in Ireland [22]. Subsequently a multidisciplinary team was established in the Charitable Infirmary, Jervis Street, to develop a renal transplantation programme [16]. The team was led by Mr. Anthony Walsh (who subsequently became President of EDTA in 1968) and Prof. W.A.L. Gowan, Consultant Vascular Surgeon at St. Laurence's Hospital. The first deceased donor renal transplant performed by this team was on 31 January 1964 [16]. Outcomes with the initial series of transplant patients were not encouraging [16], and relatively few transplants were done until 1967 when the programme recommenced. The first living donor renal transplant was performed in 1972 [16].

In 1970, a Home Haemodialysis (HHD) Programme was established [16]. An additional Nephrology Unit was established at St. Mary's Hospital Dublin in 1971 [16]. In the following year, new renal units were established in Cork and Galway, with another renal unit opening in the Meath Hospital in Dublin [16]. Continuous Ambulatory Peritoneal Dialysis (CAPD) commenced in Ireland in 1980 [44].

By 1988, there were 342 ESRD patients in Ireland treated by dialysis. Two hundred and fifty-seven patients were treated by centre-based haemodialysis (HD) in 1 of 8 renal units, 5 were treated by HHD, and 80 were treated by CAPD (by 4 of the renal units). Further expansion progressively developed over time until the current complement of 12 renal units within 7 hospital groups throughout the country was completed.

In 2002, the Minister for Health commissioned a Strategic Review of Renal Services. This multi-stakeholder review, chaired by Dr. Liam Plant, presented its report in 2006. This report has significantly influenced the subsequent strategic development of renal services. On World Kidney Day 2009, the HSE established a National Renal Office (NRO), embedded within the Clinical Strategy and Programmes Division, with responsibility for planning, coordinating and managing the strategic development of renal services across the country [23]. A key development has been the deployment of the Kidney Disease Clinical Patient Management System (KDCPMS), an electronic patient record system with a common platform, in all renal units in Ireland [24]. This system provides a framework for performance monitoring in renal care provision, comparative clinical audit, enhanced delivery and quality of care, strategic planning and effective resource utilization. It will form the base platform for an intended National Renal Registry.

## Professional and Advocacy Organisations

The Irish Nephrology Society (INS) https://www.nephrology.ie – established in 1969 – is comprised of doctors and scientists working in the care of patients with kidney disease, either at a clinical or research level. Membership extends to all parts of the island, incorporating the Republic of Ireland and Northern Ireland. Its mission is to ensure high-quality care for patients with kidney disease by promoting the highest standard of medical practice. It has an integral role in the education and training of medical practitioners and advises the government, the public and the profession on healthcare issues relating to kidney disease. The INS hosts two National Scientific Meetings each year as well as funding Young Nephrologists' research projects and recognising excellence in research by the award of specific prizes and medals.

The Irish Nephrology Nurses Association (INNA) https://www.inna-ireland.com – established in 1999 – has a mission to promote a high standard of quality care for renal patients and their families through education and research. Since its formation the association is committed to being a voice for nephrology nurses nationally and actively engaging in strategic developments in the area of renal care. The Renal Interest Group of the Irish Nutrition and Dietetic Institute (RIG/INDI) http://www.irishkidneydiet.ie/about-us/ acts as a professional organisation and forum for those practising as renal dieticians.

The primary role of the Irish Kidney Association https://ika.ie – a charitable voluntary organisation established in 1978 – is to support patients and their families who are affected by end-stage kidney disease and are being treated either by dialysis or with a functioning kidney transplant. As the only organisation representing the views of Irish kidney patients, the IKA constantly lobbies on their behalf. The priority of the association is to ensure that the unmet needs of the renal patient and family are addressed by the statutory health and education system either directly from the mainstream or via an association like itself.

## Renal Disease in Ireland

The population of Ireland in 2015 had a lower (13%) – but rapidly expanding – proportion of its population aged >64 years than the total EU population (18.9%) [14]. The vast majority of the population (92.4%) has a White ethnic background [2]. A higher proportion of the population was obese than the EU total – 18% on self-reported data and 23% based on actual measures of height and weight [14]. Between 1998 and 2015 the national prevalence of doctor-diagnosed diabetes mellitus increased from 2.8% to 5.2% [25]. This background profile has a significant influence on the incidence and prevalence of renal diseases in Ireland.

### Chronic Kidney Disease and End-Stage Renal Disease

Ireland does not have a national CKD (non-RRT) registry [26]. Incidence and prevalence studies are limited [26].

A randomly selected population based cross-sectional study of 1098 adults aged 45 years and older was conducted using data from the 2007 Survey of Lifestyle, Attitudes and Nutrition (SLÁN) [27]. Estimated Glomerular Filtration Rate (eGFR) was calculated from a single IDMS aligned serum creatinine using the CKD-EPI and the MDRD equations, and albumin to creatinine ratio was based on a single random urine sample [27]. The estimated weighted prevalence [27] of CKD-EPI eGFR<60 mL/min/1.73m$^2$ was 11.6% (95% CI 9.0–14.2%), being 12.0% (9.0–14.2%) of men and 11.2% (7.3–15.2%) of women. Ten percent (10.1%) of all subjects had albuminuria and an eGFR≥60 mL/min/1.73 m$^2$. Thus, in Irish adults aged over 45 years, the overall weighted estimated prevalence of the National Kidney Foundation (NKF)-defined CKD was 21.3% (18.0–24.6%) [27]. Twelve percent (12.4%) of subjects aged 60 to 69 years had stage 3 CKD, as had 36.2% of those aged over 70 years [27].

Another study [28] identified 207,336 adult patients, aged 18 years and over, with serum creatinine measurements recorded from a provincial database between 2005 and 2011 in the Northwest of Ireland. eGFR rates were determined using the CKD-EPI equation from standardised creatinine measurements, and the presence of CKD was defined as eGFR <60 ml/min per 1.73 m$^2$. The prevalence of CKD was 11.8% (95% CI 11.3–12.1%): 10.9% in men (10.7–11.1%) and 12.6% in women (12.4–12.8%) [28]. This corresponded to a detection rate of 4.5% (5.1% in women and 3.9% in men) [28].

The systematic review and meta-analysis of Hill and colleagues [29] suggested a global mean (95% CI) CKD prevalence of five stages to be 13·4% (11·7–15·1%) and of stages 3–5 to be 10·6% (9·2–12·2%). CKD prevalence in Ireland seems to fall within this range.

Although a formal ESRD Registry is not in place, the National Renal Office [23] has been collecting annual incidence and prevalence data for more than a decade, more recently utilising the KDCPMS platform [24]. On 31 December 2018, some 4572 adults and 80 children were living with ESRD in Ireland [7]. This equates to a prevalence of 941 pmp for adults and 16 pmp for children [7]. Over half of adults (53%) had a functioning renal transplant, as had 80% of children [7]. In 2013 [7], the incidence of ESRD in adults was 405 cases, equating to 88 pmp. Incomplete reporting since then indicates an ESRD incident rate of 85–95 pmp.

In the 2013 USRDS Report on geographic variation in the incidence of treated ESRD pmp by country, Ireland (88 pmp) fell into the lowest of four incidence groupings at <120 pmp, falling within 10 pmp of such countries as Iceland, Finland, Switzerland and Scotland [30]. An ESRD prevalence then of 862 pmp fell within the lower mid-range of countries, falling within 50 pmp of such countries as Romania, Finland, Serbia, Argentina, Scotland, Turkey, Denmark, Norway and England and Wales [30].

There is a lack of systematic data as to the causes of CKD in Ireland mostly relating to methodological variation in disease allocation and data recording. In a recent study [31] utilising the KDCPMS platform, the authors felt that for 1196 haemodialysis patients, the underlying cause of ESRD was either unknown or missing in 28% of cases. Glomerulonephritis accounted for 19.2% of cases, diabetic nephropathy for 18.6% and cystic kidney disease for 6.4%. A single-centre study [32] of all 692 incident ESRD patients between 1 January 2002 and 13 December 2015 reported that 21% of cases were due to diabetic nephropathy, 17% to glomerulonephritis, 9% to polycystic kidney disease, 7% to pyelonephritis and 5% to vascular disease. 19% of cases were attributed to a miscellaneous group of diagnoses, and 19% were of unknown or unspecified causes.

## Acute Kidney Injury

Ireland does not have a national acute kidney injury (AKI) registry. Incidence and outcome studies are limited.

A retrospective cohort study (2005–2014) used data from two regional laboratory information systems to determine incidence and severity rates of AKI [33]. The Kidney Disease: Improving Global Outcomes (KDIGO) criteria were used to identify all AKI events and subclassify each by severity grade. Incidence rates for men increased from 6.1% (95% CI 5.8–6.3%) per 100 patient-years to 13.2% (12.7–13.8%) during this period and from 5.0% (4.8–5.2%) to 10.1% (9.8–10.5%) for women [33]. Incidence rates for AKI increased in all locations of clinical supervision but much more for inpatient and emergency room settings compared with general practice [33].

At present, acute hospitals in Ireland are organised into six hospital groups covering specific geographic areas and a paediatric hospital group [34]. Within each hospital group is at least one renal unit, which acts as the regional resource for advice or direct management (sometimes following patient transfer) of cases of AKI. Not all hospitals have a renal unit on campus; some ICU units in specific hospitals have the capacity to deliver continuous renal replacement therapies; the largest (Model 4) hospitals typically have the capacity to deliver acute renal replacement therapies, either as acute haemodialysis or as continuous venovenous haemo(dia)filtration.

## Glomerulopathies

Ireland does not have a national glomerulonephritis (GN) registry. Incidence and outcome studies are limited. Ireland did not participate in the International Kidney Biopsy Survey [35]. A single-centre retrospective study has been reported [36]; 1372 native renal biopsies were performed between 2004 and 2008. Of these, 236 (17%) were performed in patients aged >64 years. The commonest indications for biopsy in those aged >64 years were AKI (32%) and nephrotic syndrome (25%). Obviously, a mix of histological features was encountered, depending on presentation. The commonest glomerular conditions reported in this series in total were pauci-immune GN (17.4%); membranous GN (8.9%); IgA GN (7.6%); minimal change disease (4.2%); and post-infectious GN (3.4%) [36]. It is probable that a different spread would be detected in younger patients and depending on presentation.

## Renal Disease in the Paediatric Population in Ireland

The Irish Paediatric Nephrology Services have evolved over the last 30 years. Specialist Paediatric Nephrology Services are provided on two campuses in Dublin, with a complement of six consultant paediatric nephrologists. The service will shortly move to the National Children's Hospital site when it is commissioned. At present 750 new patients are seen per annum, with 2500 review appointments also provided [37]. Each year 8 children develop ESRD; 15–25 are waiting for a kidney transplant; 25 develop significant haemolytic uraemic syndrome; and 200 have nephrotic syndrome [37]. Every year 1000 Irish children are born with some kind of congenital abnormality of the kidney or urinary tract [37].

About 60 children are under follow-up with a functioning kidney transplant [7, 37]. Structured adolescent to adult transition clinics are available in Dublin and Cork. In 2018 an outreach paediatric nephrology clinic was established in Cork. The future development of Paediatric Nephrology Services is incorporated into the HSE National Clinical Programme for Paediatrics and Neonatology Model of Care [37].

There has been considerable clinical and research interest in hereditary renal diseases in Ireland [38–40].

## Renal Replacement Therapy for ESRD in Ireland

All modalities of renal replacement therapies (RRT) are available in Ireland. Although some patients may elect to have private outpatient/inpatient consultations with a nephrologist, the bulk of costs, particularly the direct costs of dialysis modalities, is borne by the State. All adult ESRD patients are under the clinical governance of 1 of the 11 HSE adult renal units. All paediatric ESRD patients are under the clinical governance of the paediatric renal unit.

A formal ESRD Registry is not yet in place, but the National Renal Office [23] has been collecting annual incidence and prevalence data for more than a decade, more recently utilising the KDCPMS platform [24]. On 31 December 2018, some 4572 adults and 80 children were living with ESRD in Ireland [7]. This equates to a prevalence of 941 pmp for adults and 16 pmp for children [7]. 54% of adults had a functioning renal transplant, as had 80% of children [7].

If one focuses on RRT modalities in adults, it has been the case that, at least for the last 15 years, the majority of patients alive with ESRD each year have had a functioning transplant [7]. Between 2007 and 2017 there has been a 41% (n = 1300) increase in the number of adults with ESRD [7]. In that interval, the increase in those treated by dialysis has been 35% (n = 535) and by transplantation 47% (n = 765).

Data on patient survival from entry into ESRD is available from a single centre [32]. Six hundred and ninety-two patients entered ESRD between 1 January 2002 and 31 December 2015. If surviving for 90 days, 95% of those aged <65 years survived for 1 year and 77% for 5 years; 89% of

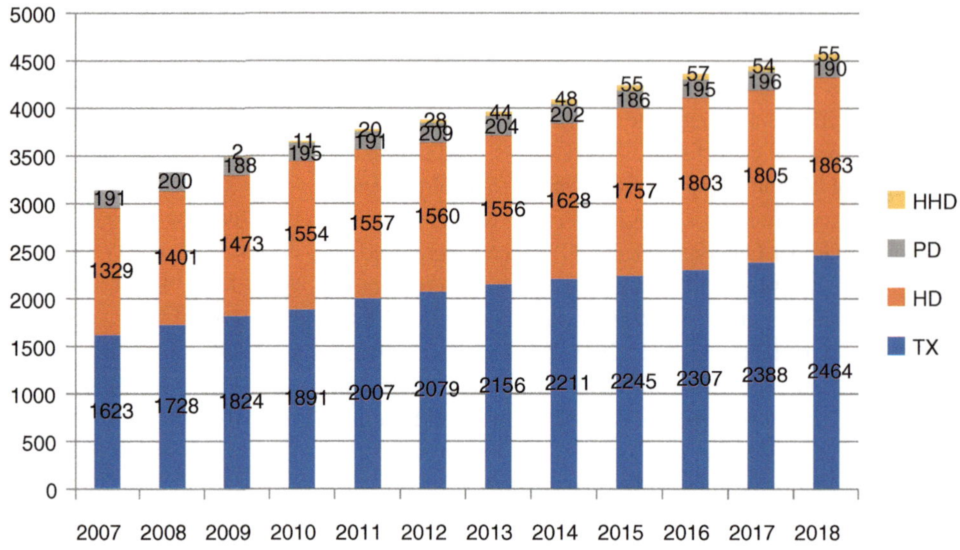


**Fig. 42.1** Increase in number of adults with ESRD 2007–2018, by modality. (HHD home haemodialysis, PD peritoneal dialysis, HD centre-based haemodialysis, TX renal transplant)

those aged >64 years survived for 1 year and 47% for 5 years [32]. As would be expected, there was a considerable survival advantage to the 30% of these who received a renal transplant [32].

As illustrated in Fig. 42.1, 54% of adults with ESRD have a functioning transplant, 41% are treated by centre-based HD and 5% by a home-based modality, either home haemodialysis (HHD) or peritoneal dialysis (PD). This percent distribution in types of RRT modalities used is very similar to that in Scotland, England and Wales [41]. The National Renal Office has set a target that 60% of ESRD patients should ideally be treated with a functioning transplant and that of those treated by dialysis, at least 20% should be treated in the home setting, either by HHD or PD. These targets are occasionally attained in individual renal units but have not yet done so consistently on a national basis [7]. As in other jurisdictions, there are increasing attributable economic and social costs between home-based, satellite centre-based and hospital centre-based therapies.

Ireland does not yet have a model to commission RRT treatments, nor an activity-based funding stream for specific therapies. Each hospital group bears the expenditure cost of RRT within its core budget; additional funding from central HSE resources is allocated based on ongoing evaluation of total activity by the NRO [7]. For a minority of patients, health insurance reimburses consultant fees for private consultations in supervising dialysis patients, but not for consumables, equipment or training – the costs of which are reimbursed from public funds. The costs per treatment of HD treatments within contracted commercial units are reimbursed by the hospital group under whose clinical governance the patient falls [7].

## Centre-Based and Satellite Centre-Based Haemodialysis (HD)

Centre-based HD (or, for a significant proportion, haemodiafiltration –HDF) is the commonest modality of dialysis delivered [7]. Not all units utilise haemodiafiltration, and the proportion varies within those that do, largely based upon the clinical judgement of the staff within the units. There is one national paediatric HD centre at the Children's University Hospital, Temple Street, Dublin. The 11 adult renal units within the 6 hospital groups supervise 22 separate HD centres. Eleven of these are directly provided on major hospital campuses; three are directly provided satellite HD centres on smaller hospital campuses; and eight are contracted satellite HD centres, staffed and provided by commercial dialysis providers (but with the parent HSE renal unit retaining clinical governance) [7]. Contracts for dialysis equipment and consumables are awarded by competitive tender within hospital groups; the provision of contracted HD centres is also awarded by competitive tender. All HD centres now host/interact with the KDCPMS [24]. Strategic development of HD services as a national integrated network is coordinated by the NRO [7].

HD centres vary in size from 10 patients or less (the paediatric HD centre) to 150–160 patients (Cork University Hospital and Beaumont Hospital Dublin) [7]. Three other HD centres treat >100 patients, but the typical HD centre caters for 60–90 patients [7]. The location of new HD centres will be decided based on the need to reduce patient travel time and avoid overcrowding in existing HD centres. In 2012, 50% of patients lived >29 km from the HD centre where they were treated [7]. Patient transport to/from HD centres is widely provided but with differences in organisation and eligibility from region to region [7].

In 2017, 29% of patients treated by centre-based HD were treated in contracted satellite HD centres (amounting to 25% of all dialysis patients and 12% of all ESRD patients) [7]. HD treatments for AKI are not delivered in these centres, and patients who are unwell will typically have the location of their treatment transferred to the parent renal unit.

Both centre-based HD units and contracted satellite HD units are predominantly staffed by registered general nurses, with smaller numbers of healthcare assistants. Dialysis technicians are not a feature in Ireland, as opposed to dialysis biotechnicians who work to introduce and maintain dialysis and other equipment. Typically the ratio of dialysis nurses to patients will vary from 1:3 to 1:4 during treatment delivery, with additional shift leaders, clinical nurse managers and other educational/administrative staff. Renal dieticians are attached to all renal units, but with a low dietician to patient ratio. Dedicated renal psychologists, renal pharmacists and renal social workers are very uncommon in Irish HD units – such services are accessed from generic resources by patients.

The vast majority of patients are treated thrice weekly. Dialysers are not reused in Ireland. Difficulties in establishing native AV access [31], and mitigating the infective risk of tunnelled HD access [42], remain an ongoing challenge. There is considerable variation (27–57%) in the proportion of those using native AV access across centres [31]. Most HD centres operate at or close to capacity, and this has implications if there are regional surges in new patients; it has also restricted easy access to holiday HD sessions both for Irish and for international patients [7].

The prevalence of blood-borne virus infections (HBV, HCV, HIV) is very low in Irish HD units (<3% of patients), but facilities for isolation are found in all units, and a standardised national policy to minimise the risk of transmission is in practice [7]. Patients infected with hepatitis C are eligible for antiviral therapies with a view to its eradication.

## Home Haemodialysis (HHD)

In Ireland, HHD and peritoneal dialysis (PD) are viewed as complementary renal home therapies. Equipment, training and protocols have a uniform structure throughout the country. There is a national competitive contract for equipment and consumables, and the six renal units providing training in HHD are linked via a National Renal Home Therapies Programme by the NRO [7].

HHD was initially provided in Ireland in 1970. Having initially been a very significant modality, it declined with the development of a wider network of regional HD centres and CAPD. A national programme was reinstituted in 2009 [43]. Analysis of the first 100 patients trained indicated that, during the period of follow-up, 29% were transplanted, 9% died and only 7% reverted to centre-based HD [43]. Twenty percent (20%) of patients were treated by nocturnal HHD (NHHD). This pattern has continued, with transplantation being the principle reason for modality change. In 2018, six renal units supervised a total of 55 HHD patients [7]. The two largest renal units in Dublin and Cork accounted for 64% of this total.

## Peritoneal Dialysis (PD)

CAPD was first delivered in Ireland in 1980 [44]. Training in both CAPD and automated PD (APD) is provided by the paediatric renal unit and eight of the adult renal units [7]. The proportion treated by APD varies, depending on patient choice and clinical considerations – typically about two thirds of all patients utilise APD. The proportion of new ESRD patients whose first modality of dialysis was PD between 2008 and 2013 was 14% [7]. In 2017, 10% of all prevalent ESRD dialysis patients were treated by PD [7], although the proportion varied considerably between hospital groups. As a proportion, this has remained relatively constant over the last decade [7], renal transplantation being amongst the commonest reasons for modality switch.

Reported outcomes [45] are similar to those reported from comparable health systems. Peritonitis rates are low. Both percutaneous and laparoscopic surgical catheter placement techniques are in use [46].

## Renal Transplantation

Renal transplantation has been performed in Ireland since the early 1960s [16, 22, 47, 48]. In that period over 4500 renal transplant procedures have been performed, and the National Renal Transplant Programme is now located in Beaumont Hospital, Dublin [47, 49]. Since 2003, the majority of paediatric kidney transplants have been performed in the Children's University Hospital, Temple Street, Dublin [47]. Having been in abeyance for some years, the National Living Donor Renal Transplant Programme was re-established in 2005 [47].

In the 5 years between 2014 and 2018, 632 kidney transplants from deceased donors were performed (including 15 simultaneous pancreas-kidney transplants), as were 240 (27.5% of the total) from living donors – 26 of these were organs transplanted within the context of a Paired Kidney Exchange Programme with the United Kingdom or desensitised in the UK [8]. Thus, there has been an average of 174 kidney transplants per annum in that interval [8]. This is illustrated in Fig. 42.2.

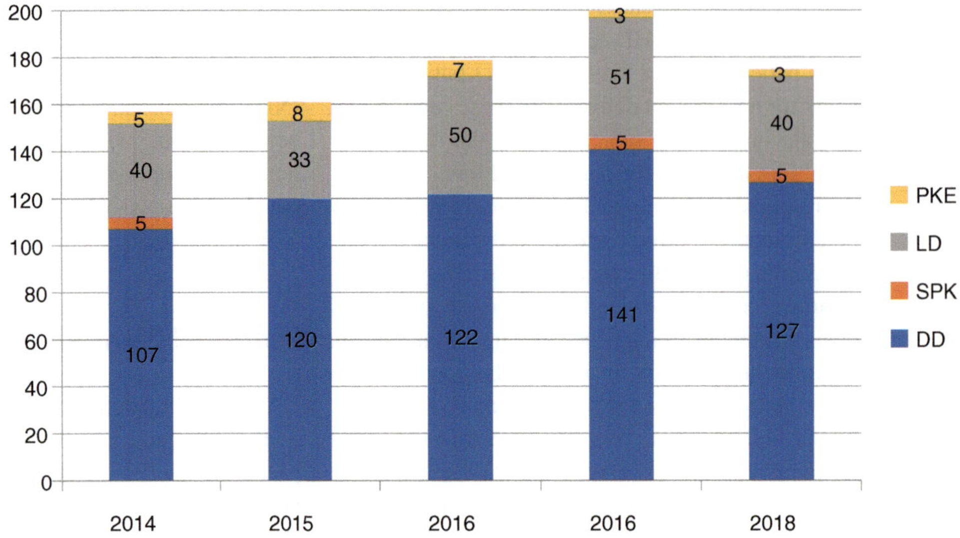


**Fig. 42.2** Renal transplants by type 2014–2018. (PKE Paired Kidney Exchange/ Desensitised in the United Kingdom, LD living donor, SPKT simultaneous pancreas-kidney transplant, DD deceased donor)

The Pancreas-Kidney Transplant Programme, previously co-located with the National Kidney Transplant Programme in Beaumont Hospital, has, since 2017, co-located with the National Liver Transplant Programme on another campus in Dublin.

Organ Donation and Transplant Ireland (ODTI) has been delegated the regulator functions assigned to the HSE in the Statutory Instrument (SI) 325 (2012), European Union (Quality and Safety of Human Organs Intended for Transplantation) Regulations 2012 [50]. Since March 2019, the Department of Health has introduced a new policy on the reimbursement of the expenses incurred by living kidney donors [51].

Currently there is no legislation relating to organ donation in Ireland [8]. It has historically functioned on the basis of voluntarism and clinical interest in organ donation [8]. A new Human Tissue Bill is anticipated, which will address, amongst other issues, the establishment of a "soft" opt-out system for deceased donor kidney procedures [8].

In the period 2014–2018, deceased organ donation came from an average of 84.5 persons per annum [8]. It is hoped that with more widespread acceptance of organs from older donors or from those with cardiac death, and with the infrastructural changes introduced by ODTI and the proposed legislative changes in the Human Tissue Bill, the numbers of deceased donors will pass above 20 pmp to a target of 26 pmp [8].

More than half (54%) of adults with ESRD in Ireland have a functioning renal transplant, a rate of just over 500 pmp [7]. This relatively high proportion reflects a relatively high organ donation rate, with a relatively low prevalence of ESRD, and good long-term transplant survival [7, 8, 48]. Between 2012 and 2016, 1-year allograft survival was 97% for deceased donor recipients and 94% for living donor recipients [8]. Ninety-eight percent (98%) of deceased donor recipients and 100% of living donor recipients were alive at 1 year [8]. Five-year allograft survival was 86% for deceased donor recipients and 89% for living donor recipients, with patient survival rates of 88% and 97%, respectively [8]. A retrospective study of 3260 transplant recipients from 1971 to 2015 indicated that 15-year allograft survival had improved from 10% for those transplanted in 1971–1975 to 45% for those transplanted between 1996 and 2000 [48].

All adult kidney transplant procedures are performed in the National Kidney Transplant Service at Beaumont Hospital, Dublin [49]; all paediatric kidney transplant procedures are performed at the Children's University Hospital, Temple Street, Dublin; all pancreas-kidney transplants are performed in St. Vincent's University Hospital, Dublin; a small number of procedures are performed in the United Kingdom as part of the Paired Kidney Exchange Programme [8]. Once stabilised, long-term follow-up for the majority (66%) of recipients is delivered by the referring renal unit [7].

In 2018, the median waiting time for a first kidney transplant was 22 months and 11 months for those who received a living donor transplant [8]. At the end of 2018, some 429 patients were on the waiting list; 167 transplants were performed during the year, and 178 new patients activated on the list [8]. This compares with a waiting list of 551 patients at the end of 2016 [8]. 156 potential living donors (for 103 potential recipients) initiated assessment, with 85 progressing to the 1-day assessment phase, and 40 living transplant procedures were performed during the year [8]. The immunosuppression protocols for patients with standard immunological risk incorporate induction with IL2ra agents, followed by long-term tacrolimus and mycophenolate mofetil maintenance therapy. Steroid withdrawal is practised in fewer than half of patients.

As in other countries, research into, and surveillance of, complications of transplantation is ongoing. In a study of 3346 Irish solid organ transplant recipients (71.2% renal transplants), the commonest cancers were squamous cell skin cancer with SIR (95% CI) 20.05 (17.97–22.31), basal cell skin cancer 7.16 (6.43–7.96), non-Hodgkin lymphoma 6.23 (4.26–8.59) and renal cell carcinoma 3.36 (1.96–5.38) [52]. New-onset diabetes after transplant (NODAT) was observed in 10.5% of patients within the first 5 years post-engraftment [53].

The survival of patients successfully transplanted (annual death rate 1.2 per 100 patient years at risk) is considerably improved (after a survival equilibrium time of 1-year post-engraftment) compared with waiting-list patients (2.4) and non-listed patients on dialysis (16.5) [54].

## Critical Care Nephrology

The nephrology services in Ireland work closely with colleagues in critical care. Many of the intensive care units (ICUs) are equipped, staffed and trained to deliver renal replacement therapy for patients with AKI and multi-organ failure. The Model of Care for Adult Critical Care of the National Clinical Programme for Critical Care identifies the need for access to continuous venovenous haemofiltration (CVVH) for level 3 ICUs and Model 4 regional and supra-regional hospitals [55].

In a 3-year retrospective single-centre study of 450 patients treated by CVVH in a Model 4 hospital, mortality in ICU was 38%, in hospital was 47%, and at 1-year was 54%. Three hundred and ninety patients had AKI, whilst 60 (13%) had pre-existing ESRD [56]. 6% of those with AKI aged <75 years who survived to discharge were RRT-dependent, as were 8.6% of those aged >74 years [56].

## Nephrology Practice in Ireland

Non-ESRD CKD care is predominantly supervised by general practitioners (GPs). In patients with identified glomerular diseases, with heavy proteinuria, with rapidly declining GFR, with hereditary nephropathies or with low clearance CKD, there is shared management with renal unit outpatient services. As complexity increases, or when patients transition to ESRD, the renal unit staff have a progressively increasing role in the long-term care pathway delivery. Other disciplines commonly participating will be, amongst others, diabetologists, cardiologists, vascular surgeons and urologists. Typically, the supervising renal unit will have a significant input into the care pathway for any other medical condition which such patients may develop (especially for those with an ESKD need) in partnership with appropriate other specialties.

Guidelines for GPs are available from the Irish College of General Practitioners [57]. Guidelines for patients are available from the HSE [58] and from the Irish Kidney Association (IKA) [59].

Management of AKI is predominantly by the in-patient medical/surgical team supervising the patient. As complexity and/or severity of AKI increases, nephrologists and/or intensive care staff will play an increasing role. Although not formally endorsed, there is widespread adherence to the recommendations of the KDIGO Clinical Practice Guideline for Acute Kidney Injury [60].

There are about 50 consultants in Ireland accredited in nephrology and appointed to clinical and/or academic posts in which at least some of their practice is in nephrology [6]. Twenty one (42%) are female [6]. The overwhelming majority are employed in the public sector, albeit with varying entitlement to private practice [6]. Many also contribute to undifferentiated general internal medicine activities; many have substantial research, teaching, administrative or leadership appointments; as a consequence of which, there are probably no more than 30 whole time equivalent (WTE) consultant sessions devoted to nephrology in Ireland – much lower than in many other countries [6, 26].

The vast majority of these consultants will have had some of their nephrology training outside of Ireland; some will have held consultant, attending or other faculty positions in other countries. These countries are typically, but not exclusively, English-speaking, such as England and Wales, Scotland, Canada, Australia, New Zealand or the United States [6].

Since 1999, Ireland has had a Higher Specialist Training in Nephrology Scheme, under the governance of the Irish Committee on Higher Medical Training [61]. Many of the alumni of this scheme have progressed to whole-time consultant appointments in Ireland, and it remains a highly desired training scheme with a very high calibre of applicant. The tradition of spending at least some time training abroad remains.

Entry to this scheme requires completion of general professional training and successful completion of the examinations needed to allow membership of the Royal College of Physicians of Ireland [61]. The duration of training is for a minimum of 5 years – 2 spent in nephrology/GIM clinical posts; 1 spent in a high-intensity GIM clinical post; 1 in a high-intensity nephrology post; and at least 1 year spent in research activities or other out-of-programme experience. On completion of this cycle, trainees are awarded a Certificate of Completion of Specialist Training and join the Specialist Register in Nephrology [61]. However, new opportunities to take up consultant posts in Ireland remain limited.

Renal nursing careers can have a focus in a variety of roles – inpatient care, delivery of haemodialysis care, outpatient care, etc. There are a number of clinical nurse specialists and advanced nurse practitioners specialising in low clearance/pre-dialysis care, in post-transplant care, in renal home therapies and in vascular access, to mention but a few. Postgraduate NFQ Level 9 (Postgraduate Diploma/MSc) courses are provided by a variety of universities and institutes of technology [62].

Renal dietitians, although few in number, are attached to renal units around the country and work together via the Renal Interest Group of the Irish Nutrition and Dietetic Institute to bring a national consistency to practice and to promote a healthy renal diet [63].

Pay scales in nephrology are the same as for other clinicians of comparable grade working in the public system. Annual salaries for consultants vary from €165,000 to €273,000, depending upon when they were appointed, where in the country they work and what proportion of their activity is exclusively devoted to public work. There is a wide variation in the amount of additional income generated by activities focussing on the care of private patients. Annual salaries for renal nurses range from €29,800 to €64,500, depending on seniority or whether they work as clinical nurse specialists, advanced nurse practitioners or clinical nurse managers. Annual salaries for renal dieticians range from €36,000 to €76,500, depending on seniority and role [64].

Irish renal units are involved in much collaborative and integrated research activities. Examples would include the Rare Kidney Disease Registry and Biobank [65]; the Vasculitis Ireland Network (VINE) [66]; the Irish Kidney Gene Project [67]; studies on the health-related quality of life of ESRD patients on dialysis [68]; and within the GEnetics of Nephropathy: An International Effort (GENIE) Consortium [69].

## Future Perspectives of Nephrology in Ireland

In Ireland, patients with kidney disease have access to a very highly trained workforce of multidisciplinary clinicians; to the most modern diagnostic equipment and medications; to the support of an active advocacy organisation (the IKA) [70]; and to a reasonably well-integrated national service with a high degree of internal concordance and collaboration. The principal challenge going forward relates to a lack of capacity within the service.

Within each of the renal units, the available HD centres continuously operate at or close to full capacity [7]. This can cause considerable problems within HD centres if there is a surge in new patient presentations or in a need to transfer patients from satellite centres to parent centres. It also restricts access to Holiday HD slots. Despite a programme of commissioning new HD centres over the last decade, demand still outstrips supply. Until this balance is restored, this item in particular introduces an unnecessary stress to care pathways.

Also reflecting capacity issues (access to vascular surgeons; access to operating theatres) is the poor proportion (27–57%) of HD patients with a functioning AV fistula. Despite an integrated national system to promote the different modalities of home-based dialysis, the national target – that at least 20% of dialysis patients should have the opportunity to avail of this – has not yet been reached. Similarly, there remains a need to maximise access to deceased donor kidneys and to those from living donors.

The KDCPMS platform needs to form the basis of a real-time Renal Registry as well as enhancing the collection of activity metrics and outcome measures.

Most deficient, however, remains the low number of clinicians. The number of consultant nephrologist WTEs varies, from 0.5 to 0.7 per 100 ESRD patients and from 3.0 to 7.0 pmp catchment population, between hospital groups. This is an unusually low proportion by international standards [26]. Expansion is needed to provide the critical mass to deliver optimum national clinical, teaching and research outputs. The same applies for renal clinical nurse specialists/advanced nurse practitioners and renal dieticians. Continued vigilance to ensure that equipment and consumable procurement obtains best value is necessary.

Easily accessible guidelines for GPs, non-renal hospital doctors and patients need to continue to be developed.

## Conclusion

Ireland has the appropriate organisation, structures, equipment and personnel to deliver top quality renal care. The principal challenges are insufficient capacity within the RRT centres and insufficient clinicians.

## References


1. The World Bank Group. Accessed in October 2019. Available from: https://databank.worldbank.org/views/reports/reportwidget.aspx?Report_Name=CountryProfile&Id=b450fd57&tbar=y&dd=y&inf=n&zm=n&country=IRL
2. Central Statistics Office. Accessed in October 2019. Available from: https://www.cso.ie/en/releasesandpublications/er/pme/populationandmigrationestimatesapril2019/
3. Central Statistics Office. Accessed in October 2019. Available from: https://www.cso.ie/en/media/csoie/newsevents/documents/census2016summaryresultspart1/Census2016SummaryPart1.pdf
4. OECD Functional urban areas. Version: January 2019. Accessed in October 2019. Available from: http://www.oecd.org/cfe/regional-policy/Ireland.pdf
5. United Nations Development Programme. Human Development Reports. Accessed in October 2019. Available from: http://hdr.undp.org/sites/default/files/2018_human_development_statistical_update.pdf

6. Irish Nephrology Society (INS) Membership data. Personal communication from President of INS. October 2019.
7. Health Service Executive National Renal Office. Programme Documents and Resources. Accessed in October 2019. Available from: https://www.hse.ie/eng/about/who/cspd/ncps/renal/resources/
8. Organ Donation Transplant Ireland Annual Report 2018. Accessed in October 2019. Available from: https://www.hse.ie/eng/about/who/acute-hospitals-division/organ-donation-transplant-ireland/publications/organ-donation-and-transplant-annual-report-2018.pdf
9. World Bank Group. The Human Capital Project. Accessed in October 2019. Available from: https://openknowledge.worldbank.org/bitstream/handle/10986/30498/33252.pdf?sequence=5&isAllowed=y
10. Government of Ireland. Department of Health. Health Policy. Accessed in October 2019. Available from: https://www.gov.ie/en/policy/c75aa0-health/
11. Government of Ireland. Department of Health. The Sláintecare Report. Accessed in October 2019. Available from: https://assets.gov.ie/22609/e68786c13e1b4d7daca89b495c506bb8.pdf
12. Government of Ireland. Health in Ireland Key Trends 2018. Accessed in October 2019. Available from: https://assets.gov.ie/9441/e5c5417ee4c544b384c262f99da77122.pdf
13. Central Statistics Office. Ireland's System of Health Accounts, Annual Results 2017. Accessed in October 2017. Available from: https://www.cso.ie/en/releasesandpublications/er/sha/systemofhealthaccounts2017/
14. European Commission. European Observatory on Health Systems and Policies. State of Health in the EU: Ireland Country Health Profile 2017. Accessed in October 2019. Available from: https://ec.europa.eu/health/sites/health/files/state/docs/chp_ir_english.pdf
15. Citizen's Information. Health System. Accessed in October 2017. Available from: https://www.citizensinformation.ie/en/health/health_system/
16. Carmody M. How the specialty of Nephrology was born. Irish Medical Times Special Souvenir Millennium Issue. 2000.
17. Kolff WJ, Watschinger B, Vertes V. Results in patients treated with the coil kidney (disposable dialyzing unit). JAMA. 1956;161(15):1433–7.
18. Walsh A, O'Dwyer WF, Woodcock JA, Doyle G, Barry AP. Earlier dialysis in renal failure. Br J Urol. 1961;33(4):430–4.
19. Barry AP, Carmody M, Woodcock JA, O'Dwyer WF, Walsh A, Doyle G. Renal failure unit: obstetrical and Gynaecological admissions. BJOG. 1964;71(6):899–907.
20. Walsh A, Carmody M, O'Dwyer WF. Dublin experience in maintenance dialysis – with a comment on bilateral nephrectomy. Br J Urol. 1966;38(6):621–2.
21. Hanson JS, Carmody M, Keogh B, O'Dwyer WF. Access to circulation by permanent arteriovenous fistula in regular dialysis treatment. BMJ. 1967;4:586–9.
22. Kennedy C, Counihan A, Magee C. Transplantation in Ireland – erratum. Transplantation. 2017;101(12):e353.
23. Health Service Executive National Renal Office. Accessed in October 2019. Available from: https://www.hse.ie/eng/about/who/cspd/ncps/renal/
24. eHealth Ireland. Kidney Disease Clinical Management System (KDCPMS). Accessed in October 2019. Available from: https://www.ehealthireland.ie/Strategic-Programmes/Kidney-Disease-Clinical-Patient-Management-System-KDCPMS-/
25. Tracey MS, Gilmartin M, O'Neill K, Fitzgerald AP, McHugh SM, Buckley CM, Canavan RJ, Kearney PM. Epidemiology of diabetes and complications among adults in the Republic of Ireland 1998-2015: a systematic review and meta-analysis. BMC Public Health. 2016;16:132.
26. Kidney Health for Life (KH4L). Chronic Kidney Disease Multinational Inventory. March 2014. Accessed October 2019. Available from: https://www.theisn.org/images/Initiatives/KH4L_-_CKD_Multinational_Inventory.pdf
27. Browne GM, Eustace JA, Fitzgerald AP, Lutomski JE, Perry IJ. Prevalence of diminished kidney function in a representative sample of middle and older age adults in the Irish population. BMC Nephrol. 2012;13:144.
28. Stack AG, Casserly LF, Cronin CJ, Chernenko T, Cullen W, Hannigan A, Saran R, Johnson H, Browne G, Ferguson JP. Prevalence and variation of chronic kidney disease in the Irish health system: initial findings from the National Kidney Disease Surveillance Programme. BMC Nephrol. 2014;15:185.
29. Health Service Executive National Renal Office. Programme Documents and Resources. Accessed in October 2019. Available from: https://www.hse.ie/eng/about/who/cspd/ncps/renal/resources/nro-year-end-statistics-2018.pdf
30. United States Renal Data System, 2015 USRDS annual data report: Epidemiology of kidney disease in the United States. Volume 2, Chapter 13 – International comparisons. National Institutes of Health, National Institute of Diabetes and Digestive and Kidney Diseases, Bethesda, MD, 2015.
31. Hussein WF, Mohammed H, Browne L, Plant L, Stack AG. Prevalence and correlates of central venous catheter use among haemodialysis patients in the Irish health system – a national study. BMC Nephrol. 2018;19:76.
32. Murray SL, Dahly DL, Canney M, Eustace J, Plant WD. Survival with ESKD in South West Ireland from 2001 to 2015. Poster SP308, 55th ERA-EDTA Congress, Copenhagen, Denmark 2018.
33. Stack AG, Li X, Kaballo M, Elsayed ME, Johnson H, Murray PT, Saran R, Browne LD. Temporal trends in acute kidney injury across health care settings in the Irish health system: a cohort study. Nephrol Dial Transplant. 2018:gfy226. https://doi.org/10.1093/ndt/gfy226.
34. Health Service Executive Acute Hospitals Division. Hospital Groups. Accessed October 2019. Available from: https://www.hse.ie/eng/about/who/acute-hospitals-division/hospital-groups/
35. O'Shaughnessy MM, Hogan SL, Thompson BD, Coppo R, Fogo AB, Jennette JC. Glomerular disease frequencies by race, sex and region: results from the international kidney biopsy survey. Nephrol Dial Transplant. 2018;33(4):661–9.
36. Brown CM, Scheven L, O'Kelly P, Dorman AM, Walshe JJ. Renal histology in the elderly: indications and outcomes. J Nephrol. 2012;25(2):240–4.
37. Health Service Executive Clinical Strategy & Programmes Division. Paediatrics and Neonatology Model of Care: Chapter 32 Paediatric Nephrology. Accessed October 2019. Available from: https://www.hse.ie/eng/services/publications/clinical-strategy-and-programmes/paediatric-nephrology.pdf
38. Connaughton DM, Kennedy C, Shril S, Mann N, Murray SL, Williams PA, Conlon E, Nakayama M, van der Ven AT, Ityel H, Kause F, Kolvenbach CM, Dai R, Vivante A, Braun DA, Schneider R, Kitzler TM, Moloney B, Moran CP, Smyth JS, Kennedy A, Benson K, Stapleton C, Denton M, Magee C, O'Seaghdha CM, Plant WD, Griffin MD, Awan A, Sweeney C, Mane SM, Lifton RP, Griffin B, Leavey S, Casserly L, de Freitas DG, Holian J, Dorman A, Doyle B, Lavin PJ, Little MA, Conlon PJ, Hildebrandt F. Monogenic causes of chronic kidney disease in adults. Kidney Int. 2019;95:914–28.
39. Cormican S, Connaughton DM, Kennedy C, Murray S, Źivna M, Kmoch S, Fennelly NK, O'Kelly P, Benson KA, Conlon ET, Cavalleri G, Foley C, Doyle B, Dorman A, Little MA, Lavin P, Kidd K, Bleyer AL, Conlon PJ. Autosomal dominant tubulointerstitial kidney disease (ADTKD) in Ireland. Ren Fail. 2019;41(1):832–41.

40. Fennelly NK, Kennedy C, Jenkinson AC, Connaughton DM, Stapleton C, Dorman AM, Doyle B, Conlon PJ. Clinical heterogeneity in familial IgA nephropathy. Nephron. 2018;139(1):63–9.
41. United States Renal Data System, 2016 USRDS annual data report: Epidemiology of kidney disease in the United States. Volume 2, Chapter 13 – International comparisons. National Institutes of Health, National Institute of Diabetes and Digestive and Kidney Diseases, Bethesda, MD, 2016.
42. McCann M, Clarke M, Mellotte G, Plant WD, Fitzpatrick F. Vascular access and infection prevention and control: a National Survey of routine practices in Irish Haemodialysis units. CKJ. 2013;6:176–82.
43. Kennedy C, Connaughton DM, Murray S, Ormond J, Butler A, Phelan E, Young J, Durack L, Flavin J, O'Grady M, O'Kelly P, Lavin P, Leavey S, Lappin D, Giblin L, Casserly L, Plant WD, Conlon PJ. Home haemodialysis in Ireland. QJM. 2018;111(4):225–9.
44. Grant G, Lombard M, Keogh B. Current problems in continuous ambulatory peritoneal dialysis. Ulster Med J. 1985;54(Suppl):S44–7.
45. Smyth A, McCann E, Redahan L, Lambert B, Mellotte G, Wall C. Peritoneal dialysis in an ageing population: a 10-year experience. Int Urol Nephrol. 2012;44(1):283–93.
46. Medani S, Hussein W, Shantier M, Flynn R, Wall C, Mellotte G. Comparison of percutaneous and open surgical techniques for first-time peritoneal Dialysis catheter placement in the unbreached peritoneum. Perit Dial Int. 2015;35(5):576–85.
47. Kennedy C, Counihan A, Magee C. Transplantation in Ireland. Transplantation. 2017;101:1–4.
48. Sexton DJ, O'Kelly P, Williams Y, Plant WD, Keogan M, Khalib K, Doyle B, Dorman A, Süsal C, Unterrainer C, Forde J, Power R, Smith G, Mohan P, Denton M, Magee C, de Freitas DG, Little D, O'Seaghdha CM, Conlon PJ. Progressive improvement in short-, medium- and long-term graft survival in kidney transplantation in Ireland – a retrospective study. Transpl Int. 2019;32(9):974–84.
49. Beaumont Hospital Kidney Centre. Accessed October 2019. Available from: http://www.beaumont.ie/kidneycentre-home
50. Health Service Executive Acute Hospitals Division. Organ Donation and Transplant Ireland. Accessed October 2019. Available from: https://www.hse.ie/eng/about/who/acute-hospitals-division/organ-donation-transplant-ireland/
51. Department of Health. Policy on the Reimbursement of Expenses of Living Kidney & Liver Donors. 12th March 2019. Accessed October 2019. Available from: https://www.hse.ie/eng/about/who/acute-hospitals-division/organ-donation-transplant-ireland/living-donor-programme/doh-policy-on-the-reimbursement-of-expenses-of-living-kidney-liver-donors.pdf
52. O'Neill JP, Sexton DJ, O'Leary E, O'Kelly P, Murray S, Deady S, Daly F, Williams Y, Dean B, Fitzgerald C, Murad A, Mansoor N, O'Neill JO, Egan J, Houlihan DD, McCormick PA, Morris PG, NiRaghallaigh S, Little D, Moloney FJ, Conlon PJ. Post-transplant malignancy in solid organ transplant recipients in Ireland, the Irish transplant Cancer group. Clin Transpl. 2019;33(10):e13669.
53. Tomkins M, Tudor RM, Cronin K, O'Kelly P, Williams Y, Little D, de Freitas DG, Denton M, O'Seaghdha CM, Conlon P, Smith D. Risk factors and long-term consequences of new-onset diabetes after renal transplantation. Ir J Med Sci. 2019;41:1–7.
54. Kaballo MA, Canney M, O'Kelly P, Williams Y, O'Seaghdha CM, Conlon PJ. A comparative analysis of survival of patients on dialysis and after kidney transplantation. Clin Kidney J. 2018;11(3):389–93.
55. Health Service Executive Clinical Strategy and Programmes Division. Critical Care Programme Model of Care. 2014. Accessed October 2019. Available from: https://www.intensivecare.ie/wp-content/uploads/2015/10/criticalcare.pdf
56. Conroy M, O'Flynn MB. Mortality and long-term dialysis requirement among elderly continuous renal replacement therapy patients in a tertiary referral intensive care unit. J Intensive Care Soc. 2019;20(2):138–43.
57. Irish College of General Practitioners. Chronic Kidney Disease Information Pack. 2007. Accessed October 2019. Available from: https://www.icgp.ie/go/library/catalogue/item?spId=B49C4B92-4CFF-4AB1-A81B86E51F816436
58. Health Service Executive. Conditions and Treatments – Chronic Kidney Disease. 2011. Accessed October 2019. Available from: https://www.hse.ie/eng/health/az/c/chronic-kidney-disease/
59. Irish Kidney Association. Patients Guides. Accessed October 2019. Available from: https://ika.ie/patient-guides/
60. Kidney Disease: Improving Global Outcomes (KDIGO) Acute Kidney Injury Work Group. KDIGO Clinical Practice Guideline for Acute Kidney Injury. *Kidney inter.*, Suppl. 2012; 2: 1–138.
61. Royal College of Physicians of Ireland. Irish Committee on Higher Medical Training. Higher Specialist Training in Nephrology. V6.0. 01 July 2018. Accessed October 2019. Available from: https://rcpi-live-cdn.s3.amazonaws.com/wp-content/uploads/2018/09/Nephrology-Curriculum-2018-19-Printable-Version.pdf
62. Irish Nephrology Nurses Association. Renal Courses currently available in the Republic of Ireland. Accessed October 2019. Available from: https://www.inna-ireland.com/education/renal-courses/
63. Irish Nutrition and Dietetic Institute Renal Interest Group. Irish Kidney Diet. Accessed October 2019. Available from: http://www.irishkidneydiet.ie
64. Health Service Executive. Payscales for HSE Staff. Accessed October 2019. Available from: https://www.hse.ie/eng/staff/benefitsservices/pay/
65. Trinity College Dublin. School of Medicine. The Rare Kidney Disease Registry and Biobank. Accessed October 2019. Available from: https://www.tcd.ie/medicine/thkc/research/rare.php
66. Trinity College Dublin. School of Medicine. Vasculitis Ireland Network. Accessed October 2019. Available from: https://www.tcd.ie/medicine/thkc/vasculitis/
67. Beaumont Hospital Kidney Centre. Irish Kidney Gene Project. Accessed October 2019. Available from: http://www.beaumont.ie/kidneycentre-aboutus-irishkidneygeneproject
68. Lowney AC, Myles HT, Bristowe K, Lowney EL, Shepherd K, Murphy M, O'Brien T, Casserly L, McQuillan R, Plant WD, Conlon PJ, Vinen C, Eustace JA, Murtagh FE. Understanding what influences the health-related quality of life of Haemodialysis patients: a collaborative study in England and Ireland. J Pain Symptom Manag. 2015;50(6):778–85.
69. Sandholm N, et al. For the FIND consortium,Godson C, et al. on behalf of the FinnDiane study group and the GENIE consortium. Chromosome 2q31.1 associates with ESRD in women with type 1 diabetes. J Am Soc Nephrol. 2013;24(10):1537–43.
70. Irish Kidney Association. Accessed October 2019. Available from: https://ika.ie

# Nephrology in the Netherlands

# 43

Pieter M. Ter Wee, Shaikh A. Nurmohamed, and Johanna A. E. Van Wijk

| | |
|---|---|
| Area[1] | 41,543 km$^2$ |
| Population[2] | 17,395,101 (2019) |
| Capital | Amsterdam |
| Three most populated cities[1] | 1. Amsterdam<br>2. Rotterdam<br>3. The Hague |
| Official language | Dutch |
| Gross domestic product (GDP)[1] | 733 billion euro (2017)<br>764 billion euro (2018) |
| GDP per capita | 38,400 euro (2017)<br>47,879 euro (2018) |
| Human Development Index (HDI)[3] | 0.931 (tenth position) |
| Official currency | Euro (€) |
| Total number of nephrologists[4] | 282 |
| National society of nephrology[4] | Netherlands Federation of Nephrology<br>www.nefro.nl |
| Incidence of end-stage renal disease[5] | 2018 – 1,965 (265 pre-emptive transplantations, 1,700 dialysis patients)<br>113 pmp |
| Prevalence of end-stage renal disease[5] | 2018 – 17,672 (11,420 transplant patients, 6,252 dialysis patients)<br>1016 pmp |
| Total number of patients on dialysis (all modalities)[5] | 2017 – 6246<br>2018 – 6252 |
| Number of patients on haemodialysis 5 | 2017 – 5369<br>2018 – 5358 |
| Number of patients on peritoneal dialysis 5 | 2017 – 877<br>2018 – 894 |
| Number of renal transplantations per year[6] | 2017 – 957<br>2018 – 972 |

[1]Google search
[2]Centraal bureau voor de statistiek: https://www.cbs.nl/nl-nl/visualisaties/bevolkingsteller
[3]United Nations Development Program. Human Development Reports. Accessed in august, 2019. Available in: http://hdr.undp.org/sites/default/files/2018_human_development_statistical_update.pdf.
[4]Nederlandse Federatie voor Nefrologie (NFN): www.nefro.nl
[5]Nefrovisie; https://www.nefrovisie.nl/nefrodata/

The authors declare that they have no conflict of interest.

P. M. Ter Wee (✉) · S. A. Nurmohamed
Department of Nephrology, Amsterdam University Medical Center, Amsterdam, The Netherlands
e-mail: pm.terwee@amsterdamumc.nl; sa.nurmohamed@amsterdamumc.nl

J. A. E. Van Wijk
Department of Paediatrics, Section of Paediatric Nephrology, Amsterdam University Medical Center, Amsterdam, The Netherlands
e-mail: jae.vanwijk@amsterdamumc.nl

## Introduction of the Netherlands

The Netherlands is a small country in the north-west of Europe, bordering the North Sea on the west side of the country, Belgium on the south side and Germany on the east side. The area is 41,543 km$^2$, 18% of which consists of water. Large parts of the area, especially in the western and northern parts of the country, lay below sea level and are reclaimed land by water management structures including dykes and dunes. The traditional Dutch windmill was developed in the Middle Ages amongst other for the purpose of pumping away water in canals and thus reclaim land from the water. The population of the Netherlands was 14.091 million in 1980 and is 17.395 million as of now, an increase of 23.4% in a 30-year period. Currently, the Netherlands are on the 29th position on the list of population density per country.

The Netherlands collaborates with Belgium and Luxembourg in an agreement called The Benelux but, more importantly, is a member of the European Union and participated in the creation of the euro, symbolized by the €. As of such, the official currency of the Netherlands is the euro, since its introduction on January 1, 2002. The Dutch gross domestic product (GDP) was 764 billion euro in 2018. On the Human Development Index, the Dutch are ranked on the tenth position, and, therefore, the Netherlands are considered to belong to the wealthier countries.


J. A. Moura-Neto et al. (eds.), *Nephrology Worldwide*, https://doi.org/10.1007/978-3-030-56890-0_43

The Netherlands declared its independency from Spain in 1581, during the 80-year war, which was internationally recognized in 1609. From 1848 on, the Netherlands has been a constitutional monarchy with a parliamentary democracy. There are 12 provinces in the country that perform local government, together with the local government of cities and communities within these provinces. The central government resides in the city of The Hague, hosting both the house of parliament and the senate. Effectively, the country is led by the prime minister; the king has a more ceremonial function but is counselled by the prime minister on certain topics. The official language is Dutch. As the Dutch have a long-standing trading tradition, most people in the country can communicate in other languages like English, German or French.

In the Netherlands, everybody is obligated to have a health-care insurance sold by several health-care insurers. People with a low income are subsidized by the government to be able to pay the fee for such an insurance. There is an excellent system of primary care or family physicians who people need to attend before being referred to a medical specialist. Only in emergency situations people can go without a referral to the emergency room of a hospital. Care provided by these family practitioners is free of charge for children up to the 18 years, and for the other people, it is covered by the health insurance policy. The fee for this insurance nowadays is around €120 per person per month. On top of that, people must pay a maximum of €385 a year in case medical care is provided or prescriptions are given. While being insured, all diagnostics, cure and care are covered by such insurance policies including full dialysis and transplant care, if needed. Patients can be referred to private clinics and hospitals as well as to academic hospitals, according to their wishes. Nowadays, the government and health-care providers push all eight academic hospitals of the Netherlands to become more and more the hospitals for complex diseases and last resort care, so-called tertiary care hospitals.

## History of Nephrology in the Netherlands

### Historical Milestones

Undoubtedly, the most important Dutch contribution to nephrology nowadays is the development of the machine with which the first successful treatment of acute kidney failure (AKI) was performed in 1945 by Doctor Willem Kolff in the city of Kampen. Dr. Kolff fabricated, out of all kinds of second-hand parts, including a Ford water pump and parts of a fallen German bomber, a wooden drum covered with cellophane (Fig. 43.1) [1]. With this machine, he started treating patients with AKI. While continuously learning from unsuccessful treatments, he finally was able to save a 67-year-old patient suffering from AKI. The treatment gave room for recovering of her own kidneys. He continued to improve the machine, and this was taken over by companies that with continuation of improvements have developed to dialysis machines nowadays. Dr. Kolff emigrated to the USA where he invented the first heart-lung machine, an artificial heart and other artificial organs and body parts. As of such, he is considered one of the best medical inventors of the last century. He also was the founder and first chairman of the American Society for Artificial Internal Organs (ASAIO). Another Dutchman who has been important for the development of renal replacement therapy (RRT) was Dr. Fred S.T. Boen. Through his research, Dr. Boen has been instrumental for the development of continuous ambulatory peritoneal dialysis (CAPD). He was one of the publishers of *Today's Art of Peritoneal Dialysis*, an issue of Contribution of Nephrology that contained the proceedings of the first international Symposium of Dialysis [2]. This symposium was the predecessor of the International Society of Peritoneal Dialysis (ISPD).Another important physician for nephrology practice nowadays is Professor Jon van Rood, an immunologist. His research contributed in the 1950s to the discovery of the HLA system [3]. Prof. Rood participated with the first performed renal transplantation in the Netherlands and was the founder of Eurotransplant. This is a non-profit organization that coordinates in eight European countries post-mortal kidney transplantation. Finally, it is worthwhile mentioning Professor Fokko van der Woude. He discovered the ANCA antibodies together with Dr. Rasmussen [4]. This boosted the research and knowledge in the field of small vessel vasculitis.

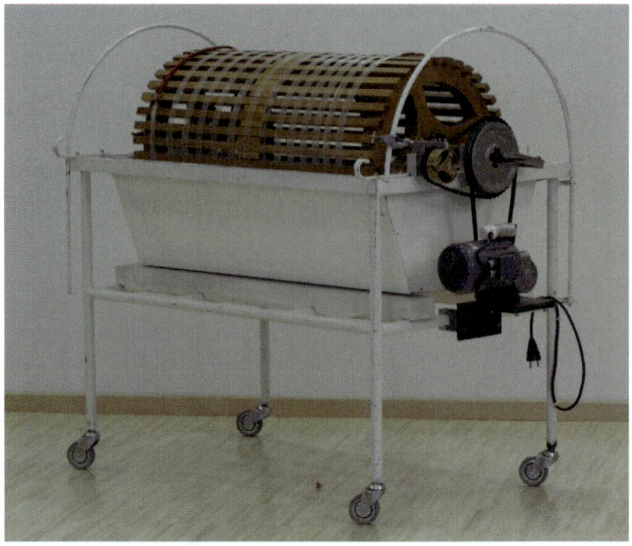

**Fig. 43.1** Artificial kidney by Willem Kolff [1]

### Organization of Nephrology in the Netherlands

In 1972, the 'Nederlandse Vereniging voor Nefrologie' was founded (NvvN = Dutch Society of Nephrology) as a scientific society for physicians and scientists with the aim of increasing the knowledge about nephrology. In the 1980s, the 'Dialyse Groep Nederland' (DGN = Dialysis Group Netherlands) was instituted by physicians to enhance the knowledge and practical care of dialysis treatment. This group of clinically working doctors initiated the first Dutch guidelines on dialysis topics like advices on laboratory tests, dialyser use, etc. In 1996, these organizations merged into the 'Nederlandse Federatie voor Nefrologie' (NFN = Netherlands Federation of Nephrology) [5]. The aim of the federation is to focus on the interests of the people working in all fields of nephrology, both scientists and clinicians. Their purpose is to achieve the highest possible quality of care for patients with renal diseases, both acute and chronic kidney disease (CKD) and dialysed and transplanted patients.

In the beginning of the 1980s, an institute called RENINE was founded for registration purposes of RRT. It was used to collect data on a number of patients being dialysed and transplanted and, in the early years of dialysis, used by the government for capacity building of dialysis in the country. The number of dialysis units, in both existing centres and new centres, was only allowed to increase after getting governmental approval. In 1999, the law ruling this capacity building was set aside by the government, which resulted in the establishment of an additional number of dialysis units in hospitals not having such a facility, as well as an increase in private and stand-alone dialysis units. Nowadays, there are 113 dialysis clinics in the Netherlands.

As mentioned before, right from the beginning of the development of dialysis treatment in the Netherlands, physicians started to collaborate in making guidelines. Thus, in the 1980s, the NvvN instituted its quality committee, which had as primary goal to develop guidelines for dialysis treatment and, later, also for CKD. In 1996, the visitation committee was established. Nephrologists started to visit each other's dialysis units for peer-to-peer review of the quality of care delivered. Shortly after, the physicians were joined by nephrology nurses while visiting as a dialysis units team. In 2003, the 'Hans Mak Instituut' (HMI) was founded with the aim of further developing the quality system for dialysis units. In order to achieve this objective, it supported especially the committee on the visits of the dialysis units as well as the quality committee of the NFN. Finally, on January 1, 2014, RENINE and HMI, together with the visitation committee, merged to the present bureau for quality and data control of the NFN, called 'Nefrovisie' [6]. This bureau hosts now web-based data on the number of dialysis and transplanted patients in the Netherlands and related topics. Annually, a 2-day conference is organized by the NFN, during which Dutch researchers and clinicians present their new data and for which local and international speakers are invited to give educational plenary lectures.

In 1997, the 'Nederlandse Transplantatie Stichting' (NTS = Dutch Transplantation Foundation) was founded. It has been licensed by the Dutch Ministry of Health and Welfare as the competent authority for execution of the organ donation law in the Netherlands. The main tasks of the NTS are appropriate maintenance of a national waiting list for patients awaiting organs or tissues, donor reporting, organ and tissue allocation, development of organ retrieval programmes in hospitals and, finally, public education with regard to donation and transplantation. The NTS has a close collaboration with the 'Nederlandse Transplantatie Vereniging' (NTV = Dutch Transplantation Society) in which all physicians working in the field of solid organ transplantation are united. The NTV has several organ-specific working groups. The heads of all eight renal transplantation centres in the Netherlands are united in the 'Landelijk Overleg Nier Transplantatie' (LONT = National Council for Kidney Transplantation). The main tasks of the LONT are to promote the quality and safety of renal transplantation; to give advices and information to the NTS, which should be embedded in international networks; and to promote and facilitate clinical trials.

In 1968, the 'Nierstichting' (= Dutch Kidney Foundation) was founded [7]. This goodwill foundation gets money from donations, a yearly door-to-door fundraiser collection and heritages. The money obtained is divided amongst several committees within the Dutch Kidney Foundation, such as the social and the scientific committees. Over the years, the social committee has served and helped numerous renal patients with practical advice, but more importantly, also financially, in particular covering additional RRT-induced additional expenses, especially for the less fortunate people. A very important issue the social committee took care of is to help out dialysis patients to go on holiday by finding suitable dialysis units in the neighbourhood of their holiday destination. In addition, financial sponsoring is also available, if needed. The scientific committee, formed by prominent Dutch basic and clinical researchers, has been responsible over the many years for the awarding of many outstanding research projects by the Dutch Kidney Foundation. As of such, the foundation has been instrumental for the development of nephrology research in the Netherlands that has been of high international quality. The foundation has a yearly income of around 20 million euros, of which 2.8 million was used to directly financially support renal patients and 8.7 million for research and innovation in 2017 [8]. Other topics that the foundation is very active in are CKD prevention and the development of a wearable dialysis machine.

Currently, around 300 nephrologists are working in the Netherlands. However, nephrology is not a recognized independent specialty. The officially recognized specialty by the Dutch Government is internist. To become a nephrologist, you do 4 years of training in internal medicine followed by a subspecialty training in nephrology for another 2 years. Thus, after 6 years of training, you become an internist-nephrologist. All eight university medical centres have the possibility to provide this subspecialty training in nephrology, often in collaboration with their nonacademic hospital partners. During these 2 years, the residents must follow 9–10 1-day training courses organized by the training committee of the NFN, covering the major topics in the field of nephrology like CKD, dialysis, hypertension, glomerulopathies, transplantation, etc. After finishing training, the internist certificate is provided by the central government and the endorsement of the subspecialty training by the NFN. Every 5 years, physicians must reapply for continuation of their permit to practice as an internist-nephrologist, both with the central government and the NFN. To have it granted, one has to show a proof of accomplishment of 40 credits per year, obtained by attending both national and international scientific or educational meetings. Further obligations to be approved for continuing working as a nephrologist are participation in a quality visitation of a renal ward and, as of January 1, 2020, having participated in InterVision sessions amongst colleagues. Likewise, for nurses there is an 18-month specialty training to become a dialysis nurse, which you must also reapply every 5 years.

As part of performing appropriate care, the nephrology community has developed a national accreditation system for dialysis units. Starting 1999, every 3 years, each unit is visited by a group of peers, nephrologists and renal nurses trained to do this. In case of doubt of the state of care, check-up visits within the 3-year period are performed. For this accreditation process, a set of rules was developed that has been updated with regular intervals and is used to follow-up the appropriateness of care in the dialysis units. Within this set of rules, it is defined that in a dialysis unit, predialysis and dialysis care are provided to patients, as well as preparation of the patients for renal transplantation. Thus, it is defined that patient care team in each unit consists of at least two nephrologists, enough renal nurses, a dietitian, a social worker, a dialysis technician and a pharmacist and that patients have 24/7 availability to vascular surgery, intervention radiology and cardiology. Stand-alone dialysis units must make agreements with neighbouring hospitals to assure this level of care. In earlier days, it was defined that for every 40 patients, one nephrologist should be available, and there had to be at least two nephrologists per centrum. In the latest version of the accreditation rules, these numbers are no longer mentioned, but more indirectly assured. Important topics that are looked after during the accreditation visits are the availability of the dialysis access team and meetings where access problems are discussed and the presence of a weekly multidisciplinary team meeting where patients are discussed with regular intervals. Furthermore, patients must have yearly full check-up by their nephrologists and must be timely prepared to receive a renal transplant, if deemed possible.

Reimbursement of dialysis is for many years in the Netherlands performed on a weekly basis for both haemodialysis (HD) and peritoneal dialysis (PD), with a slightly higher rate for automated peritoneal dialysis (APD) due the use of a cycler and higher fluid volumes. All centres nowadays use biocompatible PD fluids. At present, the weekly fee paid by the health-care providers is estimated between €1100 and €1300 for each modality. Reimbursement of care provided by nephrologists is also done on a weekly basis, with only a limited difference between HD and PD care. Thus, there is for nephrologists no financial incentive to favour one treatment modality over the other. In all cases possible, renal transplantation, preferably pre-emptive living-related renal transplantation, is the preferred treatment option for patients with end-stage renal disease (ESRD). About 50% of nephrologists are on a salary paid by the hospital. In those cases, a senior nephrologist will earn around €185,000 yearly. Nephrologists who work in private hospital setting may earn somewhat more than €250,000 per year. Senior nursing staff will earn around €60,000 yearly.

## Kidney Disease in the Netherlands

The incidence and prevalence of CKD can be estimated from community-based studies and from RRT registries. In the northern part of the Netherlands, two large community-based cohort studies have been performed: the Prevention of Renal and Vascular End-stage Disease (PREVEND) study and the Lifelines cohort study. In the study of Thio et al. [9], the investigators describe that 883 out of 6078 subjects had CKD, a prevalence rate of 14.5%. In the 5195 persons without CKD at the beginning of the study, 861 persons developed over an 11-year period CKD, an incidence rate of 17% over that period (≈1.5% a year) [9]. In the Lifelines study, 143,745 persons could be evaluated. In this group, the prevalence of early CKD (eGFR between 60 and 90 ml/min/1.73m$^2$) was 32.4% [10]. The prevalence of subjects with CKD stages 3–5 appeared to be 1.2% [10]. In another study, Brück et al. using the Lifelines study describe that the prevalence of CKD was up to 12% [11]. In 2017, the ERA-EDTA registry published data on the incidence and prevalence rates of 2014 in European countries [12]. In this report, it was documented an unadjusted incidence rate of 115 patients per million people needing RRT in the Netherlands in 2014 and an unadjusted prevalence rate of 967 patients per million people needing RRT. Altogether, these data demonstrate that CKD and RRT are a substantial health-care problem in the Netherlands.

Numbers for AKI are not readily available. RRT for AKI in the intensive care setting is usually taken care of by intensivist by means of continuous veno-venous haemofiltration (CVVH), with or without collaboration of nephrologists. When patients recover, but do not recover renal function, patients are transferred to the nephrology department and treated with intermittent HD as long as needed.

## Paediatric Nephrology in the Netherlands

Paediatric nephrologists are paediatricians with a 3-year special training in paediatric nephrology. Education and registration are strictly adapted according to the European Educational Guidelines. Paediatricians are united in the Dutch Paediatric Association where every subspecialty has its own section. Twenty to 25 paediatric nephrologists are working in one of the eight university medical centres (UMC) in the Netherlands. Every general hospital contains a paediatric department, and bigger departments can have a paediatrician with special interest in paediatric nephrology.

Every child has his or her general practitioner (GP) in the hometown. This GP can refer to a general paediatrician. Third-line referral normally goes from paediatrician to paediatric nephrologist, but in general, every doctor can make a referral to a paediatric nephrologist. Paediatric nephrologists of the UMCs and regional hospitals commonly work together in referral networks. Thus, whenever there is a possibility to cooperate with a local paediatrician, children will be referred back for local care, in close collaboration with the regional paediatric nephrologist.

The eight UMC paediatric nephrology departments have made a constitution in which relatively smaller university departments work together with a nearby larger university department. Every paediatric nephrology department can perform acute RRT at their own paediatric intensive care unit (PICU). CVVH (DF) as a treatment in AKI can be instituted in children of any age group, in close relation to paediatric intensivists and neonatologists. Small children require special equipment of dialysis machines and lines with smaller volumes. Priming is often necessary and placing small dialysis lines (double lumen, from 5 Fr onwards) can be a real challenge. Additional renal care is provided by special trained paediatric renal intensive care nurses, where one patient requires often one specialized nurse 24/7. If necessary, acute PD can be provided in these units as well.

Three university medical centres also have specialized paediatric dialysis departments, where (acute) intermittent HD can be performed outside a PICU. These departments also have facilities for a paediatric renal transplant programme, even for small children below 10 kg of weight. Although performing a kidney transplant in a child in the Netherlands is rare (about 15–20 per year), know-how and facilities have always to be up to date, including the presence of a specialized paediatric surgeon and vascular surgeon, a paediatric urologist and a paediatric nephrologist. In addition, specialized paediatric and immunology laboratories have to be available. Nephrology paediatric patients are listed in the Eurotransplant (ET) network for donor kidneys.

For children with ESRD, a kidney transplant is the treatment of choice. Chronic intermittent HD or automated PD are only seen as an option in between transplant periods, whenever necessary. In 2018, nine children were treated with intermittent HD and six with APD. Children are especially treated by pre-emptive transplantation, where the kidney is donated by one of the parents or another member of the family. These transplantations can be timed carefully, so ESRD in children is then treated without any dialysis procedure at all. Cross-over programmes are also available for children.

In four of the UMCs, the paediatric nephrologist works very closely together with paediatric urologist, creating a paediatric uro-nephrology centre. Every pregnant woman in the Netherlands is offered a 20-week prenatal ultrasound. Abnormalities in renal development are one of the most frequent pathologic findings during pregnancy. When severe pathology is suspected, the mother and baby are referred to a paediatric nephrologist and urologist in a prenatal renal centre in one of the UMCs.

The nephro-urogenital developmental disorders are known as CAKUT (congenital anomalies of kidney and urinary tract). CAKUT contains abnormalities as posterior urethral valves, mega-ureters, double kidney and ureter, ureteropelvic junction stenosis, vesicoureteral reflux, multicystic dysplastic kidney (MCDK), renal agenesis, dysplasia of one or both kidneys, horseshoe kidney, all other possible combinations and all very rare abnormalities. In most of the urological abnormalities, there is a combination with renal dysplasia, and this dysplasia is often the cause of the CKD. CAKUT can be part of any other paediatric syndrome, combining other defects and organ abnormalities, together with psychomotor development and behavioural disorders.

Genetic disorders are known in CAKUT in about 20% of cases. Increasing knowledge and specific genetic testing laboratory facilities teach us more about renal involvement in other genetic diseases. Prematurely born babies, some with extremely low body weight (ELBW), can survive with better care in neonatology, leading to specific renal damage after long-standing ICU treatment. Renal damage after specific oncology treatment, trauma care, cardio- and neurosurgical operations and other intensive care in children takes its toll for their renal future.

The underlying cause of ESRD in the paediatric transplant patients is >50% CAKUT/renal dysplasia, followed by glomerular disorders, cystic diseases, aHUS and others.

For the best preventive care, paediatric nephrologists work in a team with paediatric urologists, specialized nephrology and urology nurses, paediatric dietitians, psychologists and social workers and all other paediatric specialists needed. The goals in treating children with chronic renal disorders are to achieve normal growth and development of the child. Children may also need erythropoietin, subcutaneous growth hormone, specific paediatric hypertensive treatment and specific pharmacology (often custom made in the young age group). Young children, additionally sometimes, require tube feeding either by nose or by PEG directly into the stomach. Preventing urinary tract infections instead of treating every new infection is another important goal in children with CAKUT. Special attention must be given for gaining continence in children with urological abnormalities. Sometimes children also need intermittent catheterization for bladder disorders. In such cases, parents and children are carefully instructed to do this at home. This strong preventive strategy allows children to use their potential kidney function as good as possible, decreasing decline of the eGFR in years. Puberty with extra body growth and generating increasing waste products is often a challenging period. Sometimes kidney function deteriorates very fast, or, if not, kidney function can remain rather stable unto further in adolescence.

Transition to adult renal care is often generated in a period of life of the adolescent in which many other changes must be made. They are graduating from school, moving to another town to study, leaving the parental care and house, having their own relations and friends, etc. Transitional care starts ideally early in puberty where the children learn how to handle their own treatment and take control over their own disease and life. In most UMCs, transition to adult care is surrounded by a transition clinic.

The incidences of paediatric renal diseases in the Netherlands are not known exactly. One of the prospective incidence studies has been performed in idiopathic nephrotic syndrome (INS) [13], where INS was counted in 1.52/100,000 living children, with a male-female ratio of 2.04:1 and a median age of 3.9 years, comprising about 60 children with a de novo nephrotic syndrome/year. Congenital nephrotic syndrome is even more rare, as well as other rare glomerular diseases, for instance, C3 nephropathy, (a)HUS, membranous glomerulopathy and Alport syndrome. Acute post-streptococcal and IgA nephropathy and Henoch-Schönlein vasculitis are the most common glomerular disorders. Treating hypertension is, as in adults, an important key factor in preventing kidney function decline. Specific tubular disorders as Bartter and Gitelman syndrome, renal tubular acidosis, X-linked hypophosphatemic rachitis, nephronopthisis, congenital diabetes insipidus, cystinosis and many more rare syndromes are all treated by paediatric nephrologists. By exception, these diseases do not lead to ESRD, but it takes great effort to handle these diseases in the growing child.

Follow-up studies in the Dutch populations are not very frequent. In the KIMONO (Kidney of MONofunctional Origin) study [14], children with a single kidney were prospectively followed. About 30% of these children appeared to have one or more signs of renal damage at the age of 10 years (hypertension or hypertensive treatment, proteinuria or renal function disorders).

Follow-up of children with dialysis and transplantation years later is performed in the RICH-Q study. This study shows that these children do not grow as good as their age group, have worse bone density, have higher risk for cardiovascular disorders at young age and have more difficulty in gaining friendships, education and social contacts [15]. Working groups for paediatric nephrology in the Netherlands exist for transplantation and dialysis, nephrotic syndrome, aHUS, genetic disorders, CAKUT and some other rare diseases. Guidelines are being made and updated within these working groups. In addition, national studies are being instituted (i.e. LEARNS study, aHUS, CAKUT).

All paediatric nephrologists in the Netherlands cooperate with the European and international organizations to collect data and to do research, for example, in the IPNA/ESPN and ERA-EDTA registries [16, 17]. Studies are generated combining small numbers of patients in many more countries.

## Chronic Haemodialysis in the Netherlands

From about 2005 on, the number of patients with a functioning kidney transplant outnumbers the total number of dialysis patients. At the end of 2018, there were 11,405 patients with a kidney transplant and 6252 on dialysis [18]. The vast majority of dialysed patients is treated with chronic, in-centre intermittent HD (5076). Two hundred and eighty-two patients were treated with intermittent home HD. Of those patients, 21% were on chronic intermittent HD longer than 5 years, whereas their median time on dialysis was 2.2 years. One-year survival (with censoring for renal transplantation) of patients who had started HD in 2017 was 0.88 (95% CI: 0.86–0.90). Whereas data on vascular access are not routinely registered in the national database, it was demonstrated in a recent study that around 20% of prevalent patients in eight dialysis centres in the Netherlands had a catheter as vascular access to dialysis [19]. However, when analysing only incident patients, this was 60% of patients, despite accreditation rules that aim to have patients starting dialysis with a timely created arteriovenous fistula.

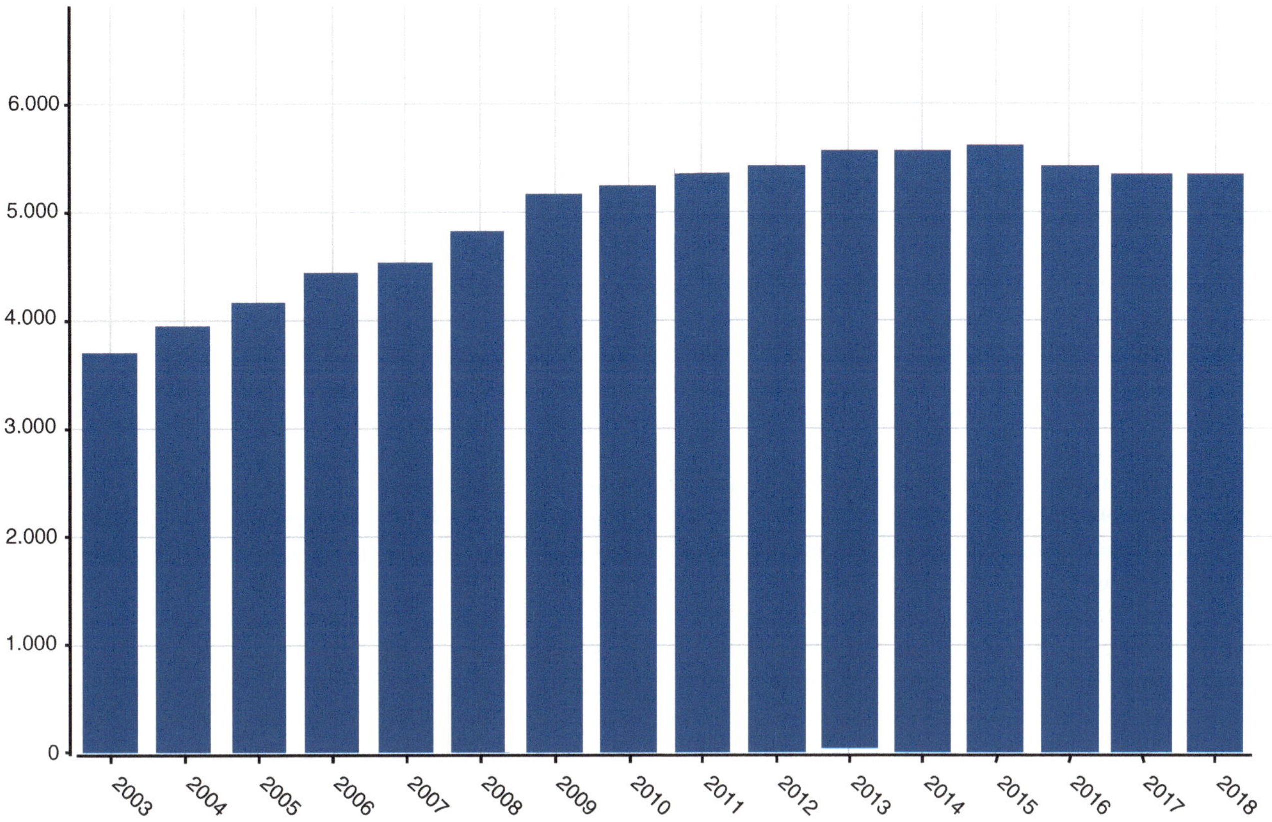


**Fig. 43.2** Prevalence of in-centre haemodialysis in the Netherlands over the period 2003–2018 [18]

At present, there are 111 dialysis facilities in the Netherlands. Most of them are hospital-based and hospital-related. A few of the dialysis units are private enterprises. Until 2013, there was a steady increase in the number of HD patients, thereafter the total number stabilized and over the last 3 years, it has even decreased (Fig. 43.2). Interestingly, this stabilization was observed in all age groups, whereas in the age group 20–44 years, even a steady decline of HD patients was observed from 2010 onwards [18]. The routine treatment regime of chronic intermittent in-hospital HD is thrice weekly 4 hours per day. The dialysate flow routinely is set on 500 ml/min with a blood flow of 250–400 ml/min. In many centres, online haemodiafiltration (HDF) is available, with the aim of achieving high convection volumes (>20 L/session) as that might be associated with better outcomes than standard HD, albeit yet not proven. On the website of the Netherlands Federation of Nephrology, 16 guidelines are available concerning several topics of appropriate dialysis treatment including guidelines about the water treatment plan, including guidelines for water quality in case of online HDF, efficacy of dialysis treatment, intervals of laboratory testing and guidelines about nutritional support and vitamin supplementation [20]. Reuse of dialysers is not allowed in the Netherlands. All costs of the HD treatment, including iron and erythropoietin supplementation if needed, and its complications are covered by the health-care insurance of the patients.

The greatest tragedy in dialysis happened in 1996 in Curacao, at that time still a full part of the Netherlands. The water company had replaced the waterlines towards the dialysis facility with cement-coated piping, ironically by the fear for development of corrosion in metal piping. As the drinking water in Curacao had been of excellent quality, dialysis had been started 26 years before that by using drinking water without a water treatment plant. Unfortunately, from the cement-coated piping, aluminium could dissipate in the water resulting in severe aluminium intoxication of dialysis patients, resulting in the death of 10 out of the 27 dialysis patients [21].

## Peritoneal Dialysis in the Netherlands

For many years, the financial reimbursement of nephrologist has been the same whether they treated patients with intermittent HD or PD. Thus, there is no financial benefit for physicians to choose one dialysis treatment modality over the other. Nevertheless, starting 2003, the number of PD patients steadily dropped until 2013; thereafter the total number of PD patients remained stable (Fig. 43.3). This decline was especially seen in the number of continuous ambulatory PD (CAPD) patients, whereas the number of APD patients has remained around 540 per year since 2003 [18]. By the end of 2018, 366 patients were treated with CAPD and 528 with APD. This drop in CAPD utilization probably has several causes, of which the rise in kidney transplantation, especially living-related kidney transplantation, during this time period is most likely the predominant cause. Another possible factor is the rise in the number of HD facilities. Of all patients treated with PD, only 5.9% were on this treatment modality for longer than 5 years, whereas their median time on dialysis treatment was 1.3 years. One-year survival (with censoring for renal transplantation) of patients who had started PD in 2017 was 0.89 (95% CI: 0.84–0.92).

Like for haemodialysis, several guidelines for peritoneal dialysis have been developed that are provided on the website of the Netherlands Federation of Nephrology. Nowadays, biocompatible peritoneal dialysis fluids are standardly used for the treatment of PD patients in the Netherlands. All costs of peritoneal dialysis treatment and its complications are covered by the health-care insurance of the patients.

## Renal Transplantation in the Netherlands

### Organ Procurement and Transplantation Network Policies

The first living renal transplantation in the Netherlands was performed in 1966 in Leiden. In 1967, Prof. van Rood founded Eurotransplant (ET), an international non-profit organization which acts as a mediator between donor hospitals and transplant centres and plays a key role in the allocation of organs. Nowadays, ET is an international collaborative including eight countries: Austria, Belgium, Croatia, Germany, Hungary, Luxembourg, the Netherlands and Slovenia. Patients in need of a kidney are put on the ET waiting list and can be offered an organ according to the allocation rules based on medical and ethical criteria. In- and cross-border organ exchange is facilitated in order to optimize matching between donor and recipient. In 1996, the organ donation law was introduced in the Netherlands. Here it was stated that you will only become a donor if you have explicitly expressed a wish to that effect. At this moment, you can decide on one of four options about donating your organs: yes, no, my partner decides and my relatives decide. Recently, the Dutch senate narrowly voted in favour of a new law to change the Dutch organ donation system to a 'yes unless' register. From July 2020, people who do

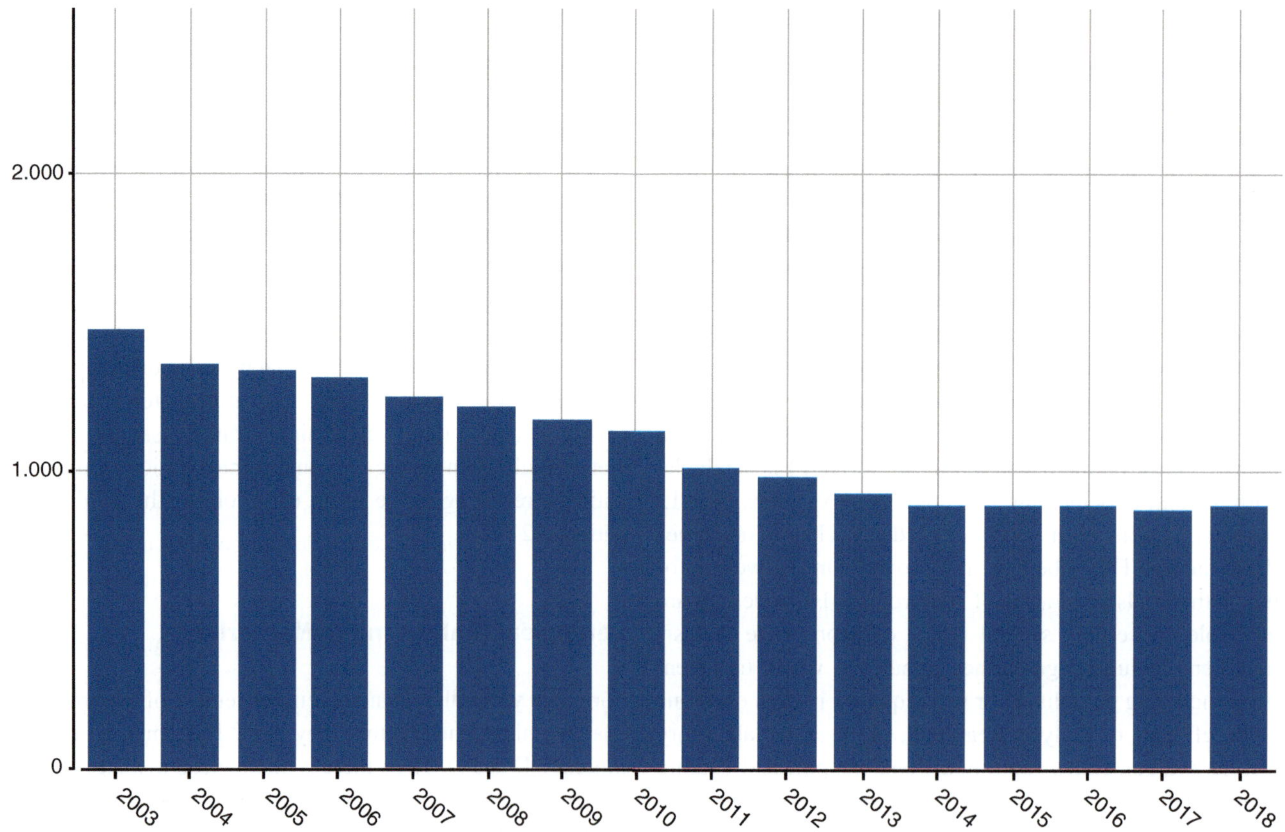


**Fig. 43.3** Prevalence of peritoneal dialysis in the Netherlands over the period 2003–2018 [18]

not opt for any of these will automatically be registered as a donor. But in any case – and this has been a contentious issue – relatives will still have the final word, even if the deceased has given permission for his organs to be used. There are approximately 100 donor hospitals and 10 renal transplant centres, including three paediatric transplant centres. For logistical reasons, the country is subdivided into two retrieval regions (East and West) and has five abdominal organ retrieval teams.

### Cadaveric Renal Transplantation

Shortly after the founding of ET, the waiting list showed a steep increase in patients waiting for a transplant, disclosing a major shortage of organs. Initially, only cadaveric kidney transplantation was performed with organs retrieved from donors after brain death (DBD; Table 43.1). Because of this shortage, other sources of organs were being sought for, and, in that search, transplant centres in the Netherlands started performing transplantation with organs from donors after circulatory death (DCD). Ever since the mid-1980s, however, the number of cadaveric transplantations performed annually is fluctuating somewhere between 350 and 500 (Table 43.1). There is an increased usage of controlled DCD donors, but the procedures with DBD donors are decreasing resulting in a more or less stable number of annually performed cadaveric transplantations. In the past years, there were more cadaveric transplantations with DCD donors than with DBD donors. By the end of 2018, 741 patients were on the active waiting list; in recent years, the waiting list has been growing disappointingly (Fig. 43.4). The median time from dialysis until transplantation is 2.7 years.

**Table 43.1** Cadaveric renal transplantation in the Netherlands

| | 2015 | 2016 | 2017 | 2018 |
|---|---|---|---|---|
| Kidney (DBD) (n) | 207 | 202 | 168 | 178 |
| Kidney (DCD) (n) | 235 | 204 | 237 | 284 |
| Total (DCD + DBD) (n) | 442 | 406 | 405 | 462 |
| Median time from dialysis to transplantation (y) | 2.7 | 2.6 | 2.3 | 2.7 |

### Living Renal Transplantation

With the increasing shortage of kidneys, some centres initiated a living kidney donor transplantation programme in the early 1980s. Few transplantations were performed with living donors, but since the late 1990s, there was a steep increase and nowadays more transplantations are performed with a liv-

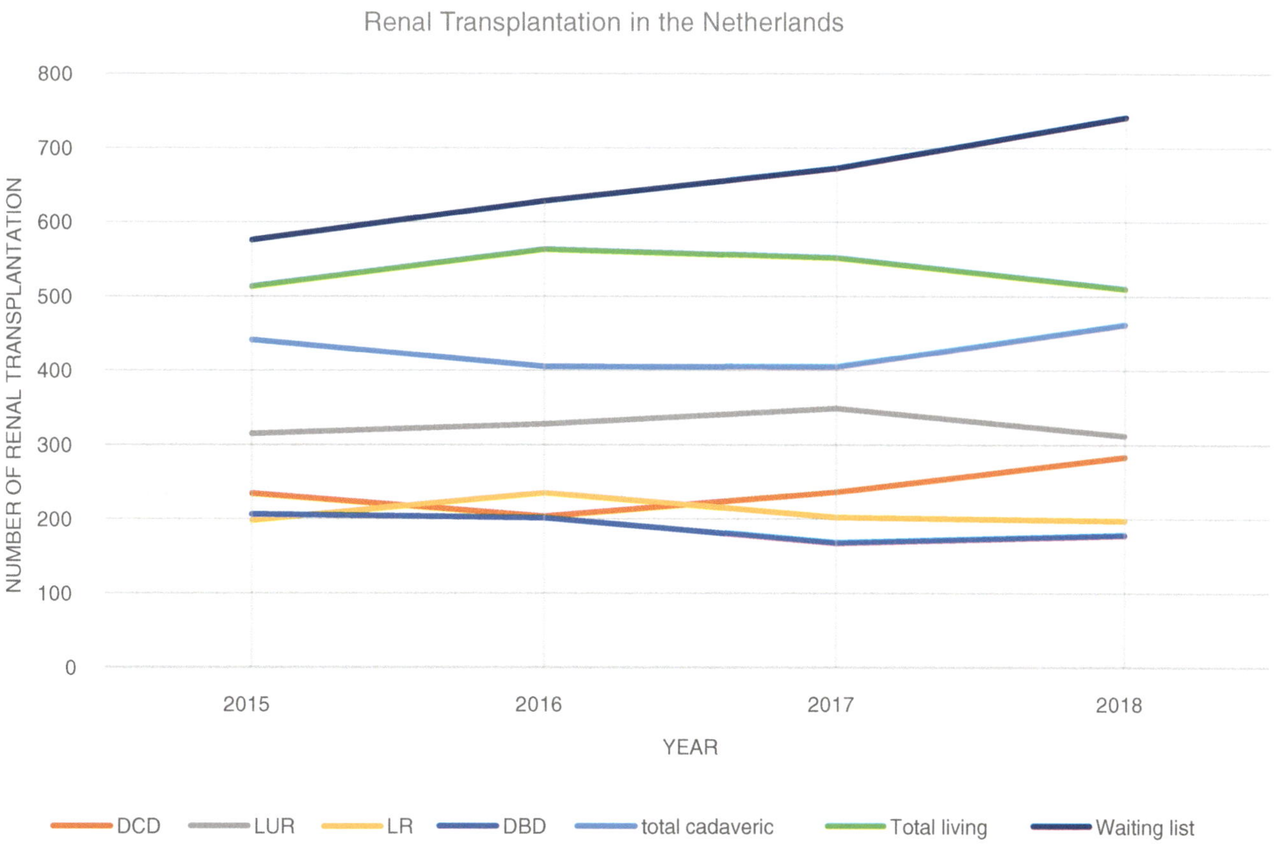


**Fig. 43.4** Overview of renal transplantations in the Netherlands in 2014–2018. DCD donors after circulatory death, LUR living unrelated, LR living related, DBD donors after brain death

ing donor (Table 43.2) as compared to transplantations with a cadaveric donor, and all centres have a successful living renal transplantation programme. Slowly, medical and ethical boundaries for living transplantation are being extended. Initially, only related donors were accepted. Then more and more unrelated donors were accepted provided that there is an emotional relationship. In 2004, a very innovative and successful nationwide paired kidney exchange programme was established for those patients with a living donor with blood group type or HLA incompatibility. For ABO-incompatible (ABOi) pairs, there is also a possibility to explore the feasibility of an ABOi transplantation. Recently one centre (Erasmus University Medical Center, Rotterdam) initiated an HLA-incompatible transplantation programme supported by all centres in the Netherlands. In recent years, there has also occurred an increase in transplantations with altruistic donors and transplantation with community solicited nondirected donors. In Fig. 43.5, the 10-year graft survival of living and cadaveric kidney transplantation is depicted [22]. As anticipated, the graft survival of living kidney donation is superior to cadaveric kidney transplantation.

**Table 43.2** Living renal donor transplantations

| | 2015 | 2016 | 2017 | 2018 |
|---|---|---|---|---|
| Living related (n) | 199 | 236 | 203 | 198 |
| Living unrelated (n) | 315 | 328 | 349 | 312 |
| Total (n) | 514 | 564 | 552 | 510 |

## Future Perspectives of Nephrology in the Netherlands

Without any doubt, the most challenging problem to deal with in the Netherlands is the shortage in workforce, especially nursing staff. The retirement of the baby boom generation and the ageing of the population due to the rise of life expectancy for both woman and man are amongst the reasons for this problem. For adequate monitoring of CKD and post-transplant follow-up, this increased burden of care time possibly can be overcome by utilizing newly developed e-health strategies. The latter requires more and better integration of current ICT systems of several health-care professionals (primary care physicians, in-hospital nephrologists) and institutes, the development of teleconsulting possibilities and easy access of laboratory testing like enhanced application of dry blood sampling in the home-based setting. Included in these changes should also be the fact that more attention should be given to the needs and wishes of indi-

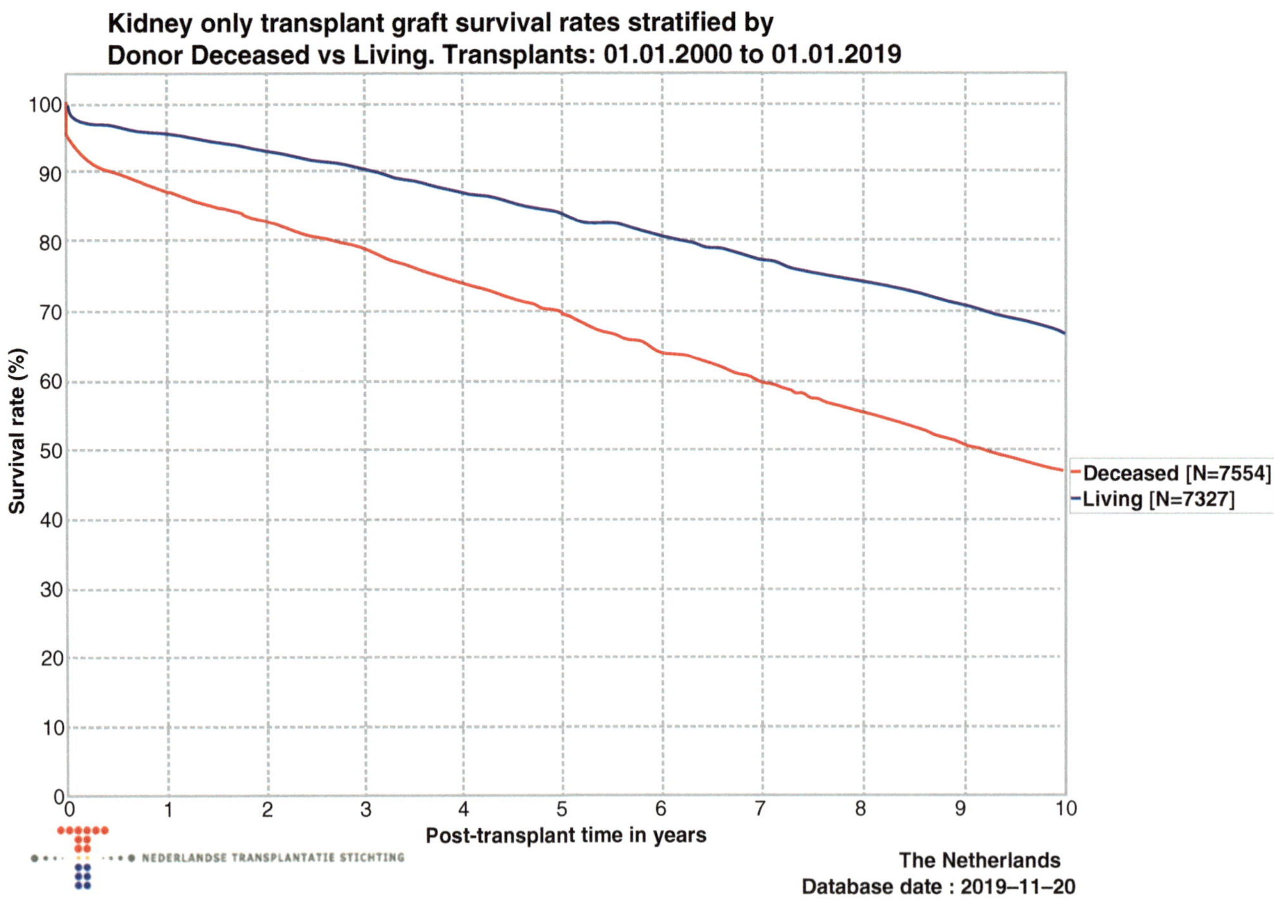


**Fig. 43.5** 10-year graft survival in living and deceased donor renal transplantation in the Netherlands [21]

vidual patients by health-care professionals. Thus, data-driven outcomes that include patient-reported outcomes (PROMS) should become standard tools to improve outcome of patients amongst others by comparing inter-physician clinical data and PROMS, aimed to achieve the best practice for all patients. On top of that, the patient's opinion should, through shared decision-making with his/her treating physician, become the leading reason for the proposal of a patient's treatment plan. Home-based dialysis treatments should be expanded, for which the availability of an easily wearable dialysis device could become a great improvement and chance for successfully achieving these goals.

## Conclusion

Nephrology in the Netherlands is well-organized. Care for CKD and RRT, including dialysis and renal transplantation, is available to everyone. There is a long-standing tradition of continuous quality improvement. This has been achieved by the early development of guidelines for HD and PD, as well as kidney diseases, and by the visits of peers to other dialysis units in order to check upon the quality of care delivered, based on standards defined by the national visitation committee in whom physicians and nurses participate on an equal basis. Things to be proud of are several historical achievements; amongst them, the development of the first haemodialysis machine by Doctor Kolff might be the most important. Furthermore, the presence of the Nierstichting has been very important for the development of nephrology in the Netherlands. Over the years, not only has this foundation helped numerous Dutch renal patients, having either a CKD or being dependent on RRT, but has also supported and facilitated the development of nephrology research, which has become well renowned and highly ranked.

## References


1. Grossw I. CC BY-SA 3.0, https://commons.wikimedia.org/w/index.php?curid=2249917
2. Boen ST. Undesired effects of peritoneal dialysis. Contrib Nephrol. 1979;17:73–6.
3. Dausset J, Brecy H. Identical nature of the leucocyte antigens detectable in monozygote twins by means of immune iso-leuco-agglutinins. Nature. 1957;180:1430.
4. Van der Woude FJ, Rasmussen N, Lobatto S, Wiik A, Permin H, van Es LA, et al. Antibodies against neutrophils and monocytes: tool for diagnosis and marker of disease activity in Wegener's granulomatosis. Lancet. 1985;23:425–9.
5. Nederlandse Federatie voor Nefrologie (NFN). https://www.nefro.nl.
6. Nefrovisie. https://www.nefrovisie.nl/nefrodata/.
7. Nierstichting. https://www.nierstichting.nl/.
8. https://www.nierstichting.nl/media/filer_public/44/e2/44e21e1f-f7f2-405a-9584-ed6518ad18d5/jaarverslag-nierstichting-2017.pdf.
9. Thio CH, Vart P, Kieneker LM, Snieder H, Gansevoort RT, Bültmann U. Educational level and risk of chronic kidney disease: longitudinal data from the PREVEND study. Nephrol Dial Transplant. 2018:1–8. https://doi.org/10.1093/ndt/gfy361.
10. Cai Q, Dekker LH, Bakker SJL, de Borst MH, Navis G. Intraregional differences in renal function in the northern Netherlands: the lifelines cohort study. PLoS One 2019; 14(10): e0223908. https://doi.org/10.1371/journal.pone.0223908.
11. Brück K, Stel VS, Gambaro G, Hallan S, Völzke H, Ärnlöv J, et al. CKD prevalence varies across the European general population. J Am Soc Nephrol. 2016;27:2135–47.
12. Pippias M, et al. The European renal association – European Dialysis and transplant association registry annual report 2014: a summary. Clin Kidney J. 2017;10:154–69.
13. El Bakkali L, Rodrigues Pereira R, Kuik DJ, Ket JC, van Wijk JA. Nephrotic syndrome in The Netherlands: a population-based cohort study and a review of the literature. Pediatr Nephrol. 2011;26:1241–6.
14. Westland R, Schreuder MF, Bökenkamp A, Spreeuwenberg MD, van Wijk JA. Renal injury in children with a solitary functioning kidney--the KIMONO study. Nephrol Dial Transplant. 2011;26:1533–41.
15. Dobrowolski LC, van Huis M, van der Lee JH, Peters Sengers H, Liliën MR, Cransberg K, et al. Epidemiology and management of hypertension in paediatric and young adult kidney transplant recipients in The Netherlands. Nephrol Dial Transplant. 2016;31:1947–56.
16. Preka E, Bonthuis M, Harambat J, Jager KJ, Groothoff JW, Baiko S, et al. Association between timing of dialysis initiation and clinical outcomes in the paediatric population: an ESPN/ERA-EDTA registry study. Nephrol Dial Transplant. 2019;34:1932–40.
17. Bonthuis M, Groothoff JW, Ariceta G, Baiko S, Battelino N, Bjerre A, et al. Growth patterns after kidney transplantation in European children over the past 25 years: an ESPN/ERA-EDTA registry study. Transplantation 2019. doi: https://doi.org/10.1097/TP.0000000000002726. [Epub ahead of print]..
18. https://ivisualz.nl/ivisualz/chartFlash/charts.
19. de kleijn HC, Uyl-de Groot CA, Hagen EC, CFM F, Schraa JA, Pasker-de Jong PCM, Ter Wee PM. Nursing care time for haemodialysis patients. J Ren Care. in press
20. https://www.nefro.nl/richtlijnen.
21. Berend K, van der Voet G, Boer WH. Acute aluminium encephalopathy in a dialysis Centre caused by a cement mortar water distribution pipe. Kidney Int. 2001;59:746–53.
22. https://members.transplantatiestichting.nl/cms/.

# Nephrology in Poland

# 44

Monika Lichodziejewska-Niemierko, Jarosław Czerwiński, Alicja Dębska-Ślizień, Ryszard Gellert, Ryszard Grenda, Jolanta Małyszko, Beata Naumnik, Michał Nowicki, Janusz Ostrowski, and Andrzej Więcek

| | |
|---|---|
| Area | 312,679 $Km^2$ |
| Population[1] | 38,386,000 (2019) |
| Capital | Warszawa (Warsaw) |
| Three most populated cities[1] | 1. Warszawa (Warsaw) 1.76 million (2018)<br>2. Kraków (Cracow) 0.77 million (2018)<br>3. Łódź (Lodz) 0.69 million (2018) |
| Official language | Polish |
| Gross domestic product (GDP)[2] | 585.664 Billion USD (2018) |
| GDP per capita[2] | 15,426 USD (2018) |
| Human development index (HDI)[3] | 0.865 (2017) |
| Official currency | Polish zloty |
| Total number of nephrologists[4] | 1100 (2018) |
| National society of nephrology | Polish Society of Nephrology www.ptnefro.pl |
| Incidence of end-stage renal disease[4] | 2018 – 201.3 pmp |
| Prevalence of end-stage renal disease (on dialysis)[4] | 2018 – 718.6 pmp |
| Total number of patients on dialysis (all modalities)[4,5] | 2017 – 21,297<br>2018 – 21,270 |
| Number of patients on haemodialysis[4,5] | 2017 – 20,171<br>2018 – 20,435 |
| Number of patients on peritoneal dialysis[4,5] | 2017 – 1126<br>2018 – 835 |
| Number of renal transplantations per year[6] | 2017 – 1059<br>2018 – 925 |

Table references:

1. GUS (Central Statistical Office) Report 2019 https://stat.gov.pl/obszary-tematyczne/ludnosc/ludnosc/ludnosc-stan-i-struktura-w-przekroju-terytorialnym-stan-w-dniu-30-06-2019,6,26.html
2. The World Bank 2018 https://data.worldbank.org/country/poland
3. United Nations Development Program. Human Development Reports. http://hdr.undp.org/sites/default/files/2018_human_development_statistical_update.pdf.
4. National Consultant in Nephrology -unpublished data on epidemiology and treatment on chronic kidney disease, 2018
5. Dębska-Ślizień A, Rutkowski B, Rutkowski P., Korejwo G, Gellert R. Aktualny stan leczenia nerkozastępczego w Polsce – 2017r. Nefrol. Dial. Pol. 2018, 22, 133–140.
6. www.poltransplant.pl

M. Lichodziejewska-Niemierko (✉) · A. Dębska-Ślizień
Department of Nephrology Transplantology and Internal Medicine, Medical University of Gdańsk, Gdańsk, Poland
e-mail: lichotek@gumed.edu.pl; adeb@gumed.edu.pl

J. Czerwiński
Department of Emergency Medicine, Medical University of Warsaw and Polish Transplant Coordinating Center Poltransplant, Warsaw, Poland
e-mail: jczerwinski@poltransplant.pl

R. Gellert
Department of Nephrology and Internal Medicine, Center of Postgraduate Education, Warsaw, Poland
e-mail: gellert@people.pl

R. Grenda
Department of Nephrology, Kidney Transplantation & Hypertension, The Children's Memorial Health Institute, Warsaw, Poland
e-mail: r.grenda@ipczd.pl

J. Małyszko
Department of Nephrology, Dialysis and Internal Medicine, Warsaw Medical University, Warsaw, Poland
e-mail: jolmal@poczta.onet.pl

B. Naumnik
1st Department of Nephrology and Transplantation with Dialysis Unit, Medical University of Białystok, Białystok, Poland
e-mail: bnaumnik@poczta.onet.pl

M. Nowicki
Department of Nephrology, Hypertension and Kidney Transplantation, Medical University of Łódź, Central University Hospital, Łódź, Poland
e-mail: nefro@wp.pl

J. Ostrowski
Department of the History of Medicine, Centre of Postgraduate Medical Education, Warsaw, Poland
e-mail: ostryjan@poczta.onet.pl

A. Więcek
Department of Nephrology, Transplantation and Internal Diseases, Medical University of Silesia, Katowice, Poland
e-mail: awiecek@sum.edu.pl



J. A. Moura-Neto et al. (eds.), *Nephrology Worldwide*, https://doi.org/10.1007/978-3-030-56890-0_44

## Introduction

Poland, officially the Republic of Poland, is a country located in Central Europe. It is divided into 16 administrative subdivisions, covering an area of 312,696 Km$^2$, and has a largely temperate seasonal climate. With a population of nearly 38.5 million people, primarily ethnic Poles, Poland is the fifth most populous member state of the European Union (EU). Poland is bordered by the Baltic Sea, Lithuania, and Russia's Kaliningrad Oblast to the north; Belarus and Ukraine to the east; Slovakia and the Czech Republic to the south; and Germany to the west [1].

Poland has a developed market and is a regional power in Central Europe, with the largest stock exchange in the East-Central European zone. It has the sixth largest economy by GDP (nominal) in the EU and the tenth largest in all of Europe. It is one of the most dynamic economies in the world, simultaneously achieving a very high rank on the human development index. Poland is a developed country, which maintains a high-income economy along with very high standards of living, quality of life, safety, education, and economic freedom. Alongside a developed school educational system, the state also provides free university education, social security, and a universal health care system [1].

## Brief History of Nephrology – Understanding How Nephrology Began in the Country

Although it was the second half of the twentieth century, which marked the significant development of nephrology in Poland, the early clinical research on the urinary tract performed in Vilnius by Jędrzej Śniadecki dates back to the beginning of the nineteenth century [2]. Then, in 1884 Józef Dietl in Krakow described the condition known as *Dietl's crisis*. Six years later, in 1900, Samuel Goldflam described a medical test currently referred to as *Goldflam's sign*. In the 1920s, Witold Orłowski examined the kidneys in the course of kidney failure and other internal organ diseases, especially those related to the heart. At the same time, Marceli Landsberg published numerous works in the field of kidney pathophysiology, and together with Henryk Gnoiński and Dawid Szenkier in the field of experimental peritoneal dialysis (PD), the area in which he is considered one of the world pioneers.

It was in 1958 when Poland's first clinic of nephrology, headed by Zdzisław Wiktor, was established at the Medical Academy of Wrocław. It took a whole decade for other medical centres to follow with the creation of their departments of nephrology. These included the clinics in Krakow (1969) headed by Zygmunt Hanicki, Gdańsk (1970) headed by Andrzej Manitius, Poznań headed by Andrzej Wojtczak and later Kazimierz Bączyk, Łódź with Zbigniew Orłowski; and finally, in 1975, Franciszek Kokot set up his centre in Katowice.

In 1961, the Society of Polish Internists established its Section of Nephrology with Zdzisław Wiktor as the first President. The Polish Society of Nephrology emerged in September 1983 during its first founding meeting in Bydgoszcz. The first President was Tadeusz Orłowski followed by Kazimierz Bączyk (Poznań) and Franciszek Kokot (Katowice).

Early activities (1964–1994) of paediatricians involved in renal diseases in children were connected with the establishment of the Section of Paediatric Nephrology by the Polish Paediatric Society in 1973. The Polish Paediatric Nephrology Association was founded and registered in 1994 with Teresa Wyszyńska as its first President.

The Polish Society of Nephrology publishes its own journals – established in 1997 *Polish Nephrology and Dialysis Treatment* (*Nefrologia i dializoterapia polska*) and the more recent creation *Forum of Nephrology* (*Forum nefrologiczne*). It was in 1984 when the structure of specialist supervision was built, initially in the form of the National Specialist Team for Renal Dialysis and Transplant Therapy, which, in 1986, was transformed into the National Team of the Medical Consultant in Nephrology. At the beginning, the team was managed by Andrzej Manitius and then by Bolesław Rutkowski. In cooperation with Irena Marcinek, an employee at the Ministry of Health, the team prepared and launched the highly successful 'Programme for Improvement and Development of Dialysis Treatment in Poland', resulting in unlimited access to this method of treatment in Poland [3].

Poland's first PD was performed in Warsaw (1953) by Jan Nielubowicz and Tadeusz Orłowski. In 1979, Zofia Wańkowicz in Warsaw and Zbylut Twardowski in Lublin launched the Continuous Ambulatory Peritoneal Dialysis programme (CAPD). Later, working in the United States, Twardowski developed the peritoneal equilibration test (PET), which is widely used all over the world today. He was also the creator of new catheters for peritoneal dialysis (PD). In children, the first intermittent PD in acute renal failure (AKI) was used in 1966 by Teresa Wyszyńska in Warsaw. A regular CAPD programme in children was introduced in 1983 by Maria Sieniawska in Warsaw. In 1980, Marta Uszycka-Karcz in Gdańsk used a device called Dialiper DA 03 for an automated dialysis.

In 1949–50, working in Krakow with Nils Alwall's prototype of the artificial kidney, Zygmunt Hanicki carried out early experimental work in haemodialysis (HD). The first HD session was performed at Jan Roguski's 2nd Clinic of Internal Medicine in Poznań, in November 1958. The medical team responsible for this historic event was headed by Kazimierz Bączyk. In early January 1959 in Warsaw, at Andrzej Biernacki's clinic, the team led by Tadeusz Orłowski initiated HD in the second centre in Poland. At that time,

Zbigniew Fałda and Mieczysław Lao also had their significant contribution in the development of the field in Warsaw. At the military dialysis centre in Łódź headed by Kazimierz Trznadel, the first HD was performed in 1962. The programme of paediatric HD was introduced in 1978 by Maria Sieniawska in Warsaw.

The kidney was the first transplanted organ both worldwide and in Poland. Polish's first, alas unsuccessful, transplant was performed by Władysław Wręźlewicz in 1965 at Wiktor Bross' 2nd Clinic of Surgery in Wrocław. The first successful operation was performed in January 1966 by the team headed by Jan Nielubowicz from the 1st Clinic of Surgery in Warsaw. Soon, in March the same year, Wiktor Bross performed the first successful transplant from a family donor and in November Józef Gasiński performed a successful operation in Katowice. In 1975, a kidney was transplanted in Krakow by Romuald Drop and, in 1980, in Gdańsk by Jerzy Dybicki. In February 1988, a Warsaw-based team headed by Jacek Szmidt performed the first successful simultaneous kidney-pancreas transplant.

In 1975, Tadeusz Orłowski facilitated the establishment of the Institute of Transplantation in Warsaw, which later played a very large role in the development of this field of medicine. Orłowski's successors were Mieczysław Lao, Magdalena Durlik and Wojciech Rowiński. The first paediatric kidney transplant (KT) was performed in 1984. The founding meeting of the Polish Transplant Society (PTT) was held in Białowieża in 1991, but it was in June 1993 when the Society was officially established during its First Congress in Warsaw and Mieczysław Lao became its first President.

Jan Roguski was a co-founder and member of the board of the International Society of Nephrology, followed by Tadeusz Orłowski and Stefan Angielski. Tadeusz Orłowski was a board member of the EDTA 1966–69, and Franciszek Kokot twice, 1978–81 and again from 1987. In 2010, he became a honorary member of the ERA-EDTA whose President in 2015–2017 was Andrzej Więcek.

Teresa Wyszyńska, Maria Sieniawska and Irena Krzeska were co-founders of the International Society of Pediatric Nephrology in 1967; and in 1984, the International Society for Peritoneal Dialysis was co-created by Kazimierz Bączyk, Przemysław Hirszel and Zbylut Twardowski.

## Renal Diseases

The exact incidence and prevalence of kidney diseases other than end-stage renal disease (ESRD) is unknown in Poland since there is no mandatory countrywide registry of urogenital diseases. There have been no endemic renal diseases identified in Poland so far, including both categories of endemic diseases, i.e. holoendemic and hyperendemic diseases. The frequency of urolithiasis, urinary tract infections and interstitial nephritis is similar to the rest of Europe. However, Poland is a country with a high prevalence of behavioural risk factors that may predispose to chronic diseases including those affecting the kidney and the urinary tract. A recent "State of Health" in EU report [4] revealed that over a third of Poland's chronic disease burden can be attributed to such risk factors as smoking, binge drinking, and obesity. In particular, obesity rates in Poland are above 17% of the adult population, resulting in a high prevalence of diabetes and atherosclerotic cardiovascular diseases that are well-recognized risk factors for kidney disease. There is also a high level of environmental pollution mostly affecting air quality in Poland that, according to the report of European Environment Agency, may result in 47,500 additional deaths in the country [5]. Since air pollution has been recently identified as a new risk factor for kidney disease, it could also contribute to the high burden of renal disease in Poland. So far, however, an impact of high level of air pollution on the incidence and prevalence of renal diseases in Poland has not been thoroughly studied.

The epidemiology of glomerular diseases in adults has been recently studied in Poland based on a countrywide non-mandatory registry of kidney biopsies [6]. The study showed that the most common renal biopsy diagnoses in adults were Ig A nephropathy (20%), focal segmental glomerulosclerosis (15%), and membranous nephropathy (11%). At the time of renal biopsy, little less than a half of the patients had nephrotic range proteinuria. In addition a subgroup of elderly patients was analyzed and it was found that primary and secondary glomerulopathies were equally common in that population.

Autosomal dominant polycystic kidney disease (ADPKD) is associated with about 5% of the ESRD cases worldwide. Recently published analysis of the prevalence of ADPKD showed a minimum number of cases of ADPKD in Poland, estimated using the data from renal registries (2012) and the published population-based data, 1486 and 6383, respectively [7].

## Chronic Kidney Disease (CKD) Epidemiology and Renal Replacement Therapy Scenario

The CKD Polish epidemiology knowledge has been mainly shaped by foreign studies; a few to be mentioned include the American NHANES III study and the European studies HUNT and INCIPE, which estimated the prevalence of CKD in 10–16% of Poles. The first Polish studies include PolNef (a pilot regional study of a medium-size town in northern Poland) and Polsenior. The authors of PolNef emphasized the screening role of albuminuria in the early detection of CKD. It was estimated that 11.9% of the studied population had albuminuria. The second cross-sectional nationwide study proved a high CKD prevalence (29.4%) in senior Polish citizens.

During the past few years, two large cross-sectional studies aimed to assess epidemiology and the risk of CKD were carried out in Poland. The first one, the NATPOL 2011 survey, examined a representative sample of 2413 Polish citizens (1245 females, 1168 males) aged 18–79 [8]. The second one, the WOBASZ Senior Survey, included 918 (466 males, 252 females) people at the age of 75 and above [9]. The criteria of CKD were: (1) drop in eGFR value <60 ml/min/1.73 $m^2$ or eGFR ≥60 ml/min/1.73 $m^2$ with albuminuria (ACR > 30 mg/g) in NATPOL 2011; (2) solely eGFR <60 ml/min/1.73 $m^2$ in WOBASZ Senior cohort. It is worth noticing a complex multi-stage respondent recruitment procedure that was managed in both studies. Its aim was to obtain the most accurate image of CKD epidemiology in Poland.

## CKD Prevalence

According to the NATPOL 2011 Survey, CKD prevalence in the Polish population was found to be 5.8% (95% CI: 4.6–7.2) [8]. Its frequency increases with age from 1.8% (group aged 18–39) to 15.3% (group aged 60–79). It was demonstrated that the majority (67.7%) of this population had the eGFR ≥60 mL/min/1.73 $m^2$ and albuminuria (ACR ≥ 30 mg/g), and fulfilled the criteria of CKD in the G1A2–3 and G2A2–3 CKD stages.

The decreased glomerular filtration rate with eGFR <60 mL/min/1.73 $m^2$ was found in 1.9% (95% CI: 1.5–2.5) of NATPOL 2011 participants. The frequency of decreased eGFR increases with age from 0.06% (group aged 18–39) to 8.1% (group aged 60–79). The overall prevalence of albuminuria was found to be at 4.5% (95% CI: 3.4–5.9). It was assessed that among adult Polish citizens (altogether over 38 million) there were approximately 1,724,960 people with CKD. The awareness of having CKD, understood as decreased GFR, was fairly low and reached 12.3%. In the population aged 18–39, the prevalence of CKD was lower than in previous surveys.

According to WOBASZ Senior Survey which included the population aged 75 and above, the prevalence of CKD (understood as decreased eGFR <60 mL/min/1.73 $m^2$) was 26.9% (95% CI: 23.1–30.9) [9]. The frequency of CKD increases with age from 24.2% in the group of 75–79 years old to 37.2% in those older than 90. The majority (70.1%) of people with CKD was in G3A stage. The population of elderly Polish citizens aged ≥75 was estimated to amount to 495,590 (95% CI: 396,363–594,817). The awareness of the disease reached around 17%. Overall, there is a particularly high prevalence of CKD in the elderly Polish population. There is a trend of an increasing prevalence of CKD associated with aging.

The cohorts mentioned in the previously described surveys were combined to find general CKD prevalence in adults aged ≥18. Based on the above-outlined criteria, the CKD 1–5 prevalence was estimated as 10.8%; 12.9% of women and 8.0% of men. A large-scale attempt to carefully characterize CKD prevalence in Europe (19 general population–based studies from 13 countries, including PolSenior study from Poland) led to the identification of a substantial variation between countries [10]. The adjusted CKD stages 1–5 (CKD-Epidemiology Collaboration equation) prevalence varied between 3.31% in Norway and 17.3% in northeast Germany. The adjusted CKD stages 3–5 prevalence varied between 1.0% in central Italy and 5.9% in northeast Germany. Stratification by risk factors further suggests that this variation in CKD prevalence across Europe is, at least, in part due to other factors than prevalence of diabetes, hypertension and obesity in the general population. Environmental factors (dietary habits, smoking, physical activity, birth weight, etc.), public health policies, genetic factors or heterogeneity of methodology used in the studies potentially contribute to these differences.

## CKD Epidemiology

The most frequent causes of CKD in Polish population include diabetes (DM; approximately 32%), glomerulonephritis (GN; about 14%) and arterial hypertension (AH; about 13%) [11].

Among adult population (18–79 years of age), DM was found to be four times more prevalent in the population with an established diagnosis of CKD in comparison to those without CKD (18.5% versus 4.5%). On the other hand, among the diabetic adults, CKD was observed in 20.3% (95% CI: 13.9–28.7) of the population. Among the elderly population (≥75 years), a similar DM prevalence was found in those with diagnosis of CKD as well as in those without CKD (11.7% and 11.4%). Furthermore, the latter range of values approximated the DM prevalence among the general elderly population.

Among the population 18–79 years of age, the sample with an established diagnosis of CKD was twice as likely to have AH than those without CKD (67.8 versus 29.0%). On the other hand, CKD was found in 12.6% of the hypertensive adults (95% CI: 9.7–16.2). The prevalence of AH in the elderly population (≥75 years old) is very high. In those with CKD, it is higher than in those without it (91.0% and 80.3%, respectively). This may be related to the aetiology of kidney injury and result from hypertensive-ischemic nephropathy, which is frequently found in this age group.

In the population 18–79 years of age, AH is found to double the chances of having CKD (OR 1.99, 95% CI: 1.11–3.54) and DM more than three times (OR 3.37, 95% CI: 1.80–6.28). The two diseases equally increase the chance of having albuminuria. Apart from AH, no other single cardiovascular pathology was found to correlate with the incidence of CKD. However, cardiovascular diseases *en bloc* are associated with an increased chance of having CKD in the elderly cohort (OR 1.87, 95% CI: 1.15–3.03).

Ageing (observed in 10-year intervals) increased the chances of the CKD development (OR 1.68, 95% CI: 1.30–2.18), decreased eGFR (OR 4.48, 95% CI: 2.71–7.38) and increased albuminuria (OR 1.42, 95% CI:1.07–1.89).

## Renal Replacement Therapy Scenario

ESRD morbidity (understood as the number of patients starting renal replacement therapy) is comparable to morbidity in many European countries. The main cause of ESRD in the dialysis patients is diabetic nephropathy. The average percentage of patients with diabetic nephropathy that start renal replacement therapy (RRT) equals to 29 (38% for HD and 25% for PD treatment). Among patients starting RRT, the vast majority consists of people older than 65.

ESRD patients have the choice among HD, PD, and preemptive KT, if eligible. Conservative care is considered only in end-stage cancer and severe dementia patients. The total number of HD, PD, and transplanted patients reaches the European average of 800 patients per million population (pmp). Based on the past few years, the total number of patients on maintenance dialysis in Poland remains constant and is estimated at around 20,000 people. Among those under RRT, a striking majority consists of HD patients. This may be partly due to a significant growth of HD units in recent years.

The percentage of KT performed in PD patients is higher than HD (over 9% vs about 4%). Among the maintenance HD patients, 13% are referred to the transplant waiting list and this number has remained constant over the past few years. Traditionally, this situation has a better outlook among the PD patients whose referral rate reaches 19% and in some centres, it exceeds 30%. Each year, among the patients who start dialysis, the number of patients who return to HD and PD after losing a KT is estimated to be 5%, for both of those methods.

## Peritoneal Dialysis

PD in the form of CAPD started to be available to all ESRD patients in Poland in the 1990s. Later, also automated PD (APD) became an RRT modality option. The detailed PD data were collected from the survey sent to all units yearly from 1995–2005 in Poland [12]. During the following 10 years, the Polish PD Registry collected the PD data. In the last few years, again aggregated data are being collected every year from all dialysis centres. The number of patients grew from 31 in 1990 to 1200 patients in 2000 [13]. In the recent years, the number of PD patients is not exceeding 1000 at the end of each year, with a steadily decreasing penetration rate from almost 11% in the turn of the century to 3.8% in 2018.

PD is offered in over 70 dialysis centres in Poland, both public and private. The treatment is fully reimbursed by the National Health Fund. Two companies, Fresenius Medical Care and Baxter, are providing equipment and solutions for the therapy. Biocompatible fluids as well as modern cyclers together with remote monitoring are available in the country. Among PD patients around 1/3 is over 65 years old, 25% are diabetic and approximately 45% are on APD. The majority (70%) of CAPD patients perform four, 2 L exchanges and around 80% use Ca 1.25 mmol/L PD solutions. There is no external help provided for assisted PD, which is solely performed by the family. All centres provide appropriate training, good adequacy of treatment and low rate of peritonitis (0.29/patient year at risk) [14]. The percentage of PD patients who are KT candidates is up to 40% in the individual units and 10–30% are transplanted every year. There is a low hospitalization rate among PD patients. The dropout to HD is mainly due to inadequate dialysis and infections and the major cause of death is of cardiovascular origin.

## Maintenance Haemodialysis

Maintenance HD in Poland is provided in 284 dialysis units [15]. Some of them, located in hospitals, also provide dialysis to patients with AKI. All hospital-based and some of the free-standing HD units provide 24/7 services. Every haemodialysis unit in Poland has to meet the rigorous technical demands defined for the provision of medical services. The compliance with these demands is verified on a regular basis by the regional delegacy of the State Sanitary Inspection. The employment guidelines define that at least one doctor has to be present at the facility when the services are provided. It is strongly advised that this is a specialist in nephrology, alternatively a trainee in the last year of internship in nephrology. The internal medicine specialists (or paediatricians at paediatric facilities) with a long record of experience in dialysis provision are also accepted, but at least one nephrologist has to be employed full time at each unit. During each shift, one nurse cares for 4–6 HD patients at the same time. The 3 × 4 h HD with the objective to reach $Kt/V > 1.2$ per session is the minimum standard treatment demanded by the National Health Fund. The service also includes regular check-up by nephrologist, laboratory and imaging examinations, and transportation to and from the dialysis unit. In more than 30% of patients, the central venous catheter (CVC) serves as the permanent vascular access. The number of patients on online haemodiafiltration (ol-HDF), as the post-dilution mode with the minimum ultrafiltration of 20.0 L/session, is very limited and only in some centres exceeds 10%. The small number of ol-HDF resulted from the fact that NHF did not contract this modality until the end of 2018. Home HD is not available in Poland yet. Most HD sessions are performed utilizing high-flux dialysers and the no-reuse policy is universal.

If needed, patients receive iron intravenously and erythopoiesis-stimulating agents (ESA) as part of the treatment, but vitamin D analogues and calcimimetics are contracted separately by the NHF. The average fee for standard HD is 110 USD per session and rises to 118 USD for the 24/7 services. The average fee for ol-HDF is 111.50 USD per session. These prices were subject to a slight increase in Q3 2019.

On 31.12.2018, there were 20,435 patients receiving HD and ol-HDF – 60% of them were males. Patients older than 65 years of age constituted 60% of this population, and every third patient was over 75 years old. Only 1/3 of the incident patients in 2018 were younger than 65 years of age. Conversion to HD from PD or after the loss of renal graft accounted for 13% of incident patients. The rate of KT in all HD modalities exceeded 5%, and the crude post 90-day mortality was 15.9% [11].

## Acute Kidney Injury and Critical Care Nephrology

AKI is an abrupt and usually reversible decline in the GFR, leading to an elevation of serum blood urea, creatinine and other metabolic waste products that are normally excreted by the kidney.

AKI not requiring RRT is usually treated in the wards where patients are admitted. In regional hospitals, where nephrology or dialysis service is not available, but nephrology consult is required due to clinical conditions, patients are usually transferred to the hospital of higher reference with appropriate facilities, including Intensive Care Unit (ICU).

In general, referral to the emergency department is due to more severe disease or life-threatening electrolyte abnormalities, stage 2 or 3 AKI as per the KDIGO criteria, patients with stage 1 AKI with an unclear aetiology, an unknown duration or trajectory of elevated creatinine, or if there is concern that the condition may not be rapidly reversible with simple interventions (such as volume expansion or removal of a potential nephrotoxin). Additionally, concomitant, uncontrolled comorbid condition (e.g. acute on chronic exacerbation of heart failure, diabetic ketoacidosis) in stage 1 AKI is another reason to ICU referral.

Patients who do not need an emergency department referral and who are managed as an outpatient should be referred for outpatient nephrology consultation if:

- Initial interventions fail to substantially improve the kidney injury.
- Glomerulonephritis (GN) is strongly suspected (such as in a patient with AKI, haematuria, and proteinuria).
- AKI occurs as a complication of treatment of an unrelated condition and future treatment depends upon nephrology input (such as AKI occurring as a complication of chemotherapy).

When medical management is ineffective, urgent RRT may be required in the following entities: pulmonary edema, hyperkalemia >6.5 mEq/L, hyperkalemia associated with symptoms or signs (ie., cardiac conduction abnormalities, muscle weakness), or hyperkalemia >5.5 mEq/L if there is ongoing tissue breakdown (eg., muscles in rhabdomyolysis) or red cells in significant gastrointestinal bleeding), signs of uremia, such as pericarditis, or an otherwise unexplained decline in mental status, severe metabolic acidosis (pH <7.1) unless it can be rapidly resolved by quickly correcting the underlying etiology (eg., diabetic ketoacidosis), hypervolemia or acute poisoning.

Multiple modalities of RRT are available in Poland. These include intermittent haemodialysis (IHD); continuous renal replacement therapies (CRRTs); and hybrid therapies, also known as prolonged intermittent renal replacement therapies (PIRRTs), such as sustained low-efficiency (daily) dialysis (SLEDD), sustained low-efficiency (daily) diafiltration (SLEDD-f), extended daily dialysis (EDD), slow continuous dialysis (SCD), and accelerated veno-venous hemofiltration (AVVH) or haemodiafiltration. Despite these varied techniques, mortality in patients with AKI remains high, exceeding 40–50% in severely ill patients.

Data do not support the superiority of any particular mode of RRT in patients with AKI. In the majority of patients, selection of modality is therefore based upon local expertise and availability of staff and equipment. CRRT represents a family of modalities that provides continuous support for severely ill patients with AKI. ICU and other emergency departments offer CRRT, while nephrology services predominantly offer intermittent HD. CRRT includes continuous hemofiltration (HF), HD and HDF, which involve both convective and diffusive therapies. Costs associated with CRRT are greater than with other modalities of RRT; however in Poland they are reimbursed for ICU, but not for nephrology. PD has a long history of use in the treatment of AKI; however, it is seldom performed for this purpose. PIRRT is a hybrid treatment that provides RRT for an extended period of time (i.e. 6–18 hours), but is intermittent (at least three times per week). PIRRT includes both convective (i.e. HF) and diffusive (i.e. HD) therapies, depending on the method of solute removal. The indication for PIRRT is dialysis-requiring AKI in a patient who is hemodynamically unstable to tolerate standard intermittent HD. SLED was introduced in early XXI century in the Department of Nephrology, Dialysis and Internal Medicine, at Warsaw Medical University (WUM). Standard intermittent HD is the modality of choice for hemodynamically stable patients with severe AKI, while in hemodynamically unstable ones CRRT or SLEDD are preferred. SLED also offers a possibility for patients' transition from CRRT to standard intermittent HD as hemodynamic stability improves. It allows for greater mobilization and rehabilitation of patients because of scheduled time off dialysis. Both SLED and intermittent HD years are reimbursed, but SLED is associated with greater cost than HD. The Genius® single-pass batch SLED was introduced as an intraoperative renal support during orthotopic liver transplantation (OLT) in the Department of Nephrology, Dialysis and Internal Medicine, WUM in 2011. The rationale behind this therapy is that patients undergoing OLT are often hemodynamically unstable and have multi-organ dysfunction with severe water, electrolyte and acid-base disorders, which can be further exacerbated by the surgery, usually necessitating massive blood products and fluid transfusions, and carries a high risk of severe acidosis, hyperkalaemia and overhydration. Since 2011, SLED during OLT has been performed in 137 patients.

Published data on RRT in AKI are extremely scarce. An alarming increase in the incidence of AKI in North America and Western Europe has been reported by Davenport and Siew [16]. Matuszkiewicz-Rowinska et al. [17] retrospectively analyzed the data obtained from individual hospital records of 774 consecutive patients with AKI, as defined by KDIGO criteria, requiring dialysis (AKI-D) in a single university hospital in Warsaw between Jan 2005 and Dec 2009. A subgroup of 126 patients, residents of three identifiable districts of Warsaw covered by the hospital with an estimated adult population of 149,687, were isolated to estimate the incidence. During the first 4 years, the incidence of AKI-D quadrupled from 52 to 202 cases per million person-years, reaching 241 per million person-years in 2009. The number of AKI-D per 1000 hospitalizations increased from 2.0 in 2005 to 4.4 in 2008. This occurred to be driven mostly by an increase in the number of patients dialyzed in different ICUs and apparently coincided with an introduction of new types of dialysis machines – Multifiltrate and Genius – which enabled performing continuous and hybrid techniques onsite. It appeared that the availability of different and more ICU-compatible RRT allowed performing dialysis in the most critically ill, and this influenced the incidence of AKI-D.

## Paediatric Nephrology

Paediatric nephrology in Poland as subspecialty gathers approximately 200 physicians, involved in renal care on different levels of reference. Paediatric nephrology care is coordinated by eleven medical centres of tertiary reference, covering the consultancy and referral requirements in relevant geographic regions. Most of them are university hospitals. All eleven centres provide general nephrology care, as well as acute and chronic dialysis program. One of the hospitals has also a position of national renal transplantation centre.

## Epidemiology of CKD

The incidence of CKD in European children is estimated to be 12 cases/pmarp (per million age-related population) for CKD stage 3–5 and 4–5/pmarp for CKD 4–5. In Poland, the incidence of RRT (equivalent to CKD 5) is 5.6 pmarp. The epidemiology of basic renal diseases in children is similar to other European countries, with CAKUT (congenital anomalies of kidney and urinary tract)-based malformations, urinary tract infections and nephrotic syndrome, as leading diseases. The epidemiology of CKD reveals the predominance of CAKUT-related renal failure up to 74% in CKD 2–4 and up to 43% in CKD 5, followed by glomerulopathies (both acquired and genetic) up to 14% in CKD 2–4 and up to 31,2% in CKD 5 and ciliopathies (PCKD and nephronophtysis) up to 5–9% in CKD 2–4 and 12% in CKD 5. Overall, approximately 2/3 of the causes of ESRD have congenital (genetic) background, which is consistent to European trends in paediatric patients [18, 19].

## Renal Replacement Therapy: Dialysis and Transplantation

Apart from data on incidence, there are data on the prevalence of RRT in children at the age of 0–14 years in Poland. Overall (age 0–14) the prevalence is 38.9 pmarp, while the detailed numbers within the age distribution are: 17.9 pmarp for the age of 0–4, 38.6 pmarp for the age of 5–9 and

61.3 pmarp for the age of 10–14 years, respectively. In regard to RRT modality, the overall prevalence (age of 0–14 years) is 27.8 pmarp for KT, 7.9 pmarp for and 2.9 pmarp for HD. In other words, approximately 73% of the children with ESRD live with functioning renal graft and the remaining live on chronic dialysis [20–22]. PD is a leading paediatric dialysis modality in Poland with the ratio between PD and HD of 2.7: 1. The overall number of children on regular PD during last decade has been between 85 and 118 per year, with the vast majority (>90%) of patients treated with APD.

## Renal Replacement Therapy in Paediatric AKI

Overall, between 2012 and 2016, out of 1156 children with AKI, 15,6% were treated with intermittent HD, 39,4% with PD and 45% with continuous veno-venous haemodiafiltration (CVVHDF) (data limited to patients reported by paediatric nephrologists; data from ICU not available).

## Renal Transplantation

Single national paediatric transplant centre runs the renal and liver-kidney transplantation program for the country. The program includes deceased-donor, living-related donor and pre-emptive KTs, as well as combined liver-kidney (CLKT), sequential kidney-after liver (SKLT) and liver-after kidney (SLKT) transplantations. The number of annual isolated KTs varies from 24 to 45, including 7–10% of living-related transplantations. Overall, 973 KTs have ever been performed. Recently (in 2018), overall 99 paediatric recipients were on active waiting list, including 13 candidates for pre-emptive transplant. The mean time on active waiting list to renal transplantation varies between 10 and 12 months [23]. Overall 25 CLKTs, 7 SKLTs and 4 SLKTs have been ever performed. The major indications (68%) were ciliopathies (autosomal recessive and autosomal dominant polycystic kidney disease; ARPKD and ADPKD), followed by primary hyperoxaluria type 1 (PH1; 24%). Overall, 90% 5-year patient survival has been achieved in this subgroup [24].

## Reimbursement

All RRT modalitites are fully refunded in Poland with no limitations. Orphan drugs, such as cysteamine (for cystinosis) and eculizumab (for aHUS), are currently refunded.

## Renal Transplantation: Living-Donor and Deceased-Donor. Organ Procurement and Transplantation Network Policies

### Renal Transplantation Policy in Poland [25]

Polish Transplant Coordinating Center "Poltransplant" is the competent authority subjected to the Ministry of Health and with main tasks as follows:

- Coordination of organ, tissues and hematopoietic cells procurement and transplantation with maintaining and financing the system of donor and transplant coordinators
- Administration and maintaining national waiting list and other registries related to transplantation medicine (National Transplants Registry, Living Donor Registry, Central Unrelated Potential Bone Marrow Donor and Cord Blood Registry)
- Monitoring and management of serious adverse reactions and events
- Evaluation and dissemination of transplantation results
- Processing applications for donation and transplant centres, in receiving ministerial permission for such activities
- Cooperation with donor and transplant centres, The National Transplantation Council, The National Center for Tissue and Cell Banking and with other national and foreign organizations related to transplantation medicine

## Donation

The activity includes deceased (the majority after brain death) and living-related kidney donation.

### Deceased Donors (DD)

In 2010, Poltransplant, thanks to funds from the National Program for Development of Transplantation Medicine, initiated a project to employ hospital donor coordinators in all hospitals where the identification of deceased donors, brain death confirmation and retrieval of organs are possible (388 hospitals met these conditions, 296 donor coordinators employed).

'Opting-out' policy was implemented for the purpose of an authorization to deceased donation. Objections to donation shall be stated in the form of: (a) registration in the Central Objection Register, (b) written statement with one's own signature and (c) oral statement made in the presence of at least two witnesses.

In 2018, the number of actual deceased organ donors was 498, which results in 13 deceased donors pmp. The numbers vary among the regions of the country.

### Living Donors (LD)

Procurement from LD constitutes a minority (10% of donors, 5% of kidney transplants). LD can be a straight-line relative (parents, grandparents, children and grandchildren), siblings, an adopted person or a spouse. Other volunteers (distant family, friends) must obtain the consent of the district court after hearing the applicant and after positive opinion of the Ethics Committee of the National Transplantation Council. Anonymous donation is not allowed.

## National Waiting List (NWL) and Kidney Allocation [26]

In 2018, 2745 patients were registered in the NWL, of which 1178 were reported de novo in 2018. Of the 1178 patients declared de novo for transplantation, 98 patients were reported in pre-emptive mode (8%). By the end of 2018, 1196 patients had an active status on NWL. The major indications for transplantation were: glomerular diseases, ADPKD and diabetic nephropathy. The mean age of the candidates was 51 years.

The average waiting time for the first DD KT was 337 days since referral to NWL and for the next KT was 630 days in 2018. Time to DD KT since initiation of dialysis was 1212 days for the first transplant. For patients referred pre-emptively, the waiting time was 168 days. For patients with urgent need for transplantation, the time to KT was 26, 21 and 16 days for the 1th, 2nd and 3rd transplantation, respectively. Data presented for 2018 are relevant to previous years.

General kidney allocation policies are as follows:

- Urgency
- Immunological compatibilities and incompatibilities (including ABO blood groups)
- Relations between donor and recipient age
- Donor-recipient weight and height matching
- Waiting time
- Expected transplantation results
- Present health status of potential recipient

In KTs, allocation system is nationwide and patient oriented. Details of allocation criteria are established by transplant centres' representatives, then implemented and supervised by Poltransplant. Some examples of mandatory transplantations are as follows: recipient without access (vascular or peritoneal) to dialysis, PRA ≥ 80%, no incompatible HLA, recipient >60 years to kidney from donor >65, paediatric recipient to kidney from paediatric donor, recipient of simultaneous kidney and other organ transplants. There are also some preference points for every lack of HLA mismatch at the locus A, B and DR, total duration of dialysis (one point for 1 year), immunization, diabetic nephropathy. Each organ donation and transplantation, as well as allocation process, must be documented in web-netted registries by donor and recipient centres.

### Immunological Work-Up in Poland

Following immunological tests are performed: complement-dependent serological (CDC), panel reactive antibody (CDC-PRA), single bead assay (SBA), virtual cross-matching (vXM), CDC-XM, flow cytometry XM.

## Renal Transplantation [26]

The program includes DD and LD kidney transplantation, combined kidney-pancreas, kidney-liver, kidney-heart and sequential kidney-after liver, kidney-after pancreas, kidney after heart as well as pancreas-after kidney and pancreatic islets-after kidney. These activities are carried out in 20 transplant centres. KTs are performed in dialyzed as well as not dialyzed yet patients (pre-emptive transplantations and re-transplantations) from NWL.

The number of annual KTs in years 2000 and 2018 varied from 674 to 1145 (Fig. 44.1) including 4–5% LD transplantations (Fig. 44.2). The total number of kidney transplants ever performed in Poland between 1966 and 2018, in various combinations, is 25,010. Currently, there are 11,703 recipients (43%) alive with an active kidney transplant. The average time of observation (partly weighted) is 14 years.

In 2018, 927 kidneys were transplanted to a total of 927 recipients (24.1 pmp) (887 from the DD (23.1 pmp); five liver-kidney transplants, one heart-kidney), and 40 from LD (1.0 pmp). Fifty-seven were performed pre-emptively (40 DD and 17 LD). One patient received islet transplantation after kidney.

Main immunosuppressive protocol consists of calcineurin inhibitor (in the recent years tacrolimus), mycophenolate mofetil and steroids. Induction therapy is given in 10 up to 59% of recipients depending on transplant unit.

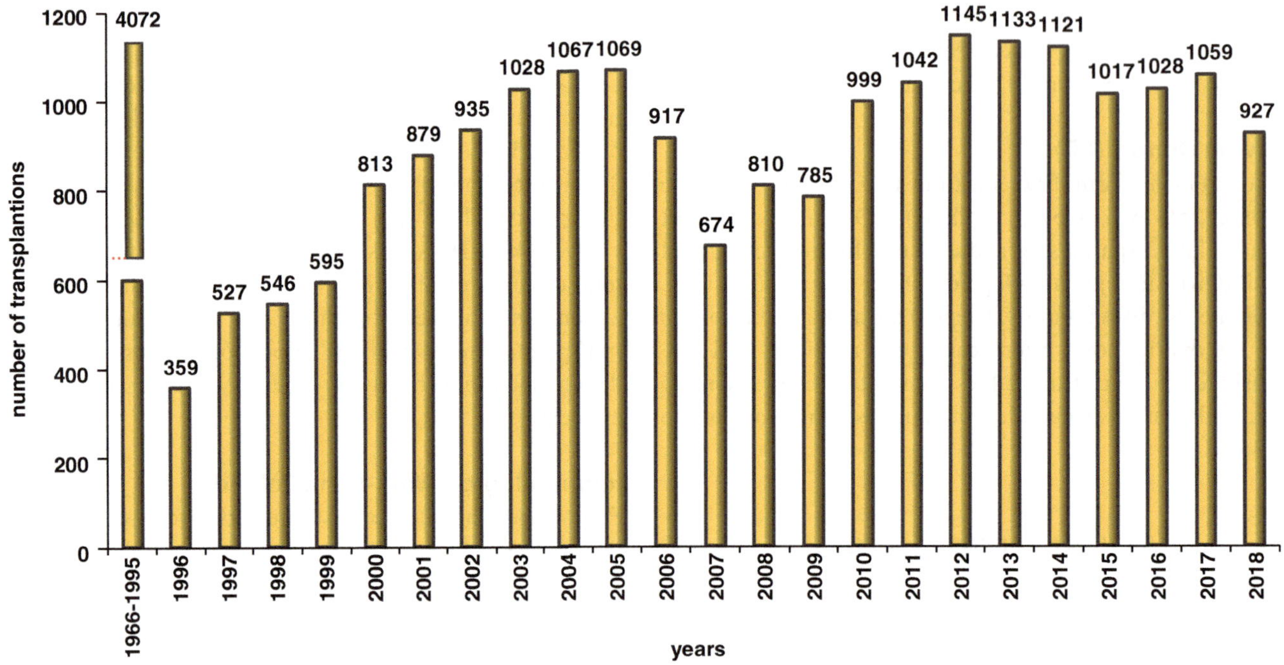


**Fig. 44.1** Number of renal transplantations in Poland in years 1966–2018

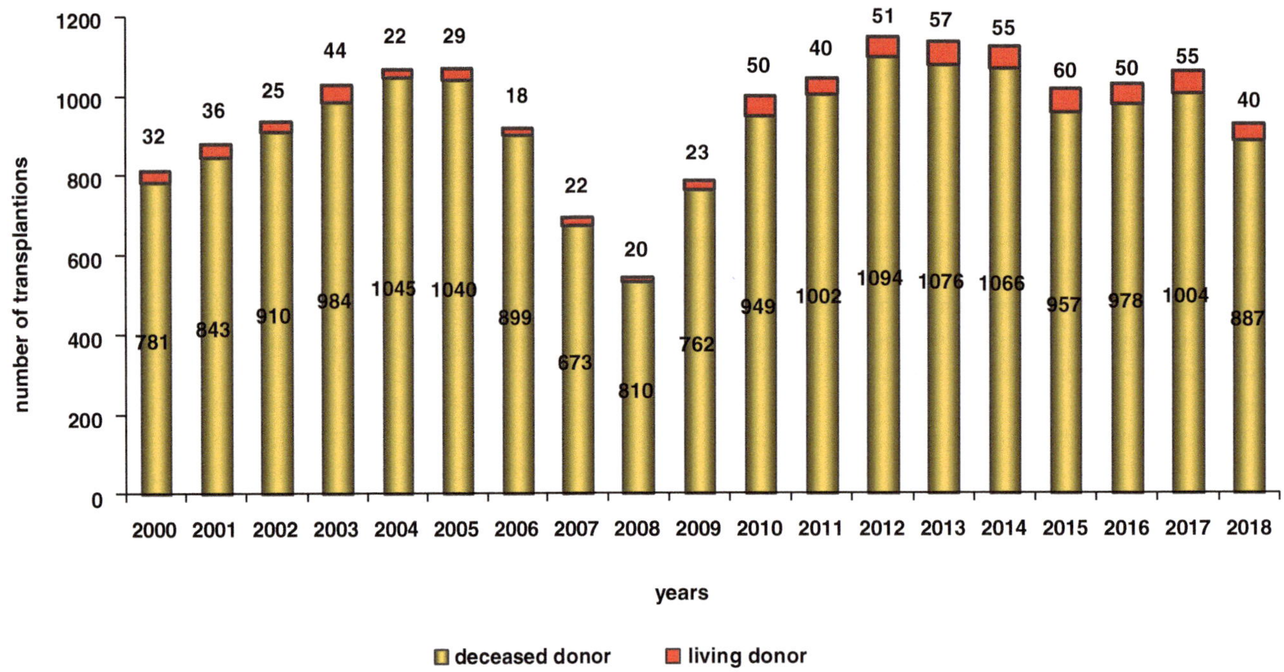


**Fig. 44.2** Number of deceased and living donor renal transplantations in Poland in years 2000–2018

## Patients and Grafts Survival [26]

In 2006, for the sake of proper monitoring and evaluation of transplantations performed, a National Transplants Registry was created. It has two main functions: gathering information on every organ transplantation performed within the country (registration function) and monitoring of quality of performed transplantations by collecting data on graft function and recipient's post-transplant survival in the short- and long-term follow-up (on the day of transplantation, 3 and 12 months after transplantation and every following year until graft loss or recipient death) (follow-up function).

Table 44.1 One-, five- and ten-year patient and graft survival in Poland

| Period | Patient survival (%) | | Graft survival (%) | |
|---|---|---|---|---|
| | 1996–2007 | 2008–2018 | 1996–2007 | 2008–2018 |
| 1 year | 95 | 95 | 89 | 91 |
| 5 years | 87 | 87 | 76 | 79 |
| 10 years | 74 | 71 | 59 | 57 |

One-, five- and ten-year patient and graft survival in Poland are presented in Table 44.1.

## Reimbursement

All organ, tissue and cell transplantation activities in Poland are financed and fully refunded (with no limitations of the number of procedures) by national health services with public resources.

## Nephrology Practice and Job Market

The system of nephrology services was split, into paediatric and adult services in Poland, only a couple of years ago [16]. The market has been developing dynamically since the end of the 1970s to reach its full availability for all those in need at the beginning of the twenty-first century.

The nephrology services system is highly fragmented and consists of 310 outpatient nephrology services, 284 dialysis units and 81 nephrology wards. This does not mean that there are no waiting lists for the outpatient CKD services – these are long and in big cities, the waiting time can exceed 1 year. The relative unavailability of outpatient services is accompanied by full and immediate access to chronic dialysis and the abundance of HD services. The waiting time for a KT for the relatively young patient on dialysis usually does not exceed 1 year.

The private sector cares for over 70% of the ESRD population. Among the largest dialysis providers are Fresenius Medical Care, Diaverum, DaVita and B. Braun networks. At the end of 2018, the number of non-public dialysis units in Poland was 182. On December 31, 2018, networks and other non-public providers took care of 13,520 HD patients (13,139) and PD (381). Of these, 6359 patients underwent dialysis in 72 Fresenius facilities, 3889 in 68 DaVita and Avitum wards (two combined in 2019) and 2208 in 24 Diaverum wards. The remaining 30% of the patients are treated in units located in public hospitals. All dialysis units are very well equipped, and the average number of patients in the dialysis unit is around 60. This situation is slightly different in big cities where the big HD units prevail. The high-flux HD and no-reuse policy are implemented universally. The PD sector is small – around 4% of dialysis patients and dominated by Fresenius and Baxter technology. The mortality on dialysis is similar to that in other European countries and the annual transplantation rate exceeds 5%. Home HD is not available in Poland.

The nephrology services market is highly regulated by the payer – the National Health Fund defines the volume of services for each treatment modality at every dialysis unit and in every outpatient nephrology service. All dialysis services are covered on the fee-for-service basis. The fee for ol-HDF is slightly higher as compared to the standard HD, but both are higher in units contracted to provide 24/7 services. Should any unit exceed the contracted volume, the surplus payment has to be negotiated separately. The hospital nephrology services are budgeted within the general hospital budget.

The dynamic rise in dialysis services at the beginning of XXI century dramatically increased the demand for trained nephrologists and nephrology nurses. The salaries exceed the country average, especially in the private sector. There is a shortage of both – nephrologists (1100 professionally active of 1400 board-certified) and dialysis nurses (777 specialists in nephrology nursing and 2346 certified dialysis and nephrology nurses).

There are enormous possibilities to master nephrological skills in Poland – there are annual meetings (congresses and symposia) of the Polish Society of Nephrology followed by the autumn Top Nephrological Trends symposium. Every year the National Kidney Foundation of Poland organizes a World Kidney Day Symposium, and every second year there is a meeting of nephrologist, nephrology nurses and technicians in Kraków (Kraków Days of Dialysis Therapy). All these national events are accompanied by numerous local scientific meetings – among them the annual cardio-nephrology symposium in Białowieża.

The Polish Society of Nephrology issues two scientific journals – 'Polish Nephrology and Dialysis Therapy' and 'Nephrology Forum'. It is also very active in preparing national guidelines for specific aspects of nephrological diagnosis and therapy.

To get the right to practice nephrology in Poland as a doctor or nurse, the applicant must become a member of the District Chamber of Physicians or the District Chamber of Nurses and Midwives, respectively. The EU certificates are recognized according to the general European rules; however, some additional training and certificate of proficiency in Polish language is also needed. For non-EU graduates, the formal recognition of diploma and skill certificates are proceeded individually.

There are two pathways to get the title of certified specialist in nephrology – one for specialists in internal medicine and the other for all the remaining. The candidate for nephrologist after completing the one-year-long postgraduate internship can either apply for residency in nephrology from the Ministry of Health or get the employer's approval to specialize during employment. The program for both is identical – 5 years of training in the accredited centre of training in hospital and outpatient general nephrology, internships in urology, transplantology and all modes of dialysis (85 weeks), and relevant courses (3,5 weeks), preceded by the three-year-long training in internal medicine and followed by the state specialization exam. Specialists in internal medicine are obliged to enter only the two-year-long specialization process. The first part of the exam, joint for all tracks to specialization, is a test of 120 questions, which, if passed, is followed by the oral exam in front of the state examination board. The separate specialization process in paediatric nephrology follows the same rules, with the exception that the internal medicine is replaced by paediatrics, and the internships and courses are performed in accredited paediatric nephrology units.

## Highlights of Nephrology in Poland

Similarly, to other Central and Eastern European countries separated after the Second World War from the Western world by the iron curtain, nephrology in Poland is a good example of how political and economic situation may influence the level of both scientific and practical aspects of nephrology. In the 1980s, Poland had a limited access to the modern methods of treatment of the acute and chronic kidney diseases and only a limited number of patients with ESRD had access to RRT. The same held true for the research possibilities and only a long-term scholarship in Western countries provided the ability to use modern research methods. For many of us, however, such a travel to the Western countries was at that time like a journey to a different planet [27]. Thirty years later, the situation in Poland has changed dramatically; and nowadays, nephrology in Poland has developed almost to the level of many Western European countries and the access to all types of RRT is unlimited for those who need them. Such an improvement was possible despite the lower financial resources spent on medical procedures in Poland in comparison to the Western countries. The number of patients with ESRD who started RRT (incidence rate) in the beginning of the 1980s (>50 pmp) and in 2016 (149 pmp) may serve as an example of our success [3]. The same is true for the prevalent patients treated with RRT in Poland in the 1980s (50 pmp) and in 2016 (812 pmp) [28]. Polish scientists who work in the field of nephrology have now access to European grants and participate in many multicentre studies. The role of Polish nephrologists in the European and international community has also been emphasized by the fact that many of us were elected for the ERA-EDTA (Council members: Andrzej Więcek, Marian Klinger, Joanna Małyszko; Andrzej Więcek also served as a Secretary-Treasurer and the President 2014–2017), International Society for Peritoneal Dialysis (Council members: Joanna Matuszkiewicz-Rowińska, Monika Lichodziejewska–Niemierko), International Association for the History of Nephrology (Presidents: Bolesław Rutkowski, Janusz Ostrowski) and EuroPD (Vice-chair: Monika Lichodziejewska-Niemierko). Earlier, Ryszard Gellert was appointed as an ERA-EDTA Registry director in London (from 1996 to 1998). This is in contrast to the 1960s and the 1980s, where only two Polish nephrologists were elected for the ERA-EDTA and ISN, namely Franciszek Kokot and Tadeusz Orłowski.

## Future Perspectives of Nephrology in Poland and Conclusion

The perspectives of nephrology in Poland are largely dependent on the reorganization of healthcare system that is being introduced and include a shift from decentralized mostly managed by local authorities to more centralized system. That change may affect a non-public sector of medical services as most of the new fundings will be directed to public healthcare services. The change of the system is not expected to generally improve the level of funding that is currently a major challenge for Polish healthcare. So far healthcare spendings in Poland have been among the lowest in EU, about two times less than an average. In 2015, public funds accounted for 72% of spendings, which was below the EU average whereas out-of-pocket spendings were higher than in most EU countries. Most of the out-of-pocket spendings of the patients are on drugs and diagnostics. They do not include most of the high-cost therapies that are reimbursed by the National Health Fund, which is a single payer for medical services for all people in Poland who have a medical insurance. RRT and KT are fully reimbursed and provided to all patients that require these therapies. That situation is not expected to significantly change in the future. More than half of all dialysis centres are non-public and for-profit, and a great majority of them are owned by large international providers. In contrast, most of nephrology wards and outpatient clinics are public.

A growing general problem of the healthcare system in Poland, including nephrology, is a shortage of professionals [29] and a high rate of a burnout among doctors [30] that reached 42% according to the results of the survey performed in 2018 by the Polish Society of Nephrology (unpublished data). The staff shortages in healthcare in Poland include mostly doctors and nurses and are caused mainly by their migration to wealthier countries in EU. Although nephrology has not been mostly affected by the staff shortages, there have already been a lack of staff in nephrology centres in public hospitals in smaller cities. A mean age of a board-certified nephrologist in Poland is now around 60 and is expected to further rise in future.

It is expected that also the current trend of the ever-increasing HD incidence in Poland will result – at the stable rates of mortality and KT – in the increasing HD prevalence not counterbalanced by the increasing PD prevalence. Since the underrepresentation of PD in chronic RRT provision is multifactorial, the National Health Fund and the Ministry of Health have been looking forward to implementing the new model of renal services – the integrated and co-ordinated value-based one [15]. The main concept behind this idea was to break the barriers resulting from the fee-for-service approach, and to merge various elements of the renal specialized care, including all forms of dialysis and referring patients to the kidney transplant waiting lists. All patients presenting with CKD stage 3B or more would meet the inclusion criteria of such a merged service – a 'NEPHRO-Unit'. The services shall be paid for from a budget allocated to the unit on per capita basis. The outcomes and quality indicators will be reported to the payer on a monthly basis. Meeting the predefined high-quality services' standards will be prized by the augmented per capita fee. Not meeting these standards for the prolonged time – the length to be decided later on – shall result in the termination of the contract. The three-year-long trial was expected to commence in autumn 2019.

It is expected that, for the population under care, every NEPHRO-Unit would create a services referral network to speed-up the access to fistula creation and servicing, physiotherapist, dietician, psychologist, and various medical specialists experienced in dealing with the CKD patients and in meeting their specific needs induced by dialysis and by the KT qualification process. It is believed that the economic effect of scale, along with the improved streaming of patients through the health system, will result in stabilization of the dialysis prevalence second to the improved pre-dialysis care, increased pre-emptive KT and cutting the waiting times for KT, as well as the appropriate conservative ESRD treatment. It should also result in the increased utilization of PD and home HD (the last is not available in Poland yet).

As a result of the aforementioned changes in the renal health system, the number of units delivering dialysis shall remain stable in the coming years. At the same time, the number of patients receiving conservative treatment of highest standards would increase and result in opening up the new outpatient renal services. This shall cut the waiting times for nephrology consultancy and shorten the time to travel to the renal consultancy room.

Due to the improved outpatient care, the number of nephrology in-hospitals beds is expected to decrease. However, this is not going to happen should the number of patients with AKI requiring dialysis rise and exceed the capacity of ICUs.

The changes in the provision of nephrology services shall increase the demand for nephrology staff. As a result, the number of nephrologists is expected to grow. This means more postgraduate training will be also needed in the long-term. As a short-term solution to the growing demand for nephrology staff, new regulations of accepting foreigners to the Polish health services are about to be issued. Second to the rising demand also nephrologists' salaries would increase, which would impose the transference of the administrative burden from the nephrologists to the specialized auxiliary staff.

It will be extremely interesting to see the coming changes happen and to participate in the process.

## References

1. https://en.wikipedia.org/wiki/Poland.
2. Ostrowski J. Nefrologia. In: Noszczyk W, editor. Dzieje medycyny w Polsce, vol. 3. Warsaw: PZWL; 2016.
3. Rutkowski B, Czekalski S, Lao M, et al. Development of renal replacement therapy in Poland. J Nephrol. 2006;19(suppl. 10):S159–64.
4. https://ec.europa.eu/health/state/country_profiles_en. Accessed 30 Jun 2019.
5. https://www.eea.europa.eu/media/newsreleases/many-europeans-still-exposed-to-air-pollution-2015/premature-deaths-attributable-to-air-pollution. Accessed 30 Jun 2019.
6. Perkowska-Ptasinska A, Bartczak A, Wagrowska-Danilewicz M, Halon A, Okon K, Wozniak A, Danilewicz M, Karkoszka H, Marszalek A, Kowalewska J, Mroz A, Korolczuk A, Oko A, Debska-Slizien A, Naumnik B, Hruby Z, Klinger M, Ciechanowski K, Myslak M, Sulowicz W, Rydzewski A, Wiecek A, Manitius J, Gregorczyk T, Niemczyk S, Nowicki M, Gellert R, Stompor T, Wieliczko M, Marczewski K, Paczek L, Rostkowska O, Deborska-Materkowska D, Bogdanowicz G, Milkowski A, Durlik M, Polish Society of Nephrology. Clinicopathologic correlations of renal pathology in the adult population of Poland. Nephrol Dial Transplant. 2017;32(suppl_2):ii209–18.
7. Willey CJ, Blais JD, Hall AK, Krasa HB, Makin AJ, Czerwiec FS. Prevalence of autosomal dominant polycystic kidney disease in the European Union. Nephrol Dial Transplant. 2017;32:1356–63.
8. Zdrojewski Ł, Zdrojewski T, Rutkowski M, Bandosz P, Król E, Wyrzykowski B, Rutkowski B. Prevalence of chronic kidney disease in a representative sample of the Polish population: results of the NATPOL 2011 survey. Nephrol Dial Transplant. 2016;31(3):433–9.
9. Zdrojewski Ł, Król E, Rutkowski B, Piotrowski W, Pająk A, Drygas W, Zdrojewski T. Chronic kidney disease in Polish elderly population aged 75+: results of the WOBASZ Senior Survey. Int Urol Nephrol. 2017;49:669–76.
10. Brück K, Stel VS, Gambaro G, Hallan S, Völzke H, Ärnlöv J, Kastarinen M, Guessous I, Vinhas J, Stengel B, Brenner H, Chudek J, Romundstad S, Tomson C, Gonzalez AO, Bello AK, Ferrieres J, Palmieri L, Browne G, Capuano V, Van Biesen W, Zoccali C, Gansevoort R, Navis G, Rothenbacher D, Ferraro PM, Nitsch D, Wanner C, Jager KJ, European CKD Burden Consortium. CKD prevalence varies across the European general population. J Am Soc Nephrol. 2016;27(7):2135–47.

11. Dębska-Ślizień A, Rutkowski B, Rutkowski P, Korejwo G, Gellert R. Actual condition of renal replacement therapy in Poland in year 2017. Nefrol Dial Pol. 2018;22:133–40.
12. Lichodziejewska–Niemierko M, Rutkowski B, Liberek T, Renke M. Peritoneal dialysis in Poland. Results from the national survey, 1995–1996. Perit Dial Int. 1999;19(2):171–3.
13. Rutkowski B, Lichodziejewska-Niemierko M, Grenda R, et al. Raport o stanie leczenia nerkozastępczego w Polsce - 2011 (Report on the renal replacement therapy in Poland -2011), Gdańsk; 2012.
14. Lichodziejewska-Niemierko M, Chmielewski M, Wojtaszek E, Suchowierska E, Golembiewska E, et al. Current epidemiology and practice patterns in prevention and treatment of PD-related infections in Poland. Int Urol Nephrol. 2019;51(2):335–41.
15. Gellert R, editor. Coordinated care over patients with chronic kidney disease. Warsaw: Nefron; 2018. ISBN:078-83-953566-0-5.
16. Siew ED, Davenport A. The growth of acute kidney injury: a rising tide or just closer attention to detail? Kidney Int. 2015;87:46–61.
17. Matuszkiewicz-Rowińska J, Zebrowski P, Kościelska M, Małyszko J, Mazur A. The growth of acute kidney injury: Eastern European perspective. Kidney Int. 2015;87:1264.
18. Harambat J, Van Stralen KJ, Kim JJ, Tizard EJ. Epidemiology of chronic kidney disease in children. Pediatr Nephrol. 2012;27:363–73.
19. Litwin M, Grenda R, Prokurat S, Abuauba M, Latoszyńska J, Jobs K, Boguszewska-Bączkowska A, Wawer ZT. Patient survival and causes of death in children on hemodialysis and peritoneal dialysis – single center study. Pediatr Nephrol. 2001;16:996–1001.
20. Harambat J, van Stralen KJ, Verrina E, Groothoff JW, Schaefer F, Jager KJ, ESPN/ERA-EDTA Registry. Likelihood of children with end-stage kidney disease in Europe to live with a functioning kidney transplant is mainly explained by nonmedical factors. Pediatr Nephrol. 2014;29(3):453–9.
21. Chesnaye NC, Schaefer F, Groothoff JW, Caskey FJ, Heaf JG, Kushnirenko S, Lewis M, Mauel R, Maurer E, Merenmies J, Shtiza D, Topaloglu R, Zaicova N, Zampetoglou A, Jager KJ, van Stralen KJ. Disparities in treatment rates of paediatric end-stage renal disease across Europe: insights from the ESPN/ERA-EDTA registry. Nephrol Dial Transplant. 2015;30(8):1377–85.
22. Chesnaye N, Bonthuis M, Schaefer F, Groothoff JW, Verrina E, Heaf JG, Jankauskiene A, Lukosiene V, Molchanova EA, Mota C, Peco-Antić A, Ratsch IM, Bjerre A, Roussinov DL, Sukalo A, Topaloglu R, Van Hoeck K, Zagozdzon I, Jager KJ, Van Stralen KJ, ESPN/ERA–EDTA Registry. Demographics of paediatric renal replacement therapy in Europe: a report of the ESPN/ERA-EDTA registry. Pediatr Nephrol. 2014;29(12):2403–10.
23. www.poltransplant.pl.
24. Szymczak M, Kaliciński P, Kowalewski G, Markiewicz-Kijewska M, Broniszczak D, Ismail H, Stefanowicz M, Kowalski A, Rubik J, Jankowska I, Piątosa B, Teisseyre J, Grenda R. Combined liver-kidney transplantation in children: single-center experiences and long-term results. Transplant Proc. 2018;50(7):2140–4.
25. The cell, tissue and organ recovery, storage and transplantation act of July 1st, 2005. The official journal of acts [dziennik ustaw] 05.169.14.
26. Poltransplant bulletin. 2019:1(27). www.poltransplant.pl/Download/Biuletyn_1_27_2019_www.pdf.
27. Holems D. Andrzej Więcek: east meets west in nephrology. Lancet. 2015;385:1937.
28. Kramer A, Pippias M, Noordzij M, Stel VS, Andrusev AM, Aparicio-Madre MI, Arribas Monzón FE, Åsberg A, Barbullushi M, Beltrán P, Bonthuis M, Caskey FJ, de la Nuez PC, Cernevskis H, De Meester J, Finne P, Golan E, Heaf JG, Hemmelder MH, Ioannou K, Kantaria N, Komissarov K, Korejwo G, Kramar R, Lassalle M, Lopot F, Macário F, Mackinnon B, Pálsson R, Pechter Ü, Piñera VC, de Pablos CS, Segarra-Medrano A, Seyahi N, Slon Roblero MF, Stojceva-Taneva O, Vazelov E, Winzeler R, Ziginskiene E, Massy Z, Jage KJ. The European Renal Associations-European Dialysis and Transplant Association (ERA-EDTA) registry annual report 2016: a summary. Clin Kidney J. 2019;12(5):702–20.
29. https://ec.europa.eu/eurostat/statistics-explained/pdfscache/37382.pdf. Accessed 01 Jul 2019.
30. Makara-Studzińska M, Załuski M, Tylec A, Panasiuk L. Do Polish doctors suffer from occupational burnout syndrome? An attempt to find an answer - Pilot study. Ann Agric Environ Med. 2019;26:191–7.

# Nephrology in Portugal

# 45

Ana Azevedo, Anabela Rodrigues, Aníbal Ferreira, Conceição Mota, Fernanda Carvalho, Fernando Macário, Helena Jardim, José António Lopes, José Diogo Barata, La Salete Martins, Manuela Almeida, Pedro Ponce, and José Vinhas

## Abbreviations

| | |
|---|---|
| ADPKD | Autosomal Dominant Polycystic Kidney Disease |
| AKI | Acute kidney injury |
| AVF | Arteriovenous fistula |
| CAPD | Continuous ambulatory peritoneal dialysis |
| CKD | Chronic kidney disease |
| CVVHDF | Continuous veno-venous haemodiafiltration |
| ERA-EDTA | European Renal Association-European Dialysis |
| ESRD | End-stage renal disease |
| FSGS | Focal segmental glomerulosclerosis |
| GDP | Gross domestic product |
| GFR | Glomerular filtration rate |
| HD | Haemodialysis |
| ICU | Intensive care unit |
| IgAN | IgA nephropathy |
| MCD | Minimal change disease |
| PD | Peritoneal dialysis |
| PTFE | Polytetrafluoroethylene |
| RRT | Renal replacement therapy |
| SLEDD | Slow low-efficiency daily dialysis |

| | |
|---|---|
| Area[1] | 92,225.61 $Km^2$ |
| Population[1] | 10,276,617 (2018) |
| Capital | Lisboa |
| Three most populated cities[1]: | (1) Lisboa<br>(2) Sintra<br>(3) Vila Nova de Gaia |
| Official language | Portuguese |
| Gross domestic product (GDP)[1] | 203.9 billion Euros (2018) |
| GDP per capita[1] | 19,826.9 Euros (2018) |
| Human Development Index (HDI)[1] | 0.847 (2017) |
| Official currency | Euro |
| Total number of nephrologists[2] | ~210 (20 pmp) |
| National society of nephrology[3] | Portuguese Society of Nephrology<br>www.spnefro.pt |
| Incidence of end-stage renal disease[3] | 2018 – 255.95 pmp |
| Prevalence of end-stage renal disease[3] (including patients with a functioning kidney transplant) | 2018 – 2,014.38 pmp |

The original version of this chapter was revised and updated. The correction to this chapter can be found at https://doi.org/10.1007/978-3-030-56890-0_54

A. Azevedo
Nephrology Department, Hospital Vila Franca de Xira, Vila Franca de Xira, Portugal

A. Rodrigues · L. S. Martins · M. Almeida
Nephrology Department, Centro Hospitalar e Universitário do Porto, Porto, Portugal

A. Ferreira
Nephrology Department, Centro Hospitalar e Universitário de Lisboa Central, Lisbon, Portugal

Nova Medical School, Universidade Nova de Lisboa, Lisbon, Portugal

C. Mota
Pediatric Nephrology Department, Centro Hospitalar e Universitário do Porto, Porto, Portugal

F. Carvalho
Nephropathology Department, Nefrolab-Clara Saúde, Paço de Arcos, Portugal

F. Macário
Chief Medical Officer, Diaverum, Portugal

H. Jardim
Pediatric Nephrology Department, Hospital CUF Porto, Porto, Portugal

J. A. Lopes
Nephrology and Renal Transplantation Department, Centro Hospitalar e Universitário de Lisboa Norte, Lisbon, Portugal

J. D. Barata
Nephrology Department, Hospital da Luz, Lisbon, Portugal

P. Ponce
Renal Unit and Intensive Care Unit, Hospital Cuf Infante Santo, Lisbon, Portugal

Fresenius Medical Care, Lisbon, Portugal

J. Vinhas (✉)
Nephrology Department, Centro Hospitalar de Setúbal, Setúbal, Portugal



J. A. Moura-Neto et al. (eds.), *Nephrology Worldwide*, https://doi.org/10.1007/978-3-030-56890-0_45

| | |
|---|---|
| Total number of patients on dialysis[3] (all modalities) | 2017 – 12,745<br>2018 – 13,014 |
| Number of patients on haemodialysis[3] | 2017 – 11,985<br>2018 – 12,227 |
| Number of patients on peritoneal dialysis[3] | 2017 – 756<br>2018 – 787 |
| Number of renal transplantations per year[3] | 2017 – 527<br>2018 – 505 |

Table references:

1. Instituto Nacional de estatística (INE). Accessed in June 2019. Available in: www.ine.pt
2. Rede Nacional de Especialidade Hospitalar e de Referenciação Nefrologia. Accessed in June 2019. Available in: https://www.sns.gov.pt/wp-content/uploads/2017/06/RNEHR-Nefrologia-Aprovada-19-06-2017.pdf
3. Gabinete de Registo da Doença Renal Crónica. Accessed in June 2019. Available in: www.spnefro.pt

## Introduction

Portugal is a country located in Southwestern Europe, being bordered to the west and south by the Atlantic Ocean and to the north and east by Spain. Its territory also includes the Atlantic archipelagos of Azores and Madeira.

The Instituto Nacional de Estatística estimates that, according to the 2011 census, the population was 10,562,178 (of which 52% was female, 48% was male). In 2018 and according to more updated data, the population decreased to 10,276,617 [1].

Portugal is a developed and a high-income country, with a GDP per capita of 19,827 euros (43rd) and a Human Development Index of 0.85 (40th). The national currency of Portugal is the euro (€), which replaced the Portuguese escudo in 2002 [2].

The Portuguese political regime is a semi-presidential representative democratic republic since the ratification of the Constitution of 1976, with Lisbon as its capital. Continental Portugal is agglomerated into 18 districts, while the archipelagos of the Azores and Madeira are governed as autonomous regions. The 18 districts of mainland Portugal are Aveiro, Beja, Braga, Bragança, Castelo Branco, Coimbra, Évora, Faro, Guarda, Lisboa, Portalegre, Porto, Santarém, Setúbal, Viana do Castelo, Vila Real and Viseu.

The average life expectancy in Portugal had reached 82 years in 2017; in 2020 it is estimated at 82.11 years [3]. The Portuguese health system is characterized by three coexisting systems: the National Health Service (Serviço Nacional de Saúde), special social health insurance schemes for certain professions (health subsystems) and voluntary private health insurance. The SNS provides universal coverage.

Nephrology is a quite recent speciality in Portugal. However, nowadays, the entire population has access to a nephrologist and to renal replacement therapy (RRT), when necessary.

Data on the incidence, prevalence and treatment of end-stage renal disease (ESRD) in Portugal is provided by the Portuguese Registry of Dialysis and Transplantation; data on the prevalence of biopsy-based diagnosis of kidney disease from the Portuguese Registry for Renal Biopsies, both sections of the Portuguese Society of Nephrology.

Portugal has no national information about the patients with the earlier stages of chronic kidney disease (CKD) followed in nephrology consultation (cohort studies) or about patients with acute kidney injury (AKI). Two cross-sectional population-based studies gave information on the prevalence of CKD stages 1–5.

## Brief History of Nephrology in Portugal

In the mid-1950s, a few Portuguese internists began to take an interest in kidney disease, and the first kidney biopsies were performed by Cerqueira Magro in Porto in 1956. Adolfo Coelho was the first to systematically focus on renal disease and pathology, and he began, in Lisbon, a regular programme to teach the fundamentals of renal physiology and kidney disease.

The first haemodialysis (HD) treatment was performed in Lisbon, in 1958, by Filipe Vaz with a Kolff rotating apparatus in a woman with AKI following a transfusion haemolysis.

The systematic access to dialysis, both peritoneal dialysis (PD) and HD, occurred in 1966 by the hand of Jacinto Simões, responsible at the time for the recently opened intensive care unit in Lisbon. The unit was equipped with a 'twin coil' artificial kidney from Travenol to perform HD and used the recently commercialized rigid stylet for PD. Initially programmed to only treat patients with AKI, this unit progressively incorporated the first patients with CKD, and it can be considered the first dialysis unit for ESRD in Portugal. In the following year, Levy Guerra in Porto and Linhares Furtado in Coimbra opened small hospital HD.

It was in Coimbra, in 1969, that Linhares Furtado performed the first living donor kidney transplant.

In the 1970s, the lack of regulation was constraining the development of both transplantation and dialysis. CKD patients were being diagnosed but still didn't receive treatment, given the scarcity of resources available in the country.

The pioneers of Portuguese nephrology and CKD treatment, who were living the day-to-day drama of following untreated patients, produced a report, in 1973, that was presented to the health authorities, with a plan for national ESRD treatment coverage.

Without a systematic public answer to the situation, the first private HD unit was built in Lisbon in 1973 by Filipe Vaz, but still didn't have the capacity to treat all the Portuguese ESRD patients. The health authorities agreed to pay the totality of the treatments in this private setting. Thenceforth, the development of the national programme for HD treatment in Portugal has been based on private initiative with full public payment coverage.

In 1974, the 'Carnation Revolution' and the consequent political instability made it difficult to issue public legislation on ESRD; both the Portuguese and the Spanish governments made an agreement to treat in Spain the incident patients that could not receive treatment in Portugal.

In 1975, the first nephrology training programme in Portugal was established. During the second half of the 1970s multiple new HD units emerged throughout the country. By June 1978 there were 294 ESRD Portuguese patients on haemodialysis, 120 of them still treated in Spain. Only in 1979 did all the patients with diagnosed CKD got access to dialytic treatment in Portugal. In 1979, a set of legislative initiatives allowed the regulation of the National Health Service and, with it, Portuguese Nephrology and the treatment of ESRD.

In the previous decade, the first steps for legal regulation of renal transplantation and cadaveric organ harvesting were done, but only in 1980 did the first complete multidisciplinary transplantation teams began to operate both in Coimbra and Lisbon.

In 1981, the Portuguese Medical Association recognized nephrology as an independent medical speciality, and Martins Prata was the first president of the Portuguese College of Nephrology. The first PD programme began first in Lisbon and then in Oporto in the year of 1981. In 1982, Eva Xavier was the first president of the recently created Portuguese Society of Nephrology, and in the same year, the first Nephrology Symposium took place.

In 1988, 10 years after the full dialytic coverage of the known ESRD patients, the national registry of the Portuguese Society of Nephrology had 2845 patients on dialysis (prevalence rate, 388 pmp), with an incidence rate of 55 patients per million population (pmp), only 25% of them were older than 65 years. This ten times increase in prevalent patients was accompanied by the growing number of nephrologists, the wider knowledge of the disease, and by the national distribution of haemodialysis units along the territory.

During the 1990s, the treatment of CKD and ESRD by dialysis or transplantation was fully regulated and reached total coverage. In 2008, a new model of ESRD Integrated Management that restructured the dialysis care and the reimbursement was introduced. This model includes bundling of payment per person per week for treatments, medication, vascular access and basic complementary exams.

Patients have now full access to dialysis treatment, and cadaveric kidney donation is universal. In the last decade, Portugal became one of the countries with the highest rates of treated ESRD patients by dialysis or transplantation worldwide [4].

## Renal Diseases in Portugal

### Introduction

Knowledge about the worldwide CKD distribution is primarily based on the analysis of kidney biopsy data from registries. Over the last two decades, published literature showed that thousands of patients have been included in world registries, ranging from single to multicentre analysis, providing useful information about the frequency of chronic nephropathies according to gender, age and clinical syndromes, based on histologic diagnosis.

IgA nephropathy is the most prevalent glomerulopathy in a major part of the world. Membranous nephropathy and focal segmental glomerulosclerosis (FSGS) are the most prevalent in some countries, being FSGS the most frequent in some regions of the USA and in Brazil. IgA nephropathy is particularly linked to Asians and FSGS to Africans including Afro-Americans [5–7].

### Portuguese Registry for Renal Biopsies

In 2009, the Portuguese Society of Nephrology created the National Registry for Renal Biopsies (NRRB-PSN) [8]. Thenceforth, records of data from all native kidney biopsies (no allograft) performed at 37 hospitals, from the continent and the Atlantic islands (Azores and Madeira), are analysed every year. Between 2009 and 2018, 7800 people underwent a kidney biopsy. Optical microscopy and immunofluorescence were applied to all biopsies. Additionally, from 2014 to 2016, electron microscopy was utilized in the evaluation of 425 *kidney biopsies*, representing 16.1% of the total kidney biopsies (2637). The number of kidney biopsies has remained stable throughout these 10 years, reaching 889 kidney biopsies in 2017. In 2017, the mean age at the time of biopsy was 53 years, with a male predominance of 56%. Distribution according to age was 4% under 18 years, 64% between 18 and 65 years and 31% above 65 years.

### Biopsy-Based Diagnosis of Kidney Disease

Nephrotic syndrome and nephrotic proteinuria were the main reasons for patients to undergo a kidney biopsy, being aligned with the Spanish registry [9], followed by AKI, non-nephrotic proteinuria and asymptomatic urinary abnormalities. The latter are mentioned as the first cause for kidney biopsy in the Italian registry [9].

Glomerular diseases were the most prevalent histopathological group. In 889 kidney biopsies, the main diagnoses

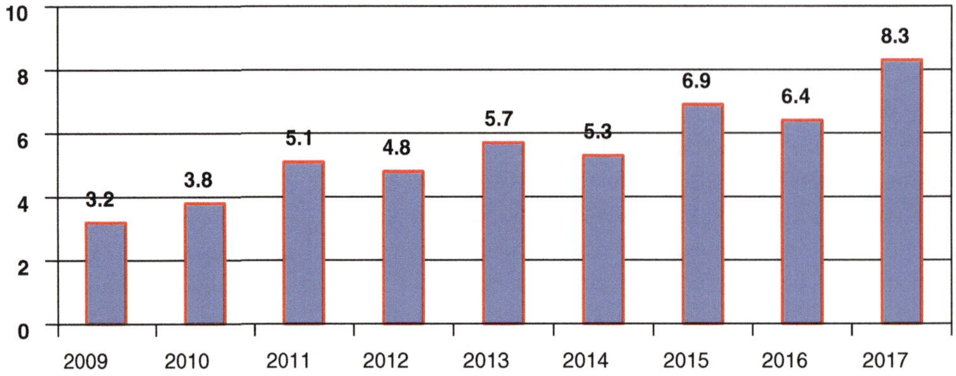


**Fig. 45.1** Biopsy-based diagnosis of kidney disease (diabetic nephropathy %) [5]

were IgA nephropathy in 107 cases (13.0%), FSGS in 94 (11.4%), diabetic nephropathy in 69 (8.3%), lupus nephritis in 66 (8.1%) and membranous nephropathy in 7 cases (6.0%).

In patients aged ≤18 years, IgA nephropathy was the most predominant (30.5%), followed by lupus nephritis (27.7%) and minimal change disease (MCD) and FSGS with 11.1% each one.

In the group aged 18–65 years, IgA nephropathy was still the most prevalent glomerulopathy (16.5%), followed by FSGS (10.6%), lupus nephritis (9.1%), membranous nephropathy (6.0%), diabetic nephropathy (5.8%), vasculitis/crescentic (4.8%) and renal amyloidosis (4.1%).

In elderly patients (≥65 years), diabetic nephropathy was the most common (12.8%), followed by FSGS (10.6%), crescentic glomerulonephritis (9.9%), renal amyloidosis (7.7%) and membranous nephropathy (4.4%).

The main primary causes of renal disease remained stable over this decade. Secondary causes such as diabetic nephropathy (Fig. 45.1) and renal amyloidosis increased their prevalence over the years and were only diagnosed in the adult and elderly population. According to 2015 registry, the main type of amyloidosis in 42 kidney biopsies was AA in 14 cases (33%), followed by Aλ in 5 cases (12%) and ATTR in 4 cases (10%); 18 cases (43%) were not classified.

## Chronic Kidney Disease in the General Population

### Epidemiology

Regarding the earlier stages of CKD, the data is scarce. In 2008, a population-based study was conducted to evaluate the prevalence of diabetes in Portugal [10] – the PREVADIAB study – and this study was an opportunity to evaluate the prevalence of CKD stages 3 and 4. The study included a nationally representative sample of 5167 subjects aged between 20 and 79 years old. In this study, CKD was classified using the National Kidney Foundation Chronic Kidney Disease classification of 2002 [11]. Glomerular filtration rate (GFR) was estimated by using the simplified (the four-variable formula) Modification of Diet in Renal Disease study equation. The prevalence of CKD stages 3 and 4 among adults aged 20–79 years was 5900 per 100,000 persons. The prevalence of CKD stages 3–5 was 6.1% (532,000 persons), with a prevalence in stage 3 of 5.6%, stage 4 of 0.3% and stage 5 of 0.18%. The prevalence was higher in older subjects, in women and in subjects with a low educational level [12]. The prevalence of risk factors associated with the development of CKD was 44.8% for hypertension, 11.7% for diabetes, 33.7% for obesity and 41.5% for metabolic syndrome. This study gave no information about CKD stages 1 and 2 as it was primarily designed to evaluate the prevalence of diabetes and did not include determination of albumin concentration in the urine [12].

Ten years later, in 2018, another study was conducted in 60 primary healthcare units, from 45 randomly selected municipalities from Portugal. This study included 3135 subjects, with at least 18 years old, and was designed to study the prevalence of CKD stages 1–5. The study showed a prevalence of CKD of 20.7%. CKD stages 1 through 5 were 0.4% for stage 1, 9.7% for stage 2, 7.9% for stage 3a, 2.1% for stage 3b, 0.5% for stage 4 and 0.1% for stage 5 (unpublished data).

## Acute Kidney Injury

### Incidence, Mortality and Causes of Acute Kidney Injury

In Portugal, the true incidence of AKI, particularly in the intensive care unit (ICU) setting, is unknown. Portuguese studies evaluating AKI incidence are quite scarce. The single-centre and retrospective nature of those studies focussing on small cohorts largely limits their generalizability and the validity of the results.

In a study performed in a tertiary teaching hospital enrolling 662 admitted to a mixed ICU, approximately 50% of patients had AKI, by AKIN criteria, during ICU stay: 21.1% with stage 1, 10.1% with stage 2 and 19.2% with stage 3 [13].

In this study, patients with AKI were more likely to be older ($p < 0.0001$), to have pre-existing cardiovascular disease ($p = 0.023$) and CKD than non-AKI patients. Using RIFLE criteria, patients with non-AKI had a mean age of 55 ± 19 years old, while patients with AKI had a mean age of 64 ± 18, 63 ± 15 and 61 ± 16 years, in the risk, injury and failure RIFLE categories, respectively. Forty-eight percent of the population without AKI had a history of cardiovascular disease, a lower proportion than that observed in the population with AKI: 63.9%, 61.6%, and 54.2%, in the risk, injury and failures RIFLE categories, respectively.

Furthermore, there was a greater proportion of patients with AKI admitted to the hospital for a medical condition, as compared to non-AKI (71.8% for non-AKI patients vs 78.4%, 80.8% and 86.7%, for the RIFLE risk, injury and failure categories of AKI, respectively; $p = 0.008$).

Patients with AKI had a higher illness severity score as compared to non-AKI (mean SAPS II in patients with non-AKI 40 ± 15, vs 48 ± 15, 51 ± 18 and 62 ± 21, in the RIFLE risk, injury and failure categories, respectively, $p < 0.0001$).

Patients with AKI were also more prone to be septic (26.6% in patients with non-AKI vs 39.2%, 61.6% and 74.2%, in the RIFLE risk, injury and failure categories of AKI, respectively, $p < 0.0001$) and to need vasopressors (21.5% in non-AKI population vs 48.5%, 63.0% and 76.7%, in the RIFLE risk, injury and failure categories of AKI, respectively, $p < 0.0001$).

In addition, AKI patients had longer hospital stay and increased in-hospital mortality (41% vs 11%). In fact, AKI carried a threefold increased risk for hospital death (odds ratio 2.78, 95%CI 1.74–4.45, $p < 0.0001$). In this study, 79 patients (27.2%) received RRT.

Another Portuguese study which included 457 critically patients with severe sepsis or septic shock showed that in-hospital mortality was 38.3% in patients with AKI using AKIN definition, a twofold increase in mortality risk (odds ratio 2.3, 95% CI 1.2–6.2, $p = 0.021$) as compared to patients with non-AKI [14].

A recent study performed in a Portuguese unit, including 450 patients undergoing major non-vascular abdominal surgery showed an incidence of 22.4% of postoperative AKI. In this study, AKI was associated with increased in-hospital mortality (20.8% vs 2.3%, $p < 0.0001$) [15].

Portuguese studies have also shown that AKI has a detrimental impact on long-term mortality and on long-term risk for progressing to CKD in septic patients and in patients undergoing major abdominal surgery [16, 17].

## Clinical Practice Patterns

Clinical practice patterns in Portugal are possibly quite similar to that of other countries. Serum cystatin C is widely available and can be easily ordered if considered necessary. Urinary dipstick is performed at admission in all medical and some surgical and cardiac ICUs. Further blood and urinary tests and renal ultrasound are offered to some patients, according to three parameters: clinical history, physical examination and routine blood and urinary tests. Renal ultrasound is normally performed with three goals: to exclude urinary tract obstruction, to exclude renal abscesses and to exclude ESRD with small kidneys (if an earlier value of serum creatinine concentration is not available). Renal biopsy is offered to only a minority of ICU patients due to the high risk of complications associated with this technique in critically ill patients and is only offered when the potential for benefit and the expected impact on treatment is considered high.

## Treatment Modalities for Acute Kidney Injury

Therapeutic approach is performed according to the aetiology of AKI and broadly follows the Kidney Disease Improving Global Outcomes (KDIGO) guidelines of AKI [18]. A particular emphasis is made on the optimization of haemodynamics and fluid balance, with avoidance of nephrotoxins. Of interest, in ICU AKI patients requiring RRT, slow low-efficiency daily dialysis (SLEDD) is only offered in very few hospitals, and the vast majority of those patients undergo intermittent HD or continuous modalities. Continuous veno-venous haemodiafiltration (CVVHDF) is the most used continuous modality.

## The Role of the Nephrologist in the ICU

The role of the nephrologist in the ICU has changed over the years and varies according to the hospitals and the expertise of the intensive care specialists. Until recently, intensive care medicine in Portugal was considered a subspecialty, with admission from other specialities occurring following completion of the primary specialty training, in most cases, internal medicine or one of its branches (pulmonology, cardiology or nephrology) or anaesthesiology. In 2018, intensive care medicine was considered a speciality in its own right without a second or a base speciality, and this may change the future role of the nephrologist in the ICU. For the time being, many ICUs are primarily ruled by medical doctors which are not so familiar with the therapeutic approach of AKI and, namely, the dialysis prescriptions, and, therefore, their multidisciplinary approach usually includes a nephrologist. In the units where the management is essentially intensivist-based, the main reasons for asking for nephrology collaboration are the prescription of intermittent dialysis (as opposed to CRRT where most intensivists are autonomous), prescription of therapeutic apheresis and the diagnosis and therapeutic approach to glomerulopathies. Globally, the relationship between nephrologists and intensivists is positive, and constructive and national joint meetings are occasionally organized.

## Renal Replacement Therapy in Portugal

### Introduction

Portugal has one of the highest incidence and prevalence of RRT in Europe as reported by the European Renal Association-European Dialysis and Transplantation Association (ERA-EDTA) that provides information about RRT across Europe [19].

Access to RRT is universal in Portugal, and there is a good network of facilities. This network and the referral to nephrology and RRT have been revised in an official document published by the health authorities in 2017 [20]. According to this document, the number of nephrologists per 1000 population in 2015 was 0.02, and the number of nephrologists per 1000 ESRD patients was 11.5 [20]. The Portuguese Registry of Dialysis and Transplantation from the Portuguese Society of Nephrology [21] provides aggregated data regarding RRT and will be used in this description of RRT in Portugal. The Portuguese Registry retrieves data from questionnaires sent yearly to both public and private dialysis units in Portugal, with 100% response rate since 1997. The latest report (2018) gathered data from 124 HD units, 25 PD units and 9 (eight adult and one paediatric) kidney transplant units and reported a high ESRD incidence of 256 pmp representing a total of 2634 patients starting RRT during 2018 (Fig. 45.2). The majority of incident patients started HD (90.3%), with the remaining patients initiating PD (8.7%) or receiving a pre-emptive kidney transplantation (1%).

As of December 31, 2018, 20,730 patients were being treated for ESRD in Portugal, giving a point prevalence of 2014 pmp. The majority of the patients were treated by HD (58.9%) with the remaining patients living with a functioning renal graft (37.3%) or treated by PD (3.8%) (Fig. 45.3).

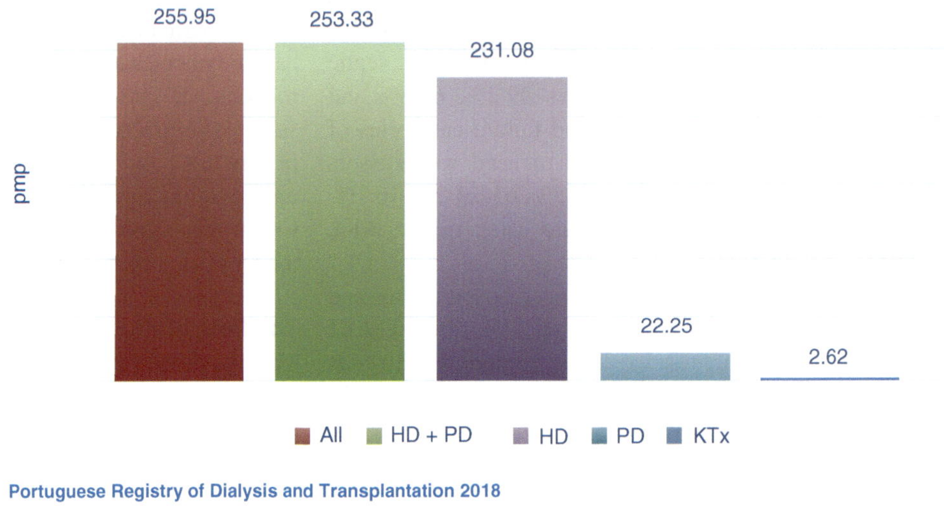


**Fig. 45.2** Incident patients accepted for RRT during 2018

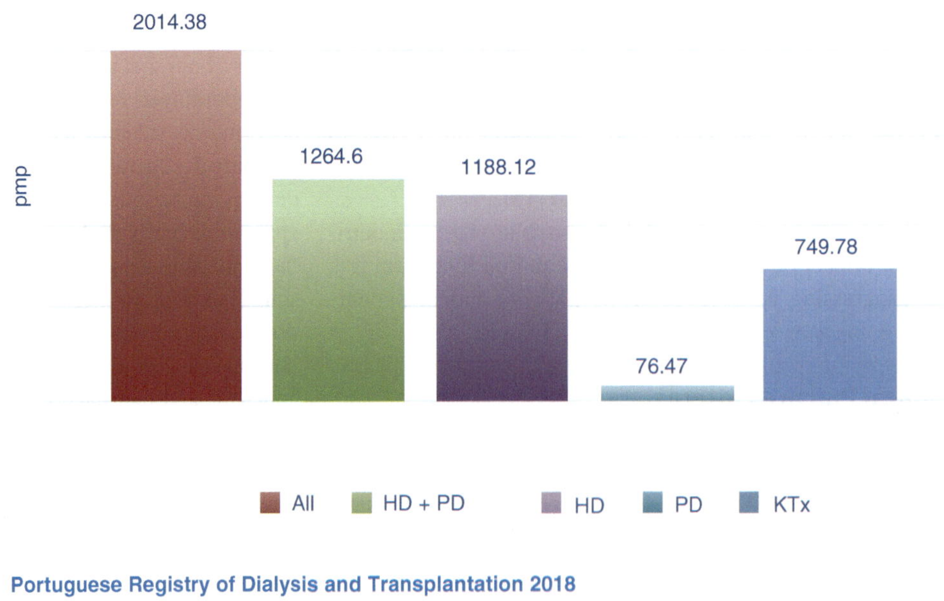


**Fig. 45.3** Prevalent patients on RRT by modality as of December 31, 2018

All hospitals are required to have a multidisciplinary consultation for patients in the later stages of CKD, whose goal is to inform patients of all RRT modalities that are available and about the alternative, conservative management for kidney failure. Prior to initiation of RRT, patients must sign an informed consent form authorizing to receive the selected treatment modality. The directorate-general of health regularly audits this process.

## Haemodialysis

### Incidence and Prevalence

The data on the treatment of ESRD presented in this section was mostly extracted from the 2018 Registry of the Portuguese Society of Nephrology, last updated on March 31, 2019 [21].

As mentioned earlier, ESRD patients are treated in 124 haemodialysis units, with a good geographical coverage of the whole country.

The overall incidence of patients accepted for RRT during 2018 was 255.9 pmp, 231.1 for HD, 22.3 for PD and 2.6 pmp for renal transplant, meaning that, in 2018, 2378 incident patients began their RRT by HD and 229 pts by PD. Compared to other European countries included in the 2016 EDTA registry, an unadjusted incidence of 236 pmp observed at day 1 was only exceeded by the Czech Republic and Greece [19].

Of all HD patients beginning RRT, only 21% had more than 3 months of follow-up in a nephrology clinic (35% in 2008). On admission to a HD unit, 35.4% were aged 18–65 years old, 40% were 65–80 years old and 24.4% were older than 80 years.

In patients who initiated HD treatment in 2018, the causes of renal disease were diabetes mellitus 32.5%, hypertension 14.2%, chronic glomerulonephritis 10.3%, autosomal dominant polycystic disease (from now on, polycystic kidney disease) 5.2% and an unknown cause 18.2%.

As of December 31, 2018, ESRD point prevalence was 2014 pmp, 1188 pmp being treated by HD, 76.5 pmp by PD and 749.8 pmp by renal transplant (Fig. 45.3). The annual growth of prevalent patients on dialysis is clearly dropping from numbers ranging between 4% and 8% yearly until 2008 to figures below 2% yearly ever since. The annual growth in 2017 and 2018 was 2.1% (Fig. 45.4). Based on the EDTA-ERA registry, at the end of 2016, Portugal had the largest prevalence of all European countries registered (1906 pmp) and the fifth position in the world after Taiwan, Japan, the USA and Singapore [19]. In 2018, the mean age of prevalent patients was 68 years.

For prevalent patients, in 2018, diabetes (27.8%), hypertension (13.8%), chronic glomerulonephritis (13.8%) and polycystic kidney disease (6.2%) were the main causes of ESRD.

### Vascular Access

In 2018, 51.6% of incident patients were using a tunnelled catheter, 7.3% a transient catheter, 39.1% a native arteriovenous fistula (AVF) and 1.9% grafts (PTFE). The catheter rate in the first HD session steadily rose from 51.4% in 2008 to 58.9% in 2018.

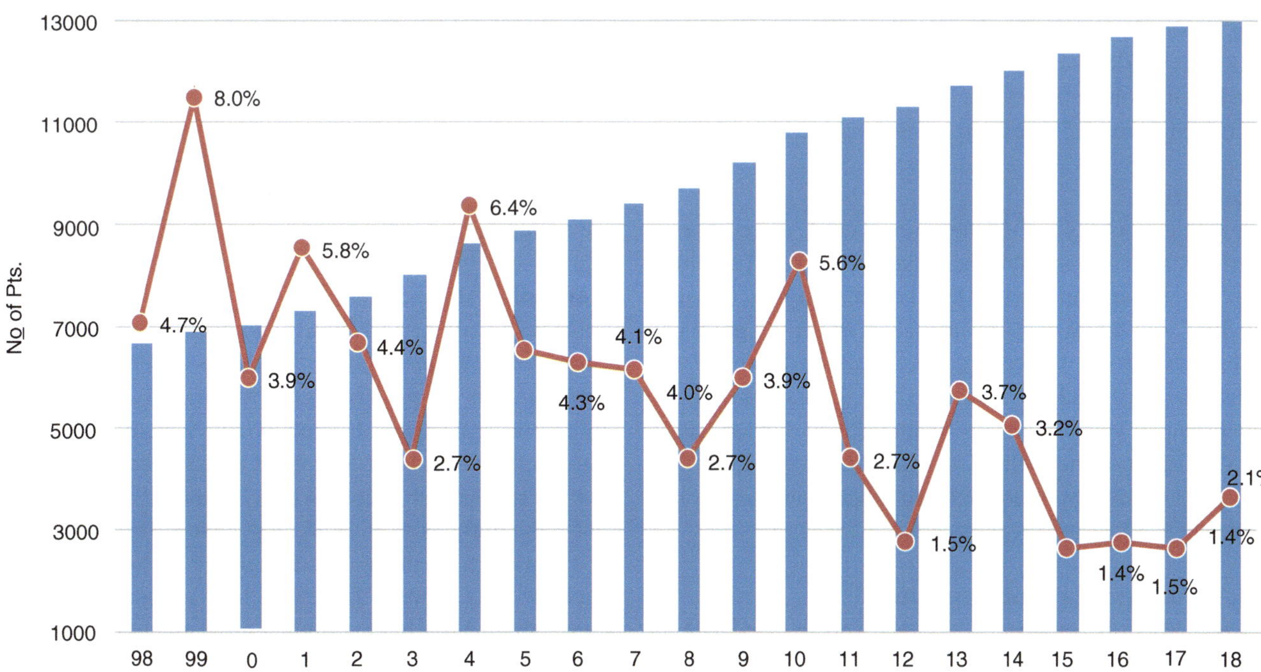


**Fig. 45.4** Yearly growth of the patients' pool on dialysis

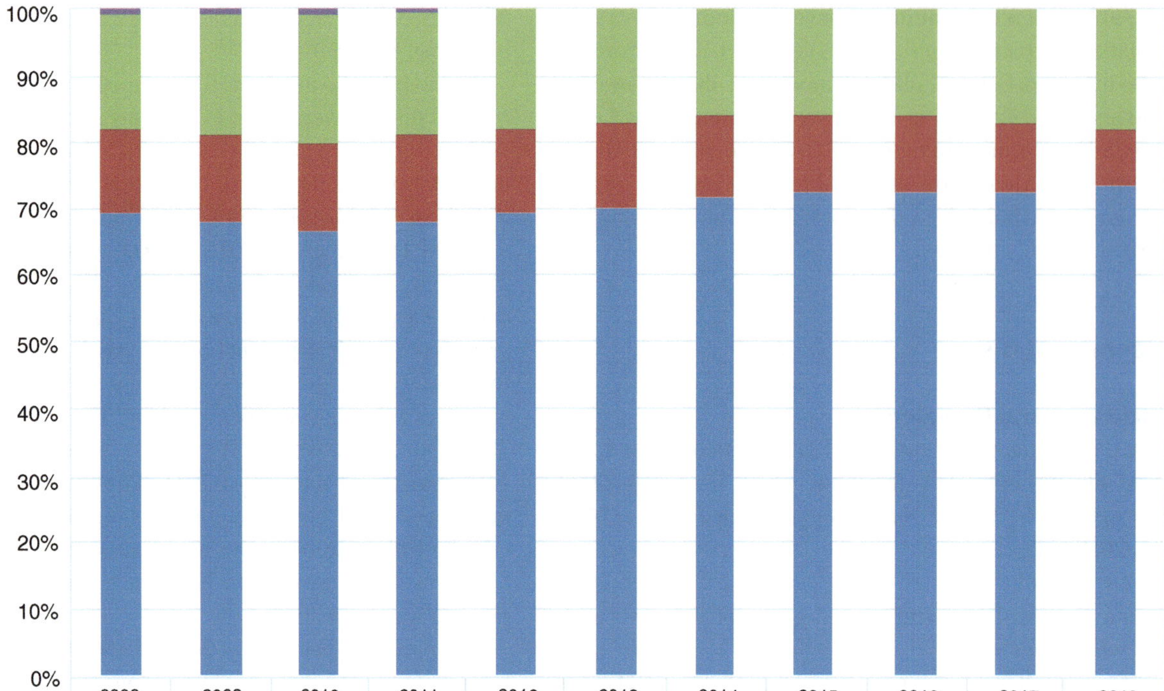


| | 2008 | 2008 | 2010 | 2011 | 2012 | 2013 | 2014 | 2015 | 2016 | 2017 | 2018 |
|---|---|---|---|---|---|---|---|---|---|---|---|
| Non-Tunneled Cat | 76 | 39 | 42 | 25 | 16 | 23 | 15 | 24 | 2 | 10 | 35 |
| Tunneled Catheter | 1572 | 1769 | 1953 | 1905 | 1889 | 1834 | 1770 | 1804 | 1895 | 1971 | 2109 |
| Graft | 1191 | 1256 | 1365 | 1402 | 1349 | 1258 | 1317 | 1273 | 1239 | 1216 | 1101 |
| AVFistula | 6464 | 6538 | 6788 | 7077 | 7257 | 7750 | 8202 | 8434 | 8598 | 8782 | 8978 |

**Fig. 45.5** Vascular access type on use in prevalent HD patients

By December 31, 2018, the proportion of prevalent patients with an AVF for vascular access was 73.5%, with a PTFE graft was 9% and with a tunnelled catheter was 17.3%. The prevalence of AVF increased from 66.9% in 2010 to 73.5% in 2018, a constant rising trend, with an opposite trend being observed in the proportion of grafts, which decreased from 13.5% in 2010 to 9% in 2018 (Fig. 45.5).

### Mortality

Regarding mortality in HD, the national crude mortality rate was 13.8%, 20.7% in public hospital units and 13.1% in private outpatient units in 2018. The mortality in the first 90 days was 4.8%, and the annual mortality of prevalent patients (since day 91) was 12.7%. Of all the 1660 patients deceased in 2018, 82.1% were older than 65 years and 44.2% older than 80 years. Causes of death were cardiovascular in 24.8%, infection not related to vascular access in 21.6% (23.3% if all infections are included), malignancy in 11.6%, cachexia in 8.0% and sudden death in 8.5%.

### Haemodialysis Patient Disposition

During 2018, the number of patients who initiated HD as their first RRT was 2378. In the same year, 2636 patient initiated HD, and this figure includes 159 renal transplant failures and 99 patients transferred from PD.

During the same year, 2271 patients went out of the 'HD pool': 1660 deaths, 394 transplanted, 54 patients moving into PD, 94 patients withdrawn from dialysis treatment and 69 who recovered renal function.

### Waiting List for Renal Transplantation

Of the whole pool of prevalent HD patients, 20.8% were in active waiting list for kidney transplantation.

### Haemodialysis Facilities

Portuguese College of Nephrology define in *Manual das Boas Práticas de Diálise Crónica* (*Good Practice Guidelines on Chronic Dialysis*) the dialysis facility setting in Portugal. All units need to have a medical director (who must have at least 5 years of experience as nephrologist), a head nurse, nephrologists and doctors responsible for the dialysis shift (who must have at least 3 months of experience treating these patients). Nephrologists should work 1 h/week for every four assigned patients. Nurses should not have assigned more than five patients per shift [20].

### Private For-Profit Share of Haemodialysis Facilities

As of December 31, 2018, considering the prevalent HD population, 91% (12,227) were being treated in an outpatient dialysis unit ran by the private sector, while 9.1% (1146 pts) were dialysed in public hospitals.

By the end of 2018, 80.5% of HD patients received treatment in units owned by large dialysis providers, with 43.1% of all patients being treated in HD units ran by Fresenius/NephroCare, 27.9% Diaverum units and 9.5% in units ran by DaVita.

### Treatment Modalities

As of December 2018, as far as treatment modality is concerned, 2.2% (270 patients) of the patients were receiving low-flux dialysis, 40.4% (4944 patients) were receiving high-flux dialysis and 57.4% (7013 patients) were receiving haemodiafiltration.

### Haemodialysis Reimbursement System

To control for the ever-rising costs of the ESRD treatment programme, the Portuguese health authorities negotiated in 2008 with all providers a bundled services prospective payment arrangement, denominated comprehensive price, a capitated system in which the dialysis unit reimburses a fixed predefined weekly rate per patient and provides all services included in the negotiated bundle. The bundle presently includes (a) the dialysis treatment itself and all related supplies; (b) regular clinical follow-up by the attending nephrologist; (c) all needed laboratory, imaging and other diagnostic tests related to the care of CKD patients; (d) all medications indicated for the treatment of anaemia, metabolic bone disease, blood pressure and cardiovascular disease and parenteral antibiotics for intra-dialytic administration; (e) blood transfusions; and (f) implantation, surveillance and correction of vascular access malfunction. In this system, the provider accepts the risk of a prospective payment and optimizes care management so that its cost remains below the fixed reimbursement rate. An auto-regulated system in which cost control and the demonstration of the quality of care become the responsibility of the provider that benefits from more process autonomy in exchange for substantial financial risk. Predefined quality indicators, covering structure, process, outcomes and patient satisfaction, are closely monitored and monthly uploaded in an official data base. A dialysis unit that repeatedly does not reach indicators' targets is at risk of losing its license.

In Portugal, the weekly reimbursement rate suffered, since its beginning in 2008, a continuous depreciation, currently ranking much below, in absolute terms and after adjustment for the per capita GDP, the reimbursement rates in countries such as the USA, France, Canada, Germany or Belgium. Furthermore, this occurs in spite of the fact that the number of services included in the Portuguese bundle is much higher than those provided by those countries (Figs. 45.6 and 45.7). Data from large HD providers shows that, despite this adverse economic environment, and following the initiation of the comprehensive price in 2008, a sustained decrease in dialysis treatment costs was registered, as well as in medication expenditures, which was paired with a continuous drop in

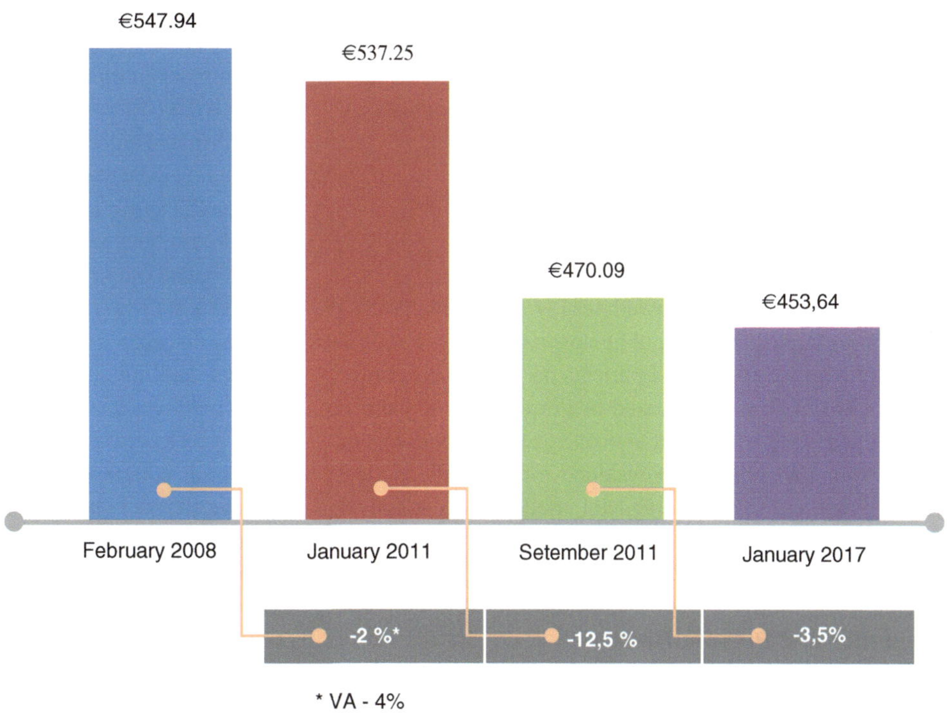


**Fig. 45.6** Trends in the haemodialysis reimbursement rates in Portugal

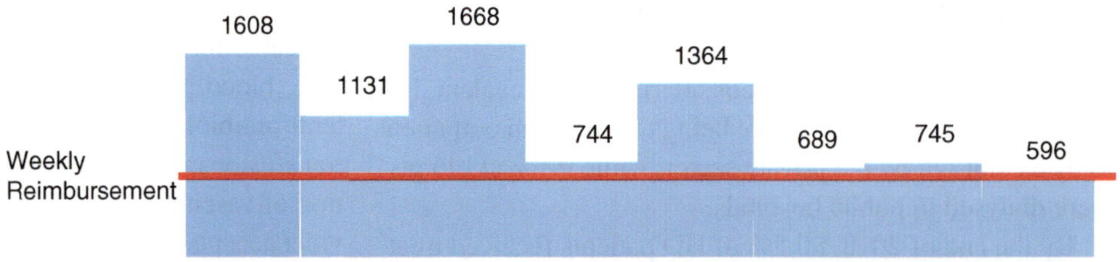


| Items | BEL | GER | NL | UK | FRA | USA | CAN | POR |
|---|---|---|---|---|---|---|---|---|
| ESA | N | N | Y | N | N | Y | N | Y |
| Iron IV | N | N | Y | N | Y | Y | Y | Y |
| Vit. D IV | N | N | Y | Y | Y | Y | Y | Y |
| Oral meds | N | N | N | N | N | N | N | Y |
| LAB | N | N | N | N | N | Y | Y | Y |
| Nephrologist | Y | N | Y | N | N | N | N | Y |
| Vasc. Acces. | N | N | N | N | N | N | N | Y |

* In US $

**Fig. 45.7** Haemodialysis reimbursement: items included in the bundled payment in different countries. Y means no separate payment for this factor. (Adapted from Vanholder R, Davenport A, Hannedouche T, et al. Reimbursement of dialysis: a comparison of seven countries. J Am Soc Nephrol. 2012;23:1291–8)

morbidity and mortality, a reduction in variance among dialysis units and a continuous improvement in key performance indicators such as dialysis adequacy, time on dialysis, haemoglobin, phosphate and albumin levels.

Noteworthy, reuse of dialysers is not allowed in Portugal. Furthermore, there are no reports on the cost of a HD patient per month treated at public hospitals or private providers.

## Peritoneal Dialysis

### Background

PD patients are only followed in PD units integrated in nephrology departments in public hospitals. It is not possible for private providers to enrol patients on PD in their clinics.

PD use has slowly increased in Portugal, mostly during the last decade. Portugal remains one of the European countries with the highest prevalence of dialysis patients (1265 pmp), but allocation to RRT modalities is massively asymmetric with 236 pmp incident patients in HD and 22 pmp in PD [21].

### Incidence and Prevalence

The data presented in this section was extracted from the 2018 Registry of the Portuguese Society of Nephrology on the treatment of ESRD [21]. Portuguese ESRD patients are treated in PD units, with a good geographical coverage of the whole country.

The overall incidence of patients accepted for RRT during 2018 was 255.9 pmp, but the incidence rate for PD was only 22.3 pmp, meaning that, in 2018, 229 incident patients began their RRT by PD (Fig. 45.2). Of all PD patients beginning RRT, 88% had more than 3 months of follow-up in a nephrology clinic, as compared with 21% in HD patients. On admission to a PD unit, 21 patients pmp were younger than 65 years old, 29 pmp between 65 and 80 years old and 16 pmp more than 80 years old.

In patients who initiated PD treatment in 2018, the causes of renal disease were chronic glomerulonephritis in 27.1%, diabetes mellitus in 19.2%, polycystic kidney disease in 10.0% and hypertension in 9.6%.

As of December 31, 2018, PD point prevalence was 77 pmp, as compared with 1188 pmp being treated by HD, meaning that the prevalent PD population represented 3.8% of the ESRD population, as compared with 58.9% for the HD population (Fig. 45.3).

In prevalent PD patients, in 2018, chronic glomerulonephritis (26.7%), diabetes (15.5%), polycystic kidney disease (11.4%) and hypertension (7.8%) were the main causes of ESRD.

### Peritoneal Dialysis Access

In 2018, the peritonitis rate was 0.31 episodes/patient. PD access problems were the reason for withdrawal in 50.8% of the patients, 33.3% due to infection and 17.5% due to mechanical problems. Other reasons for PD withdrawal included non-compliance (8.8%) and ultrafiltration problems or inadequate dialysis (28.9%).

### Mortality

Regarding mortality in peritoneal dialysis patients, in 2018, 46 patients died, making a crude mortality rate of 5.5%. The mortality rate in the first 90 days was 2.7%. Causes of death were cardiovascular 44.2%, infection not related to PD 14.0% (25.6% if all infections are included), sudden death 14.0%, malignancy 9.3% and cachexia 4.7%.

### Waiting List for Renal Transplantation

Of the whole pool of prevalent PD patients, 49.3% were in active waiting list for kidney transplantation, as compared with 20.8% in the HD population. There are notorious differences in demographic and clinical characteristics between the HD and the PD populations that explain the differences in mortality and proportion of patients in the waiting list. The median age was 68 years in HD patients and 55 years in PD patients. The aetiology of CKD in HD patients was attributed to diabetes in 28% of the cases and to hypertension in 13.9%, compared to 15.5% and 7.8% in PD patients, respectively. Glomerulonephritis (26.7 vs 12.8%) and ADPKD (11.4 vs 5.8%) were more frequent in PD patients [21].

### Treatment Modalities

As of December 2018, as far as treatment modality is concerned, 415/787 patients (52.7%) were receiving continuous ambulatory peritoneal dialysis (CAPD), while 372/787 patients (47.3%) were receiving automated peritoneal dialysis (APD).

### Peritoneal Dialysis Reimbursement System

The PD reimbursement system is similar to that for HD. It is a capitated system in which the dialysis unit reimburses a fixed predefined weekly rate per patient and provides all services included in the negotiated bundle. The bundle presently includes (a) the dialysis treatment itself and all related supplies; (b) regular clinical follow-up by the attending nephrologist; (c) all needed laboratory, imaging and other diagnostic tests related to the care of CKD pts; (d) all medications indicated for the treatment of anaemia, metabolic bone disease, blood pressure and cardiovascular disease and parenteral antibiotics for intra-dialytic administration; (e) blood transfusions; and (f) implantation, surveillance and correction of peritoneal dialysis access malfunction. There is no data on the monthly cost of a PD patient in Portugal. PD companies charge an average of 350 euros per week for the PD products. The PD reimbursement per week is the same as that for haemodialysis, which is 453.64 euros.

### Final Remarks

Percentage of patient allocation to PD increased from 5.6% in 1997 to 8.7% in 2018. Despite this modest increment, the positive trend in Portugal is the result of a set of measures that are showing favourable results towards individualized dialysis treatments.

*Science* From incipient or residual PD prescription in the early 80s, the steadily increase in admitted patients to reference centres under the lead of motivated clinicians became persuasive of the good outcomes with the technique. Clinical investigation was then the track to capture attention and make the modality renowned, both in the wards and in national forums. Research is an attractive field for younger nephrologists, and, therefore, an active work of promoting studies and academic investigation was a winning strategy.

*Education* Task forces in institutional groups, as the Portuguese Society of Nephrology and the College of Specialists of Nephrology, promoted two important directives: allowance of nephrology departments to admit trainees was dependent on the capacity of centres to offer PD treatment, and PD training core curriculum was extended from 3 to 6 months. During this period, trainees can upgrade their knowledge by experiencing successful PD programmes both in Portugal and abroad.

*Knowledge diffusion* The wave of interest in the PD technique was accompanied by an increase in the number of PD sessions in the congresses and in dedicated symposiums. Exposition and continuous education were basilar to increase PD awareness and updated prescription. This strategy was also followed by the Group for Peritoneal Dialysis of the Portuguese Society of Nephrology – meant to influence PD uptake and promote the modality. A movement of sharing experiences, knowledge and protocols was put forward. Motivated clinicians and opinion leaders fulfilled the mission of promoting patient-centred home PD.

*Economy* The increasing costs of healthcare services challenge its sustainability. The bundled price reimbursement, applied to HD providers since 2008, has suffered progressive cuts, but quality remained high with gains of efficacy and efficiency. In the field of HD, scale economy with highly protocolized procedures, minor variability and high reproducibility, allowed a steady increase in the number of HD centres. These are clearly competitive in terms of cashflows, by opposition to the lack of focussed dialysis management in public hospitals, lagging a backbone in structure and resources.

The Portuguese Health Ministry signed a set of legislative measures that gave an opportunity for hospital-based home dialysis programmes, but pale initiatives were visible. The institutional policy of signed consent for the RRT modality was an important ethical input, but the Option Process (modality choice) remains insufficient. There is also lack of assisted PD programmes to offer the desired modality to patients unable to self-dialysis. Around 10% of the total cost of HD treatment is related with patient transportation to centre haemodialysis, supported by the National Health Service, but there is no support to home-assisted PD.

So, to conclude, several issues have shown to influence the choice of the treatment modality by patients in Portugal:

1. Investigation and academy interest on PD
2. Physician's PD education and knowledge diffusion
3. Expanded PD core curriculum for the nephrology trainees
4. Increase in the number of PD patients depending exclusively on PD offer capacity of the public hospitals
5. Nephrology society PD groups lobbying
6. Signed consent policy and improved Option Process (selection of treatment modalities by patients)
7. HD bundled price reimbursement
8. Scale economy and the opportunity for expanding services in the HD setting

## Renal Transplantation

### Background

Kidney transplantation has begun in Portugal on July 20, 1969, in Coimbra, with a living donor kidney transplant. The first deceased donor transplant was performed in 1980, after legislation approval defining brain death criteria and the creation of histocompatibility centres in 1976. Over the next decades, renal transplant activity was boosted by immunosuppression and surgical technique improvements. Five coordination and organ procurement offices (two in Porto, one in Coimbra and two in Lisbon) and nine renal transplant centres are currently active in Portugal (two in the north, one in the centre and the remaining six in the south).

To understand the situation of kidney transplantation in Portugal, it is crucial to acknowledge the existence of a high ESRD prevalence in Portugal. The incidence of patients accepted for RRT in Portugal was 253 pmp, whereas the rate of prevalent patients on dialysis was 1265 pmp on December 31, 2018, which are among the highest in the world [21, 22]. At that time, the point prevalence of patients with a functioning renal graft was 750 pmp.

About 500 kidney transplants are performed annually, at 8 renal transplant units, reaching the mark of 49 pmp in 2018, one of the world's top rates. Nevertheless, a shortage of organs for transplantation remains a significant problem: 1926 patients were still in the waiting list at the end of 2018, being 27% of them candidates to a second or subsequent renal transplant and 348 patients having a calculated PRA over 98% (according to loci HLA-ABDR).

The most common primary renal diseases of renal transplanted patients are chronic glomerulonephritis and diabetic nephropathy.

### The Kidney Allocation System

According to the current allocation system, implemented in Portugal since 2007 [23], deceased donor kidneys are primarily allocated via ABO-identical and a score system based on a combination of HLA mismatching and time on dialysis. The score system also accounts (candidates received additional prioritization points) for sensitized candidates, patients' ages and prior transplants.

Transplant candidates can be listed on the waiting list of two of the renal transplant units available in the country, according to their choice. Portugal has three histocompatibility centres (north, centre and south), and the allocation is regional, except for prioritized patients with 'super urgent' inscription and multiorgan transplants which are nationally allocated.

The waiting time depends on blood group, although it can reach more than 5 years from the start of dialysis. Blood group O recipients have longer time on dialysis than patients from other groups [24].

### Deceased Donor Transplant

Portugal is among the countries where consent is presumed for organ donation when a person dies, unless they have previously manifested opposition in the form of a legal document stating that they do not want to be considered for donation after death. RENNDA – the National Registry for Non-Donors – was created in 1994 to be signed by anyone living in Portugal and wanting to be out of the 'Presumed Consent' law [24]. This option can be reviewed if the patient changes his desires. In practice, though, consent of relatives is often sought.

Increased awareness to detect potential and possible donors is mandatory, as well as efforts to maintain the donor under the ideal conditions for organ retrieval. Most of deceased donor organs are from donors after brain death. Donors' characteristics have significantly changed during the last decades: less organs are retrieved from road traffic victims and more come from neurocritical patients. Increased use of expanded criteria donor organs (older, several comorbidities) is a reality. The acceptance criteria are defined by each transplant unit and usually combine clinical and anatomical data with blood tests and preimplantation renal biopsy, to ensure organ quality.

Viable recipients are then contacted, after selection through computer algorithms, by the Portuguese Institute for Blood and Transplantation. The transplant procedure is usually performed by the transplant unit that made organ retrieval and where the patient is listed. Current results are excellent, with less than 5% acute rejection episodes registered and less than 20% delayed graft function. Overall 5-year patient and kidney graft survival are 93.7% and 85.0%, respectively [25].

Possibility of organ donation after uncontrolled circulatory death (Category II of the Maastricht classification) has been legislated in Portugal in 2013, and organ retrieval from theses donors (DCD) has begun 1 year later in one of the transplant centres. Increased rates of delayed graft function and primary graft non-function have been recorded, as described in international registries. Decreasing ischaemia times in these organs is of paramount importance. Other units are beginning this programme. Uncontrolled DCD, although requiring more complex organization, provides an opportunity to significantly expand the pool of potential deceased organ donors.

### Living Donor Transplant

Living kidney donor transplant (LKDT) has been initiated in Portugal in 1969. Thenceforth, thousands of LKDT have been performed, although rates are still low and represent less than 15% of the renal transplants performed annually over the last 10 years. About half of these transplants are performed in one centre, in which living donor transplants represent about 30% of kidney transplant activity. The rate of living donor transplant was 7.5 pmp in 2017 and has a potential to increase.

In agreement with the evidence that even unrelated donors lead to increased patient and graft survival, the legislation has been changed in 2007 [26], allowing non-genetically related transplantation, with good results. Most of these were performed between spouses.

More recently, living donor kidney transplantation embraced new challenges. Strategies to overcome major blood group incompatibility and a positive T-cell cross-match have been developed, combining desensitization techniques and kidney paired donation.

Transplant programmes with living kidney paired exchange have been created in 2010 [27, 28], and the first exchange between incompatible pairs has been performed in 2013. However, the program has increased very slowly, with less than 40 pairs active in the program at the end of 2018, and 19 transplants performed. The participation of one centre in the South Alliance Programme is expected to improve the rate of successful transplantation of Portuguese pairs.

Living donor ABO-incompatible transplantation has been performed in Portugal since 2014. Ten pairs have already been transplanted with excellent results. Pairs are considered according to the isoagglutinin titer pre-desensitization and after excluding the possibility of a kidney paired exchange.

Recent studies on donor population have described an increased, although still low, risk of adverse outcomes, including ESRD and complications during pregnancy. Living donors who develop ESRD should be prioritized on the transplant waiting list, if they need a kidney transplant. New allocation policies are being discussed and will include this issue.

### Hypersensitized Patients

Access to kidney transplantation for hypersensitized patients is a major challenge, as it is worldwide. These patients remain on the waiting list for long periods without benefiting from a kidney transplant. A working group is developing a program with the purpose of detecting possible donors for those patients in a national priority allocation system based on virtual cross-match. For patients with HLA-incompatible living kidney donors, paired exchange donation can also be considered.

### Conclusion

Portugal has a highly relevant activity in the field of kidney transplantation, but the shortage of organs for transplantation is a limiting factor for further increase. Living kidney transplantation should be amplified, always in parallel with maximized deceased donor transplantation, in order to reduce the waiting time for a renal transplant.

## Renal Replacement Therapy in the Paediatric Population

### Brief History of Paediatric Nephrology in Portugal

Paediatric nephrology (PN) as a clinical and biomedical discipline arose in the early 1940s with the pioneer studies of the newborn immature kidney. Clinical knowledge and management of renal diseases, including RRT, introduced in the adult population in the second half of twentieth century, were progressively extended to children. PN units emerged in most countries by the 1970s and in Portugal; to the best of our knowledge, the first one was created in 1975. Back then, the skills acquired in the management of both adults and children with renal diseases were used in paediatrics.

In Portugal, the first PN meeting was held in Lisbon in 1979, with a great success, gathering the most prominent Portuguese paediatricians and nephrologists dedicated to PN. This meeting led to the launch of the Portuguese Paediatric Nephrology Nucleus that united physicians from all five PN units created in our country over the decade of 1975–1985.

In Europe and the USA, PD was widely used in children since 1980 and recognized as a technique of particular value. Portugal accompanied this practice with the first PD in a newborn in 1978 at Santa Maria Hospital, shortly after the beginning of CAPD.

HD in children was first performed in 1983 at Maria Pia Children's Hospital, and the first paediatric kidney transplants were successfully performed in 1984, at the Transplantation Unit of Hospital Santo António, both in Porto.

In 1992, the Paediatric Nephrology Cycle of Special Studies, a Portuguese fellowship, was approved by the Portuguese Ministry of Health, open to paediatricians and nephrologists interested in this subspecialty. The first editions were held at Hospital Santa Maria in Lisbon and at Hospital Maria Pia in Porto. Later, in 2000, the Portuguese Board of Physicians recognized officially PN as a subspecialty with the agreement of both the Paediatric and Nephrology Specialties Boards and with open access to paediatricians and nephrologists detaining the PN cycles completion.

The country has five PN units created during the decade of 1975–1985 and two Paediatric Renal Transplant Referral Centres (Centro Hospitalar do Porto and Hospital de Santa Maria, Lisbon) that are included in the European Reference Networks, approved in 2016, by the European Union.

## Incidence and Prevalence of ESRD in the Paediatric Population

As mentioned earlier, Portuguese paediatric ESRD patients are treated in five PN units in public hospitals, with a good geographical coverage of the whole country.

Data from 2017 [29] showed that, over the year, 13 paediatric patients initiated RRT, 7/13 patients (53.8%) received PD, 2/13 patients (15.4%) received HD and 4/13 patients (30.8%) received a pre-emptive renal transplant. The mean age of the incident patients was 10.3 ± 6.1 years.

The overall incidence of patients accepted for RRT during 2018 was 7.1 pmp, 2.5 pmp for HD and 4.6 pmp for PD.

On December 31, 2017, there were 23 prevalent dialysis patients, 16/23 patients (69.5%) on PD and 7/23 patients (30.5%) on HD. As of December 31, 2018, dialysis point prevalence in the paediatric population was 16.7 pmp, 7.1 pmp being treated by HD and 9.6 pmp by PD.

During 2017, 13 patients received a kidney transplant, of which 3 patients received a living donor kidney transplant and 10 patients a deceased donor kidney transplant. As of December 31, 2017, there were 95 patients with a functioning kidney transplant, giving a transplant point prevalence of 106 pmp.

## Nephrology Practice in Portugal

To apply for the specialty of nephrology, the candidate needs to take the competitive National Examination for application for postgraduate training posts.The Examination will rank the candidate at the national level according to his/her mark and thus his/her position in the competition for training posts. Each year the number of training positions is announced at http://www.acss.min-saude.pt. This opening takes place, usually, in August, and the deadline for the application is by the end of September. The application can be made online [30].

Nephrology specialization is provided exclusively in public hospitals. Training programmes in nephrology are long (5 years), including 1 year internal medicine and 6 month modules in transplantation, PD, HD and ICU. Trainees have to apply for a specialty certificate examination in nephrology, which is a three-step examination, including a discussion on the information included in the curriculum vitae, an oral presentation of selected topics in nephrology and a discussion of a clinical case based on a patient's history and physical examination collected by the candidate. Twelve percent of Portuguese nephrologists hold the European Certificate in Nephrology (the highest rate in Europe) [31].

The contract offered to training posts is unfixed term, 40 hours a week. On-call times usually last for 12 hours. The salary is 1835.42 euros per month in the first year and 1937.39 euros in the following years. Some of the trainees, after finishing the residency, find employment in public hospitals. The monthly salary at the beginning of the career is 2746.24 euros and is 5063.38 euros at the top of the career.

However, the majority of novel specialists in nephrology find only work at private HD units. The application for work at private HD units is made at site. Currently, there is no unemployment for nephrologists in Portugal. Most nephrologists work simultaneously in the public and private sector.

## Conclusion

Some of the most relevant characteristics of the Portuguese nephrology are:

- High incidence of CKD risk factors, according to the Organisation for Economic Co-operation and Development (OECD) reports: fourth oldest population, first diabetic prevalence and third hypertension prevalence, in Europe.
- Very high incidence and prevalence of the dialysis population (respectively, fifth and ninth world ranking).
- Dialysis and transplantation care (including medication and transportation) are freely available to all patients from stage 3 CKD.

- First country in the world to introduce, 10 years ago, a national capitation payment for dialysis treatments (including dialysis sessions, medication, vascular access care, laboratory and image exams), with excellent results [32, 33].
- Very high kidney and pancreas transplant rate (second European, in both cases). In Portugal, everyone is a potential deceased organ donor (unless expressly stated otherwise).
- Private HD facilities represent 70% of total units but covering 94% of total patients. National health authorities control price and quality. Transplant and PD units are performed exclusively at public hospitals.
- Specialization in nephrology is very attractive and on the top of young Portuguese doctors' choice, different from what is observed in the majority of European and North American countries [34].
- In Portugal, interventional radiology on vascular access is performed almost exclusively by nephrologists. Portuguese nephrologists are distinguished by the many technical skills retained by its specialists (e.g. tunnelled catheters, kidney and bone biopsies, continuous dialysis in ICU). Most nephrologists work simultaneously in the public and private sector.

**Conflict of Interest** The authors declare that they have no conflict of interest.

## References


1. Instituto Nacional de Estatística. Redução da população residente em 2018 menor que a de 2017–2018. Accessed in February 2020. Available in: www.ine.pt.
2. Monetary International Fund. Report for selected countries and subjects. Accessed in February 2020. Available in: https://www.imf.org/external/index.htm.
3. Instituto Nacional de Estatística. Esperança de vida mais elevada à nascença na região norte e aos 65 anos na Área Metropolitana de Lisboa. Accessed in February 2020. Available in: www.ine.pt.
4. 2018 USRDS Annual data report, vol 2, Chapter 11: International comparisons. Accessed in June 2019. Available in: https://www.usrds.org/2018/download/v2_c11_IntComp_18_usrds.pdf.
5. Pesce F, Schena FP. Worldwide distribution of glomerular diseases: the role of renal biopsy registries. Nephrol Dial Transplant. 2010;25(2):334–6.
6. Sim JJ, Batech M, Hever A, Harrison TN, Avelar T, Kanter MH, et al. Distribution of biopsy-proven presumed primary glomerulonephropathies in 2000-2011 among a racially and ethnically diverse US population. Am J Kidney Dis. 2016;68(4):533–44.
7. Korbet SM, Genchi RM, Borok RZ, Schwartz MM. The racial prevalence of glomerular lesions in nephrotic adults. Am J Kidney Dis. 1996;27(5):647–51.
8. National Registry for Renal Biopsies of Portuguese Society of Nephrology. Accessed in June 2019. Available in: https://www.spnefro.pt/biopsias_renais.
9. Rivera F, López-Gómez JM, Pérez-García R. Glomerulonephritis SRo. Clinicopathologic correlations of renal pathology in Spain. Kidney Int. 2004;66(3):898–904.
10. Gardete-Correia L, Boavida JM, Raposo JF, Mesquita AC, Fona C, Carvalho R, et al. First diabetes prevalence study in Portugal: PREVADIAB study. Diabet Med. 2010;27(8):879–81.
11. Foundation NK. K/DOQI clinical practice guidelines for chronic kidney disease: evaluation, classification, and stratification. Am J Kidney Dis. 2002;39(2 Suppl 1):S1–266.
12. Vinhas J, Gardete-Correia L, Boavida JM, Raposo JF, Mesquita A, Fona MC, et al. Prevalence of chronic kidney disease and associated risk factors, and risk of end-stage renal disease: data from the PREVADIAB study. Nephron Clin Pract. 2011;119(1):c35–40.
13. Lopes JA, Fernandes P, Jorge S, Gonçalves S, Alvarez A, Costa e Silva Z, et al. Acute kidney injury in intensive care unit patients: a comparison between the RIFLE and the Acute Kidney Injury Network classifications. Crit Care. 2008;12(4):R110.
14. Pereira M, Rodrigues N, Godinho I, Gameiro J, Neves M, Gouveia J, et al. Acute kidney injury in patients with severe sepsis or septic shock: a comparison between the 'Risk, Injury, Failure, Loss of kidney function, End-stage kidney disease' (RIFLE), Acute Kidney Injury Network (AKIN) and Kidney Disease: Improving Global Outcomes (KDIGO) classifications. Clin Kidney J. 2017;10(3):332–40.
15. Teixeira C, Rosa R, Rodrigues N, Mendes I, Peixoto L, Dias S, et al. Acute kidney injury after major abdominal surgery: a retrospective cohort analysis. Crit Care Res Pract. 2014;2014:132175.
16. Lopes JA, Fernandes P, Jorge S, Resina C, Santos C, Pereira A, et al. Long-term risk of mortality after acute kidney injury in patients with sepsis: a contemporary analysis. BMC Nephrol. 2010;11:9.
17. Gameiro J, Neves JB, Rodrigues N, Bekerman C, Melo MJ, Pereira M, et al. Acute kidney injury, long-term renal function and mortality in patients undergoing major abdominal surgery: a cohort analysis. Clin Kidney J. 2016;9(2):192–200.
18. Khwaja A. KDIGO clinical practice guidelines for acute kidney injury. Nephron Clin Pract. 2012;120(4):c179–84.
19. Kramer A, Pippias M, Noordzij M, Stel VS, Afentakis N, Ambühl PM, et al. The European Renal Association - European Dialysis and Transplant Association (ERA-EDTA) registry annual report 2015: a summary. Clin Kidney J. 2018;11(1):108–22.
20. Rede Nacional de Especialidade Hospitalar e de Referenciação Nefrologia. Accessed in February 2020. Available in: https://www.sns.gov.pt/wp-content/uploads/2017/06/RNEHR-Nefrologia-Aprovada-19-06-2017.pdf.
21. Portuguese Registry of Dialysis and Transplantation from the Portuguese Society of Nephrology. Accessed in June 2020. Available in: https://www.spnefro.pt/tratamento_da_doenca_renal_terminal.
22. NEWSLETTER TRANSPLANT International figures on donation and transplantation 2017, EDQM Volume 22, 2018.
23. Diário da República. Accessed in June 2020. Available in: www.spt.pt/download/nova_lei_do_dador-20140113-212949.pdf.
24. Instituto Português do Sangue e da Transplantação.Plano Estratégico 2017-2019. Accessed in June 2020. Available in: http://www.ipst.pt/files/IPST/INTRUMENTOS_GESTAO/Plano_Estrategico_2017_2019_IPST_homologado.pdf.
25. Gabinete de registo - Sociedade Portuguesa de Transplantação. Accessed in June 2020. Available in: https://norahsevents.eventkey.pt/Ficheiros/SPT/RSPT%202018_compressed.pdf.
26. Diário da República n.° 124/2007, Série I de 2007-06-29. Accessed in June 2020. Available in: https://data.dre.pt/eli/lei/22/2007/06/29/p/dre/pt/html.
27. Diário da República n.° 163/2010, Série I de 2010-08-23. Accessed in June 2020. Available in: https://data.dre.pt/eli/port/802/2010/08/23/p/dre/pt/html.
28. Programa Nacional de Doação Renal Cruzada. Accessed in June 2020. Available in: http://www.ipst.pt/files/TRANSPLANTACAO/CN_ASST_1_2011.pdf.

29. Registo IRCT - Sociedade Portuguese de Pediatria, secção Nefrologia Pediátrica. Accessed in June 2020. Available in: https://www.spp.pt/UserFiles/file/Seccao_Nefrologia/registo_IRCT_%202018.pdf.
30. European Medical Mobility. Accessed in June 2020. Available in: http://www.medicalmobility.eu/portugal.
31. Cannata-Andía JB, Weinstein T, Slotki I, Ferreira A, Zoccali C, Lappin D, et al. The European Certificate in Nephrology: towards harmonization and excellence in training. Clin Kidney J. 2019;12(2):167–71.
32. Coelho AP, Sá HO, Diniz JA, Dussault G. The integrated management for renal replacement therapy in Portugal. Hemodial Int. 2014;18(1):175–84.
33. Ponce P, Marcelli D, Guerreiro A, Grassmann A, Gonçalves C, Scatizzi L, et al. Converting to a capitation system for dialysis payment--the Portuguese experience. Blood Purif. 2012;34(3–4):313–24.
34. Sharif MU, Elsayed ME, Stack AG. The global nephrology workforce: emerging threats and potential solutions! Clin Kidney J. 2016;9(1):11–22.

# Nephrology in Russia

# 46

Boris T. Bikbov

| | |
|---|---|
| Area | 17 million km² |
| Population | 146.8 million (2019) |
| Capital | Moscow |
| Three most populated cities | 1. Moscow<br>2. Saint-Petersburg<br>3. Novosibirsk |
| Official language | Russian |
| Gross domestic product [1] | 1.578 trillion USD (2017) |
| GDP per capita[1] | 10,749 USD (2017) |
| Human development index [2] | 0.816 (49° position, 2017) |
| Official currency | Ruble |
| Total number of nephrologists | 2802 (19.1 pmp) |
| National society of nephrology | Russian Nephrology Society www.nonr.ru |
| Incidence of end-stage kidney disease accepted to renal replacement therapy | 2017 – 66.6 pmp (9425 patients) |
| Prevalence of end-stage kidney disease (including patients with a functioning kidney transplant) | 2017 – 333.3 pmp |
| Total number of patients on dialysis (all modalities) | 2017 – 36,495 |
| Number of patients on hemodialysis | 2017 – 34,074 |
| Number of patients on peritoneal dialysis | 2017 – 2421 |
| Number of patients with functioning kidney transplant | 2017 – 9169<br>2018 – 10,851 |
| Number of renal transplantations per year | 2017 – 1175<br>2018 – 1361 |

General Table. Core indicators of nephrology care in Russia
1. The World Bank. https://data.worldbank.org/country/russian-federation
2. United Nations Development Programme. Human Development Reports. http://hdr.undp.org/en/countries/profiles/RUS

## Geographic and Economic Features of Russia

The territory of Russia covers more than 17 million square kilometers – about one seventh of the world's land mass – and is home to almost 147 million people [1]. Population density is extremely non-uniform, being low in many areas of Siberia and Asian parts of the country, while in European Russia and the Urals the density is close to the Western European level. A quarter of the population lives in rural settlements, and almost 16% of citizens live in small towns and settlements with a population of less than 50 thousand people. Of note, the vast majority of dialysis facilities are situated in bigger cities, and considerable distances between home and hospital, especially in regions with low population density, impede treatment. The travel time to the nearest cities could exceed 5 hours in many areas of Siberia, Far East and North European parts of Russia, and in some areas exceeds 10 hours [2].

The Russian Federation is composed of 85 territorial entities, each administrated by its own regional government with a separate budget. The latter defines the disparities in RRT acceptance rates, since funds for dialysis treatment come from regional budgets. Kidney transplantation (KT) is mainly supported by the federal budget, and each year all regions receive a certain quota for the number of transplantations which could be covered by the federal budget. However, it is possible to state that many regions faced with a shortage of both dialysis provision and KT activity, and a substantial proportion of end-stage kidney disease (ESKD) patients are not able to start treatment, even if the situation has been significantly ameliorated in the last few decades.

The gross domestic product (GDP) of Russia in 2017 was 92,089 trillion Rubles (1.578 trillion USD, 3783 trillion PPP int$). The total state budget income in 2018 accounted for 19,454 trillion Rubles (267 trillion Euros, 302 trillion USD), with 46.3% formed by oil and gas export [1], making the budget very sensitive to global fluctuations in their prices. Only 3.2% of state federal expenditures were allocated to healthcare, and the total state healthcare expenditures (both

B. T. Bikbov (✉)
Academician V.I.Shumakov Federal Research Center of Transplantology and Artificial Organs, Moscow, Russian Federation
e-mail: boris@bikbov.ru


J. A. Moura-Neto et al. (eds.), *Nephrology Worldwide*, https://doi.org/10.1007/978-3-030-56890-0_46

federal and regional) in 2018 were about 3605 trillion rubles (49.6 trillion Euro, 55.9 trillion USD). Thus, the average GDP per capita was 10,749 USD (25,763 PPP int$), and the total health care spending per capita was 380 USD (910 PPP int$). A substantial part of these funds should cover the deficit of regional healthcare budgets and the planned increase of medical personnel salaries; however, the proportion of funds for different financial tasks is not detailed enough in official statistics. As much as 40% of current health expenditures in 2017 were covered by out-of-pocket payments (with only 30% in 2005 and 35% in 2010) [3], which represents the real hurdle for the population with low income. Indeed, 13.2% of the entire population was living below the poverty line in 2017 (29.0% in 2000, 12.5% in 2010) [4], and national household surveys performed in 2019 revealed that only 35% of families were able to make financial savings, other 35% of families could afford to buy durable goods, and 21.1% could not buy fruit even in the summer season [5]. Healthcare is also suffering from economic troubles, and accumulated depreciation of hospital infrastructure and equipment has reached 56%, 31% of medical organizations had no piped water supply, 35.5% had no centralized canalization, and 40.5% had no centralized heating in 2016 [6]. Nevertheless, in spite of persisting troubles in economics, the life expectancy at birth is constantly increasing in the recent decades and has reached 72.1 years in 2017 (68.8 in 1990, 65.5 in 2005, 68.8 in 2010) [4], although it could vary up to 18 years between regions. However, the age-standardized mortality rate from NCDs remains almost twofold higher than in Europe or North America [7].

Russia is ranked at 31st (from 190) position in Doing Business [8] and 138th (from 180) in Corruption Perceptions Index [9]. In the Human Development Index, the country is ranked at 49th (from 187) place with index 0.816 [10].

## Brief History of Nephrology in Russia

Many bright individuals have contributed to kidney care development in Russia since its beginning. In this chapter, it is only possible to highlight some of their names and roles. Several prominent breakthroughs were made by Russian scientists and doctors in the early era of studying pathophysiology and treatment of kidney diseases. Of note, the Russian medical society has had good connections with European medical schools from the seventeenth century, and many works and studies were performed within close international collaboration. Thus, Russian physician Alexander Schumlansky, at obtaining his doctoral degree in Strasburg in 1783, published the dissertation "De structura renum" which, in addition to the detailed description of intra-renal blood vessels and kidney structure, contained the description of experiments proving that the glomerulus is connected with the tubule. This finding was documented again by Bowman only 59 years later with much more advanced optical equipment [11]. Tragically, after returning to Russia, Schumlansky could not obtain recognition from authorities and peers, and died in poverty. Later, after the increase of scientific world's interest in kidney diseases driven by the landmark work of Richard Bright published in 1827, Russian physicians also became more attentive to clinical aspects of kidney damage that occur in different diseases. One of the prominent findings was discovered by Alexey Polunin who published in 1853 an article documenting kidney involvement in patients who died of cholera [12], which could now be interpreted as a description of advanced acute kidney injury (AKI). In 1860, the first Russian translation of the English monograph "On the Diseases of the Kidney" by George Johnson (originally dated 1852) was published in Saint-Petersburg. Historical evidence traced dissertations written on a wide range of topics, with some of them prepared in French or German, according to the scientific background and rules of those times. Dissertations focused on "anatomo-pathological changes in kidney parenchymal inflammation" (1862) [12], "globulinuria during chronic inflammation of kidneys" (1886) [13], "excretion of gelatin by kidneys" (1903) [14], "excretion of salt and importance of low-salt diet in nephritis" (1910) [15], "reverse absorption in kidney" (1913) [16], "morphological changes in bone marrow" (1897) [17], and "malpigian glomeruli" (1889) [18] in "inflammatory kidney diseases" could be interpreted as precursors of modern studies in morphology and pathophysiology of kidney diseases. The amazing power of clinical observation in constellation with pathology studies has led to evaluation of relationships between the kidneys and other organs in dissertations on "changes in arteries in chronic nephritis" (1883) [19], "pathologo-anatomical changes in heart muscle at interstitial kidney inflammation" (1885) [20], "evaluation of arterial media in patients with wrinkled kidneys" (1890) [21], kidney involvement in diabetes (1894) [22], and common diseases those days, typhoid fever (1888) [23] and tuberculosis (1894) [24]. Distinct popularity was given to the textbooks *Diseases of Kidneys* by Herman Senator translated from German and published in 1896, and *Therapy of Kidney Diseases* by Ernest Gaucher translated from French in 1898. However, kidney diseases, as a part of non-communicable disease family, did not play a primary role in the disease burden in that époque; the major impact on morbidity and mortality was given by infectious disease and the extremely high rate of injuries among factory workers which accompanied the Industrial Revolution at the end of nineteenth century in Russia. Of note, mortality from occupational injuries was as high as those during war conflicts [25], and the awful labor and life conditions became one of the major drivers of the forthcoming socialistic revolutions. In 1901, Vladimir Lindeman for the first time in the history induced immune nephritis in rabbits by injecting serum from guinea pigs which were preliminarily sensitized by the injection of rabbits' kidney suspension [26]. The first nephrology textbook *Clinic of Nephrosis, Nephritis, and Atherosclerotic Kidneys* written by Russian physician Georg Gustav Jawein (he was born in a family of ethnic Germans in Saint-Petersburg, studied and worked in Russia, performed a fellowship in Pasteur Institute in Paris, and contributed to prevention and treatment of both infectious and non-communicable diseases in Russia) was published in Saint-Petersburg in 1917 and was followed by four more editions. This year radically and irreversibly changed the history of the country, since in February, and then in October, the Revolution demolished the political monarchical system, and a new communistic regime bringing a profound shock to all the strata of the Russian society. Formation of the Soviet Union was accompanied by civil war, severe shortage of food, economic devastation, total expropriation of private property, and several waves of immigration, with them all weakening the country, and exhausting also the clinical and scientific medicine. Nevertheless, even in those hard times, the new Soviet government had invested outstanding resources to provide universal health and pension coverage, improve public health, support education, increase quality of life, enhance the role of scientific institutions, and industrialize the country. But much darker times came with the tyrannical governance of Stalin and his henchmen who ruled bloodily in Russia with means of repression over 29 years until 1953. Unskilled policy led to several waves of starvation, even in most fertile regions, and more than 6 million people died from starvation. Repressive mechanism constructed by Stalin and military representatives resulted in almost 21 million citizens incarcerated in the concentration camps of the Soviet GULAG system, of which 1.7 million died due to unbearable living conditions [27]. Even the exact numbers are still not clear; reliable estimates indicate that about 5 million people were arrested due to political reasons (sometimes only due to a light joke about communist regimen), and about 1 million of them were shot without any juridical trial [28]. Historical estimates suggest that more than 6 million representatives of different ethnic minorities were deported from their original settlements, and almost one in fifth of them died in exile. Stalin's terror touched all layers of society, and substantial part of intellectuals. Medical and biological science suffered from doctrinism with the domination of only several officially accepted theories. Contacts with foreign colleagues and publication in English language journals were almost impossible, and even communication about foreign achievements could be considered as "cosmopolitism" with a high risk for career damage and danger of confinement to GULAG camps, precluding exchange of clinical and experimental experience with the rest of the world. World War II took the lives of almost 27 million Soviet citizens, many of whom could have survived if the internal terror organized by Stalin and his numerous henchmen had not deprived the Soviet army of commanding officers, and if unskilled policy had not exhausted agriculture. The total number of victims of this regime is almost impossible to perceive, and these crimson-dark pages narrate about one of the most monstrous genocides to a country's own population in human history.

Some prominent Soviet nephrologists lived in this period, and continued to work for the benefit of the people. Moreover, during this period the first kidney transplantation in the world from deceased donor was performed by the Soviet surgeon Yurii Voronoy in Kherson (territory of modern Ukraine) in 1933 as an attempt to treat AKI provoked in a young woman by sublimate poisoning [29]. Even if this first kidney transplantation did not lead to saving the patient's life and resulted in acute rejection, Dr. Voronoy published the results in Russian and Spanish, and performed four more kidney transplantations in subsequent years. It was only in 1954 that the first successful kidney transplantation was performed by Dr. Joseph Murray in Boston between identical twins. However, due to the iron curtain dividing the Soviet Union from the rest of the world, Dr. Murray never knew about the work performed by Dr. Voronoy, nor were Soviet surgeons aware about the achievement of Dr. Murray for a long time.

Kidney physiology was extensively studied by Alexander Ginetsinsky who made a substantial contribution to the understanding of osmoregulation and action of antidiuretic hormone. He had the courage to advocate scientific principles in physiological studies and not to agree with officially implanted obscurantism during Stalin's period. As a consequence, he was exiled from the institute where he had worked for almost 20 years, and forced to relocate to Novosibirsk city situated almost 3000 kilometers away [30].

One of the most profound influences on nephrology development in Russia has been provided by Evgeniy Tareev, who was an outstanding physician with a wide range of interests also covering hepatology, rheumatology, cardiology, to name a few. He made an outstanding contribution in studying kidney disease, popularization of nephrology, organization of national professional society, and founding the nephrology scientific school that still represents one of the strongest clinical and scientific bodies in the country.

In 1953, the Soviet repressive system with its anti-semitic internal policy initiated the fabricated judicial trial against outstanding physicians of that time, who were accused of health damnification to higher ruling party representatives. Fortunately, Stalin died soon after that and the political atmosphere in the country ameliorated, including the cessation of the trial. International contacts became possible again, providing the opportunity to exchange knowledge and experience; even though the memory of fear during Stalin's terror, the "iron curtain", and the insufficient knowledge of foreign languages have continued to block comprehensive participation of Russian clinicians and scientists in the global community. For decades, Soviet researchers predominantly communicated and published abroad in countries of the former socialistic camp (socialistic part of Germany, Hungary, etc.), and were poorly represented in English literature. Nevertheless, many big events in nephrology were held in parallel in Russia and other countries.

Maria Ratner, who started her career in 1945, actively participated in clinical and experimental work, initiating her activity in cardiology and hypertension, and eventually transferred to a closely related nephrology field. She has published a series of articles with results of experiments demonstrating how renin regulates blood pressure starting since 1953, and with clinical and morphological analysis exploring the impact of tubular dysfunction on glomerulonephritis progression since 1966 in Russian language (and only in 1985 she was published the major results in English) [31]. Morphological analysis for the latter publications was done by the pathologist Viktor Serov, who actively studied morphogenesis of nephropathies, and also collaborated with Prof. Tareev. Prof. Ratner was among the pioneers who used steroids in nephrology, and was the first to apply it in the Soviet Union at the end of 1950s for a child with severe nephrotic syndrome.

The first specialized beds for kidney patients were introduced in 1957 by an initiative of Miron Vovsy at the internal diseases unit of Moscow's Hospital 52, and he invited Prof. Ratner to manage them. In 1964, Prof. Ratner transformed these beds into the first nephrology unit in the Soviet Union where in the same year the first kidney biopsy in the country was performed, and in 1965 she also had led the establishment of the pediatric nephrology unit. They remained the only nephrology units for the whole country until 1971, when other nephrology departments were set up initially in Moscow and Saint-Petersburg (then named Leningrad) and after in other big cities [32]. The first chair of nephrology was established in Moscow's Botkin Hospital in 1983 under the leadership of Gert Kulakov [33]. The first HD procedure was performed in 1958 by Anton Pytel for AKI treatment using the "Moeller" dialysis machine. The first Soviet HD machine "AKA-60" was manufactured by Jury Kozlov with colleagues in 1957, and it was used in the clinic in 1962 [33]. A first specialized facility for maintenance HD in adults was established in 1967 and in 1976 Vyacheslav Timokhov and Aida Melikyan performed the first arteriovenous fistula surgery in the country that soon replaced initially used shunts [32]. The first pediatric dialysis department was organized in 1976, led by Dmitry Zverev who performed the first peritoneal dialysis (PD) procedure in the Soviet Union in 1991.

Natalia Tomilina, who from the very start of her clinical activity was supervised by Prof. Ratner and who also worked in the first nephrology unit in the country from its very start in 1964, has had a long and productive nephrology career. Prof. Tomilina has contributed a lot in studying the pathophysiology and morphology of kidney diseases, spreading the practice of kidney biopsy, establishing the Russian Dialysis Society and RRT Registry, developing a nephrology service in Moscow city and facilitating it in many Russian regions, improving international collaboration, organizing nephrology education events all over the country, being the founder and the chief editor of one of the Russian nephrology journals, and providing mentorship for several generations of nephrologists.

The first successful kidney transplantation (KT) in the Soviet Union was performed by Boris Petrovsky from a living related donor in 1965. This provided the foundation to establish a KT program in the country both from living related and non-heart beating deceased donors. The first official instruction defining brain death was issued in 1987, and the first law regulating transplantation was accepted in 1992, which led to an increase in transplantation activity and the start of multi-organ donation [34]. The Research Institute of Transplantology and Artificial Organs has played a leading role in Russia from the beginning (first director Boris Petrovsky) and up to now (director Sergey Gautier). For 34 years this institute was led by Valery Shumakov, who had an outstanding impact on the development of transplantation, introducing to Soviet practice methods of kidney graft conservation, proposing several innovative surgery operations, establishing an experimental animal unit for studying diverse aspects of transplantation, advocating legislative regulation, and also contributing to cardiac surgery, invention of several heart valve prostheses, and heart transplantation. The first dual kidney transplantation was performed in 2008 by Oleg Reznik with collaborators, but up to now only a few such operations have been done [35]. Transplantation in Russia was developed also by many other brilliant physicians; one of them is Yan Moysyuk who has been profoundly involved in transplantation programs in many regions, has performed a dozen of kidney and liver transplantations, and has mentored many specialists until now. Russian law assumes the presumed consent ("opt-out") for deceased donation. Historically the law prohibited organ retrieval from donors under 18 years old, and even though since 2015 the donation from a child deceased donor is possible based on the authorization from parents, this practice is not widespread – decreasing opportunities for KT in children. Living unrelated transplantation is prohibited by law in Russia. The Istanbul declaration on organ trafficking and transplant tourism is translated to Russian and accepted by Russian professional societies.

The aforementioned achievements during the Soviet époque revolutionized the practice of renal replacement therapies (RRT) and increased the availability of nephrology service in the country, even though it remained limited for the majority of the population due to both organizational and financial reasons. The beginning of "Perestroyka" in 1985 has dramatically changed the social and political landscape in Russia. On one hand, during this turbulent period poverty and social inequality increased sharply, the country's economy fell into a profound collapse, healthcare was faced with severe funding shortages (to the extent of hospitalized patients themselves needing to buy basic medications and gauze medical bandage rolls), and everyday life became impregnated with unprecedented criminal influence, the outbreak of several local war conflicts on the territory of the country, the decadence of scientific institutes, and mass emigration. On the other hand, "Perestroyka" and subsequent reforms have brought freedom of speech, political diversity, returned legislative concept of private property to the country, initiated rapid development of business, allowed the establishment of independent mass media, and led to decentralization of governance and healthcare financing. The latter has served to increase RRT provision in many regions, possibility to acquire modern dialysis machines and water purification systems, and establishment of nephrology departments according to local needs. However, even now general nephrology care is substantially underdeveloped, especially in outpatient services.

There are several landmark items to be mentioned in educational, networking, and scientific achievements. The specialized journal *Urology and nephrology* has been published since 1965 (up to 1998 when it returned its historical title to "Urology"). Currently there are five professional Russian journals, of which three cover the full spectrum of topics in nephrology and two are dedicated primarily to transplantation [36]. The Soviet Nephrology Society (becoming later as the Russian Nephrology Society) was established in 1969, the Russian Dialysis Society and the Creative Society of Pediatric Nephrologists in 1998, and the Russian Transplantology Society in 2008. There are also several regional nephrology societies performing important work at the local level. The Russian Registry of Renal Replacement Therapy was established in 1998 on the initiative of Prof. Tomilina, the Russian Pediatric Nephrology Registry in 1999 on the initiative of Elena Molchanova, and the Russian Transplantology Registry in 2008 on the initiative of Prof. Moysyuk and Prof. Gautier. Boris Bikbov has actively contributed to the management and development of the Russian Renal Replacement Therapy Registry for 15 years, and has provided a strong impact evaluating the kidney disease burden from a global health perspective in the framework of the Global Burden of Disease Study [37–39].

## Medical and Epidemiological Highlights Relevant to Kidney Care

Soon after the fall of the Soviet Union, the social value of the medical profession decreased, as a consequence of low salaries, high work load, and excessive administrative pressure in comparison with other activities. Unfortunately, all these factors are relevant up to now [40] and resulted in the deficit of medical specialists. According to the Ministry of Health, in all specialties a deficit in human resources accounted for 3.2% (22,5 thousand) of physicians and 9.0% (133 thousand) of nurses, but a lack of personnel in out-of-patient clinics achieves almost 20% [1]. In addition to absolute shortage of human resources, healthcare in Russia has also been faced with increased median age of health personnel, due to a deficit of young specialists starting careers, and a substantial proportion of medical universities graduates not proceeding with the career as a physician. There are no official data on human resources shortages in nephrology, but it is possible to assume that many patients have difficulties in accessing kidney care specialists.

Several categories of people have extremely limited access to specialized medical service, including nephrology care. This primarily concerns labor migrants (17.7 million persons were accounted as migrants during 2018, with only 1.7 million official working patents issued in the same period [1] – the difference between these numbers reflects a proportion of migrants not covered by the social security and medical insurance) and prisoners (546.4 thousand persons were incarcerated in Russia at beginning of 2019 [1]). Poor economic conditions in some regions limited the development of secondary and tertiary care hospitals, and insufficient transport infrastructure impedes access to existing medical care units, which hamper access to nephrology (and other specialized care) facilities for residents of rural areas and small towns. Indeed, while the proportion of the rural residents in the general Russian population is 25.0%, in the dialysis population it reaches 20.8%, and 15.5% among KT patients [41]. Moreover, prevalent HD patients from rural areas had significantly higher prevalence of anemia, secondary hyperparathyroidism, and hypertension [42].

National Health Priority Project does not include kidney care, and is mainly concentrated on cardiovascular and oncology. The Essential Drug List, which contains medicines guaranteed by the federal government, covers erythropoiesis-stimulating agents, parenteral iron, low molecular weight heparin, maintenance immunosuppression, anti-CMV and anti-HBV agents, vitamin D analogues, calcimimetics, non-calcium phosphate binder, and ketoanalogues of amino acids. However, some patients have bought these medicines (this mainly refers to immunosuppression) due to periodic drug shortages or state acquisition of commercial drugs having different pharmacokinetics compared with previously used ones.

Chronic kidney disease (CKD) risk factors are highly prevalent in the population, including raised high fasting blood glucose in 10%, diabetes mellitus in 3%, raised blood pressure in 35%, obesity in 35%, and smoking in 40% of adult population [7]. Alcohol abuse and binge drinking are also very frequent, with almost 50,000 annual deaths according to official statistics [1], and could provoke alcohol kidney injury. The majority of medicines (including NSAID, antibiotics, etc.) could be bought without a physician's prescription, which could lead to high rates of tubulo-interstitial nephritis and analgetic nephropathy; however, this issue has never been studied at the population level. Counterfeit drugs have been revealed in the general Russian medications market, even if it never involved kidney-specific medications. Environmental pollution is high, especially in industrialized regions of Ural and Siberia, where air quality is far from ideal. Recently, many regions have suffered from lack of modern waste recycling technologies. These factors could affect not only the development of CKD or AKI in the population, but also influence the embryonal development of the kidneys.

CKD screening has been included in the national screening plan for high-risk populations since 2014, but its results have not yet been published. Since 2018 the estimated GFR is automatically calculated upon the availability of serum creatinine in the United Medical Information and Analytical System of Moscow, but not in other regions.

Historically, dialysis was based in state public hospitals, but the facilities working in the framework of state-private partnership are rapidly increasing (since the first such facility was established in 1999). Patients do not pay for the treatment, and all expenses for private centers are reimbursed by the regional government.

## Financial Indicators of Kidney Care

Medical care financing strongly depends on the regional budget that resulted in contrast RRT rates between Russian regions. Laws and legislative acts which regulate dialysis provision change rather frequently for adjusting to economic realities and accounting to a wide range of medical procedures related to kidney care. The price for one HD session was defined by Federal Social Security Fund as 5949 Rubles (84 Euro, 94 USD), but the application of regional coefficients by local health authorities leads to its reimbursement rate from 3557 to 6779 Rubles. Reimbursement for PD accounting for "one day of treatment" was defined by Federal Fund as 4529 Roubles (64 Euro, 72 USD), but due to regional coefficients it varies from 2200 to 5270 Rubles. Creation of access for HD is reimbursed with about 40,000 Rubles, and implantation of PD catheter – about 26,000 Rubles. Pharmaco-economic analysis accounting for all expenses, including social security support for invalidity, has found that in Russia the annual cost of PD was almost 14% lower compared with HD treatment [43]. However, PD still represents the minor treatment modality in the country, and even completely absent in some regions. KT has separate financing in Federal Fund that covers high-technology treatments, and one operation performed in any Russian region is reimbursed with 923,200 Rubles (13,000 Euro, 14,654 USD). The Federal Fund for high-technology treatment covered 76% of all transplantations in 2017 (58% in 2010), while 24% of operations were supported by other sources [44].

On the whole country level, the cost of CKD (including RRT treatment) has been estimated as 451 trillion Rubles (10 trillion Euro, 13 trillion USD by the exchange rate at the 2013 year of analysis) [45].

## Nephrology Taskforce and Practice in Russia

Nephrology as specialty is presented in the education curriculum during the 6 years of medical university studies, although to a limited extent. Further comprehensive nephrology specialization according to the Ministry of Health standards could be done in the form of 2-year residence program. However, taking into account the deficit of nephrology specialists, some universities proposed shorter programs varying from 6 months in case of primary specialization to 3.5 months in case of secondary specialization for physicians already having clinical practice experience. In addition to this, a wide range of postgraduate certification courses, with duration from 2 to 8 weeks, are available for physicians already working in nephrology. Recently, distance education has also been approved in the health sector, and there are online lectures and remote courses accessible for physicians and nurses. During each year several congresses and workshops are held at federal and regional levels with participation of Russian and foreign lecturers, and with the provision of educational credits.

The Federal State Statistics Service accounted for 2802 nephrologist physicians (1820 of them working in state clinics) in 2017, corresponding to 19.1 per million population, whereas in 2013 there were 2075 nephrologists [1]; however, the number of nephrology nurses is not known.

Professionals working in kidney care are represented by 4 major labor groups. The majority of the nephrologists (>70%) work in dialysis facilities, and usually do not manage pre-dialysis patients. The Russian RRT registry reported 1567 physicians, 3617 nurses, and 565 technicians working only in dialysis facilities in 2013 [41]. The second group consists of nephrologists who treat the whole spectrum of kidney disease. The majority of them perform clinical activity in inpatient clinics, while the number working in outpatient sector is small. There are relatively few nephrologists specialized in the complex management of KT patients after the discharge from transplantation surgery units. The Ministry of Health (MoH) has reported 7007 nephrology beds [1], but this number seems to include both true nephrology beds in inpatient wards, as well as dialysis places in some hospitals reporting them as beds. The third group consists of transplant surgeons who predominantly perform only surgical activity and follow-up patients in early post-transplant period, and more rarely extend follow-up also to long-term post-operative care. Renal pathologists are very rare in Russia, working in the framework of general pathology service. The forth group provides the treatment of advanced forms of AKI requiring dialysis is performed either in general or specialized (burn, obstetric, etc.) intensive care units (ICU), or in some dialysis units which provide both acute and chronic maintenance dialysis. There are also very few physicians specialized in the treatment of intensive care patients with AKI.

Every 5 years all physicians and nurses have to renew their professional certificates.

## Chronic Kidney Disease in Russia

Official nation-wide statistic, accounting for ICD-10 codes as a reason of either primary hospitalization or outpatient consultation in 2018, identified 426.8 thousand incident and 2487.9 thousand prevalent patients with kidney or urological diseases (290.8 and 1694.7 per 100,000 population, or 0.29% and 1.69% of adult population, respectively), and accounted for 97.5 thousand people with prevalent CKD [1]. Census statistics revealed 16,251 persons died from AKI and CKD in 2018 (11.1 per 100,000 population, 0.9% of all deaths) [1]. However, these metrics have strong limitations due to the nature of any administrative database, merging statistic for urological and kidney disease, inability to attribute markers of kidney damage to acute or chronic disease in case of outpatient coding, and low attribution of immediate cause of death due to CKD.

The Global Burden of Disease Study [37–39], which applies advanced modeling approaches with the inclusion of all possible data, estimated the burden of CKD in Russia much higher in 2017: 11,360 deaths directly resulted from ESKD (7.8 deaths per 100,000 population, 22nd in the rank among all causes of death in the country), and 111,270 deaths (76.1 per 100,000 population) occurred indirectly due to cardiovascular disease (CVD) associated with low GFR or albuminuria. Thus, in total CKD was responsible for 122,630 deaths (83.9 per 100,000 population), making it the 9th leading mortality cause. The number of deaths (both directly related to ESKD and indirectly to CVD) increased by 16.7% and the death rate increased by 20.8% since 1990, but the age-standardized death rate, also accounting to changes in the population structure, decreased by −20.1% from 1990 to 2017. The total number of disability-adjusted life-years (DALYs) due to CKD as both direct cause of kidney morbidity and mortality, and indirect cause related to the acceleration of CVD was 2247.6 thousand (with rate 1537.5 per 100,000 population), ranking CKD as 11th leading cause of disease burden among all risk factors. Over 27 years, the DALYs all-ages rate increased by 8.4%, but decreased by −19.5% considering age-standardized rate. The decrease in age-standardized rate has been observed not only in Russia, but in the majority of countries, and is related to population aging.

Several local screening programs and registries have provided important insights on CKD prevalence and nosology structure. Kidney disease registries were established in several regions starting from 1980s, and collect information based on active patients' referral to nephrology service. Comparison and interpretation of prevalence data obtained before unification of CKD classification by K/DOQI and later by KDIGO is rather difficult, and below only modern results are presented.

Moscow city nephrology registry (established in 1995) reported that 0.3% of population (3000 pmp) was being followed up by nephrologists in 2013; however, in the city district with the highest number of out-patient nephrologists, this figure increased to 0.6% (5767 pmp) [46]. Chronic glomerulonephritis (GN) and tubule-interstitial nephritis (TIN) were the leading causes of referral to kidney care (435 and 790 pmp, respectively), followed by hypertensive nephropathy, type 2 and type 1 diabetes nephropathy (344, 308 and 123 pmp, respectively), and a distinct proportion of congenital and inherited diseases (101 pmp) as well as polycystic kidney disease (93 pmp). Among patients with low eGFR, over the recent 5 years, the percentage of diabetic nephropathy, hypertensive nephritis, and TIN have almost doubled, for each of these nosologies. Many patients started RRT due to urgent indications, with 53% of all these patients initiating dialysis within less than 3 months of pre-dialysis nephrology care (PDNC), and only 36% greater than 1 year of PDNC [47]. Shorter duration of PDNC resulted in substantially lower survival rates after dialysis initiation, mainly due to increased mortality during the first month in diabetic patients [48].

According to different registries, prevalence rates of patients followed up by nephrologist with CKD stages 3–5 have been reported to be 1181 pmp in Moscow [46], 818 pmp in Irkutsk region [49], whereas patients with CKD stages 2–5 defined by K/DOQI classification has been 516 pmp in Novosibirsk region [50].

A screening performed in one of Moscow's districts, among almost 78,000 patients referred to an outpatient clinic due to any reason, revealed the prevalence of low GFR as 3.9% (3.76% with GFR grade 3, 0.16% grade 4 and 0.023% grade 5) [51]. Similar in screening design a report from the Krasnodarsky region indicated a low GFR prevalence of 7.4% (10.1% in males and 5.2% in females) in almost 1000 adult participants [52]. Screenings performed among only elderly populations revealed low GFR prevalence of 34.1%

in 1000 patients >60 years (and a total CKD prevalence of 57.9%) in Moscow [53], and of 18.9% of 611 patients >65 years in Saint-Petersburg [54]. The reasons for differences in CKD prevalence rate between aforementioned studies are not clear, and a national health survey with random selection of participants is needed for better planning of the national kidney care.

Endemic diseases with kidney involvement play a role in some regions, and limited evidence from Central European part of the country suggests that the difference in the incidence rates of hemorrhagic fever with renal syndrome between forest and steppe provinces is correlated with the number of chronic renal failure patients in these areas [55]. Genetic factors may influence the regional prevalence of some kidney diseases, especially in areas traditionally isolated by landscape features or in small ethnic groups. Thus, the prevalence of Schönlein-Henoch purpura and associated glomerulonephritis was more than two-fold higher in Buryat ethnic group than in the closely situated multiethnic regional center [56]. Historical data suggest that prevalence of eGFR <30 ml/min/1.73 m$^2$ was almost twice higher in the Republic of Tuva (Siberia) than in two regions of the European part of Russia [57]. Last but not least, different occupational and unfavorable labor conditions could impact CKD development in working age persons; for example, 33% of 490 miners presented with abnormal urine analysis upon ascending from the coal mine (18% had hematuria, 11% had proteinuria, and 4% had both) [58].

Russian nation-wide diabetes registry provides important insights on CKD patterns in this high-risk population [59]. In 2016, CKD prevalence was 2303 in type I, and 687 per 10,000 type II diabetic patients, with substantial increase over recent years, mainly related to better diagnostic and more accurate CKD registration. The mean age of diabetic nephropathy diagnosis was 40.4 in type I and 66.8 years in type II patients, and the mean duration of diabetes before CKD diagnosis was 14.2 and 8.2 years, respectively. According to the registry analysis, angiotensin-converting enzyme inhibitors or angiotensin-II receptor blockers were administered only in 22.3% of type I and 47.7% of type II diabetics with CKD, but these numbers should be interpreted cautiously because they most probably reflect incomplete filling of the administrative database. Impaired eGFR <60 ml/min/1.73 m$^2$ was diagnosed in 23% of type I and 39% of type II patients with incident diabetic nephropathy. According to the Russian diabetes registry, regular urinalysis for the detection of microalbuminuria was performed only in 18.9% of patients with diabetes [60]. Moreover, microalbuminuria prevalence was reported only in 10.8% of the registry patients, whereas a focused screening was able to detect it in 35.0% of diabetic patients [61]. These data indicate an important demand for improving CKD diagnostic and treatment in high-risk populations.

## Renal Replacement Therapy in Russia

In 2016, RRT was provided in 534 facilities (there were 377 facilities in 2012 and 300) situated in 83 (out of 85) regions [41, 62], with. 8521 patients initiated RRT (92.2% of them HD, 7.8% PD) and accounting to incidence rate of 58.1 pmp (53.5 pmp for HD, 4.5 pmp for PD), representing a substantial increase from 46.8 pmp in 2012 to 27.8 pmp in 2006 (General Table). The median age of the incident population increased up to 57.0 years (52.9 years in 2013, 50.9 in 2011), and the proportion of patients with diabetic nephropathy reached 17.5% (13.8% in 2013). This rapid growth and increase in percentage of older patients and diabetics are related to the establishment of new and enlargement of existent facilities, which were able to accept a substantial part of the ESKD persons. However, the heterogeneity in the aforementioned metrics indicates areas where RRT is still severely shortened: among the regions, the incidence rate varied from 1 to 175 pmp, mean age differing for almost 8 years, and percentage of diabetics almost two-fold [41, 63].

At the end of 2016 (Table 46.1 and Fig. 46.1), the total number of patients receiving RRT reached 44,544, that corresponded to the prevalence rate 303.4 pmp (219.1 pmp in 2012, 127.1 in 2006). Of them, 8537 (19.2%, 58.1 pmp) had functioning kidney graft, 33,671 (75.6%, 229.4 pmp) were treated by HD or HDF, and only 2336 (5.2%, 15.9 pmp) by PD. Prevalence rates varied between regions from 100 to 500 pmp (Fig. 46.2), and the proportion of RRT modalities was extremely non-uniform. Almost 24 million persons (17% of the population) lived in regions with RRT prevalence rates higher than 400 pmp, and 22 million (15% of population) in regions where it was 100–200 pmp. These contrasts reflect the lack of a federal state program for dialysis co-financing, and its dependence on regional healthcare budgets. Private-

**Table 46.1** RRT core indicators

| | Number of patients | Per million population | Mean annual percent change[a] |
|---|---|---|---|
| RRT incidence, 2016 | 8521 | 58.1 | 6.9% |
| RRT prevalence, 2016 | 44,544 | 303.4 | 8.8% |
| Hemodialysis, 2016[b] | 33,671 | 229.4 | 9.8% |
| Peritoneal dialysis, 2016[c] | 2336 | 15.9 | 3.6% |
| Functioning kidney graft, 2016[d] | 8537 | 58.1 | 7.0% |
| Kidney transplantations, 2017[d] | 1175 | 8.0 | 4.6% |

[a]Mean over last 5 years
[b]Including hemodialysis, hemodiafiltration, and hemofiltration
[c]Including continuous ambulatory peritoneal dialysis and automated peritoneal dialysis
[d]Including transplants from deceased and living related donors

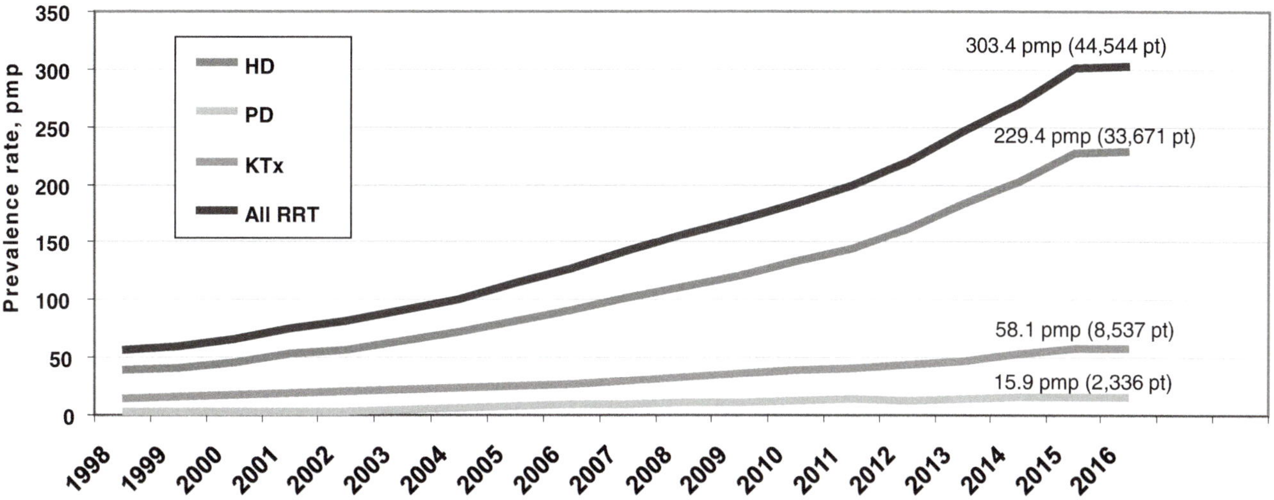


**Fig. 46.1** Prevalence rates of all RRT modalities, 1998–2016. HD hemodialysis, hemodiafiltration and hemofiltration, PD continuous ambulatory peritoneal dialysis and automated peritoneal dialysis, KTx functioning kidney graft from deceased and living related donors

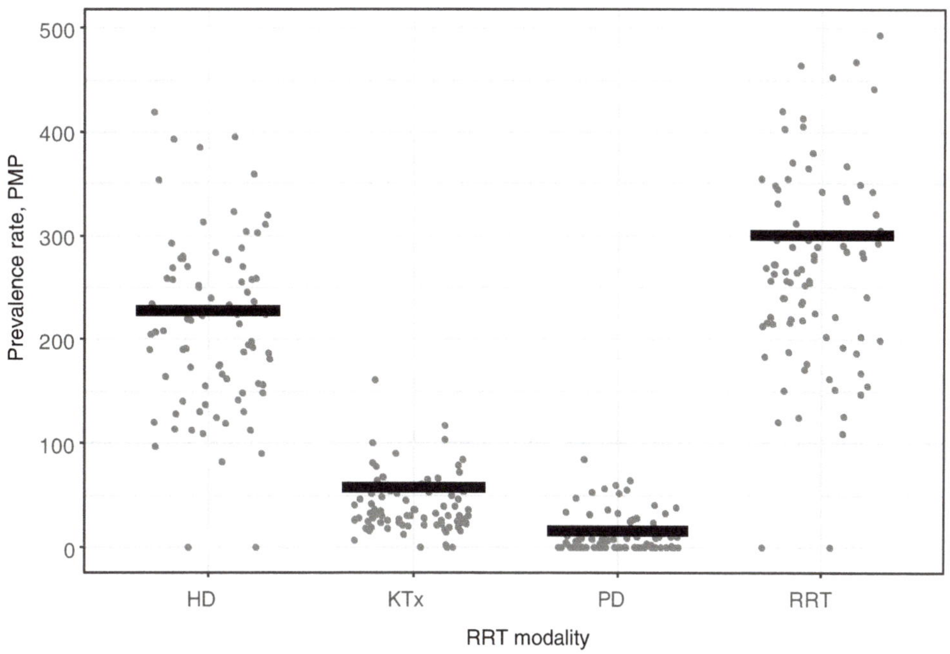


**Fig. 46.2** Regional differences in provision of RRT modalities in 2015 (each dot at the figure represents regional RRT prevalence rate, line indicates mean Russian prevalence rate)

public partnership facilities play an important role in dialysis provision, treating almost 65% of HD and 30% of PD patients in 2015 (35% and 18% in 2012, respectively).

Dialysis patients in case of complications may be hospitalized either at in-patient beds which were presented in 20% of the dialysis facilities or at nephrology unit beds available in 50%, whereas the other facilities were able to treat hospitalized patients only in units of other therapeutic profiles. The rapid growth of private-state partnership dialysis facilities was not accompanied with the proportional increase in nephrology beds, and this remains one of the public health areas which require improvement. Another problem is represented by a deficit of specialists which should be involved in patient care: only 10% of all dialysis facilities had a consultant dietitian and 16% a psychologist.

## Hemodialysis

HD has predominated in the RRT structure, even if the proportion of HDF is steadily rising (20% of all sessions were HDF in 2015, 15% in 2013). In 2016, a rate of dialysis facilities achieved 3.0 per million population, and 2.6 per 100,000 sq.km (2.5 and 2.1 in 2012, respectively), that is several times lower than in Europe or the United States. In some regions of Siberia there were less than one facility per 100,000 sq.km, but in some areas in the European part of Russia this indicator achieved 25–50. As much as 7% of patents missed, at least one HD session during a month, which was higher than in Europe, but lower than 12.2% in the United States [64]. Such high rate could be explained by long travel time from home to hospital and insufficient development of public transport in some regions. However, 97.5% of patients received 3, and 0.6% more than 3 sessions per week on a regular basis, while the prescribed treatment with 2 sessions per week was applied for only 1.9% of patients. Duration of each session was 3.5 hours or less in 2.6%, 4 hours in 68.2%, 4.5–5 hours in 28.9%, and greater than 5 hours in 0.3% of patients in 2015. The majority of sessions were performed by dialyzers with synthetic membranes (98.4%), and high-flux (65.8%), or high-efficiency (25.0%) dialyzers. Bicarbonate buffer was used in 99.4% of all sessions; and reuse was applied only in one facility. The predominant vascular access type was arteriovenous fistula (AVF) (88.0% in 2015, 91.8% in 2006), with much lower proportion of tunnel catheter (5.4% and 0%, respectively), vascular graft (3.6% and 4.4%, respectively), and temporary catheter (3.0% and 3.7%, respectively). The rate of catheter implantations was lower than that of primary or reconstructive AVF operations, indicating appropriate early diagnostic of VA dysfunction. Almost 65% of prevalent patients were treated with the use of primary AVF, and 35% had secondary or reconstructed AVF [41].

HD prevalent population is rapidly changing by an increase of patients >65 years and with diabetes. The leading cause of ESKD was chronic GN (35%), though rarely verified by biopsy. The second leading cause since 2012 has been diabetic nephropathy (now almost 16% compared to 5% in 2000), and hypertensive nephritis has also increased rapidly (8% recently, 2% in 2000). TIN and polycystic kidney disease accounted each for almost 13%, while congenital abnormalities of kidney and urinary tract were recognized as the primary ESKD etiology in 3% of patients (but 33% of the pediatric population). Men represented 53.2%, and this proportion has not changed substantially over the years [65].

The availability of laboratory facilities for the diagnosis of metabolic disturbances substantially varied both for a given biochemistry analysis, and for the same analysis between regions. Even if laboratory services have become substantially more accessible over the past years, and markers of mineral and bone disorder, hemoglobin, albumin, and ferritin determined in 90–100% of all patients, inflammatory markers and transferrin analysis were available to only 75%, whereas acid-base indicators and glycated hemoglobin to only about 50% of patients. However, in the Caucasus and Far East regions this availability was much lower.

In 2013, the prevalence of hepatitis B was 6.0%, hepatitis C – 9.5%, and both HBV and HCV – 2.1%, while in 2003 these numbers were equal to 9.8%, 17.2%, and 5.3%, respectively. HBV vaccination was performed in 78.3% of the facilities in 2013 (in 58.7% in 2003), and dialyzer reuse performed only in 0.5% of facilities (14% in 2003).

In almost 90% of patients spKt/V was 1.2 or greater (in 30% it exceeded 1.6) in 2013, and this percentage has increased when compared with previous years; that could be correlated with the increase of high-flux membranes use. However, in some regions spKt/V > 1.2 was achieved only in 70% of patients, what could be explained by inappropriate dialyzer choice, problems with VA, and sometimes shorter session duration. High blood pressure (>= 140/90 mm Hg) was diagnosed in almost 60% of patients, and while this proportion remained almost the same, the diastolic blood pressure had a tendency to lower at the population level over the last 10 years. The majority of laboratory parameters improved over the recent years, especially serum hemoglobin which was lower than 90 g/L in only 11% of patients in 2013 but in 42% of patients in 2003. However, in spite of the progress in the correction of metabolic abnormalities, less than half of the HD patients achieved the recommended target levels, and about 10% of patients had exceptionally abnormal biochemistry (Fig. 46.3). Almost 10% of patients did not require ESA, while about 60% received ESA regularly and 30% received ESA not regularly due to some problems with the centralized supply. Parenteral iron was indicated in almost 80%, whereas oral iron medicines were used in 4% of patients [65]. Even if the practice patterns for anemia treatment were rather different from Europe and the United States, patients in Russia had achieved similar levels of serum hemoglobin [7]. Calcium-based and non-calcium based phosphate-binders were used in 55% and 17% of patients, respectively; vitamin D metabolites in 37.6%, cinacalcet in 9%, and paricalcitol in 3% of patients. Almost 30% had high serum cholesterol and 40% any form of dyslipidemia, with almost 50% of them being treated for these disturbances [65]. Mean physical and mental component score for HD patients were comparable with European results [66].

Survival rates among HD patients who started treatment in 2009–2013 were 89.9% (95% CI 89.4–90.3) for 1 year, 79.1% (95% CI 78.3–80.0) for 3 years, and 69.7% (95% CI 67.8–71.6) for 5 years of follow-up. The mortality rate among prevalent HD patients was 7.2 (95% CI 6.9–7.4) per 100 patient-years [65].

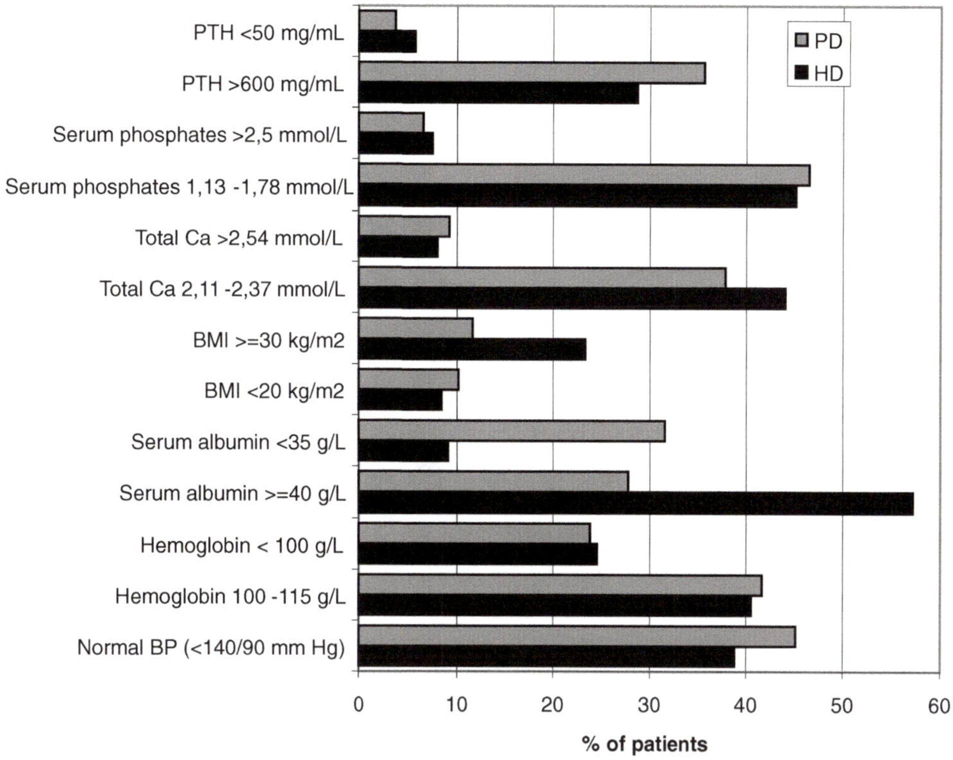


**Fig. 46.3** Clinical and biochemical abnormalities in prevalent dialysis patients, 2013. HD hemodialysis, hemodiafiltration and hemofiltration, PD continuous ambulatory peritoneal dialysis and automated peritoneal dialysis

## Peritoneal Dialysis

PD was available in 111 facilities situated in 51 regions in 2015, but only half of them treated more than 10 patients. The two biggest cities, Moscow and Saint-Petersburg, accounted for 26% of all incident and 22% of all prevalent PD patients in Russia. Paradoxally, PD was used insufficiently in the regions with low population density and high proportion of rural population. PD catheters were implanted by mini-laparotomy in 71%, and by laparoscopy in 29% of the cases. Automated PD (APD) was used in 12.9% of the patients. Peritonitis frequency was 1 per 23.0 patient-months [41, 63, 65].

During the year, 19.4% of PD patients were switched to HD treatment, due to peritonitis, PD inadequacy, technical complications, catheter dysfunction, and necessity of surgical interventions in the abdominal cavity accounting for 49.3%, 28.0%, 5.3%, 4.9%, 4.1%, respectively. While the indications for switch have remained almost the same over the last years, the percentage of PD patients requiring transfer to HD substantially increased (in 2009–2013 only about 9% of PD patients were transferred to HD), suggesting an urgent need in education of patients and staff, first of all in facilities with low number of PD patients.

PD differed from HD population in some traits: there were more children on PD with relation to the higher proportion of CAKUT, and 55% of PD patients were represented by women. Latest available data concerning 2013 [65] suggest that, when compared with HD, more PD patients had normal blood pressure and PTH >600 pg/mL, while less PD patients had albumin >40 g/L and recommended serum calcium levels (Fig. 46.3). Kt/V was >2.1 in 44.6%, 1.7–2.09 in 43.9%, and <1.7 in 11.5%. Among the cohort initiating PD treatment in 2009–2013, patient survival rates at 1, 3, and 5 years were 90.3% (95% CI 88.7–91.9), 76.0% (95% CI 72.7–79.5), and 66.1% (95% CI 60.1–72.7). PD technique survival rates were 89.2% (95% CI 87.5–90.9), 70.6% (95% CI 67.2–74.2), and 56.2% (95% CI 48.8–64.7), respectively. Mortality rate among prevalent PD patients was 8.2 (95% CI 7.4–9.0) per 100 patient-years [65].

## Kidney Transplantation

According to the 2017 published data [44], medical programs dedicated to deceased organ donation functioned only in 26 regions with a population of 89 million (thus, in 30% of all regions in which lived 61% of the country's population),

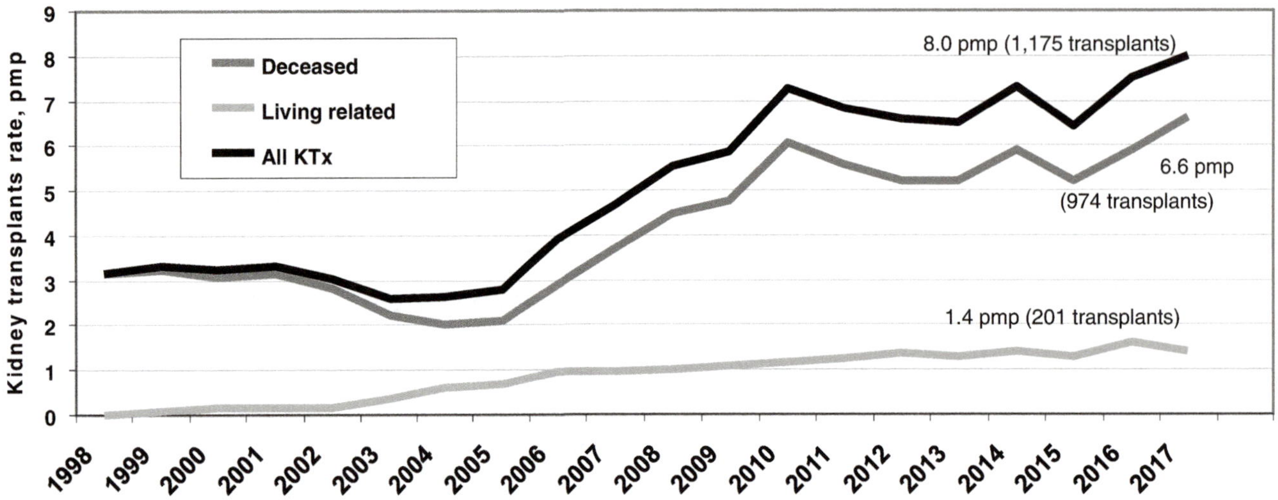


**Fig. 46.4** Kidney transplantation rate, 1998–2017

and only three regions had programs for living related transplantation. Overall, the number of effective donors accounted to 564 (3.8 pmp considering the whole country, and 6.3 pmp considering only the population of the regions with donation programs), with almost half of them restricted to Moscow and Moscow region. Donors with brain death represented 91.5% (with substantial increase from 48.3% in 2007), and multi-organ donors represented 66.5% (26.7% in 2007).

During 2017, 1175 (8.0 pmp) KT (Fig. 46.4) were performed in 41 centers (with 10 centers in Moscow and Moscow region performing 53.5% of all KT). Kidney grafts were obtained from deceased donors in 82.9%, and from living related donors in 17.1% (with the percentage of living related donors remaining rather stable since 2007). Only 105 KT have been done in children under 18 years old in ten centers, with 92% of them being performed in Moscow's centers for children from different regions. Preemptive KT is very rare. The number of KT is increasing steadily (from 935 in 2013 and 782 in 2008) to 1175 in 2017, although still much lower than needed. Kidney waiting list included 5531 patients (12% of the dialysis population) in 2017, and rapidly growing (4360 in 2013). Of note, more than other 2000 patients could be considered as potential recipients according to dialysis facilities personnel but were not enrolled in the waiting lists, primarily because they lived in regions without transplantation centers. Median duration of stay in waiting list before receiving kidney graft was 4.7 years in 2017, and is substantially increased compared with 3.7 years in 2012. These data highlight the very positive dynamic of transplant activity in Russia, but also indicate persisting major problems. Particularly, surgical centers performing KT are absent in 56 out of 85 Russian regions, which are home for 55.4 million people, the number of effective deceased donors is disproportionately low to the potential donors (14,000 people die in traffic accidents and 133,000 from stroke each year in Russia), the appointment of transplant coordinators is lacking, financial coverage of induction immunosupression is insufficient, the credibility of the population to transplantation is poor, and different social institutions (church, etc) are not actively involved in its popularization, and still there are some legislative contradictions in the field of organ donation. Mathematical modeling suggests a possibility to increase the annual number of KT to 2060-7160, based on different scenario considering the resolution of the aforementioned obstacles [67].

The total number of patients with functioning kidney graft achieved 9658 (65.7 pmp) in 2017 (6651 patients, 47.8 pmp in 2013), which are being followed up in 96 centers. Almost 15% had a living related donor graft [44]. Regional prevalence rates varied from <10 to 160 pmp, with the highest rate in Moscow. Compared with the dialysis population, kidney graft recipients were younger with a higher percentage of CAKUT (9.7%), 58.8% were men. Adult recipients with eGFR >60 ml/min/1.73 m$^2$ represented 40.8% of the prevalent patients in 2003, and eGFR grade 3a was diagnosed in 28.6% and 3b in 20.7%, while eGFR grades 4 and 5 were found in 8.6% and 1.3%, respectively [65]. Recipients of graft from living related donor had, at average, 10 ml/min/1.73 m$^2$ higher eGFR, independently of the follow-up duration. Annual slope of eGFR, based on only two eGFR values, was negative and exceeded −10 ml/min/1.73 m$^2$ in 21.9%, and was positive with greater than 10 ml/min/1.73 m$^2$ in 6.1% of patients [68].

Immunosupression was presented by three medicines in 74.1% and two medicines in 25.4% of the patients. Cyclosporine A and tacrolimus were used each in 47.2% of patients in 2013 (66.5% and 28.8% in 2010, respectively), everolimus in 4.2%, and sirolimus in 0.5%. Mycophenolate was administered to 85.4%, azathyoprin to 1.7%, and steroids to 88.9%. These percentages remaining rather stable compared with 2010, except for azathyoprin and everolimus which were then used in 5.6% and 1.7, respectively [65]. Tuberculosis rate in prevalent patients may achieve 3.9% in some regions [69], while there is no nation-wide data on this topic.

Mortality rate among prevalent recipients of cadaveric graft during 2009–2013 was 1.0 (95% CI 0.9–1.2) per 100 patient-years, and it substantially decreased compared to 2.4 (95% CI 2.2–2.7) during 2004–2008 period. Among living related donor recipients, mortality rates were 0.8 (95% CI 0.6–1.1) and 1.9 (95% CI 1.3–2.5), respectively. Data about earliest post-transplantation period and related graft losses are not provided from substantial part of facilities, whereas data about graft and patient survival after discharging from surgery units are routinely collected. Due to this, based on the Registry data, it is only possible to calculate survival starting from 90 days after transplantation, which is described below. In recipients of graft form deceased donor, patient survival rates at 1, 3, and 5 years were 98.4 (95% CI 97.9–99.0), 96.8 (95% CI 95.9–97.6), and 96.4 (95% CI 95.4–97.4). Death-censored graft survival rates were 97.7% (95% CI 97.1–98.4), 91.8% (95% CI 90.3–93.3), and 86.8% (95% CI 84.1–89.7), respectively. Patient-graft survival rates were 96.2% (95% CI 95.4–97.0), 88.8% (95% CI 87.2–90.5), and 83.7% (95% CI 80.9–86.6), respectively. In recipients of living related graft, patient survival rates were 98.0 (95% CI 96.8–99.3), 96.4% (95% CI 94.7–98.2), and 94.1% (95% CI 89.3–99.1), respectively. Graft survival rates were 98.0% (96.8–99.2), 94.2% (95% CI 91.6–96.8), and 82.0% (95% CI 68.6–97.9), respectively. Patient-graft survival rates were 96.1% (95% CI 94.4–97.8), 90.8% (95% CI 87.9–93.9), and 77.1% (95% CI 64.1–92.8), respectively [65].

## Acute Kidney Injury and Critical Care Nephrology in Russia

Epidemiology of early AKI stages is studied insufficiently, and more data are available for advanced AKI forms. Russian RRT Registry also collects AKI treatment data, reported by 339 facilities providing care for AKI in 2012, with a regional variability in terms of both population supply per million population (median 2.2 facilities, IQR 1.6–3.5) and geographical availability per 100,000 sq.km (median 3.9 facilities, IQR 1.8–9.6). During 2008–2012, 10,886 patients were treated in these facilities, mainly with advanced forms of AKI: 86.5% received HD (with a median of 5.5 (IQR 3.6–7.6) sessions) and PD was used in 1.4% of patients, while simultaneous use of HD and PD in the same patient accounted for 0.9% of cases, and conservative treatment without dialysis was used in 11.2% of patients.

The leading causes of AKI were the use of nephrotoxic substances (15.3%), sepsis (9.5%) and urosepsis (2.9%), shock (6.4%), acute interstitial nephritis (5.9%), and crush-syndrome (6.2%). A substantial proportion of patients had AKI superimposing over existing CRF (11.5%) that could be explained by the characteristics of the facilities providing the information. Overall, short-term mortality reported by facilities reached 27.3%. Mortality was substantially higher in patients with advanced AKI and need for dialysis treatment (30.8% among those treated by HD and 18.8% by PD) in comparison with those not requiring dialysis (5.6%) [70, 71]. Even if this analysis does not cover non-nephrology units, it highlights substantial inter-regional differences and need for improving access to AKI treatment and prevention.

## Pediatric Nephrology

Nation-wide administrative accounting based on ICD-10 codes estimated that there were 346.000 prevalent children aged 0–14 years, and 93.000 teenagers of 15–17 years of age with kidney or ureter diseases in 2017 (1354 and 2311 per 100,000 population of a given age group). Among them, CKD was prevalent in 1760 and 1074 children, respectively (6.9 and 26.7 per 100,000 population of a given age group) [1]. Similarly to the adult population, these administrative data have substantial limitations.

Nation-wide pediatric nephrology registry revealed that among almost 1500 children with CKD stages 3–5, 41.0% had congenital obstructive uropathies, 20.8% kidney hypo- or dysplasia, 12.3% primary GN, 6.6% polycystic disease, 5.2% TIN, 4.7% inherited kidney diseases, 4.4% HUS, 4.0% secondary kidney diseases [72]. Analysis performed in 625 children followed up by nephrology services in the Chuvashia region estimated the total CKD prevalence as 2450 per million of pediatric population, with 11.2% of them having low eGFR. Etiology of CKD was presented by obstructive uropathies in 33%, congenital abnormalities in 25%, single kidney in 15%, and GN in 9.9% [73].

Of note, the Russian Murmansk regional birth registry found that the CAKUT rate in newborns was higher compared to Europe (5.4–5.6 vs. 3.4–3.5 per 1000 newborns), with congenital hydronephrosis being the most frequent pathology. The reasons for higher CAKUT rates in Russia are not completely understood, especially keeping in mind earlier childbearing age in Russia, but several risk factors were identified, including gestational diabetes, medications use during pregnancy, and evidence of alcohol abuse [74].

In 2016, there were 77 incident and 440 prevalent children 0–14 years old receiving RRT (3.6 and 20.4 pmp, respectively) [75]. The number of children under age 18 receiving RRT increased from 493 in 2013 to 626 in 2015, although the prevalence rate, accounted for children population, remained almost the same (18.0 and 20.2 pmp, respectively) [41, 63]. Only 45% of under-18 children had kidney graft, 30% were treated by HD, and 25% by PD. Prevalence rates for these treatment modalities were 9.1, 6.0, and 5.0 pmp, respectively. Unadjusted survival of children in Russia was similar to European for HD, much lower for PD [65] and for KT [76] in Russia. The overall RRT mortality among children in Russia was 35.2 compared to 15.8 deaths per 1000 patient-years in Europe [77]. The large analysis of KT outcomes in children revealed a high incidence of infectious complications followed by fatal outcomes (41% of all fatal outcomes), loss of allograft due to primary dysfunction (in 19%), and longer duration of cold ischemia. Even if the situation has been ameliorated recently, much more improvement should be done for matching donor and recipient, control of immune system status, appropriate follow-up in pubertal period, and other aspects of care [76].

Structure of AKI was studied, in the unit which first started the provision of RRT to children in Russia (see "History"), by the analysis of 245 patients admitted during 2011–2015 years from all regions of the country. As only the most difficult patients were referred to this center, pediatric RIFLE classification identified risk category in 4.5%, injury in 14.3%, and failure in 81.2%. Newborns and toddlers 1–12 months accounted for 10.6% each, the majority of patients (27.3%) were 1 year, and 13.8% – 2 years old, with every other age group not exceeding 7% of studied population. Renal causes were the reason of AKI in 94.7%, postrenal – in 3.3%, and prerenal – in 2.0% of cases. Typical diarrhea-associated HUS resulted in 53.1%, atypical HUS in 6.5%, AKI associated with sepsis, shock, or intra-natal hypoxia accounted for 22.9% and interstitial nephritis for 6.9% of all AKI patients [78].

## Conclusion

Kidney disease burden is high in Russia, in terms of morbidity, mortality, and economic expenses. Substantial progress has been made for the treatment of ESKD and development of RRT facilities, even if the population of many regions still has limited access to this life-saving therapy. KT should be enhanced by the establishment of surgery centers in all regions, introduction of transplant coordinators institute, and active involvement of civil society and social institutes in its popularization. Inequalities in dialysis provision between regions could be overcome by introducing central federal government co-financing. In advance to KT transplantation, development of PD program should become one of the priorities, taking into account that almost a quarter of the population live in rural areas.

Relatively little attention has been paid to improving outpatient nephrology care, and this area needs urgent public health actions since it is the only way to detect and prevent CKD progression. Complex actions are required to educate more kidney care specialists, provide adequate financial incentives for staff, support laboratory facilities and fulfill automatic calculation of eGFR, disseminate educational materials for patients, sustain screening in high-risk populations for early CKD detection, finance scientific work and epidemiological studies, and cover the cost of nephroprotective therapy for all patients with government programs.

Russia is a very diverse country with rich history, with many parts of it requiring economic improvement and investment in human capital that would secure the future of the country. Healthcare infrastructure in general and delivery of kidney diseases prevention and treatment should be better addressed in both federal and regional health policies. The most vulnerable layers of society (poor households, rural citizens, labor migrants, prisoners) have to obtain special attention. Multiple interventions for effective correction of risk factors have to be done, including both anti-tobacco and anti-alcohol efforts, and providing people with alternatives and possibilities to realize their true potential and follow a healthy life style. There is a need to establish a comprehensive national care plan that would support evaluation, prevention, treatment, and research of both AKI and CKD.

**Acknowledgments** The author thanks Ellie Maslin for editorial assistance during preparation of the manuscript.

## References

1. Federal State Statistics Service. http://www.gks.ru.
2. Weiss DJ, Nelson A, Gibson HS, Temperley W, Peedell S, Lieber A, et al. A global map of travel time to cities to assess inequalities in accessibility in 2015. Nature. 2018;553(7688):333–6.
3. Global Health Expenditures Database. WHO. https://apps.who.int/nha/database.
4. World Bank. https://data.worldbank.org/country/russian-federation.
5. RosBusinessConsulting. https://www.rbc.ru/.
6. Interview of Chairwoman of the Accounts Chamber of Russia. Vedomosti. https://www.vedomosti.ru/economics/characters/2017/11/29/743589-mi-kopim.
7. Bikbov B, Bieber B, Andrusev A, Tomilina N, Zemchenkov A, Zhao J, et al. Hemodialysis practice patterns in the Russia Dialysis Outcomes and Practice Patterns Study (DOPPS), with international comparisons. Hemodial Int. 2017;21(3):393–408. Available from: https://doi.org/10.1111/hdi.12503.
8. The World Bank Group. Doing business. 2019. http://www.doingbusiness.org/en/data/exploreeconomies/russia.
9. Transparency International. Corruption perceptions index. 2018 https://www.transparency.org/country/RUS.
10. United Nations Development Programme. Human development index. 2018. http://www.hdr.undp.org/en/countries/profiles/RUS.
11. Gottschalk CW. Alexander Schumlansky 's De structura renum. Am J Nephrol. 1994;14(7155):320–4.
12. Polunin A. Anatomo-pathologic changes in those died from cholera epidemy. Moscow Physician J. 1853;IV:85.

13. Kamenskiy DA. Materials for studying clinical significance of globulinuria in chronic kidney inflammation. Saint-Petersburg; 1886. p. 39.
14. Gavrilov PI. On excretion of gelatin by kidneys. Kiev; 1903. p. 153.
15. Kastanayan EM. On excretion of salt and significance of the low-salt diet in nephritis and oedema in general. Rostov-on-Don; 1910. p. 10.
16. Vashetko NP. On reverse absorption in kidney. Kiev; 1913. p. 86.
17. Rabynovich IG. On pathologo-anatomical changes in bone marrow at chronic kidney inflammation. Saint-Petersburg; 1897. p. 54.
18. Ivanovsky NP. On changes in malpigian glomeruli in inflammatory kidney diseases. Saint-Petersburg; 1889. p. 26.
19. Kuskov NI. On issue of arterial changes in chronic nephritis. Saint-Petersburg; 1883. p. 53.
20. Pismenniy N V. Materials on issue of pathologo-anatomical changes in heart muscle at interstitial kidney inflammation. Moscow; 1885. p. 100.
21. Smirnov GA. On changes of arterial media in idiopathyc heart hypertrophy and wrinkled kidney. Saint-Petersburg; 1890. p. 49.
22. Polunosov-Jarusov SN. On issue of kidney changes in diabetic polyuria. Moscow; 1894. p. 8.
23. Konyaev VS. On bacterial kidney damage in typhoid fever. Saint-Petersburg; 1888. p. 48.
24. Pletner VI. On hystological changes in tuberculosis. Saint-Petersburg; 1894. p. 63.
25. Erisman FF, Chloponin G V. Medicine and public health in Russia. In: Russia, its present and past. Saint-Petersburg; 1900. p. 889.
26. Lindeman VK. Cytolysins as a reason of toxic nephritis. Moscow; 1901.
27. GULAG map. https://gulagmap.ru/.
28. Chronology, statistics, and geography of repressions. Memorial. https://www.memo.ru/ru-ru/history-of-repressions-and-protest/chronology-stat/.
29. Matevossian E, Kern H, Hüser N, Doll D, Snopok Y, Nährig J, et al. Surgeon Yurii Voronoy (1895–1961) - a pioneer in the history of clinical transplantation: in memoriam at the 75th anniversary of the first human kidney transplantation. Transpl Int. 2009;22(12):1132–9.
30. Natochin YV. Formation of nephrology – to the 120th anniversary of the birth A.G. Ginetsinsky, H.W. Smith, E.M. Tareev. Nephrology. 2015;19:9–16.
31. Tomilina N. Professor Maria Ratner. Nephrol Dial Transpl. 1999;14:510–1.
32. Zakharova E. History, current advances, problems, and pitfalls of nephrology in Russia. Kidney Dis. 2018;4:238–45.
33. Lashutin SV. History of hemodialysis in Russia. Alm Clin Med. 2009;20:59–65.
34. Shumakov VI, Moisiuk YG, Tarabarko NV, Kozlov IA, Sechkin AV, Dolbin AG. Multiorgan donation program in the Moscow Region of the USSR - present status and future prospects. Transpl Proc. 1991;23(5):2526–7.
35. Reznik ON, Bagnenko SF, Ananev AN, Skvortsov AE, Loginov IV, Ulyankina IV. First experience of dual kidney transplantation in Russian Federation. I I Grek Vestn Surg. 2009;6(168):82–5.
36. Russian nephrology and urology journals. https://boris.bikbov.ru/2011/01/03/russkoyazyichnyie-zhurnalyi-po-nefrologii/.
37. Roth GA, Abate D, Abate KH, Abay SM, Abbafati C, Abbasi N, et al. Global, regional, and national age-sex-specific mortality for 282 causes of death in 195 countries and territories, 1980–2017: a systematic analysis for the Global Burden of Disease Study 2017. Lancet. 2018;392(10159):1736–88.
38. Kyu HH, Abate D, Abate KH, Abay SM, Abbafati C, Abbasi N, et al. Global, regional, and national disability-adjusted life-years (DALYs) for 359 diseases and injuries and healthy life expectancy (HALE) for 195 countries and territories, 1990–2017: a systematic analysis for the Global Burden of Disease Study 2017. Lancet. 2018;392(10159):1859–922.
39. Bikbov B, Purcell C, Levey AS, et al. Global, regional, and national burden of chronic kidney disease, 1990–2017: a systematic analysis for the Global Burden of Disease Study 2017. Lancet. 2020;395:709–33. https://doi.org/10.1016/S0140-6736(20)30045-3.
40. Price of promisses. Kommersant. https://www.kommersant.ru/doc/3812301.
41. Bikbov BT, Tomilina NA. Renal replacement therapy for ESRD in Russian Federation, 1998–2013 (Report of the Russian Renal Replacement Therapy Registry. Part 1). Nephrol Dial. 2015;17(3 Suppl):5–111. Available from: http://journal.nephro.ru/index.php?r=journal/downloadPdfFile&articleId=1935.
42. Bikbov B, Tomilina N. Treatment patterns among city and rural prevalent hemodialysis patients: a cross-sectional study. Nephrol Dial Transpl. 2016;31(Suppl 1):287. Available from: https://doi.org/10.1093/ndt/gfw175.21.
43. Abdarashitova GT, Yagudina RI, Serpik VG. Pharmacoeconomic analysis of medical care for patients with chronic kidney disease requiring renal replacement therapy. Pharmacoeconomy Theory Pract. 2015;3(3):103–10.
44. Gautier SV, Khomyakov SM. Organ donation and transplantation in Russian Federation in 2017 - 10th report of the national registry. Russ J Transplantology Artif Organs. 2018;20(2):6–28.
45. Yagudina RI, Serpik VG, Abdarashitova GT, Kotenko ON. Econoomic burden of chronic kidney disease in Russian Federation. Pharmacoeconomy Theory Pract. 2014;2(4):34–9.
46. Tomilina NA, Bikbov BT. Prevalence and structure of chronic kidney disease in Moscow according to the City Nephrology Registry data. Nephrol Dial. 2011;13(3):361–3.
47. Bikbov B, Tomilina N. Influence of pre-dialysis nephrology care duration on clinical and biochemical parameters at the dialysis initiation. Nephrol Dial Transpl. 2015;3(Suppl 3):494–5. Available from: https://doi.org/10.1093/ndt/gfv192.15.
48. Bikbov B, Tomilina N. Mortality patterns among incident hemodialysis diabetic patients: a cohort study. Nephrol Dial Transpl. 2016;31(Suppl 1):296–7. Available from: https://doi.org/10.1093/ndt/gfw175.48.
49. Kisileva NN. Prevalence of chronic kidney disease in Irkutsk region. Sib Mediacal J. 2009;3:98–9.
50. Dunicheva OV. Role of registry in organization of service for patients with chronic kidney failure. Novosibirsk; 2006. p. 24.
51. Dudko MY, Kotenko ON, Malkoch AV. Significance of screening in revealing chronic kidney disease. Lech physician. 2019;1:50–2.
52. Bolotova EV, Samorodskaya IV, Dudnikova AV, Kartavenkov SA. Prevalence of risk factors for chronic kidney disease among the able-bodied population of Krasnodar. Profil Med. 2014;5:60–4.
53. Antonova TN, Bikbov BT, Gal IG, Tomilina NA. Prevalence of chronic kidney disease in elderly population of Moscow and its relationship with cardiovascular pathology. Nephrol Dial. 2011;13(3):353–4.
54. Van Pottelbergh C, Gurina N, Degryse J, Frolova E. Prevalence of impaired renal function in the elderly in the St. Petersburg District: results of the Crystal study. Advances in Gerontology. 2011;24:108–13.
55. Shutov A, Maximova E, Potrashkova K, Bruzgacheva O. Haemorrhagic fever with renal syndrome and chronic renal failure. Lancet. 1996;348(9041):1594–5.
56. Egorova TV. Prevalence and clinic of postcapillaro-toxic glomerulonephritis in Prybaikalye. Sib Med J. 2011;6:297–9.
57. Smirnov AV, Dobronravov VA, Bodur-Oorzhak AS, Zverkov RV, Kayukov IG, Sanchi MN, et al. Incidence and prevalence of late stages of chronic kidney disease in the republic of Tuva. Nephrology. 2005;4:25–9.
58. Kozyr' VI, Plotkin VI. Diseases of the kidneys and urinary tract and possibilities of their active detection in miners. Klin Med. 1992;70(3–4):44–6.
59. Shamkhalova MS, Vikulova OK, Zheleznyakova AV, Isakov MA, Shestakova MV, Dedov II. Trends in the epidemiology of chronic

kidney disease in Russian Federation according to the federal diabetes register (2013–2016). Diabetes Mellit. 2018;21(3):160–9.
60. Kalashnikova MF, Suntsov YI, Belousov DY, Kantemirova MA. Analysis of epidemiological indices of type 2 diabetes mellitus in the adult population of Moscow. Diabetes Mellit. 2014;3:5–16.
61. Dedov II, Shestakova MV, Suntsov YI, Peterkova VA, Galstyan GR, Mayorov AY, et al. Results of "Diabetes mellitus" program realization. Diabetes Mellit. 2013;16(Suppl 2):1–48.
62. ERA-EDTA Registry: ERA-EDTA registry annual report 2016. Amsterdam UMC, location AMC, Department of Medical Informatics, Amsterdam, the Netherlands; 2018.
63. Renal replacement therapy for End Stage Renal Disease in Russian Federation, 2010–2015. Part 1. Nephrol Dial. 2017;19(4):2–94.
64. Al Salmi I, Larkina M, Wang M, Subramanian L, Morgenstern H, Jacobson SH, et al. Missed hemodialysis treatments: international variation, predictors, and outcomes in the dialysis outcomes and practice patterns study (DOPPS). Am J Kidney Dis. 2019;72(5):634–43. Available from: https://doi.org/10.1053/j.ajkd.2018.04.019.
65. Bikbov BT, Tomilina NA. The contingent and treatment quality indicators in patients on replacement therapy of end stage renal disease in the Russian Federation in 1998–2013 years (Report of the Register of Renal Replacement Therapy of the Russian Dialysis Society. Part II). Nephrol Dial. 2016;18(2):98–164. Available from: http://journal.nephro.ru/index.php?r=journal/downloadPdfFile&articleId=1952.
66. Vasilieva IA. Quality of life in chronic hemodialysis patients in Russia. Hemodial Int. 2006;10(3):274–8. Available from: http://www.ncbi.nlm.nih.gov/pubmed/16805889.
67. Gautier SV, Khomyakov SM. Assessment of requirement of the population in the organ transplantation, the donor resource and planning of the effective network of the medical organizations (the centers of transplantation). Russ J Transplantology Artif Organs. 2013;15(3):11–24.
68. Bikbov B, Tomilina N. Trajectory of eGFR changes among kidney transplant recipients: a cohort study. Nephrol Dial Transpl. 2016;31(Suppl 1):583–4. Available from: https://doi.org/10.1093/ndt/gfw200.60.
69. Yaremin BI, Starostina AA, Tsygankov IL. Tuberculosis after kidney transplant in the Samara region of Russia: possible solutions to diagnosis and treatment. Exp Clin Transplant. 2017;Suppl 1:68–70.
70. Bikbov BT, Tomilina N. Epidemiology of acute kidney injury in Russian Federation: analysis of the Russian registry of renal replacement therapy, 2008–2012. Nephrol Dial. 2014;16(4):453–64. Available from: http://journal.nephro.ru/index.php?r=journal/downloadPdfFile&articleId=1870.
71. Bikbov B, Tomilina N. Epidemiology of acute kidney injury in Russia: a registry data. Nephrol Dial Transpl. 2015;30(Suppl 3):459–60. Available from: https://doi.org/10.1093/ndt/gfv190.57.
72. Molchanova EA. Registry of children with chronic kidney failure. In: Ignatova MS, editor. Pediatric nephrology. MIA: Moscow; 2011. p. 601–3.
73. Ivanova IE, Rodionov VA, Trefilov AA, Lavrentyeva IN. Regional features of chronic illness of kidneys at children of Chuvashiya. Vestn Chuvashian Univ. 2010;3:109–14.
74. Postoev VA, Grjibovski AM, Kovalenko AA, Anda EE, Nieboer E, Odland JØ. Congenital anomalies of the kidney and the urinary tract : a murmansk county birth registry study. Birth defects Res (Part A). 2016;106:185–93.
75. ESPN/ERA-EDTA Registry 2016 report, Amsterdam. 2018. https://www.espn-reg.org/files/AR2016_final.pdf.
76. Sushkov AI, Molchanova EA, Kaabak MM, Moysyuk YG. Pediatric kidney transplantation: early and long-term outcomes following 1187 procedures. Khirurgiya Zhurnal im NI Pirogova. 2019;1:14–26.
77. Chesnaye NC, Schaefer F, Bonthuis M, Holman R, Baiko S, Baskın E, et al. Mortality risk disparities in children receiving chronic renal replacement therapy for the treatment of end-stage renal disease across Europe: an ESPN-ERA / EDTA registry analysis. Lancet. 2017;389:2128–37.
78. Muzurov AL, Zverev DV, Abaseeva TY, Generalova GA, Pankratenko TE, Emirova HM, et al. Epidemiology of an acute renal injury in children. Russ J Pediatr Surgery Anesth Intensive Care. 2017;7(1):30–9.

# Nephrology in Spain

# 47

Belén Marrón, Miguel González-Molina Alcaide, Domingo Hernández Marrero, Juan Carlos Martínez-Ocaña, José Manuel Gil-Cunquero, J. Emilio Sánchez Alvárez, and Alberto Ortíz

| | |
|---|---|
| Area[1] | 505,990 Km$^2$ |
| Population[2] | 46,934,632 (2019) |
| Capital | Madrid |
| Three most populated cities: | 1. Madrid<br>2. Barcelona<br>3. Valencia |
| Official languages | Spanish, Catalonian, Valencian, Basque, Galician |
| Gross domestic product (GDP)[3] | 1.864 trillion international $ (2018, PPP) |
| GDP per capita[3] | 40,290 international $ (2018, PPP) |
| Human Development Index (HDI)[3] | 0.891 (2018) |
| Official currency | Euro (€) |
| Total number of nephrologists | ~1800 |
| National society of nephrology | Sociedad Española de Nefrologia (S.E.N.)<br>www.senefro.org |
| Incidence of end-stage renal disease[4] | 2017 – 141 pmp<br>2018 – 147 pmp |
| Prevalence of end-stage renal disease[4] (including patients with functioning kidney graft) | 2017 – 1284 pmp<br>2018 – 1322 pmp |
| Total number of patients on dialysis[4] (all modalities) | 2017 – 27,629 pmp<br>2018 – 27,998 pmp |
| Number of patients on hemodialysis[4] | 2017 – 24,522 pmp<br>2018 – 24,900 pmp |
| Number of patients on peritoneal dialysis[4] | 2017 – 3107 pmp<br>2018 – 3098 pmp |
| Number of patients with functioning kidney graft[4] | 2017 – 32,181 pmp<br>2018 – 33,766 pmp |
| Number of renal transplantations per year[4] | 2017 – 3269 pmp<br>2018 – 3313 pmp |

1. Anuario Estadístico de España. At: http://www.ine.es/prodyser/pubweb/anuario08/anu08_01entor.pdf
2. Instituto Nacional de Estadística. At: https://www.ine.es/en/prensa/cp_e2019_p_en.pdf
3. EAE Business School. At: https://www.imf.org/external/pubs/ft/weo/2018/01/weodata/weorept.aspx?pr.x=70&pr.y=7&sy=2018&ey=2018&scsm=1&ssd=1&sort=country&ds=.&br=1&c= 193,946,122,137,124,546,156,181,423,138,935,196,128,142,939,182,172,359,132,135,134,576,174,936,532,961,176,184,178,144,436,146,136,528,158,112,542,111,941&s=NGDPD,PPPGDP,NGDPDPC,PPPPC&grp=0&a=
4. Spanish Registry of Spanish Renal Patients (REER). At: https://www.senefro.org/contents/webstructure/SEN_2019_REER_modificada.pdf

## Introduction

Spain is a Western and Mediterranean European country, which is expected to have the longest life expectancy in the world by 2040 [1]. The successful prolongation of life expectancy is already resulting in an aging population, and chronic kidney disease (CKD) is expected to be more frequent, becoming the second most common cause of death in Spain in the near future [2]. Tackling this problem will require a huge investment in Nephrology research and care, offering job opportunities for smart problem-solving-oriented healthcare professionals. Spain has a long history of Nephrology,

B. Marrón (✉)
Corporate Diaverum Home Therapies, Diaverum Madrid Clinic, Madrid, Spain
e-mail: belen.marron@diaverum.com

M. González-Molina Alcaide · D. Hernández Marrero
Department of Nephrology, Carlos Haya Regional University Hospital, Málaga, Spain

J. C. Martínez-Ocaña
Department of Nephrology, Parc Tauli University Hospital, Sabadell, Barcelona, Spain
e-mail: jcmartinez@tauli.cat

J. M. Gil-Cunquero
Department of Nephrology, University Hospital of Jaén, Jaén, Spain
e-mail: jmgilc@senefro.org

J. E. Sánchez Alvárez
Department of Nephrology, University Hospital of Cabueñes, Gijón, Asturias, Spain

A. Ortíz
Department of Nephrology and Hypertension, Fundación Jiménez Díaz University Hospital, Madrid, Spain
e-mail: aortiz@fjd.es



J. A. Moura-Neto et al. (eds.), *Nephrology Worldwide*, https://doi.org/10.1007/978-3-030-56890-0_47

dating from the 1950s, and is a world leader in kidney donation and transplantation. Indeed, a majority of patients on renal replacement therapy (RRT) in Spain have a functioning kidney graft. However, Spanish Nephrology will have to reinvent itself to successfully face the growing CKD epidemic.

## Brief History of Nephrology in Spain

### First Milestones

Two sites co-share the origin of Nephrology in Spain and were key in the expansion of Nephrology to Latin America. Professor Luis Avendaño (1926–2018†) is considered as the father of Spanish Nephrology. His dream to publish the History of Spanish Nephrology became live in 2012 [3]. The following text is mainly extracted from it.

In 1957, Emilio Rotellar and his team built a modified Kolff artificial kidney by themselves. However, the first acute and chronic hemodialysis were delivered in 1959 at his Clinic University Hospital in Barcelona, while the first known Spanish kidney biopsy was performed in 1960. This early nephrology embryo run in parallel with the hospital Urology service, whose main objective was to develop a kidney transplant program.

The Jiménez Díaz Foundation Nephrology Department in Madrid was the first in Spain, providing humoral and dialysis care, as well as comprehensive nephrology care, similar to current Nephrology departments. Professor Luis Hernando Avendaño led the institution for more than four decades. Milestones included the first acute dialysis in Madrid (1959), first ward and outpatient clinic for kidney disease patients (1962), first acute and chronic peritoneal dialysis program (1962), first large-scale chronic hemodialysis program (1964), first kidney transplant in Madrid (1966), as well as a research laboratory studying renal physiology and pathology that is still one of the most relevant research institutions within the country.

The first Society of Nephrology in Spain was the Catalonian Society founded in 1963. However, back in 1960 during the IV Congress of the Spanish Internal Medicine Society, Professor Hernando and Gerardo de Río proposed the creation of a Nephrology section. In 1964, the *Sociedad Española de Nefrología*/Spanish Society of Nephrology (S.E.N) was born. Forty delegates attended the first Congress (1965). Today, over 2000 delegates from Spain and Latin America attend the yearly meeting.

During the late 1960s and 1970s, the creation of new nephrology services accelerated and included Puerta de Hierro (Madrid, 1964), Navarra University Hospital (Pamplona, 1967), Hospital Central Asturias (Oviedo, 1967), La Paz Hospital (Madrid, 1968), the Air Force Hospital (Madrid, 1968), La Fe Hospital (Valencia, 1968), Gregorio Marañón University Hospital (Madrid, 1970), and Vall d'Hebron which also founded the first pediatrics nephrology service in Spain (Barcelona, 1970).

The more extended use of hemodialysis to treat patients with chronic renal failure started in 1970, but it was not consolidated at least until 1976. New Nephrology services, outpatient nephrology and hypertension clinics, and 24 hour emergency attendance were started, while a wider number of patients were offered chronic dialysis. However, demand exceeded resources, and subsegments of the population were prioritized for therapy. Similarly, there was no universal healthcare coverage as we know today, and end-stage renal disease (ESRD) patients died without getting access to RRT.

At the end of the 1970s, a national system was created called National Social Security, and Puerta de Hierro Hospital was the first offering universal care. However, not all ESRD patients could be offered RRT until the 1980s. By then, many hospitals across the country offered RRT, and private dialysis centers emerged in response to the shortage of dialysis posts in public hospitals.

Many of these early private hemodialysis centers were founded by pioneer nephrologists and then gradually sold to big multinational companies by the end of 1990s and early 2000s.

As a result, while transplant and peritoneal dialysis are exclusively linked to the national public sector, the hemodialysis population is nowadays attended in a mix model of public hospitals and private providers tenders.

### Early Kidney Transplantation Experiences

The history of kidney transplantation in Spain dates from 1960, though it was not until 1965 when first transplants were successful.

The first attempt between brothers by the urologist Jose Antonio Martinez Piñeiro at the current Gregorio Marañón University Hospital (Madrid) in May 1960 resulted in a non-functioning graft, and the patient died 4 days after surgery. Two further unsuccessful attempts were performed resulting in the death of both recipients transplanted from their fathers at the Madrid Paloma Clinic (by Carlos Younger de la Peña) in 1961 and at the Clinic University Hospital, Barcelona (by Jose Mª Gil-Vernet and nephrologist Antonio Caralps), in 1965.

Failures resulted in media hostility towards urologists, nephrologists, and kidney transplantation. Moreover, the

Royal Academy of Medicine in Barcelona hosted a conference titled "Kidney transplantation: a utopia" requesting the prohibition of kidney transplantation.

Despite this setback, and likely influenced by successful experiences in the United States and France, the Barcelona Clinic University Hospital achieved in July 1965 a 2-year survival in a 35-year-old woman who received a cadaveric graft from a brain death donor. The hospital went on to perform 45 transplants in 1965–1970, and 20 were performed at Fundación Jiménez Díaz in Madrid. This later institution was led by the urologists Carlos Alférez and later Remigio Vela Navarrete and the nephrologist Luis Hernando who was on duty in Boston on the day of the first kidney transplant. Further hospitals starting transplant programs were Puerta de Hierro in Madrid (1968), University of Navarra Clinic (1969), and La Paz University Hospital in Madrid (1970) among others.

Contributors to the growth of transplantation included the discovery of the HLA system (not before 1969), therapy with antilymphocyte serum, and improvements in organ perfusion and conservation techniques with the Collins solution to prevent ischemic injury.

Legal challenges negatively influenced the development of kidney transplantation. The Law of December 18, 1950, and its modification in 1955 only allowed donation after heart and lung inactivity. Recommendations from University of Harvard Expert Committee in 1968 accepting as death when no vital signs were observed in other organs such as the brain [4] were not uniformly accepted causing inequity in kidney donation and transplantation. This situation dramatically changed after the First Transplantation Law was published in 1979 and later extended by a Royal Decree in 1980.

Further progress was made when combined kidney-pancreas transplant was possible in type 1 diabetes, first at Clinic University Hospital in Barcelona led by the urologist Jose Maria Gil-Vernet, the surgeon Laureano Fernández Cruz, and nephrologists Antonio Caralps and Jordi Andreu (1983) [5]. The recipient survived 11 years. Other hospitals successfully developing such transplant programs were Reina Sofía University Hospital in Córdoba, Carlos Haya Regional University Hospital in Málaga, Doce de Octubre University Hospital in Madrid, and Tenerife and Santiago de Compostela University Hospitals.

## Renal Diseases in Spain

The Dialysis and Transplant Registry of the Spanish Society of Nephrology (S.E.N) was created in 1975 and works closely with European Renal Association/European Dialysis and Transplantation Association (ERA/EDTA), which was constituted in 1964. The first report of the Spanish Registry was published in 1979. At that time, the incidence of dialysis was 1045 patients [28 per million population (pmp)], and dialysis prevalence was 4244 patients (114 pmp).

Since then, the Spanish Registry has evolved to become in 2006 the Spanish Registry of Renal Patients (REER) as we know it today. The Scientific Committee of the Registry is formed by the S.E.N., the National Transplant Organization (ONT), and various regional Registries from Spanish Autonomous Communities. Every year, during the October annual S.E.N meeting, the REER makes public and publishes online the previous year data. This information is easily accessed through the S.E.N. (www.senefro.org) and REER websites (www.registrorenal.es). Last available open-access data on REER are from 2018 [6] and are described below.

### Incidence of RRT

In 2018 (latest data available as of January 2020), the annual incidence of RRT in Spain was 6883 patients (147 pmp). This is an average European rate, far from the top countries such as the Czech Republic and Mediterranean countries such as Greece and neighboring Portugal that hover around 200–250 pmp [7].

The progressive aging of the population means that the most advanced age groups are those with the fastest-growing incidence of RRT. Specifically, 60% of the patients who started RRT in 2018 were older than 65 years (30% were older than 75 years).

Globally, diabetes mellitus (DM) is the most frequent cause of ESRD (almost 25% of cases); however, there are wide variations between age groups and regions, with the Canary Islands topping the ranking for both RRT and diabetic kidney disease. In younger patients, congenital hereditary diseases and glomerulonephritis are frequent, while DM and vascular kidney disease predominate later in life.

Hemodialysis is the most frequent modality of incident RRT and accounts for 79% of cases, peritoneal dialysis (PD) for 16%, and preemptive transplantation for 5% of cases. PD is registering a slow but continuous increase as an initial modality of RRT.

The implementation of live renal donation programs about 10 years ago led to a progressive increase of this modality of preemptive transplantation that has slowed down in the last 3 or 4 years. Additionally, some very active transplant centers are providing cadaveric preemptive transplantation after waiting lists of patients already on RRT have become depleted.

## Prevalence of RRT

RRT prevalence is increasing in Spain; at the end of 2018, 63,086 patients (1322 pmp) were on RRT. The increasing prevalence reflects both the increased incidence and the improved survival. The current prevalence of RRT in Spain is at the forefront of Europe with other six countries [7].

Also among prevalent patients, the elderly are overrepresented. More than 45% of patients are over 65 years old, while 34% are 45- to 64-year-olds. Since 2011, renal transplantation is the most frequent prevalent RRT modality, representing 54% of these, higher than hemodialysis (41%) and PD (5%) combined.

The increase in PD as an incident modality is not transferred to prevalence. This is linked to the profile of patients choosing PD: they are frequently younger, have less comorbidity, and are rapidly transplanted.

The transplant activity in Spain is very prominent. Spain leads the world ranking in adjusted rates both in kidney transplantation and in all-organ transplantation. In 2018, 3313 transplants were performed in Spain. Every year, the previous year record is beaten. Most organs are from brain death donors, but in the last 5 years, there has been an exponential increase in controlled asystole or Maastricht type III donors. As previously discussed, living donation experienced a rapid growth in the 2000s, but in the last 4 years, it has declined.

Despite a high number of annual transplants, waiting lists are still long. In 2018, the ratio of transplant patients to the waiting list exceeded 84%.

Cardiovascular disease remains the leading cause of death among patients on RRT but is closely followed by cancer, especially among transplant patients on immunosuppressant.

Survival in over 67,000 patients on RRT was 92, 82, and 59% at 1, 2, and 5 years, respectively, better than in most references. In a multivariate analysis of the limited number of variables available in the REER, age and DM are associated with worse general survival and female gender and PD were associated with better survival [6].

## Renal Replacement Therapy in Spain

For several decades, Spain has been offering all RRT modalities in a universal free at the point-of-care manner as part of the National Health System portfolio. Care is almost exclusively provided by Nephrology departments at public hospitals (university and/or secondary and local hospitals). While PD and transplantation can only be provided at hospital from the public network, hemodialysis is provided by hemodialysis units within public hospitals and by extrahospitalary dialysis clinics (EDC) called satellite hemodialysis units that are usually private but ascribed to a public referral hospital.

As a consequence, nephrologists that work in PD and transplantation can only work in the public sector, but those working on hemodialysis may be ascribed to public (most) or to private providers through EDCs. As a consequence, it is unusual for nephrologists who actively work at public hospitals to also do in private providers.

Nephrologist salaries vary with Autonomous Community, but within the same public hospital or region, salaries are similar for nephrologists working on hemodialysis, PD, or transplantation, as no incentives exist to switch patients between dialysis modalities. However, some salary differences may apply depending on regions and by professional career, and some hospitals provide incentives to kidney transplantation that may be shared by all nephrologists in the hospital.

A 2011 S.E.N survey [8] disclosed the existence of 363 EDC (half of them run by private multinational providers such as Fresenius, Diaverum, B. Braun, and Baxter, mainly), 120 public hospitals (university or locals) with Nephrology Departments, and 69 pure private clinics or hospitals. The mean number of patients per dialysis unit was 72 (range 11–212), but it was lower at hospital-based units. Most centers worked in 3 shifts, with a mean ratio of 39 patients/physician, 4.7 patients/nurse, and 9 patients/nurse assistant [9]. Up to 64% of the EDCs employed non-nephrologists as medical staff (this can only be done when no nephrologist can be found), and almost half of this medical staff had also duties at their referral hospital [10]. New tenders, such as the 2018 Madrid Region tender, applied a lower ratio of patients per nurse or nurse assistants (four patients/nurse and eight per nurse assistant).

## Hemodialysis

### Hemodialysis Structures

Since 2007, healthcare is run independently in each of 17 autonomous communities and 2 extra peninsular cities. While the umbrella of renal care is similar across the country, differences do exist across regions, especially regarding reimbursement schemes or amounts for health providers and tender models.

However, renal care in Spain is publically driven, and there is almost no private setting in hemodialysis, PD, or transplantation care. Therefore, different private renal providers (mainly multinational companies) apply for public tenders that allow them to provide patient care for a certain number of years and to be reimbursed for that. In any case, patients do not pay for RRT nor for associated medications such as erythropoietin (EPO), vitamin D analogues, certain phosphate binders, cinacalcet, or etecalcetide.

Generally speaking, 45% of patients receive hemodialysis in public hospitals and 55% in EDCs [11].

*Hospital Dialysis Units* are integrated in the hospital Nephrology departments. They attend acute kidney injury patients and chronic hemodialysis patients (especially those with higher comorbid and complex clinical situations) but also deliver techniques such as plasmapheresis, therapeutic apheresis, or hemoperfusion. Hospital units must have associated vascular surgeons and interventional radiologists. They are responsible for kidney transplantation listing and some even for transplantation itself and are usually the referral hospital for the non-hospital hemodialysis clinics.

*Extrahospitalary Dialysis Centers (EDC)*, also called satellite hemodialysis clinics. These clinics are always ascribed to a referral hospital with nephrology department. EDCs are almost exclusively driven by public tenders and supervised by regional health authorities [12]. A strong bidirectional communication between referral hospital and EDC is strongly advised, as well as the existence of common procedures, protocols, and electronic medical records systems [8]. As a difference to other countries, these EDC do not provide predialysis care nor PD as they only function as hemodialysis providers when patients have been redirected mostly from public care hospitals and/or from former private physicians in very limited cases. Therefore, modality choice and predialysis care usually take place in the public hospital environment.

## Hemodialysis Epidemiology

According to the 2018 REER report [6], 79% of patients started on hemodialysis while as a prevalent RRT modality is second to kidney transplantation, with 24,900 patients. However, wide differences were observed in modality prevalence by regions probably due to the different use of PD and access to kidney transplantation [13, 14]. While the absolute hemodialysis prevalence increased from 2006 to 2018, the relative prevalence decreased from 46 to 40.3% of RRT patients in the same period, as a result of the increasing prevalence of functional kidney transplants.

As in other parts of the world, the mean age of patients on hemodialysis is increasing; more than 30% of patients are above 75 years of age [13]. Nevertheless, different patterns are observed among regions that likely reflect different criteria at the time of dialysis start for the elderly [14]. On average the mean estimated glomerular filtration rate at the onset of hemodialysis was 9.6 ml/min/1.73m$^2$ in 2017 [15].

Diabetic nephropathy remains as the main cause to ESRD starting RRT on hemodialysis, being 24.6% of patients (80–90% due to type 2 diabetes). Vascular diseases (14%), glomerular (12.4%) and interstitial nephropathy, polycystic kidney disease, and systemic diseases (6–7% each) complete the most frequent causes, while in 22% of cases, the cause is unknown [13]. Recent Catalonian Registry data suggest that the incidence of diabetic kidney disease may be decreasing and survival rates increasing in recent years, which may reflect improved diabetes and cardiovascular risk factors management [16]. Apart from diabetes, another challenge is the increasing comorbidity index of patients at the start of hemodialysis, with average values of 5.7, generally higher than in PD and transplant patients [15].

During 2018, the annual mortality in the adult hemodialysis population was 16% and higher (23.8%) for those >75 years of age. A recent increase has been observed probably due to the older age of incident patients. Mortality causes were cardiovascular (25%), infectious (19%), psychological or social (including withdrawal of hemodialysis, 11%), cancer (9%), sudden death (6%), and unknown causes (14%) [6].

## Hemodialysis Prescription

The length of hemodialysis sessions has increased in recent years, and dialysis adequacy has improved [9, 17, 18]. Almost 90% of patients were dialyzed at least 12 hours per week and reached an equilibrated Kt/$V_{urea}$ > 1.2 in 2017 [15]. High Kuf biocompatible membranes are widely used [9], filters are not reused, and ultrapure dialysis fluid is the standard, as more than 90% of patients are on high flux and/or online hemodiafiltration (OL-HDF) [19].

According to some surveys, use of OL-HDF is close to 30% (data on file non-published from the Madrilian Society of Nephrology), but may be higher in regions such as Catalonia in which OL-HDF use has increased from 31% in 2011 to 70% in 2017 [15]. Remarkably, over 95% of patients on OL-HDF (mostly on postdilution) achieved convective volumes higher than 20 liters per session [15]. Erythropoiesis-stimulating agents [15–17], non-calcium-based phosphate binders, and calcimimetics [17] are widely used.

## Vascular Access

An important issue of hemodialysis treatment is vascular access. Data from the Catalonian Registry [20] show that only 50% of incident patients has a functioning arteriovenous fistula (AVF) and this remained stable for 2000–2011. Higher AVF rates were found for patients followed in predialysis care for at least 2 years before initiation of dialysis and lower rates for those with higher comorbidities [20]. One year after starting hemodialysis, 67% of patients with non-tunneled catheters and 60% with tunneled catheters had switched to AVF [20]. However, the percentage of patients starting hemodialysis with a functioning AVF has decreased from 2011 on, probably due to higher comorbidities and older age. Thus, in 2017 40% of incident patients had AVF, 2% grafts and 59% catheters [15]. The same year, 5% of prevalent patients had a non-tunneled catheter, 20% tunneled catheters, 4% grafts, and 62% AVF (50% radiocephalic and 50% brachiocephalic/brachiobasilic AVF) [15].

DOPPS (2012–2015) data show a higher frequency of catheters in incident patients in Spain than in Italy, Germany, or Japan and similar rates to the UK but lower than in the USA, Canada, or Belgium [18]. A higher percentage of prevalent patients was dialyzed through catheters in Spain than in the UK, Germany, or Australia; rates were similar to Italy and Sweden and lower than in Belgium or Canada [21].

This alarming scenario has fostered different initiatives from the Spanish scientific societies seeking to:

- Improve management of advanced chronic kidney disease
- Create working groups on interventional Nephrology [22]
  - Establish multidisciplinary groups of nephrologists, vascular surgeons, and radiologists.
  - Develop Spanish Clinical Guidelines on Vascular Access for Hemodialysis, which were recently published [23].
  - Improve nephrologist training in vascular access monitoring and increase the use of Doppler ultrasound [24].

## Blood-Borne Virus Infections

Another worldwide challenge at hemodialysis units is the control of blood-borne virus infections. The prevalence of hepatitis B (HBV), hepatitis C (HCV), and human immunodeficiency virus (HIV) infections has markedly dropped in Spain. According to REER, in 2018 the prevalence of HBV infection was 1.9%, HCV 4.3%, and HIV infection <1%) [6]. HBV vaccination is recommended since early stages of predialysis care or immediately after hemodialysis start. More recently, the widespread use of direct antiviral agents for HCV has decreased the prevalence of HCV, with some units achieving cure of all patients.

Data from 2008 indicated that 79% of dialysis units had HCV-infected patients (50% of them with isolation measures) while 14% units had HBV-infected patients and 4% HIV patients (some under complete isolation) [9]. Though new blood-borne virus infection management guidelines are expected soon, isolation measures for HCV or HIV patients may differ among regions depending on regional regulations or applications of tenders according to regional health authorities. This has created some confusion as to how to deal with cured HCV patients that remain anti-HCV positive.

## Home Hemodialysis

The use of home hemodialysis is still limited in Spain (less than 0.3% of prevalent hemodialysis patients or 0.1% in Catalonia), but it has grown recently in some Spanish hospitals such as the Navarra University Clinic [25, 26]. Low prevalence may be related to lack of economic incentives, structural reasons, hospital facilities and resources suitable to train patients, patient choice, socioeconomic factors, but especially the closeness of hospitals and EDC to patient homes [27]. In the infrequent case of remote places, such as the Canary Islands or extensive, mountainous, low populated provinces, patients may join home hemodialysis programs but more often are encouraged to initiate PD [27]. Different initiatives are aimed at boosting home hemodialysis in Spain [26]. It should be mentioned that when dialysis first became available in Spain, home hemodialysis was the only option of patients living outside Madrid or Barcelona and the first hospitals to offer hemodialysis had large home hemodialysis programs [3], with patients living hundreds of kilometers away and lacking what we would now consider basic facilities such as water treatment plants.

## Pediatric Hemodialysis

There are no recent published data on Spanish pediatric hemodialysis. According to Dr. Angel Alonso (La Paz University Hospital), the incidence of RRT among patients aged <18 years is 3.7 pmp. In 2016, there were 454 prevalent patients, most on them with functioning kidney graft ($n$ = 400), 32 on hemodialysis, and 22 on APD. More detailed information is available from the Catalonian Registry for the period 2014–2017 [15]. These data cover Catalonia and close regions ascribed to Barcelona referral centers. In this period, 50 (11.4 pmp) pediatric patients started RRT in Catalonia: 42% started on hemodialysis and 16% on PD, and 42% got a preemptive transplantation. As of December 31, 2017, RRT prevalence was 100 children: 7% hemodialysis, 2% PD, and 91% with a functioning kidney transplant (84% from cadaveric donors and 16% from living donors). Mean time to first kidney transplant was 5.4 months after dialysis start. The relatively short time between dialysis start and the transplantation explains the high rate of central catheters; 71% tunneled and 29% percutaneous. The causes of primary kidney disease in incident children were tubulointerstitial nephropathy (31%), glomerular (29%), hereditary or familial diseases (16%), and unknown (20%).

## Costs

Publications on hemodialysis costs are relatively old [28, 29]. In 2013, a Spanish study [29] estimated the hemodialysis costs to be 53,289 €/year for in-hospital hemodialysis and 44,971 €/year for private service providers via EDC. However, the cost may differ according to regional health authorities.

The Catalonian model applies an "all-inclusive cost," in which private EDC providers provide dialysis sessions, medications, transport, and nutritional-psychological support for a fix amount per month. However, the most extended model applies a payer reimbursement on service, mostly related to the hemodialysis treatment. In this model, medications and transport are usually excluded. Medications available at external pharmacies are prescribed by Primary Care physicians and bought by patients at discount prices. Medications only available through hospital pharmacies (e.g., EPO, parenteral vitamin D analogues, or cinacalcet) will be covered by referral hospitals.

In conclusion, high-quality hemodialysis is provided in Spain, with no restrictions on access or reimbursement and no direct costs for the patient, as the National Health System has universal public coverage. However, there are issues that can be improved, such as promoting home hemodialysis or reducing the use of catheters as vascular access. In this regard, several initiatives aim at improving hemodialysis quality in Spain including the standards and recommendations of the Ministry of Health [11], the Guideline for Dialysate Quality of the Spanish Society of Nephrology [19], the search for quality indicators in hemodialysis [30, 31], the recommendations for the coordination of outpatient hemodialysis centers and reference hospitals [32], the creation of the Working Group on Diagnostic and Interventional Nephrology of the Spanish Society of Nephrology [22], or the publication of the Spanish Clinical Guidelines on Vascular Access for Hemodialysis [23].

## Peritoneal Dialysis

### Background

The first PD were performed at Fundación Jiménez Díaz from 1962; however, PD was dwarfed by the hemodialysis program [3]. Some Prof. Hernando disciples exported PD to other hospitals such as Puerta de Hierro University Hospital (Madrid), Asturias General Hospital (Oviedo), La Paz University Hospital (Madrid), Vírgen del Rocío Hospital (Seville), and Clinic University Hospital in Barcelona. PD development ran in parallel with the expansion of nephrology departments throughout the country and international events. *Peritoneal Dialysis Bulletin* was published from 1980 and later evolved to *Peritoneal Dialysis International*, the referral journal on PD. International courses such as the Vicenza course from 1982 and the International Society for Peritoneal Dialysis (ISPD), founded in 1984, contributed to expand PD. Technical advances such as the "Y connection" in 1980 [33], double bag systems (1988), and the "flush before fill" technique (1999) contributed to improve PD outcomes.

Spanish Nephrology contributed to PD knowledge through figures such as Prof Rafael Selgas who characterized peritoneal membrane failure [34, 35] or Francisco Coronel who pioneered PD in the diabetic population [36].

### Incidence and Prevalence

According to the 2018 REER [6], PD incidence was 24.1 pmp and prevalence 66.5 pmp (5%). However, there are large interregional and interhospital differences depending on local expertise, patient populations, predialysis care, and hemodialysis availability.

The incidence of PD has continuously increased from 2007 (15.1 pmp) to 2018 (24.1 pmp) [6]. Potential contributors include the creation of the Spanish Group for the Promotion and Development of PD (GADDPE) lobby in 2009. GADDPE has generated health economic models and scenarios and has estimated that huge cost savings to the payer and a more cost-efficient model would result from increasing PD incidence to 30% of RRT and planned dialysis start increased from 50% to 75% of patients [37–40]. However, the impact has been limited by healthcare authorities not promoting a "PD first approach" and because existing healthcare structures favor the hemodialysis start even for non-planned dialysis start patients. The situation may still change since GADDPE is supported by the Spanish Society of Nephrology Nursing (SEDEN) and by renal patient associations (FRAE, ALCER) which are strong stakeholders.

GADDPE also generated "*Decision making aids*" to be used at the time of patient modality choice, which are increasingly used by key referral hospitals and even promoted by Regional Health Authorities such as in Andalucía. Use of these tools increased PD choice to 45% of patients who used them and PD incidence to 48% [41].

Similar to hemodialysis, actual prevalent patients on PD are older and with higher comorbidity than some years ago [6]. Actual annual death is 9.6% vs. 15.9% in HD [6].

### PD in Congestive Heart Failure

Spanish PD nephrologists are interested in using PD to treat refractory congestive heart failure [42, 43]. A Nephrology-Cardiology consensus document has been generated to offer PD to NYHA IV heart failure patients [44, 45].

### Decreasing Rates of Peritonitis

As in other parts of the world, advances in connectology, new Y systems, and perhaps a general use of non-lactate solutions have decreased the rate of peritonitis [46]. As an example, the Andalusian registry reported a decrease from 0.7–0.5 episodes/patient/year (2000–2010) to 0.58–0.40 (2011–2016) [47]. Similar trends were observed in other regional registries [48–50].

### PD Solutions

There is not much information on the relative use of different PD solutions in Spain. There are only two providers (Baxter and Fresenius Medical Care). However, glucose-free osmotic agents (Nutrineal® and Extraneal®) are widely used, especially for patients potentially benefiting from glucose-sparing regimes such as diabetics, malnourished, hyperlipidemic, or morbidly obese patients or during acute peritonitis episodes [51].

Similarly, non-lactate solutions are widely used since 2009, when Baxter limited the production of lactate-based solutions due to manufacturing issues. Low glucose degradation products (GDP) solutions are also widely used. According to the Andalusian registry, 87% of patients are prescribed bicarbonate solutions and 50% icodextrin [47].

### Automated Peritoneal Dialysis (APD)

The APD share has decreased from over 50% of PD patients (e.g., 66% in the Catalonian 2003–2005 registry or 54% in the Andalusian 2009 registry) to around 45–50% today [47]. Factors contributing to this decline may include local key opinion leaders' publications on the faster loss residual renal function [52, 53], or the controversial results on peritonitis rates [46, 54–56].

### New Technologies: Telemedicine and Connectivity

Telemedicine has been pioneered by groups such as the Severo Ochoa Hospital in Leganés, which reported increased patient confidence and transport cost savings [57, 58]. However, the short distance between patient home and referral hospitals as well as the frequent advanced age of PD patients has limited its use. However, the population use of digital platforms is evolving, and telemedicine may allow to conciliate a larger and more demanding patient population with limited hospital staff resources [59].

More recently, systems have been developed that allow to export daily treatment outcomes in a bidirectional manner to the hospital PD staff. This would allow immediate problem-solving (especially true in alarms during therapy), improving patient monitoring and outcomes while reducing costs by decreasing the number of hospital visits [60, 61].

### Cost

PD is free for patients as part of their universal healthcare coverage. PD patients are trained in public hospitals on an ambulatory basis. They are followed at the hospital where they may be admitted or transferred to another RRT modality. PD providers supply materials and devices at home every other fortnight. Providers are ruled by hospital or regional tenders.

PD cost estimation differs from other countries, in that it is not assigned per bag but rather it is a fixed cost per day of therapy depending on modality and solutions used. Roughly speaking, the daily price on continuous ambulatory PD is 45 €/day, and on APD 67 €/day. Use of non-lactate solutions increases the daily cost in 12 €/day and icodextrin in 6 €/day. This means that it is not a single product buying as in other latitudes. There are no specific incentives to offer PD, and PD does not impact staff salaries. In fact, PD may be a money-losing enterprise for hospitals, since healthcare authorities pay directly the cost of PD to providers of PD materials and hospitals assume the costs of PD personnel and patient follow-up. By contrast, the costs of in-hospital hemodialysis are payed directly to the hospital, and an optimized management of hemodialysis units may result in a net benefit for the hospital.

## Renal Transplantation

Kidney transplantation is considered the RRT of choice in Spain as it generally provides better quality of life and survival at a lower cost [62–65]. Therefore, a large public policy effort is aimed at increasing kidney transplantation rates and acceptance of donation by the population.

### Spanish Legislation Favors Renal Transplantation

During the 1970s, the lack of enough hemodialysis facilities and the improving results of kidney transplantation aligned medical and surgical teams with patient associations to demand legislation changes to favor organ transplantation. These changes included brain death as an accepted cause of death that allows donation. This was included in the first organ transplant law published on November 6, 1979 (Law 30/1979), later extended and detailed by the Royal Decree 426/1980. The Decree included new legislation for release, extraction, conservation, and exchange of organs if therapeutic purposes applied but also the following important features:

1. No economic compensation could be received for the donation of organs.
2. The Ministry of Health and Social Security will authorize those Medical Centers that can extract human organs.
3. Organs can be obtained from living donors for implanting in another person provided the donor is of legal age, is in full possession of mental faculties, has been informed of the consequences, and gives express free and conscious consent in written form to the public authority and that the organ itself is destined for a particular person.
4. Extraction of organs from deceased persons can be done after verifying death based on the presence of irreversible data of brain lesions incompatible with life, determined

by a neurologist or neurosurgeon and the Head of Service of the medical unit, or their substitute. No member of the transplant team can participate in this process.

5. Extraction of organs can be performed in deceased persons provided they have not stated their express opposition. Persons who die in road accidents can also be considered donors if the deceased person has left no record of express opposition, although in this case authorization must be obtained from a judge and in last years after first grade family member's consent to provide.
6. The person responsible for the Medical Unit can only give their agreement if the recipient is aware of the process after receiving the pertinent information and giving written consent.

The law establishes that help will be given to Regional and National Organizations as well as collaboration with international entities to encourage and facilitate the exchange and circulation of organs for transplant.

Royal Decree 2070/1999 published in 1999 allowed organ donation after cardiac arrest.

Royal Decree 1723/2012 published on December 29, 2012, regulated activities related to the procurement, clinical use, and territorial coordination of human organs destined for transplant with the relevant requirements for quality and safety.

## Creation of the National Transplant Organization (ONT)

The ONT was created in 1989 and became the coordinating institution for organ transplant teams, as well as for consensus measures favoring organ donation and extraction and any other measure encouraging organ transplantation. The ONT also created a transplant registry for Spain.

The ONT depends on the Ministry of Health and is headquartered in Madrid. The nephrologist Rafael Matesanz was the first and longest-serving director and was a key driving force for the success of the Spanish transplant programs. He was succeeded by Blanca Miranda and, currently, by Beatriz Domínguez-Gil, both also nephrologists.

The post of regional coordinator was created, along with a network of hospital coordinators, thereby having three levels of organ transplant coordinators: national, regional, and hospital. These posts are appointed by the national and regional governments and by the managing director or medical director of the hospital from among qualified health personnel (physician, technical medical assistant, or registered nurse) entrusted with the tasks of orientation, coordination, support, and promotion of organ donation. This organizational system for the optimization of organ donation fits perfectly into the infrastructure and universal public model of healthcare in Spain. What is popularly known as the "Spanish Model of Organ Donation and Transplantation" is the combination of laws, measures, and teams to encourage organ transplantation. It includes the legislator, ONT, coordinating teams, emergency services, intensive care specialists, neurologists, neurosurgeons, anesthetists, and members of the hospital transplant units.

## Healthcare Infrastructure

Given that kidney transplantation is considered the treatment of choice for ESRD, all patients who have an indication for kidney transplantation must be included on the waiting list for transplant from a deceased donor, unless they have the opportunity of a living donor transplant. National Healthcare Service approves hospitals that provide kidney transplantation.

In general, all hospitals have a predialysis unit for advanced CKD (G4/G5) patients. The possibility of living donation should be raised and encouraged in this unit. One aim is to encourage living donation for children and preemptive transplants, be it from living or deceased donors, by wait listing when glomerular filtration rate (GFR) is ≤15 ml/min/1.73 $m^2$. The predialysis unit also deals with patients with type 1 diabetes mellitus and ESRD who have an indication for a combined kidney-pancreas transplant. Indeed, for this latter group of patients, the ONT oversaw the creation of a protocol in 2005 drawn up with the participation of transplant team professionals [66].

Pre- and posttransplant follow-up is done by the Nephrology Service of the reference hospital in collaboration with non-transplanting hospitals in the same area.

## Optimization of Deceased Donor Donation

Most transplants in Spain during the initial stages of kidney transplantation programs came from brain death donors. However, the number of patients on dialysis kept growing, while the number of annual transplants did not surpass 3000 and the waiting list did not fall below 4000 [67]. Mortality in patients on the waiting list is higher than for those who received a kidney transplantation [62, 68–70]. As donors resulting from road traffic accidents decreased (43% in 1992 to 4.2% in 2015), alternative donor sources allowed a continuous increase in donations to 48 donors pmp in 2018.

Two key strategies to increase the donor pool were as follows.

### Old Donors for Old Recipients

Renal transplant recipients receiving a kidney from an expanded criteria donor have improved survival compared with wait-listed patients [71]. It is evident that kidneys from older donors show changes characterized by increased glomerular, vascular, and tubular senescence [72]. To determine whether the graft is suitable for kidney transplantation, in addition to checking its gross appearance and main vessels, a protocol biopsy is first done, the scores for which determine whether the graft is suitable for implantation, either as a single or a dual implant [73]. Kidneys from older donors are preferentially assigned to older recipients who have lower life expectancies.

### Non-Heart-Beating Donors

The Report of Medical Consultants on the President's Commission for the Study of Ethical Problems in Medicine and Biomedical and Behavioral Research on Guidelines for the Determination of Death was published in 1981. This document, in line with that previously published by Harvard University, proposed that all jurisdictions in the USA should follow a protocol for the diagnosis of death and take into account that, although the traditional concept of death was based on the irreversible loss of heart and lung functions, it is now possible to maintain both functions mechanically, despite the loss of all brain functions. Accordingly, an individual with irreversible cessation of circulatory and respiratory functions is dead; and an individual with irreversible cessation of all functions of the entire brain, including the brain stem, is dead [74]. This document therefore endorses donation from non-heart-beating donors. Notwithstanding this, and bearing in mind the previous criteria for brain death from the Harvard Committee, an article was published in 1975 concerning the in situ preservation of cadaver kidneys for transplantation by perfusion of a cold solution using a double-balloon triple-lumen catheter designed for cases of non-heart-beating donors. This was introduced into the aorta via the femoral artery [75], and in 1989 the Japanese reported their experience with organ extraction after cardiac arrest [76]. This same year saw the start at the San Carlos University Hospital in Madrid of an organ procurement program from non-heart-beating donors [77]. From 1989 to 1998, 144 kidneys were procured from non-heart-beating donors of which 95 were transplanted. The organs procured were classified according to Maastricht donor categories and most were type I [78]. The kidney grafts were maintained from the moment of the diagnosis of cardiac arrest until the time of procurement by cardiopulmonary bypass. The results, published in 2000, compared these donors with heart-beating donors. The non-heart-beating donor organs had a 5.73-fold increase in the incidence of delayed graft function. At 5 years there were no differences in renal function (estimated by serum creatinine and creatinine clearance) or graft survival (82.7% vs. 83.9%; respectively, $p = 0.576$). In 1996, this center signed an agreement with the Madrid emergency facilities (SAMUR 061, SERCAM) and established a protocol for the procurement of organs from persons with sudden death outside the hospital after irreversible cardiac arrest (Maastricht type I donors) who were taken to the hospital. This protocol does not affect any cardiovascular pulmonary resuscitation maneuvers, and the assessment as a potential donor is done when the cardiac arrest is considered irreversible after a minimum period of resuscitation attempts of 30 minutes or when the lesions provoking the cardiac arrest are incompatible with life. The reasons for exclusion as a donor were also established, together with the usual laboratory tests for organ transplantation. Once death has been confirmed, the femoral artery and vein are cannulated to perfuse the organs connected to a cardiopulmonary bypass machine with external oxygenation and hypothermia [79].

A consensus conference on non-heart beating donation was held at the headquarters of the ONT on November 27, 1995. A consensus document was elaborated by 69 specialists on organ procurement from non-heart-beating donors. Various points of agreement were reached about non-heart-beating donors who undergo unsuccessful resuscitation attempts (Maastricht types I and II), considering two groups [80]:

(a) Outside the hospital, attended by the Out of Hospital Emergency Services who transfer the potential donor to the hospital, applying cardiopulmonary compression and ventilatory support
(b) Inside the hospital, with immediate resuscitation measures.

The requirements and protocol to follow included estimation of the time of arrest, 30 minutes of unsuccessful cardiopulmonary resuscitation, and transfer to the reference hospital for admission to the Intensive Care Unit. After 5 minutes with no pulse or the absence of an electrocardiogram trace, death is certified and resuscitation measures are initiated with a cardiac compressor.

Although the Spanish Law of 1979 on kidney transplantation and its subsequent Decree in 1980 specify the conditions for brain death, no reference is made to death after cardiac arrest. Accordingly, the authorities were encouraged to make legal provision for this particular situation, even though Spanish legislation considers any deceased person to be a potential donor provided no express opposition against donation has been made. This is why from the legal point of view, it can be considered acceptable to initiate organ conservation measures with a view to donation, and the law includes a series of ethical measures to follow. The Royal Decree 2070/1999 that allows organ donation after cardiac arrest was published in 1999. This contemplates the use of preservation techniques to ensure organ viability while reporting to the competent Court of First Instance so that, if necessary, any restriction or approval for donation can be established. Donation from non-heart-beating donors rose from 2.2% of all kidney transplants in 1995 to 25.8% in 2018.

### Living Donor Transplantation

Since its start, the percentage of transplants from living donors has always been much lower than that from deceased donors. The percentage of living donor transplants in the kidney transplantation registry of the ONT has risen from 1.2% when the registry was started in 1991 to 9% in 2018. For many years only two centers, Fundación Jiménez Díaz in Madrid and Clinic Hospital in Barcelona, regularly performed living donor transplantation. Some other centers considered this unethical, given the availability of cadaveric donors.

A survey undertaken in 2005 found that 59% of patients on dialysis had no information about a kidney transplantation from a living donor and 83% stated that their medical team had not mentioned the possibility of this treatment. The main reason for not offering this possibility was that the physician considered that deceased donor transplant activity was sufficient in Spain [81].

In 2009 the ONT, in its living donor initiative, created a program for the exchange of organs (crossed donation) between pairs whose ABO group was incompatible or who had a positive crossmatch. Up until 2018 almost 200 crossed-donation kidney transplants had been done. For this, once donors and recipients have been studied, an agreement is reached on the same day of surgery for all donor-recipient pairs, and after extraction, each organ is transferred to the relevant recipient center, either by land or by air, depending on the distance.

### General Results of Kidney Transplantation in Spain

Observational studies of the US registry show only a marginal increase in the real kidney graft survival between 1988 and 1995 [82–84], while comparative single-center studies in Spain [85, 86] for the periods before and after 1995 show a significant increase in death-censored and uncensored graft survival with effect from 1996. The uncensored real graft half-life was 10.25 years in the first period, and the actuarial graft half-life was 14.58 years in the second period ($p < 0.001$). The attrition rates, censored and uncensored, showed a significantly lower graft loss in the most recent period. This difference remained after excluding the first year from the analysis ($p = 0.0018$ and $p = 0.0001$, respectively). Similar data have been reported in a Spanish multicenter study [87] and worldwide [88]. This encouraged us to compare the US and Spain Caucasian populations. The study included 9.609 US and 3.808 Spanish recipients who received a deceased donor kidney transplant in 1990, 1994, 1998, and 2002 with a follow-up to September 2006. Among recipients alive with graft function 1 year after transplant, the 10-year graft survival was 71.3% for Spanish and 53.4% for US recipients ($p < 0.001$). The 10-year death-censored graft survival was 75.6% vs. 76.0% for Spanish and US recipients, respectively ($p = 0.73$). The 10-year recipient survival was 86.2% vs. 67.4% ($p < 0.001$) for Spanish and US recipients. In patients with diabetes mellitus as the cause of ESRD, the adjusted death with graft function rates at 10 years were 23.9 and 53.8 per 1000 person-years for Spanish and US recipients, respectively ($p < 0.001$), and among recipients whose cause of ESRD was not diabetes mellitus, the adjusted 10-year rates were 11.0 and 25.4 per 1000 person-years for Spanish and US recipients, respectively. The conclusion of this study is that US kidney transplant recipients had more than twice the long-term hazard of dying with a functioning graft than Spanish kidney transplant recipients and similar levels of death-censored graft function. Pre-transplant medical care, comorbidities such as cardiovascular disease, and their management in each country health system are possible explanations for the differences between the two countries [89].

Other obligatory analyses of graft and patient survival are those involving cases of non-heart-beating donation and "old-for-old" transplantations. Concerning non-heart-beating donation, the group from San Carlos University Hospital in Madrid analyzed their experience between 1989 and 2004 with non-heart-beating ($n = 320$) and heart-beating donors ($n = 584$). Five-year graft survival was 73.3% vs. 85.5% ($p < 0.001$), respectively; and a similar analysis but just with donors in both groups younger than 60 years of age gave figures of 82.1% vs. 87.4% ($p = 0.22$). The 5-year patient survival was 90% vs. 87.4% ($p = 0.22$), respectively [79].

Concerning the impact of donor age on results of renal transplantation, a Spanish multicenter study of 3.365 kidney transplants performed between 1990 and 1998 compared the results between those who received their graft from donors older or younger than 60 years of age ($n = 478$ vs. $n = 2.887$, respectively). The mean serum creatinine at 3 and 12 months was significantly higher in the group with older donors, and graft and patient survival were significantly lower. Also, a linear increase in the risk of graft loss and patient death was noted when donor age was divided into subsets of 10-year increments [90]. More recently, the group from the Hospital del Mar in Barcelona has reported satisfactory results in terms of survival using deceased donors older than 75 years of age, thus confirming the benefit of this treatment option over dialysis, even in an aged population [91, 92].

## Nephrology Practice in Spain

Nephrology human resources structures are almost exclusively at the public sector.

To become a nephrologist within Spain, it is mandatory to overpass a "national all disciplines in medicine exam" in Spanish language, called MIR, that is held once every year. After a 4-year training, a place in the public health service networking is not guaranteed, and already degree nephrologists must undertake another exam to get a permanent position. These exams may differ among regions and so do the frequency in which these exams are announced.

Being a nephrologist via MIR (or commutation of same degree within the European Union) is also a requirement to work at EDC; however, other specialists may apply if a position remains vacant, as an "in clinic physician" is a must to have according to regulatory bodies. Outside Europe nephrologists may be able to work at EDC without performing the MIR exam and training, if a previous commutation of general medicine diploma has been obtained through the Health and Education Ministries. Achieving the commutation of a nephrology title may get longer and up to 6 years.

Private nephrology practice is very limited but has recently been enlarged due to the recent appearance of private hospitals across the country that provide care through different private insurances used by some citizens as a volunteer complementary care to the universal national health cover.

Salaries for healthcare professionals in Spain are low: this is the basis of affordable universal health coverage. As far as we are aware, no public references state how much nephrologists may earn. In any case, salary for degree nephrology staff depends on regions, professional career, and number of days on call (average 4–5 days on duty) and/or if part of a transplantation team program. Roughly speaking, salaries at the public hospitals may range from 70,000 to 100,000 €/year (tax included), while for nephrologists at the EDC would be much lower on 43,000–50,000 €/year, varying in accordance with being nephrologists or if extra medical director responsibilities take place.

As a consequence, Spain exports locally formed nephrologists and nurses, while it imports healthcare professionals from Latin America and other countries with lower GDP.

## Highlight of Nephrology in Spain

The main highlight of Spanish Nephrology is its successful kidney transplant program led by the ONT. Year after year, Spain tops the list of kidney donations per million population and is one of few countries having more patients carrying a functional kidney graft than dialysis patients. This is quite in line with one of the best and more comprehensive healthcare systems in the world. Spain regularly features among the world countries with longest life expectancy, and it has been predicted to lead this ranking by 2040 [1]. However, this success is also leading to a progressive aging of the population, and CKD is expected to become the second most common cause of death after Alzheimer before the end of the century [2].

## Future Perspectives of Nephrology in Spain

There is discrepancy between interest in the specialty by doctors in training and expected increasing burden of CKD in the next few decades. Spain has a national exam, the MIR, which ranks candidates to specialty training. In the 1980s, Nephrology was one of the top specialties chosen. However, from the 1990s, a decline in interest by specialist training candidates has been observed. Specifically, in 2009, nephrology was ranked 29 of 47 specialties. According to Bernis et al. [93], the average position of the Nephrology MIR dropped from 1199 in 1990 to 2007 in 2000 and 3457 in 2008 (Fig. 47.1). Indeed, in 2008 Nephrology could still be chosen by candidates ranked 5485 (out of 6000 specialization places). This is not an exclusively Spanish phenomenon, as it is also observed in other countries. We believe that it is due to very diverse causes:

- Lack of information, incomplete or low quality at University.
- Complex pathophysiology of renal diseases.
- Exaggerated exposure to dialysis patients and chronic patients with high comorbidity.
- Excessive care burden.
- Too much emotional pressure.
- Lack of significant private practice: dialysis centers or on-duty nights as initial job opportunities.
- Loss of autonomy of the nephrologist. In many Units, renal biopsies are performed by radiologists, peritoneal catheter inserted by surgeons, acute renal failure is in the hands of intensivists, and vascular access is provided by radiologists or surgeons.

In contrast to the decline in interest by trainees, the burden of CKD continues to increase. According to GBD 2016 estimates, CKD was the 8th cause of death in Spain in 2016 [94]. Among the top ten causes of death, CKD was the fastest growing from 2006 to 2016, after Alzheimer's disease [2] (Fig. 47.2a). Additionally, among

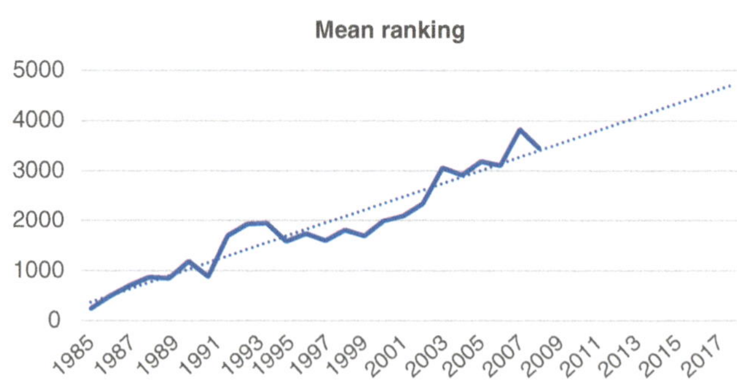


**Fig. 47.1** Annual average position of the Nephrology MIR fellows over time. From the 1990s, a decline in interest by specialist training candidates has been observed. The average position of the Nephrology MIR dropped from 1199 in 1990 to 2007 in 2000 and 3457 in 2008 [93]

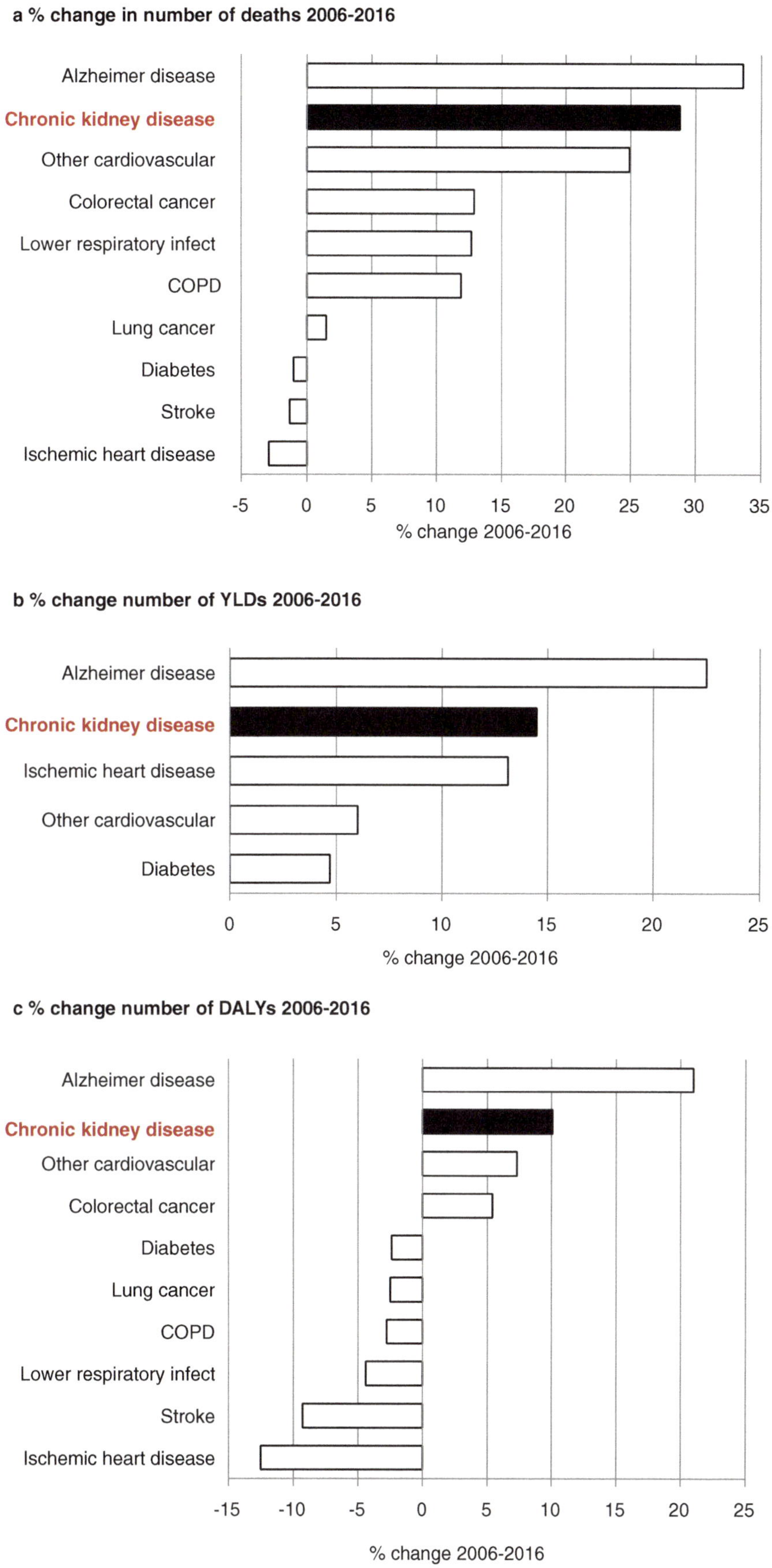


**Fig. 47.2** Trends in top ten causes of death in Spain, 2006–2016. The top ten causes of death in 2016 in Spain in terms of number of deaths and their impact on YLDs and DALYs are shown. (**a**) % change in number of deaths 2006–2016. (**b**) % change in number of YLDs 2006–2016. Data for top ten causes of death in 2016 which are also among the top 30 causes of YLDs are shown. (**c**) % change in number of DALYs 2006–2016. COPD chronic obstructive pulmonary disease, YLDs Years Lived with Disability, DALYs Disability Adjusted Life Years [2]

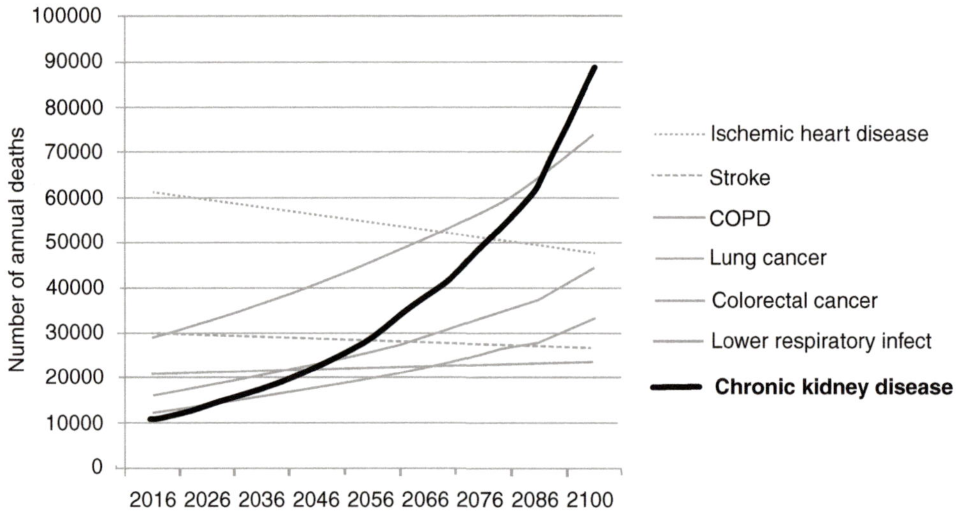


**Fig. 47.3** Predicted growth of the top eight causes of death from 2016 to 2100 in Spain, based on growth from 2006 to 2016 according to the GBD 2016 study. Alzheimer is predicted to become the most frequent cause of death by 2026 and is not represented in the graph due to its magnitude, which would preclude appreciating details for the other causes of death. The 2006 to 2016 change in number of deaths was extrapolated to predict annual number of deaths up to 2100. COPD chronic obstructive pulmonary disease, YLDs Years Lived with Disability, DALYs Disability Adjusted Life Years [2]

the top ten causes of death, it also ranked second only to Alzheimer as the fastest growing cause of Years Lived with Disability (YLDs) (Fig. 47.2b) and Disability Adjusted Life Years (DALYs) [2] (Fig. 47.2c). DALYs are the sum of years of potential life lost due to premature mortality and the years of productive life lost due to disability. At the current pace, CKD is set to become the second most frequent cause of death in Spain by 2100, after Alzheimer's disease [2] (Fig. 47.3). This should be a call to action for the medical community, healthcare authorities, and the population at large. Without a significant increase in funding for such activity that dramatically changes the 2006–2016 trend, CKD is set to become the second cause of death in Spain for future generations.

## Conclusion

Nephrology in Spain has over 60 years of history and deals with one of the longest life expectancies in the world that may impact in the sustainability of the actual universal National Public Health System. All renal replacement therapy modalities are widely used across the country being more than half of prevalent patients with a functioning kidney graft. Therefore, the National Transplant Organization is one of the most admired and awarded Spanish institutions. In terms of dialysis, hemodialysis is largely used providing high flux and/or online hemodiafiltration in more than 90% of all patients. The recent growth of peritoneal dialysis incidence is promising and likely driven by a larger use of decision-making aids. Different challenges need to be addressed by the Spanish Society of Nephrology, such as lack of interest in nephrology training, reduction of the worrisome use of central vein catheters, the continuous growth of patients on the kidney transplant waiting list, and the potential inequity that may bring a national healthcare system with transfer of competencies into 17 different regions.

**Acknowledgments** This manuscript was supported in part by the Spanish Ministry of Economy and Competitiveness (MINECO) (grant ICI14/00016 and grants PI17/02043, PI16/02057, DTS18/00032) from the Instituto de Salud Carlos III co-funded by the Fondo Europeo de Desarrollo Regional (FEDER), RETICS (REDINREN RD16/0009/0006 and 0001), and ERA-PerMed-JTC2018 (KIDNEY ATTACK AC18/00064 and PERSTIGAN AC18/00071). The authors thank the transplant team of Carlos Haya Regional University Hospital and Beatriz Dominguez-Gil, director of the ONT, for their collaboration. We also thank Ian Johnstone for linguistic assistance in the preparation of the text.

## References

1. Foreman KJ, Marquez N, Dolgert A, Fukutaki K, Fullman N, McGaughey M, et al. Forecasting life expectancy, years of life lost, and all-cause and cause-specific mortality for 250 causes of death: reference and alternative scenarios for 2016–40 for 195 countries and territories. Lancet. 2018;392(10159):2052–90.
2. Ortiz A, Sanchez-Niño MD, Crespo-Barrio M, De-Sequera-Ortiz P, Fernández-Giráldez E, García-Maset R, et al. The Spanish Society of Nephrology (SENEFRO) commentary to the Spain GBD 2016 report: keeping chronic kidney disease out of sight of health authorities will only magnify the problem. Nefrologia. 2019;39(1):29–34.

3. Hernando Avendaño L, editor. Historia de la Nefrología en España. Barcelona: Grupo Editorial Nefrología de la Sociedad Española de Nefrología; 2012. At: http://www.revistanefrologia.com/files/Libro_historia_SEN_web.pdf.
4. A definition of irreversible coma. Report of the Ad Hoc Committee of the Harvard Medical School to examine the definition of brain death. JAMA. 1968;205:337–40.
5. Fernandez-Cruz L. Trasplante de páncreas. Med Clin. 1983;80:723–8.
6. Registro Español de Enfermos Renales. Informe de Diálisis y Trasplante 2018. At: https://www.senefro.org/contents/webstructure/SEN_2019_REER_modificada.pdf. Last accessed date: 8 Jan 2020.
7. ERA-EDTA Registry; annual report 2016. At: https://www.era-edta-reg.org/files/annualreports/pdf/AnnRep2016.pdf.
8. de Francisco ALM, Piñera C. Nephrology around Europe: organization models and management strategies: Spain. J Nephrol. 2011;24(4):438–45.
9. Albalate M, Arenas MD, Berdud I, Sanjuan F, Postigo S. Encuesta sobre los centros de hemodiálisis extrahospitalaria en España. Nefrologia. 2007;27(2):175–83.
10. Arenas MD, Bernat A, Ramos R, Berdud I, Blanco A. Investigation into the relationship between outpatient haemodialysis centres and referring hospitals in Spain. Nefrologia. 2009;29(5):439–48.
11. Palanca Sánchez I, Conde Olasagasti J, Elola Somoza J, Bernal Sobrino J, Paniagua Caparrós J, Grupo de Expertos. Unidad de depuración extrarrenal: estándares y recomendaciones. Madrid: Ministerio de Sanidad, Política Social e Igualdad; 2011.
12. Departamento de Salud. Generalitat de Catalunya. Orden SLT/167/2018, de 1 de octubre, por la que se establecen para el año 2018 las tarifas máximas de los servicios de diálisis realizados por los centros y establecimientos sanitarios de ámbito no hospitalario que contrate el Servicio Catalán de la Salud. DOGC. 2018;(7723):1–2.
13. Martín Escobar E. Registro Español de Enfermos Renales (REER). Registro Español de Enfermos Renales. Informe 2013 y evolución 2007–2013. Nefrologia. 2016;36(2):97–120.
14. Helve J, Kramer A, Abad-Diez JM, Couchoud C, de Arriba G, de Meester J, et al. Factors associating with differences in the incidence of renal replacement therapy among elderly: data from the ERA-EDTA registry. Nephrol Dial Transplant. 2018;33(8):1428–35.
15. Statistical Report 2017. Registre de malalts renals de Catalunya. Barcelona: Organització Catalana de Trasplantaments. Registre de malalts renals de Catalunya; 2019.
16. Comas J, Arcos E, Castell C, Cases A, Martínez-Castelao A, Doñate T, et al. Evolution of the incidence of chronic kidney disease stage 5 requiring renal replacement therapy in the diabetic population of Catalonia. Nephrol Dial Transplant. 2013;28(5):1191–8.
17. Pérez-García R, Palomares-Sancho I, Merello-Godino JI, Aljama-García P, Bustamante-Bustamante J, Luño J, et al. Epidemiological study of 7316 patients on haemodialysis treated in FME clinics in Spain, using data from the EuCliD® database: results from years 2009–2010. Nefrologia. 2012;32(6):743–53.
18. Robinson BM, Akizawa T, Jager KJ, Kerr PG, Saran R, Pisoni RL. Factors affecting outcomes in patients reaching end-stage kidney disease worldwide: differences in access to renal replacement therapy, modality use, and haemodialysis practices. Lancet. 2016;388(10041):294–306.
19. Pérez-García R, García Maset R, Gonzalez Parra E, Solozábal Campos C, Ramírez Chamond R, Martín-Rabadán P, et al. Guía de gestión de calidad del líquido de diálisis (LD) (segunda edición, 2015). Nefrologia. 2016;36(3):e1–52.
20. Roca-Tey R, Arcos E, Comas J, Cao H, Tort J, Feixas J, et al. Vascular access for incident hemodialysis patients in Catalonia: analysis of data from the Catalan Renal Registry (2000–2011). J Vasc Access. 2015;16(6):472–9.
21. Port FK, Morgenstern H, Bieber BA, Karaboyas A, McCullough KP, Tentori F, et al. Understanding associations of hemodialysis practices with clinical and patient-reported outcomes: examples from the DOPPS. Nephrol Dial Transplant. 2017;32(suppl_2):ii106–12.
22. Rivera Gorrín M, Cornago Delgado I, Betriu Bars À, Lanuza Luengo M, Ceballos Guerrero M, Paraíso Cuevas V, et al. Creation of the Working Group on Diagnostic and Interventional Nephrology of the Spanish Society of Nephrology. Nefrologia. 2016;36(3):325–6.
23. Ibeas J, Roca-Tey R, Vallespín J, Moreno T, Moñux G, Martí-Monrós A, et al. Guía Clínica Española del Acceso Vascular para Hemodiálisis [Spanish Clinical Guidelines on Vascular Access for Haemodialysis]. Nefrologia. 2017;37(Suppl 1):1–191.
24. Sosa Barrios RH, Ibeas J, Roca Tey R, Ceballos Guerrero M, Betriu Bars A, Cornago Delgado I, et al. Diagnostic and interventional nephrology in Spain: a snapshot of current situation. J Vasc Access. 2019;20(2):140–5.
25. Vega A, Sequí MJ, Abad S, Yuste C, Santos A, Macías N, et al. Daily home hemodialysis is an available option for renal replacement therapy in Spain. Ther Apher Dial. 2016;20(4):408–12.
26. Pérez-Alba A, Barril-Cuadrado G, Castellano-Cerviño I, Martín-Reyes G, Pérez-Melón C, Slon-Roblero F, et al. Home haemodialysis in Spain. Nefrologia. 2015;35(1):1–5.
27. Pérez Alba A, Slon Roblero F, Castellano Gasch S, Bajo Rubio MA. Barriers for the development of home haemodialysis in Spain. Spanish nephrologists survey. Nefrologia. 2017;37(6):665–8.
28. Moncasi EP, Jiménez MDA, Alonso M, Martínez MF, Pardo AG, Rebollo P, et al. Multicentre study of haemodialysis costs. Nefrologia. 2011;31(3):299–307.
29. Conde Olasagasti JL, Garcia Diaz JE, Carrasco Benitez P, Mareque Ruiz MÁ, Parras Partido MP, Moreno Alia I, et al. Cost analysis of integrated renal replacement therapy program in the province of Toledo (2012–2013). Nefrologia. 2017;37(3):285–92.
30. Arenas Jiménez MD, Lorenzo S, Álvarez-Ude F, Angoso M, López-Revuelta K, Aranaz J. Implantación de sistemas de gestión de calidad en las unidades de nefrología españolas. Nefrologia. 2006;26(2):234–45.
31. Alcázar JM, Arenas MD, Alvarez-Ude F, Virto R, Rubio E, Maduell F, et al. Preliminary results of the Spanish Society of Nephrology multicenter study of quality performance measures: hemodialysis outcomes can be improved. Nefrologia. 2008;28(6):597–606.
32. Berdud I, Arenas MD, Bernat A, Ramos R, Blanco A. Appendix to dialysis centre guidelines: recommendations for the relationship between outpatient haemodialysis centers and reference hospitals. Opinions from the Outpatient Dialysis Group. Nefrologia. 2011;31(6):664–9.
33. Buoncristiani U, Bianchi P, Gozzari M, et al. A new, safe, simple connection system for CAPD. Int J Nephrol Urol Androl. 1980;1:50–3.
34. Yáñez-Mó M, Lara-Pezzi E, Selgas R, et al. Peritoneal dialysis and epithelial to mesenchymal transition of mesothelial cells. N Engl J Med. 2003;30(5):403–13. 348.
35. Selgas R, Fernandez-Reyes MJ, Bosque E, Bajo MA, Borrego F, Jimenez C, et al. Functional longevity of the human peritoneum: how long is continuous peritoneal dialysis possible? Results of a prospective medium long term study. Am J Kidney Dis. 1994;23:64–73.
36. Coronel F, Cigarrán S, Herrero JA. Morbimortalidad en pacientes diabéticos en diálisis peritoneal. Experiencia de 25 años en un solo centro. Nefrologia. 2010;30(6):626–32.
37. Lamas Barreiro JM, Alonso Suárez M, Saavedra Alonso JA, Gándara MA. Costes y valor añadido de los conciertos de hemodiálisis y diálisis peritoneal. Nefrologia. 2011;31(6):656–63.

38. Arrieta J, Rodríguez-Carmona A, Remón C, Pérez-Fontán M, Ortega F, Sánchez Tomero JA, et al. La diálisis peritoneal es la mejor alternativa coste-efectiva para la sostenibilidad del tratamiento con diálisis. Nefrologia. 2011;31(5):505–13.
39. De Francisco ALM. Sostenibilidad y equidad del tratamiento sustitutivo de la función renal en España. Nefrologia. 2011;31(3):241–6.
40. Márquez-Peláez S, Caro-Martínez A, Adam-Blanco D, Olry-de-Labry-Lima A, Navarro-Caballero JA, García-Mochón L, et al. Eficiencia de la diálisis peritoneal frente a hemodiálisis para el tratamiento de la Insuficiencia Renal. Agencia de Evaluación de Tecnologías Sanitarias. Escuela Andaluza de Salud Pública. Consejería de Igualdad, Salud y Políticas Sociales. Junta de Andalucía. At: http://www.juntadeandalucia.es/salud/servicios/contenidos/nuevaaetsa/up/Aetsa_2010_7_DialisisPeritoneal.pdf.
41. Prieto-Velasco M, Quiros P, Remon C, Spanish Group for the Implementation of a Shared Decision Making Process for RRT Choice with Patient Decision Aid Tools. The concordance between patients' renal replacement therapy choice and definitive modality: is it a utopia? PLoS One. 2015;10(10). At: https://www.ncbi.nlm.nih.gov/pmc/articles/PMC4605797/.
42. Portolés Pérez J, Cuevas BX. Síndrome cardiorrenal. Nefrologia. 2008;supl 3:29–32.
43. Montejo JD, Bajo MA, Del Peso G, Selgas R. Papel de la diálisis peritoneal en el tratamiento de la insuficiencia cardíaca refractaria. Nefrologia. 2010;30(1):21–7.
44. Sánchez JE, Rodríguez C, González I, Fernández-Viña A, Núñez M, Peláez B. Análisis de las ventajas de la diálisis peritoneal en el tratamiento de la insuficiencia cardíaca refractaria crónica. Nefrologia. 2010;30(5):487–9.
45. Quirós-Ganga PL, Remón-Rodríguez C, Tejuca-Marenco M, De la Espada-Piña V. La diálisis peritoneal permite el trasplante cardíaco con éxito en paciente con insuficiencia cardíaca refractaria. Nefrologia. 2015;35(1):121–4.
46. Rodriguez–Carmona A, Perez Fontán M, Garcia Falcon T, Fernandez Rivera C, Valdes F. A comparative analysis on the incidence of peritonitis and exit-site infection in CAPD and automated peritoneal dialysis. Perit Dial Int. 1999;19:253–8.
47. Remón C, Quirós P. Registro de pacientes en diálisis peritoneal de Andalucía: período 1999–2016. At: https://nefrosan.com/san/index.php/2017?download=258:registro-andaluz-modulo-dialisis-peritoneal.
48. Pérez-Fontán M, Rodríguez-Carmona A, García-Naveiro A, et al. Peritonitis-related mortality in patients undergoing chronic peritoneal dialysis. Perit Dial Int. 2005;25:274–84.
49. Remón C, Quirós PL, Pérez-Bañasco V, et al. Informe del registro de pacientes con insuficiencia renal crónica en tratamiento con diálisis peritoneal de Andalucía: periodo 1999–2004. Nefrologia. 2006;26(1):45–55.
50. Remón-Rodríguez C, Quirós-Ganga P, Portolés-Pérez J, Gómez-Roldán C, Miguel-Carrasco A, Borrás-Sans M, et al. Resultados del trabajo cooperativo de los registros españoles de diálisis peritoneal: análisis de 12 años de seguimiento. Nefrologia. 2014;34(1):18–33.
51. Arrieta J, Bajo MA, Caravaca F, Coronel F, García-Pérez H, González-Parra E, et al. Sociedad Española de Nefrología. Guidelines of the Spanish Society of Nephrology. Clinical practice guidelines for peritoneal dialysis. Nefrologia. 2006;26(Suppl 4):1–184.
52. Rodriguez-Carmona A, Pérez-Fontan M, García-Naveiro R, Villaverde P, Peteiro J. Compared times profiles of ultrafiltration, sodium removal, and renal function in incident CAPD and automated peritoneal dialysis patients. Am J Kidney Dis. 2004;44(1):132–45.
53. Pérez Fontan M, Remon Rodríguez C, Borrás Sans M, Sánchez Alvarez E, da Cunha NM, Quirós Ganga P, et al. Compared decline of residual kidney function in patients treated with automated peritoneal dialysis and continuous ambulatory peritoneal dialysis: a multicenter study. Nephron Clin Pract. 2014;128(3–4):352–60.
54. De Fijter CW, Oe LP, Nauta JJ, van der Meulen J, Verbrugh HA, Verhoef J, et al. Clinical efficacy and morbidity associated with continuous cyclic compared with continuous ambulatory peritoneal dialysis. Ann Intern Med. 1994;120:264–71.
55. Locatelli AJ, Marcos GM, Gomez MG, Alvarez SA, DeBenedetti LC. Comparing peritonitis in continuous ambulatory peritoneal dialysis patients versus automated peritoneal dialysis patients. Adv Perit Dial. 1999;15:193–6.
56. Huang JW, Hung KY, Yen CJ, Wu KD, Tsai TJ. Comparison of infectious complications in peritoneal dialysis patients using either a twin-bag system or automated peritoneal dialysis. Nephrol Dial Transplant. 2001;16:604–7.
57. Gallar P, Gutiérrez M, Ortega O, Rodríguez I, Oliet A, Herrero JC, et al. Utilidad de la Telemedicina en el seguimiento de los pacientes en diálisis peritoneal. Nefrologia. 2006;26(3):365–71.
58. Gallar P, Vigil A, Rodríguez I, Ortega O, Gutierrez M, Hurtado J, et al. Two-year experience with telemedicina in the follow-up of patients in home peritoneal diálisis. J Telemed Telecare. 2007;13(6):288–92.
59. Alvillo-Arbizu J, Roa-Romero LM, Milán-Martín JA, Aresté-Fosalba N, Tornero-Molina F, Macía-Heras M, Vega-Díaz N. Methodological approach to designing a telecare system for pre-dialysis and peritoneal dialysis patients. Nefrologia. 2014;34(2):149–57.
60. Culleton B. Bettering the lives of patients with end-stage renal disease with HomeChoice Claria with ShareSource: an interview with Dr. Bruce Culleton. Expert Rev Med Devices. 2015;12(5):501–3.
61. Clark WR, Garzotto F, Neri M, Lorenzin A, Zaccaria M, Ronco C. Data analytics for continuous renal replacement therapy: historical limitations and recent technology advances. Int J Artif Organs. 2016;39(8):399–406.
62. Wolfe RA, Ashby VB, Milford EL, et al. Comparison of mortality in all patients on dialysis, patients on dialysis awaiting transplantation, and recipients of a first cadaveric transplant. N Engl J Med. 1999;341:1725–30.
63. Schnuelle O, Lorenz D, Trede M, et al. Impact of renal cadaveric transplantation on survival in end-stage renal failure: evidence for reduced mortality risk compared with hemodialysis during long-term follow up. J Am Soc Nephrol. 1998;9:2135–41.
64. Rebollo P, Ortega F, Baltar JM, et al. Health related quality of life (HRQOL) of kidney transplanted patients: variables that influence it. Clin Transplant. 2000;14:199–207.
65. Lorenzo-Sellares V, Pedrosa MI, Santana-Expósito B, et al. Cost analysis and sociocultural profile of kidney patients. Impact of the treatment method. Nefrologia. 2014;34(4):458–68.
66. Documento de consenso sobre trasplante de páncreas e islotes. Organización Nacional de Trasplantes. ISBN 84-7885-397-9; 2005.
67. de la Rosa G, Domínguez-Gil B, Matesanz R, et al. Continuously evaluating performance in deceased: the Spanish quality assurance program donation. Am J Transplant. 2012;12:2507–13.
68. Schold JD, Buccini LD, Goldfarb DA, et al. Association between kidney transplant center performance and the survival benefit of transplantation versus dialysis. Clin J Am Soc Nephrol. 2014;9:1773–80.
69. Hernandez D, Castro P, Muriel A, et al. Clinical assessment of mortality risk in renal transplant candidates in Spain. Transplantation. 2014;98:653–9.
70. Hernandez D, Muriel A, Castro P, et al. Survival in southern European patients wait-listed for kidney transplant after graft failure: a competing risk analysis. PLoS One. 2018;13(3):e0193091.
71. Ojo AO, Hanson JA, Meier-Kriesche HU, et al. Survival in recipients of marginal cadaveric donor kidneys compared with other recipients and wait-listed transplant candidates. J Am Soc Nephrol. 2001;12:589–97.

72. Anderson S, Brenner BN. Effects of aging on renal glomerulus. Am J Med. 1986;80:435–42.
73. Del Castillo D, Posada G, Anaya F, et al. Utilización racional de donantes renales de cadáver de edad avanzada (>60 años). Nefrologia. 1998;18(Supl 5):33–7.
74. Barber J, Becker D, Behrman R, et al. Guidelines for the determination of death. Report of medical consultants on the president's commission for the study of ethical problems in medicine and biomedical and behavioral research. JAMA. 1981;246:2184–6.
75. Garccia-Rinaldi R, Le Frak EA, De Fore WW. In situ preservation of cadaver kidneys for transplantation. Ann Surg. 1975;182:576–84.
76. Fujita T, Matsui M, Yanekoa M, et al. Clinical application of in situ renal cooling: experience with 61 cardiac arrest donors. Transplant Proc. 1989;21:1215–7.
77. Sanchez-Fructuoso A, Prats D, Torrens J, et al. Renal transplantation from non-heart beating donors: a promising alternative to enlarge the donor pool. J Am Soc Nephrol. 2000;11:350–8.
78. Kootstra G, Daemen JH, Oomen AP. Categories of non-heart-beating donors. Transplant Proc. 1995;27:289–2894.
79. Sanchez-Fructuoso A, Marques M, Prats D, et al. Victims of cardiac arrest occurring outside the hospital: a source of transplantable kidneys. Ann Intern Med. 2006;145:157–64.
80. Matesanz R. Documento de consenso español sobre extracción de órganos de donantes en asistolia. Nefrologia. 1996;16(Supl 2):48–53.
81. Alvarez M, Martin E, Garcia A, et al. Opinion survey on renal donation from living donor. Nefrologia. 2005;Supl 2:57–61.
82. United States Renal System. USRDS annual data report: atlas of end-stage renal disease in the United States. Bethesda: National Institute of Health, National Institute of Diabetes and Digestive Kidney Diseases; 2003.
83. Meier-Krieske HU, Schold JD, Kaplan B. Long-term renal allograft survival. Have we made significant progress or is it time to rethink our analytic and therapeutic strategies? Am J Transpant. 2004;4:1289–95.
84. Meier-Krieske HU, Schold JD, Srinivas TR, et al. Lack of improvement in renal allograft survival despite a marked decrease in acute rates over the most recent era. Am J Transplant. 2004;4:378–83.
85. Sola E, González-Molina M, Cabello M, et al. Long-term improvement of deceased donor renal allograft survival since 1996: a single transplant center study. Transplantation. 2010;89:714–20.
86. González-Molina M, Burgos D, Cabello M, et al. Impact of immunosuppression treatment on the improvement in graft survival after deceased donor renal transplantation: a long-term cohort study. Nefrologia. 2014;34(5):570–8.
87. Moreso F, Alonso A, Gentil MA, et al. Improvement in late renal allograft survival between 1990 and 2002 in Spain: results from a multicentre case-control study. Transpl Int. 2010;23:907–13.
88. Hernández Marrero D, González-Molina M. Resultados Globales del Trasplante Renal. In: Lorenzo V, López Gómez JM, editors. Nefrología al Día. At: http://www.revistanefrologia.com/es-monografias-nefrologia-dia-articulo-resultados-globales-del-trasplante-renal-58.
89. Ojo AO, Morales JM, Gonzalez-Molina M, et al. Comparison of long-term outcome of kidney transplantation: USA versus Spain. Neprol Dial Transplant. 2013;28:213–20.
90. Oppenheimer F, Aljama P, Peinado CA, et al. The impact of donor age on the results of renal transplantation. Nephrol Dial Transplant. 2004;19(Suppl 3):11–5.
91. Pérez-Sáez MJ, Arcos E, Comas J, et al. Survival benefit from kidney transplantation using kidneys from deceased donors aged ≥75 years: a time-dependent analysis. Am J Transplant. 2016;16:2724–33.
92. Pérez-Sáez MJ, Montero N, Redondo-Pachón D, et al. Strategies for an expanded use of kidneys from elderly donors. Transplantation. 2017;101:727–45.
93. Bernis Carro C, Ortega Suárez F, Quereda Rodríguez-Navarro C, Martínez Castelao A, Górritz Teruel JL, Matesanz Acedos R, et al. Comisión Nacional de la Especialidad de Nefrología en España. Trends in resident positions offered in nephrology (1985–2008). Nefrologia. 2011;31(2):155–61.
94. Soriano JB, Rojas-Rueda D, Alonso J, Antó JM, Cardona PJ, Fernández E, Colaboradores de GBD en España, Lista de colaboradores de GBD en España, et al. The burden of disease in Spain: results from the Global Burden of Disease 2016. Med Clin (Barc). 2018;151(5):171–90.

# Nephrology in Sweden

# 48

Staffan Schön, Maria Stendahl, Max Bell, José Carolino Divino-Filho, Helena Rydell, Olof Heimbürger, Torbjörn Lundgren, Mårten Segelmark, and Gunilla Welander

| | |
|---|---|
| Area[a] | 450,295 km$^2$ |
| Population[a] | 10.3 million (2019) |
| Capital[a] | Stockholm |
| Three most populated cities[a]: | 1. Stockholm<br>2. Gothenburg<br>3. Malmö |
| Official languages[b] | Swedish, Sami, Meänkieli, Finnish, Romani, and Yiddish |
| Gross domestic product (GDP)[c] | 551.135 billion US dollars (2018) |
| GDP per capita[c] | 54,459 US dollars (2018) |
| Human Development Index (HDI)[d] | 0.937 (2018) |
| Official currency[e] | Swedish krona |
| Total number of nephrologists[f] | ~300 |
| National society of nephrology[f] | Svensk Njurmedicinsk Förening (The Swedish Society of Nephrology) |
| Incidence of end-stage renal disease[g] | 2018 – 107 pmp |
| Prevalence of end-stage renal disease[g] (including patients with a functioning kidney transplant) | 2018 – 980 pmp |
| Total number of patients on dialysis[g,h] (all modalities) | 2017 – 4101<br>2018 – 4074 |
| Number of patients on hemodialysis[g,h] (including hemodiafiltration and hemofiltration) | 2017 – 3209<br>2018 – 3245 |
| Number of patients on peritoneal dialysis[g,h] (APD and CAPD) | 2017 – 892<br>2018 – 829 |
| Number of renal transplantations per year[g,h] | 2017 – 464<br>2018 – 435 |

Table references:
[a]Statistics Sweden, Swedish Government Agency
[b]https://www.riksdagen.se/en/, The Swedish Parliament
[c]https://countryeconomy.com/gdp/sweden
[d]http://hdr.undp.org/en/2018-update
[e]https://www.riksbank.se/en-gb
[f]https://njurmed.se/, The Swedish Society of Nephrology
[g]Swedish Renal Registry, Annual Report 2019 (Svenskt Njurregister 2019)
[h]Swedish Renal Registry, Annual Report 2018 (Svenskt Njurregister 2018)

The authors declare that they have no conflict of interest.

S. Schön (✉) · M. Stendahl
Swedish Renal Registry, Jönköping County Hospital, Jönköping, Sweden
e-mail: snr@rjl.se; maria.stendahl@rjl.se

M. Bell
Perioperative Medicine and Intensive Care Medicine, Karolinska University Hospital, Stockholm, Sweden
e-mail: max.bell@sll.se

J. C. Divino-Filho
Division of Renal Medicine, CLINTEC, Karolinska Institutet, Stockholm, Sweden
e-mail: jose.divino@ki.se

H. Rydell
Swedish Renal Registry, Jönköping County Hospital, Jönköping, Sweden

Division of Renal Medicine, CLINTEC, Karolinska Institutet, Stockholm, Sweden

Department of Nephrology, Karolinska University Hospital, Stockholm, Sweden
e-mail: helena.rydell@sll.se

O. Heimbürger
Division of Renal Medicine, CLINTEC, Karolinska Institutet, Stockholm, Sweden

Department of Nephrology, Karolinska University Hospital, Stockholm, Sweden
e-mail: olof.heimburger@ki.se

T. Lundgren
Swedish Renal Registry, Jönköping County Hospital, Jönköping, Sweden

Department of Transplantation Surgery, Karolinska University Hospital, Stockholm, Sweden

Department of Clinical Science, Intervention and Technology, Karolinska Institute, Stockholm, Sweden
e-mail: torbjorn.lundgren@sll.se

M. Segelmark
Swedish Renal Registry, Jönköping County Hospital, Jönköping, Sweden

Department of Clinical Sciences, Division of Nephrology, Skane University Hospital and Lund University, Lund, Sweden
e-mail: marten.segelmark@med.lu.se

G. Welander
Swedish Renal Registry, Jönköping County Hospital, Jönköping, Sweden

Nephrology Unit, Central Hospital Karlstad, Karlstad, Sweden
e-mail: gunilla.welander@regionvarmland.se


J. A. Moura-Neto et al. (eds.), *Nephrology Worldwide*, https://doi.org/10.1007/978-3-030-56890-0_48

## Introduction

The Kingdom of Sweden is one of three Scandinavian countries, in addition to Sweden also Denmark and Norway, located in the northern part of Europe. More broadly Scandinavia refers to the Nordic countries, including also Finland, Iceland, and the Faroe Islands [1]. Sweden is the fifth largest country in Europe with an area of 450,295 km$^2$ and with a population of 10.3 million people [2]. An increase in immigration during the last decades has resulted in a large proportion, 2.5 million, of the population having a foreign background, i.e., foreign born or born in Sweden with two foreign-born parents [2].

Sweden has three levels of government: national, regional, and local (municipalities). Being a constitutional monarchy, all legislative power belongs to the parliament (Swedish: Riksdag) with its elected 349 members. Members are elected on the basis of proportional representation to a 4-year term [3].

The country's regions and municipalities are responsible for providing a significant proportion of all public services [4]. There are 21 geographically defined healthcare regions in Sweden, usually referred to as counties. The counties are government bodies led by a council appointed by general elections held, as for the national parliament, every fourth year. The counties have the responsibility to provide equal and good-quality medical care for all inhabitants, and they have taxation authority. Most hospitals are owned and run directly by the counties [5]. 65 units are identified as nephrology units, all reporting to the Swedish Renal Registry (SRR) [6], most of them operated by the counties. There are a few private dialysis clinics that perform in-center hemodialysis (HD) after being contracted by the counties. Except for Visby Hospital, all peritoneal dialysis (PD), home hemodialysis, and in-hospital care for acute kidney injury (AKI) are managed at county-operated hospital departments. Many chronic kidney disease (CKD) patients, especially those in the earlier stages, are managed by general practitioners or other specialists in internal medicine, of whom a minor proportion are private.

## A Brief History of Nephrology in Sweden

On March 15, 1965, the first meeting of what was then called "The Swedish Society of Urology" was held in Stockholm. This society was acknowledged by the Swedish Medical Society on May 30, 1967, by the name "Swedish Society of Nephrology," and nephrology was approved as a specialty by the Swedish Medical Association [7]. The first HD treatment in Sweden was performed in Lund already in 1946 by the legendary pioneer Dr. Nils Alwall (please see "Highlights of Nephrology in Sweden"), and the first renal transplantation was performed in 1964 in Stockholm by the renowned surgeon Curt Franksson [8]. For many years now, dialysis treatment is a well-established procedure and carried out in about 65 facilities throughout the country, whereas kidney transplantation activity is centralized to four university clinics.

## Renal Diseases in Sweden

The most common group of diseases among patients on renal replacement therapy (RRT) is glomerulonephritis, followed by diabetic nephropathy. Concerning incidence rates, diabetes has been the most common cause of end-stage renal disease (ESRD) for many years [6]. However, the number and hence the incidence rate of diabetes type 1 as cause of uremia are not increasing, rather the opposite, and the age at start of RRT has increased [9]. Some diseases are continuously decreasing as causes of uremia, especially infectious diseases such as pyelonephritis, as well as obstructive uropathy in men.

Although the pattern of kidney diseases in Sweden is in general the same as in other countries in the West, there are a few endemic diseases in Sweden affecting the kidneys. The most remarkable might be the hereditary transthyretin amyloidosis (hATTR), a serious multisystem disease engaging the autonomic and sensory-motor nervous system, the heart, the eyes, the brain, and the kidneys. It is a hereditary autosomal dominant disease caused by a mutation in the transthyretin gene, resulting in defect proteins that are uploaded as extracellular deposits of amyloid in body organs [10]. However, the penetrance and the symptomatology differ between individuals, and few of these patients will be in need for RRT.

hATTR is spread over the world, but clusters of patients can be found in Portugal, Brazil, Japan, and the north of Sweden. In studies performed in 2014 by Norgren et al. at Umeå University, 912 carriers of the gene were identified. Genealogy showed that 73% of the carriers of the mutation in Sweden are linked to six ancestors from the 17th and 18th centuries, thus showing that the Swedish type of mutation is at least 400 years old [11]. As the protein is synthesized in the liver, liver transplantation is the major current treatment. However, new ways of treatment are under development [11].

### Acute Kidney Injury

Acute kidney injury (AKI) is a common condition, complicating 10–25% of hospital admissions [12]. The etiology of AKI is complex; it is not a disease, but rather a collection of syndromes, ranging from kidney-specific diseases, such as interstitial nephritis, to those that are part of systemic pathologies, like sepsis and heart failure, or those that arise from treatments such as major surgery or chemotherapy [13].

Severe AKI is treated with acute RRT, almost always in intensive care units (ICU). The yearly number of patients treated for AKI in ICUs with continuous RRT between November 2018 and October 2019 in Sweden was 1840, equaling 4.4% of the ICU population [14]. In larger academic ICUs, the proportion is over 10%, reflecting the severity of the critical illness in those populations. In a cohort study between 1995 and 2004, Bell et al. examined 2202 patients with AKI from 32 ICUs, treated with RRT [15], and 85.7% of patients in the study received treatment with continuous renal replacement therapy (CRRT), whereas 14.3% were given intermittent hemodialysis (IHD) treatment. Half (1102) of the patients were alive after 90 days of treatment, with no difference between the treatment groups. Renal survival was better in the CRRT group, in which 8.3% were still in need of chronic RRT at the end of the study, compared to 16.5% in the IHD group.

In another study, Rimes-Stigare et al. investigated 103,363 patients treated in ICUs between 2005 and 2011, using data from the Swedish Intensive Care Registry [16]. Patients were divided into five groups, where patients with no prior renal dysfunction and no AKI were controls. Among the total number of patients, 4192 had pre-existing CKD, 1389 had ESRD, 5273 developed AKI, and 998 patients with CKD developed acute-on-chronic kidney disease (AoC). One-year mortality was the highest in AoC patients (54%) followed by AKI (48.7%), CKD (47.6%), and ESRD (40.3%) ($P < 0.001$). Five-year mortality was the highest for the CKD and AoC groups (71.3% and 68.2%, respectively) followed by ESRD (62.9%) and AKI (61.8%) ($P < 0.001$). ESRD incidence was the greatest in the AoC and CKD groups (adjusted incidence rate ratio (IRR) 259 (95% confidence interval [CI] 156.9–429.1) and 96.4 (95% CI 59.7–155.6), respectively) and elevated in AKI patients when compared with controls (adjusted IRR 24 (95% CI 3.9–42.0); $P < 0.001$).

## Renal Replacement Therapy in Sweden

RRT, also known as dialysis and transplantation, was established in Sweden in the 1960s and since then has developed and improved. Today, all patients who are considered having a clear indication for RRT are offered suitable treatment. The largest expansion in the number of patients occurred in the 1990s, but even today we see an expansion, although much smaller (2% in 2017) [6]. This means that the number of dialysis patients has increased by 43% during the 2000s, whereas the number of transplanted patients increased by 78% during the same period.

The Swedish Renal Registry (SRR) was founded in 2007. It has a unique structure as it follows patients on an individual level from the debut of CKD until death. The RRT epidemiology is the core of the registry, and it dates back to 1991 when the precursor the Swedish Registry for Active Treatment of Uraemia started [17]. The registry contains information regarding demographic variables at RRT onset, cause of kidney disease, RRT modality, and survival status. The registry performs cross-sectional investigations of dialysis quality, and since 2014, it also harbors data on dialysis access.

At the end of 2018, the number of patients on RRT in Sweden was 10,025, corresponding to a prevalence of 980 per million population (pmp). The yearly incidence rates have been very stable for the past 20 years. During 2018, the national incidence rate was 107 pmp. The incidence rates have been unchanged for two decades and now seem to be decreasing. The continuous increase in the number of patients on RRT is mainly due to an increase in the number of transplanted patients and an improved survival among patients on RRT. The incidence rate differs between regions due to a varying age spectrum across the country. In general, areas or cities with a younger population have lower incidence and prevalence rates [3, 18].

In order to illustrate the flow of patients throughout RRT, a figure was created (Fig. 48.1). During 2017, a total of 1170 patients initiated RRT and were added to the already-existing patient pool. The majority of the patients started with HD (715), second came PD (363), and, finally, 92 patients were pre-emptively transplanted. A few patients moved to Sweden during the year: two transplanted and five on HD. The total number of deaths while on RRT was 953, of those 785 were treated with dialysis and 168 had a functioning renal transplant [6].

The mean age for patients on treatment has been increasing for the RRT population as a whole, although nowadays this increase is only attributed to transplanted patients and patients on peritoneal dialysis.

## Hemodialysis

All of the information in this section originates from the SRR [6]. Among Swedish patients starting RRT, including renal transplantation, around 60% start on HD, while the proportion of patients on HD among prevalent patients is only 30%. Each year, around 7% of patients on HD receive a renal transplant, 2% switch to PD, and the annual mortality rate is about 19%. Patients on HD are older compared to patients on PD and patients with a renal transplant. During recent years, the mean age for patients on HD has been 66 years.

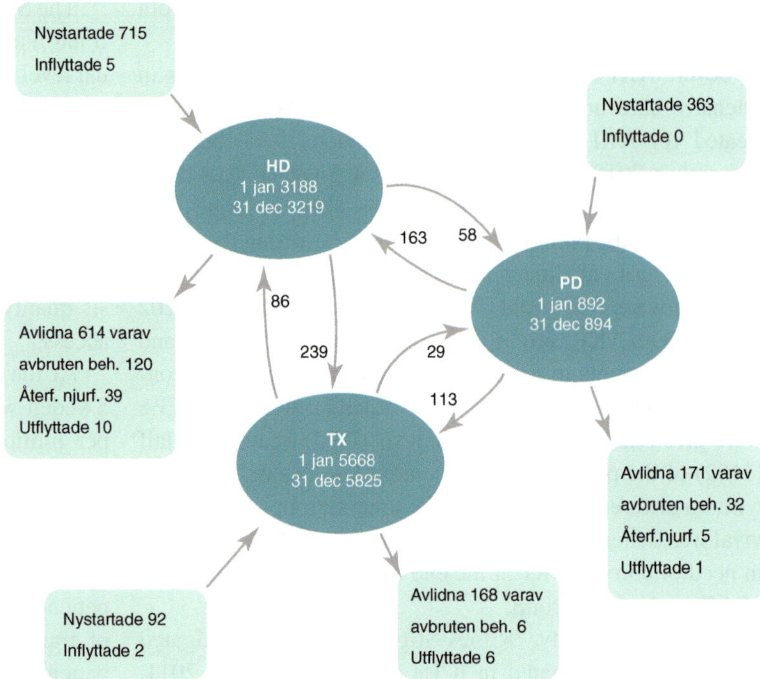


**Fig. 48.1** Flowchart of how patients move among the different RRT options

| Translation | |
|---|---|
| Nystartade | new to the therapy |
| Inflyttade | transferred to |
| Utflyttade | transferred from |
| Avlidna 171 varav avbruten beh.32 | 171 deaths from which 32 suspended therapy |
| Återf.njurf | renal function recovery |

The majority of the Swedish patients have in-center HD, but the aim is to increase the proportion of patients with home HD and self-care HD. The proportion of patients on home HD is 4%, while around 6% have self-care HD, and 8% have self-care HD with some assistance from healthcare personnel. Most patients with home HD are linked to clinics at university hospitals, but there are also smaller clinics taking care of a few patients. Around 60% of the dialysis clinics have self-care HD units. In those units, patients gain a great deal of trust and have a lot of responsibility. As an example, a patient may be the first person to enter the clinic in the morning, starting the water treatment system and the dialysis machine. Only a minority of Swedish patients on HD are treated in private dialysis provider clinics, 6%, in 2018.

Around 70% of the prevalent patients have a functioning AV fistula (AVF) or graft. An important factor for vascular access intervention is right timing, and it is a challenge to reach the goal of 65% of patients starting HD or hemodiafiltration (HDF) with a functioning AVF. When comparing the results of 2017 (50%) with 2015 (60%), we unfortunately observe a negative trend in the achieved result from the expected goal. However, it should be noted that it is a difficult task to create an AVF with enough margin to provide time for a possible need of re-intervention and, at the same time, avoid unnecessary and costly interventions for the patient. In Sweden as a whole, the number of central dialysis catheters (CDC) inserted during 2017 was unchanged in relation to the numbers in the years before (about 1200). There is still a significant difference between the choice of AVF or CDC as first access at initiation of HD/HDF within the country. In 2017, only one region achieved the goal of 65% AVF at first dialysis. Even though such a high percentage of patients start HD/HDF with a CDC, AVF is the most common access for the majority of the patients during total dialysis therapy time.

The mean blood flow rate is 294 ml/min, with 62% with a blood flow rate of >250 ml/min and 34% with >350 ml/min. Most Swedish patients on HD, 71%, have dialysis sessions thrice weekly, while 13% have less frequent dialysis, mostly twice weekly. More frequent dialysis is prescribed as every other day for 2% of the patients and as more than that for 14% of the patients. Regarding the length of an HD session, the weekly dialysis duration is 12 hours for 29% of the patients, whereas 25% of the patients are prescribed <12 hours and 46% >12 hours. The mean urea reduction ratio (URR) is 74%.

About 80% of the HD/HDF patients have received a weekly Kt/V of around 2.0 (in accordance with KDOQI guidelines) since 2008. For HD patients, the average spK/V is 1.52 and the eKt/V is 1.35. The corresponding data for HDF are 1.67 and 1.49, respectively.

Online HDF is common in Sweden, 50–55% of the total number of HD patients are prescribed convective treatment, but there are only a small number of patients with online hemofiltration (0.2%). The average convective volume per session is 23.4 l. HDF is prescribed more frequently in patients younger (52–58%) than in patients older (43%) than 75 years.

Bicarbonate dialysate and reverse osmosis water treatment are universal, while HD machines are supplied by a limited number of companies. No reuse of dialyzers is performed in Sweden.

Eighty-four percent (84%) of patients are on erythropoietin treatment (median dose 8000 U per week, median Hb 11.3 g/dL), and 69% are on intravenous iron.

Median serum phosphate level for HD patients is 1.5 mmol/L with a range of 1.2–1.8 mmol/L, whereas for PTH the median serum level is 26 pmol/L and range 14–53 pmol/L.

## Peritoneal Dialysis

Most of the information in this section originates from the SRR [6]. Intermittent peritoneal dialysis (IPD) for the treatment of renal failure was introduced in Sweden in the 1960s. One of the early pioneers was Jon Gjessing, an anesthesiologist in the town of Sundsvall, who was the first to use dextran and amino acids as osmotic agents [19]. In his PhD thesis in Uppsala in 1967, he already described osmotic agents like amino acid and dextran, new indications for PD like severe hemorrhagic pancreatitis, pharmacokinetics of drugs administered intraperitoneally and as a diagnostic test in acute abdominal conditions, as well as the use of PD in the treatment of acute poisoning (more specifically barbiturates, salicylates, and methyl alcohol) [20–24]. His conclusions arose from a series of investigations over 5 years, during which a total of 460 patients were treated with PD for a variety of conditions. These conditions ranged from the treatment of overdosage, notably barbiturate and salicylate, to chronic renal failure. PD was found to be an easy method requiring simple apparatus and the minimum of skilled technical help. It was also found that the judicious addition of other compounds to the dialysate frequently conferred major advantages depending upon the clinical circumstances. The associated problems of infection and protein loss were largely overcome, thus extending the range of usefulness of this technique.

For ESRD treatment, few patients were treated with IPD until CAPD was introduced in Stockholm in 1978, and the treatment spread rapidly in the country. The use of PD has been relatively constant since the 1990s with about 20–25% of the dialysis patients treated with PD [6]. A lot of clinical research in PD has been performed in Sweden, particularly in peritoneal transport physiology [25–27], PD solutions (transport, biocompatibility, and alternative osmotic agents) [27, 28] and metabolism in PD patients [29, 30].

At present, PD is available all over Sweden with 892 of the 4101 dialysis patients being treated with PD (21.8%) [6]. On average, 35% of PD patients are treated with APD, but variation is very large (3–76% in different centers). APD is more prevalent than CAPD in the younger age group, 67% among children and teenagers and 60% in patients between 45 and 64 years old.

In the SRR, PD quality data, including catheter data, are being fully registered since 2017. In 2017, 468 PD catheters were inserted, most commonly by laparotomy (184), percutaneous (162), laparoscopy (91), and others (2). The precise insertion technique varies a lot within the country, and to collect specific information on that is an important goal for the SRR in the future. All patients are treated with biocompatible glucose-based PD solutions as the old non-biocompatible glucose-based PD solutions are not available anymore in Sweden. However, the use and prescription of PD vary between regions (use of PD 10–40%) [6]. Icodextrin is used by on average 54% (5–100%).

Assisted PD (either CAPD or APD) also varies a lot between different regions, mainly due to different reimbursement policies. The number (and percentage) of patients has increased from 88 (11%) in 2010 to 145 (17%) in 2017. Most patients receiving assisted PD are over 75 years of age (57%), and only 4% are younger than 45 years of age [6].

Data from the SRR show that 86% of patients have a weekly Kt/V urea >1.7 [6], an increase of about 6% when compared to 2014. There is a significant difference in achieved goals, between 50% and 100%, among PD centers across the country; however, collected data is missing for 30–40% of the PD patients during follow-up, making interpretation difficult. Moreover, the proportion of patients with palliative care indication might influence the degree of dialysis dose goal achievement.

Three hundred eighteen APD patients are prescribed on average 12.8 l total infusion volume per day, with 91 (29%) of them with a dry day dwell and 227 (71%) with a wet day. Most CAPD patients, 411/538 (76%), perform 4 exchanges per day, and the most common total infusion volume per day is 8 l, 326/538 (61%). Assisted PD is performed in 16% of the CAPD and 13% of the APD patients.

On January 1, 2017, there were 892 patients (prevalent) on PD and by December 31 (same year) 894; during the year 113 of those PD patients were transplanted (13%), 163 were transferred to HD (18%), 171 died (19%), 32 interrupted treatment, 5 recovered renal function, and 1 moved to another country. During the same period, 363 new patients (incident) started on PD, 58 transferred from HD, and 29 came from renal transplantation.

Eighty percent (80%) of patients are on erythropoietin, median dose 5000 U per week, and the median Hb is 11.4 g/dL. Intravenous iron is prescribed to 24% of the PD patients [6].

## Renal Transplantation

Following the first kidney transplantations in Boston, Swedish surgeons went to the USA in the late 1950s and early 1960s to learn the new techniques. The first transplantation in Sweden was performed in Stockholm in April 1964 when a young man received a kidney from his father. Soon after this, three more programs opened, in Gothenburg (1965), Malmö (1968), and Uppsala (1969), with Gothenburg becoming the center with the largest volumes. Scandiatransplant, the organ procurement organization of Scandinavia, was started in 1969. Of the 15,984 kidneys transplanted in Sweden 1964–2018, 4696 have been from living donors (29%). Improvements in technique, organ preservation, and pharmacological treatment now allow us to expect an almost 90% 5-year uncensored graft survival in transplantations from deceased donors and even better from living donors [6]. The total number of transplants has recently been around 450 per year (45 per million inhabitants). Swedish research achievements that have or in the near future might change our treatment include the studies that have made it possible to perform ABO-incompatible living donor transplants with similar results as in ABO-compatible couples [31]. Today, 15% of living donor transplantations are done with ABO-incompatible donor and receiver. To allow even more living donor transplantations, a Swedish exchange program has been initiated with the first transplants performed in 2018 [32]. Within the upcoming year, this will be expanded to the Nordic countries within Scandiatransplant.

All centers now use a low-dose tacrolimus immunosuppression protocol based on the "Symphony study" [33]. Type 1 diabetes has a very high incidence in Sweden and is the underlying disease in a large portion of patients needing RRT. Combined pancreas-kidney transplantation is recommended for most of these patients [34], and more than 700 pancreas transplantations have been performed. In the near future, we also hope to be able to transplant more patients with pre-existing anti-donor HLA antibodies. If long-term results from ongoing studies [35] will confirm that this can be done safely with acceptable efficacy, this could serve well a special population that today has problems getting a transplant.

## Nephrology Practice in Sweden

There were about 39,000 physicians working in Sweden in 2016, according to statistics from the Swedish Medical Society (Läkarförbundet) and Swedish Board of Health and Welfare (Socialstyrelsen) [5, 36]. Gender distribution is nearly equal, a few more men than women. However, there is a predominance of women below 50 years of age women; in the age group 30–35, they make up 60% of the total physician workforce [36].

Nephrologists constitute less than 1% of all specialists in the country or in absolute number around 300. The age and gender distributions are similar to doctors in general (40% women). Even if there is a shortage of nephrologists, salaries are not substantially different from most other specialties. In 2018, the median yearly salary for a qualified nephrologist was around € 90,000 before taxes. On top of that, there is in most cases extra payment for being on-call, averaging an addition of 5–20%; any income originating from on-call work deducts, at least, 50% taxes. The shortage of nephrologists will most probably continue for several years since the number under training is too low, both to fill the vacancies and to replace predicted retirements. For doctors living in other European Union (EU) countries, the language is the major barrier; for those moving to Sweden from non-EU countries, their education, training, and other credentials first need to be verified by the Board of Health and Welfare, and then they are required to take an exam before receiving a license to practice.

At the specialized nephrology units, multi-professional teams take care of the patients. At larger units there are separate teams for HD, PD, home hemodialysis, pre-dialysis, and post-transplantation follow-up, while at smaller units a single team perform all these duties. The teams include physicians, nurses, help nurses, technicians, physiotherapists, occupational therapists, dieticians, and social workers. Overall, nurses dominate numerically over other healthcare professionals, especially in institutional HD teams, where it is common with a ratio of 10 nurses or more per doctor. The relative proportion of physiotherapists, occupational therapists, dietitians, and social workers are highly variable. Local traditions and attitudes regarding the relative importance of diet restrictions, physical exercise, and coping strategies for the survival of CKD patients highly influence these proportions. There is also a shortage of nurses in Sweden, and as for doctors, language is a major barrier for nurses from other EU countries. A yearly salary for a nurse in Sweden is around € 35,000, with around 10–15% extra for those frequently working weekends and night shifts.

The role nephrologists take in the care of AKI and in ICUs is variable. CRRT is usually prescribed directly by the anesthesiologists responsible for the ICUs, but in some hospitals, all severe AKI cases render consultations and daily follow-up visits by nephrologists. At other centers, the nephrology involvement is restricted to providing intermittent HD on demand. In a similar fashion, there are great differences in the involvement of nephrologists in plasma exchange and other forms of extracorporeal apheresis therapies. At some hospitals all apheresis service is provided by clinical immunology departments or specialized apheresis units, while at other hospitals all apheresis is performed by the dialysis departments under the auspice of nephrologists. At the four transplantation centers, there are special nephrologists employed who participate both in pre- and postoperative medical decisions. After the postoperative period, stable patients are referred to their local nephrologists for follow-up. In uncomplicated cases this typically happens after a week.

## Highlights of Nephrology in Sweden

### Dialysis Access in the Swedish Renal Registry: A Unique Combination of Practical Clinical Use and a National Quality Parameter Follow-Up

Dialysis access is an area of challenge and a factor that can improve quality of dialysis and reduce patient mortality. Follow-up of quality parameters is important locally as well as nationally.

A previously regional registry for vascular access became national in 2011, and, in 2014, it became an integrated part of the SRR [6]. By combining data from different parts of the registry, it allows the opportunity to follow the whole patient flow process from uremia progress, planning for dialysis as well as the functional status and complications of different types of access and treatments. The registry covers both vascular and peritoneal dialysis (PD) access.

All registration is done by nurses and help nurses at the renal units. Data concerning fistulas, central venous catheters (CVC), and PD catheters are recorded, including placement, function, complications, and interventions. Readymade reports make it easy to obtain data, and since the registry is web-based, each facility can have their reports in seconds. The usefulness of easy access to the number of CVC days and the corresponding infection rate is an example. Each patient's access history is also available. The practical clinical use motivates registration. Each unit can also create their own reports, useful for sharing with the multidisciplinary team.

The annual report of national data demonstrates a widespread difference in contemporary access care and gives an assessment of quality and time trends. New techniques and devices can be evaluated. Vascular surgeons requested a better follow-up of fistulas and a yearly report is now provided for surgeons, and locally each surgeon and interventionist can get their results.

### Nils Alwall

More than 2 million people suffering from kidney failure are currently being kept alive by dialysis. But when Nils Alwall was a young doctor 80 years ago, medicine had little to offer patients with kidney diseases other than bed rest and tasteless diets, measures that only added new burdens, on top of those imposed by the uremic state. Alwall was one of the pioneers determined to change this.

Born in 1904, Nils Andersson (his name at birth) came from a farming family without academic traditions. His uncle Jöns, who had no children, sponsored him throughout the studies until high school graduation (in the classic line, including Latin and Greek) in June 1923. He had the second-best school grade at the final exams. He was registered as a medical student at Lund University on December 4, 1923. It must have been during 1923 that Nils decided to choose medicine as his profession; and there is a suspicion that Alf Sjövall, his classmate and son of the school principal, was the one who influenced him to become a medical doctor. Many years later, they both would become professors at Lund University where they studied medicine. On August 31, 1927, he finalized his basic medical student exams, and 3 weeks later, he (and his brother Edvin) got permission to change their family name from Andersson to Alwall.

As a top student at the medical faculty, he was offered an assistant teaching position in the Department of Physiology while also carrying on with his studies. The teaching position opened the opportunity for research, and he received thorough training in medical chemistry, pharmacology, and physiology.

The departments of physiology and medical chemistry at Lund University were both located in a brick building outside the main campus and hospital area. These departments must have constituted a highly creative and competitive cluster where three Nobel Prize laureates spent important years in their early careers; and at least one of them (Arvid Carlsson, 2000, dopamine) had the same mentor and supervisor as Alwall, namely, Gunnar Ahlgren.

Alwall obtained his PhD in 1935, evaluating the relation between thyroxin and metabolism-influencing substances, such as dinitrophenol. In the fall of 1936, he was appointed by Prof. Sven Ingvar as junior physician in the Department of Medicine of the Lund University Hospital. Among his junior colleagues, there was another future successful Swedish medical doctor, Erik Ask-Upmark. He became touched by the difficult existence and gloomy fate of those patients with ESRD. In a memory book 45 years later, he wrote about a young woman with proteinuria and generalized edema whose only treatment was a strict diet and bed rest for 1 year. Chronic renal failure patients were not usual in the medicine clinic in Lund, probably because most of them died at home. During his first 7 years working there, he saw 80–90 patients per year with the diagnosis uremia or chronic/acute renal failure. From 1947 on, the number suddenly doubled – that most likely due to improved diagnosis and also to the energetic and well-recognized doctor who attracted more patients to the University Hospital. The correct diagnosis was usually not made before the patient's death at those times. In Denmark, they had started doing liver biopsies, and Alwall decided to use the same new technique to take kidney tissue samples. He performed the first 13 kidney biopsies in the world in 1944, and the technique proved to be useful.

However, a fatal complication with the 13th patient made him consider the procedure not ethical to pursue at that time. Some years later (in the 1950s), the method became a routine diagnostic procedure.

He was a visionary man with great passion, and seeing how uremic patients suffered, he felt the need to do something about it. He had some very creative ideas. He obtained access to an area in the basement of the hospital, and there, on evenings and weekends when not working in the hospital wards, he began to carry out experiments on rabbits. Instrument technicians in the department of physiology constructed the necessary devices; and he used heparin and cellophane to overcome problems with inadequate surface area and coagulation, obstacles that had hampered previous attempts to keep anuric animals alive with dialysis. Heparin molecule structure was identified by a chemist, Erik Jorpes, in Stockholm right before the Second World War. This made it possible for the first heparin product to be manufactured and released for intravenous use by the Swedish company Vitrum AB in 1936. Alwall's first try to build an artificial kidney, around the end of the Second World War, utilized some plex-glass from an American bomber plane that had made an emergency landing in South Sweden. He was convinced that there should exist a physiological method to replace the kidneys' function.

Alwall was very much aware of the crucial aspects of water removal, and his machines were designed to allow negative pressure to be applied across the cellophane membrane, in order to remove excess fluid. There is no doubt that Kolff and Alwall worked independently of each other during the Second World War. Alwall had Kolff as a good example, as the pioneer in treating patients with dialysis. On the other hand, he had different opinion of how a dialysis machine should be built. He insisted first in performing animal (rabbits) experimental dialysis and based on the observations collected, to establish fundamental conditions for harmless and effective dialysis. Only thereafter he took the next step, to start dialysis in patients. He wanted, first of all, to try dialysis in patients with acute renal failure, whereas patients with an acute worsening of a chronic renal failure condition or poisoning (e.g., sleeping pills) could become a second possibility.

In September 1946, about 3 years after Willem Kolff had performed his first dialysis, Alwall treated the first ever patient with acute renal failure by combining dialysis with controlled ultrafiltration. The patient was a 49-year-old man with an old pulmonary disease (silicosis), who then was dying with renal failure and pneumonia and almost in coma. The patient improved dramatically, and even though he died of pneumonia a few days later, it was recognized as a major success. He immediately persuaded the hospital administrators to designate a special unit for dialysis treatment, and before the end of the same year, he had become the head of the first dialysis department in the world.

In January 1947, a 54-year-old woman with a chronic kidney inflammation became suddenly much worse, anuric, and with a blood urea concentration of 235 mg/dL. Hemodialysis goes well, she recovers quickly, urine production resumes, and the patient can go home after 2 weeks and could live 15 more years after that! The third patient had an important psychological impact for him, as his childhood's friend Alf Sjövall, who was known as a good and ethical physician besides being the Professor of Gynecology and Obstetrics, asked him to treat one of his cancer patients with bilateral ureteral obstruction. The woman woke up after the second session of dialysis and asked for a cup of coffee right away! Blood urea went down from 346 mg/dL to normal 77 mg/dL.

He had explained the differences between Kolff's and his apparatus as follows: (a) In Kolff's, the blood is not all the time in contact with the dialysate, requiring much longer blood lines, and the apparatus becomes bulky. (b) There is no obstacle to the 30–40-m-long line to dilate itself, figuratively speaking, swallowing too much of the patient's blood. For this last comment, Alwall's apparatus was better: the bloodlines were on both sides covered by a wire netting so that they could not dilate. This also provided the possibility to apply a positive pressure within the bloodlines (or suction pressure on the outside), so that filtration could be controlled within the bloodlines wall.

Alwall and a younger colleague, Anders Lunderquist, observed, both in experiments with rabbits and also with patients, that when they "pressed fluid out" with ultrafiltration, the lung changes seen in X-rays went into regress rapidly. This observation changed completely the medical approach for patients with acute renal failure who earlier would be treated with rapid large fluid infusions. Another important observation from their study also remain until today, that the best way to control dialysis patient's water balance is a weight scale! It is interesting to note that in his application for Professorship, one of the recommendation's letter was written by John P. Merrill from Harvard Medical School and the dialysis pioneer in the USA in 1948. He certifies that Kolff and Alwall led the development of dialysis therapy. Merrill also mentions, among Alwall's unique achievements, ultrafiltration in order to remove fluid out of the patients, daily weighing of the patients, and dialysis therapy for sleeping pills' intoxication. He became Professor of Medicine, particularly Renal Diseases, at Lund University on July 1, 1957.

The technique, the equipment, and medical care continued to improve, and Alwall's reputation skyrocketed. In the 1950s, patients from all over Europe and the Middle East were sent to southern Sweden by airplane to receive dialysis by the "miracle man with the artificial kidney" in Lund. The dialysis unit at the University Hospital in Lund has now provided 74 years of continuous front-end treatment for renal failure. In order to move from treatment of AKI to ESRD renal replacement therapy, Alwall had to overcome two major obstacles: the problem of vascular access and the limited capacity to treat large numbers of patients on a continuous basis. He struggled on both fronts. Beginning with his animal experiments in the early 1940s, he had designed an external arteriovenous shunt made of silicone-coated rubber and in heparinized rabbits was able to use it repeatedly for up to a week. In the late 1940s, he used a similar shunt for humans but had to abandon the technique because of clotting problems. When Belding Scribner solved the problem of clotting by making his shunts of Teflon and Silastic, Alwall was quick to adopt this technique. In 1960, he began to treat patients with ESRD using the Scribner shunt and within 2 years was able to achieve long-term survival for his patients.

At a private dinner in 1961, Alwall met Holger Crafoord, the CEO of Tetra Pak AB, a company making packaging machines for the food industry. They struck up a lively discussion, and this was the first step in the founding of Gambro AB, which soon became a global supplier of "disposable kidneys" and other dialysis equipment. When shortage of dialysis equipment was no longer a problem, the lack of other resources became the new bottleneck. A shortage of designated units with trained staff now hindered patients from getting life-saving treatments. To alleviate this, Alwall sent out his younger co-workers to start dialysis units all over the country and invited colleagues from all over the world to come and train in his department. In order to get more resources for dialysis and other aspects of renal care, Alwall engaged himself politically. He joined the ruling Social Democratic Party and became a representative in the county council. He used his contacts within the party to approach the national government and persuaded the Board of Health (Medicinalstyrelsen) to put the expansion of dialysis on their agenda. EDTA was established in 1964 and Alwall was one of the founders. It is said that at the beginning, most of the founders wanted the organization to be named WEDTA with the W standing for West, meaning that only members of the West Europe would be allowed. Alwall protested, as he was the only one of the founders who had close contact with colleagues from Eastern Europe. On the global level, he participated in the organization of conferences and formation of international societies and became one of the first presidents of the International Society of Nephrology.

Alwall's political activities, however, also gave him many enemies. Conservative professors in other disciplines disliked his unconventional ways of getting a large share of the limited resources. On the international level, his contacts with university hospitals in Prague, Warsaw, and Rostock in East Germany attracted antipathy in Western Europe and across the Atlantic. Contrasting with his political stands, he lived a traditional family life with his wife Ellen and their three children. His wife Ellen was a descendant of Jonas Alströmer, the founder of Swedish industrialism.

Dialysis was not Alwall's only interest in nephrology. In 1944, he had already begun performing kidney biopsies, and toward the end of his career, he started a large screening program for the early CKD detection. A handful of patients who participated in that project and never developed ESRD are still followed in Lund University Hospital's department of nephrology.

One can summarize his innovation activities within renal care in five items:

1. He was the first one, in theory and practice, who could perform ultrafiltration and, with the help of pressure variation within the dialyzer in- and outside, steer water flow in the dialyzer. His device was the first that could be named "artificial kidney" and not only dialysis machine. Ultrafiltration is the central process in urine formation. He was also the first to clarify the mechanisms for lung edema in uremia and establish that weighing the patient was a simple but important method to control body water balance.
2. He was the first to indicate the principle of arteriovenous shunt for repeated sessions of HD.
3. His ward in Lund was the first unit for dialysis treatment in the world; it became in many respects germinal for other dialysis units.
4. He performed the first 13 kidney biopsies in the world in 1944, and the technique proved to be useful.
5. His political-organizational work for the Swedish renal care gave important impulses also to other countries' renal care.

In November 1971, Alwall got a surprising letter from his old friend Wilhelm Kolff, then professor in Santa Lake City, inviting him for a guest-professorship at his Division; they would work together in a NIH research project about utilization of gamma globulin to prevent hepatitis in HD patients. However, in May 1972, Kolff got the news that the research project did not get the funding. Alwall and Kolff were friends for almost 40 years.

Nils Alwall was able to take his vision of treating ESRD with an artificial kidney from animal experiments to the bedside and further to worldwide implementation. To accomplish his goal, he had to be able to collaborate with and seek help from instrument technicians, physicians from different specialties, hospital administrators, industrialists, international academic peers, and politicians. In doing so he became part of the creation of a new discipline, nephrology. Alwall had a myocardial infarction and passed away on February 2, 1986, leaving a legacy behind as one of the giants in the history of nephrology [37–40].

## Future Perspectives of Nephrology in Sweden

During the last two decades, the incidence rate of patients in need for RRT has been stable; if anything, a small decrease has been seen. One important reason for the levelling off of the incidence rates is a delayed progression toward ESRD, which has been shown among diabetic patients in particular. This trend is expected to continue due to an increased awareness of the importance of a meticulous conservative treatment in patients with CKD.

The increase in the number of prevalent patients in dialysis can be attributed to immigration and an improved survival among patients on treatment. Transplanted patients make up an increasing proportion of patients, and this trend will probably continue.

The number of home HD patients has not increased substantially over the last decade. The age distribution together with the large proportion of transplanted patients may be one explanation for this. Older patients are mostly not suitable for transplantation and not healthy enough to manage HD at home, whereas younger patients have a great possibility to get a renal transplant. Also, self-care HD and PD make up a substantial proportion of patients that perform much of the treatment themselves, although with assistance from nephrology personnel.

A large majority of nephrology departments and dialysis clinics are managed by public healthcare providers. There is no trend toward a growing number of clinics run by private companies, and those few that are working today are doing so contracted by public authorities, according to tenders every 5 years.

The shortage of nephrologists will probably be solved by an increase in the number of medical students as well as of doctors immigrating to Sweden.

## Conclusion

Nephrology in Sweden has a long and beautiful history. It began with the pioneer work and achievements by Nils Alwall, creating the artificial kidney. His work led to the creation of Gambro, one of the major innovators and producers of dialysis equipment and water treatment systems in the world. Scientific work regarding CKD, PD, and transplantation has also been successful, bringing Swedish insights into the nephrology community worldwide. During the last decades, Swedish nephrology has developed rapidly, nephrology units are spread over the country, and today all patients considered suitable for RRT are offered treatment. Healthcare in Sweden is managed by public authorities, although a few privately run clinics are working on behalf of these authorities. The patient's own costs are low as healthcare is largely publicly financed.

Today around 10,000 patients are on RRT, giving a prevalence of around 1000 pmp. The percentage of transplanted patients has increased, and the majority of RRT patients today have a functioning transplant. The RRT incidence rate is around 120 pmp and not increasing. The growth of the RRT population is thus a function of an improved survival, and of an increase of the general population, especially due to immigration.

The pattern of diseases leading to ESRD is in accordance with other countries in the West, glomerulonephritis and diabetic nephropathy being the most prevalent. Thanks to an active CKD care, there are signs of a slower progression toward ESRD for some groups of patients, especially diabetics, which has been shown in studies.

The nephrology future in Sweden is bright. If the increase in the number of patients on RRT will continue to be mostly due to an increase in the number of transplanted patients, the costs will be affordable, and the resources of society will cover the needs.

## References


1. https://web.archive.org/web/20180208124953/http://www.norden.org/en/fakta-om-norden. [Facts about the Nordic countries]. Swedish.
2. Statistics Sweden. https://www.scb.se/en/.
3. https://www.riksdagen.se/. Swedish.
4. https://skr.se/tjanster/englishpages.411.html.
5. National Board of Health and Welfare. https://www.socialstyrelsen.se/statistik-och-data/statistik/statistikamnen/halso-och-sjukvardspersonal/. Swedish.
6. Swedish Renal Registry. Annual report 2018. Swedish.
7. Grefberg N. [Anniversary book, The Swedish Society of Nephrology] Jubileumsbok, Svensk Njurmedinsk Förening. https://njurmed.se/wp-content/uploads/2017/04/SNF-Jubileumsbok.pdf. Swedish.
8. Groth C.-G. https://www.lakartidningen.se/OldWebArticlePdf/1/17666/LKT1203s111_112.pdf. Läkartidningen. Swedish.
9. Toppe C, Möllsten A, Waernbaum I, Schön S, Gudbjörnsdottir S, Landin-Olsson M, Dahlquist G. Decreasing cumulative incidence of end-stage renal disease in young patients with type 1 diabetes in Sweden: a 38-year prospective nationwide study. Diabetes Care. 2019;42(1):27–31.
10. Plante-Bordeneuve V, Said G. Familial amyloid polyneuropathy. Lancet Neurol. 2011;10:1086.
11. Norgren N. Hereditary transthyretin amyloidosis – from genes to genealogy. Ph.D. thesis, Umeå University, ISBN: 978-91-7459-786-8.
12. Al-Jaghbeer M, et al. Clinical decision support for in-hospital AKI. J Am Soc Nephrol. 2018;29:654–60.
13. Kellum JA, Prowle JR. Paradigms of acute kidney injury in the intensive care setting. Nat Rev Nephrol. 2018;14:217–30.
14. https://portal.icuregswe.org/utdata/home.
15. Bell M, SWING, Granath F, Schön S, Ekbom A, Martling CR. Continuous renal replacement therapy is associated with less chronic renal failure than intermittent haemodialysis after acute

renal failure. Intensive Care Med. 2007;33(5):773–80. https://doi.org/10.1007/s00134-007-0590-6. Epub 2007 Mar 16

16. Rimes-Stigare C, Frumento P, Bottai M, Mårtensson J, Martling CR, Bell M. Long-term mortality and risk factors for development of end-stage renal disease in critically ill patients with and without chronic kidney disease. Crit Care. 2015;19:383. https://doi.org/10.1186/s13054-015-1101-8.
17. Schön S, Ekberg H, Wikström B, Odén A, Ahlmén J. Renal replacement therapy in Sweden. Scand J Urol Nephrol. 2004;38(4):332–9.
18. Statistics Sweden, SCB. https://www.statistikdatabasen.scb.se/pxweb/sv/ssd/.
19. Gjessing J. Addition of aminoacids to peritoneal-dialysis fluid. Lancet. 1968;2(7572):812.
20. Gjessing J. The effect of glucose and THAM in peritoneal dialysis. Opusc Med. 1966;11:250–3.
21. Gjessing J. [Peritoneal dialysis adding Tris (hydroxymethyl) ominate – THAM – in the PD fluid in barbiturate intoxication] Peritoneal dialysis med Tris (hydroxymethyl) ominaten-THAM-i dialysvätskan vid barbitursyreintoxikation. Opusc Med. 1965;10:153–6. Swedish.
22. Blomberg R, Cronstedt J, Lundberg S. [Some cases of methanol poisoning]. Några fall av metanolförgiftning. Svenska Läkartidningen. 1963;60:1937. Swedish.
23. Gjessing J. Absorption of aminoacids and fat: from the peritoneum. Opusc Med. 1968;13:251–2.
24. Gjessing J, Nilsson L. [Peritoneal dialysis in acute severe pancreatitis]. Peritoneal dialys vid akut grav pankreatit. Svenska Läkartidningen. 1965;62:3706. Swedish.
25. Rippe B, Stelin G. Simulations of peritoneal solute transport during CAPD. Application of two-pore formalism. Kidney Int. 1989;35:1234–44.
26. Heimbürger O, Waniewski J, Werynski A, Tranaeus A, Lindholm B. Peritoneal transport in CAPD patients with permanent loss of ultrafiltration capacity. Kidney Int. 1990;38:495–506.
27. Park MS, Heimbürger O, Bergström J, Waniewski J, Werynski A, Lindholm B. Peritoneal transport during dialysis with amino acid-based solutions. Perit Dial Int. 1993;13:280–8.
28. Rippe B, Simonsen O, Heimbürger O, Christensson A, Haraldsson B, Stelin G, Weiss L, Nielsen FD, Bro S, Friedberg M, Wieslander A. Long-term clinical effects of a peritoneal dialysis fluid with less glucose degradation products. Kidney Int. 2001;59:348–57.
29. Bergström J, Fürst P, Alvestrand A, Lindholm B. Protein and energy intake, nitrogen balance and nitrogen losses in patients treated with continuous ambulatory peritoneal dialysis. Kidney Int. 1993;44:1048–57.
30. Nordfors L, Heimbürger O, Lönnqvist F, Lindholm B, Helmrich J, Schalling M, Stenvinkel P. Fat tissue accumulation during peritoneal dialysis is associated with a polymorphism in uncoupling protein 2. Kidney Int. 2000;57:1713–9.
31. Tydén G, Kumlien G, Genberg H, Sandberg J, Lundgren T, Fehrman I. ABO incompatible kidney transplantations without splenectomy, using antigen-specific immunoadsorption and rituximab. Am J Transplant. 2005;5(1):145–8.
32. Wennberg L, Lindnér P, Linders J, Bengtsson M, Sedigh A, Andersson T. First donations and transplantations performed in Swedish kidney exchange program. [Article in Swedish]. Lakartidningen. 2019;116:FL4A.
33. Ekberg H, Tedesco-Silva H, Demirbas A, Vítko S, Nashan B, Gürkan A, Margreiter R, Hugo C, Grinyó JM, Frei U, Vanrenterghem Y, Daloze P. Halloran PF; ELITE-Symphony Study. Reduced exposure to calcineurin inhibitors in renal transplantation. N Engl J Med. 2007;357(25):2562–75.
34. Tydén G, Bolinder J, Solders G, Brattström C, Tibell A, Groth CG. Improved survival in patients with insulin-dependent diabetes mellitus and end-stage diabetic nephropathy 10 years after combined pancreas and kidney transplantation. Transplantation. 1999;67(5):645–8.
35. Jordan SC, Lorant T, Choi J, Kjellman C, Winstedt L, Bengtsson M, Zhang X, Eich T, Toyoda M, Eriksson BM, Ge S, Peng A, Järnum S, Wood KJ, Lundgren T, Wennberg L, Bäckman L, Larsson E, Villicana R, Kahwaji J, Louie S, Kang A, Haas M, Nast C, Vo A, Tufveson G. IgG endopeptidase in highly sensitized patients undergoing transplantation. N Engl J Med. 2017;377(5):442–53. https://doi.org/10.1056/NEJMoa1612567.
36. Facts about the medical profession. Läkarfakta Swedish. https://slf.se/publikationer/lakarfakta-2016/.
37. Alwal N, et al. Therapeutic and diagnostic problems in severe renal failure. Lund: Berlingska boktryckeriet; 1963.
38. Alwal N. Historical perspectives on the development of artificial organs. Lund: Gambro AB, Education Department; 1985. Reprint of lecture.
39. Westling H. [The artificial kidney – a book about Nils Alwall]. Konstgjord njure – En bok om Nils Alwall. Stockholm: Bokförlaget Atlantis; 2000. Swedish.
40. Segelmark M. Nils Alwall – one of the founding fathers of nephrology. Hektorama (https://hekint.org/hektorama/)|Nephrology (https://hekint.org/nephrology/).

# Nephrology in Switzerland

# 49

Michel Burnier, Rebecca Winzeler, Patrice Ambühl, and Olivier Bonny

| | |
|---|---|
| Area | 41,285 Km$^2$ |
| Population | 8.48 million (2018) |
| Capital | Bern |
| Three most populated cities: | 1. Zurich<br>2. Geneva<br>3. Basel |
| Official languages | German, French, Italian, and Romantsch |
| Gross domestic product (GDP) | 705.5 billion USD (2018) |
| GDP per capita | 78,816 USD (2018) |
| Human Development Index (HDI) | 0.946 (2018) |
| Official currency | Swiss Francs (CHF) |
| Total number of nephrologists | 286 |
| National society of nephrology | Swiss Society of Nephrology www.swissnephrology.ch |
| Incidence of end-stage renal disease[1] | 2017 – 97.5 pmp |
| Prevalence of end-stage renal disease[1] | 2017 – 937.9 pmp |
| Total number of patients on dialysis[2] (all modalities) | 2017 – 3683<br>2018 – 3796 |
| Number of patients on hemodialysis[2] | 2017 – Home-HD:50, In-Center-HD:3205, Self-Care:85<br>2018 – Home-HD:50, In-Center-HD:3294, Self-Care:89 |
| Number of patients on peritoneal dialysis[2] | 2017-APD: 171, CAPD: 172<br>2018- APD: 177, CAPD: 181, Unknown: 5 |
| Number of renal transplantations per year[3] | 2017 – 360<br>2018 – 358 |

*Data from:*

1. Kramer A, et al. The European Renal Association – European Dialysis and Transplant Association (ERA-EDTA) Registry Annual Report 2016: a summary. Clinical Kidney Journal, 2019, 1–19
2. The SWISS RENAL REGISTRY AND QUALITY ASSESSMENT PROGRAM (srrqap)
3. Swisstransplant at www.swisstransplant.org

M. Burnier (✉)
Service of Nephrology and Hypertension, Departments of Medicine, University Hospital, Lausanne, Switzerland
e-mail: michel.burnier@chuv.ch

R. Winzeler
Service of Nephrology and Hypertension, Departments of Medicine, University Hospital, Lausanne, Switzerland

Service of Nephrology, Stadspital Waid, Zürich, Switzerland

P. Ambühl
Service of Nephrology, Stadspital Waid, Zürich, Switzerland

O. Bonny
Department of Pharmacology and Toxicology, University of Lausanne, Lausanne, Switzerland

## Introduction

Switzerland is a small country located in the center of Europe with borders with Germany, France, Italy, and Austria. The population is 8.5 million, and there are four official languages (French, German, Italian, and Romantsch). The official currency is the Swiss Franc. Its actual value is close to 1.0 USD and 0.9 Euro. The gross domestic product (GDP) is 705.5 billion USD in 2018, and the GDP per capita was 78,816 USD in 2018.

Switzerland is both a direct and representative democracy. At any time, the population can contest a law due to a system of popular initiatives. It is a confederation of 26 states (Cantons) with different languages. The Federal State is directed by a group of 7 ministers, of whom one serves as president for a 1-year term. There are two chambers of Congress, one in which each state is represented by two persons elected in their canton and another chamber in which the representation is distributed according to the number of inhabitants in each canton. Laws are defined at three levels: federal, cantonal, and community level. At each level, there are three powers: executive, legislative, and judiciary.

Regarding the healthcare system, laws are defined by the Federal State and the cantons. Medical insurance is obligatory but is based on a private system. There is no state insurance like in many European countries.



J. A. Moura-Neto et al. (eds.), *Nephrology Worldwide*, https://doi.org/10.1007/978-3-030-56890-0_49

## The Swiss Society of Nephrology

The Swiss Society of Nephrology (SSN) is a medical society member of the Swiss Medical Association (FMH). Its mission is to represent its members toward the population, authorities, and various institutions. In particular, the SSN guarantees quality of the medical practice of nephrology in Switzerland. The SSN encourages and supports basic and clinical research of the kidney and its associated diseases, and the SSN defends the interest of its members.

Today, a board consisting of ten members leads SSN. The three major linguistic regions as well as the university and non-university centers are represented. Colleagues in private practices and research centers in addition to nephro-pediatrics are also represented.

The SSN created the Swiss Renal Foundation (SRF) in 2003 to support renal research activities, kidney donation, and patients' information. SSN works in close collaboration with the Swiss Transplant Society.

A Swiss renal registry and quality assessment program (SRRQAP) was established in 2006 by the SSN. All chronic dialysis patients in Switzerland are captured and characterized in the dialysis registry. The registry not only reflects the demographic situation and the development of the Swiss dialysis population but also allows the assessment of important epidemiological and health policy issues prospectively. Thereby, it contributes significantly to the medical care of these patients and to the gain of new insights into disease mechanisms in chronic renal failure (CKD). Quality control and continuous quality improvement are other aims, which are achieved mainly by the comparison of individual centers with Swiss and with other ERA-EDTA registry countries benchmarks. Thus, the SRRQAP publishes the annual figures, puts together benchmark analyses among individual centers, and submits a minimum data set to the ERA-EDTA for further comparisons.

Other registries are supported by the SSN, such as the Renal Biopsy Registry, the Lupus Registry, and the Swiss Kidney Stone cohort, and a close collaboration with the Swiss Transplantation registry is maintained.

The main goals of the SSN are the following:

- To establish the 6-year curriculum for obtaining the FMH title of specialist in nephrology, in accordance with federal laws
- To validate and control the continued education for the FMH title in nephrology
- To support financially the Swiss Renal Foundation which funds research projects
- To organize the annual meeting based on high standards
- To organize two annual sessions for continued medical education (CME)
- To organize since 2008 courses for kidneys, urinary tracts, and dialysis shunts

SSN is represented in the Swiss Medical Council of the FMH, in the Institute for postgraduate and continued education (SIWF), in the Swiss Academy for Quality in Medicine (SAQM), SwissDRG, TarMed, etc.

## Brief History of Nephrology in Switzerland

The SSN was established in Bern by 17 members in 1969. The first hemodialysis (HD) was performed in the early 1960s. The two first kidney transplantations were performed in Bern and in Zurich in 1964. SSN has created the SRF in 2003.

Switzerland was also the cradle of the International Society of Nephrology (ISN). Indeed, the ISN was created in 1960 following the 1st International Congress of Nephrology held that year in Geneva (Switzerland) and Evian-les-Bains (France).

Several famous internationally renowned nephrologists were members of the SSN. Among them, one can cite; Prof Reubi who created the nephrology center of Bern; Prof. G. Thiel in Basel in the field of transplantation; Prof. H. Murer in Zurich who is a leader in renal transport systems; Prof. B. Rossier in Lausanne, who cloned the epithelial sodium channel and was a leader in the regulation of tubular sodium transport; Prof. H.R. Brunner in Lausanne, who was pioneer in the field of hypertension and the renin-angiotensin system; Prof. J.P. Guignard from Lausanne, an internationally recognized pediatric nephrologist; and Prof. MJ Mihatsch in Basel, who is still a very active and renowned renal pathologist.

## Renal Diseases in Switzerland

The overall prevalence of CKD in Switzerland is 10.4% [1]. The prevalence in the low, moderate, high, and very high risk KDIGO categories are 89.6%, 8.4%, 1.6%, and 0.5%, respectively. The prevalence of CKD is similar in all linguistic regions. In the Swiss population, a higher prevalence of CKD was found in three subgroups: participants older than 60 years (25%), diabetic (37%), and hypertensive (23%) subjects. There is no actual endemic renal disease in Switzerland. In the past, analgesic nephropathy was particularly prevalent in Switzerland. Today, diabetes and vascular nephropathy (including hypertension) are still the most prevalent causes of CKD [1, 2].

In a single center study performed in Geneva, patients with a community-acquired acute kidney injury (CA-AKI) represented 4% of all admissions to the emergency department during a 8-week period. Most of these patients were elderly, with major comorbidities and potentially nephrotoxic medications. CA-AKI in this population was predominantly pre-renal and KDIGO stage 1 at presentation [3].

In 2017, the adjusted incidence of end-stage renal diseases in Switzerland was 97.5 per million population (pmp), and the prevalence was 937.9 pmp. Kidney disease deaths in Switzerland reached 982 or 1.76% of total deaths. The age-adjusted death rate from kidney diseases is 5.14 per 100,000 of the Swiss population [4].

## Renal Replacement Therapy in Switzerland

In 2012, changes in epidemiology of patients undergoing RRT by either HD or peritoneal dialysis (PD) over four decades have been examined in the Zurich area [5]. In this study, incident mean age progressively increased from 48 ± 14 to 64 ± 15 years from first to fourth quartile ($p < 0.001$), with a concomitant decrease in 3- and 5-year survival from 72.2 to 67.7%,and 64.1 to 54.8%, respectively. Nevertheless, life span continuously increased from 57 ± 13 to 74 ± 11 years ($p < 0.001$). Patients transplanted, at least once, were significantly younger at dialysis initiation, with significantly better survival.

In 2015, data for the Swiss Renal Registry indicated that the mean age in dialysis was 67.9 years old, but half of the patients were older than 70.8 years and 40.7% were older than 75 years. The first-year survival rate of a dialysis patient is 90.7%. The dialysis population is characterized by a very high rate of comorbidities, mainly cardiovascular diseases and diabetes. In incident dialysis patients (hemo- or peritoneal dialysis; $N = 3567$) from the Swiss dialysis registry followed up from 2014 on until December 31, 2017, 18.8% of the patients died representing a yearly average below 10% [6].

### Hemodialysis

HD represents 90% of all RRT and is fully reimbursed by insurances, which are obligatory for all individuals living in Switzerland (private insurances). Some drugs and interventions during dialysis are included in the global prize of a dialysis session (bundle). All types of hemodialysis are available in the country (HD, HDF), but there are not yet numbers on the prevalence of each technique. A HD session in Switzerland costs between 480 and 530 Swiss Francs depending on the percentage of patients on autonomous dialysis programs (see section on PD). There are no defined numbers of nurses or physicians per patients on HD in Switzerland. Filters reuse is allowed but rarely used in the country because of the low price of HD filters today in regard to the costs and quality control obligations necessary for the reuse of filters.

**Table 49.1** Prevalence of hepatitis B, hepatitis C, and HIV in dialysis patients in Switzerland

| | Hepatitis B | Hepatitis C | HIV |
|---|---|---|---|
| Home HD, % | 0.02 | 0.02 | 0.00 |
| Center HD, % | 2.35 | 2.26 | 0.78 |
| PD, % | 0.19 | 0.09 | 0.02 |
| Total, % | **2.56** | **2.37** | **0.80** |

Data from the SRRQAP 2018

For hospitalized patients, acute or chronic dialyses are paid separately in the context of the patient clinical case (DRG). In intensive care, the management of ESRD varies from center to center. In some centers, nephrologists are fully in charge of ESRD patients. In some others, there is a collaboration, intensive care physicians being independent to perform continuous hemofiltration whereas intermittent dialysis is performed by nephrologists only.

The typical HD prescription has a dialysate flow of 500 ml/min and a blood flow rate that varies from 300 to 400 ml/min, depending on the patient and the vascular access. The conventional in-center, 4-hour, thrice-weekly session schedule is the standard in Switzerland. Home HD is low (1.2%). Nighttime dialysis is provided in very few centers. Regarding vascular accesses, the distribution is the following: AV fistulas, 56.1%; grafts, 11.3%, catheter, 32.4% (temporary, 2.9%, long term, 97.1%), and others, 0.2%. Kt/V is widely adopted as the main indicator of dialysis adequacy, and target laboratory values are those recommended by KDIGO.

The prevalence of hepatitis B, hepatitis C, and HIV in Swiss dialysis patients is the following (Table 49.1):

In HD, the main causes of death are cardiac arrest/sudden death (12.6%), followed by patient refusing further dialysis (10.2%) and unknown cause of death (9.7%). Recent data from the Swiss registry indicate that dialysis patients in Switzerland have an 8% and 14% higher survival in the first and second year, respectively, compared to other European countries [6, 7].

### Peritoneal Dialysis

PD is available in all university centers in Switzerland as well as in many non-university centers since the end of the 1970s. The prevalence of PD is low in Switzerland and was 7.3% of all RRT in 2014 and 9.5% in 2017 [8].

However, there has been a slight increase to about 9–10% in the last years, due to the newest version of the dialysis reimbursement contract. According to the new contract, the value of the HD reimbursement is modulated depending on the percentage of new incident patients with ESRD who start their dialysis in an autonomous program, i.e., PD, home HD, or a self-care program. Over two consecutive periods of 6 months, this percentage must be greater than 20%. If not, the reimbursement of the HD session is reduced by about 10% in the center, which does not achieve the target.

So far, this approach has led to a modest increase in the prevalence of PD and a greater increase in the incidence of home dialysis (from 9% to 26.8%) and self-care programs in centers although the prevalence of home and self-care program remain low (about 1.5–2%).

## Dialysis in the Pediatric Population

There are five pediatric centers in Switzerland in which 21 children were dialyzed in 2018.

## Renal Transplantation

In Switzerland, renal transplantation is performed in six centers, i.e., Basel, Bern, Lausanne, Geneva, St. Gallen, and Zurich. The attribution of organs is centralized and Switzerland is connected to Eurotransplant. A new transplantation law was enforced in 2007, requiring a mandatory lifelong follow-up of all transplanted patients in Switzerland. In a collaborative effort with the Federal Office of Public Health, the Swiss transplant cohort discussed below ensures compliance with the requirements of the law.

The transplant rate in 2016 was 36 pmp (22 for deceased donor and 14 for living related donors) [4]. In 2018, 949 patients were on the waiting list to receive a renal transplant with a slight decrease in the waiting list (1198 cases in 2014), and 250 kidneys were transplanted. The number of deceased donors slightly increased (157) in 2018, but the trend goes toward a greater increase in the number of living related donors. ABO incompatible and cross-over transplantation is performed in some, but not all centers. In Switzerland, all immunosuppressive agents are available. The most frequently used as chronic therapy are calcineurin inhibitors (96.9%), mycophenolate mofetil (97.6%), mTOR inhibitors (1.1%), and steroids. The protocol depends on the centers [9]. Drugs are paid 90% by the insurance.

On October 1, 2018, Swiss Transplant created a National Registry of Organ donation which enables any citizen older than 18 years to register his/her wish to donate in case of death. The main political discussion regarding transplantation in general in Switzerland is the national implementation of the presumed consent, which is in place in some but not all Swiss Cantons.

## Nephrology Practice in Switzerland

The nephrology and dialysis network in Switzerland is based on institutional and private practices. About 30% of the centers offering dialysis in Switzerland are private institutions. In addition to patient care, they are themselves responsible for the infrastructure of their centers. In the SSN a working group of "Freipraktizierende Nephrologen" was founded to share experiences and to advise the requests of these smaller units.

Currently, the official curriculum in Nephrology is 6 years (3 years of internal medicine or another specialty and 3 years specifically in Nephrology). Hospitals providing nephrology training are classified in three categories: (A) university hospitals with renal transplantation, (B) large hospitals without transplantation, and (C) smaller centers with a dialysis unit. The duration of the possible training is defined for each category: 2 years for A, 1 year for B, and 3–6 months for C centers. Trainees have to do at least 2 years in A center and must go in a Bor C center to have their training recognized. Swiss trainees now have to perform the European exam of the Nephrology board. Physicians from other countries than Switzerland can perform their training in a Swiss Nephrology center, but the conditions are defined essentially by the local hospital and the Canton.

Once Swiss certified, physicians either can continue to work in a hospital or established themselves on their own. The conditions to open a dialysis center or a private practice are defined by the Cantonal laws. There are special conditions of acceptance for countries of the EU and non-EU defined by a Swiss Federal commission (MEBEKO). In addition to the recognition of the certificates, physicians must have a sufficient knowledge of the local language (French, German or Italian) with at least a B2 level. Thus, there is both a Cantonal and a Federal level of acceptance. Salaries of nephrologists are very heterogeneous. They depend on the Canton, the level of competence (from fellow to professorship), and public versus private. Thus, the yearly salary can range from 50 K to more than 250 K CHF. Salaries are higher in private practice but depend on the activity and the area of practice. The same is true for nurses. For them, the training, number of years of practice, and the site (private vs public) determine the level of salary. In that case, the difference between public and private is often in favor of the public. Nurse salaries can range between 40 and 90 K CHF.

Job opportunities for specialized dialysis nurses are handled by the dialysis centers themselves in collaboration with their administration and the Canton. The market for specialized nurses in dialysis is relatively open in Switzerland because of the high need. Job offers are usually available on the Hospitals' websites. A sufficient level of German, French, or Italian is necessary as well.

## Highlights of Nephrology in Switzerland

### The Swiss Transplantation Cohort

In Switzerland, solid organ donor evaluation and organ allocation have been well organized at the level of six transplant centers since 1985. Each transplant program collected its own data and no monitoring or auditing was performed. No country-wide structure existed to systematically monitor transplant outcomes and to coordinate multicenter studies for the post-transplant process.

In 2006, several Swiss investigators from different disciplines decided to launch a prospective multicenter cohort project, the Swiss Transplant Cohort Study (STCS), aiming at a nationwide comprehensive and structured data collection in all solid organ transplant (SOT) recipients. After a 2-year set-up period, the STCS started patient enrolment in May 2008.

The main objectives of the STCS are:

1. To record all SOTs within one unique database system in order to have a complete assessment of all patient-, transplant-, and center-specific activities in Switzerland.
2. To collect prospectively high-quality longitudinal clinical and laboratory data of transplant recipients at the Swiss national level, to evaluate the quality, effectiveness, and efficiency of SOT in order to support patients, health care professionals, and policy makers with informed decision-making
3. To implement a biobank sampling scheme to integrate biological and clinical information
4. To reflect the complexity of the post-transplant patient care in an appropriate data model and integrate this complexity into research hypothesis and methodology
5. To collect selected psychosocial and behavioral data at time of listing and during follow-up
6. To systematically capture relevant infectious diseases episodes.
7. To record and periodically update specific risk profiles to reflect changes in disease and treatment status
8. To assess determinants of poor short- or long-term outcome and allow studying alternative pathways that contribute to the understanding of patient – and allograft survival

For more information, see https://www.stcs.ch/about/study-description.

### National Centre of Competence in Research

The Swiss National Centre of Competence in Research (NCCR) Kidney Control of Homeostasis (Kidney.CH) is a nationwide research network bringing together leading specialists in experimental and clinical nephrology from all Swiss universities teaching medicine and from corresponding university hospitals. The Swiss National Science Foundation supports it.

The long-term objective of our national research network is to advance knowledge and understanding of the renal homeostatic mechanisms controlling body composition in health and disease. Knowledge and technology transfer and the education of the next generation of scientists and promotion of women are essential features and give this long-term research project strategic importance.

More on: https://www.nccr-kidney.ch/

### The Swiss Kidney Stone Cohort (SKSC)

SKSC is a longitudinal multicentric observational cohort of stone formers, aiming at fostering research on kidney stones and at collecting epidemiological data and biological samples from stone formers. It was launched in 2014 and involves five university centers and one State hospital covering most of Switzerland. Kidney stone formers with recurrent events or single stone former with risk factors (osteoporosis, intestinal diseases, age <25 year, etc.) are included. However, children are not included.

The investigation protocol is identical in all recruiting centers. At baseline, patients collect two consecutive 24 h urine samples and complete a 2-day food diary that helps answering two 24 h structured recall interviews performed by trained dieticians using the software Globodiet. Validated food frequency and physical activity questionnaires are also filled. Fresh morning urine is examined for crystalluria. Biological samples (2 × 24 h urine and blood) are analyzed centrally and biobanked (native, acidified, or alkalinized urine; serum or plasma). DNA is extracted and stored. Based on this initial baseline evaluation, patients either are given nutritional counsels (by nephrologists or dedicated dieticians) and/or are treated with specific drugs appropriate to their condition. A follow-up visit at 3 months (blood and 1 × 24 h urine are collected) provides evidence of adherence to the proposed intervention and allows further therapeutic refinement. Further annual follow-ups during 3 years (blood and 2 × 24 h urine collections) are meant to boost adherence, check for cardiovascular and metabolic risk factors over time, and allow evaluation of the remaining stone burden. Then, follow-up phone calls every other year is continued for up to 10 years in order to keep track of stone and/or cardiovascular events.

By June 2019, 782 patients had been included in the SKSC.

Started in 2018, a control group of 250 matched-for-age-and-sex-individuals without kidney stone (as demonstrated by native abdominal CT-scan) completes the study by offering data collected with the exact same protocol of non-stone formers.

SKSC is open to researchers interested in kidney stones. Its strengths uncover strong nutritional phenotype, longitudinal follow-up, and standardized protocols coupled to biobanking. SKSC sets the stage for further clinical interventional trials or for basic genetic, molecular, or omics studies. More on http://sksc.nccr-kidney.ch/

## Future Perspectives of Nephrology in Switzerland

Recently, at the request of the Swiss Academy of Medical Sciences, and noting the interest of the Swiss Academy for Quality in Medicine and a similar initiative of the Swiss Society of Internal Medicine, the Board of the Swiss Society of Nephrology joined the international campaign "Choosing Wisely." The campaign aims at promoting doctor-patient dialog and contains medical guidelines in case of unfavorable individual risk-benefit balance.

In the field of dialysis, there is a strong incentive to augment the number of PD patients on or performing home HD. Programs of daily dialysis and night dialysis have started.

In the field of transplantation, there is strong political debate to find solutions to increase deceased donors and hence increase the overall renal transplantation capacities.

## Conclusion

Swiss Nephrology is very active and continuously adapting to fulfill the clinical tasks defined by the State and the SSN in the face of a growing population of elderly patients with ESRD. There is an important need to contain the costs of dialysis by favoring renal transplantation and home dialysis.

**Conflict of Interest** The authors declare that they have no conflict of interest.

## References

1. Forni Ogna V, Ogna A, Ponte B, et al. Prevalence and determinants of chronic kidney disease in the Swiss population. Swiss Med Wkly. 2016;146:w14313.
2. Lu Y, Stamm C, Nobre D, et al. Changing trends in end-stage renal disease patients with diabetes. Swiss Med Wkly. 2017;147:w14458.
3. Stucker F, Ponte B, De la Fuente V, et al. Risk factors for community-acquired acute kidney injury in patients with and without chronic kidney injury and impact of its initial management on prognosis: a prospective observational study. BMC Nephrol. 2017;18:380.
4. Kramer A, Pippias M, Noordzijet M, et al. The European Renal Association – European Dialysis and Transplant Association (ERA-EDTA) Registry Annual Report 2016: a summary. Clin Kidney J. 2019;12(5):702–20.
5. Rhyn Lehmann P, Ambuehl M, Corleto D, Klaghofer R, Ambuehl PM. Epidemiologic trends in chronic renal replacement therapy over forty years: a Swiss dialysis experience. BMC Nephrol. 2012;13:52.
6. Winzeler R, Ambühl P. Survival on dialysis: Switzerland in comparison with other countries. Swiss Med Wkly (Supplementum 234). 2018;148:32S.
7. Kramer A, , Pippias M, Noordzijet M et al. The European Renal Association - European Dialysis and Transplant Association (ERA-EDTA) Registry Annual Report 2015: a summary. Clin Kidney J 2018; 11(1):108–122.
8. Scotti Gerber J, et al. Incidence and prevalence of home dialysis treatment in the Swiss dialysis population between 2013 and 2017. Swiss Med Wkly (Supplementum 234). 2018;148:9S.
9. Lengwiler E, Stampf S, Zippelius A, et al. Solid cancer development in solid organ transplant recipients within the Swiss Transplant Cohort Study. Swiss Med Wkly. 2019;149:w20078.

# Nephrology in Ukraine

# 50

Mykola Kolesnyk, Natalia Stepanova, Iryna Dudar, Ingretta Bagdasarova, and Svitlana Fomina

| | |
|---|---|
| Area[1] | 603,550 Km$^2$ |
| Population[2] | 42,216,766 (2019) |
| Capital | Kyiv |
| Three most populated cities | 1. Kyiv<br>2. Kharkiv<br>3. Odesa |
| Official language | Ukrainian |
| Gross domestic product (GDP)[3] | 130.832 billion USD (2018) |
| GDP per capita[3] | 3,095.174 USD (2018) |
| Human development index (HDI)[4] | 0.75 (88o position) |
| Official currency | Ukrainian Hryvnia (UAH) |
| Total number of nephrologists[5] | 459 |
| National society of nephrology | Ukrainian Association of Nephrologists & Kidney Transplant Specialists www.uankts.com.ua |
| Incidence of the end-stage renal disease[5] | 2018 – 48 pmp |
| Prevalence of the end-stage renal disease[5] | 2018 – 229 pmp |
| Total number of patients undergoing dialysis (all modalities)[5, 6] | 2017 – 7645<br>2018 – 8290 |
| Number of patients on hemodialysis [5, 6] | 2017 – 6759<br>2018 – 7426 |
| Number of patients on peritoneal dialysis [5, 6] | 2017 – 886<br>2018 – 864 |
| Number of renal transplantations per year[5, 6] | 2017 – 112<br>2018 – 122 |

1. World Atlas. https://www.worldatlas.com/webimage/countrys/europe/ukraine/ualand.htm (2018). Accessed 20 Jan 2020
2. State Statistics Service of Ukraine. https://ukrstat.org/en/operativ/menu/menu_e/ds.htm (2019). Accessed 20 Jan 2020
3. The World Bank. https://data.worldbank.org/country/ukraine (2020). Accessed 20 Jan 2020
4. United Nations Development Program. Human Development Reports. http://hdr.undp.org/en/countries/profiles/UKR (2020). Accessed 20 Jan 2020
5. Kolesnyk M, Kozliuk N, Razvazhaieva O, National Registry of Patients with Chronic Kidney Disease and Patients with Acute Kidney Injury. State Institution «Institute of Nephrology of the National Academy of Medical Sciences»; 2019. [In Ukrainian]
6. Kolesnyk M, Kozliuk N, Razvazhaieva O, National Registry of Patients with Chronic Kidney Disease and Patients with Acute Kidney Injury. State Institution «Institute of Nephrology of the National Academy of Medical Sciences»; 2018. [In Ukrainian]

M. Kolesnyk (✉) · N. Stepanova
State Institution «Institute of Nephrology of the National Academy of Medical Sciences», Department of Nephrology and Dialysis, Kyiv, Ukraine

Ukrainian Association of Nephrologists & Kidney Transplant Specialists, Kyiv, Ukraine
e-mail: director@inephrology.kiev.ua

I. Dudar
Ukrainian Association of Nephrologists & Kidney Transplant Specialists, Kyiv, Ukraine

State Institution «Institute of Nephrology of the National Academy of Medical Sciences», Department of Efferent Technology, Kyiv, Ukraine

I. Bagdasarova · S. Fomina
Ukrainian Association of Nephrologists & Kidney Transplant Specialists, Kyiv, Ukraine

State Institution «Institute of Nephrology of the National Academy of Medical Sciences», Department of Pediatric Nephrology, Kyiv, Ukraine
e-mail: sfomina@meta.ua

## Introduction

Ukraine is the largest country in Europe and has more than one thousand years of history and traditions. Ukraine is located in the geographical center of Europe at the intersection of the main transport routes from Europe to Asia and from the Scandinavian states to the Mediterranean region. The Carpathians (where over 73,000 rivers are located) and the Black and Azov Seas are at the territory of Ukraine. Administratively our country is divided into 24 provinces (regions) and the Autonomous Republic of Crimea.

Ukraine is a unitary republic with the parliamentary-presidential system, meaning that our head of state, President, and legislators are elected on the national level. The official currency is the Ukrainian Hryvnia (UAH), introduced in 1996. Currently (2019), UAH 1.00 is worth 0.042 USD and 0.038 euros.



J. A. Moura-Neto et al. (eds.), *Nephrology Worldwide*, https://doi.org/10.1007/978-3-030-56890-0_50

Ukraine is a member of numerous international and regional international organizations, including the United Nations, the Council of Europe and the European Union (EU) Energy Community. Ukraine is currently taking steps to accede to the EU and has a special partnership with the organization. The main information for Ukraine is summarized in the general table [1–6].

On April 26, 1986, Ukraine survived the Chernobyl nuclear accident, which was the largest uncontrolled radioactive release in history. 115,000 innocent people, who lived in the area and, thus, had to be evacuated, received an average effective radiation dose of 30 mSv. For comparison, the total worldwide average effective dose from natural background radiation is around 2.4 mSv per year [7]. Nevertheless, the ultimate health consequences, besides the acute effects, are still unknown.

At present, the country is characterized by a decreasing level of income. The armed conflict, or "hybrid war," on the territory of the country's eastern regions and the annexation of Crimea by Russia have been deepening the difficult economic and social situations of the country.

Another devastating issue for Ukraine is the significant outflow of population and labor force, which includes highly skilled professionals. In 2019, the population of Ukraine was 42,216,766, which represents a decrease of approximately 25% over the last 25 years. Emigration from Ukraine not only contributes to the decreasing population but also to a "brain drain." People who leave Ukraine primarily fall into the age group of 20–49 years, so the working-age population is being reduced. Another serious problem is the emigration of highly skilled specialists, including medical professionals [8]. The war, lack of jobs, or decently paid jobs in Ukraine are the main push factors behind migration.

According to the Constitution, health care in Ukraine is free of charge and it should be ensured through the state funding. However, in practice, the Ukrainian health network comprises not only state medical institutions (hospitals, polyclinics, research institutions, maternity homes, women's consulting centers, first aid stations), but private clinics, which frequently come with more comfortable service. Moreover, many medical professionals work in state and private clinics at the same time. Therefore, the majority of people tend to prefer paying for private healthcare services.

In August 2014, the Ukrainian Ministry of Health initiated the development of National Strategy on Health Reform to revitalize and speed up the process of reform implementation in the health sector through improving the quality and access to health care and ensuring the mitigation of financial risks for the population [9]. In 2017, the re-modeling of the Ukrainian health care system started, providing a new approach to the financing of healthcare institutions and individual healthcare practitioners. The introduction of the new system on the primary level took place in 2018, while the implementation of the whole reform will have been finished by the end of 2020 [9].

## Brief History of Nephrology in Ukraine

Professor Feofil Yanovskiy (1860–1928) was the founder of clinical nephrology in Ukraine. His work "Diagnostics of kidney diseases according to their pathologies" (1927) was the first textbook used for studying nephrology in Ukraine.

In 1933, Yurii Voronoy (1895–1961), the native of the Poltava region performed the first human kidney allotransplantation in the world. In Kherson, Voronoy made the first human kidney transplantation without immunosuppression with the intention of bridging to allow the treatment of acute renal failure. He published his results in 1936 in a Spanish journal; this decision reflects Voronoy's complicated political situation as he was Ukrainian living in the Soviet Union [10, 11].

Further development happened with the establishment of the first Nephrology Department in Ukraine at the Institute of Kidney and Urinary Tract Diseases in 1965. Thereafter, new departments were opened in Dnipropetrovsk (1967), Lugansk (1968), Donetsk, Odesa, Kharkiv, and Cherkasy (1970), followed by the openings in all regional hospitals.

Nephrology became a medical specialty in 1970, and medical doctors performed their nephrology training at the Department of Nephrology of the Institute of Kidney and Urinary Tract Diseases.

Professor Viktor Karpenko (1923–2003), a representative of the Kyiv Scientific Research Institute of Urology and Nephrology, conducted successful renal transplantation from an alive family donor in 1972 and one from a cadaver on September 4, 1973 [12]. In 1977, the first department of hemodialysis (HD) and kidney transplantation was established in the Institute of Kidney and Urinary Tract Diseases (Kyiv).

At the beginning of the current millennium, the status of nephrology in Ukraine remained at the same level as of 1950 – even a common classification of kidney disease was absent. For example, internists in Kyiv, Kharkiv, Odesa, or Lviv had their own classifications of glomerulonephritis (GN); therefore, no single classification existed. Nephrology began and finished within each regional hospital and there were no unified conventions in the country.

The defining moment of the development of Ukrainian nephrology was the establishment of the Institute of Nephrology as a part of the Academy of Medical Sciences of Ukraine in 2001. Then, a new stage of development of nephrology was initiated in Ukraine. The Institute of Nephrology is the nation's scientific and clinical center, and it serves as a coordinator in the field. The Institute of Nephrology consists of the following departments: nephrology and dialysis, critical care nephrology, efferent technologies, pediatric nephrology, scientific-organizational, and patent licensing, as well as laboratories of biochemistry, immunology, microbiology, and pathomorphology. There are eight doctors of medical sciences, five professors, and seventeen PhDs present in the staff [13].

Because of the efforts of the Institute's team led by prof. M. Kolesnyk, a national program of nephrological care was created. Indeed, it is constantly being improved. Today, nephrology in Ukraine complies with all the modern requirements by structure and organization of scientific and clinical parts. The main reason for its inability to provide adequate nephrological care is the lack of financial resources. The present organizational structure of nephrological care in Ukraine is shown in Fig. 50.1.

In 2003, the National Coordination Committee (headed by Prof. M. Kolesnyk) was created as a part of the Institute of Nephrology. This committee together with regional coordinators established national and provincial registers of patients with chronic kidney disease (CKD) and patients with acute kidney injury (AKI); since 2007, the Ukrainian Renal Date System (URDS) Registry has become a part of the ERA-EDTA Registry [13].

In January 2004, the Specialized Academic Nephrology Council was created, and it granted the right to conduct the acceptance of consideration regarding thesis defense for the doctoral and PhD degrees in nephrology.

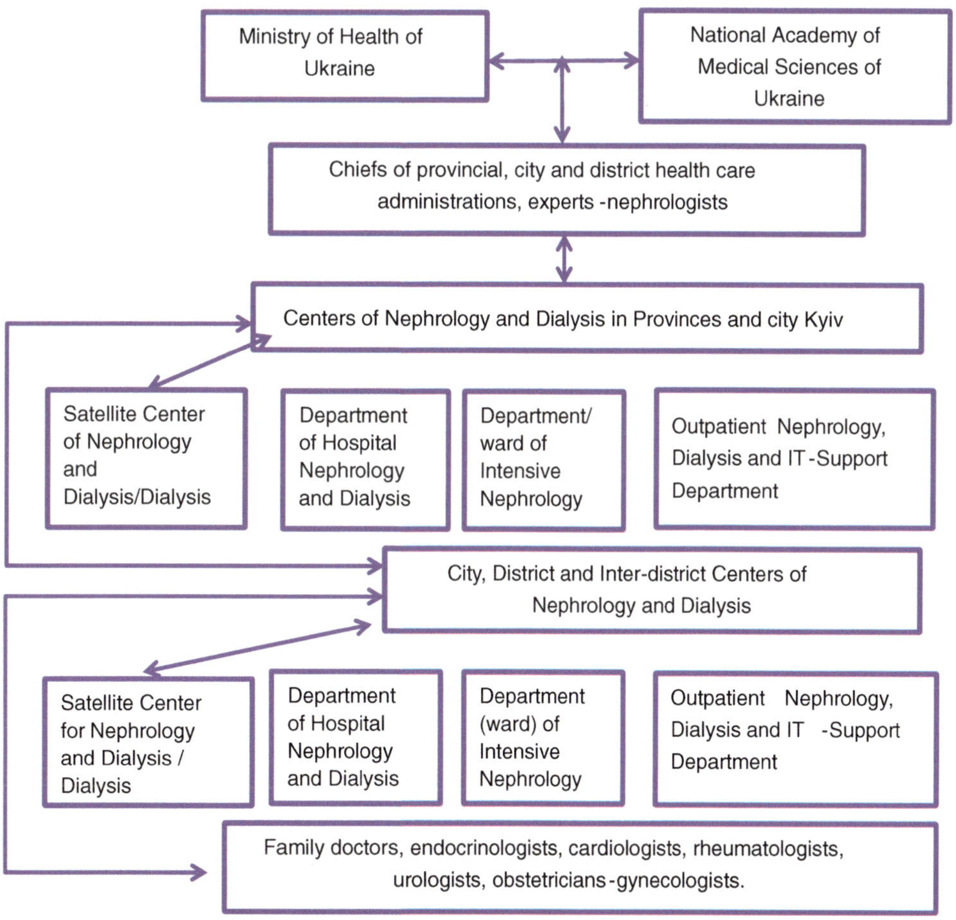


Fig. 50.1 The present organizational structure of nephrological care in Ukraine

In 2004, the scientific and practical quarterly edition called the "Ukrainian Journal of Nephrology and Dialysis" was established. It has provided readers with a wide range of publications of practical and experimental nephrology and related disciplines. It has been certified by the Higher Attestation Commission of the Ministry of Education and Science of Ukraine. The *Ukrainian Journal of Nephrology and Dialysis* is referenced and indexed in the Crossref Registration Agency (DOI prefix 10.31450), the Directory of Open Access Journals (DOAJ), the National repository Vernadsky National Library of Ukraine, and the Ulrich's international periodicals directory. The site of the journal is http://www.ukrjnd.com.ua.

Created by the employees of the Institute of Nephrology, the urinary system disease classification for nephrological practice was approved by the second National Nephrology Congress (Kharkiv 2005). This classification made it possible to unify the terminological concepts, approaches to diagnosis, treatment, and prevention as well as the creation of national and regional CKD patient registries.

In 2007, the Department of Intensive Nephrology was opened along with the National Institute of Cardiovascular Surgery. In 2009, a similar department was created at the provincial center of nephrology and dialysis in Ivano-Frankivsk. Wards of intensive nephrology are functioning in some provincial hospitals.

The Institute is a co-founder of the National Renal Fund of Ukraine, the main objective of which is to provide charitable assistance in the development of nephrological science and practice, as well as to promote the level of social rehabilitation of patients with a nephrological profile [13].

Since 2010, professional dialysis, intensive nephrology, and pediatric nephrology improvement courses have been launched for nephrologists, general practitioners, and nurses. CKD 5 stage medical care guidelines and protocols were developed and published in 2016. In the same year, the rating evaluation method of the main components of specialized medical care to nephrological patients was implemented [13].

The Ukrainian Association of Nephrologists (UAN) was founded in 1982, and it was reorganized into the Ukrainian Association of Nephrologists and Kidney Transplant Specialists (UANKTS) in 2017. Since 1982, congresses with the participation of all Ukrainian nephrologists and invited international speakers have been organized annually by the UAN and UANKTS.

## Renal Diseases in Ukraine

### Chronic Kidney Disease

Disadvantages of medical care for CKD patients reflect the state of the health care system in Ukraine in general. According to the URDS Registry, there were 36,973 patients with CKD 3–5 stages at the end of 2018. This indicates a very low level of CKD diagnosis in Ukraine [5]. Incidence and prevalence in the years 2017–2018 clearly demonstrate an insufficient level of CKD diagnostics in Ukraine (Table 50.1).

As presented in Table 50.1, the incidence of CKD stages 3, 4 and 5 combined was 112.4 pmp [5]. The main causes of CKD were pyelonephritis (25.89%), diabetic nephropathy (25.3%), and glomerulonephritis (23.93%) (Table 50.2).

The pyelonephritis overdiagnosis is associated with the number of the nephrologist in different regions of Ukraine: the higher the number of the nephrologist in the region is, the lower pyelonephritis prevalence is observed.

Qualified nephrologists are available only in big cities/regional centers, and this fact is reflected in the annual

**Table 50.1** Incidence and prevalence of CKD 3–5 stages

| Year | | CKD 3–5 (pmp) | CKD 3 (pmp/%) | CKD 4 (pmp/%) | CKD 5 (pmp/%) | RRT (pmp/%) |
|---|---|---|---|---|---|---|
| 2017 | Prevalence | 821.7 | 462.2/56.2% | 116.5/14.2% | 243.0/29.6% | 204.7/84.3% |
| | Incidence | 118.1 | 55.2/46.7% | 18.6/15.7% | 44.4/37.6% | 35.2/79.4% |
| 2018 | Prevalence | 875.8 | 486.2/55.5% | 122.1/13.9% | 267.5/30.5% | 229/83.0% |
| | Incidence | 112.4 | 45.5/40.5% | 19.3/17.1% | 47.6/42.4% | 38.6/81.1% |

**Table 50.2** Primary renal disease as underlying cause of CKD

| Year | | CKD 3–5 pmp | DM DM I % | DM II % | GN % | HN % | PN % | PKD % | Other % | Un-known % |
|---|---|---|---|---|---|---|---|---|---|---|
| 2017 | Prevalence | 821.7 | 14.56 | 10.43 | 23.97 | 10.38 | 26.25 | 6.74 | 7.16 | 0.22 |
| | Incidence | 118.1 | 6.57 | 22.87 | 22.87 | 12.04 | 21.54 | 6.47 | 7.19 | 0.46 |
| 2018 | Prevalence | 875.7 | 14.06 | 11.25 | 23.93 | 10.35 | 25.89 | 6.87 | 7.31 | 0.33 |
| | Incidence | 112.4 | 6.60 | 23.22 | 24.68 | 12.29 | 16.67 | 7.31 | 8.05 | 1.18 |

Abbreviations: *DM* diabetes mellitus, *GN* glomerulonephritis, *HN* hypertensive nephropathy, *PN* pyelonephritis, *PKD* polycystic kidney disease diagnostics of CKD. Lack of experienced nephrologists leads to later stages of CKD diagnosis. Approximately 60% of CKD patients fall into nephrologists' hands at the third CKD stage and begin renal replacement therapy (RRT) on time. However, many ESRD patients with a late referral to nephrologist have multiple complications and have to start an urgent HD. Most ESRD patients start RRT with GFR < 10 mL/min/m$^2$, regardless of CKD cause and without previous nephrological consultation (62% in 2018). It means that nearly 60% of ESRD patients do not have any pre-dialysis education.

Based on the URDS Registry, the total number of patients undergoing dialysis in Ukraine was estimated to be 8290 in 2018 [5]. The prevalence of dialysis was 229 patients pmp, with the highest rate in Ivano-Frankivsk province (399 pmp) and the lowest in the Lugansk province (31 pmp). Similarly, the incidence of new patients with CKD on RRT also varied significantly (from 0 to 82 pmp) in the different provinces of Ukraine. Nevertheless, since 2013 there has been a significant increase in the prevalence (159–229 pmp) and absolute number of patients undergoing dialysis (7214–8290) [14].

## Acute Kidney Injury and Critical Care Nephrology

According to the 2018 URDS Registry, there were 946 (22.4 pmp) patients with AKI. However, it is important to note that the registry only includes data from dialysis centers. Unfortunately, there are no exact data from resuscitation, cardiology, surgical, and other clinics.

The main causes of AKI among these patients were interstitial nephritis of different etiologies (30%), sepsis (11.3%), hepatorenal syndrome (10%), hypovolemia (9.3), and obstruction (9.3%) (Table 50.3) [5].

In the vast majority of cases, patients fell into the nephrologists' hands at the third stage of the AKI (67.3%). The distribution of patients according to the AKI stages is presented in Table 50.4.

Different RRT modality options are usually available in the critical care nephrology units. The choice of the RRT method for AKI varies according to the locality and its different peculiarities, such as the availability of conventional HD, HDF, or continuous renal replacement therapy (CRRT) equipment, and the experience of the nephrology team.

For the treatment of AKI patients at the third stage, intermittent HD (12.1 pmp) and hybrid (1.1 pmp) dialysis therapy were used. Continuous veno-venous hemofiltration (CVVH) was used to treat 27 patients at the third stage of AKI (0.6 pmp) [5]. It is important to point out the fact that not all the country's dialysis centers usually receive AKI patients. The general incidence of RRT treatment for AKI patients at the third stage was 13.8 pmp in 2018 [5].

The ICU mortality rate for patients with the third stage of AKI was 0.6 pmp in 2018 [5]. The outcomes' profile of AKI patients at the third stage is demonstrated in Table 50.5.

The establishment of databases has added some information about AKI prevalence and its outcomes in Ukraine. Unfortunately, our all-cause ICU mortality rate is higher than the one of the international standards. However, important information about the prevalence and mortality of AKI patients among different ICUs is missing. These data could guide decisions regarding the burden of treatment and success rates in our country. Moreover, the AKI treatment results might be improved by creating a department or, at least, a ward for intensive nephrology care in the regional hospitals.

## Renal Replacement Therapy in Ukraine

Since its independence in 1992, the country remains in the transitional stage, not only politically and economically, but also in terms of health care, which results in unpleasant consequences for RRT availability. Unfortunately, RRT is generally a low-priority area for healthcare planners in Ukraine. Currently, only 437 nephrologists, 92 of whom are pediatric nephrologists, provide medical care in Ukraine (9 pmp). The ESRD dialysis treatment is carried out by 115 regional, district, inter-district, and city centers of nephrology and dialysis [5]. Expenses for the dialysis ESRD treatment during 2018 resulted in almost three billion UAH (about 12 million USD). Reimbursement from the state budget formed just over one billion UAH (6 million USD) [15].

In terms of RRT modalities, Ukraine follows the pattern of Eastern and South European countries where HD is prescribed for the majority of patients. Meanwhile, the HD share in Western European countries reaches only 50%. This is due to an active increase in kidney transplant rates.

**Table 50.3** Incidence and etiology of AKI

| Year | AKI N/pmp | Sepsis % | Hypovolemia % | CRS1 % | HRS % | IN % | RPGN % | Obstruction % | Unknown % |
|---|---|---|---|---|---|---|---|---|---|
| 2017 | 803/18.9 | 12.5 | 8.3 | 12.1 | 7.3 | 33.4 | 2.4 | 7.1 | 17.7 |
| 2018 | 946/22.4 | 11.3 | 9.3 | 7.8 | 10.0 | 30 | 2.1 | 9.3 | 20.1 |

Abbreviations: *CRS* cardiorenal syndrome, *HRS* hepatorenal syndrome, *IN* interstitial nephritis, *RPGN* rapidly progressive glomerulonephritis

**Table 50.4** AKI by stages

| | AKI | AKI stages (%) | | |
|---|---|---|---|---|
| Year | N/pmp | 1 | 2 | 3 |
| 2017 | 803/18.9 | 24.2 | 19.4 | 56.4 |
| 2018 | 946/22.4 | 13.4 | 19.2 | 67.3 |

**Table 50.5** Outcomes of the AKI 3 stage treated with IHD or CVVH

| 2017 | Outcomes | IHD ($n$ = 346) | | CVVH ($n$ = 24) | |
|---|---|---|---|---|---|
| | | N | % | N | % |
| | Complete remission | 124 | 35.8 | 8 | 33.3 |
| | Partial remission | 117 | 33.8 | 4 | 16.7 |
| | CKD V | 21 | 6.1 | 3 | 12.5 |
| | ICU mortality | 48 | 13.9 | 7 | 29.2 |
| | Hospital mortality | 17 | 4.9 | 0 | 0.0 |
| | Prolongation RRT | 19 | 5.5 | 2 | 8.3 |
| 2018 | | ($n$ = 511) | | ($n$ = 72) | |
| | Complete remission | 217 | 42.5 | 20 | 27.8 |
| | Partial remission | 166 | 32.5 | 20 | 27.8 |
| | CKD V | 15 | 2.9 | 4 | 5.5 |
| | ICU mortality | 73 | 14,3 | 20 | 27,8 |
| | Hospital mortality | 22 | 4,3 | 4 | 5,5 |
| | Prolongation of RRT | 18 | 3,5 | 4 | 5,5 |

Abbreviations: *IHD* intermittent hemodialysis, *CVVH* continuous veno-venous hemofiltration, *ICU* intensive care unit

**Table 50.6** Changes in renal care over the last 5 years in Ukraine

| | Years | |
|---|---|---|
| The indicators | 2013 | 2018 |
| The dialysis center's number | 97 | 115 |
| State-funded dialysis facilities, % | 97.7 | 94.6 |
| For-profit dialysis facilities, % | 2.3 | 5.4 |
| Dialysis machines number, pmp | 2.3 | 3.5 |
| Nephrologist coverage, pmp | 9 | 9 |
| RRT prevalence, pmp | 159 | 229 |
| RRT patients' number, abs | 7214 | 9659 |
| PD patients' number, abs | 966 | 886 |
| HD patients' number, abs | 5236 | 5365 |
| HDF patients' number, abs | 99 | 2061 |
| KT patients' number, abs | 913 | 1364 |
| Prevalence of PD, % | 13.4 | 9.2 |
| Prevalence of HD, % | 72.6 | 55.4 |
| Prevalence of HDF, % | 1.4 | 21.4 |
| KT prevalence, % | 12.7 | 14.2 |

Ukraine's percentage of PD utilization is relatively high in comparison with Western European countries, although this may also reflect our underdeveloped kidney transplant program with the lowest yearly rate in Europe [16].

However, despite all the existing problems, it is absolutely necessary to note that there has been significant progress in the field of medical care over the last 5 years. A substantial increase in the number of RRT patients has occurred as a result of the increasing number of dialysis centers in Ukraine. Changes in renal care over the past 5 years are shown in Table 50.6.

More than 90% of all ESRD patients were 20–64 years old, while the oldest age group (75 years and older) accounted for only 6% of the total number of patients. Although the majority of dialysis patients were between 45 and 64 years old, most of the transplant recipients were 20–44 years old [5].

As one can see in Table 50.3, the RRT prevalence was 229 pmp in 2018 and the annual increase in dialysis patients was approximately 40 pmp. The proportion of ESRD patients on RRT in Ukraine varies from 31 to 399 pmp, depending on the region (Fig. 50.2).

The smallest number of such patients is observed in Donetsk and Lugansk regions. First of all, this is related to the armed conflict in those areas, yet the war is not the only cause of serious regional differences in the number of RRT patients. Naturally, the RRT prevalence is directly associated with the gross regional domestic product (GRDP) and the number of nephrologists. Moreover, the long distance between the patients living in the rural or mountainous areas (including occupied territories) and dialysis centers is an important geographical factor, which contributed to the absence and irregular dialysis treatment.

Thus, the obstacles for the RRT implementation in low-gross-income regions are associated with the lack of qualified medical specialists, geographical restrictions, infrastructure, and inadequate administrative support of regional administrations.

## Hemodialysis

Traditionally, HD is the leading RRT modality in Ukraine. 7426 (77%) of ESRD patients were treated with HD in 2018 (176 pmp). Among them, there were 5365 (72%) patients who received HD and 2061 (28%) patients who received hemodiafiltration (HDF) [5]. In the majority of cases, HDF is available only in regional dialysis centers and private clinics because of the technical and financial barriers.

Only 5.4% of the total dialysis sessions are funded by private dialysis centers, while the great majority (94.6%) is state-funded. The cost of HD treatment varies among the Ukrainian regions. The average cost of 1 HD session in 2018 was 2215 UAH (93 USD), while 1 HDF session costed 2270 UAH (95 USD) [15].

The typical HD prescription in Ukraine does not differ from the generally accepted one. It includes a dialysate flow rate of about 500 ml/min with a blood flow rate from 300 to 400 ml/min, depending on the patient and vascular access. Four-hour sessions conducted three times per week are standard in Ukraine [15, 16].

Kt/V is used as the main indicator of dialysis adequacy in Ukraine. Kt/V, blood phosphate and calcium levels, parathyroid hormone (PTH), serum urea before dialysis session, hemoglobin, and serum albumin concentrations are included

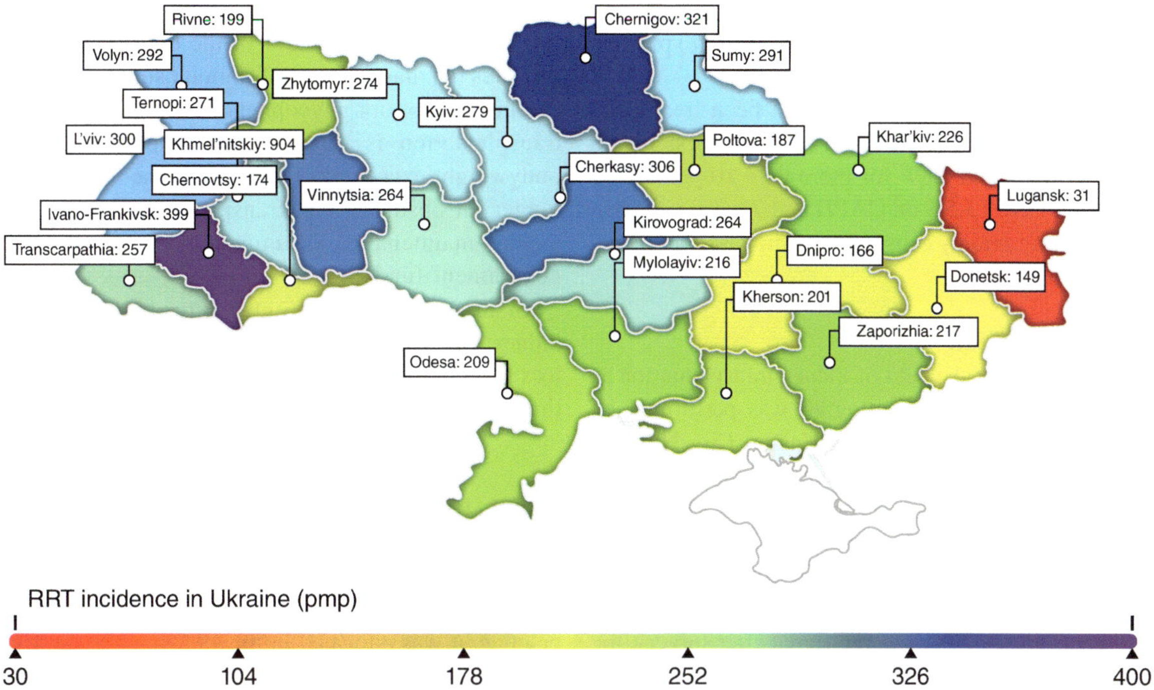


**Fig. 50.2** The prevalence of RRT in Ukraine in 2018

in the rating criteria [17]. These target levels were achieved for 60% of the HD patients in 2018 [5].

Reuse of dialyzers is forbidden in Ukraine. The seroprevalence of hepatitis B, hepatitis C, and HIV are 4.5%, 3.8%, and 0.06%, respectively. Despite the high hepatitis C level, its seroprevalence decreased from 6.1% in 2013 to 3.8% in 2018 [5, 6].

There were 707 deaths of patients who were treated by chronic HD and HDF in 2018; the mortality rates on HD and HDF were 10.9% and 7.4%, respectively. Cardiovascular diseases were the main causes of death (77.6%) [5, 14].

## Peritoneal Dialysis

PD is a well-established treatment modality for ESRD patients [18]. Currently, there are approximately 9% (21 pmp.) of ESRD patients maintained on PD in Ukraine. As 13.4% (22 pmp) of patients received this treatment in 2013, a downward trend is observed [5, 14, 18]. Such factors as the high costs of PD in comparison to HD, lack of adequate PD education of practicing nephrologists, and the patient's PD awareness might be the main causes of the low implementation of PD in Ukraine.

First of all, the annual costs per patient for continuous ambulatory PD (CAPD) and automated PD (APD) were 374,980 UAH (15,625 USD) and 559,677 UAH (23,320 USD), respectively. However, the annual cost for HD treatment was significantly lower and formed 345,509 UAH (14,396 USD) [15].

Secondly, not all dialysis centers can provide PD services in Ukraine. The main reason lies in the lack of any interest in either local authorities and nephrologists or solving this problem. In addition, the lack of laboratory tests availability for surveilling PD-associated complications has made the choice toward HD.

Finally, the decision concerning the choice of RRT modality should be based on both clinical considerations and patient preferences. However, this opportunity is not always available in Ukraine because of two reasons. The first one is the lack of capacity and desire to implement PD in the dialysis centers. The second one is the fact that urgent initiation of dialysis therapy in recently diagnosed patients often determines its choice.

As in the case of HD, government funds cover CAPD and APD treatments without imposing direct costs for the patients. However, an extremely low number of PD patients were taken into consideration in 2018 (864 on CAPD and 79 on APD) [5].

Despite the existence of the "Clinical Practice Guideline on Peritoneal Dialysis in Adults" [19], there is a wide variation in PD peritonitis rates in Ukraine. While the best rate achieved was 0.002 incidents/year in one center, it depends on the dialysis center. Overall, there were 120 (13.8%) PD patients who presented with peritonitis episodes during

2018. Among those who had peritonitis, PD catheter removal was performed in 13 (10.8%) cases, while 20 (15%) patients were transferred to HD [5].

The majority of patients (39.8%) had been treated by PD for up to 3 years in 2018; 19.45% for 5 years; 14.6% from 6 to 10 years, and 2.8% for more than 10 years. The mortality rates were 13.5% on CAPD and 7.4% on APD in 2018; deaths were mainly caused by cardiovascular events (80%) [5].

### Renal Transplantation

Ukraine is a pioneer in the field of kidney transplantation as the first clinical human renal allograft was performed by Ukrainian surgeon Yurii Voronoy in Herson City Hospital (1933) [10]. Voronoy transplanted a human kidney of blood group B to a patient with the blood group O and AKI, which was a result of mercuric chloride poisoning. The donor's kidney was obtained from a patient, who died from a head injury and transplanted to the thigh vessels of the recipient. Although some urine output was registered after surgery, the patient died 2 days later [11]. In the modern era, the first successful kidney transplantation in Ukraine was performed in Kyiv Institute of Urology in 1972 by Professor V.S. Karpenko and his team.

Currently, there are 7 transplantation centers in the country where they perform such surgical procedures: Kyiv, Zaporizhzhya, Kharkiv, Dnepr, Lviv, Odesa, and Kovel. The transplantation program has just started in Kovel, and doctors have already grafted two deceased donor kidneys successfully.

In 2018, there were 1369 kidney transplanted patients in the country. The prevalence of patients living with a functioning renal graft was 32 pmp in 2018 [5]. Unfortunately, the number of transplants in Ukraine per year is very small (120–130) and does not meet the needs: the majority of grafts being transplanted from living related donor [5, 6]. That causes patients to look for kidney transplantation abroad, often in Belarus. The reason for this is the lack of appropriate by-laws and regulatory acts. A new transplantation law, passed by Ukrainian Parliament in 2018, may change the situation for the better, as it introduces the transplant coordinator service, with the head at the National Coordination Center, and the nationwide registry of recipients and people willing to become organ donors in case of their sudden death. These changes may contribute to the development of deceased organ donation and significantly increase the number of transplanted organs.

Kidney transplantation surgery and posttransplantation management are carried out in accordance with European guidelines. Immunosuppression protocol includes induction of basiliximab in the cases of immunologically low risk and thyroglobulin in the high-risk ones. It also includes the maintenance of immunosuppression with calcineurin inhibitors, mycophenolates and steroids. Kidney transplantation is done to adults and children whose bodyweight exceeds 8–10 kg; ABO incompatibility is no longer an obstacle. The transplantation surgery, as well as the maintenance of immunosuppression, is mostly government-funded.

In 2018, the worst outcomes were observed in 94 (6.9%) kidney transplanted patients. The main cause of transplant loss was chronic graft rejection (67%). Infectious complications were observed in 2.1% of cases only [5].

## Renal Disease in the Pediatric Population

Pediatric nephrology in Ukraine was part of general pediatrics for many years. As a separate discipline and clinical practice, it was allocated in the 1970s, while the Ukrainian Association of Pediatric Nephrologists (UAPN) was founded only in 2017.

### Renal Diseases

Epidemiological studies and population surveys in pediatric CKD have not been conducted in Ukraine. Local annual reports, published by the Ministry of Public Health, are not personalized and include general analysis of the urogenital system diseases [20]. Unfortunately, CKD incidence and prevalence among the Ukrainian pediatric population is unknown.

According to the 2012 Annual Report, there were 431,698 children and adolescents with kidney disorders [20]. The revised data, conducted by the Ukrainian Ministry of Health (2018), revealed the increasing rate of the urinary system disease incidence among children during the last 20 years (+116.3%) [21].

In 2014, the "Institute of Nephrology of the National Academy of Medical Sciences of Ukraine" established the Pediatric CKD Registry, which became a part of the ESPN/ERA-EDTA Registry [22].

The Registry included 2043 children who were less than 18 years old, by the end of 2018, this number representing 0.026% of the corresponding population. Patients with CKD stages 1–2 make up 79.6%, whereas those with CKD stages 4–5 make up 12.0% [23].

Congenital malformations and dysplasia congenital anomalies of the kidney and urinary tract (CAKUT) (36.3%), glomerulonephritis (25.3%), polycystic kidney disease (7.8%), other cystic (2.9%), and renal (10.4%) dysplasia are the most frequent diagnoses in the Ukrainian children with CKD [23].

CAKUT is dominated in CKD 4–5 stages (36.1%). Also, an increasing trend of polycystic kidney disease and other renal dysplasia (13.0% and 18.1%, respectively) is observed [23, 24].

### Renal Replacement Therapy

The National Model of Pediatric RRT includes all the modalities (kidney transplant, HD, and PD). According to the legislation, government funding in this area should cover all costs; however, limited resources and actual special conditions contribute to the shift of the responsibility and financial liability on parents or caregivers.

According to the Register, the prevalence of ESRD among Ukrainian children and adolescents was 23.2 per million age-related population (pmarp) on May 1, 2018 [23], being stable since 2014 [22].

Although there are five pediatric dialysis centers in the country (Kyiv, Kharkiv, Odesa, Lviv, Zaporizhzhya), predialysis training (modality and access) is performed only in National Children Hospital "OHMATDYT" (Kyiv). Dialysis in AKI is carried out only in the National Children Hospital "OHMATDYT" with an annual rate of 30–40 children.

The information is, unfortunately, the only one on the prevalence and incidence of RRT in Ukraine.

### Hemodialysis

In 2018, the HD share of RRT was 30.1% among children and adolescents. The HD incidence among pediatric patients ranged from 12.0 to 16.0 pmarp in 2013–2018. The HD prevalence among the patients who are 0–17 years old was 7.0 pmarp (only adolescents constituted 56,6%) in 2018 [23].

### Peritoneal Dialysis

The PD's share in pediatric RRT was 13.6% with the incidence rate of 1–2 pmarp. The prevalence was 3.2 pmarp in 2018 (adolescents: 12.5%) [23].

### Kidney Transplantation

Kidney transplantation occupies the first position among RRT for Ukrainian children (56.3%). The prevalence among the 0–17 years old patients was 13.0 pmarp, whereas the majority were younger than 15 years of age (67.8%) [23, 24].

Since 2005, kidney transplantation has been performed in 158 pediatric patients. In most cases (67.7%), they were with living-related donors [20]; the youngest child was 9 months old. The largest number of transplants (66.3%) has taken place in recent years (2014–2018), whereas one-third of people underwent KT abroad (mainly in Belarus).

To sum up, the incidence and prevalence of RRT in the Ukrainian pediatric population are too low compared to those of other countries. An increase in the number of certified pediatric nephrologists and specialized centers can help to improve the situation in Ukraine.

## Nephrology Practice in Ukraine

Nephrology is not rated as a priority specialty among young professionals in Ukraine because of its association with a low salary (120–150 USD per month). As a result, specialized medical care for adults is provided by 437 nephrologists in Ukraine whereas there are only 94 certified pediatric nephrologists in Ukraine, although this number fluctuates throughout the year.

In order to obtain a degree in nephrology, one must graduate from a medical school (6 years), a complete residency of internal medicine (2 years), and go through 6 months of specialization. Subsequently, nephrologists in Ukraine have to confirm their qualification every 5 years, just like the ones in many European countries.

There are no issues with further employment for nephrologists in Ukraine. Nevertheless, the interest in nephrology among graduating students is extremely low because of the aforementioned salary. Surprisingly, the wages of nurse practitioners are about the same as those of doctors. A nephrologist, working in a private center, could earn 2–3-fold greater than in a state hospital.

Overall, one nephrology care team in Ukraine includes a nephrologist, advanced nurse practitioners, clinical laboratory specialists, and dialysis technicians. Regional dialysis centers typically include vascular surgeons and microbiological laboratories. Unfortunately, there are no dietitians, social workers, or pharmacists in the Ukrainian nephrology care teams. The Ministry of Health suggests one nephrologist, one nurse, and one dialysis technician for every eight HD machines per one dialysis shift. The Hospital Nephrology Unit comprises one nephrologist for 20 beds and one nephrologist for 25 PD patients.

## Highlights of Nephrology in Ukraine

### The Chernobyl Tragedy

Ukraine is affected significantly by the Chernobyl tragedy of 1986. In 2016, the data of the urinary system pathology among children born after 1995 were analyzed by their residence zones with different radioactive levels in 1986. The prevalence of urinary system pathology due to official statistics was 57.2 per 1000 children among the residents of the "compromised" zone (the most affected zone according to the maps of radioactive contamination in 1986) vs. 51.6 among those from the "clean" zone [25].

The study of 560 Ukrainian patients who have CKD 2–5 stages, congenital malformations, or dysplasia (single kidney, renal duplication, dystopia, hydronephrosis, cystic dysplasia, hypoplasia, others) found that the highest incidence was observed among the subjects born in 1995–2000 (59.5%). The portion of affected children who were from the "compromised" zones and born in 1995–2000 was lower than that of children from non-polluted areas (53.0% vs. 62.3%, $p = 0.009$) [25].

### The Restart of Nephrology in Ukraine

Although nephrology became a medical specialty in Ukraine in 1970, its active development began only 30 years later. Despite the imperfect CKD clinical scenario and other difficulties mentioned above, the number of RRT patients is constantly increasing year after year.

### World Kidney Day in Ukraine

In order to popularize the knowledge related to kidney disease among the Ukrainian population, the UANKTS team holds annual World Kidney Day activities in different regions of Ukraine.

## Future Perspectives of Nephrology in Ukraine

In Ukraine, perspectives of nephrology vary depending on the changes in the general medical care system. If the aim of the State Institutes is to build a modern healthcare system based on the partnership of the public and private hospitals, the situation will change for better as a result of:

- Increased number of nephrologists (at least 25–30 pmp)
- Implementation of the national CKD screening program
- Organization of AKI patients care system
- Creation of new centers of nephrology and dialysis
- Increased capacity in the existing centers
- Creation of a system that ensures implementation of KT
- Creation of multidisciplinary CKD Academic Center
- Organization of online consultations conducted by the Institute of Nephrology for patients from different Ukrainian regions
- Use of IT technologies for the optimization of diagnostics and treatment of complicated cases in regional and municipal departments of nephrology and dialysis

In terms of pediatric nephrology care, the need to create multidisciplinary working groups on the problems of pediatric nephrology is urgent. They would include urologists, pediatricians, transplantologists, and managers of the Ministry of Public Health. Other issues are connected to the amateur responsibility for personalized databases (registers) and connection to state programs.

Finally, it is appropriate to plan and conduct epidemiological studies related to ethnic homogeneity and the effects of special factors, particularly of indirect radiation exposure after the Chernobyl tragedy.

## Conclusion

The history of nephrology in Ukraine is 100 years old. Despite this, the availability and quality of nephrological assistance of patients are significantly lower in Ukraine than in the countries of the European Union. The low incidence and prevalence of RRT in the country suggest that the need is not satisfied. Considering the low transplantation rate and young dialysis population in Ukraine, it is suggested that strategies to reduce the RRT deficit in Ukraine should be the development and improvement of transplantation as well as home-based dialysis programs.

For the Ukrainians who are affected by the armed conflict, the hope for a better future derives first of all from the peace agreements, to which we are looking forward. Moreover, we hope for the creation of a modern medical care program for nephrology patients, a program based on transparent diversification of expenses. It can be created with the united efforts of the state, private individuals, and healthcare companies.

## References

1. World Atlas. 2018. https://www.worldatlas.com/webimage/countrys/europe/ukraine/ualand.htm. Accessed 20 Jan 2020.
2. State Statistics Service of Ukraine. 2019. https://ukrstat.org/en/operativ/menu/menu_e/ds.htm. Accessed 20 Jan 2020.
3. The World Bank. 2020. https://data.worldbank.org/country/ukraine. Accessed 20 Jan 2020.
4. United Nations Development Program. Human development reports. 2020. http://hdr.undp.org/en/countries/profiles/UKR. Accessed 20 Jan 2020.
5. Kolesnyk M, Kozliuk N, Razvazhaieva O. National registry of patients with chronic kidney disease and patients with acute kidney injury. State Institution «Institute of Nephrology of the National Academy of Medical Sciences»; 2019. [In Ukrainian].
6. Kolesnyk M, Kozliuk N, Razvazhaieva O, National registry of patients with chronic kidney disease and patients with acute kidney injury. State Institution «Institute of Nephrology of the National Academy of Medical Sciences»; 2018. [In Ukrainian].
7. Socol Y. Reconsidering health consequences of the chernobyl accident. Dose Response. 2015;13(1):14–40. https://doi.org/10.2203/dose-response.14-040.Socol.
8. Coupe T, Vakhitova H. Costs and benefits of labour mobility between the EU and the eastern partnership partner countries: Ukraine Country Study Kyiv. 2013. https://case-research.eu/sites/default/files/Ukraine%20country%20study%20-%20final.pdf. Accessed 20 Jan 2020.

9. Ministry of Health of Ukraine. National health reform strategy for Ukraine 2015–2020. http://healthsag.org.ua/wp-content/uploads/2015/03/Strategiya_Engl_for_inet.pdf. Accessed 20 Jan 2020.
10. Matevossian E, Kern H, Hüser N, Doll D, Snopok Y, Nährig J, Altomonte J, Sinicina I, Friess H, Thorban S. Surgeon Yurii Voronoy (1895–1961) – a pioneer in the history of clinical transplantation: in Memoriam at the 75th Anniversary of the First Human Kidney Transplantation. Transpl Int. 2009;22:1132–9. https://doi.org/10.1111/j.1432-2277.2009.00986.x.
11. Barker CF, Markmann JF. Historical overview of transplantation. Cold Spring Harb Perspect Med. 2013;3(4):a014977. https://doi.org/10.1101/cshperspect.a014977.
12. Kobza I, Chopyak V, Zhuk R, Petrov V. Organ transplantation in Ukraine – history in personalities and events. Proc Shevchenko Sci Soc Med Sci. 2018;52(1):25–32. https://doi.org/10.25040/ntsh2018.01.02.
13. Kolesnyk M, Driianska V, Liksunova L, Kozliuk N. Analysis of results and forecast of activities SI "Institute of Nephrology of the NAMS of Ukraine". Ukr J Nephrol Dial. 2019;3(63):3–16. https://doi.org/10.31450/ukrjnd.3(63).2019.01.
14. Kolesnyk M, Kozliuk N, Nikolaenko S, Kulizskyi M. National registry of patients with chronic kidney disease. State Institution «Institute of Nephrology of the National Academy of Medical Sciences»; 2014. [In Ukrainian].
15. Kolesnyk M, Liksunova L, Selezneva T, Maistrenko T. The cost of dialysis renal replacement therapy for end-stage renal disease patients in Ukraine. Ukr J Nephrol Dial. 2019;4(64):4–10. https://doi.org/10.31450/ukrjnd.4(64).2019.01.
16. Kolesnyk I, Noordzij M, Kolesnyk M, Kulyzky M, Jager KJ. Renal replacement therapy in Ukraine: epidemiology and international comparisons. Clin Kidney J. 2014;7(3):330–5. https://doi.org/10.1093/ckj/sfu037.
17. Clinical Practice Guideline on hemodialysis in adults. 2016. https://dec.gov.ua/wp-content/uploads/2019/11/2016_89_akn_xxn.pdf. Accessed 20 Jan 2020. [In Ukrainian].
18. Stepanova N, Burdeyna O. Association between dyslipidemia and peritoneal dialysis technique survival. Open Access Maced J Med Sci. 2019;7(15):2467–73. https://doi.org/10.3889/oamjms.2019.664.
19. Clinical Practice Guideline on peritoneal dialysis in adults. 2016. https://dec.gov.ua/wp-content/uploads/2019/11/2016_89_akn_pd.pdf. Accessed 20 Jan 2020. [In Ukrainian].
20. Bagdasarova IV, Fomina SP. Chronic kidney disease in children and renal replacement therapy in Ukraine. Ukr J Nephrol Dial. 2015;1:3–7. https://doi.org/10.31450/ukrjnd.1(45).2015.01.
21. Indicators of public health and use of health resources in Ukraine for 2012–2013. Center of Medical Statistics of the Ministry of Health of Ukraine. Kyiv; 2014. [In Ukrainian].
22. ESPN/ERA-EDTA registry: European registry for children on renal replacement therapy. 2016. https://espn-reg.org/index.jsp?p=pua. Accessed 20 Jan 2020.
23. Ukrainian Pediatric CKD Registry: 2011–2019 (unpublished data).
24. Antipkin YG, Volosovets OP, et al. Status of child population health – future of the country (part 1). Zdorov'e Rebenka. 2018;13(1):1–11. https://doi.org/10.22141/2224-0551.13.1.2018.127059.
25. Fomina SP, Bagdasarova IV. Urinary tract anomalies in children born in the years 1995–2012. The abstracts' book of the IV Congress of the Association Nephrologists of the Newly Independent States, September 29–30, Minsk, Belarus; 2016:125–126. [In Russian].

# Nephrology in the United Kingdom

# 51

Andrew J. P. Lewington

| | |
|---|---|
| Area[1] | 243,305 Km$^2$ |
| Population[2] | 67,530,172 (2019) |
| Capital | London (England)<br>Edinburgh (Scotland)<br>Cardiff (Wales)<br>Belfast (Northern Ireland) |
| Three most populated cities[3] | London – 9,750,500<br>Birmingham – 2,453,700<br>Manchester – 1,903,100 |
| Official language | English |
| Gross domestic product (GDP)[4] | £522,247 million (2019 Q3) |
| GDP per capita[5] | £33,251.59 (2019) |
| Human development index (HDI)[6] | 0.922 |
| Official currency | Pound Sterling |
| Total number of nephrologists[7] | 754 |
| National society of nephrology | Renal Association UK<br>British Renal Society<br>www.renal.org and www.britishrenal.org |
| Incidence of end-stage renal disease (Adult)[8, 9] | 2016 – 118 pmp<br>2017 – 121 pmp |
| Incidence of end-stage renal disease (Paediatric)[8, 9] | 2016 – 9 pmarp (per million age-related population)<br>2017 – 7.9 pmarp |
| Prevalence of end-stage renal disease (Adult)[8, 9] (including patients with a functioning kidney transplant) | 2016 – 962 pmp<br>2017 – 983 pmp |
| Prevalence of end-stage renal disease (Paediatric)[8, 9] | 2016 – 64.1 pmarp (per million age-related population)<br>2017 – 64.8 pmarp |
| Total number of (adult) patients on dialysis[8, 9] (all modalities) | 2016 – 28,876<br>2017 – 29,064 |
| Total number of (paediatric) patients on dialysis[8, 9] (all modalities) | 2016 – 964<br>2017 – 966 |
| Number of (adult) patients on haemodialysis[8, 9] | 2016 – 25,261<br>2017 – 25,553 |
| Number of (adult) patients on peritoneal dialysis[8, 9] | 2016 – 3615<br>2017 – 3531 |
| Number of (adult) renal transplantations per year[10] | 2017 – 3351<br>2018 – 3596 |

Table references:

1. www.thecommonwealth.org. Accessed 30/11/2019 13.55 hrs
2. www.worldometers.info. Accessed 30/11/2019 14.00 hrs
3. www.citymetric.com. Accessed 30/11/2019 14.02 hrs
4. www.ons.gov.uk/economy. Accessed 30/11/2019 14. 10 hrs
5. www.tradingeconomics.com. Accessed 30/11/2019 14.13 hrs
6. http://hdr.undp.org/sites/all/themes/hdr_theme/country-notes/GBR.pdf. Accessed 30/11/19 14.18 hrs
7. https://www.rcpmedicalcare.org.uk/developing-physicians/specialties/renal-medicine/workforce. Accessed 03/12/2019 22.59 hrs
8. UK Renal Registry 20th Annual Report 2018 (Data for 2016) www.renalreg.org. Accessed 16/02/20 22.20 hrs
9. UK Renal Registry 21st Annual Report 2019 (Data for 2017) www.renalreg.org. Accessed 16/02/20 23.27 hrs
10. https://nhsbtdbe.blob.core.windows.net/umbraco-assets-corp/12256/nhsbt-kidney-transplantation-annual-report-2017-2018.pdf. Accessed 30/11/2019 14.50 hrs

## Introduction

The United Kingdom (UK) is formed from the countries England, Scotland, Wales and Northern Ireland. The National Health Service (NHS) was founded on 5 July 1948 by Aneurin Bevan to provide free health care at the point of need [1]. It was the first time anywhere in the world that completely free health care was made available on the basis of citizenship rather than the payment of fees or insurance. Hospitals, doctors, nurses and dentists were brought together to work under one service. It includes NHS England, NHS Scotland, NHS Wales and the affiliated Health and Social Care in Northern Ireland and employs over 1,700,000 people with a budget of £139.3bn in 2019/20. All nephrology services in the UK are provided for free at the point of need, with very little private practice.

Nephrology in the UK has grown from its early beginnings into an established specialty with 84 renal units (71 adult and 13 paediatric) located in tertiary referral hospitals

A. J. P. Lewington (✉)
Renal Department, St. James's University Hospital, Leeds Teaching Hospitals Trust, Leeds, UK
e-mail: andrew.lewington@nhs.net



J. A. Moura-Neto et al. (eds.), *Nephrology Worldwide*, https://doi.org/10.1007/978-3-030-56890-0_51

across the country. More recently there has been a growth in the number of nephrologists working in the smaller district general hospitals that surround and refer in to the larger more specialised nephrology units. The population in the UK is relatively underserved with nephrologists compared to comparable European countries with 8.5 per million population [2]. The Renal Association (RA) was founded in 1950 to represent the profession [3]. The British Renal Society (BRS) was formed later in 2001 developing on from The British Renal Symposium as it was recognised a society was needed that embraced all of the specialist groups caring for patients with kidney disease [4]. Scotland has its own independent Renal Association. The British Association of Paediatric Nephrology (BAPN) was founded in 1973 [5].

Haemodialysis became established in the UK in the 1950s, and the first kidney deceased donor transplant was performed in Leeds in 1959 [6]. Home therapies including peritoneal dialysis (PD) and home haemodialysis remain less well developed in the UK. In 2009 the National Confidential Enquiry into Patient Outcomes and Death (NCEPOD) Acute Kidney Injury (AKI) 'adding insult to injury' report was published. The report led to a national programme to improve the outcomes of patients with AKI in the UK [7].

In 2017, 8001 adult patients commenced renal replacement therapy (RRT) for end-stage renal disease (ESRD), which represented an overall incidence rate of 121 per million population (pmp). The majority of patients were male (64.1%) with a median age of 63.7 years. Diabetes was the leading cause of ESRD in patients starting RRT (29.4%) in 2017. At the end of 2017, there were 64,887 adults receiving RRT for ESRD in the UK, representing an increase of 3.0% from 2016 and a UK prevalence rate of 983 pmp. Most patients on RRT had a functioning transplant (55.2%) followed by in centre haemodialysis (37.3%), peritoneal dialysis (5.4%) and home haemodialysis (2.0%) [8].

In the UK, the NHS established a Clinical Reference Group (CRG) to cover the delivery of treatment for acute kidney injury, dialysis and kidney transplantation for patients with ESRD. These are referred to as specialised services and are funded by NHS England and have to meet a defined set of standards. These standard specifications have been developed by specialised clinicians, commissioners, expert patients and public health representatives to describe both core and developmental service standards. Core standards are those that all funded providers should be able to demonstrate, with developmental standards being those which may require further changes in practice over time to provide excellence in the field [9].

In recent years, the importance of the patient voice and the need for shared care and decision-making have been increasingly recognised within the NHS. There are a number of national (and local) influential patient charities including Kidney Care UK, the National Kidney Federation and the Polycystic Kidney Disease Charity. These charities play an important role in working with the renal societies to lobby commissioners and the government for further investment and development of nephrology services. Research into kidney disease in the UK like many other countries is grossly underfunded by the government but is well supported by the main charity Kidney Research UK (KRUK) along with many local charities.

Some of the main challenges for UK nephrology include slowing the progression of chronic kidney disease (CKD) in native and kidney transplants and preventing AKI. The clinical pressure on nephrology services is ever-increasing which has undoubtedly had an effect on trainee recruitment in some areas due to the intensity of work. Initiatives from the societies and local units to attract and retain trainees have been successful in some centres. There is a long tradition of overseas trainees studying in UK Renal Units adding an international perspective and leading to long-lasting collaborations. Currently all nephrology units are running at capacity reinforcing the need to offer more remote patient care through telemedicine and increase the numbers of kidney transplants and patients on home therapies. With an aging population, there is increasing interest in how to approach multi-morbidity and frailty in patient care.

## Brief History of Nephrology in the United Kingdom

The earliest accounts of nephrology in the UK described in the Renal Association (RA) archives date from the 1950s of Robert Platt and Arthur Ellis who worked on nephritis and chronic renal failure and Clifford Wilson who specialised on hypertension, diabetes and nephritis [3].

Haemodialysis was first performed on a dozen patients in the UK by Eric Bywaters and Mark Joekes in London at the Hammersmith Hospital in 1946–1947 [10]. They were the third team in the world to use the artificial kidney. However, there was little evidence that the treatment was superior to conservative therapy, and the program closed down. It was not until 1956 that haemodialysis was reintroduced into the UK in Leeds, followed by five new units opening across the UK in 1959. Regional dialysis units were opened in the mid- to late 1960s. There was then very little further expansion of nephrology services for almost 20 years in the UK. The first deceased donor kidney transplant was performed at the Leeds General Infirmary in 1959, and the first live donor kidney transplant was performed between identical twins in Edinburgh in 1960.

The Renal Association was formed on 30 March 1950 in London at a meeting of a diverse group of specialists. It is one of the oldest renal societies in the world second only to the Société de Pathologie Rénale that held its first meeting in Paris in February 1949 [11]. There were 30 attendees at the first meeting of the Renal Association that included urologists and obstetricians as well as physiologists and physicians. Arnold Osman was the first president of the Renal Association and is still recognised by the Osman lecture at the annual conference. In 1953 the Renal Association organised the first international meeting on all aspects of kidney function and disease.

Nephrology was slow to establish itself as a specialty in the UK and was not recognised as such by the Royal College of Physicians until 1967. The Ministry of Health also failed to recognise the specialty until a survey of manpower in nephrology units was performed and published in the British Medical Journal in 1976 [12].

The British Renal Society (BRS) was established in 2001 to represent the whole multiprofessional nephrology team evolving from the British Renal Symposium, an annual meeting started in 1989 which focused on research and education in the care of patients with kidney disease. The BRS is a federation of the various professional groups representing those involved in nephrology.

In 1996 the UK Renal Registry (UKRR) was established by the Renal Association under the guidance of Terry Feest, with the primary aim of collating data centrally from all adult UK nephrology centres to improve the care of patients with ESRD [13]. The first UKRR report was published in 1998. The UKRR achieved complete UK wide electronic data collection on 100% of patients receiving dialysis in 2009. The UKRR reports are recognised as authoritative and provide crucial data for the NHS and the Department of Health.

There are 62 Renal units in England, 10 units in Scotland, 6 in Wales and 6 in Northern Ireland. Today most data are collected from nephrology centres via automatic quarterly downloads. English, Welsh and Northern Irish centres send their data directly to the UKRR. The UKRR identifies and resolves errors and inconsistencies before detailed statistical analyses are performed. Scottish data are collected, validated and published by the Scottish Renal Registry before they are shared with the UKRR. The UKRR collects, analyses and reports on data from 71 adult and 13 paediatric renal centres. Participation is mandated in England through the NHS National Service Specification, and the Chief Executive of each Trust is responsible for adherence to this contract.

The UKRR is funded through an annual capitation fee levied on patients receiving dialysis which in 2016 was £27.50 per patient in England and £22.50 in Wales and Northern Ireland. The Renal Registry Dataset Specification (RRDSS) is available on its website and defines the data currently collected. The data are published annually in the UKRR Annual Report. The report acts as a source of data for audit and benchmarking against the quality of care standards created by the Renal Association and other organisations such as the National Institute of Health and Care Excellence (NICE). The data is a shared resource and used to develop further research into kidney disease and improve the quality of care for patients.

The British Association for Paediatric Nephrology (BAPN) was founded by Richard White with the first meeting on 22 February 1973 in London [5]. Over the last decade, the BAPN has worked increasingly closely with the Renal Association. In 2010 the BAPN ceased to be an independent entity and became a 'chapter' of the Renal Association.

The Renal Association was one of the first national societies to develop clinical standards against which quality of care could be audited locally and also nationally through the UKRR. The standards were then developed as clinical practice guidelines and overseen by an appointed chair [14]. The Clinical Practice Guidelines applied and were successful in achieving the much converted NICE accreditation in 2011. As a result, the guidelines are hugely influential in shaping national policy and delivery of services. More recently, in recognition of many different guideline bodies, there has been an attempt to avoid repetition and where another respected guideline body such as NICE or KDIGO issues a guideline the Renal Association will produce a commentary to highlight any specific considerations relevant to UK practice. There are a number of other committees with one of the most recent being the Equal Opportunities in Nephrology Committee. This was created to demonstrate the Renal Association's commitment to support and develop equality of opportunity in nephrology in the UK. The committee aims to improve access to mentoring and career advice for nephrologists and also encourage women in leadership.

The importance of the patient voice and the need for shared care and decision- making have been increasingly recognised within the NHS. There are a number of national (and local) influential patient charities including the National Kidney Federation [15] and the Polycystic Kidney Disease (PKD) Charity [16]. Kidney Care UK [17] is an organisation whose main purpose is support quality improvement in kidney care as part of implementation of the National Service Framework. There has been an expansion in the role of the multidisciplinary team and specialised clinics to care for patients with kidney disease.

Research into kidney disease in the UK like many other countries is grossly underfunded by the government but is well supported by the main charity Kidney Research UK (KRUK) along with many local charities [18]. Kidney Research UK has collaborated with the Renal Association and British Renal Society to from the UK Kidney Research

Consortium (UKKRC) in 2007. The UKKRC was established in 2007 and is jointly supported by the Renal Association, Kidney Research UK and the British Renal Society. The aim is to facilitate the best collaborative clinical research for health in kidney disease.

## Renal Diseases in the United Kingdom

Kidney disease can be broadly considered as acute kidney injury (AKI) or chronic kidney disease (CKD) and represents an underappreciated UK public health challenge facing the NHS [19].

### Chronic Kidney Disease

Chronic kidney disease can be considered as a gradual loss of kidney function over time [20]. Kidney disease may be detected by routine testing in people with diabetes or hypertension. Diabetes is the most common cause of CKD in the UK and has been associated with increased rates of obesity. CKD is classified in five stages, according to the level of kidney function and the presence of albumin in the urine. Patients with CKD stages 3–5 have moderate to severe kidney disease. As kidney disease progresses, they are become less effective at removing waste products from blood resulting in the accumulation of water, waste and toxic substances in the body. The kidneys are also important endocrine organs involved in blood pressure regulation, the secretion of erythropoietin to stimulate red blood cell production and bone metabolism. In the earlier stages of CKD, there are no symptoms. A relatively small proportion of patients with CKD will develop complete kidney failure and require dialysis or a kidney transplant. CKD is associated with a significant increased risk of stroke, heart disease, bone disease and anaemia [21]. It is estimated that there are 40,000–45,000 premature deaths each year in people with CKD [20]. CKD has been shown to be associated with reduced quality of life.

Chronic kidney disease is a major cause of mortality and morbidity which consumes a substantial healthcare resource [22]. CKD substantially reduces quality of life and can lead to premature death. It was estimated that in England in 2014, there were 2.6 million adults (6.1% of the population) aged over 16 years living with CKD stage 3–5 [23]. The cost of CKD to the NHS in England was estimated at 1.44–1.45 billion pounds in 2009–2010, which is equivalent to nearly 1.3% of the annual NHS budget [24]. The cost includes both treatment directly associated with CKD and also treatment for excess non-kidney problems such as strokes, heart attacks and infections in people with CKD. In 2009–2010, there were an estimated 7000 extra strokes and 12,000 extra heart attacks in people with CKD, relative to the expected number in people of the same age and sex without CKD. The cost to the NHS of health care related to these strokes and heart attacks is estimated at £174–178 million [25]. Patients with CKD have an increased length of hospital stay, averaging 35% longer. With increased life expectancy and multimorbidity, the prevalence of CKD will continue to increase [26].

A number of national policy initiatives have been introduced in England that may have had an impact on the prevention, detection and management of CKD over the past decade [27]. In 2004–2005, the National Service Framework for Renal Services promoted the national reporting of frequency of CKD [28]. A new Quality Outcomes Framework (QOF) for primary care introduced payments linked to targets for CKD (2006), hypertension and diabetes management [29]. Major improvements in the management of hypertension have subsequently been demonstrated [30]. In 2014 the National Institute of Health and Care Excellence (NICE) published Chronic Kidney Disease in Adults: Assessment and Management Clinical Guideline (CG182) [31].

There are very few proven therapeutic interventions to slow the progression of CKD beyond tight blood pressure control. In the England, NICE published a favourable assessment of the use of tolvaptan in 2015 for patients meeting defined criteria to slow the progression of polycystic kidney disease [32]. A number of nephrology units have established specialised clinics to assess patient's suitability for the treatment and monitor response if commenced on tolvaptan.

### Acute Kidney Injury

Acute kidney injury (AKI) can be considered as a rapid reduction in kidney function occurring over hours to days [33]. Newer definitions are based on rises in serum creatinine and/or reductions in urine output [34]. The severity of AKI is staged on a scale of 1–3 based on the rise in creatinine from baseline or the reduction in urine output. Higher AKI scores are associated with increased morbidity, mortality, length of stay and a risk of CKD [35]. It has been estimated that AKI costs the NHS in England £1.02 billion [36]. AKI is a syndrome with multiple causes. The most common causes in the UK occur in acutely ill patients with sepsis, toxins, hypovolaemia, hypotension and/or obstruction. Other rarer causes include vasculitis, interstitial nephritis, glomerulonephritis and myeloma.

The Department of Health launched the National Service Framework (NSF) for Renal Services. Part one of the NSF for Renal Services was published in 2004 and established five standards for dialysis and transplantation for people with established renal failure. In 2005 Part two of the NSF for

Renal Services set out a new framework of standards identified four quality requirements covering chronic kidney disease, acute renal failure and end of life care [37]. In 2007 Donal O'Donoghue became the first National Clinical Director for Kidney Care for England. On behalf of The Renal Association, John Feehally submitted a proposal to the National Confidential Enquiry into Patient Outcomes and Death (NCEPOD) to examine the care of patients who died with a diagnosis of acute kidney injury. In 2009 the NCEPOD Acute Kidney Injury 'adding insult to injury' report was published [7]. The report identified multiple deficiencies in the care of patients that died from a diagnosis of AKI. The report was discussed in the House of Parliament, and a national programme of work was established by Donal O'Donoghue to improve the outcomes of patients with AKI. The Renal Association, the Royal Colleges and NHS Kidney Care worked together to promote improvements in care in this previously neglected area of nephrology.

The Department of Health established an AKI Delivery Board with a multiprofessional membership in recognition of the nature of the breadth of specialties involved in caring for patients with AKI. There were a number of initiatives that included the AKI UK Consensus Conference on the Management of acute kidney injury: the role of fluids, e-alerts and biomarkers held at Royal College of Physicians of Edinburgh on November 2012 [38]. This was soon followed by the publication of the Acute Kidney Injury: Prevention, Detection and Management Clinical Guideline (CG169) by NICE in 2013 [39]. The NCEPOD report highlighted that education on AKI was poor, and Mike Jones led on introducing formal education on AKI in the national post-graduate curriculum.

Further work was continued by the Think Kidneys national programme led by Richard Fluck, which was set up to continue to improve the care of patients with AKI and provide educational resources [40]. NHS England produced a patient safety notice that mandated all UK NHS trusts to implement the NHS AKI warning algorithm into their laboratories [41]. The AKI warning was initially launched in secondary care in April 2016 and then rolled out into primary care. The NHS AKI algorithm was based on the Kidney Disease: Improving Global Outcomes (KDIGO) AKI criteria, which is universally accepted as a biochemical definition for AKI [42]. The AKI warning is transmitted as an AKI e-alert that should prompt a clinical review to determine whether the patient has a clinical diagnosis of AKI. All AKI alerts are submitted to the UK Renal Registry by the laboratories which are linked with the master patient index and provide an opportunity to better characterise AKI epidemiology and associated morbidity and mortality and to develop AKI risk prediction models.

It has been reported that 6–8% of hospital admissions have AKI [43]. Further analysis has identified 60% of these patients have AKI when they reach hospital [35] This has led to the distinction of community-acquired AKI (c-AKI) from hospital-acquired AKI (h-AKI). Patients with c-AKI admitted to hospital have a mortality of 19.6% during hospitalisation (lower than h-AKI), which increases to 45% 14 months post-discharge [43]. The incidence of c-AKI detected in primary care and not admitted to hospital within 7 days using the official NHS AKI algorithm was reported as 1.4% in a Scottish registry [44]. This study showed that these patients were of similar age but suffered fewer comorbidities than patients with c-AKI that were admitted to hospital. The mortality rates were 17% and 42.3%, respectively, at 1 year. Patients with c-AKI who were not admitted to hospital were also less likely to make a full recovery of kidney function when compared with those who were admitted with c-AKI. In response to these important publications the Royal College of General Practitioners (RCGP) has produced an AKI toolkit [45].

In England the Commissioning for Quality and Innovation (CQUIN) provide payment targets to improve health care provided by care providers. In 2016 a national AKI CQUIN was developed that mandated the diagnosis and severity of AKI was included in a patient's discharge summary to improve the transition of care. It has been proposed that AKI and CKD are intertwined bidirectional clinical syndromes with CKD being a risk factor for AKI and AKI a risk factor for subsequent episodes of AKI and development of CKD [46]. The aim of the CQUIN was to improve the recognition of new cases of CKD and highlight patients at risk of further AKI events.

## Renal Replacement Therapy in the United Kingdom

### Haemodialysis

It was during the bombing of London in the second world war that Eric Bywaters at the Hammersmith Hospital became interested in the histopathology of the acute kidney injury (AKI) caused by crush injury. Towards the end of the war whilst Mark Joekes was researching a new treatment for malaria at the Hammersmith Hospital, he received a copy of one of Willem Kolff's earliest papers on the artificial kidney. Joekes recognised the potential for dialysis and set up a unit under the supervision of Eric Bywaters. Willem Kolff had successfully hid an artificial kidney from the occupying forces in Holland which was transported to the Hammersmith Hospital by Bywaters in 1946. Between 1946 and 1947, a dozen patients at the Hammersmith Hospital received haemodialysis [3]. The initial results failed to demonstrate any advantage of dialysis over conservative treatment with diet and electrolytes, and the unit was closed.

Interest in haemodialysis was not revisited until the mid-1950s. Leslie Pyrah was a surgeon at the Leeds General Infirmary and had played a leading part in the establishment of urology as a specialty in the UK. He arranged for his registrar, Frank Parsons, to study in Chicago in 1955. Whilst in the USA, Parsons spent the last 3 months at the Peter Bent Brigham Hospital, Boston, to learn about the drum-coil artificial kidney. Frank Parsons managed to convince the Leeds Infirmary Board of Governors to purchase a Kolff-Brigham dialyser for £5500 from Boston. In 1956 Parsons transported the dialyzer to Leeds, although as the dialyzer was en route across the Atlantic, he was summoned to the Medical Research Council and told 'Our advisors tell us there is no place for an artificial kidney in British medicine' and 'Parsons, try it, but remember the country is against you'. Despite the lack of support, Frank Parsons established haemodialysis for AKI at Leeds General Infirmary in 1956 [3]. Parsons demonstrated the utility of dialysis through treating 70 patients with AKI [47]. At this time, patients were transported from across the UK to receive treatment in Leeds.

Following Parson's success, urologist Ralph Shackman opened a haemodialysis unit at the Hammersmith Hospital using the French Usifroid version of the rotating drum dialyser in 1957/1958. Mark Joekes was now supporting Group Captain Ralph Jackson to deliver haemodialysis using the new Travenol twin-coil kidney at the RAF unit based at Halton hospital in Buckinghamshire. Further acute dialysis units were subsequently set up in Edinburgh, Belfast, Glasgow, Newcastle and the London hospital during 1959.

The first haemodialysis unit for chronic kidney disease (CKD) in the UK was established by Stanley Shaldon at the Royal Free Hospital, London. Shaldon was later the first to introduce home dialysis to the UK in 1964, and The Royal Free has also been credited as the first unit to train and employ nurse technicians to oversee dialyses [48].

Haemodialysis units across the country have developed along a hub and spoke model with haemodialysis provided in satellite units adjacent or within smaller district general hospitals who are served by the larger tertiary referral teaching hospitals with nephrology units. The 21st UK Renal Registry Report on the 2017 data returns from across the UK reported that there were 25,553 patients receiving haemodialysis or haemodiafiltration in the UK. The majority of patients (94.5%) in the UK on in centre HD receive dialysis three times a week with 74.5% of patients having dialysis for 4–5 hours per session, and 86.8% achieved dialysis adequacy as defined by a urea reduction ratio of >65%. Of the prevalent haemodialysis population in 2017, approximately 32% had a tunnelled or non-tunnelled catheter and approximately 68% had an arteriovenous fistula or graft (rarely). In 2017 the overall death rate was 91 per 1000 prevalent RRT patients with an overall relative risk of death of 7.6 [8].

## Peritoneal Dialysis

It is not well documented when peritoneal dialysis (PD) was first used in the UK. There are reports from 1959 that a number of patients underwent PD in preparation for receiving a kidney transplant. Peritoneal dialysis became very popular in the UK throughout the 1980s and 1990s in the face of significant limitations in the provision of hospital and satellite haemodialysis facilities. Over the recent years, PD programmes have gradually shrunk and vary between 5% and 30% of the total dialysis population. In 2016 there were 3615 patients on peritoneal dialysis [49]. Automated PD has become increasingly popular and is the most common modality in many units. In 2017, 40% of PD patients were on continuous ambulatory PD, and 60% were on automated PD. In 2016–2017, the PD peritonitis rate in England was 1 : 26.7 months. The leading cause of death in patients on PD < 65 years was cardiac disease (30.1%) and in older patients on PD > 65 years was treatment withdrawal (25.1%) [8]. PD continues to be offered as a self-care home-based therapy. Assisted PD in the home supported by helpers other than relatives is now available for some patients, and PD delivered by nursing home carers has assumed an increasing role for older frailer PD patients. Further research is ongoing to improve patient self-monitoring in the community.

## Kidney Transplantation

Peter Raper was a urologist at Leeds General Infirmary (LGI) who had previously worked with Frank Parsons in treating renal artery stenosis. Raper is credited to have performed the first deceased donor kidney transplant in Leeds on 13 July 1959. He went on to perform a total of nine deceased donor kidney transplants up to 1966 [3]. At this time, little was known about the immune system or the medication required to prevent rejection. The first patient received total body irradiation preoperatively and died perioperatively; the next two had cyclophosphamide alone, and in the remainder a combination of cyclophosphamide and steroids. One patient survived for 8 months with a functional transplant sadly to die of a viral infection [50].

On 30 October 1960, Michael Woodruff performed the first UK living donor kidney transplant between 49 years old identical twins. The recipient lived for a further 6 years before dying of an unrelated illness [51]. At the Royal Free in London, three kidney transplants were performed between 1959 and 1960. The first two were deceased donor kidney transplants and failed. The third transplant was a live kidney donor transplant from father to son performed on 1 November 1960 [3]. The recipient survived 41 days, dying with tuberculosis. This was the first organ transplant from a live related non-sibling donor in the world using chemotherapy (6-mercaptopurine and prednisolone) to prevent rejection.

NHS Blood and Transplant reported that 4757 patients were waiting for a kidney transplant in 2018 [52]. In 2018, 408 patients died in the UK whilst on the transplant waiting list. There have been a number of initiatives over the years in the UK to increase the number of kidney transplants and reduce the number of patients on the waiting list. There has been an increase in the number of units able to provide donation after circulatory death (DCD) and efforts to increase living kidney donation.

In 2017/2018, there were 3272 adult kidney only transplants performed in the UK an increase of 7% compared to 2016/17. Of these, 1380 were from donation after brain death (DBD) donors, 940 were from DCD donors and 952 were from living donors. There were 130 paediatric kidney transplants performed in 2017/2018, representing a 2% increase from the previous year [52]. The UK kidney transplant survival rate at 5 years after first adult deceased donor kidney only transplant is 86%. These rates vary between centres, ranging from 76% to 91% (risk adjusted). The equivalent rate after first paediatric deceased donor kidney only transplant is 85%, ranging from 75% to 100%. The UK kidney transplant survival rate at 5 years after first adult living donor kidney only transplant is 93%. These rates vary between centres, ranging from 87% to 96% (risk adjusted). The equivalent rate after first paediatric living donor kidney only transplant is 86%, ranging from 78% to 100%.

The UK Living Kidney Sharing Scheme (UKLKSS) was launched in April 2007 to allow patients with friends and family who were not able to donate because of incompatible blood group or tissue (HLA) type [53]. The scheme allows a patient to enter the sharing scheme with their friend or family member and then awaits a matching run (performed four times per year) to see if they are matched with another couple in the scheme. If matching occurs, each recipient receives a kidney from the other's friend or family member. This kidney exchange programme increases the number of people who can receive transplants from living kidney donors and the opportunities for patients who wait a long time for a transplant. In March 2019, the UKLKSS performed the 1000th kidney transplant. Since the scheme was created.

Nondirected altruistic donation of an organ from a live donor to a stranger was made legal in by the Human Tissue Act 2004 and Human Tissue (Scotland) Act 2006. Since this time, there has been a slow but steady increase in the number of altruistic donors in the UK. Six people donated in 2007 increasing to 107 donors in 2018 [54]. A recent change in allocation practice in the UK means that one altruistic donor can start a chain of three transplants between incompatible pairs in the UKLKSS. In 2017/18, 22% of all UK adult kidney transplants and 11% of kidney transplants in children were from nondirected altruistic or paired exchange donations. As of January 2018, all those who come forward to be a nondirected altruistic donor are registered in the UKLKSS, unless there is a high priority recipient on the waiting list.

In 2019 a new kidney offering scheme was introduced by NHS Blood and Transplant in the UK to reflect the changing donor pool and to address some of the inequities observed in the previous scheme [55]. The new kidney offering scheme will allocate all kidneys from both deceased brain dead (DBD) and deceased after circulatory death (DCD) donors and will more effectively match kidney transplant life expectancy with patient life expectancy.

From spring 2020, an 'opt out' system will be implemented whereby all adults in England will be considered an organ donor when they die unless they have recorded a decision not to donate on the Organ Donor Register or are in one of the excluded groups. This is referred to as an 'opt out' system [56]. People under 18, people who have lived in England for less than 12 months or who are not living here voluntarily and people who lack the capacity to understand the change will be excluded. Evidence from Wales suggests that consent rates have increased significantly since they introduced the opt out system in 2015.

## Nephrology Practice in the United Kingdom

### Adult Care

In the UK, there are 71 adult renal units located in teaching hospitals. Patients with kidney disease are cared for on dedicated nephrology wards with specialised nephrology teams. In hospitals without renal units, patients with kidney disease will be admitted to general medical wards. In many of these hospitals, there are nephrologists who will also cover internal medicine. Patients within these hospitals needing dialysis or other specialised kidney care will need to be transferred to the local renal unit if stable. Unstable patients requiring urgent dialysis will have to receive care in the intensive care unit.

In the UK, many renal unit wards are not plumbed for haemodialysis, and patients will need to be transferred to the main dialysis unit for treatment. A smaller number of renal units are plumbed, and patients can receive haemodialysis whilst staying on the ward. Some units in the UK have their own high dependency units and can provide haemodialysis, although in most hospitals, patients are frequently managed on general high dependency units. These units are typically not plumbed for haemodialysis, and patients may have to be moved through the hospital to the dialysis unit. With respect to vascular access and the insertion of peritoneal dialysis access, practice is fairly varied in the UK. Traditionally the kidney transplant surgeons would create arteriovenous fistulas and insert PD catheters. Over the recent years, the vascular surgeons have taken on this responsibility. Temporary dialysis catheters are more usually inserted by nephrologists under ultrasound guidance with the more challenging cases referred to radiology. As kidney biopsy is no longer a required skill for nephrology trainees, it is now increasingly performed by radiology.

There are 24 NHS specialist kidney transplant centres in the UK with 6 in London [57]. There is variation in the models of patient care with some centres preferring a more surgical-led approach to both the inpatient and outpatient care, whilst other units prefer a joint medical and surgical approach. Some centres have separate kidney transplant wards, and others care for patients with kidney transplants on general nephrology wards. After discharge from the specialist kidney transplant centre following the surgery, patients are reviewed in their own local renal units. All centres are now working as multidisciplinary teams in the assessment and care of patients.

Over the recent years, there has been an expansion in the number of specialised clinics in renal units to match the increase in patients with kidney disease. These clinics include low clearance clinics, to include low clearance transplant clinics, ADPKD clinics, adolescent transition clinics, vasculitis clinics, joint obstetric/renal clinics, joint diabetes/renal clinics, joint rheumatology/renal clinics and joint urology/renal stone clinics. Many of these clinics are delivered by a multiprofessional team including nurse specialists, dieticians and pharmacists.

Patients admitted to the intensive care unit (ICU) in the UK will be cared for by the intensivists, nephrology or by both teams depending on whether the ICU is an open or closed ICU. An online survey of all general adult UK ICU was performed 2009–2010. There was a 72% response rate from the 233 ICUs approached [58]. In 40% of ICUs, the nephrology team is never or rarely consulted about patients with AKI. The most commonly used form of dialysis is either continuous venovenous haemofiltration (CVVH) or continuous venovenous haemodialysis (CVVHD). Continuous forms of dialysis are performed by the ICU nurses and overseen by the intensivists. Intermittent haemodialysis (IHD) is rarely used and is managed by nephrologists. The practice of critical care nephrology whereby the nephrology team manage the patient on ICU is less common now partly due to shortages of nephrology trainees and the development of closed ICUs where the intensivists do not welcome other specialties managing patients.

## Paediatric Care

There are 13 tertiary paediatric renal units in the UK which are equipped to provide peritoneal dialysis (PD) and haemodialysis (HD). Ten of these centres also perform kidney transplantation. Young people aged 16–18 years may be managed in either paediatric or adult services. This is variable across the UK and dependent on local practices, social factors and patient/family wishes. In the UK, in 2015, the prevalence rate of children and adolescents aged 16 years receiving treatment for end-stage kidney disease was 62.7 per million age-related population (pmarp), and the incidence rate was 10.2 pmarp [59].

## Training

Over recent years, in the UK, there has been a declining interest in training in nephrology. It has been proposed that the lack of interest in nephrology as a specialty is multifactorial. Nephrology is recognised as a demanding profession and is considered by some trainees to have a poor work-life balance. The opportunities for private practice are also restricted in comparison with other specialties such as cardiology and dermatology. With an increase in female graduates, there is a pressing need to develop more imaginative and flexible training posts within nephrology [60].

Currently, it is possible to qualify as a consultant nephrologist in 3 years following 4–5 years training in internal medicine. However, most trainees prefer to combine their training with another specialty such as general internal medicine, intensive care medicine or clinical pharmacology over a 5-year period. Nephrology training programmes in the UK will cover all aspects of kidney disease including acute kidney injury, glomerular and interstitial diseases, chronic kidney disease and the management of end-stage kidney disease with dialysis and transplantation. The training has a strong emphasis on clinical leadership and multidisciplinary teamworking, with opportunities to undertake practical procedures such as the insertion of dialysis catheters. Kidney biopsy is no longer a mandatory requirement, and the opportunities to perform are more restricted. Some trainees choose to take an academic or educational period out of training (OOP) to perform research or develop leadership skills. Involvement in clinical research is now encouraged as it has been recognised that NHS hospitals that engage in clinical research have better patient outcomes [61].

All doctors intending to practise medicine in the UK are required to be registered with the General Medical Council (GMC). Doctors qualifying from outside the UK may be eligible to apply directly for full registration if they hold an acceptable primary medical qualification and have completed a period of postgraduate clinical experience (internship). To practice as a specialist consultant in nephrology, a doctor must be on the specialist register of the GMC. To be eligible to apply for specialist registration with the GMC, doctors must have successfully completed a GMC-approved training programme and been granted one of the following certificates: Certificate of Completion of

Training (CCT) or a Certificate confirming Eligibility for Specialist Registration (CESR). Doctors who have not completed a full GMC-approved training programme and wish to have their training, qualifications and experience assessed for eligibility for entry onto the specialist register must make an application under The General and Specialist Medical Practice Order for a CESR. It is not possible to hold specialist registration without also holding full registration [62].

## Nephrology Working Practice

The NHS employs 8.5 nephrologists per million population to manage kidney disease in the UK, which is at the lower end of the scale among European countries. More than half of nephrologists will also contribute to general internal medicine, thereby reducing the time available for specialised nephrology care [63]. Nephrologists may practice in many different ways, e.g. general nephrologists, transplant nephrologists, academic nephrologists, interventional nephrologists, haemodialysis and peritoneal dialysis nephrologists. Nephrologists in the UK work in teams, sharing responsibilities with each other and with multiprofessional colleagues. Most nephrology units in the UK now have multiple specialist clinics, e.g. clinics for people with diabetes, pregnancy, lupus and vasculitis and transition clinics for young adults transferring from paediatric clinics.

In the UK, the inpatient workload has become very 'consultant heavy' and requires a significant commitment. In renal units, patients with renal disease are cared for on dedicated nephrology wards with appropriate nursing expertise. The nephrology team will also review patients outside of the renal unit across the hospital with kidney-related disease, e.g. AKI, and kidney patients under the care of other clinicians, including intensive care. Ward rounds are performed every day of the week, including weekends, and may include 40–50 patients. Consultants will cover different areas of the service for a variable number of weeks and then rotate to other duties. Additionally, consultants will be rostered for night time and weekend cover with a variable number of trainees. Many nephrologists travel to outlying dialysis units and hospitals to facilitate care closer to the patient's home. The profile of AKI has increased significantly in recent years, which has led to a major increase in referrals for specialist nephrological opinion. This has led to the need to expand nephrology expertise in the smaller district general hospitals. A newly appointed consultant nephrologist will commence on a salary of £79,860 per year which can rise to a maximum of £107,668 after 19 years service to the NHS, over 8 increments. By comparison a newly qualified Band 5 nurse will commence on £22,128 per year and reach a maximum of £28,746 over 8 increments, and a Band 6 nurse will start on £26,565 rising to £35,577 over 9 increments.

## Highlights of Nephrology in the United Kingdom

### Acute Kidney Injury

The UK has a long history of recognizing and furthering the clinical management of AKI dating back to the first descriptions of crush injury during the bombing of London in the Second World War [10]. Leeds then set up the first renal unit for the treatment of patients with AKI [3]. In 2009 the NCEPOD AKI report led to a national NHS campaign to improve the care of people at risk of, or with, AKI [7]. This initiative has produced a wide range of guidance and information for people working in all healthcare sectors to help with the prevention, detection, management and treatment of AKI. In 2014 the NHS mandated that all NHS hospitals introduced an AKI warning into the biochemistry departments that was transmitted to the clinical team as an AKI-alert. The UKRR has developed a master patient index of people who have had a blood test that triggered AKI alert across England. The master patient index will link with the NHS Hospital Episode Statistics (HES) to allow hospital specific reporting of AKI rates. More recent work in the UK has demonstrated an improvement in the quality of care of patients with AKI and a reduced length of stay when a care bundle supported by an education package was linked to the AKI alert [64]. The UK is now recognised as having the most advanced systems in place for the detection and management of AKI in the world.

### UK Kidney Research Consortium and the NIHR Clinical Research Network

The Renal Association and BRS took the initiative with Kidney Research UK (KRUK) to establish a UK Kidney Research Consortium (UKKRC). The Consortium established 12 clinical specialty groups (CSGs) to develop national clinical trials in nephrology. The UKKRC has also gone on to establish three renal networks – the UK Renal Imaging Network, the Kidney Patient Involvement Network and the UK Renal Trials Network.

The NHS established the NIHR Clinical Research Network (CRN) for most specialties across England. Nephrology was identified as a research priority in 16 of 20 local CRNs in England, and nephrology leads were appointed. The purpose of the NIHR CRN was to support the delivery of clinical research within the NHS. Meetings of the UKKRC are held twice a year in conjunction with the meeting of the NIHR CRN Renal Disorders Specialty Group.

To date, there have been a number of successful research studies that have been developed within UKKRC CSGs and then delivered through the NIHR CRN Renal Disorders Specialty Group. These include PIVOTAL, led by Iain

Macdougall, which was a study in patients on haemodialysis which demonstrated that a high-dose intravenous iron regimen administered proactively was superior to a low-dose regimen administered reactively and resulted in lower doses of erythropoiesis-stimulating agent being administered [65]. Another recently completed project was NURTuRE (the National Unified Renal Translational Research Enterprise) led by Maarten Taal, which has collected a biorepository of patient tissue, samples and linked clinical data from 3000 patients with CKD and over 800 patients with idiopathic nephrotic syndrome (INS). It is the first and unique kidney biobank for INS covering England, Scotland and Wales. In the long term, it will provide a strategic resource for fundamental and translational research in the UK. It will hopefully accelerate new advances in the understanding of the pathophysiology of kidney disease that will benefit kidney patients, their treatment and care [66].

The Rare Diseases CSG developed a rare diseases register (RaDaR) in 2009, initially recruiting paediatric patients with steroid resistant nephrotic syndrome and membranoproliferative glomerulonephritis (MPGN). In 2012 it expanded to other conditions in paediatric centres and then to adult centres in Autumn 2013. RaDaR now recruits both adult and paediatric patients for over 70 conditions and is reaching 25,000 recruits [67]. This registry will allow important future research into too often overlooked rare disease.

## Green Nephrology

In 2009 Sir Muir Gray on behalf of the Campaign for Greener Healthcare laid down a challenge to the Renal Association to reduce the carbon footprint of renal medicine. In partnership with the British Renal Society, with funding from NHS Kidney Care, a Green Nephrology trainee was recruited. The Renal Association has adopted a sustainability policy, committing itself to a reduction in carbon output as a result of its activities.

## PatientView

Nephrology in the UK has led the initiative to allow patients to view their own blood results both online and via a mobile phone through a system known as PatientView. It began as a renal project developed by a group of Renal Association members led by Neil Turner from Edinburgh and Keith Simpson from Glasgow. PatientView was launched in 2004 and now covers 90% of UK renal units. In 2014 other specialties began to use the PatientView system, starting with inflammatory bowel disease and diabetes [68].

## Future Perspectives of Nephrology in United Kingdom

Some of the main challenges lying ahead for UK nephrology include slowing the progression of chronic kidney disease in native and kidney transplants and preventing AKI. The clinical pressure on nephrology services is ever increasing which has contributed to poor medical and nursing trainee recruitment in some areas. Initiatives from the societies and local units to attract trainees have been successful in some units.

The recent NHS 10-year plan did not include nephrology as a stand-alone area but instead challenged the nephrology community to work closely in partnership with other specialties such as cardiology and diabetes [69]. There is a recommendation to offer more near patient clinics and home care for patients. The improvements in digital technology and development of artificial intelligence will be important to enabling nephrology to deliver these aspirations. With an aging population and growing multi-morbidity and frailty, there is a real need to work together with other specialties to improve patient care.

## Getting It Right First Time (GIRFT)

Getting It Right First Time (GIRFT) is a national programme designed to improve medical care within the NHS by reducing unwarranted variations. The initiative aims to tackle variations in the way services are delivered across the NHS and by sharing best practice between trusts. In the UK, Graham Lipkin and Will McKane are leading on GIRFT for the nephrology community. They have visited all nephrology units to review practice and produce reports to identify changes to improve care and patient outcomes, as well as highlighting increased efficiencies and cost savings [70].

## The Kidney Quality Improvement Partnership (KQuIP)

There has been an explosion in interest in quality improvement within the NHS. The Kidney Quality Improvement Partnership (KQuIP) was launched in 2016 as a network of kidney health professionals, patients and carers who are committed to developing, supporting and sharing quality improvement (QI) in kidney services to enhance outcomes and quality of life for patients with kidney disease [71]. The organisation has achieved major engagement within the UK nephrology community and has set up three national priority QI projects. These projects are: Transplant First, improving access to pre-dialysis transplant listing and kidney transplantation; Home Therapies, improving access to home dialysis therapies; and Managing Access by Generating Improvements in Cannulation (MAGIC): improving arteriovenous fistula rates by improving needling techniques. KQuIP has a central repository of resources called the KQuIP Hub [72]. This is a growing resource to make QI accessible to clinicians and multidisciplinary team members, as well as patients. Material includes QI tools, sharing of best practice, case studies, abstracts from the Renal Association/British Renal Society UK Kidney Week and other major renal events.

## Conclusion

The NHS allows all UK citizens with kidney disease to receive free medical care at the point of need. The NHS provides all aspects of kidney care to include chronic kidney disease specialist care, acute kidney injury, dialysis in hospital and at home and kidney transplantation. Nephrology is a well-established specialty in the NHS, but the patient population is relatively underserved with only 8.5 Nephrologists per million population. The Renal Association and British Renal Society are the main professional bodies and are moving closer together reflecting the increasing delivery of care to patients by the multidisciplinary team.

More recently there has been a drive to increase the rate of kidney transplantation with the introduction of a national opt out consent system in 2020. Funding for research into kidney disease has been limited, which has therefore restricted progress in new diagnostics and specific therapies compared with other more well-known specialties. Coordinated effects led by the RA and BRS along with the major UK kidney charity, Kidney Research UK have led to a more cohesive strategy and some significant successes more recently. The patient voice is well represented within nephrology with a number of charities playing an influential role in NHS policy. Nephrology in the UK has led the way with patient self-care and empowerment with PatientView allowing patients to view their own results. Nephrology in the UK has embraced quality improvement, and the specialty is now in a strong position to embrace the new digital age and artificial intelligence to continue to provide excellent patient care [73].

## References


1. https://www.nationalarchives.gov.uk/cabinetpapers/alevelstudies/origins-nhs.htm. Accessed on 01/12/2019 at 08.05 hrs.
2. Hole B, et al. UK renal registry 20th annual report: chapter 1 UK renal replacement therapy adult incidence in 2016: national and centre-specific analyses. Nephron. 2018;139(suppl1):13–46.
3. https://renal.org/history/. Accessed on 01/12/2019 at 08.32 hrs.
4. https://britishrenal.org/aboutus/. Accessed on 01/12/2019 at 08.36 hrs.
5. https://renal.org/bapn/about-the-bapn/. Accessed on 01/12/2019 at 08.54 hrs.
6. A history of clinical specialties in leeds teaching hospitals NHS Trust 1767–2018.
7. https://www.ncepod.org.uk/2009aki.html. Accessed on 01/12/2019 at 21.19 hrs.
8. UK Renal Registry 21st annual report 2019. www.renalreg.org. Accessed 16/02/20 23.27 hrs.
9. https://www.england.nhs.uk/commissioning/spec-services/npc-crg/group-a/a06/. Accessed 17/02/20 at 08;00 hrs.
10. Bywaters EGL, Joekes AM. Artificial kidney: its application to treatment of traumatic anuria. Proc R Soc Med. 1948;41:420–6.
11. Richet G. La Société de Pathologie Rénale (1948–1959). Nephrologie. 2000;21:23–6.
12. Anonymous. Distribution of nephrological services for adults in Great Britain. Report of the Executive Committee of the Renal Association. Br Med J. 1976;ii:903–6.
13. https://www.renalreg.org/about-us/. Accessed on 01/12/2019 at 08.42 hrs.
14. https://renal.org/guidelines/. Accessed on 12/12/2019 at 08.07 hrs.
15. https://www.kidney.org.uk/. Accessed on 12/12/2019 at 08.09 hrs.
16. https://www.kidneycareuk.org/about-kidney-health/conditions/polycystic-kidney-disease-pkd/. Accessed on 12/12/2019 at 08.10 hrs.
17. https://www.kidneycareuk.org/. Accessed on 12/12/2019 at 08.11 hrs.
18. https://kidneyresearchuk.org/research/. Accessed on 12/12/2019 at 08.14 hrs.
19. Barat A, Goldacre MJ, Lambert TW. Career choices for nephrology and factors influencing them: surveys of UK medical graduates. J R Soc Med Open. 2018;9(8):1–10.
20. https://www.england.nhs.uk/improvement-hub/wp-content/uploads/sites/44/2017/11/Chronic-Kidney-Disease-in-England-The-Human-and-Financial-Cost.pdf. Accessed on 03/12/2019 at 22.36 hrs.
21. Roth M, Roderick P, Mindell J. Kidney disease and renal function. In: Craig R, Mindell J, editors. Health survey for England – 2010: respiratory health, vol. 1. Leeds: The Health and Social Care Information Centre; 2011.
22. Stevens PE, O'Donoghue DJ, de Lusignan S, et al. Chronic kidney disease management in the United Kingdom: NEOERICA project results. Kidney Int. 2007;72:92–9.
23. The Information Centre for health and social care. Prevalence data tables. Leeds: The NHS Information Centre for health and social care; 2011.
24. Kerr M, Bray B, Medcalf J, et al. Estimating the financial costs of chronic kidney disease in the NHS in England. Nephrol Dial Transplant. 2012;27(suppl 3):iii73–80.4.
25. Verhave JC, Hillege HL, Burgerhof JG, et al. The association between atherosclerotic risk factors and renal function in the general population. Kidney Int. 2005;67:1967–73.
26. de Lusignan S, Tomson C, Harris K, et al. Creatinine fluctuation has a greater effect than the formula to estimate glomerular filtration rate on the prevalence of chronic kidney disease. Nephron Clin Pract. 2011;117:c213–24.
27. http://healthsurvey.hscic.gov.uk/media/63736/HSE2016-Adult-kid-liv.pdf. Accessed 03/12/2019 at 22.41 hrs.
28. The National Service Framework for Renal Services. Part two: chronic kidney disease, acute renal failure and end of life care. London: Department of Health; 2005.
29. NHS digital quality and outcomes framework – prevalence, achievements and exceptions report England 2016–17. http://digital.nhs.uk/catalogue/PUB30124.
30. Falaschetti E, Mindell JS, Knott C, et al. Major improvements in hypertension management in England. Serial cross-sectional data from 1994 to 2011. Lancet. 2014;383:1912–9.

31. https://www.nice.org.uk/guidance/cg182. Accessed 09/12/2019 at 08.25 hrs.
32. https://www.nice.org.uk/guidance/ta358/chapter/1-Guidance. Accessed 09/12/2019 at 08.31 hrs.
33. Tollitt J. Acute kidney injury in primary care: where are we now and where are we going? Br J Gen Pract. 2017;67:394–5.
34. NHS England in partnership with UK Renal Registry. Acute Kidney Injury (AKI) in primary care. https://www.thinkkidneys.nhs.uk/aki/. Accessed 12/12/2019 at 08.49 hrs.
35. Selby NM, Crowley L, Fluck RJ, et al. Use of electronic results reporting to diagnose and monitor AKI in hospitalized patients. Clin J Am Soc Nephrol. 2012;7(4):533–40.
36. Kerr M, Bedford M, Matthews B, O'Donoghue D. The economic impact of acute kidney injury in England. Nephrol Dial Transplant. 2014;29(7):1362–8.
37. The National Service Framework for renal services part two: chronic kidney disease, Acute renal failure and end of life care; 2005.
38. https://renal.org/event/acute-kidney-injury-uk-consensus-conference/. Accessed 2/12/2019 at 17.51 hrs.
39. https://www.nice.org.uk/guidance/cg169. Accessed on 09/12/2019 at 08.42 hrs.
40. https://www.thinkkidneys.nhs.uk. Accessed 09/12/2019 at 08.32 hrs.
41. https://www.england.nhs.uk/2014/06/psa-aki/. Accessed on 12/12/2019 at 17.56 hrs.
42. Kellum JA, Lameire N, KDIGO AKI Guideline Work Group. Diagnosis, evaluation, and management of acute kidney injury: a KDIGO summary (part 1). Crit Care. 2013;17(1):204.
43. Wonnacott A, Meran S, Amphlett B, Talabani B, Phillips A. Epidemiology and outcomes in community-acquired versus hospital-acquired AKI. Clin J Am Soc Nephrol. 2014;9(6):1007–14.
44. Sawhney S, Fluck N, Fraser SD, et al. KDIGO based acute kidney injury criteria operate differently in hospitals and the community—findings from a large population cohort. Nephrol Dial Transplant. 2016;31(6):922–9.
45. https://www.rcgp.org.uk/clinical-and-research/resources/toolkits/acute-kidney-injury-toolkit.aspx. Accessed on 12/12/2019 at 18.10 hrs.
46. Chawla LS, Eggers PW, Star RA, Kimmel PL. Acute kidney injury and chronic kidney disease as interconnected syndromes. N Engl J Med. 2014;371(1):58–66.
47. Parsons FM, Hobson SM, Blagg CR, Mccracken BH. Optimum time for dialysis in acute reversible renal failure. Description and value of an improved dialyser with large surface area. Lancet. 1961;7169:129–34.
48. https://bts.org.uk/wp-content/uploads/2016/09/BTS_EarlyHistoryRenalFailure-1.pdf. Accessed 12/12/2019 at 21.02 hrs.
49. MacNeilla SJ, et al. UK renal registry 20th annual report: chapter 2 UK renal replacement therapy adult prevalence in 2016: national and centre-specific analyses. Nephron. 2018;139(suppl1):47–74.
50. Parsons FM, Fox M, Anderson CK, Markland C, Clark PB, Raper FP. Cyclophosphamide in renal homotransplantation. Br J Urol. 1966;38:673–6.
51. 15. http://www.nhsgraduates.co.uk/about-the-nhs/history/1960s/first-kidney-transplant-1960/. Accessed on 01/12/2019 at 14.13 hrs.
52. https://nhsbtdbe.blob.core.windows.net/umbraco-assets-corp/12256/nhsbt-kidney-transplantation-annual-report-2017-2018.pdf. Accessed on 12/12/2019 at 21.19 hrs.
53. https://www.odt.nhs.uk/living-donation/uk-living-kidney-sharing-scheme/. Accessed 12/12/2019 at 21.30 hrs.
54. https://www.organdonation.nhs.uk/become-a-living-donor/. Accessed on 12/12/2019 at 21.32 hrs.
55. https://nhsbtdbe.blob.core.windows.net/umbraco-assets-corp/16915/kidney-allocation-policy-pol186.pdf. Accessed on 03/12/2019 at 22.08 hrs.
56. https://www.organdonation.nhs.uk/helping-you-to-decide/about-organ-donation/faq/what-is-the-opt-out-system/. Accessed 03/12/2019 at 21.50 hrs.
57. https://www.odt.nhs.uk/transplantation/transplant-units-in-the-uk/. Accessed 12/12/2019 at 21.42 hrs.
58. Jones SL, Devonald MA. How acute kidney injury is investigated and managed in UK intensive care units--a survey of current practice. Nephrol Dial Transplant. 2013;28(5):1186–90.
59. Hamilton AJ, Braddon F, Casula A, Inward C, Lewis M, Mallett T, Maxwell H, O'Brien C, Tse Y, Sinha MD. UK renal registry 18th annual report: chapter 4 demography of patients receiving renal replacement therapy in paediatric centres in the UK in 2014. Nephron. 2016;132(suppl 1):99–110.
60. Sharif MU, Elsayed ME, Stack AG. The global nephrology workforce: emerging threats and potential solutions! Clin Kidney J. 2016;9(1):11–22.
61. Boaz A, Hanney S, Jones T, Soper B. Does the engagement of clinicians and organisations in research improve healthcare performance: a three-stage review. BMJ Open. 2015;5(12):e009415.
62. https://www.healthcareers.nhs.uk/explore-roles/doctors/information-overseas-doctors. Accessed 17/02/20 at 23.18 hrs.
63. https://www.rcpmedicalcare.org.uk/developing-physicians/specialties/renal-medicine/workforce. Accessed 03/12/2019 at 23.05 hrs.
64. Selby NM, Casula A, Lamming L, Stoves J, Samarasinghe Y, Lewington AJ, Roberts R, Shah N, Johnson M, Jackson N, Jones C, Lenguerrand E, McDonach E, Fluck RJ, Mohammed MA, Caskey FJ. An organizational-level program of intervention for AKI: a pragmatic stepped wedge cluster randomized trial. J Am Soc Nephrol. 2019;30(3):505–15.
65. Macdougall IC, White C, Anker SD, Bhandari S, Farrington K, Kalra PA, McMurray JJV, Murray H, Tomson CRV, Wheeler DC, Winearls CG, Ford I, PIVOTAL Investigators and Committees. Intravenous iron in patients undergoing maintenance hemodialysis. N Engl J Med. 2019;380(5):447–58.
66. https://www.nurturebiobank.org/. Accessed on 12/12/2019 at 22.40 hrs.
67. https://rarerenal.org. Accessed 04/12/2019 at 12.15 hrs.
68. http://help.patientview.org/patientview2/about/history/#early. Accessed 02/12/2019 at 06.07 hrs.
69. https://www.longtermplan.nhs.uk. Accessed on 12/12/2019 at 22.51 hrs.
70. https://gettingitrightfirsttime.co.uk/what-we-do/. Accessed 03/12/2019 at 23.21 hrs.
71. Evans K, Pyart R, Steenkamp R, Whitlock T, Stannard C, Gair R, McCann J, Slevin J, Medcalf J, Caskey F. UK renal registry 20th annual report: introduction. Nephron. 2018;139(suppl1):1–12.
72. https://www.thinkkidneys.nhs.uk/kquip/kquip-hub/. Accessed 12/12/2019 at 23.00 hrs.
73. Tomašev N. A clinically applicable approach to continuous prediction of future acute kidney injury. Nature. 2019;572:116–9.

# Part V

# Oceania

# Nephrology in Australia

# 52

Pedro Henrique Franca Gois, Helen G. Healy, Dwarakanathan Ranganathan, Andrew John Mallett, Angela C. Webster, John Kanellis, Katherine Barraclough, Marina Wainstein, David W. Johnson, and Peter G. Kerr

| | |
|---|---|
| Area[a] | 7,688,287 km$^2$ |
| Population[b] | 25,101,900 (2018) |
| Capital | Canberra |
| Three most populated cities: | 1. Sydney<br>2. Melbourne<br>3. Brisbane |
| Official language | English |
| Gross domestic product (GDP)[c] | 1.386 trillion USD (2017)<br>1.419 trillion USD (2018) |
| GDP per capita[c] | 55,966 USD (2017)<br>56,555 USD (2018) |
| Human Development Index (HDI)[d] | 0.938 (3rd, 2018) |
| Official currency | Australian dollar (AUD) |
| Total number of nephrologists[e] | 598 |
| National society of nephrology | Australian and New Zealand Society of Nephrology – ANZSN<br>www.nephrology.edu.au |
| Incidence of end-stage renal disease[f] | 2017 – 125 pmp<br>2018 – 124 pmp |
| Prevalence of end-stage renal disease[f] (including patients with a functioning kidney transplant) | 2017 – 1002 pmp<br>2018 – 1026 pmp |
| Total number of patients on dialysis[f] (all modalities) | 2017 – 13,051<br>2017 – 13,032<br>2018 – 13,399 |
| Number of patients on haemodialysis[f] | 2017 – 10,624 (9.6% on home HD)<br>2017 – 10,624 (9.6% on home HD)<br>2018 – 10,983 (9.6% on home HD) |
| Number of patients on peritoneal dialysis[f] | 2017 – 2,427<br>2017 – 2,427<br>2018 – 2,416 |
| Number of kidney transplantations per year[f] | 2017 – 1,109<br>2018 – 1,149 |

Table references:

[a]Geoscience Australia. Available at http://www.ga.gov.au/scientific-topics/national-location-information/dimensions/area-of-australia-states-and-territories

[b]Australian Demographic Statistics, September quarter 2018. Available at https://www.abs.gov.au/AUSSTATS/abs@.nsf/mf/3101.0

[c]Australian Government. Department of Foreign Affairs and Trade. Available at https://dfat.gov.au/trade/resources/Documents/aust.pdf

[d]Human Development Indices and Indicators Statistical Update. United Nations Development Programme. 2018 Statistical update

[e]2017 ANZSN Workforce Report. Available at https://www.nephrology.edu.au/workforce-report.asp

[f]Australia and New Zealand Dialysis and Transplant Registry (ANZDATA) Annual Report 2018 and 2019. Available at http://www.anzdata.org.au/v1/index.html

P. H. F. Gois (✉)
Nephrology Department, Royal Brisbane & Women's Hospital, Brisbane, QLD, Australia

University of Queensland School of Clinical Medicine - Royal Brisbane Clinical Unit, QLD, Australia
e-mail: pedrogoismd@usp.br; Pedro.francagois@health.qld.gov.au

H. G. Healy · M. Wainstein
Nephrology Department, Royal Brisbane & Women's Hospital, Brisbane, QLD, Australia

D. Ranganathan
Nephrology Department, Royal Brisbane & Women's Hospital, Brisbane, QLD, Australia

School of Medicine, Griffith University, Brisbane, QLD, Australia

A. J. Mallett
Department of Renal Medicine, Townsville University Hospital, Douglas, QLD, Australia

A. C. Webster
Centre for Transplant and Renal Research, Westmead Hospital, Westmead, NSW, Australia

J. Kanellis
Department of Nephrology, Monash Health and Centre for Inflammatory Diseases, Department of Medicine, Monash University, Monash Medical Centre, Clayton, VIC, Australia

K. Barraclough
Nephrology, Royal Melbourne Hospital, Parkville, VIC, Australia

D. W. Johnson
Department of Nephrology, University of Queensland at Princess Alexandra Hospital, Brisbane, QLD, Australia

P. G. Kerr
Nephrology, Monash Health and Monash University, Clayton, VIC, Australia

## Introduction

Australia is the smallest continent and one of the largest countries on Earth. The Australia's mainland extends from west to east for nearly 4000 km and from Cape York Peninsula in the northeast to Wilsons Promontory in the southeast for



J. A. Moura-Neto et al. (eds.), *Nephrology Worldwide*, https://doi.org/10.1007/978-3-030-56890-0_52

nearly 3200 km. Australian jurisdiction extends 500 km further to the southern extremity of the island of Tasmania [1].

Global isolation, low relief and the aridity of much of its surface are few of the most prominent characteristics of the vast country. Australia's isolation from other continents explains much of its unique plant and animal life. Isolation is also a pronounced feature of the social landscape beyond the large coastal cities as most of Australia's population is concentrated on or around the coastal areas [1]. As of 1 December 2019, the resident population of Australia is projected to be 25,538,835 [2]. In 2011, over 85% of the population lived within 50 km of the coastline of Australia, mostly in capital cities [3].

An equally significant characteristic of modern Australian society is multiculturalism, stemming from immigration that is transforming the Anglo-Celtic orientation of Australian culture [1]. Strikingly, there are more than 300 different ancestries in Australia, and 28% of the resident population is born overseas [4].

Historically part of the British Empire and now a member of the Commonwealth, Australia is a prosperous independent country. Australia has a federal system of government, with a national government for the Commonwealth of Australia and individual state governments (i.e. New South Wales, Victoria, Queensland, South Australia, Western Australia and Tasmania). Each state has a constitution, and its government exercises a limited degree of sovereignty. There are also two internal territories: the Northern Territory, a self-governing territory since 1978, and the Australian Capital Territory (including the city of Canberra), which attained self-governing status in 1988. In addition, there are seven external territories: Ashmore and Cartier Islands, Australian Antarctic Territory, Christmas Island, Coco (Keeling) Islands, Coral Sea Islands, Heard Island and McDonald Islands and Norfolk Island [1, 5].

Australia has completed 28 consecutive years of annual economic growth, one of the few economies in the Second World War period to achieve this. Australia's gross domestic product (GDP) was 1.419 trillion USD in 2018 and according to the Global Wealth Report (Credit Suisse) is the wealthiest nation in terms of median wealth per adult. Australia ranks in the top 20 countries across a wide range of indexes including the economy, international trade, investment, education and other global indexes [6].

## Brief History of Nephrology in Australia

Renal medicine flourished in Australia in the years following the end of the Second World War, with the first haemodialysis (HD) performed in Australia at the Brisbane General Hospital, Queensland, on 10 February 1954 in a 36-year-old woman with retained placental products who developed severe acute kidney injury (AKI) in the setting of sepsis [7], with the artificial kidney built by Dr. John Dique. She survived. The specialty continued to differentiate from the broader specialty of internal medicine, and leading practitioners formed the Australasian Society of Nephrology (later the Australian and New Zealand Society of Nephrology) with the first scientific meeting held in 1965. The young Society embarked on the ambitious undertaking of systematically reporting on all patients receiving renal replacement therapy (RRT) annually. The first report of the Australian and New Zealand Data Registry (ANZDATA) was produced in 1977 and annually thereafter. Reports are accessible to the public at anzdata.org.au. Figure 52.1 illustrates the milestones of Australian nephrology.

## Renal Diseases in Australia

### Acute Kidney Injury

The Australian Institute of Health and Welfare reports that AKI was the principal and/or additional diagnosis in 131,780 hospitalisations between 2012 and 2013, representing 1.6% of total hospital admissions across the country [8]. Hospitalisations attributed to AKI are increasing at an average 6% per annum. The average length of stay doubles in the presence of AKI, respectively, 11.4 vs. 5.6 days in those without AKI. Mortality is higher, with 14,590 (11% of all hospital admissions) deaths in 2012–2013 where AKI was the principal diagnosis and an additional 5160 deaths where AKI was recorded as the underlying or associated cause of death [8]. AKI-related mortality rates have remained relatively stable from 2000 to 2013, notwithstanding the rise in hospitalisations [8]. Hospitalisation rates attributable to AKI are higher among males, the elderly (≥85 years old) and those living in socioeconomically disadvantaged areas as well as in very remote areas [8].

The aetiology of AKI precipitating hospitalisation is subject to source bias. Data from 200 consecutive AKI episodes in a major tertiary hospital in Sydney showed volume depletion and reduced cardiac output as the most common causes of AKI [9]. In a larger cohort of 2367 patients with underlying chronic kidney disease (CKD) enrolled in the CKD Queensland registry, from the Logan and Royal Brisbane and Women's Hospitals, the leading aetiology of AKI was obstructive nephropathy (36.5%), followed by glomerulonephritis (18%) and acute interstitial nephritis (10%) [10]. CKD was attributed to AKI in 6.7% (159 patients), as opposed to 7.4% (179 patients) where AKI was superimposed on pre-existing CKD [10]. By contrast, sepsis/septic shock was the most common cause of AKI in the intensive care unit (ICU) setting with 28.4% of these cases so severe that RRT was required [11].

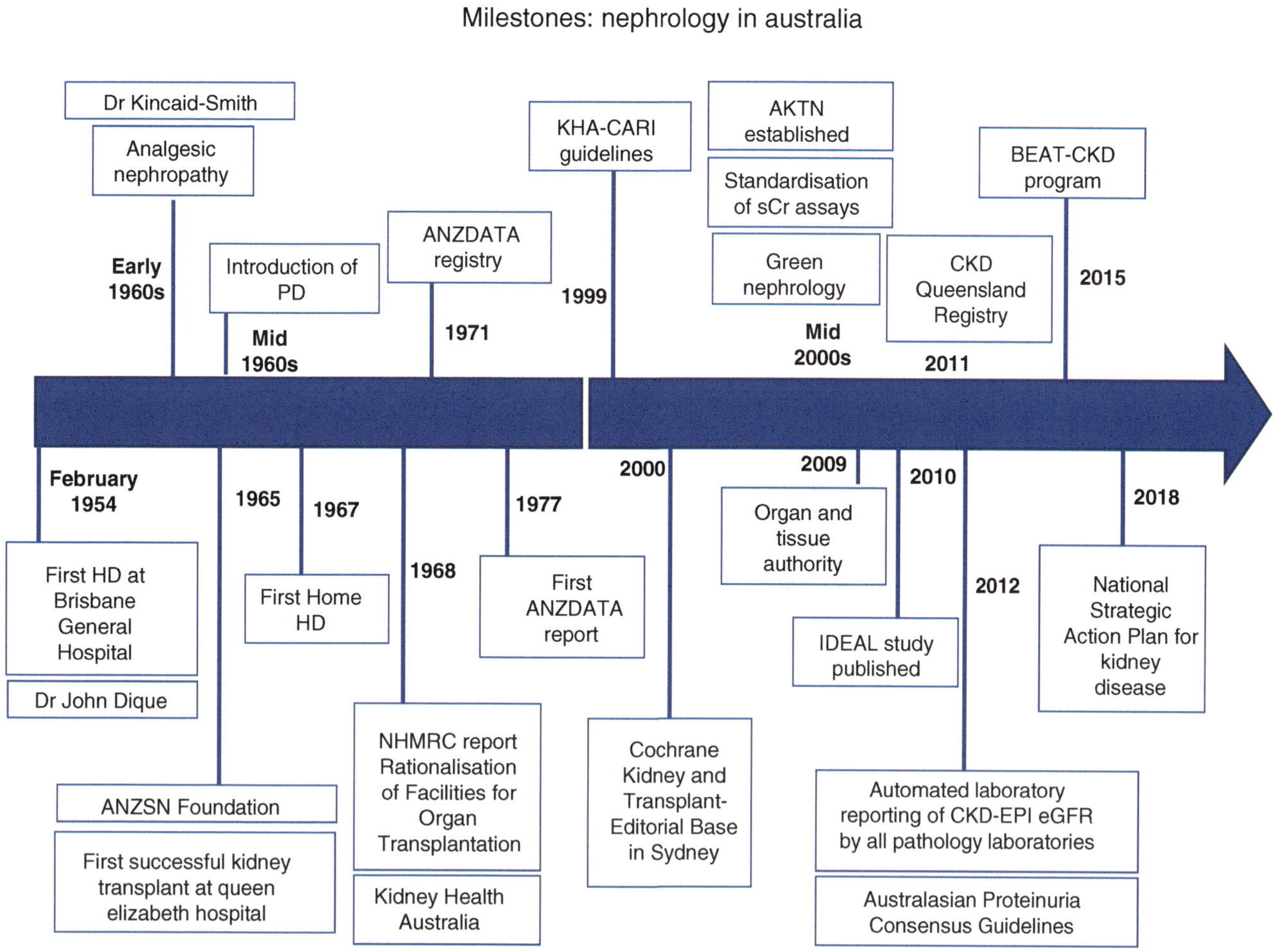


**Fig. 52.1** Milestones of Australian nephrology. HD haemodialysis, ANZSN Australian and New Zealand Society of Nephrology, PD peritoneal dialysis, NHMRC National Health and Medical Research Council, ANZDATA the Australia and New Zealand Dialysis and Transplant Registry, KHA-CARI Kidney Health Australia-Caring for Australasians with Renal Impairment, AKTN Australasian Kidney Trials Network, sCr serum creatinine, IDEAL study Randomized, Controlled Trial of Early versus Late Initiation of Dialysis, BEAT-CKD Better Evidence and Translation in Chronic Kidney Disease

In Australia, the vast majority of hospitalised severe AKI cases are managed by critical care physicians and nurses and not nephrologists. In a prospective audit of all ICUs performing RRT across Australia ($n$ = 81 units), 299 patients with AKI requiring RRT were admitted in a 3-month period. RRT via a double lumen catheter was started at median of 1 day (range 0–44 days) after ICU admission. In all but 14 patients (4.7%), operation and set-up of RRT were exclusively carried out by critical care nurses. Nephrologists were consulted in only 42.1% of patients, notwithstanding that the majority had underlying CKD. In-hospital mortality rate was 46.8% with no difference in outcome between the cohort managed with nephrologists and those who are not [11].

All 34 Australian and New Zealand ICUs in 1 survey selected continuous renal replacement therapy (CRRT) as the support dialysis modality of choice [12]. Among the CRRT techniques, continuous veno-venous haemodiafiltration (CVVHDF) was most commonly used, typically using prefilter fluid replacement in a 1:1 ratio of dialysate to replacement fluid volumes [12]. All 34 units used a fixed-dose regimen, but the rate ranged from 1.5 to 4 L/h, and CRRT dosing was not modified according to patient's body weight [12]. The majority (23/34) continued CRRT until kidney recovery, discharge from the ICU, or death [12]. The remaining 11 ICUs (constituting <10% patients) converted CRRT to either sustained low-efficiency dialysis (SLED) or intermittent HD (IHD), conditional on haemodynamical stable patients and those approaching ICU discharge [12]. Intensivists continued to prescribe SLED, delivered by ICU nursing staff, and nephrologists IHD, delivered by dialysis nursing staff [12]. All ICUs handed over management of RRT to nephrologists when the patients were discharged from the ICU [12].

## Chronic Kidney Disease

Two groups have profiled CKD cross-sectionally in the Australian population, using the framework of the KDIGO 2012 Clinical Practice Guideline for the Evaluation and Management of CKD (first published in 2002) [13, 14]. The first, AusDiab Study [15], was a statistically random selection of 11,247 non-institutionalised Australians over the age of 24 years who attended physical screening during the Aus Diab survey. The sampling systematically excluded Indigenous Australians. The results of the initial analyses were published in 2003 and the data re-analysed in 2010 in response to contemporary shifts in the methodology of estimating glomerular filtration rate, from the Modification of Diet in Renal Disease (MDRD) to the Chronic Kidney Disease Epidemiology Collaboration (EPI-CKD) [16]. The second is an ongoing national dataset of prevalence, demographics and outcomes of people who participate in the National Health Measures survey conducted by the Australian Institute of Health and Welfare (AIHW) (last reported on 30 August 2019) [17].

Prevalence of CKD in Australia is age and sex dependent, varying from 4.5% of men under 45 years to 43.3% of men over the age of 74 years [18]. Most are unaware of their kidney disease, with less than one in ten in the 2011–2012 Australian Health Survey [19]. Hospitalisation where CKD is listed as the principal diagnosis (excluding dialysis) is common and has risen 44.4% since 2000 – from 126 people per 100,000 population in 2000–2001 to 182 people per 100,000 in 2016–2017, the latest year for which data are available [17]. The analyses of the National Mortality Database by AIHW found death, where CKD was an underlying or associated cause, has remained around 56 people per 100,000 since 1997, representing 10.9% of all deaths in 2017 [20].

More granular data are difficult to source, with management of CKD fragmented across healthcare jurisdictions and internal medicine specialities, including general physicians, geriatricians and cardiologists among others as well as nephrologists. The most comprehensive Australian CKD dataset is the CKD.Qld Registry, a cohort of >9000 people biased towards the more advanced CKD that is managed by specialists nephrology practices in the public health system in Queensland [21]. In this cohort opportunities still exist for better control of blood pressure [22]. The Registry found poorer outcomes among the cohort that developed superimposed AKI, with higher likelihood of deaths, transition to dialysis and higher hospitalisation costs compared to those who do not have additional AKI [23]. The Registry also has the capacity to profile across the geography of this large Australian state [24]. Among publications to come is a description of patterns of progression of CKD.

Anecdotally progression has changed over the decades, from a predictable and straight trend line that could be described by the reciprocal of creatinine to stepwise progression that tracks episodes of AKI. The changes in patterns of progression mirror the ageing of the population and the changes in the most common causes of CKD, from patterns like glomerulonephritis still present in younger people with CKD to metabolic causes like diabetes and renovascular diseases found in the older age groups.

## Inherited and Genetic Kidney Diseases

The research and subspecialty practice development of inherited and genetic kidney disease in Australia has progressed significantly and rapidly over the past decade. Epidemiologically, approximately 10% of Australian adults with chronic kidney disease [25] and ESRD [26] have a potential genetic renal disease. Among Australian children, this has been quantified as 70.6 children per million age-representative population [27]. These lines of enquiry have been reflected by multiple lines of research as well as modifications to clinical practice.

A long-standing and leading area of research has been around Alport syndrome and collagen 4-related glomerular basement membrane disorders. Seminal work around the relationships between Alport syndrome and de novo anti-GBM disease post-transplantation [28, 29] has laid a foundation for significant contribution to global research, opinion and guidelines in Alport syndrome [30] and thin basement membrane nephropathy [31]. In other specific genetic renal diseases, guidelines for autosomal dominant polycystic kidney disease have been generated [32, 33] for both local and international application incorporating patient and consumer perspectives [34]. Further innovative clinical trials are underway locally to further identify new and novel therapies [35].

Seminal research in the field of renal regeneration and model systems, specifically kidney organoids [36] and induced pluripotent stem cell approaches [37], has resulted in new approaches to research of genetic kidney diseases [38, 39]. This body of work continues to both enable new ways of understanding these kidney diseases and give hope to patients of new approaches to renal replacement therapy in the coming decades.

In the clinical domain, specific renal genetics clinics around Australia have formed [40] and are now identifying applications and utility of both genetic and genomic clinical testing in this context [41, 42]. As this is a relatively new and emerging field in nephrology, it has become critical to ensure that there are appropriate opportunities for both genomic training and upskilling [43], as well as information dissemination. This approach is delivering real-world change to clinical care and outcomes for individual patients and families whilst also subtly changing and progressing the practice of nephrology in Australia. The ability to have ensured connection between clinical research, fundamental research and clinical care is strategically placing the Australian healthcare system to deliver iteratively improved patient outcomes from a nephrological perspective. In addition, in the future this may have more generalised effects in terms of understanding kidney health, kidney disease mechanisms and future therapies for a broader group of patients than just those with genetic or inheritable kidney disease. It is critical to dissect hype from hyperbole, but the approach to genetic kidney disease in Australia is seeking further understanding whilst delivering a more personalised approach to healthcare for affected patients and families.

## Indigenous Kidney Health

The Indigenous people of Australia, also known as Aboriginal and Torres Strait Islander peoples, are one of the oldest surviving Indigenous cultures in the world having populated Australia approximately 50,000 years ago after leaving Africa and crossing into eastern Asia [44]. They were traditional hunter-gatherers of the land and later established long-distance trade by sea with the Indigenous people of Papua New Guinea and Indonesia. Like other First Nations peoples, their population was decimated during times of British colonisation as a result of disease, war and massacres and remained a subjugated and marginalised group for many years. In recent times, however, the recognition of their rights and interests to land and waters through the "Native Title Act" of 1993 and a formal process of reconciliation has healed some wounds and seen the population increase to 649,171 in the latest census, comprising 2.8% of the population of Australia [45, 46].

Kidney disease is very common among Indigenous Australians. In 2017, the number of new Indigenous patients reaching end-stage renal disease (ESRD) was ~450 per million population, representing a slow but persistent increase compared to a stable ~100 per million population among non-Indigenous patients [47]. Indigenous women are 15 times more likely to develop ESRD than non-Indigenous women in the fourth and fifth decades of life, whilst a similar increased risk is observed in younger men. The aetiology of kidney disease is predominantly diabetic (~70%) with smaller contributions from glomerulonephritis – often infectious – and hypertension. The excessive and comparatively higher prevalence of kidney disease in this population is complex and results from a number of factors including reduced kidney capacity at birth from maternal malnutrition and a maladaptive metabolic response to a Western diet rich in saturated fats leading to the accelerated development of diabetes [48]. A majority of Indigenous patients are treated with facility-based haemodialysis (76%) with very few able to access and successfully engage with long-term peritoneal dialysis (PD) (9%) or home haemodialysis (HHD) [47]. The remoteness of the towns and communities many Indigenous Australians live in, particularly in the Northern Territory and Western Australia, means they must relocate to urban centres for dialysis leading to a social, geographic and cultural dislocation that is thought to be responsible for much of the morbidity and mortality observed during the first year of dialysis. In this context, promotion of home therapies such as PD and transplantation is key.

Unfortunately, the rate of kidney transplants among Indigenous Australians is very low. At the end of 2017, Indigenous patients with ESRD accounted only for 3% of all kidney transplants done in that year, despite representing ~14% of all patients on dialysis [47]. Living donation is extremely rare due to the endemically high levels of diabetic disease and a cultural reluctance to donate. The reasons for the disproportionately low rate of transplantation in this population have been the subject of much debate in recent years and have been attributed, among others, to difficulties progressing through the stages of activation to the deceased donor list as well as poorer graft and patient outcomes influencing clinicians' willingness to view them as appropriate transplant candidates [49]. The latest ANZDATA report shows that 5 years after transplantation, 84% of Indigenous patients were alive compared to 90% of non-Indigenous patients and graft function was recorded in 71% vs. 83% of transplant recipients, respectively; higher rates of infection, poor HLA matching, increased steroid exposure and lack of compliance with prescribed immunosuppressive medications are some of the factors thought to explain these differences [47, 50].

Despite the reality of these figures, an enormous amount of work is being dedicated by passionate advocates of Indigenous kidney health through innovative, holistic and multidisciplinary care strategies that strive to understand and harmonise the social, cultural and spiritual context of this ancient population with the traditional, Western model of healthcare. Moving forward, supporting them must be one of Australia's main priorities.

## Renal Replacement Therapy in Australia

### Haemodialysis and Haemodiafiltration

#### Evolution and Epidemiology of Haemodialysis in Australia

Although haemodialysis was introduced in Australia in the early 1950s, initially this was for treatment of acute kidney injury, and not for people with irreversible ESRD. In tandem with the development of kidney transplantation in Australia, the need for maintenance haemodialysis was clear by the late 1960s, and the National Health and Medical Research Council formed a committee to address the rationalisation of transplantation and dialysis in 1968. Following the committee report, coordinated maintenance haemodialysis programmes commenced, with patient outcomes aggregated and recorded in what eventually became the ANZDATA registry [51].

The number of people receiving maintenance haemodialysis has increased annually ever since. In 1990, 611 people started haemodialysis for ESRD in Australia for the first time; by 2000 this was 1283, and by 2010 1752. In 2018, there were 2193 incident haemodialysis patients treated. There are much larger numbers of prevalent patients. In 1990, there were 2034 people in Australia receiving regular haemodialysis, which grew to 4669 by the year 2000. In 2010, the number of prevalent haemodialysis patients was 8659, and in the end of 2017, there were 10,983 people receiving haemodialysis. The steady growth in prevalent haemodialysis patients in Australia is because incident patients exceed the number of people ceasing haemodialysis (either by getting a transplant, switching to PD, withdrawing from treatment or dying on treatment) [52].

Over time, the haemodialysis population in Australia has aged. In 2018, 49% of incident patients were over 65 years of age, but the average age of prevalent patients was 58 years. Other characteristics are more stable. About 40% of people receiving haemodialysis are female, and this proportion has been the same for over 20 years [53]. The incidence of haemodialysis is approximately fivefold higher for Indigenous Australians, compared to other Australians, and the magnitude of this difference has not changed in the last decade [47].

The underlying cause of ESRD for people receiving dialysis has evolved. In 2000, 37% of people on haemodialysis had underlying glomerulonephritis, but this had fallen to 20% by 2017, although in absolute terms the number of people with glomerulonephritis-related ESRD remained relatively stable (between 1800 and 2000 prevalent patients). The greatest contribution to growth in haemodialysis patient numbers has been due to diabetic nephropathy. In 2000, diabetic kidney disease was the underlying pathology in 17% of prevalent people receiving haemodialysis. By 2017, this proportion had grown to 39% [52, 53].

Overall, currently approximately 88–90% receive haemodialysis in a dedicated facility, and 10–12% at home. These proportions have been stable over the last decade. Approximately 6% of people are dialysed in private dialysis facilities. The majority (67%) of prevalent haemodialysis patients live in major Australian cities, with only 4% in remote settings [54].

The use of high flux haemodialysis has increased markedly in Australia over time and is now the recommended standard [55]. Haemodiafiltration (HDF) prescription has also increased over time, but initially at a relatively slower rate than some other countries (including New Zealand). Between 2000 and 2014, 14.4% of patients in Australia received periods of HDF [54], although in recent years there has been a sharp increase; by 2017, 32% of dialysis patients were receiving HDF [53]. Use of HDF was more likely for males (odds ratio [OR] 1.13, 95% CI 1.03–1.24) and less likely with older age (reference <40 years; 40–54 years OR 0.85, 95% CI 0.72–0.99; 55–69 years OR 0.79, 95% CI 0.67–0.91; >70 years OR 0.48, 95% CI 0.41–0.56). In Australia, HDF use is correlated with some comorbidities; increasing obesity increases the likelihood of HDF use (BMI <18.5 kg/m$^2$ OR 0.62, 95% CI 0.46–0.84; 18.5–29.9 kg/m$^2$ reference; >30 kg/m$^2$ OR 1.46, 95% CI 1.33–1.61), but other comorbidities make HDF use less likely: chronic lung disease (OR 0.84, 95% CI 0.76–0.94, $p < 0.001$), cerebrovascular disease (OR 0.76, 95% CI 0.67–0.85, $p < 0.001$) and peripheral vascular disease (OR 0.77, 95% CI 0.70–0.85, $p < 0.001$). There is no association with HDF use and race. Neither living remotely nor having a lower socioeconomic status is associated with HDF use in Australia ($p > 0.05$) (Fig. 52.2) [54].

#### Haemodialysis in Practice

The median eGFR for adult patients (calculated using the CKD-EPI formula) starting haemodialysis in Australia is 7.4 mL/min/1.73 m$^2$ and has remained unchanged over the last decade. Of patients referred "late" to nephrology services (defined as within 3 months of requiring ESRD treatment), the majority start on haemodialysis. As a proportion of all new patients, later referrals comprise 18%, which has remained unchanged in recent years [56].

Approximately 43% of new starts on haemodialysis start with an arterio-venous fistula or graft, 40% with a tunnelled catheter, and the remainder with a non-tunnelled catheter. Chances of starting dialysis without permanent access were increased for younger patients (80% under 25 years) and late referrals (90% without fistula). Average blood flow rates achieved are 300–349 mL/min, slightly lower when access is a central venous catheter [53].

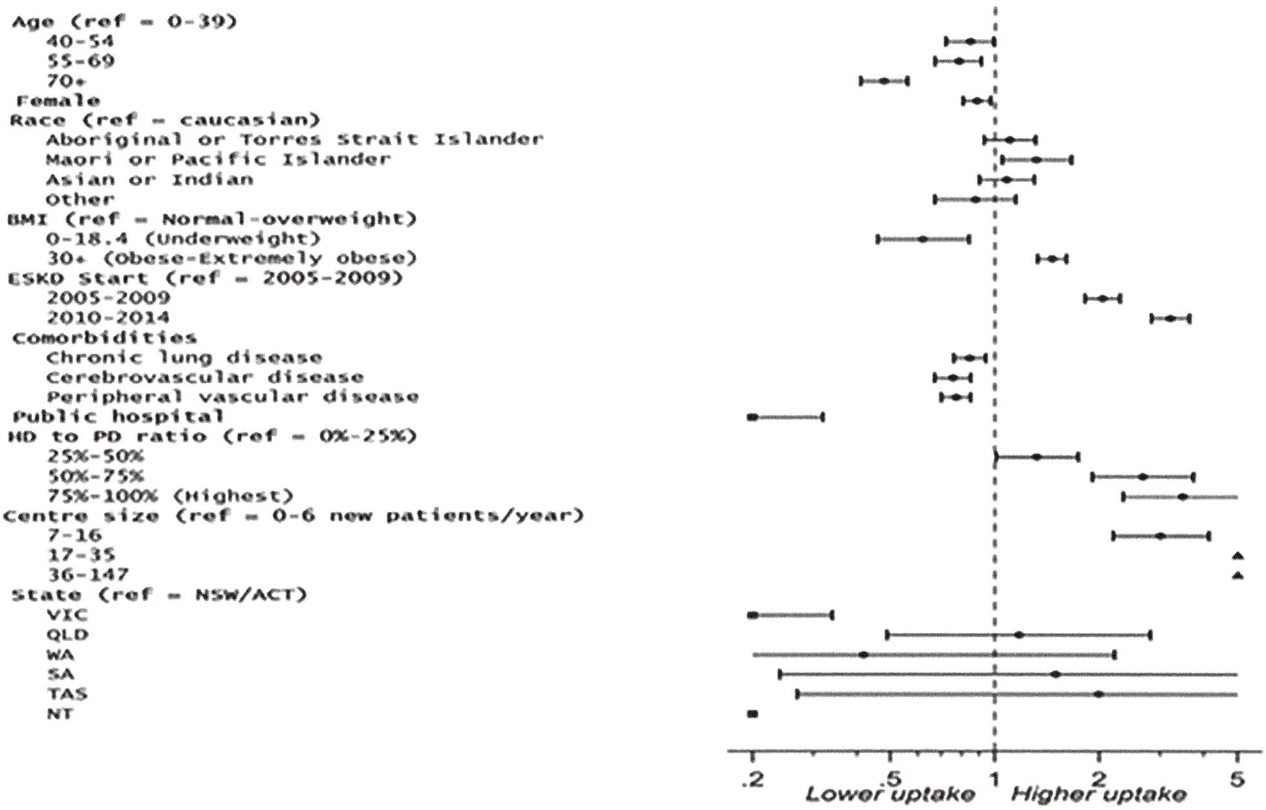


**Fig. 52.2** Associations (odds ratios) with HDF uptake in Australia between 2000 and 2014. Multivariable models: (▲) OR (odds ratio) > 5, (●) OR < 0.2. (Adapted from Mac et al. [54])

Haemodialysis is usually started at a frequency of three times a week, with occasional patients starting twice weekly ("incremental dialysis"). Incremental haemodialysis starts are infrequent (3%) but more common in older people and those without diabetes [57]. The majority of patients, once established, dialyse for 4–5 hours per session, three times a week. Fewer than 10% of haemodialysis patients undertake quotidian dialysis (>3 sessions per week OR > 5 hours per session), and this proportion is falling over time [53]. According to the Therapeutic Goods Administration (TGA) regulations, dialysers are single-use medical devices and, therefore, not for reuse [58].

Dialysis adequacy (as measured by achieving a urea reduction ration (URR) >70%) is achieved by 72% of people on haemodialysis in Australia and is more likely for those with longer dialysis sessions. The median URR for those dialysing three times a week varies by dialysis centre from 65% to 88% [53].

A recent study showed some differences between the haemodialysis population using HDF compared with standard dialysis, although as this is observational registry data, these differences may be due to selection bias of those chosen for HDF treatment [59]. Compared to patients receiving standard haemodialysis, a greater proportion of HDF patients had a blood flow rate ≥ 350 ml/min and used a high flux dialyser, although fewer did quotidian (3.5+ sessions per week) or extended hour (>5 hours per session) dialysis, and fewer required erythropoietin. Vascular access and phosphate control were comparable between new starters after 12 months [59].

Treatment centres account for 36% of the variability in use of HDF in Australia. In a recent study, people receiving dialysis at centres with a higher proportion of patients on HD (as compared to PD) had a higher likelihood of receiving HDF ($p < 0.001$), and there was a graded incremental association with increasing HD:PD patient ratios ($p < 0.001$). People dialysed in larger centres were more likely to receive HDF ($p < 0.001$), and the chances of HDF increased with centre size ($p < 0.001$). Although private dialysis units had higher proportion of patients on HDF (23%) compared with public units (15%), this was not significantly associated with HDF use ($p = 0.7$). However, differences in use of HDF by state/territory were seen ($p < 0.001$). There were lower odds of receiving HDF in the Northern Territory (OR 0.01, 95% CI <0.01–0.11) and Victoria (OR 0.13, 95% CI 0.05–0.34), compared with New South Wales [54].

### Haemodialysis Outcomes

Survival on haemodialysis has remained unchanged over the last decade in Australia. Overall, after 6 months of haemodialysis, 97% (95% CI 96–97) survive, but this falls to 92% (95% CI 91–93) by 1 year. Survival varies by age, presence of diabetes and cardiovascular disease. A person <40 years, without diabetes or cardiovascular disease, can expect an 85% 5-year dialysis survival, where someone similar but older would have poorer prognosis (aged 60–74 when starting dialysis, 5-year survival is 60%). In the presence of diabetes and cardiovascular disease, expected 5-year survival for the under 60s is <60% [53].

Those treated with HDF in Australia have improved survival, but this may reflect the types of people able to access HDF rather than a direct treatment effect (i.e. selection bias). In a recent paper, in adjusted analysis, HDF was independently associated with a significantly lower risk of death (hazard ratio, HR, 0.63, 95% CI 0.57–0.68), with no differences across patient subgroups. This benefit may be lessening over time ($p = 0.09$). There was no difference in the risk of cardiovascular death (HR 1.01, 95% CI 0.84–1.23, $p = 0.90$), compared to patients managed with standard haemodialysis (Fig. 52.3) [59].

## Haemodialysis at Home

### History and Epidemiology

HHD was initiated simultaneously in the USA and UK [60–63] in 1964 and is claimed to have been underway even earlier in Japan [64]. In 1967, the first Australian patient was started on HHD [63], and a year later, the NHMRC report on rationalisation of facilities for organ transplantation in 1968 supported HHD as a suitable method for the treatment of ESRD [65]. There was then a progressive rise in the number of patients utilising HHD, increasing from 17% to 52% between 1971 and 1977. Subsequently, the percentage of HHD patients in Australia fell to 23% in 1987 and later 12% by 1997 following an increase in satellite HD and PD [51]. After the turn of the century, there was a resurgence on HHD with growing interest in nocturnal HHD [66]. Since this time, the utilisation rate of HHD remained stable at 11–12% though there is considerable interstate variation in its use. Globally, the prevalence of HHD is highest in New Zealand, and this is followed by Australia [67].

### Selection of Patients and Training

A multidisciplinary team assess the suitability of patients who could undergo HHD training. There are several tools available that may help to decide home suitability including the Jo-Pre-training Assessment Tool (JPAT) [68] for Home Dialysis (version 2.1) or Method to Assess Treatment Choices for Home Dialysis (MATCH-D) [69]. Once a patient is deemed suitable for HHD, nurses provide training at a dialysis centre. Most HHD units have their own training procedures. The training period is usually 4–12 weeks and tailored to the individual's learning skills. Patients, if elected, can also be trained to undergo nocturnal HD. Patients are trained to set up the machine, self-needle and self-dialyse. Patients are also encouraged and trained to self-administer intravenous erythropoietin and iron and self-centrifuge pre- and post-dialysis blood for biochemistry every 4–6 weeks depending on unit practices. Rarely, though usually discouraged, partners or family members are trained to assist with the procedure. Patients on HHD require a strong support system to resolve problems either intra-dialytically or inter-dialytically. Currently remote monitoring of dialysis using modem technology is not practised in Australia. "On-call nursing" and technical maintenance officers can give advice for troubleshooting and equipment problems. HHD training

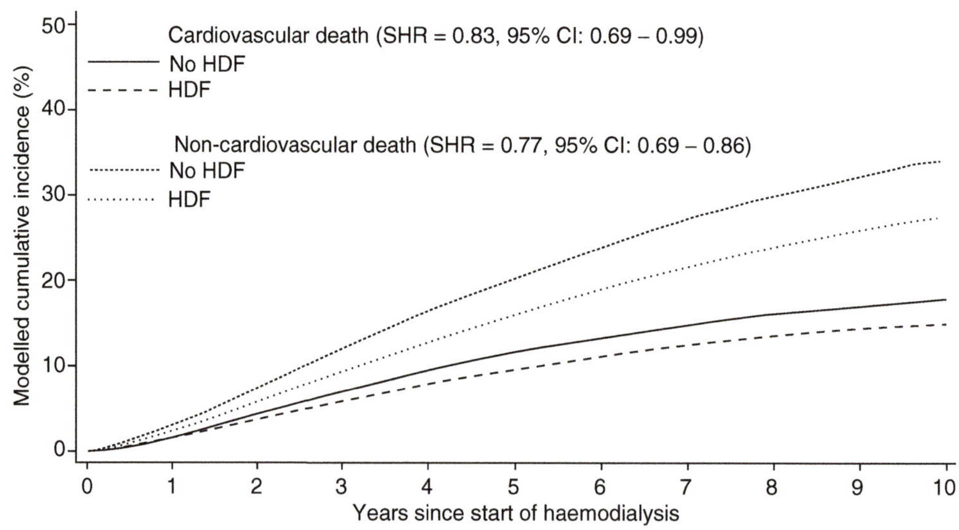


**Fig. 52.3** Cause-specific cumulative mortality curves comparing cardiovascular and non-cardiovascular deaths for people managed with haemodiafiltration and standard haemodialysis in Australia. (Adapted from See et al. [59])

nurses and technicians visit patients' homes periodically at approximately quarterly intervals. Patients attend outpatient clinic every 2 to 3 months for review.

### Equipment and Access

The proportion of HD patients undergoing HHD differs by state (4–13%). Ninety-one centres offer HD and about half of them offer HHD. In 2017, 53 centres train patients, with the number of centres varying between states, for example, 21 in New South Wales versus 1 from the Australian Capital Territory [53]. The proportion of patients undertaking HHD also varied by treating centres (2–26%). Most of these centres train the patients on conventional single pass HD systems and volumetric controlled. About 10% of them provide transportable, water source-independent HD systems (e.g. the NxStage System) to their patients for regular use or when they travel (Chris Davies, Senior Biostatistician, ANZDATA, Personal Communication). Water treatment and reverse osmosis units are required when patients use standard HD system. The cost of machines, home modifications including plumbing and power source to install the machines are borne by the dialysis units. Agencies subsidise water and power costs of HHD patients. Dialysis units regularly perform water quality testing, which may add further costs.

All patients perform dialysis using high-performance dialysers and bicarbonate dialysate. Many of them are dialysing on alternate day schedule – 7 sessions every 2 weeks. The proportion of patients dialysing 3 days and 4.5 hours or longer and the proportion dialysing more than 12 hours a week plateaued recently (89% in 2017). The proportion of patients dialysing >5 sessions a week continues to fall, and at the end of 2017, only 2% dialyse for this number of sessions. Vascular access is predominantly arterio-venous fistulas (AVF) or grafts. Rarely (<6%) patients are trained to use central venous catheters, i.e. permcaths (Chris Davies, Senior Biostatistician, ANZDATA, Personal Communication). Centres train the patients to adopt either rope ladder (RL) or buttonhole (BH) technique for AVF puncture. Each centre chooses the technique best suited to their patients. The BH technique is used in patients with limited access length or when undergoing daily or nocturnal HHD.

### Outcome

Last reported HHD patient survival rates (censored at first transplant, renal recovery or lost to follow-up) at 1, 3 and 5 years were 99% (95% CI 97–99%), 93% (95% CI 88–96%) and 82% (95% CI 72–88%), respectively (Chris Davies, Senior Biostatistician, ANZDATA, Personal Communication). Technique survival rates for the same period were 83% (95% CI 81–85%), 67% (95% CI 63–70%) and 48% (95% CI 43–53%); death-censored technique survival rates were 86% (95% CI 83–88%), 75% (95% CI 72–78%) and 64% (95% CI 59–69%). Death as the cause of technique failure in HHD patients is 29% (Chris Davies, Senior Biostatistician, ANZDATA, Personal Communication). ANZDATA do not capture access-related infection rates routinely, but one centre reported an infection rate of 0.10 events per 1000 AVF days associated with RL and 0.39 events per 1000 AVF days associated with BH approach [70].

### Barriers to Home HD

Barriers to patients undertaking HHD include anxiety, particularly with respect to needle insertion perceived complex and the challenging nature of the treatment and fear about isolation from medical and social support [71]. Financial barriers include home suitability, high out-of-pocket costs and time away from employment to undergo training. There is evidence that low-income and indigenous patients have reduced access to HHD [72]. Recognising and addressing these barriers can expand the HHD programmes in Australia and elsewhere. In Australia HHD is exclusively funded by the government, and it is one of the major reasons for increased uptake compared with other Western countries [73, 74].

## Peritoneal Dialysis

### Epidemiology

PD was introduced in Australia in the mid-1960s [75, 76]. Its popularity increased markedly in the late 1970s and 1980s after continuous ambulatory treatment became available [77]. Over the last decade, despite steady increases in the absolute numbers of PD patients in Australia, the proportion of patients with ESRD treated with PD has progressively fallen slightly from 21% ($n$ = 862) in 2009 to 19% in 2017 ($n$ = 2440) [26, 78]. During this time period, there have been progressive increases in the proportions of male, Indigenous and obese patients with higher comorbidity burdens [79]. Australia has the fifth highest utilisation of PD in the world with a treatment prevalence of 99 per million population (pmp) that is higher than both the global average (38.1 pmp) and the high-income country average (53 pmp) [80]. Like New Zealand and Finland, Australia follows a "home dialysis first" model rather than a "PD first" model [81]. Indeed, a number of Australian states specify targets for the proportion of dialysis patients receiving treatment at home (either PD or HHD) as a key performance indicator (e.g. Queensland specifies a target of 50%).

### Practice

PD is organised into "hub and spoke" models with parent services being responsible for clinical governance. There are 55 PD centres in Australia equating to 2.3 per million population, which is higher than the global average of 1.3 PD centres pmp [80]. Approximately two-thirds (67%) of Australian PD patients receive automated PD (APD), which is higher than the average APD utilisation by developed countries (42.4%, 95% CI 34.4–50.5) [26, 82]. Icodextrin prescription in 2016 was 45%, which has remained stable for the past decade [26]. In contrast, utilisation of neutral pH, low degradation production solutions has steadily increased from 4% in 2009 to 18% in 2016 [26], following the publication of the balANZ trial in 2012 [83]. Surgeons insert PD catheters in 78% of units using laparoscopy-only (34%), laparoscopy or open insertion (34%), open insertion-only (17%) or some other approach (15%) [84]. Despite evidence that coiled PD catheters have inferior outcomes, 45% of Australian PD units still use these catheters [84]. Two-thirds of units use a titanium connector, and 84% routinely flush the PD catheter during periods of PD rest ranging from alternate daily to monthly [84]. The median doctor/patient and nurse/patient ratios are 10:1 and 12:1, respectively, and 44% of units undertake multidisciplinary patient review [85]. In terms of infection control practices, 83% of Australian PD units prescribe antibiotic prophylaxis prior to PD catheter insertion, 22% routinely screen for nasal *S. aureus* carriage, 56% prescribe daily topical exit site mupirocin, 33% prescribe nasal mupirocin, and 89% coprescribe antifungal prophylaxis with antibiotic courses [85]. The most common initially prescribed antibiotics for the treatment of PD-related peritonitis are gentamicin (70%) and vancomycin (40%) [26]. PD training is provided by nursing staff and most commonly takes 4–5 days to complete with an average of 4–6 hours spent per day [86]. Eighty-six per cent of units have a written PD training curriculum, but only 37% undertake competency assessments following initial training [86].

### Outcomes

The most recently reported PD patient survival rates in Australia at 1, 3 and 5 years were 99% (95% CI 98–99%), 95% (95% CI 94–96%) and 64% (95% CI 61–66%), respectively [26]. Corresponding figures for technique survival (including death) were 84% (95% CI 82–85%), 41% (95% CI 37–46%) and 20% (95% CI 17–22%), whilst those for death-censored technique survival were 88% (95% CI 86–89%), 59% (95% CI 54–63%) and 37% (95% CI 33–41%) [26]. There have been progressive improvements in patient and technique survival rates over the last 15 years. The most common cause of technique failure is death (36%), followed by infection (21%), inadequate dialysis (11%), mechanical (10%), social (9%) and other (13%) [26, 87]. Peritonitis rates in Australia have fallen dramatically following a national quality improvement project (vide infra) and averaged 0.31 episodes per patient year at the end of 2016 [26]. However, there remains a sevenfold variation in observed peritonitis rates between different centres, which appears to be largely driven by centre factors rather than patient factors (case mix) [88, 89]. The most common organism responsible for PD-related peritonitis is coagulase-negative staphylococci followed by Gram-negative organisms [26]. Approximately three-quarters of patients with PD-related peritonitis are hospitalised, and 16% have their PD catheters removed [26, 90].

### Quality Improvement Initiative

The establishment of the Australian Peritonitis Registry on 1 October 2003 led to the generation of important information that clearly demonstrated that Australian PD units had variable and often poor PD infection control practices, which led to variable and unacceptably high peritonitis rates, which in turn led to variable and unacceptably high PD technique failure rates [91, 92]. These concerning data provided the impetus for the establishment of a national PD continuous quality improvement initiative in 2009 [91]. As part of this initiative, a national PD-related peritonitis key performance indicator project was established in which quarterly unit peritonitis data were fed back to individual units and benchmarked against all other units in an identified fashion. Other strategies included publishing two call to action papers [93, 94], conducting randomised controlled trials of novel PD-peritonitis prevention interventions through the Australasian Kidney Trials Network (AKTN) [83, 95], identifying barriers and enablers to adhering to ISPD peritonitis prevention and treatment guidelines through a KHA-CARI guideline implementation project [96], targeting education of early career nephrologists through the Australian PD Academy, developing local key opinion leaders to champion PD infection control, establishing a standardised PD training programme [97] and development of a Home Dialysis Network to educate, enable and empower home dialysis patients (http://homedialysis.org.au/). As a result of these projects, national peritonitis rates fell by one-third, and between-centre variation was halved within a period of 4 years and has been sustained thereafter (Fig. 52.4).

## Dialysis Reimbursement

Access to dialysis is universal to Australian residents who hold a current Medicare Card [98]. Australian public health system is predominantly based on the delivery and reimbursement of defined activities. The Australian government reimburses state and territory hospitals for the type and mix of services delivered, and the provision of dialysis is the responsibility of each state or territory [99]. Activity Based Funding (ABF) is one type of health funding in line with the August 2011 National Health Reform Agreement. Funding for public dialysis services comprises an ABF to cover dialysis services, including consumables and coordination costs [100].

Each in-centre (hospital-based) HD session counts as an admitted patient episode and is classified and funded under the admitted acute model. This payment applies only to

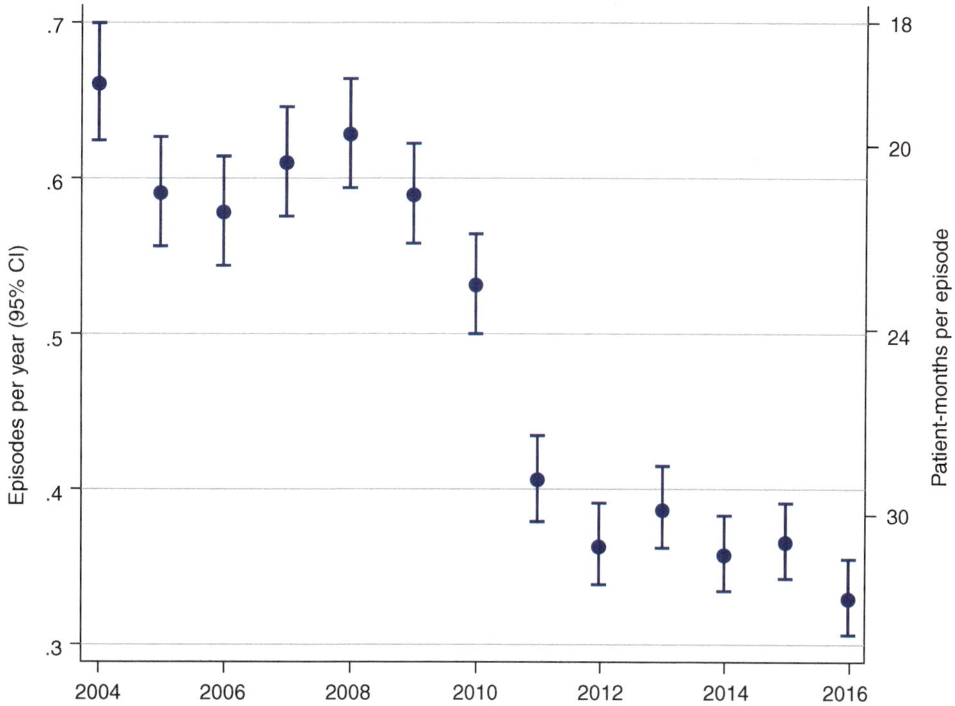


**Fig. 52.4** PD-related peritonitis rates in Australia 2004–2016. (Reproduced with permission of the Australia and New Zealand Dialysis and Transplant Registry)

activity measured by episode of care which is defined as a period of care with the principal clinical intent provided by a healthcare provider with a defined starting time and finish time. The episode of acute admission for HD is the same-day Australian Refined Diagnosis Related Groups (AR-DRG) code L61Z, with International Classification of Diseases 10th revision Australian Modification (ICD) principal diagnosis code Z49 [101, 102]. However, this does not apply to a patient undergoing dialysis whilst an inpatient for other conditions. In these circumstances, dialysis will be reimbursed as part of the hospital admission costs.

Dialysis sessions performed in satellite units are under the governance of hospital health services. Health services providing satellite dialysis are required to make a mandatory payment, comprising two components, per L61Z dialysis separation to their specialist hub to cover equipment, consumables and specialist services (i.e. 24 hour on-call/emergency service and other specialist renal coordination and services) [102]. On the other hand, home dialysis therapies (HHD and PD) are funded as a non-admitted service event based on relevant coding [101].

The annual cost of each dialysis modality per patient was estimated by the New South Wales Dialysis Costing Study, indexed to 2008–2009 Australian dollars. The total costs (including direct dialysis service provision, medical costs, ongoing out-of-pocket costs to patients and transplant work-up for those on waiting list) of hospital HD, satellite HD, HHD and PD were, respectively, $85,128, $70,409, $53,268 and $56,910 [103]. More recently, a micro-analysis study in Australia's Northern Territory urban and rural areas reported that the average annual cost of PD per patient (indexed to 2017 Australian dollars) was $87,250 in the first year, dropping to $58,489 in the second and subsequent years [99].

## Renal Transplantation

The first successful kidney transplant in Australia was performed in February 1965 at the Queen Elizabeth Hospital in Adelaide using a living donor. Successful living donor kidney transplants followed in both Melbourne and Sydney in that same year [104]. Much progress has been made since that early period as it has internationally. As with many other countries where kidney transplantation has become part of the routine care of patients with end-stage kidney failure, Australia has long ago developed a successful deceased donor programme whilst continuing to rely on living donation. In the last decade, a highly successful national paired kidney donation programme has also been established to assist those with incompatible living donors and to improve HLA matching using living donors [105].

Increased governmental efforts to improve organ donation rates have occurred through the establishment of a national Organ and Tissue Authority (OTA) in 2009. The OTA's responsibilities include the identification of as many donors as possible in hospitals, improving donor family consent rates and supporting donor coordination services. As a consequence, since 2009 Australia has experienced a doubling in the number of deceased organ donors. Deceased donation rates reached 22.2 donors per million population (dpmp) in 2018, compared to the pre-reform historic mean of 10.2 dpmp (2000–2008) [106]. In 2018 there were 897 kidneys transplanted from deceased donors and 238 kidneys transplanted from living donors [106]. Approximately one-third of all deceased kidney donations are now from donors with circulatory death (DCD) with two-thirds coming from donors with brain death (DBD). The average age of deceased donors has also increased in recent years with an increased use of older donors with various comorbidities. In 2017, 14.7% of donors were 65–74 years of age, and 1.8% were aged 75 years or older. The mean age of deceased donors was 46.4 years [107]. Of interest, the living donor rate in Australia has fallen as the number of deceased donors has increased and the waiting time for transplantation has improved.

National sharing of kidneys has been a feature of the Australian programme since kidney transplant units were first established in 1967. Kidneys are allocated to recipients that are blood group compatible and have a negative T cell cross match test with the donor. The cross match is currently based on a cytotoxicity assay, but Luminex identified HLA antibodies and a virtual cross match are also taken into account. In general, kidneys are matched and allocated either at a national level if there is a well-matched kidney especially for a sensitised recipient anywhere in the country or at a state level where more weight is given to time on the list. The national algorithm favours HLA matching with 0, 1 or 2 HLA mismatches whilst also prioritising the sensitised (based on panel reactive antibody score). Paediatric recipients (<18 years old) are also prioritised. If national criteria are not met for allocation, kidneys are then allocated according to a regional (state-based) algorithm which relies mostly on waiting time but also on some degree of HLA matching in most states [108]. Each state can also promote rare patients to an urgent category, usually those who become nearly impossible to dialyse due to difficult dialysis access. The current national and state-based kidney allocation system is coordinated through custom built computer software known as OrganMatch (released in May 2019). The principles and rules of allocation are defined by the national Renal Transplant Advisory Committee (RTAC), a committee of the Transplantation Society of New Zealand (TSANZ). The allocation rules and protocols are publicly available at the TSANZ website [108].

Individuals with ESRD have access to the kidney transplant waiting list and to transplantation if they are eligible for Medicare, the national public health support scheme. This is generally the case for all Australian citizens and permanent residents. Investigations, hospitalisation and surgery are all covered by the national scheme. Immunosuppressive medication costs are heavily subsidised by the government. Transplantation generally occurs in the public hospital system and not in private hospitals. Equity of access is an important basic principle, allowing candidates access to the waiting list and a transplant on the merits of their overall medical, surgical and psychological suitability, regardless of their level of private insurance, social status or race. Kidney transplant programmes follow national guidelines in the form of the Transplantation Society of Australia and New Zealand's (TSANZ) Clinical Guidelines [108] and the NHMRC Ethical Guidelines for Organ Transplantation from Deceased Donors [109].

Waiting time for kidney transplantation has shortened through increased deceased donation from a median of 5–6 years at its peak in the early 2000s to 2.4 years currently [110]. The total number of patients waiting for a kidney in Australia has also fallen from 1580 at its peak in 2002 to just under 1000 currently. Despite these significant improvements, challenges remain, especially for potential transplant recipients who have been sensitised to HLA antigens. Approximately 25–30% of the waiting list have moderate-high levels of anti-HLA antibodies making it difficult for them to find a compatible donor.

Living donation has always been an important component of kidney transplantation programmes in Australia. In recent years, recipients relying most heavily on living kidney donation are the sensitised, the paediatric population and those wishing to avoid dialysis. Currently, acceptance onto the deceased donor waiting list requires patients to have commenced dialysis; therefore, a pre-emptive (pre-dialysis) transplant is generally only possible with a living donor. Living donor assessment generally follows fairly strict guidelines, usually excluding potential donors with significant comorbidity such as vascular disease, suboptimal renal function, obesity, glucose intolerance, diabetes and past or current malignancy. Living donation is fully supported in the public hospital system under Medicare. Depending on their work circumstances, living donors also have access to a financial support scheme which partly covers their income so they can donate.

Blood group incompatible living donor transplants are performed either directly or as part of the paired kidney donation programme. Sensitised patients with incompatible living donors are also entered into the paired kidney donation programme as are some compatible pairs that are hoping to obtain an improved HLA or epitope match. Improving the immunological match is particularly important for younger patients who are likely to need a further transplant in the future. Non-directed (altruistic) living donors who are deemed suitable to donate are generally entered into the paired kidney donation programme to assist those who are sensitised. In this way, paired kidney donation domino chains can be generated with the last donor kidney in the sequence going to a recipient on the deceased donor waiting list. Otherwise paired kidney donations occur in closed-loop configurations consisting of 2–6 pairs in each chain.

Immunosuppressive drugs are heavily subsidised by the government significantly reducing the cost to recipients. In the current era, the majority of patients are on triple therapy maintenance immunosuppression with tacrolimus, mycophenolate mofetil and low-dose prednisolone. Steroid-free protocols are sometimes used, but these are less common over the last 15–20-year period. In the last decade, some patients are treated with mTOR inhibitors (sirolimus or everolimus) as one of their 2–3 agents. Cyclosporin and azathioprine are still used on occasion. Recipients with allografts surviving more than 15–20 years are more likely to still be on these older drugs and possibly be steroid-free. Induction agents commonly used include basiliximab as well as polyclonal antithymocyte antibodies.

The majority of units in Australia monitor patients with protocol biopsies especially within the first-year post-transplant. Often these are performed at 1, at 3–6 months and then at 12 months. At this stage, monitoring allografts with molecular techniques (e.g. gene arrays) is very uncommon due to the cost and lack of general availability of these methods.

As reported through the ANZDATA, overall Australian 5-year kidney transplant recipient survival is approximately 90%, with 5-year kidney survival at approximately 80% [111]. There is a five- to tenfold reduction in mortality for patients who have received a kidney transplant compared to those who remain on dialysis [112].

With the implementation of Australia's new allocation software, OrganMatch, in May 2019, survival matching or longevity matching of donor organs to recipients is currently under consideration. The broadened spectrum of both donors and recipients over the last decade requires a more sophisticated approach of allocation than we have had to date. Good-quality kidneys from younger, healthier donors have a longer predicted life span, and logically these should be allocated to recipients with longer predicted life expectancy. Kidneys with a shorter predicted life span are better allocated to older patients also with a shorter predicted life span. In the near future, Australia is likely to adopt an approach using Kidney Donor Prognosis Index (KDPI) to assist in the allocation process. It is hoped that this will allow for better overall outcomes from the entire available donor pool and avoid wasted life years of kidney function [113].

## Nephrology Practice in Australia

The practice of nephrology in Australia is similar that in other developed economies globally. Specific aspects in some ways are reflected by the somewhat unique organisation, funding and governance structures of Australian healthcare more broadly [114]. In 2019, Australia is a commonwealth of six states, two internal territories and several smaller external territories that came into being as a single country on 1 January 1901. The division of responsibilities as they pertain to healthcare between federal and state or territory governments gives insights as to specific structural and operational differences to other health systems [115]. In general and in terms of delivery, community-based healthcare has become the responsibility of the national federal government where public hospital-based healthcare is the responsibility of state/territorial governments. Overarching this however is the principle of a universal healthcare system underpinned by public hospitals and an additional private healthcare system with partially publicly reimbursed and incentivised private health insurance. Despite this apparent complexity, healthcare access and outcomes are enviable within a global context [116].

Kidney healthcare delivery is no exception. Resourcing of kidney health and workforce development deliver nephrological care effectively, even in spite of increasing numbers of renal replacement therapy-treated patients [26, 117]. Chronic kidney disease more generally is being understood with greater clarity, including the variation in its incidence, prevalence and characteristics around Australia [118]. The significant geographical and environmental challenges that can occur further add a depth to this complexity.

The nephrology workforce in Australia is developed via a training pathway nationally accredited and regulated by the Australian Medical Council in concert with Australian Health Practitioner Regulation Agency, both operating under the auspices of the Australian Federal Government. This pathway commences after medical school training and a 1-year accredited internship. It is administered by the Royal Australasian College of Physicians which is the professional college for adult physician and paediatrician training across both Australia and New Zealand. After an initial 3 years of basic physician training, both a written and clinical examination are undertaken, success at which enables progress to a further 3 years of advanced training. At present this requires all 3 years to be core training time and must include acute kidney transplantation and kidney biopsy exposure and experience. At the completion of the 6-year programme in either adult or paediatric medicine, Fellowship is granted in Nephrology or Paediatric Nephrology which enables one to enter nephrology practice. This training pathway has resulted in a nephrology workforce which compares favourably both regionally and globally [119].

At present, the supply of nephrologists and nephrology trainees in Australia is favourable in terms of domestic supply [119], resulting in some challenges in terms of post-training employment [120]. In public employment after completion of nephrology training, specialist nephrologists in Australia are remunerated at approximately $300,000 Australian dollars/year/full time equivalent, though there may be variation by location, state, specific duties and other role-specific elements.

The practice of nephrology in Australia as a specialist is not significantly different to that of other comparable Commonwealth countries such as New Zealand, Canada or the UK. Whilst some regional variations clearly can occur, they are not likely generalised in nature. Patients and their priorities and outcomes are the key focus of Australian nephrologists, and this is reflected by the SONG (Standardised Outcomes in Nephrology) initiative which has been initiated and based from Australia. The enthusiastic and functional nature of Australian nephrological practice is likely to continue as the specialty evolves internationally.

## Highlights of Nephrology in Australia

### Green Nephrology

The twenty-first century has seen accelerating climate change and biodiversity loss, which together pose unprecedented risks to human health [121–123]. The world over, this has led to growing appreciation of the need for all sectors to start "thinking and doing" in more environmentally conscious ways.

The healthcare sector is a significant contributor to resource depletion and greenhouse gas emissions [124, 125], with the environmental impact of kidney care delivery (particularly dialysis) appearing to be especially high [126]. This suggests the nephrology community has a major role to play in exploring environmentally responsible healthcare practice.

The concept of "green nephrology" was first pioneered in Australia, where over 15 years ago, the Barwon Health Renal Service, led by Professor John Agar, began to critically analyse and document the vast resource usage and carbon footprint of haemodialysis procedures [127, 128]. This was followed by detailed chemical and microbial testing of reverse osmosis reject water to prove its quality and then the installation of the necessary infrastructure to allow for its capture and reuse [127, 129]. The ability of renewable energy generation to offset haemodialysis-related power usage was also investigated, with both feasibility and cost-effectiveness demonstrated [130].

Since that time, a limited number of other individual dialysis services in Australia have taken similar important steps towards monitoring and improving the environmental profile of dialysis. However, efforts have been piecemeal, and overall progress has been slow, as has been the case elsewhere in the world.

More recently, however, signs of more wide-ranging, substantive change have appeared. The Australian and New Zealand Society of Nephrology (ANZSN), in partnership with the Renal Society of Australasia and Kidney Health Australia, has developed a position statement on green nephrology. The ANZSN is also now funding prizes to encourage research in the environmental space, the first known national body to do so. Research is underway examining the utility of adding shredded, sterilised waste plastic from haemodialysis procedures into concrete, with preliminary results suggesting this may improve the quality and durability of the end product [131, 132]. The implications of this are potentially far-reaching not only for waste management in dialysis but also in the broader healthcare sector. An existing Australian "Green Dialysis" website (htpps://www.greendialysis.org) has been expanded and upgraded to provide practical information for those wishing to implement changes in their own facilities, whilst social media platforms for posting and discussing ideas are slowly building.

Outside Australia, other national and regional societies have also begun to demonstrate leadership. The European Renal Association-European Dialysis and Transplant Association has recently committed to a broad range of initiatives aimed at "greening" the renal sector [133]. In Brazil, a "call to action" has been made by the national kidney society to the nephrology community [134]. Nephrology journals are also increasingly seeking and publishing papers in the environmental space [135–137].

Is there more to do? With awareness still low, changes far from widespread and dialysis patient numbers and thereby resource usage exponentially rising across the developed and developing world, the answer to this question is a categorical "yes". The need for the nephrology community to quantify, to document and to adopt resource conservation measures becomes ever-more important, in Australia and elsewhere.

### The Big Red Kidney Bus: An Australian Dialysis Holiday

The Big Red Kidney Bus (BRKB) is a heavily modified bus equipped to offer HD at remote locations. It has been fitted out with full water purification (pre-filtration and reverse osmosis) and 3 HD machines, thus offering 12 patients per week the opportunity of undertaking dialysis on holiday. Staffed by a fully trained dialysis nurse, it offers two shifts of dialysis per day typically in a "caravan park" (=trailer park in the USA) at a desirable location such as by the seaside or in the mountains (Fig. 52.5). Water and power are provided on-site by the parks (including three-phase power). The bus remains on-site for typically 6–8 weeks, and patients are able to book in for 1-week blocks – they organise their own accommodation, most typically in on-site cabins. They are then able to take advantage of the local touristic attractions.

Care is coordinated through a single public hospital. Initially, patients book through the patient advocacy group Kidney Health Australia (KHA) either on-line or over the phone, and then the Hospital "Bus Coordinator" ensures the patient meets the acceptance criteria (e.g. no temporary lines, stable cardiovascular status, non-infective status). The

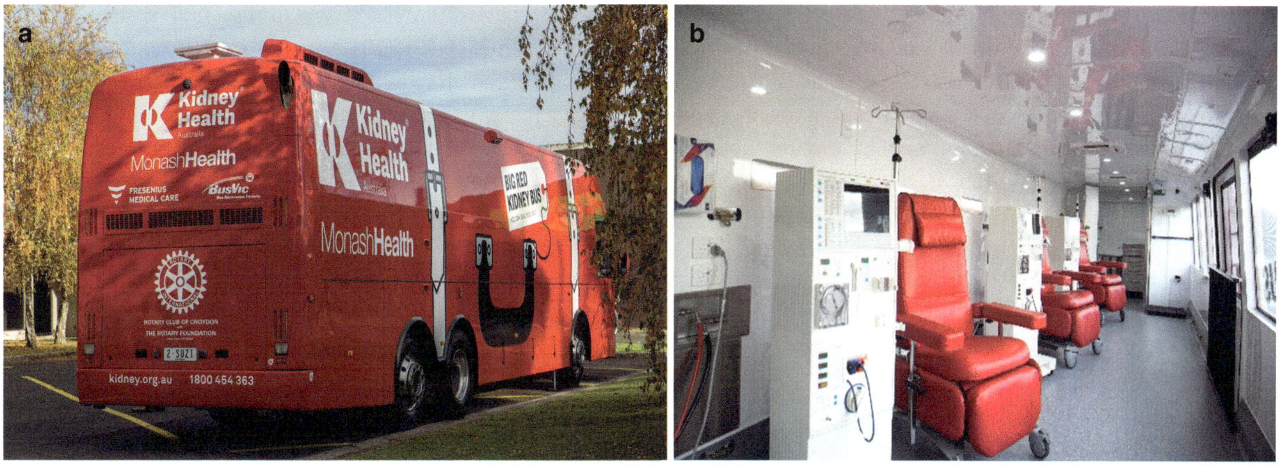


Fig. 52.5 The Big Red Kidney Bus

Hospital provides the dialysis consumables and is funded via the public hospital system, considering the dialysed patients as hospital patients. The patients bring their own medications, including anti-coagulation for dialysis. On-site dialysis nurse staffing is also provided by the Hospital.

The Bus Coordinator then juggles the schedules and staffing to optimise use of the facilities. Medical supervision is remote only – with the on-site dialysis nurse being able to contact a nephrologist from the Hospital whenever required. If there is a nearby dialysis facility, they are always notified of the Bus's presence in case of need. Technical services are provided by the coordinating hospital, which includes assistance with set-up and pack-up. Typically, a week is allocated to pack-up, moving to a new site and subsequent set-up.

The BRKB has been a great success, offering holiday and respite dialysis to a large group of patients from around Australia. The response from patients and their families has been universally positive. The model began in the state of Victoria but has since expanded to a second Bus in New South Wales. The model began as the initiative of a group of patients in Victoria who approached both KHA and the Hospital with the suggestion of the Bus. KHA raised the money to obtain and refit the Bus through charitable endeavours.

## The Keeping Kidneys Programme: A General Practitioner with Special Interest Model of Care for Community Kidney Health

Intervention in early-stage CKD slows rate of progression [138]. First-contact healthcare providers like general practitioners (GPs) are ideally positioned to detect and manage the early stages of CKD, with >80% of Australians attending a GP each year. Keeping Kidneys in the Community (KK) was developed to leverage this high prevalence of patient contact. The programme was implemented in 2018 in a less-privileged socioeconomic area of Queensland, Australia, where access to specialised kidney care was not available. The aim of the programme is to augment a specific subset of GP kidney care skills in a two-phase curriculum. The longer-term aim is taking these skills back to local practices managing people with CKD in their communities [139].

In the proof of concept, two GPs were recruited and trained in a two-phase curriculum. The first phase focused on augmenting present knowledge and skills in CKD, specifically screening for kidney disease, developing a diagnostic approach to CKD aetiologies and formulating management plans. The second phase was a 6-month period of clinical detailing with a consultant nephrologist.

Patients are streamed to the KK clinic if they are (1) referred for kidney care to the parent specialty kidney service, (2) have at least one indicator of kidney disease, (3) live in the surrounding community and (4) do not have an exclusion criterion. Exclusion criteria include rapid deterioration of kidney function (eGFR decline >8 ml/min p.a.), kidney transplant recipient, receiving dialysis or expected to start within 6 months and/or on immunomodulatory therapies targeting kidney disease. Goals of care include:

- Establishing a (putative) diagnosis
- Developing a management plan and the decision of who and where follow-up care will be – discharged back to their GPs, managed in shared care with their GPs or managed in shared care with a specialist

Figure 52.6 illustrates patients' timeline and pathways of KK [139].

One hundred and forty patients were referred to KK in the first 8 months of its operation. Median age was 76 years (67–81). Most patients were in CKD stage 3B (54%) or 3A (22%). Hypertension and diabetes were the leading CKD causes, but 33% had no aetiological diagnosis at entry. Most patients had low-average scores for CKD knowledge

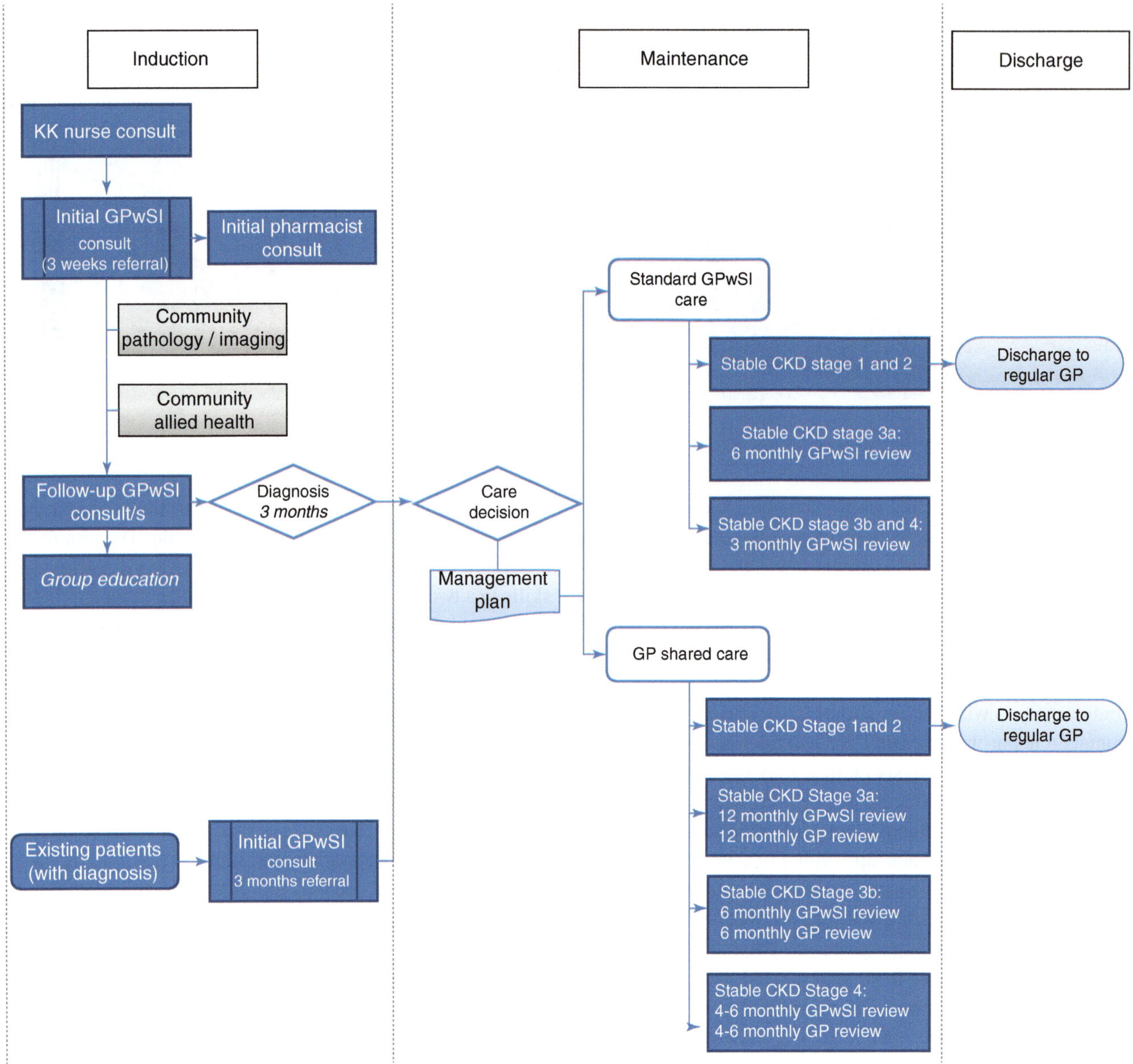


**Fig. 52.6** Patient timeline and pathways of the Keeping Kidneys (KK) Programme. GP general practitioner, KHS Kidney Health Service, OPD outpatient department, GPwSI general practitioner with special interest, RRT renal replacement therapy

(13 ± 14/28) and CKD self-management (46 ± 6/116). Median Charlson comorbidity score, which quantifies an individual's burden of disease, was 7 and predicted a survival of <10 years. CKD complications, e.g. anaemia and bone mineral disease, were not largely prevalent in this cohort. Mean haemoglobin (Hb) was 12.6 ± 2 g/dL but 5% had Hb <10 g/dL. Mean parathyroid hormone, calcium and phosphate were, respectively, 94 ± 81 pg/mL, 9.6 ± 0.5 and 3.4 ± 0.5 mg/dL. Prevalence of hypocalcaemia and hyperphosphataemia were, respectively, 1% and 2%. Median urine albumin/creatinine ratio was 38 (12–75) mg/g. One patient was referred for renal biopsy due to nephrotic range proteinuria and one for bone marrow biopsy with a differential diagnosis of multiple myeloma. Patients travelled, on average, 25 minutes less for their appointments, with 72% seen within 15 km of their homes. Patients were generally satisfied with the care they receive with 90% agreeing or strongly agreeing that they "have confidence and trust in the doctor they saw". Furthermore, the local district health service noted a 25% reduction in the outpatient waiting list for specialty kidney services during this time [139, 140].

KK is a new model of care that focuses on the interface between patients, GPs and specialists, with a strong emphasis on the pivotal role of GPs in the health system in Australia. Trained GPs were capable of staging severity of kidney disease, initiating the work-up of the cause(s) of the kidney disease and screening for complications. They managed a cohort of patients with CKD that were elderly and had intermediately advanced CKD and complex comorbidities in their communities. KK also released capacity in public kidney specialty services.

Many cases of CKD may be preventable through the control of modifiable risk factors [141]. All the opportunities to change the burden of CKD lie in the better recognition, knowledge and management of CKD at earlier, less severe stages of disease. Furthermore, delaying the onset of ESRD reduces the huge and escalating cost on our society. Therefore, additional training and education is warranted to better equip GPs to directly impact on CKD complications and disease progression. KK presents a unique opportunity to explore a new model of care aiming to deliver better healthcare outcomes.

## Future Perspectives of Nephrology in Australia

An ageing population, increasing prevalence of diabetes mellitus and the burden of CKD challenge the capacity of health jurisdictions across Australia [142]. Kidney disease utilises approximately 15% of all hospitalisations in Australia [103]. Furthermore, the demand for dialysis has significantly increased in Australia over recent decades [53]. The cost of treating ESRD from 2009 to 2020 is estimated to be around $12 billion to the Australian government [103]. In recent years, state-wide commissions and networks have proposed evidence-based initiatives and actions to address current and future challenges to renal services [142–148]. Each state has its own commission for strategic planning. Nevertheless they share several common goals and priorities such as:

- Investment in early detection and management of CKD particularly engaging local primary care physicians
- Integration of renal and palliative care for patients with chronic renal disease through kidney supportive care programmes
- Increasing accessibility – renal care closer to home
- Decentralisation of services with increased utilisation of telehealth
- A shift towards less inpatient activity to well-supported outpatient home-based care, including HHD and PD
- Increasing renal transplantation

The future of nephrology in Australia is optimistic given how engaged the many stakeholders, necessary to product different outcomes in chronic diseases, like kidney disease, are. At a system level, our federal legislators have enacted enablers like the national Organ and Tissue Authority in the parliament; health planners in multiple states continue to engage in the challenges of delivering CKD services, with the Advancing Kidney Care 2026 in Queensland but one example; and we have reliable and robust platforms for ongoing data collections and reporting in the Australian Bureau of Statistics, the Australian Institute of Health and Welfare and ANZDATA. Australia has a vibrant kidney research community of academics, clinician-scientists and clinicians delivering measurable impacts across the spectrum of types of research. In recent times research funders have emphasised the translational impact of their granting, with clinical trials, implementation science and service delivery research. Innovations like green nephrology and different models of care are springing from these environments. The immediate future promises to be an incubator for nephrology clinicians who have ideas to test in our clinical spaces.

## References


1. Australia|history, cities, capital, map, & facts|Britannica. https://www.britannica.com/place/Australia. Accessed 2 Dec 2019.
2. Population clock. https://www.abs.gov.au/AUSSTATS/abs@.nsf/Web+Pages/Population+Clock?opendocument&ref=HPKI. Accessed 2 Dec 2019.
3. 1301.0 – year book Australia, 2004. https://www.abs.gov.au/Ausstats/abs@.nsf/Previousproducts/1301.0Feature. Article 32004. Accessed 2 Dec 2019.
4. Interesting facts about Australia's population. https://www.abs.gov.au/websitedbs/D3310114.nsf/home/Interesting+Facts+about+Australia's+population. Accessed 2 Dec 2019.
5. Remote offshore territories|geoscience Australia. https://www.ga.gov.au/scientific-topics/national-location-information/dimensions/remote-offshore-territories. Accessed 2 Dec 2019.
6. Australia is a top 20 country – Department of Foreign Affairs and Trade. https://dfat.gov.au/trade/resources/publications/Pages/australia-is-a-top-20-country.aspx. Accessed 2 Dec 2019.
7. Dique JC. The artificial kidney in the treatment of severe puerperal infection due to Clostridium welchii, with report of a case. Med J Aust. 1955;42:781–9.
8. Acute kidney injury in Australia: a first national snapshot – Australian Institute of Health and Welfare. https://www.aihw.gov.au/reports/chronic-kidney-disease/acute-kidney-injury-in-australia/contents/table-of-contents. Accessed 7 Aug 2019.
9. Teo S, Kotwal S, Campbell C, Liu Z, Herath S, Horvath AEZ. Outcome and management of acute kidney injury (AKI) detected using electronic alerts – a prospective study from an Australian Tertiary Care Centre. Nephrology (Carlton). 2018;23:71.
10. Wilson GJ, Mallett A, Kark A, Tan AK, Cameron A, Wang Z, Healy HG, Hoy W. Rates and characteristics of acute kidney injury (Aki) in the chronic kidney disease in Queensland (Ckd. Qld) registry. Nephrology. 2017;22:53.
11. Silvester W, Bellomo R, Cole L. Epidemiology, management, and outcome of severe acute renal failure of critical illness in Australia. Crit Care Med. 2001;29:1910–5.
12. The RENAL Study Investigators. Renal replacement therapy for acute kidney injury in Australian and New Zealand intensive care units: a practice survey. Crit Care Resusc. 2008;10:225–30.
13. Levin A, Lamb EJ, White CT, Stevens PE, Bilous RW, Coresh J, De Francisco ALM, De Jong PE, Griffith KE, Hemmelgarn BR, Iseki K, Levey AS, Riella MC, Shlipak MG, Wang H, Winearls CG. KDIGO 2012 clinical practice guideline for the evaluation and management of chronic kidney disease. Kidney Int Suppl. 2013;3:1–150.

14. National Kidney Foundation. K/DOQI clinical practice guidelines for chronic kidney disease: evaluation, classification, and stratification. Am J Kidney Dis. 2002;39:S1–266.
15. Chadban SJ, Briganti EM, Kerr PG, Dunstan DW, Welborn TA, Zimmet PZ, Atkins RC. Prevalence of kidney damage in Australian adults: the AusDiab kidney study. J Am Soc Nephrol. 2003;14:S131–8.
16. White SL, Polkinghorne KR, Atkins RC, Chadban SJ. Comparison of the prevalence and mortality risk of CKD in Australia using the CKD Epidemiology Collaboration (CKD-EPI) and Modification of Diet in Renal Disease (MDRD) Study GFR estimating equations: the AusDiab (Australian Diabetes, Obesity and Lifestyle) study. Am J Kidney Dis. 2010;55:660–70.
17. Australian Institute of Health and Welfare. Chronic kidney disease. Cat. no. CDK 16. Canberra: AIHW; 2019. https://www.aihw.gov.au/reports/chronic-kidney-disease/chronic-kidney-disease. Accessed 23 Sep 2019.
18. National health survey: first results, 2017-18. https://www.abs.gov.au/ausstats/abs@.nsf/Lookup/bySubject/4364.0.55.001~2017-18~MainFeatures~Kidneydisease~65. Accessed 23 Sep 2019.
19. Australia Bureau of Statistics. Australian health survey: biomedical results for chronic diseases, 2011-12. Canberra: ABS; 2013. https://www.abs.gov.au/AUSSTATS/abs@.nsf/DetailsPage/4364.0.55.0052011-12. Accessed 23 Sep 2019.
20. AIHW. National mortality database. https://meteor.aihw.gov.au/content/index.phtml/itemId/395084. Accessed 23 Sep 2019.
21. Venuthurupalli SK, Hoy WE, Healy HG, Cameron A, Fassett RG. CKD.QLD: establishment of a chronic kidney disease [CKD] registry in Queensland, Australia. BMC Nephrol. 2017;18:189.
22. Zhang J, Healy HG, Venuthurupalli SK, Tan K-S, Wang Z, Cameron A, Hoy WE. Blood pressure management in hypertensive people with non-dialysis chronic kidney disease in Queensland, Australia. BMC Nephrol. 2019;20:348.
23. Zhang J, Healy HG, Baboolal K, et al. Frequency and consequences of acute kidney injury in patients with CKD: a registry study in Queensland Australia. Kidney Med. 2019;1:180–90.
24. Venuthurupalli SK, Healy H, Fassett R, Cameron A, Wang Z, Hoy WE. Chronic kidney disease, Queensland: profile of patients with chronic kidney disease from regional Queensland, Australia: A registry report. Nephrology. 2019;24:1257.
25. Mallett A, Patel C, Salisbury A, Wang Z, Healy H, Hoy W. The prevalence and epidemiology of genetic renal disease amongst adults with chronic kidney disease in Australia. Orphanet J Rare Dis. 2014;9:98.
26. ANZDATA 40th annual report 2017 – ANZDATA. https://www.anzdata.org.au/report/anzdata-40th-annual-report-2017/. Accessed 7 Aug 2019.
27. Fletcher J, McDonald S, Alexander SI. Prevalence of genetic renal disease in children. Pediatr Nephrol. 2013;28:251–6.
28. Savige JA. The gene corresponding to the putative Goodpasture antigen is present in Alport's syndrome. Clin Exp Immunol. 1991;85:236–9.
29. Savige JA, Mavrova L, Kincaid-Smith P. Inhibitable anti-GBM antibody activity after renal transplantation in Alport's syndrome. Transplantation. 1989;48:704–5.
30. Savige J, Gregory M, Gross O, Kashtan C, Ding J, Flinter F. Expert guidelines for the management of alport syndrome and thin basement membrane nephropathy. J Am Soc Nephrol. 2013;24:364–75.
31. Savige J, Rana K, Tonna S, Buzza M, Dagher H, Wang YY. Thin basement membrane nephropathy. Kidney Int. 2003;64:1169–78.
32. Rangan GK, Savige J. Introduction to the KHA-CARI guidelines on ADPKD. Semin Nephrol. 2015;35:521–3.
33. Rangan GK, Alexander SI, Campbell KL, et al. KHA-CARI guideline recommendations for the diagnosis and management of autosomal dominant polycystic kidney disease. Nephrology. 2016;21:705–16.
34. Tong A, Tunnicliffe DJ, Lopez-Vargas P, et al. Identifying and integrating consumer perspectives in clinical practice guidelines on autosomal-dominant polycystic kidney disease. Nephrology. 2016;21:122–32.
35. Wong ATY, Mannix C, Grantham JJ, et al. Randomised controlled trial to determine the efficacy and safety of prescribed water intake to prevent kidney failure due to autosomal dominant polycystic kidney disease (PREVENT-ADPKD). BMJ Open. 2018;8:1–13.
36. Takasato M, Er PX, Chiu HS, et al. Kidney organoids from human iPS cells contain multiple lineages and model human nephrogenesis. Nature. 2015;526:564–8.
37. Howden SE, Thomson JA, Little MH. Simultaneous reprogramming and gene editing of human fibroblasts. Nat Protoc. 2018;13:875–98.
38. Haynes JM, Selby JN, Vandekolk TH, et al. Induced pluripotent stem cell–derived podocyte-like cells as models for assessing mechanisms underlying heritable disease phenotype: initial studies using two Alport syndrome patient lines indicate impaired potassium channel activity. J Pharmacol Exp Ther. 2018;367:335–47.
39. Forbes TA, Howden SE, Lawlor K, et al. Patient-iPSC-derived kidney organoids show functional validation of a ciliopathic renal phenotype and reveal underlying pathogenetic mechanisms. Am J Hum Genet. 2018;102:816–31.
40. Jayasinghe K, Quinlan C, Stark Z, Patel C, Mallawaarachchi A, Wardrop L, Kerr PG, Trnka P, Mallett AJ. Renal genetics in Australia: kidney medicine in the genomic age. Nephrology. 2019;24:279–86.
41. Mallett AJ, McCarthy HJ, Ho G, et al. Massively parallel sequencing and targeted exomes in familial kidney disease can diagnose underlying genetic disorders. Kidney Int. 2017;92:1493–506.
42. Mallett A, Fowles LF, McGaughran J, Healy H, Patel C. A multidisciplinary renal genetics clinic improves patient diagnosis. Med J Aust. 2016;204:58–9.
43. Jayasinghe K, Quinlan C, Stark Z, Patel C, Sampson MG, Saleem M, Mallett AJ. Meeting report of the 2017 KidGen Renal Genetics Symposium. Hum Genomics. 2018;12:5.
44. Rasmussen M, Guo X, Wang Y, et al. An aboriginal Australian genome reveals separate human dispersals into Asia. Science. 2011;334:94–8.
45. Australian Bureau of Statistics Census of Population and Housing: Australia revealed, 2016. https://www.abs.gov.au/ausstats/abs@.nsf/0/63230DE0557F3B83CA2581470023C559?Opendocument. Accessed 26 Sep 2019.
46. Broome R. Aboriginal Australians: a history since 1788. Auckland: Allen & Unwin; 2010.
47. ANZDATA Registry. 41st report, chapter 10: end stage kidney disease in Indigenous peoples of Australia and Aotearoa/New Zealand. Adelaide: Australia and New Zealand Dialysis and Transplant Registry; 2018. http://www.anzdata.org.au. Accessed 28 Sep 2019.
48. Hoy WE, Hughson MD, Bertram JF, Douglas-Denton R, Amann K. Nephron number, hypertension, renal disease, and renal failure. J Am Soc Nephrol. 2005;16:2557–64.
49. Lawton PD, McDonald SP, Snelling PL, Hughes J, Cass A. Organ transplantation in Australia: inequities in access and outcome for Indigenous Australians. Transplantation. 2017;101:e345–6.
50. Rogers NM, Lawton PD, Jose MD. Kidney transplant outcomes in the Indigenous population in the Northern Territory of Australia. Transplantation. 2006;82:882–6.
51. George CR. History of home haemodialysis in Australia. Nephrology. 2005;10:215–21.
52. ANZDATA 42nd annual report 2019 – ANZDATA. https://www.anzdata.org.au. Accessed 28 Sep 2019.
53. ANZDATA Registry. 41st report, chapter 4: haemodialysis. Adelaide: Australia and New Zealand Dialysis and Transplant Registry; 2018. http://www.anzdata.org.au. Accessed 22 Aug 2019.

54. Mac K, Hedley J, Kelly PJ, et al. Effect of centre- and patient-related factors on uptake of haemodiafiltration in Australia and New Zealand: a cohort study using ANZDATA. Nephrology. 2019;25:63.
55. Kerr PG, Toussaint ND, Kidney Health Australia, Caring for Australasians with Renal Impairment. KHA-CARI guideline: dialysis adequacy (haemodialysis): dialysis membranes. Nephrology. 2013;18:485–8.
56. ANZDATA Registry. 41st report, chapter 1: incidence of end stage kidney disease. Adelaide: Australia and New Zealand Dialysis and Transplant Registry; 2018. http://www.anzdata.org.au. Accessed 28 Sep 2019.
57. Wolley MJ, Hawley CM, Johnson DW, Marshall MR, Roberts MA. Incremental and twice weekly haemodialysis in Australia and New Zealand. Nephrology (Carlton). 2019;24:1172.
58. Australian regulatory guidelines for medical devices (ARGMD), V1.1|Therapeutic Goods Administration (TGA). https://www.tga.gov.au/publication/australian-regulatory-guidelines-medical-devices-argmd-v11. Accessed 2 Dec 2019.
59. See EJ, Hedley J, Agar JWM, et al. Patient survival on haemodiafiltration and haemodialysis: a cohort study using the Australia and New Zealand Dialysis and Transplant Registry. Nephrol Dial Transplant. 2019;34:326–38.
60. Curtis FK, Cole JJ, Fellows BJ, Tyler LLSB. Hemodialysis in the home. Am Soc Artif Intern Organs. 1965;11:7–10.
61. Merrill JP, Schupak E, Cameron E, Hampers CL. Hemodialysis in the home. JAMA. 1964;190:468–70.
62. Baillod RA, Comty C, Ilahi M, Konotey-Ahulu FID, Sevitt LSS. Overnight haemodialysis in the home. Proc Eur Dial Transpl Assoc. 1965;2:99–103.
63. Dawborn JK, Marshall VC. Home dialysis: a case report. Med J Aust. 1968;2:837–40.
64. Nosé Y. Home hemodialysis: a crazy idea in 1963: a memoir. ASAIO J. 2000;46:13–7.
65. Report of the ad-hoc committee on rationalisation of facilities for organ transplantation and renal dialysis. Med J Aust. 1968;2:1200–8.
66. Agar JWM, Somerville CA, Dwyer KM, Simmonds RE, Boddington JM, Waldron CM. Nocturnal hemodialysis in Australia. Hemodial Int. 2003;7:278–89.
67. United States renal data system. https://www.usrds.org/2018/view/v2_11.aspx. Accessed 19 Aug 2019.
68. Chow J. A pre-training assessment tool for home dialysis (JPAT). EDTNA ERCA J. 2005;31:19–23.
69. Home Dialysis Central|MATCH-D. https://homedialysis.org/match-d. Accessed 19 Aug 2019.
70. Muir CA, Kotwal SS, Hawley CM, Polkinghorne K, Gallagher MP, Snelling P, Jardine MJ. Buttonhole cannulation and clinical outcomes in a home hemodialysis cohort and systematic review. Clin J Am Soc Nephrol. 2014;9:110–9.
71. Walker RC, Hanson CS, Palmer SC, Howard K, Morton RL, Marshall MR, Tong A. Patient and caregiver perspectives on home hemodialysis: a systematic review. Am J Kidney Dis. 2015;65:451. https://doi.org/10.1053/j.ajkd.2014.10.020.
72. Walker R, Howard K, Morton R. Home hemodialysis: a comprehensive review of patient-centered and economic considerations. Clin Outcomes Res. 2017;9:149–61.
73. Kidney Health Australia. Financial support for home dialysis patients in Australia 2. https://kidney.org.au/cms_uploads/docs/home-dialysis-financial-assistance-electricity-water-and-subsidies.pdf. Accessed 19 Aug 2019.
74. Independent Hospital Pricing Authority Home delivered dialysis costing study to inform the National Efficient Price 2015. 2014. Final Report.
75. Gurr F. Peritoneal dialysis. Med J Aust. 1954;2:653–5.
76. Wood T. Experiences with peritoneal dialysis. Med J Aust. 1965;2:150–3.
77. George CRP. Caring for kidneys in the antipodes: how Australia and New Zealand have addressed the challenge of end-stage renal failure. Am J Kidney Dis. 2009;53:536–45.
78. ANZDATA Registry. 33rd report, chapter 6: peritoneal dialysis. Adelaide: Australia and New Zealand Dialysis and Transplant Registry; 2010.
79. Li PKT, Chow KM, Van De Luijtgaarden MWM, Johnson DW, Jager KJ, Mehrotra R, Naicker S, Pecoits-Filho R, Yu XQ, Lameire N. Changes in the worldwide epidemiology of peritoneal dialysis. Nat Rev Nephrol. 2017;13:90–103.
80. Bello AK, Levin A, Lunney M, et al. (2019). Global Kidney Health Atlas: A report by the International Society of Nephrology on the Global Burden of End-stage Kidney Disease and Capacity for Kidney Replacement Therapy and Conservative Care across World Countries and Regions. International Society of Nephrology, Brussels, Belgium.
81. Liu FX, Gao X, Inglese G, Chuengsaman P, Pecoits-Filho R, Yu A. A global overview of the impact of peritoneal dialysis first or favored policies: an opinion. Perit Dial Int. 2015;35:406–20.
82. Jain AK, Blake P, Cordy P, Garg AX. Global trends in rates of peritoneal dialysis. J Am Soc Nephrol. 2012;23:533–44.
83. Johnson DW, Brown FG, Clarke M, et al. Effects of biocompatible versus standard fluid on peritoneal dialysis outcomes. J Am Soc Nephrol. 2012;23:1097–107.
84. Cho Y, Boudville N, Palmer SC, et al. Practice of peritoneal dialysis catheter flushing in Australia and New Zealand: multi-center cross-sectional survey. Perit Dial Int. 2018;38:98–103.
85. Boudville N, Johnson DW, Zhao J, et al. Regional variation in the treatment and prevention of peritoneal dialysis-related infections in the peritoneal dialysis outcomes and practice patterns study. Nephrol Dial Transpl. 2018;34:2118.
86. Boudville N, Cho Y, Equinox KL, et al. Teaching peritoneal dialysis in Australia: an opportunity for improvement. Nephrology. 2018;23:259–63.
87. Lan PG, Clayton PA, Johnson DW, McDonald SP, Borlace M, Badve SV, Sud K, Boudville N. Duration of hemodialysis following peritoneal dialysis cessation in Australia and New Zealand: proposal for a standardized definition of technique failure. Perit Dial Int. 2016;36:623–30.
88. Htay H, Cho Y, Pascoe EM, et al. Center effects and peritoneal dialysis peritonitis outcomes: analysis of a National Registry. Am J Kidney Dis. 2018;71:814–21.
89. Nadeau-Fredette AC, Johnson DW, Hawley CM, et al. Center-specific factors associated with peritonitis risk—a multi-center registry analysis. Perit Dial Int. 2016;36:509–18.
90. Ghali JR, Bannister KM, Brown FG, Rosman JB, Wiggins KJ, Johnson DW, McDonald SP. Microbiology and outcomes of peritonitis in Australian peritoneal dialysis patients. Perit Dial Int. 2011;31:651–62.
91. Nataatmadja M, Cho Y, Johnson DW. Continuous quality improvement initiatives to sustainably reduce peritoneal dialysis-related infections in Australia and New Zealand. Perit Dial Int. 2016;36:472–7.
92. Cho Y, Johnson DW. Peritoneal dialysis-related peritonitis: towards improving evidence, practices, and outcomes. Am J Kidney Dis. 2014;64:278–89.
93. Jose MD, Johnson DW, Mudge DW, Tranaeus A, Voss D, Walker R, Bannister KM. Peritoneal dialysis practice in Australia and New Zealand: a call to action. Nephrology. 2011;16:19–29.
94. Mudge DW, Boudville N, Brown F, et al. Peritoneal dialysis practice in Australia and New Zealand: a call to sustain the action. Nephrology. 2016;21:535–46.
95. Johnson DW, Badve SV, Pascoe EM, et al. Antibacterial honey for the prevention of peritoneal-dialysis-related infections (HONEYPOT): a randomised trial. Lancet Infect Dis. 2014;14:23–30.

96. Campbell DJ, Brown F, Craig J, Gallagher M, Johnson DW, Kirkland G, Kumar SK, Lim WH, Ranganathan D, Saweirs W, Sud K, Toussaint ND, Walker RG, Yehia MMD. Assessment of current practice and barriers to antimicrobial prophylaxis in peritoneal dialysis patients. Nephrology. 2014;19:42.
97. Chow JSF, Cho Y, Equinox K-L, et al. An intervention design: supporting skills development for peritoneal dialysis trainers. Perit Dial Int. 2019;39:134–41.
98. Medicare benefits schedule book. http://www.health.gov.au/mbsonline. Accessed 2 Dec 2019.
99. Gorham G, Howard K, Zhao Y, et al. Cost of dialysis therapies in rural and remote Australia – a micro-costing analysis. BMC Nephrol. 2019;20:231.
100. State of Queensland (Queensland Health). Health funding principles and guidelines 2017–18 financial year. https://www.health.qld.gov.au/__data/assets/pdf_file/0021/707133/funding_guidelines.pdf. Accessed 2 Dec 2019.
101. Zhao Y, Poppe S, Lawton P, Hutchings J, You JQ, Annesley K, Cameron N, Guthridge S. Satellite dialysis costs in the top end, 2011-2013. In: Dep. Heal. Darwin, 2014. https://digitallibrary.health.nt.gov.au/prodjspui/bitstream/10137/1316/1/Satellite%20Dialysis%20Costs_Renal%20costing%20report.pdf. Accessed 2 Dec 2019.
102. Funding for renal services in Victoria – health.vic. https://www2.health.vic.gov.au/hospitals-and-health-services/patient-care/rehabilitation-complex-care/renal-health/funding-for-renal-services. Accessed 2 Dec 2019.
103. Cass A, Chadban S, Gallagher M, Howard K, Jones A, Mcdonald S, Snelling P, White S. The economic impact of end-stage kidney disease in Australia. Projections to 2020. Melbourne: Kidney Health Australia; 2010.
104. Chapman JR. Transplantation in Australia – 50 years of progress. Med J Aust. 1992;157:46–50.
105. Australian and New Zealand Paired Kidney Exchange (ANZKX) Program|DonateLife. https://donatelife.gov.au/about-donation/living-donation/australian-and-new-zealand-paired-kidney-exchange-anzkx-program. Accessed 7 Aug 2019.
106. Australian Donation and Transplantation Activity Report. 2018. www.donatelife.gov.au. Accessed 1 Dec 2019.
107. ANZOD Registry. 2018 annual report, section 4: deceased organ donor profile. Adelaide: Australia and New Zealand Dialysis and Transplant Registry; 2018. www.anzdata.org.au. Accessed 8 Jul 2019.
108. Transplantation Society of Australia and New Zealand. TSANZ clinical guidelines version 1.3 May 2019. www.tsanz.com.au/organallocationguidelines/index.asp. Accessed 8 Jul 2019.
109. National Health and Medical Research Council. Ethical guidelines for organ transportation from deceased donors. Canberra: National Health and Medical Research Council; 2016. www.nhmrc.gov.au/guidelines/publications/E76. Accessed 8 Jul 2019.
110. ANZDATA Registry. 41st report, chapter 6: Australian transplant waiting list. Adelaide: Australia and New Zealand Dialysis and Transplant Registry; 2019. www.anzdata.org.au. Accessed 8 Jul 2019.
111. McDonald SP. Australia and New Zealand dialysis and transplant registry. Kidney Int Suppl. 2015;5:39–44.
112. McDonald SP. Survival of recipients of cadaveric kidney transplants compared with those receiving dialysis treatment in Australia and New Zealand, 1991-2001. Nephrol Dial Transplant. 2002;17:2212–9.
113. Clayton PA, McDonald SP, Snyder JJ, Salkowski N, Chadban SJ. External validation of the estimated posttransplant survival score for allocation of deceased donor kidneys in the United States. Am J Transplant. 2014;14:1922–6.
114. Hall J. Australian Health Care — the challenge of reform in a fragmented system. N Engl J Med. 2015;373:493–7.
115. Peabody JW, Bickel SR, Lawson JS. The Australian health care system. Are the incentives down under right side up? JAMA. 1996;276:1944–50.
116. Fullman N, Yearwood J, Abay SM, et al. Measuring performance on the Healthcare Access and Quality Index for 195 countries and territories and selected subnational locations: a systematic analysis from the Global Burden of Disease Study 2016. Lancet. 2018;391:2236–71.
117. Australian Institute of Health and Welfare. End-stage kidney disease in Australia: total incidence, 2003–2007. Cat. no. PHE 143. Canberra: AIHW; 2011. www.aihw.gov.au. Accessed 7 Aug 2019.
118. Australian Institute of Health and Welfare. Chronic kidney disease: regional variation in Australia. Cat. no. PHE 172. Canberra: AIHW; 2013. www.aihw.gov.au. Accessed 7 Aug 2019.
119. Osman MA, Alrukhaimi M, Ashuntantang GE, et al. Global nephrology workforce: gaps and opportunities toward a sustainable kidney care system. Kidney Int Suppl. 2018;8:52–63.
120. Glenn D, Ocegueda S, Nazareth M, Zhong Y, Weinstein A, Primack W, Cochat P, Ferris M. The global pediatric nephrology workforce: a survey of the International Pediatric Nephrology Association. BMC Nephrol. 2016;17:83.
121. Costello A, Abbas M, Allen A, et al. Managing the health effects of climate change. Lancet. 2009;373:1693–733.
122. Watts N, Adger WN, Agnolucci P, et al. Health and climate change: policy responses to protect public health. Lancet. 2015;386:1861–914.
123. Foley JA, Monfreda C, Ramankutty N, Zaks D. Our share of the planetary pie. Proc Natl Acad Sci. 2007;104:12585–6.
124. Eckelman MJ, Sherman J. Environmental impacts of the U.S. health care system and effects on public health. PLoS One. 2016;11:e0157014.
125. Malik A, Lenzen M, McAlister S, McGain F. The carbon footprint of Australian health care. Lancet Planet Heal. 2018;2:e27–35.
126. Agar JWM. Green dialysis: the environmental challenges ahead. Semin Dial. 2015;28:186–92.
127. Agar JWM. Reusing and recycling dialysis reverse osmosis system reject water. Kidney Int. 2015;88:653–7.
128. Lim AEK, Perkins A, Agar JWM. The carbon footprint of an Australian satellite haemodialysis unit. Aust Health Rev. 2013;37:369–74.
129. Agar JW. Conserving water in and applying solar power to haemodialysis: "green dialysis" through wiser resource utilization: original article. Nephrology. 2010;15:448–53.
130. Agar JWM, Perkins A, Tjipto A. Solar-assisted hemodialysis. Clin J Am Soc Nephrol. 2012;7:310–4.
131. Win-win as dialysis waste reinforces concrete|Engineers Australia. https://www.engineersaustralia.org.au/News/win-win-dialysis-waste-reinforces-concrete. Accessed 7 Aug 2019.
132. This innovative concrete recipe doubles as a way to recycle medical waste – Create digital magazine. https://www.createdigitalmagazine.org.au/concrete-doubles-recycle-medical-waste/. Accessed 7 Aug 2019.
133. Blankestijn PJ, Arici M, Bruchfeld A, et al. ERA-EDTA invests in transformation to greener health care. Nephrol Dial Transplant. 2018;33:901–3.
134. Moura-Neto JA, Barraclough K, Agar JWM. A call-to-action for sustainability in dialysis in Brazil. J Bras Nefrol. 2019;41:560.
135. Barraclough KA, Holt SG, Agar JWM. Climate change and us: what nephrologists should know. Nephrology. 2015;20:760–4.
136. Barraclough KA, Blashki GA, Holt SG, Agar JWM. Climate change and kidney disease—threats and opportunities. Kidney Int. 2017;92:526–30.
137. Blankestijn PJ, Bruchfeld A, Capasso G, et al. Lancet countdown paper: what does it mean for nephrology? Nephrol Dial Transplant. 2019;34:4–6.

138. Wouters OJ, O'Donoghue DJ, Ritchie J, Kanavos PG, Narva AS. Early chronic kidney disease: diagnosis, management and models of care. Nat Rev Nephrol. 2015;11:491.
139. Gois P, Purtell L, Bonner A, Chang GK, Lal V, Cation A, Kark AL, et al. The keeping kidneys program: baseline results form a new model of care for community kidney health. J. Am. Soc. Nephrol. Abstr. Suppl. 2019;30;1180. American Society of Nephrology Kidney Week 2019 Nov 5–10; Washington DC.
140. Charlson ME, Pompei P, Ales KL, MacKenzie CR. A new method of classifying prognostic comorbidity in longitudinal studies: development and validation. J Chronic Dis. 1987;40:373–83.
141. Kazancioğlu R. Risk factors for chronic kidney disease: an update. Kidney Int Suppl. 2013;3:368.
142. Queensland Government. Queensland statewide renal health services plan, 2008–17, part one: the way forward. Brisbane: Queensland Government; 2007.
143. Renal integrated care pathway guide for Victorian renal services – June 2016 – health.vic. https://www2.health.vic.gov.au/about/publications/policiesandguidelines/renal-integrated-care-pathway. Accessed 6 Sep 2019.
144. Tasmanian Government. Tasmanian state plan for renal services 2010-2020, part one: overview and action plan. Hobart: Tasmanian Government; 2009.
145. Renal Network NSW. https://www.aci.health.nsw.gov.au/networks/renal. Accessed 6 Sep 2019.
146. Statewide Renal Clinical Network. South Australian statewide renal key performance indicators statewide renal clinical network. 2014. https://www.sahealth.sa.gov.au/wps/wcm/connect/9010bd80453022288e54de005ba75f87/SA-Renal-KPI%27s-Feb-2014-final.pdf?MOD=AJPERES&CACHEID=ROOTWORKSPACE-9010bd80453022288e54de005ba75f87-mN5EgMd. Accessed 6 Sep 2019.
147. Northern Territory Renal services strategy 2017 – 2022. https://digitallibrary.health.nt.gov.au/prodjspui/handle/10137/1438. Accessed 6 Sep 2019.
148. Renal Health Network Western Australia. https://ww2.health.wa.gov.au/Articles/N_R/Renal-Health-Network. Accessed 6 Sep 2019.

# Nephrology in New Zealand

53

Robert James Walker, Kelvin Lewis Lynn, and Ian Dittmer

| | |
|---|---|
| Area | 268,000 km$^2$ |
| Population | 4,793,358 (2018) |
| Capital | Wellington |
| Three most populated cities | 1. Auckland<br>2. Wellington<br>3. Christchurch |
| Official language | English |
| Gross domestic product (GDP)[1] | 205.59 billion US Dollar (2018) |
| GDP per capita[1] | 38,000.7 US Dollar (2018) |
| Human Development Index (HDI)[2] | 0.921 (14th position) |
| Official currency | New Zealand Dollar |
| Total number of nephrologists | 61 |
| National society of nephrology | Australian and New Zealand Society of Nephrology www.nephrology.edu.au |
| Incidence of end-stage renal disease[3] | 2018 – 127 pmp |
| Prevalence of end-stage renal disease[4] | 2018 – 985 pmp |
| Total number of patients on dialysis[4] (all modalities) | 2017 – 2779<br>2018 – 2846 |
| Number of patients on haemodialysis[4] | 2017 – 1917<br>2018 – 1978 |
| Number of patients on peritoneal dialysis[4] | 2017 – 862<br>2018 – 868 |
| Number of renal transplants per year[4] | 2017 – 187<br>2018 – 182 |

1. https://tradingeconomics.com/new-zealand/gdp-per-capita accessed December 2019
2. United Nations Development Programme Human Development Reports accessed December 2019. http://hdr.undp.org/sites/all/themes/hdr_theme/country-notes/NZL.pdf
3. ANZDATA Registry. 42nd Report, Chapter 1: Incidence of Renal Replacement Therapy for End Stage Kidney Disease. Australia and New Zealand Dialysis and Transplant Registry, Adelaide, Australia. 2019. Available at: http://www.anzdata.org.au accessed December 2019
4. ANZDATA Registry. 42nd Report, Chapter 2: Prevalence of Renal Replacement Therapy for End Stage Kidney Disease. Australia and New Zealand Dialysis and Transplant Registry, Adelaide, Australia. 2019. Available at: http://www.anzdata.org.au accessed December 2019

## Introduction

New Zealand has a population of almost five million people, with Auckland being the largest and most ethnical diverse city in New Zealand with a population of about 1. Four million individuals. Māori, the indigenous population, make up 15% of the New Zealand population with Pacific People 7.4% and Asian people contributing 11% [1]. Māori first came to New Zealand from the Pacific around 1200 AD. Abel Tasman was the first European to discover New Zealand in 1642 but did not actually set foot on New Zealand. Captain James Cook was the first European to set foot on New Zealand in 1769. He subsequentially circumnavigated New Zealand drawing detailed maps of the coastline. With his discovery, New Zealand was claimed as a British Colony. However, unlike many other British Colonies, the indigenous population (Māori) actually signed a treaty with the English Crown – the Treaty of Waitangi – which was meant to protect the rights of Māori to their land and sovereignty (see below). Whilst the initial settlers of New Zealand were predominantly from the United Kingdom, more recently, New Zealand has seen a much more multi-cultural society develop with immigrants from Asia, India and Europe.

R. J. Walker (✉)
Department of Medicine, University of Otago, Dunedin, New Zealand
e-mail: rob.walker@otago.ac.nz

K. L. Lynn
Department of Nephrology, Christchurch Hospital, Christchurch, New Zealand

I. Dittmer
Department of Nephrology, Auckland City Hospital, Auckland, New Zealand
e-mail: Idittmer@adhb.govt.nz


J. A. Moura-Neto et al. (eds.), *Nephrology Worldwide*, https://doi.org/10.1007/978-3-030-56890-0_53

New Zealand's main economy is related to farming and the production of primary produce, which is exported worldwide. New Zealand has a democratically elected parliament which has a fairly strong focus on the social welfare of its people, such that education and healthcare are publicly funded. Although it is a relatively small country, it plays an important role in the international arena. The country's sports teams particularly in rugby, sailing, cricket and softball are highly regarded.

The healthcare system in New Zealand is based on a publicly funded healthcare system with substantially subsided access to primary healthcare and freely funded hospital care. As such, the provision of nephrology services comes under the publicly funded hospital system. The government oversight of the health system is provided by the Ministry of Health. An important component of the delivery of healthcare in New Zealand is the Treaty of Waitangi (English version) and Te Tiriti o Waitangi (Māori language version) which recognises the sovereignty of Māori in New Zealand. Within New Zealand law, the health sector is required to work to eliminate health inequalities between Māori and other New Zealanders [2]. This involves a partnership between government (Ministry of Health) working with iwi (tribe), hapū (sub-tribe), whānau (extended- families) and Māori communities to develop strategies for Māori health gain and appropriate health and disability services. Māori participation is required at all levels of the health and disability sector, including in decision-making, planning, development and delivery of health and disability. Under the Treaty obligations, the government has to ensure Māori have at least the same level of health as non-Māori and safeguard Māori cultural concepts, values and practices [2, 3]. However further work is required to ensure the government continues to fulfil their obligations to the Treaty [2].

There are a small number of nephrologists who provide some general nephrology in a private (fee paying) capacity. The majority of nephrologists in New Zealand are salaried full time or part time hospital physicians. Salaries range from about 160,000 to 240,000 NZ dollars per annum. At present, there are 61 consultant nephrologists and 29 advanced nephrology trainees (fellows) around New Zealand. There are nephrology services based in all of the tertiary hospitals in New Zealand. Within Auckland, there is Auckland City Hospital, Middlemore Hospital, North Shore Hospital and Waitakere Hospital. There are nephrology units at Whangarei (Northland), Hamilton (Waikato), Hastings (Hawkes Bay), Palmerston North (Manawatu), New Plymouth (Taranaki) and Wellington, which are all in the North Island (See map). In the South Island, there are nephrology units based at Christchurch and Dunedin Hospitals. There are a number of regional units where nephrology services are provided by physicians who are dual trained in Internal Medicine and Nephrology. The majority of these have satellite dialysis facilities and collaborate with their regional hospital nephrology service (listed above). In addition, there is a national paediatric nephrology service based at the Starship Children's Health, which is part of Auckland Hospital, with four paediatric nephrologists (Fig. 53.1).

## History of Dialysis

Prior to 1960, there were occasional isolated instances where acute peritoneal dialysis or acute haemodialysis using a Kolff kidney had been used to treat acute kidney injury. During the 1960s, renal units were established in Auckland, Hamilton, Wellington, Christchurch and Dunedin with the appointment of the first nephrologists in New Zealand [4].

In the early days, haemodialysis was solely a bridge to maintain the individual in a stable state until they could be transplanted. Dialysis was not seen as a long-term proposition. The units utilised different dialysis systems; either a Multiple Artificial Kidney System (MAKS) from Bio/Systems Inc. of Santa Monica CA or Kolff/Travenol dialysis machines. Dialysis with Kiil flat plate dialysers was for 4–5 hours, two or three times a week during the day/evening and up to 10 hours twice a week overnight for those who were working [4].

In 1966, Dr. Peter Little was appointed as Canterbury's (Christchurch Hospital) first nephrologist, and he instigated the home haemodialysis programme in New Zealand in 1969. The development of the Drake-Willock dialysis machines and Kiil dialysers meant there was affordable, relatively simple technology that could be mastered by patients. With this equipment, patients could be trained to carry out overnight dialysis at home. Initially, home dialysis training and support was provided by the Christchurch unit for patients from throughout the country (see Fig. 53.2). Key elements of the training programme were training patients in a building separate from the hospital, reintegration of the patient back into the community to manage their own care and close liaison with their general practitioners, local hospital, laboratory, pharmacy, employers, and schools [4]. These patients were often residing long distances from the training unit (Fig. 53.2).

Home dialysis training units were subsequently set up in Auckland (1970), Dunedin (1974), Wellington (1975) and Waikato (1976) and Middlemore Hospital in South Auckland (1983). Home dialysis is still the main form of dialysis, particularly in the South Island of New Zealand [4].

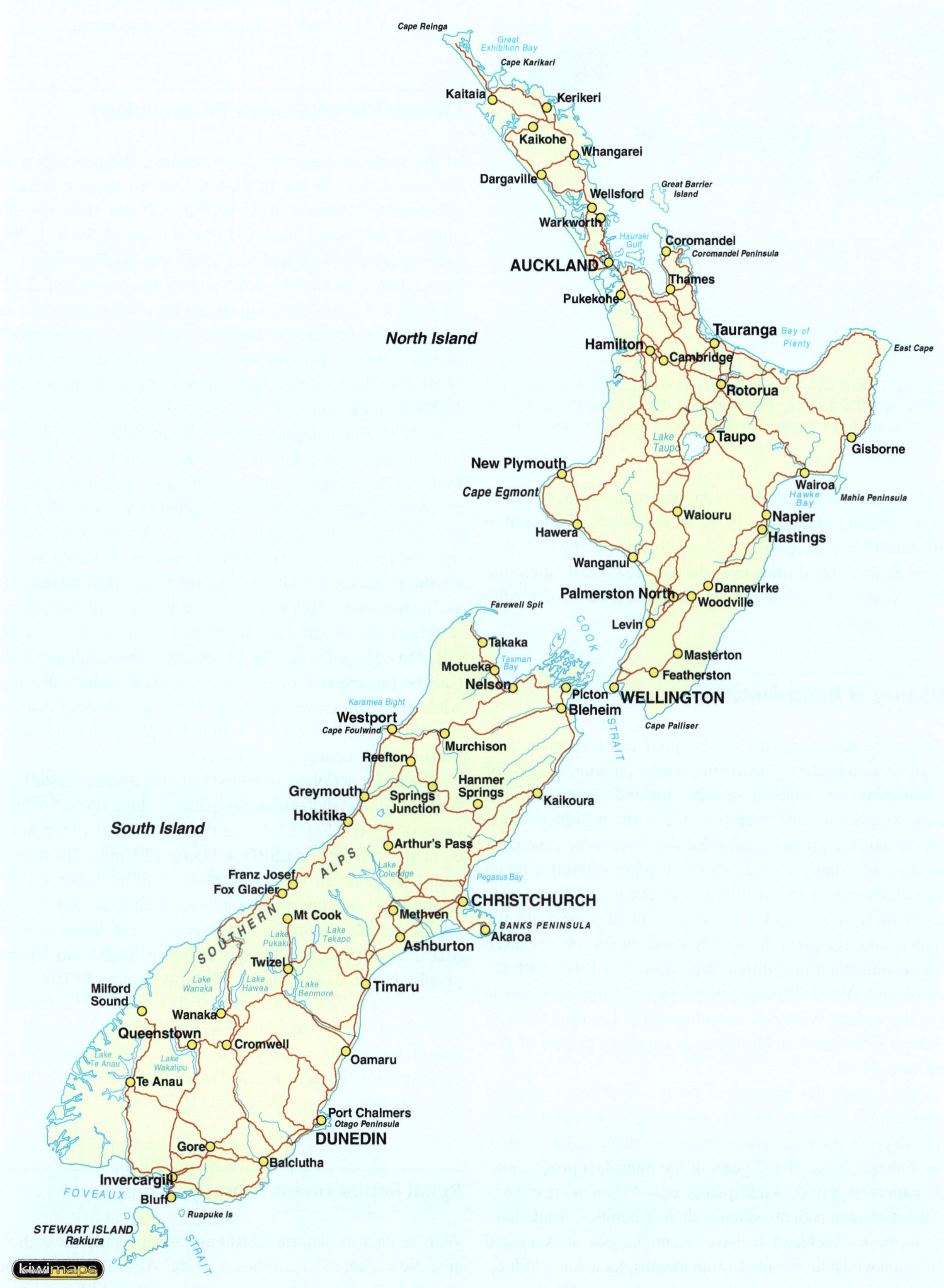


Fig. 53.1 Map of New Zealand. (Supplied by Kiwimaps Ltd. Copyright. All rights reserved)

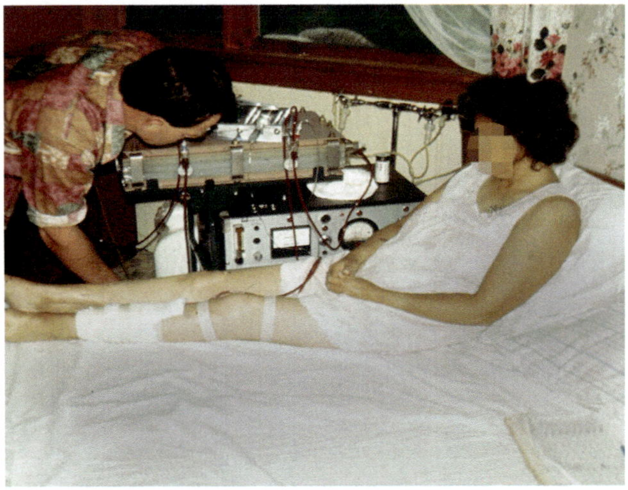

**Fig. 53.2** Neil and Gloria Herrick. Home dialysis Orepuki, rural Southland 1972 Left leg AV shunt, Kiil dialyser and Drake-Willock machine. (Picture reproduced with the permission of the family [4])

Continuous ambulatory peritoneal dialysis (CAPD) in New Zealand started in 1978, at the Waikato (Hamilton Hospital) Unit [4]. CAPD was rapidly adopted by the other New Zealand renal units over the next few years, such that New Zealand now has one of the highest rates of CAPD internationally.

## History of Transplantation

The early nephrologists and hospital administrators saw dialysis as a bridging treatment, whilst patients waited for a transplant and dialysis services for end-stage renal disease would not have been possible without kidney transplants being available in New Zealand. As is the case now, in the early days, a successful transplant offered a much superior survival and quality of life. The first kidney transplant in New Zealand was carried out in 1965 with the donor and recipient being identical twins. A deceased donor transplant programme was started in 1966, with the Auckland Blood Transfusion Service setting up a tissue typing service. New Zealand adopted the Harvard Medical School Committee definition of brain death as part of this process [4–6].

The criteria for acceptance on the Auckland transplant programme were restrictive by today's standards; aged 15–45 years, no other serious health problems and absolutely no diabetes. In the first 2 years of the transplant programme, 35 patients received 44 transplants: only 4 from living donors. All out of town patients, often with their families, would have to move to Auckland to have haemodialysis at Auckland Hospital whilst they waited, often months, for a donor kidney. All transplant surgery took place in Auckland until Wellington (1969), Christchurch (1972) and Waikato (1974) started their own programmes [4]. Now, transplantation services are provided from Auckland, Wellington and Christchurch.

## Chronic Kidney Disease Epidemiology

In the southern region of New Zealand, the prevalence of chronic kidney disease (CKD), as defined as an estimated Glomerular Filtration Rate (eGFR) of less than 60 ml/min/1.73 m$^2$, was estimated to be at least 11.8% [7]. The same study demonstrated that CKD was more prevalent in Māori (OR 1.56, CI 1.45–1.69) and Pacific people (OR 2.62, CI 2.28–3.01) even after adjustment for confounding factors including the presence of diabetes mellitus. Given the much greater number of Māori and Pacific people resident in the North Island, prevalence rates are probably even higher than 11.8% nationwide [7, 8].

In New Zealand, glomerulonephritis (GN) is the second most frequent cause for progressive chronic kidney disease. In the 1970s, a total of 765 individuals with a biopsy-proven diagnosis of primary GN were enrolled in a prospective registry. Membranoproliferative GN and IgA nephropathy were the most prevalent forms of GN. Of interest, in the Māori and Pacific population, acute proliferative GN (post infectious) and membranoproliferative GN were more common, whereas in this ethnic group, IgA nephropathy was uncommon [9, 10]. Patients with rapidly progressive glomerulonephritis had the highest risk of reaching end-stage kidney disease, whilst the cumulative incidence of end-stage kidney disease was 20% and 30% for those with IgA nephropathy and membranous nephropathy, respectively.

The major aetiology of end-stage renal disease (ESRD) in New Zealand is diabetic nephropathy making up 54% of the cases of ESRD (Fig. 53.3), but there is marked variation by ethnicity with 68% of ESRD in Māori, 72% in Pacific people and 43% in Asian New Zealanders, due to diabetes [11]. There is a disproportionate representation of Māori and Pacific people requiring renal replacement therapy, with Māori almost twice as likely to develop ESRD and Pacific people over three times more likely to develop ESRD compared to New Zealand Europeans (Fig. 53.4) [11]. Among Māori and Pacific peoples, disparities in the incidence of ESRD are evident as early as ages 15–24 years and remain evident across all age groups. There is no indication of gender differences in New Zealand [11].

## Renal Replacement Therapy

With respect to data on ESRD and renal replacement therapy, New Zealand contributes to the Australian and New Zealand Dialysis and Transplant (ANZDATA) registry (http://www.anzdata.org.au) which records all individuals who have commenced renal replacement therapy for more than 90 days. In 2017, there was a total of 4658 patients receiving renal replacement therapy: 2768 on dialysis and 1890 with a functioning renal transplant. The number of patients commencing dialysis was 615 (128 per million population). New Zealand has one of the highest rates of home dialysis with 1291 (47%) of the 2768 individuals on a home dialysis therapy. Of the 1291 individuals on home dialysis, 34% are on home haemodialysis, and the rest are on peritoneal dialysis [11, 12] (Fig. 53.5). In the South Island, over 85% of the dialysis population are on a home dialysis therapy.

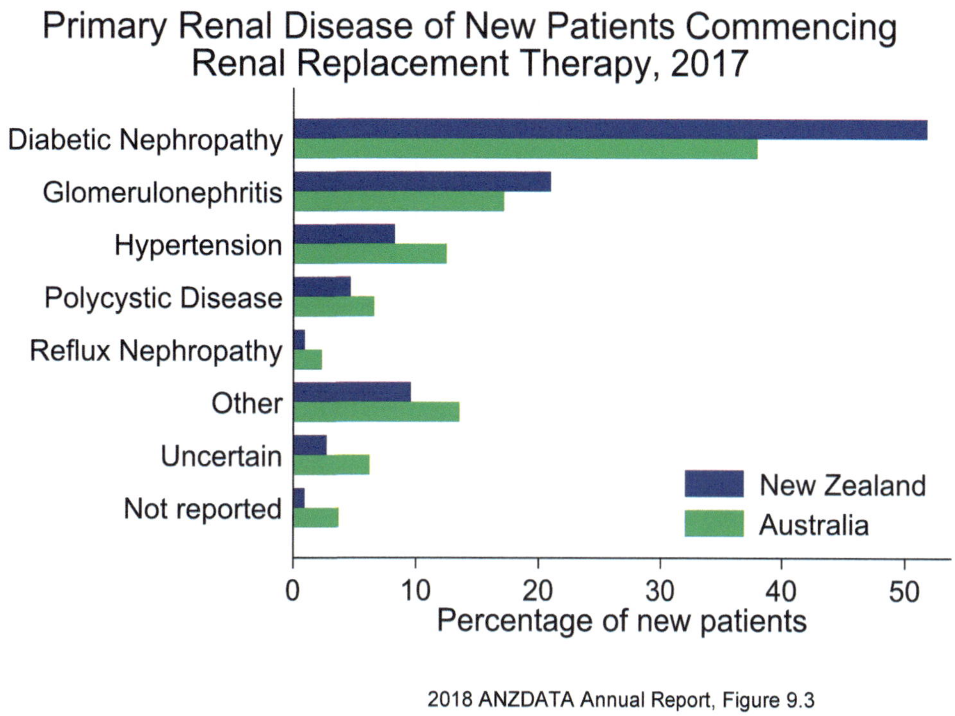


**Fig. 53.3** Primary renal disease of new patients commencing renal replacement therapy, 2017. (Reproduced with permission. ANZDATA Registry [18])

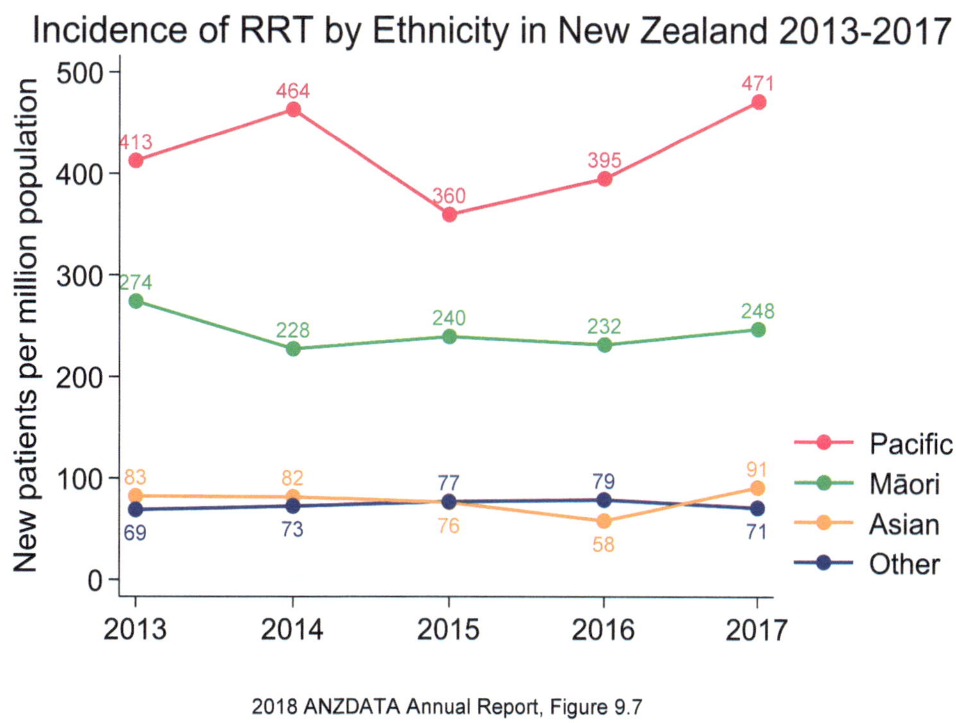


**Fig. 53.4** Incidence of renal replacement therapy by ethnicity in New Zealand 2013–2017. (Reproduced with permission: ANZDATA Registry [18])

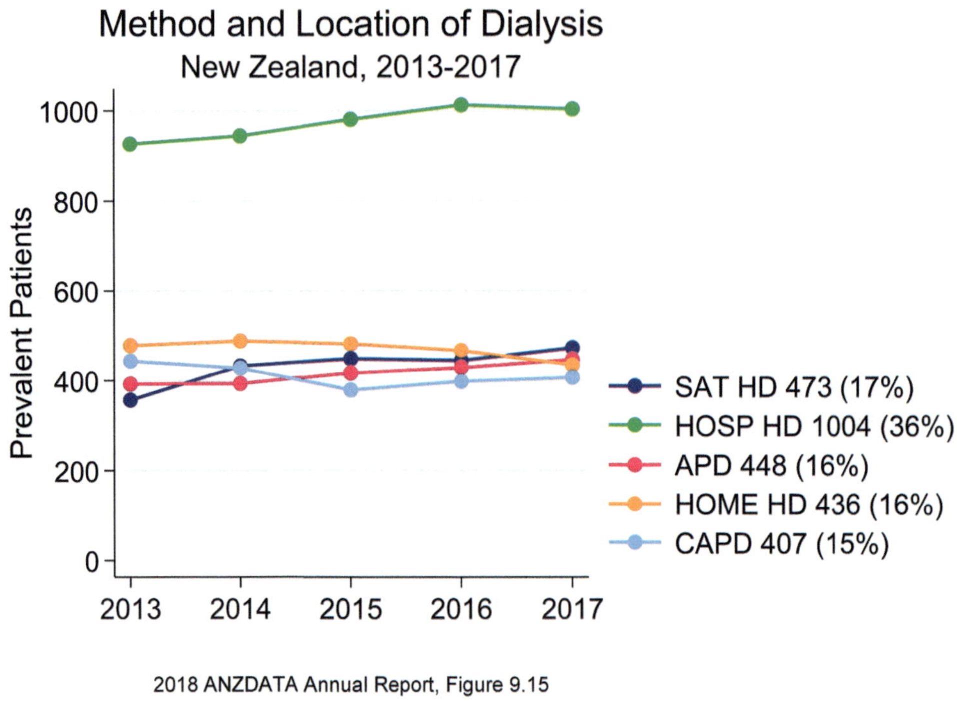


**Fig. 53.5** Method and location of dialysis – New Zealand 2013–2017. (Reproduced with permission: ANZDATA Registry [18])

As New Zealand has a fully funded public hospital system, the cost of renal replacement therapies is covered by the government. The provision of dialysis is largely determined by individual patient choices along with nephrology multidisciplinary team input. There is a strong focus in New Zealand on a 'home first' dialysis policy. As all nephrologists, as well as allied health staff, are salaried staff, there are no physician-related reimbursement costs for dialysis, and there are no private dialysis programmes in New Zealand. There are no financial incentives that may influence decisions to commence dialysis. Likewise there is no pre-specified staffing requirement for dialysis units, either in hospital or satellite units.

In New Zealand, the majority of haemodialysis is with high flux membranes (91%), with 22% using haemodiafiltration, with predominantly pre-dilutional fluid substitution. Average blood flow speed is between 300 and 350 ml/minute. Seventy-seven percent (77%) of individuals dialyse three times a week for 4.5 hours or longer at a time. Overall, the majority of individuals are dialysing between 13.5 and 20 hours a week. There is no dialyzer reuse in New Zealand.

In New Zealand, the majority of haemodialysis access is via arteriovenous fistulae (71%) with 28% via a tunnelled dialysis catheter. One-year dialysis survival is 90% and 5-year survival is 55% (censored for transplantation) [13].

Of the patients on peritoneal dialysis, 53% are on APD and 47% on CAPD. Icodextrin usage is high with 60% on those on CAPD and 74% of those on APD using icodextrin [14]. PD survival rates (censored for transplantation) are 95% at 1 year, 76% at 3 years and 53% at 5 years [14]. Peritoneal dialysis-related peritonitis rates are currently 1 episode per 24.1 patient months (NZ Peritoneal Dialysis Registry – personal communication).

New Zealand has one of the highest rates of home dialysis per million population in the world. The two nephrology centres in the South Island of New Zealand, based in Christchurch and Dunedin, have an almost exclusive home dialysis policy, which is unique in the world. Of the total dialysis population in New Zealand, 47% are on home dialysis, which is broken down to 16% APD, 15% CAPD and 16% home haemodialysis [11]. The majority of the home haemodialysis patients are in the South Island. Those on home haemodialysis either self-dialyse or have a support person where needed. A significant proportion of those on home haemodialysis dialyse long hours (8 or more) overnight at least three times a week. The longest home haemodialysis patients have been dialysing at home for over 35 years. It is also important to note that there is no remote monitoring – the patients are not linked up to any sort of monitoring systems back to the dialysis unit.

Active conservative care programmes are also an integral part of nephrology services. Several of the larger units in New Zealand now have combined clinics with their palliative care physician colleagues to help manage those individuals who chose an active conservative care pathway or who decide to withdrawal from dialysis. Throughout the country, palliative care services and hospices collaborate with nephrology services. Withdrawal from renal replacement therapy now accounts for 20–25% of deaths in ESRD population [12].

## Acute Kidney Injury and Critical Care Nephrology

In New Zealand, all acute kidney injury patients are managed predominantly by the nephrology services. They provide acute haemodialysis as required. Patients are only admitted to the intensive care units if there are additional requirements for circulatory and respiratory support. In all the main hospitals, acute dialysis in the intensive care unit is provided by the intensivists, with varying support provided by the nephrology service. The modality of acute dialysis treatment used depends upon individual unit preferences and experience. These range from continuous venovenous haemodiafiltration (CVVHD) to sustained low efficiency haemodiafiltration (SLED-HDF).

## Paediatric Nephrology

New Zealand has a national paediatric nephrology service based at the Starship Children's Health, Auckland Hospital with four paediatric nephrologists. In addition to their inpatient services, they provide a national outreach service with paediatric nephrology clinics in the main centres of New Zealand. Renal replacement therapies for paediatric patients are overseen by the national service, with the majority of patients dialysing in their own region or their transplant follow-up in close liaison with local paediatricians.

## Renal Transplantation

Renal transplantation takes place at three major centres. Auckland City Hospital provides the transplant services for the top half of New Zealand, which contains the largest population base. It is also centre for the national liver, pancreas, heart and lung transplantation services. Wellington provides transplantation for the lower North Island and Christchurch is the transplant centre for the South Island. In New Zealand, transplant recipients are managed by the nephrologists in both the pre-transplant assessment phase and post-operatively: initially in conjunction with the transplant surgical team in the immediate post-operative phase (first 5–7 days), with subsequent follow-up entirely undertaken by the nephrologists.

There are clear national guidelines related to assessment and acceptance onto the deceased donor transplant waiting list. All organ retrieval is undertaken by the Auckland Intra-abdominal Transplant Service with organs allocated according to a nationally agreed algorithm overseen by the New Zealand Renal Transplant Leadership Team (https://www.health.govt.nz/system/files/documents/pages/nrts-nz-kidney-allocation-scheme-feb2019-final.pdf). Organ Donation New Zealand is responsible for co-ordinating retrievals and transport of organs to the recipient operating centres.

Immunosuppression therapy is fully funded by the government, as is all approved medications. Anti-CD25 induction therapy is standard along with calcineurin inhibitors (cyclosporin A 72% and tacrolimus 22%) mycophenolate mofetil (99%) and prednisone (99%) as initial immunosuppressive therapy [15].

In 2017, there were 187 transplants (40 per million population), 69 of which were from live donors. New Zealand has recently expanded its deceased donor pool and now uses deceased cardiac donors as well. Donor rates have been increasing steadily over recent years. Long-term transplant survival rates compare favourably with those of other western countries. For primary deceased donor grafts, patient survival is 99% at 1 year and 88% survival at 5 years with graft survival at 1 year at 98% and 83% at 5 years. For living donor transplants, patient survival is 97% at 1 year and 97% at 5 years, with graft survival 96% at 1 year and 91% at 5 years. As of 2017, 12% of prevalent transplants have functioned for at least 20 years [15].

In New Zealand, death with a functioning transplant (62%) or chronic allograft nephropathy (22%) are the two most common causes of graft loss [15]. Of note and concern is the alarming increase in cancers, particularly skin cancers, in long-term transplant recipients. Malignancy is now the second most common cause of death in our transplant recipients and match cardiovascular deaths [12, 15].

ABO blood group incompatible transplantation was first undertaken at Auckland Hospital in 2008 and is now available at all three transplant centres. There has been a kidney exchange scheme operating for patients whose live donor is incompatible either for ABO blood group or a positive crossmatch. This has contributed a small number of transplants each year since inception. On August 18, 2019, the scheme joined with its Australian counterpart, and it is expected that this will significantly increase the number of transplants performed.

## Nephrology Practice in New Zealand

### Medical and Nephrology Education

New Zealand has two medical schools, the University of Otago and the University of Auckland, with an annual intake of medical students around 480 per year. The course is a 6-year undergraduate programme. Once undergraduate study is completed, New Zealand graduates spend the next 2 years in supervised attachments in metropolitan and regional hospitals in order achieve full registration with the Medical Council of New Zealand. These attachments are predominantly medical and surgical attachments, with other specialties being options in the second year of provisional registration.

Nephrology training comes under the auspices of the Royal Australasian College of Physicians' (RACP) programme for medical training (https://www.racp.edu.au/). All trainees undertake basic physician training covering various medical disciplines. At the end of the second year of basic training, they are able to sit the RACP Part One written examination. Upon passing the written examination, there are clinical examinations to pass. It is only once a trainee has passed these examinations, that they can undertake specialty (advanced) training in Nephrology. Nephrology training is a supervised 3-year programme with requirements to cover core competencies related to nephrology. Training is supervised in each nephrology unit by senior nephrologists. The overall training programme and review of the trainees' progress is undertaken by the Advanced Training Committee – Nephrology which is run by the RACP (independent of the hospitals). It is expected that that trainee will undertake a broad range of attachments in order to get a wide exposure to all aspects of nephrology. Any specialty area of interest is usually undertaken as part of a post fellowship attachment.

In New Zealand, nephrologists generally cover all areas of nephrology in their clinical practice. In the larger tertiary units, the nephrologists may have a sub-specialty interest such as transplantation or dialysis, but they maintain their general nephrology practice as well.

The Australian and New Zealand Society of Nephrology (ANZSN) contributes substantially to the training programme with provision of a number of trainee educational programmes which trainees are required to attend over their 3-year training programme. Details of these courses are available on the ANZSN website: https://www.nephrology.edu.au.

Once advanced training is completed and the trainees have been awarded their fellowship, they can apply to the Medical Council of New Zealand for vocational registration as a specialist nephrologist. For overseas trained doctors, there are several requirements to be fulfilled in order to be registered with Medical Council, to undertake clinical practice. The exact details are listed on the Medical Council of New Zealand website (https://www.mcnz.org.nz/registration/getting-registered/). Requirements will depend upon the country of origin and the training programme undertaken.

There are a number of countries that are recognised as having comparable health systems. If an individual has trained in one of these countries, their specialist registration is usually recognised. These overseas trained doctors may need to undertake a year of supervised clinical practice before being granted full vocational registration. The obligation is upon the individual to check their qualifications and status with the Medical Council of New Zealand before arriving in New Zealand to commence practice.

## Dialysis and Allied Health Staff

New Zealand now has a few clinical nurse specialists in nephrology who lead low GFR (CKD 4 and 5 pre-dialysis) clinics, who are actively involved in pre-dialysis education as well as transplantation education and assessment (both recipients and potential donors). Most dialysis units around the country are staffed by trained dialysis nurses; however, there is an increasing number of trained renal physiologists who oversee the dialysis training and on-going supervision of dialysis patients. The training, on-going supervision and maintenance of clinical practice standards are overseen by the Clinical Physiologist Registration Board (www.cprb.org.nz) in conjunction with the New Zealand and Australia Society of Renal Dialysis Practice (https://www.nzasrdp.com/).

In New Zealand, there are no specific Ministry of Health stipulations as to the staffing of dialysis units. In all units, there is a multi-disciplinary support team of dieticians, social workers, clinical psychologists and dialysis technicians. However, there is considerable variability around the country as to the actual extent of staffing related to these support staff, with no specific standards available.

## Nephrology Research

New Zealand nephrologists actively contribute to many clinical studies, both investigator-initiated as well as pharma-sponsored studies. New Zealand nephrologists contribute actively to the Australasian Kidney Trials Network (AKTN – https://aktn.org.au/). There are a number of clinical trials sponsored by the Health Research Council of New Zealand (HRC-NZ) and the National Health and Medical Research Council of Australia (NH&MRC) that have been designed and managed by the AKTN. In addition, there is good collaboration with the George Institute (Sydney, Australia) with regard to international studies such as CREDENCE, ACHIEVE and REDUCCTION.

At a translational science level, Professor Alan Davidson (University of Auckland) has established a developmental biology laboratory focusing on (1) understanding the embryonic development and regeneration of the kidney, which mostly involves the zebrafish model, and (2) using human-induced pluripotent stem cells to model kidney diseases and injury, such as the lysosomal storage disease cystinosis and acute kidney injury caused by toxins.

Professor Suetonia Palmer (Christchurch) has an internationally recognised research programme involving meta-analyses and systematic network analyses of trials in kidney disease. She is the principal investigator on a number of clinical trials in conjunction with the AKTN sponsored by the Health Research Council of New Zealand. She is also an active member of the 'Kidney in Health and Disease' research theme based at University of Otago.

The Kidney in Health and Disease' research theme is directed by Professor Robert Walker and is a broad collaboration of investigators with interests in kidney physiology, pathophysiology from bench to bedside, as well as a strong focus on patient related outcomes in CKD (https://www.otago.ac.nz/kidney/). The theme holds three meetings each year, which is a forum for young researchers just establishing their research programmes, as well as presentations by more senior researchers. In addition, the theme holds a biannual research meeting with the Renal Scientists group of the ANZSN to further encourage basic translational research in nephrology in this region.

## Australian and New Zealand Society of Nephrology (ANZSN)

The ANZSN has been in existence since 1965 and has been an important collaborative and collegial organization of Australian and New Zealand Nephrology, which represents the interests of health professionals committed to the prevention and treatment of kidney disease. The ANZSN and its membership support a range of research, education and clinical care initiatives to promote evidenced-based practice and quality outcomes for patients in Australia, New Zealand and our wider region (https://www.nephrology.edu.au).

Within the ANZSN, there is a New Zealand Chapter which meets annually, separate to the main ANZSN annual scientific meeting. It serves an important role to promote specific research, educational and clinical initiatives that are focused on New Zealand's needs. Almost all of the New Zealand nephrologists and nephrology trainees belong to the ANZSN.

## Ministry of Health and Regulatory Standards

The National Renal Advisory Board (NRAB) is a committee that works with the Ministry of Health to implement renal work plans throughout the country. Membership includes renal physicians, renal nurse specialist, clinical physiologists, managers and a consumer representative in addition to ex officio members from allied groups. NRAB meets quarterly and the agenda includes a summary from each of the renal units outlining challenges, successes and any critical incidents. Recent workstreams include ensuring that all unit's disaster management plans are visible on the national Emergency Management system (EMIS), providing advice on technical issues for monitoring and management of viruses in haemodialysis units, formation of guidelines for immunisations for renal patients, and setting up a national late Chronic Kidney Disease database. NRAB receives the annual ANZDATA and Key Performance Indicator (KPI) reports from the responsible workgroups (https://www.health.govt.nz/about-ministry/leadership-ministry/expert-groups/national-renal-advisory-board).

The National Renal Transplant Service (NRTS) was set up in September 2014. It is responsible for leadership, oversight and support of renal transplantation nationally. A specific workstream is to increase the number of live donor transplants performed in NZ. Membership includes a physician, surgeon and manager from each of the transplant units and transplant co-ordinators. A larger oversight committee includes consumer representatives and members from supporting organisations such as *Organ Donation NZ* and *the NZ Blood Service*. Protocols pertaining to policies for listing patients for transplantation and allocation of organs are overseen by NRTS. There has been a significant increase in the number of transplants performed during the last 5 years. In particular, each renal unit has been funded to employ a live kidney donor co-ordinator, and it is expected that this will become business as usual from 2020. A number of quality improvement metrics have been formulated to monitor the success of this programme.

## Future Perspectives of Nephrology in New Zealand

Like many countries, although the incidence of ESRD is possibly slowing down, New Zealand is facing an increased prevalence of CKD & ESRD in our indigenous population, the Māori, as well as our Pacific people. In particular, this is related to the rising rates of type 2 diabetes and our obesity epidemic [16]. Unfortunately, this is also associated with significant health and social inequalities including access to healthcare, adequate housing and education. These issues are not unique to nephrology, rather they are problems related to healthcare in general. Critical components in starting to address these issues are the cultural aspects to healthcare that are important to Māori. This is reflected in Hauora Māori, which is a concept that combines the physical, mental and emotional, social, and spiritual dimensions of health from a Māori perspective [17]. *Taha tinana* is the physical well-being and relates to the body and how to care for it. *Taha hinengaro* is the mental and emotional well-being of the individual which acknowledges thought and being, feelings and the positive responses to this. *Taha whanau* is the social well-being of both the individual and the family (whanau). This feeling of belonging and supporting each other is a very strong and important concept for

Māori. *Taha wairua* is the spiritual well-being of the individual that incorporates the beliefs, identity and personal awareness of the person [17]. All four components are closely linked and important as a total health concept for Māori well-being.

These concepts are taught in New Zealand medical schools and continue throughout postgraduate training. For overseas trained doctors, understanding and incorporating these values into their clinical practice is part of the supervised training they need.

## Conclusion

New Zealand nephrology is delivered under a publicly funded hospital system with nephrology units based in all the major cities of New Zealand. All nephrologists are salaried employees of the district health boards they work for. All units provide a comprehensive nephrology service from general nephrology through to renal replacement services. New Zealand faces an epidemic of obesity and diabetes with diabetes the leading cause of CKD and ESRD. In New Zealand, the indigenous population – Māori as well as Pacific people – have disproportionately higher rates of CKD along with inequities in accessing healthcare which need to be addressed. Nephrology training in New Zealand is overseen by the Royal Australasian College of Physicians and registration as a nephrologist is also regulated by the Medical Council of New Zealand. As New Zealand is a relatively small country, the nephrology community is very collegial and contributes to the high level of standards for care in conjunction with the Ministry of Health for New Zealand.

## References

1. Stats NZ. https://www.stats.govt.nz/. Last accessed 29 July 2019.
2. Came H, Cornes R, McCreanor T. Treaty of Waitangi in New Zealand public health strategies and plans 2006–2016. N Z Med J. 2018;131:1469.
3. Ministry of Health New Zealand. https://www.health.govt.nz/our-work/populations/maori-health/he-korowai-oranga/strengthening-he-korowai-oranga/treaty-waitangi-principles. Last accessed 1 Aug 2019.
4. Lynn KL, Buttimore AL, Hatfield PJ, Wallace MR, editors. The treatment of kidney failure in New Zealand: National Library of New Zealand Cataloguing-Publication Data. ISBN PDF - 978-0-473-45293-3.
5. Richmond DE, Miller TE, Murphy J. In the beginning. A history of the Medical Unit at Auckland Hospital and the formative years of the Department of Medicine, The University of Auckland. 2013. p. 33. http://librarysearch.auckland.ac.nz/UOA2_A:Combined_Local:uoa_alma21160494770002091.
6. Doak PB, Duke AJ, Maclaurin CH, Montgomerie JZ, North JD. Two years' experience with renal transplantation. N Z Med J. 1968;68:221–7.
7. Lloyd H, Li G, Tomlin A, Tilyard MW, Walker R, Schollum J. Prevalence and risk factors for chronic kidney disease in primary health care in the southern region of New Zealand. Nephrology. 2019;24:308–15.
8. Walker RJ, Tufunai M, Krishnan A. Chronic kidney disease in New Zealand Māori and Pacific people. Semin Nephrol. 2019;39:297–9.
9. The New Zealand Glomerulonephritis Study: Introductory report. Clin Nephrol. 1989;31:239–46.
10. Chembo CL, Marshall MR, Williams LC, Walker RJ, Lynn KL, Irvine J, Pilmore HL. Long-term outcomes for primary glomerulonephritis: NZ Glomerulonephritis Study. Nephrology. 2015;20:899–907.
11. ANZDATA Registry. 41st Report, Chapter 9: End stage kidney disease in Aotearoa New Zealand. Australia and New Zealand Dialysis and Transplant Registry, Adelaide, Australia. 2018.
12. ANZDATA Registry. 41st Report, Chapter 3: Mortality in end stage kidney disease. Australia and New Zealand Dialysis and Transplant Registry, Adelaide, Australia. 2018.
13. ANZDATA Registry. 41st Report, Chapter 4: Haemodialysis. Australia and New Zealand Dialysis and Transplant Registry, Adelaide, Australia. 2018. Available at: http://www.anzdata.org.au.
14. ANZDATA Registry. 41st Report, Chapter 5: Peritoneal dialysis. Australia and New Zealand Dialysis and Transplant Registry, Adelaide, Australia. 2018. Available at: http://www.anzdata.org.au.
15. ANZDATA Registry. 41st Report, Chapter 7: Kidney transplantation. Australia and New Zealand Dialysis and Transplant Registry, Adelaide, Australia. 2018. Available at: http://www.anzdata.org.au.
16. Mann J, Taylor R, Cutfield W. The diabesity crisis. N Z Med J. 2017;130:1459.
17. Durie M. Whaiora: Māori health development. Auckland: Oxford University Press; 1994.
18. ANZDATA Registry. 41st Report, Chapter 9: End-stage renal disease in Aotearoa New Zealand. Australia and New Zealand Dialysis and Transplant Registry, Adelaide, Australia. 2018. Available at: http://www.anzdata.org.au.

# Correction to: Nephrology in Portugal

Ana Azevedo, Anabela Rodrigues, Aníbal Ferreira, Conceição Mota, Fernanda Carvalho, Fernando Macário, Helena Jardim, José António Lopes, José Diogo Barata, La Salete Martins, Manuela Almeida, Pedro Ponce, and José Vinhas

## Correction to:

Chapter 45 in: J. A. Moura-Neto et al. (eds.), Nephrology Worldwide, https://doi.org/10.1007/978-3-030-56890-0_45

The original version of chapter 45 had an incorrect affiliation for co-author, Pedro Ponce. This has now been corrected as below.

Pedro Ponce
Renal Unit and Intensive Care Unit, Hospital Cuf Infante Santo, Lisbon, Portugal.
Fresenius Medical Care, Lisbon, Portugal.

The updated version of this chapter can be found at https://doi.org/10.1007/978-3-030-56890-0_45



J. A. Moura-Neto et al. (eds.), *Nephrology Worldwide*, https://doi.org/10.1007/978-3-030-56890-0_54

# Index




J. A. Moura-Neto et al. (eds.), *Nephrology Worldwide*, https://doi.org/10.1007/978-3-030-56890-0

**O**

GPSR Compliance

*The European Union's (EU) General Product Safety Regulation (GPSR) is a set of rules that requires consumer products to be safe and our obligations to ensure this.*

*If you have any concerns about our products, you can contact us on ProductSafety@springernature.com*

In case Publisher is established outside the EU, the EU authorized representative is:

Springer Nature Customer Service Center GmbH
Europaplatz 3
69115 Heidelberg, Germany

**Batch number: 10731665**

Printed by Printforce, the Netherlands